HANDBOOK OF DISABILITY STUDIES

EDITED BY

GARY L. ALBRECHT
KATHERINE D. SEELMAN
MICHAEL BURY

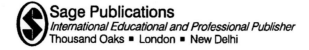

Sage Publications
International Educational and Professional Publisher
Thousand Oaks ▪ London ▪ New Delhi

Cover Illustration: Raphael, *The Fire of Borgo*. Courtesy of the Vatican Museums.

For information:

 Sage Publications, Inc.
2455 Teller Road
Thousand Oaks, California 91320
E-mail: order@sagepub.com

Sage Publications Ltd.
6 Bonhill Street
London EC2A 4PU
United Kingdom

Sage Publications India Pvt. Ltd.
M-32 Market
Greater Kailash I
New Delhi 110 048 India

Printed in the United States of America

Library of Congress Cataloging-in-Publication Data

Albrecht, Gary L.
    Handbook of disability studies / by Gary L. Albrecht, Katherine D. Seelman,
and Michael Bury.
        p.   cm.
Includes bibliographical references and index.
    ISBN 0-7619-1652-0 (cloth: alk. paper)--ISBN 0-7619-2874-X (pbk.)
    1. Disability studies—Handbooks, manuals, etc.   2. Sociology of
disability—Handbooks, manuals, etc.   I. Seelman, Katherine D.
II. Bury, Michael.   III. Title.
    HV1568.2.A42   2000
    362.4—dc21   00-012353

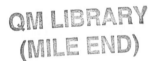
06   07   08   09   8   7   6   5

Acquiring Editor:	Rolf Janke
Editorial Assistant:	Karen Wiley
Production Editor:	Diana E. Axelsen
Editorial Assistant:	Candice Crosetti
Copy Editor:	Gillian Dickens
Typesetter/Designer:	Janelle LeMaster
Indexer:	Mary Mortensen
Cover Designer:	Ravi Balasuriya

Contents

Part II: EXPERIENCING DISABILITY

Part III: DISABILITY IN CONTEXT

Acknowledgments

The ideas for this handbook germinated in the American civil rights movement of the 1960s and took root in the international human rights impetus of the past 25 years. The handbook represents the tensions between academic scholarship and the passion of activists; the different perspectives of disability studies and rehabilitation sciences; the uneasy coalition of disabled people with health professionals, technicians, and policymakers; and the value conflicts between aggressive capitalism, social welfare states, and the poor who struggle for survival in industrial and developing countries. We acknowledge and thank those who first broke the ground in this fertile and important field.

Development of multidisciplinary, international projects takes place in extensive social networks. As a consequence, many individuals contributed to the evolution of the handbook project. Our enthusiasm to produce the handbook became focused in animated conversations with colleagues, activists, members of the silent majority of disabled people, policymakers, government leaders, and Sage Publications over a period of years in England, France, and the United States. Chris Rojek and Stephen Barr provided the opportunity to produce a book prospectus and extensive feedback from anonymous international reviewers, which helped us hone the original concept into a more complete and representative whole. Rolf Janke continuously supported the project with vision and marshaled the forces at Sage to ensure a high-level product.

Many individuals and organizations helped shape the field of disability studies over the years. While we have an enormous intellectual debt to all of them, it is impossible to remember everyone who contributed to the field and movement. However, we would like to acknowledge the special contributions over the years of Irv Zola, Judy Heumann, Ed Roberts, Marca Bristo, Philip Wood, Margot Jefferys, Mike Oliver, Paul Longmore, Richard Smith, David Pfeiffer, Corrine Kirchner, Jane West, Lois Verbrugge, David Grey, Dudley Childress, Catherine Barral, Henry Betts, Carl Granger, Bob Gris, Jimmy Carter, Kathy Charmaz, Anselm Strauss, Eliot Freidson, Jonathan Mann, Ray Fitzpatrick, Mary Boulton, Jerry Ross, Norman Denzin, Isabelle Baszanger, John McKinlay, Paul Higgins, Gerald Dworkin, Patrick Devlieger, Lu Ann Aday, Robert Atchley, Donald Light, Ed Laumann, Sander Gilman, Russ Bernard, Jack Kemp, Byron Hamilton, Claude Hamonet, Henri Paicheler, Claudine Herzlich, and Derek Wade, who displayed vision, offered insights into the disability world, and raised innumerable theoretical, policy, and real-life issues.

The International Advisory Editorial Board members were an invaluable help in reviewing the book prospectus, suggesting authors, and reviewing manuscripts. Their high standards, diversity of background and opinions, and insights into the critical issues of the field improved the conception of the book and individual chapters. The distinguished authors also gave freely of their time and advice in offering suggestions to improve the book and in reviewing manuscripts. In addition, many other colleagues eagerly engaged in debates, offered ideas, and reviewed individual manuscripts.

Academic visits by Gary Albrecht to Nuffield College, the University of Oxford, Maison des Sciences de l'Homme in Paris, and as a lecturer in disability studies to Australia provided the time and atmosphere to conceive the project, engage colleagues, and test ideas. David Cox and Anthony Atkinson set a scholarly tone at Nuffield College, and the Fellows provided the encouragement to persist in a daunting undertaking. Jean-Luc Lory and colleagues at the Maison des Sciences de l'Homme opened the world of French intellectual life and provided contacts and perspectives to deepen the thinking in the book. In Australia, Wendy Seymour, Roy Brown, Karen Nankeris, Barrie O'Conner, Greg Murphy, and Trevor Parmenter orchestrated a three-week moving seminar on disability studies in Adelaide, Melbourne, and Sydney. Bedirhan Üstün, Jerome Bickenbach, and Alan Lopez at the World Health Organization in Geneva and Serge Moscovici and Robert Castel at the l'École des Hautes Études en Sciences Sociales in Paris provided welcome insights into disability in developing countries.

The immediate impetus for the project came in May 1995 when the U.S. Department of Education's National Institute on Disability and Rehabilitation Research (NIDRR) Steering Committee on Disability Studies recommended the development of a "seminal handbook on disability studies." During the entire production process, the unwavering support of the entire NIDRR staff made this enormous task possible.

David Mitchell and Sharon Snyder were the source and inspiration for the book cover. Their interest in the depiction of disability in art and literature over the years led them to study Raphael's painting, *The Fire of Borgo,* in context at the Vatican Museum. They are to be credited with selecting this painting for the cover and helping with its meaningful interpretation. Ravi Balasuriya, the art director at Sage, translated the concept into reality.

The administration, faculty, and staff of the Department of Disability and Human Development at the University of Illinois at Chicago were encouraging at every stage of the project. Special thanks go to David Braddock for his vision, belief, and administrative support. The production of the book was coordinated by our editorial assistant, Reena Verghese, whose management skills, attention to detail, and cheerful reminders of deadlines helped move the book from a dream to a reality. Maggi Lunde at the School of Public Health, University of Illinois, handled innumerable phone calls, e-mail files, and express mail packages that kept the project efficiently moving. Pamela Ippoliti was a sage adviser in organizing the project. Gigi Thomas and Sharla Willis de Lopez set up the original project files. Glenn Fujiura and Dale Mitchell cheerfully solved numerous budgetary problems. Kiyoshi Yamaki was ever present to solve computer glitches, especially those dealt by nasty worms and viruses from all over the world that sneaked through virus protection software. We also thank our technical editor, Phyllis Crittenden, who reviewed all chapter manuscripts for form and technical consistency, and William Sayers, who translated the Ravaud and Stiker chapter. Finally, we thank our families, who provided unwavering support during the exciting but difficult process of bringing this book into being. In sum, the handbook was a worldwide effort made possible by generous people from multiple social networks.

To disabled people

Introduction

The Formation of Disability Studies

GARY L. ALBRECHT
KATHERINE D. SEELMAN
MICHAEL BURY

Disability is an enigma that we experience but do not necessarily understand. While some people are born with or experience disability as children, most of us become familiar with disability later in life. For the majority, then, what was once deemed as foreign, something outside of our bodies and experience, frequently becomes an intimate part of our lives as we age. As our parents reap the blessings of hard work and long lives, disability enters as a companion affecting their cognitive, intellectual, physical, and social functioning. In today's world, our children and their friends are more vulnerable to violence-triggered impairment, exposed to environmentally produced asthma, and diagnosed with learning disorders and hyperactivity deemed to require control by drugs. At work and in public spaces, universal design, accessible buildings, and broadened public laws have made disabled people a ubiquitous presence. World news highlights how ongoing civil wars, natural catastrophes, and environmental disasters around the globe leave an inordinate amount of disability in their aftermath. Disability is a worldwide phenomenon with global consequences (Albrecht and Verbrugge 2000).

Science has contributed to this transition in disability incidence, prevalence, and awareness by making life with serious and chronic impairments increasingly feasible. The result is that debates about technologies and medical ethics catch the public interest. The good news is that disability is in the public consciousness and increasingly on the political agenda. The bad news is that with all of this exposure, we do not necessarily know what disability is, what it implies, or what to expect for ourselves, others, society, or our environment (Bowker and Star 1999). The anomaly is starkly apparent that affluence, better medical care, and the wonders of science, together with long lives, have brought us all closer to the daily experience of disability.

Disability is both a private and public experience. For some, disability represents a personal catastrophe to be avoided if at all possible, a shameful condition to be denied or hidden if present and negotiated within the sanctuary of one's family and personal space. For others, disability is a source of pride and empowerment—a symbol of enriched self-identity and self-worth and a central force coalescing a community intent on extolling the fundamental values of life,

1

human rights, citizenship, and the celebration of difference. Disability for many reasons is a re-defining experience, adding value to individual lives and clarifying what it means to be human. Disability as difference enriches society and creates new sets of powerful social bonds, responsibilities, and opportunities for individuals, families, and society (Crozet et al. 2000).

At the same time that disability is receiving worldwide attention, a major paradigm shift is occurring in social institutions, communications, national identities, and world culture that will dramatically affect how disability is defined, encountered, and interpreted (Friedman 1999; McNeill 2000). Changes in epidemiology, improved health status, and medical care imply that every family in the world will likely be confronted with disability but will not necessarily know how to respond. The virtual world of communications, with instant access to and sharing of information and explosion of health sciences in a borderless world, offers promise to everyone confronting the prospect of chronic illness or disability. Yet, the pace of life and sheer barrage of people and information intruding in our lives leave most breathless and feeling "out of control." Whom can we trust? Where do we turn for support, advice, and security? Who is in control? We are citizens of what nations and members of what institutions? What values are driving the system?

Social analysts discuss these questions in terms of social institutions, economics, values, culture, tradition, and quality of life. Richard Sennett (1998) has recently examined the consequences for individuals of living and working in a global society where nations and institutions are merged, acquired, disappear, or restructured at a moment's notice. To what nation does a firm belong? How long will it exist in its present form? What security do people have in this environment, and what happened to the reciprocal obligations of contracts, citizenship, and implied loyalty? These issues are exacerbated by the persistent emphasis on short-term profits and pleasures and the mistaken assumption that individuals in our society ought to be continually happy (Bruckner 2000).

Guéhenno (1993) suggests that democracy as we know it is undergoing a radical structural reorganization as fewer people vote, elections are overturned, political oligarchies and multinational corporations covertly rule countries, and a homogenized American culture is marketed worldwide (Miller and Hoffmann 1999). Bernstein (1994) points out that the global movement of people and capital redefines cultural identity and loyalty, weakening individual ties to nations and institutions. The implications are that people are not certain whom to trust or how to behave on the individual, community, or national level (Fukuyama 1995). Giddens (1998), a major architect of Tony Blair's "Third Way" in the United Kingdom, advocates that democracy can be redefined to meet these challenges in a creative way that preserves the safety net provided through social welfare systems while also being fiscally responsible and accountable in a world economy. These societal questions and debates frame our daily lives and drive the way that we conceive of and respond to disability. This book takes up these issues and faces the challenges presented.

The *Handbook of Disability Studies* was conceived in the context of these major historical, economic, social, value, and institutional issues. Disability studies is an emergent field with intellectual roots in the social sciences, humanities, and rehabilitation sciences. The theoretical and conceptual armamentaria of these disciplines provide frameworks to address the persistent themes addressed in the volume, raise the critical issues in need of attention, better understand the problems of the field, and suggest integrative approaches to uniting the field. Equally important to the conception of disability studies is the inclusion of the disability community and those with disabilities who do not actively participate in the community or discourse. A persistent question raised here and throughout the volume is the following: Who are disabled people, and who should speak for them? These multiple issues and voices are included in the volume.

The book, then, is aimed at an academic audience, disabled people, and those interested in forming social welfare policies. These multiple perspectives, diverse voices, and different goals combine to shape the emerging field of disability studies. They are represented by the rapid expansion of Rehabilitation International; the Society for Disability Studies; the British Council of Disabled People; the development of the Australian Disability Strategy; the influence of the Leeds group in England, especially through its Internet discussion groups and Web sites; the strong support of the National Institute on Disability and Rehabilitation Research in the United States; and the emergence of academic disability studies programs offering degrees in disability studies, such as those in the College of Health and Human Development Sciences at the University of Illinois at Chicago and at the University of Leeds (Pfeiffer and Yoshida 1995). The formation of disability studies, then, has strong theoretical, applied, and social policy origins, emphases, and goals. At present, the field is in the process of cohering around fundamental issues. We hope that this volume situates the field, raises the critical issues, sharpens the debate, and helps to take the field to another level of inclusion, integration, and sophistication.

In planning the volume, we were acutely aware of the considerable challenges faced by the emerging field of disability studies. The first challenge focuses on the controversies surrounding the importance of language, symbol, and representation in discussing disability. At this point in the dialogue, diverse historical, theoretical, advocacy, political, and cultural forces influence how disability is expressed and represented. These issues become increasingly contentious as the discourse moves across national boundaries, disability types, and societal reactions. In the United States, for example, a controversy has raged over preferred linguistic usage. One group historically advocated people-first language, expressed in the term *people with disabilities,* emphasizing the historical roots of American exceptionalism, the importance of the individual in society, and disability as being something *not* inherent in the person. An equally vocal group has more recently denounced people-first language as offensive, claiming that it was promoted by powerful nondisabled people, particularly advocates for persons with developmental disabilities. This second group prefers the term *disabled people,* emphasizing minority group identity politics. It should be noted that the evolution and accepted practice of linguistic usage has changed as much in response to political positions and pressures as to conceptual and theoretical developments. This heated discourse struggles with expressing values that acknowledge individual difference and inclusion in a society based on civil rights.

In the United Kingdom, the choice is the term *disabled people,* signifying in some instances the importance of community and group identity and oppression experienced in the social environment. In French, *les handicapés* points to constraints imposed on groups of individuals who experience limits from some health condition or accident and from the environment. In French culture, the emphasis continues to be placed on groups and on the obligation and support of the welfare state equipped with reasonable safety nets to support "les handicapés." In Spanish, *inhabilidad* refers to the inability of people to perform certain activities and roles, again with emphasis being on the community or state to provide support. Disability language certainly is rooted in history, nationality, culture, and ideology. The importance and signification of language are at the center of an ongoing discussion.

The complexity of the concepts used in disability studies and the permeability of meaning between different words used to reflect disability are expressed at this moment in the interactive Internet discussions about what language to use in referring to disability and persons in this world. Then there are more focused exchanges about the terms to be used in discussing specific conditions such as mental retardation, mental illness, intellectual and cognitive disabilities, low vision, deafness, learning difficulties, developmental disabilities, hidden disabilities, environmentally based disabilities, and neurological and orthopedic conditions and impairments (that may or may not be disabling). The discussions are lively and heated. Numerous chapters in the handbook present the reasoned positions that lead to one interpretation over another. The important point is that the discussion needs to continue, be respectful, and aim at understanding. Ultimately, the field will mature as theory, concepts, appreciation of differences, and acknowledgment of political implications are refined and incorporated into the discourse.

Visual representations and images of disability are likewise the source of much discussion (Stafford 1993). For example, a presentation of artistic images of disability at the meetings of the Society for Disability Studies in Oakland, California, in 1998 by Henri-Jacques Stiker provoked a lively debate that continues in the field to this day over disability representations among a multidisciplinary and multinational audience. The critical issue persists: Why are so many depictions of disability in art and literature negative in character, portraying disabled people as dependent, "nonhuman," "freaks," marginal, or even dangerous? As Deutsch and

Nussbaum (2000), Mitchell and Snyder (1997), Thompson (1997), Longmore (1997), and Darke (1998) have noted in their work on stigma, image, and representation, positive visual and verbal imagery of disability is practically nonexistent. Sensitive to this debate, we selected a classical painting for the cover of the handbook that represents some of the key issues in the discussion. Raphael's *The Fire of Borgo* was selected as the cover for the handbook because of its classic imagery and "gravitas" but also because it raises many crucial issues in disability representation that are addressed in literature, art, and painting throughout the book. Raphael (1483-1520) was commissioned by Leo X (Giovanni de'Medici, the son of Lorenzo the Magnificent) to paint four works in the papal apartments in Rome depicting events in the lives of previous popes named Leo (Paoletti and Radke 1997). Raphael began this work in 1514 in the Stanza dell'Incendio, which takes its name from one of these four paintings, *The Fire of Borgo* (Vasari 1998).

The Fire of Borgo commemorates an event in the life of Leo IV (847-855), who extinguished a fire in front of the old St. Peter's Church in Rome, but it includes allegories and symbolism that transcend history. The painting becomes a commentary on the periodic and actual ritual of the sacking of Rome, symbolizing multiple threats to the established order. In Raphael's stylistic development, *The Fire of Borgo* breaks with previous harmony in his painting by presenting one figure that deviates from the classic form. As Snyder and Mitchell (2001) thoughtfully point out, Raphael draws on Virgil's story of the founder of Rome who refuses to leave his blind and lame father, Anchises, behind in Troy. In the left foreground, Aeneas is carrying his father to safety and the future.

The critic could argue that the painting is male, traditional, Eurocentric, and negative in that it gives agency to a nondisabled person caring for a disabled person and thus confirms a distasteful stereotype. While these objections have merit, we chose *The Fire of Borgo* for the cover to emphasize the salience of the debate and simultaneously reinforce the importance of considering representations in context. Every image is bounded; it has limitations, strengths, and insights. Works of art are by their nature situated, allegorical, and often provocative, and they require a reading. Our values today cannot alter past history and culture, so we try to understand that which was left to us. In fact, we cannot fully understand the place of disability in society unless we analyze images across time, space, and context. This painting signifies that disabled people have a value and place in society, that disability and intergenerational relations have been important across history, and that disability is to be understood in its historical and cultural context. The painting celebrates difference and the multiple values and interpretations of life. Continuity and hope are expressed in the painting by Aeneas taking the life experiences, wisdom, values, and family with him represented in the form of his father.

A second challenge to our understanding of disability studies is to determine what should be included and excluded from the field. If disability studies has no clear boundaries and no firm agreement about core concepts, theories, perspectives, and content, it will not be a coherent field. This is a problem with many traditional disciplines today as problems and paradigms shift (Smith-Lovin 1999; Wolf 1999). For disability studies to be taken seriously, we must describe and analyze the phenomena of interest—disability. This leads to numerous epistemological and methodological problems that are present in all of science and the humanities. Stephen Jay Gould (2000:259) attempts to debunk the purported "science wars" between the realists and the relativists by arguing that this is an artificial and overly simplistic distinction made to describe the process of doing science. He suggests that "useful knowledge . . . must record an improving understanding of an objective external world" but that this work is undertaken by fallible human beings in a historical, social, and ideological context. "Progress" in knowledge is achieved by being curious and observant, asking the important questions, developing different explanations and testing them, and taking both the objectivist and subjectivist perspectives into account. In disability studies, these "science wars" are characterized by the chasms observed between traditional rehabilitation interventions based on the medical model, rehabilitation sciences focusing on the application of technology and engineering to improve accessibility and the built environment, social sciences and the humanities, and the experientialists who find validity only in the subjective experience of disability.

Aware of these considerations, we reasoned that the field would be well defined and integration of frameworks possible only if our intellectual net were cast wide. All three editors have a longstanding interest in disability studies but considerably different backgrounds in the social sciences, humanities, and technology and a diverse range of experiences in academic institutions, government agencies, research projects, social policy experience, and government service in the United States and England. The editors also had short-term experiences in European, Middle Eastern, Asian, and African countries and, in one form or another, had personal experiences with chronic illness and disability. At this stage in the development of the field, we opted for inclusion but emphasized the social sciences, humanities, and perspectives of persons with disabilities.

An extensive book prospectus was prepared and sent for blind review by our publisher to 31 experts in the field representing many countries and constituencies. The feedback from the reviewers was longer than the original proposal; most of it was very insightful and helpful. These many suggestions were incorporated into the conception of the handbook. We tried to make the book as international as possible by including members of the International Advisory Editorial Board and authors from North America, the United Kingdom, the European continent, Australasia, and those with experience in Third World countries. We attempted to include scholars of different persuasions, people with and without disabilities, activists, policymakers, service deliverers, and consumers. Some of these contributors were based in traditional academic settings, while others were situated in institutes, agencies, and governmental settings. We used a series of meetings and focus groups of individuals from various disciplines, nations, and perspectives to identify the issues in the emerging field, the important paradigms, and who was doing some of the most interesting work. These meetings and contacts were used to identify the most appropriate authors to write on diverse topics. With few exceptions, every author invited to write a chapter agreed to do so. To add to the quality and depth of the book, two knowledgeable experts in that area and the editors reviewed each draft manuscript. Extensive revisions were made grounded in this feedback. While one book cannot include every theory and perspective, a serious attempt was made to reflect the diversity and depth of disability studies in this volume. In short, this was a thoughtful exercise drawing on the expertise of more colleagues than we could name—some known to us, others anonymous. We acknowledge their many contributions but take full responsibility for whatever shortcomings there might be in the final product.

A third challenge concerned the organization and content of the book. The book is divided into three major sections, each representing an overarching theme: The Shaping of Disability Studies as a Field (Part I), Experiencing Disability (Part II), and Disability in Context (Part III). These three themes organize the critical work that has been done in the past, resonate with current developments in the field, and, we expect, will serve as the key foci for the future evolution of the field.

By concentrating the first theme on the shaping of disability studies as a field, we highlight the importance of examining the historical roots, critical questions, and theoretical frameworks that define disability studies. The history of disability studies in the Western world reveals that from early times, disability has raised questions of normality, theories of difference, the perceived threat of difference to the established social order, and institutions and mechanisms of social control (Heaney 2000; Stiker 1999). Who were these people, what did they mean in a society, and what should be done about them? These questions were applied particularly to people with mental illness and intellectual and cognitive disabilities. In each case, disabilities were identified, defined, and dealt with in a specific social, economic, and cultural context (Huizinga 1949). Physical disabilities were present, as evidenced by literature, historical accounts, art, and archeological remains. For the most part, however, people with physical disabilities were more often absorbed into the community, even though infanticide and abandonment were common in some cultures and historical periods. On the other hand, people with mental conditions were more probably institutionalized or separated from the community in some other way. At a deep level, with the development of civil society, disability evoked the question of citizenship and its rights and responsibilities (Glenn 2000). In turn, considerations of citizenship and disability forced philosophers and ethicists to consider issues of social inequality, human rights, right to life, and participation. These issues resonate through debates over social welfare and social security in any society and stimulated the development of social theory and policy.

Disability theory engaged the Cartesian question of the separation/integration of mind and body, later to be expanded into an entire area of investigation: body and society. The question of social differences and problems of social support forced societies to articulate disability definitions and develop methods to assess, count, and understand disability. This led to disability definitions based on organic problems embodied in the medical model, social construction of difference theories, social models of disability, environmental and genetic models, Foucaultian and other postmodern interpretations, and modern political economic theories of welfare. These themes, issues, theories, and related social policies are addressed in the first part of the book. They provide the history and frameworks that undergird an understanding of disability studies.

The second part of the book revolves around the theme of experiencing disability. In this section, disability is weighed in terms of subjective experience and interpretations. The level of analysis is often that of the individual. Here, disabled people and their families speak about the disability world from the inside looking out. The formation of restructured identities is explored in the context of personal histories, trajectories, and living with chronic health conditions. This section expresses disability as a corporeal and social experience in a cultural context. The interface of disabled people and their friends and families with the larger community is examined in terms of social network and social support theory. From these analyses, we see that disability rearranges social worlds and positions disabled people in new relationships with their families, communities, and health and social professionals, giving their lives new meanings. Self-empowerment occurs, if they make their own decisions and consistently take control over their own lives as much as possible. Additional self-empowerment can occur through exercising the power of the vote in democratic societies. Inaccessible health care, traditional institutional procedures, and professional attitudes, along with recalcitrant bureaucracies, are the impediments to the full exercise of freedom for disabled people.

The third part of the book examines disability in context. The level of analysis here shifts from the individual to the organizational and institutional arrangements that shape and redefine the experience of living with a disability. More recent analyses of disability have added to our knowledge by examining how the effect of cultural history, structural forces, institutional procedures, the environment, types of accessible goods, services, and opportunities affect disabled people. Of particular concern in postindustrial countries are the pervasive managed care and managed competition dynamics that reward service providers for avoiding high-cost patients such as disabled people who are most in need of integrated and consistent care (Bodenheimer 2000). In another context, there has been an implicit assumption on the part of the medical providers, medical supply corporations, the pharmaceutical establishment, and health policymakers in developed countries that disability was an area in which they were well informed and had the expertise to disseminate their knowledge effectively within countries and around the world. Rooted in this context, most responses to disability have been reactive based on traditional and Western social welfare models rather than aimed at prevention, enabling disabled people with an accommodating environment, or taking local cultures and the level of economic resources into account. The chapters in this section explore these assumptions, theories, and practices.

Through its institutions, mainstream society acts to deal with the issues of inclusion and exclusion, human rights, laws, access to education, the physical and social environment, employment opportunities, disability benefit programs, and science and technology as applied to disabled people. The private and governmental institutions organized to manage these issues are situated in political economic systems that place values on disabled people and treat them accordingly. To effect change in institutional behavior requires a deep understanding of the ideology, power, and dynamics of these key social actors. For disabled people to take a more participatory role in affecting their daily lives and become more self-empowered, they must understand the history of disability policy and practice and the institutional stakeholders with whom they must deal. The chapters in this section analytically take these issues on board.

A fourth challenge confronted by the editors involved trying to look beyond the horizon and pointing to the future. Recent World Health Organization and World Bank studies point to the projected global increase in disability over the next 20 years and its impact on the economic growth and political stability of entire nations (Murray and Lopez 1996). Disability due to HIV/AIDS is expected to affect more than 30 percent of the entire population of many African and Asian countries. Increases in neuropsychiatric conditions such as unipolar depression, the effects of continuing civil wars, drug-resistant endemic diseases, and the lack of health infrastructures, medicine, and assistive technologies in poor nations only add to the problem. The World Bank increasingly recognizes that increases in global disability are a serious threat to economic development and political stability. Taking these forces into account, we felt that it was imperative not only to provide a balanced and deep understanding of the history, concepts, theories, issues, and practices that ground and constitute the field of disability studies but also to gaze into the future.

We asked each set of authors to take this task seriously by giving suggestions and indicating directions for future work in the field. This exercise involves pointing out the critical issues that have not received sufficient attention to permit the field to mature, focusing on ways to integrate balkanized portions of the field, and indicating that interrelated work is required on the analytical, social policy, and practice levels to imagine how to include disabled people as key participants in forming their own destinies. Even this ambitious exercise is limited in a global world, if the focus of attention is on Western culture and industrial countries. In a world population of 6 billion people, 80 percent of all disabled people reside in developing countries. Almost nothing is systematically known about these people and their life circumstances. We do know that the problems of disabled people in developing countries are closely related to issues of resources, development, and human rights. The following question is raised: How can the disability studies field understand and contribute to our knowledge of this world and offer perspectives on how to ameliorate the lives of disabled people worldwide? Clearly, one response is to develop a true global vision of our interconnected world. We confronted these issues by inviting contributors from different perspectives and national origins, asking authors to make their chapters as international as possible, and pointing to the importance of making their analyses of the field global in perspective. We also asked them to select well-chosen international examples of their arguments and to provide useful bibliographies that would serve as a basis for further work.

While the book is not definitive, it represents a creative work in progress. We hope that the handbook broadens our knowledge of disability studies and stimulates others to take on the challenge of advancing the field in understanding and practice. After taking pause and reflecting on the field, let the next wave of work begin.

REFERENCES

Albrecht, G. and L. Verbrugge. 2000. "The Global Emergence of Disability" Pp. 293-307 in *The Handbook of Social Studies in Health and Medicine,* edited by G. Albrecht, R. Fitzpatrick, and S. Scrimshaw. Thousand Oaks, CA: Sage.

Bernstein, R. 1994. *The Dictatorship of Virtue: Multiculturalism and the Battle for America's Future.* New York: Knopf.

Bodenheimer, T. 2000. "California's Beleaguered Physician Groups: Will They Survive?" *New England Journal of Medicine* 342:1064-68.

Bowker, G. and S. Star. 1999. *Sorting Things Out: Classification and Its Consequences.* Cambridge: MIT Press.

Bruckner, P. 2000. *L'Euphorie perpétuelle.* Paris: Grasset.

Crozet, Y., D. Bolliet, F. Faure, and J. Fleury. 2000. *Les grandes questions de la Société Française.* Paris: Nathan.

Darke, P. 1998. "Understanding Cinematic Representations of Disability." Pp. 181-97 in *The Disability Reader*, edited by T. Shakespeare. London: Cassell.

Deutsch, H. and F. Nussbaum, eds. 2000. *"Defects": Engendering the Modern Body*. Ann Arbor: University of Michigan Press.

Friedman, T. 1999. *The Lexus and the Olive Tree: Understanding Globalization*. New York: Farrar, Straus and Giroux.

Fukuyama, F. 1995. *Trust: The Social Virtues and the Creation of Prosperity*. London: Hamish Hamilton.

Giddens, A. 1998. *The Third Way*. London: Polity.

Glenn, E. 2000. "Citizenship and Inequality: Historical and Global Perspectives." *Social Forces* 47:1-20.

Gould, S. 2000. "Deconstructing the 'Science Wars' by Reconstructing the Old Mold." *Science* 287:253-61.

Guéhenno, J. -M. 1993. *La Fin de la démocratie*. Paris: Flammarion.

Heaney, S., trans. 2000. *Beowulf*. New York: Farrar, Straus and Giroux.

Huizinga, J. 1949. *The Waning of the Middle Ages*. New York: Doubleday Anchor.

Longmore, P. 1997. "Conspicuous Contribution and American Cultural Dilemmas: Telethon Rituals of Cleansing and Renewal." Pp. 134-58 in *The Body and Physical Difference: Discourses of Disability*, edited by D. Mitchell and S. Snyder. Ann Arbor: University of Michigan Press.

McNeill, W. 2000. "Goodbye to the Bison." *New York Review of Books* 47:23-25.

Miller, A. and J. Hoffmann. 1999. "The Growing Divisiveness: Culture Wars or a War of Words?" *Social Forces* 78:721-52.

Mitchell, D. and S. Snyder. 1997. "Introduction: Disability Studies and the Double Bind of Representation." Pp. 1-31 in *The Body and Physical Difference: Discourses of Disability*, edited by D. Mitchell and S. Snyder. Ann Arbor: University of Michigan Press.

Murray, C. and A. Lopez. 1996. *The Global Burden of Disease*. Boston: Harvard University Press.

Paoletti, J. and G. Radke. 1997. *Art in Renaissance Italy*. New York: Henry N. Abrams.

Pfeiffer, D. and K. Yoshida. 1995. "Teaching Disability Studies in Canada and the USA." *Disability and Society* 10:475-500.

Sennett, R. 1998. *The Corrosion of Character: The Personal Consequences of Work in the New Capitalism*. New York: Norton.

Smith-Lovin, L. 1999. "Core Concepts and Common Ground: The Relational Basis of Our Discipline." *Social Forces* 78:1-23.

Snyder, S. and D. Mitchell. 2001. "An 'Infinity of Forms': Disability Figures in Artistic Traditions." In *Enabling the Humanities: A Disability Studies Sourcebook*, edited by S. Snyder, B. Brueggeman, and R. G. Thompson. New York: Modern Language Association.

Stafford, B. 1993. *Body Criticism: Imaging the Unseen in Enlightenment Art and Medicine*. Cambridge: MIT Press.

Stiker, H.-J. 1999. *A History of Disability*. Ann Arbor: University of Michigan Press.

Thompson, R. 1997. "Integrating Disability Studies into the Existing Curriculum." Pp. 295-306 in *The Disability Studies Reader*, edited by L. Davis. New York: Routledge.

Vasari, G. 1998. *The Lives of the Artists*. Oxford, UK: Oxford University Press.

Wolf, J. 1999. "Sociology and Border Disciplines: Opportunities and Barriers to Intellectual Growth." *Contemporary Sociology* 28:499-507.

THE SHAPING OF
DISABILITY STUDIES
AS A FIELD

An Institutional History of Disability

1

DAVID L. BRADDOCK
SUSAN L. PARISH

The primary objective of this chapter is to describe the institutional history of disability in Western society, establishing explicit connections between the social context in which people have lived and the ways in which disability has or has not been identified and addressed as a social problem. Our central thesis is that changing social and political perspectives on poverty during the seventeenth and eighteenth centuries, coupled with the development of increasingly medicalized interpretations of disability during the nineteenth and twentieth centuries, contributed to increasing segregation and stigmatization of persons with disabilities. However, a related thesis is that the congregation of people with similar disabilities for treatment and services also made possible the development of group identities, which ultimately facilitated the rise of political activism in the modern era.

Impairment and Disability

Throughout Western history, disability has existed at the intersection between the particular demands of a given impairment, society's interpretation of that impairment, and the larger political and economic context of disability. The contrast between disability and impairment informs a key underlying premise of this chapter: Disability exists as it is situated within the larger social context, while impairment is a biological condition. Lennard Davis (2000) has succinctly described the relationship between disability and impairment as follows:

AUTHORS' NOTE: This chapter initially grew out of the American Association on Mental Retardation Distinguished Lecture, given by the first author at the 123rd national convention of the Association in New Orleans, Louisiana, on May 26, 1999. Research support for the further development of this work was provided during academic year 1999-2000 by the National Institute on Disability and Rehabilitation Research under the auspices of a Mary Switzer Research Fellowship to the first author. The second author, a doctoral student in the University of Illinois at Chicago's School of Public Health, was partially supported on a grant from the Administration on Developmental Disabilities, U.S. Department of Health and Human Services for the State of the States in Developmental Disabilities Project in the Department of Disability and Human Development at the University of Illinois at Chicago (UIC). The authors express their gratitude to Professors David Mitchell and Gary Albrecht in the UIC Department of Disability and Human Development and to Professor Paul Longmore of the Department of History at San Francisco State University for their comments on earlier drafts of the chapter. We also thank Mary Catherine Rizzolo, Leslie Chapital, and Stephen Rubin at UIC for research assistance.

Disability is not so much the lack of a sense or the presence of a physical or mental impairment as it is the reception and construction of that difference.... An impairment is a physical fact, but a disability is a social construction. For example, lack of mobility is an impairment, but an environment without ramps turns that impairment into a disability ... a disability must be socially constructed; there must be an analysis of what it means to have or lack certain functions, appearance and so on. (P. 56)

Davis notes that disability was not constituted as a social category prior to the eighteenth century, even though impairments were no doubt quite prevalent in the general population.

Writing a history of disability in the West is a challenging undertaking. We will comment briefly on just three of the key problems facing researchers. First, the utilization of primary source evidence, the gold standard of historical research (Brundage 1989; Schafer 1980), is extremely limited in the literature, especially for periods preceding the nineteenth century (Brockley 1999). Recent historical accounts of disability have relied more heavily on primary source documentation but have generally limited their focus to the institutional nature of service delivery in the United States, beginning in the nineteenth century (Bredberg 1999; Brockley 1999; Ferguson 1994; Trent 1995; Wright and Digby 1996). While the constraints of writing a disability history within the confines of a concise book chapter have forced us to use secondary sources frequently, primary sources have been used when possible to reveal the rich historical fabric of a diverse and varied existence.

A second limitation of many published historical accounts is that the archive mainly describes formal services and treatment approaches from the standpoint of the professionals who controlled the delivery of services (e.g., Barr 1904; Earle 1898; Obermann 1968; Scheerenberger 1983; Sheldon 1921); this institutional perspective has often eclipsed the perspectives of persons with disabilities and even their families. The reliance on professionals' records has reflected and legitimated professional behavior (Hirsch 1995). Historians, for example, have tended to rely on the public record of residential institutions while largely ignoring lay perspectives toward disability (Jackson 1998). Such a practice has occurred even though only a small fraction of the entire disabled population has ever been institutionalized, particularly prior to the twentieth century. Moreover, people with disabilities have only infrequently recorded accounts of their experiences, so historians are left to interpret "lived experience" vicariously through the filter of professionals who did leave extensive records (Porter 1987b; Rushton 1988). Thus, historians are often put in the perilous position of interpreting the history of people with disabilities based on the claims of professionals, although this posture has been soundly rejected in recent years by the disability movement (Anspach 1979; Carabello and Siegel 1996; Shapiro 1993; Ward and Schoultz 1996), which today advances the philosophy of "nothing about us without us" (Charlton 1998).

The third limitation is that histories of disability are rarely representative of a broad cross-disability perspective that depicts the historical interconnections across the full spectrum of mental, physical, and sensory disability. In this chapter, we will address disability history across this broad spectrum, but we will also explicitly examine the history of mental disability in greater depth.

Overview of the Chapter

The chapter begins with a discussion of the extensive presence of people with impairments in ancient times and moves forward chronologically to the present day. Ancient Western notions of impairment in Greece and Rome accepted the belief that persons with congenital impairments embodied the wrath of the gods and should be killed. Yet this view coexisted with the fact that those who acquired their disabilities later in life were often integrated into society as workers, citizens, and soldiers. During the Middle Ages, widespread belief in demonology as an etiology of impairment was counterbalanced by religious movements preaching compassion and support toward persons with disabilities. Development of the first residential institutions for persons with disabilities is traced to the Middle Ages as well.

In the early modern period through the close of the eighteenth century, disability was strongly influenced by the rise of the scientific method during the Renaissance and by changing public perceptions toward poverty and disability. The radical intellectual revolution born of the Enlightenment, including scientists' subsequent emphasis on distinguishing mental illness from intellectual disability, is considered in some depth in this section of the chapter. Enlightenment thinking transformed fundamental concepts about the essential relationships between humans, nature, and God. This transformation involved the increasing legitimacy of science in society and led to the ascendancy of physicians, educators, and caretakers in the lives of persons with disabilities. Scientific inquiry into the medical aspects of impairment has been characterized by the development and application of increasingly complex diagnostic and etiological classification schemes. This process of categorizing persons with disabilities into the minutiae of their impairments resulted in the development of specialized treatments and residential and educational services but also established and reinforced notions of the boundaries between normalcy and aberrance in Western society.

Disability in the American colonies during the seventeenth and eighteenth centuries is examined along with the subsequent development and proliferation across Europe of institutions for persons with mental disabilities and schools for the deaf and blind. In the American colonies, and later in the United States, persons with impairments were often perceived to menace the economic well-being of the community. The practices of auctioning off the care of disabled persons to the highest bidder or running them out of town with threatened or real violence reflected an intimate connection between poverty and disability in this period of history.

Our discussion of disability history in the nineteenth century acknowledges the significance of political organization by deaf advocates—the first rumblings of activism by people with disabilities. That nascent movement sharply contrasted with the contemporaneous exploitation of people with disabilities as freak show attractions and the ascendancy of the eugenics era. The onset of the twentieth century was marked by a dramatic expansion of residential institutions for persons with mental disabilities and by the rapidly increasing segregation of children and youth with disabilities in public schools. We trace developments for persons with physical disabilities, independent living, and the emergence of family, community, and consumer advocacy, and we discuss litigation that forged a constitutional right to treatment for persons with mental disabilities in the United States. The chapter also discusses international disability rights initiatives such as the United Nations' *Standard Rules,* the Americans with Disabilities Act, and various European antidiscrimination legislation such as Great Britain's Disability Discrimination Act of 1995. The chapter concludes with a consideration of disability priorities in the twenty-first century.

ANTIQUITY

Prehistory

Individuals with physical impairments have been part of the social order since well before the evolution of humans. There is also anthropological evidence of impaired members living in prehistoric subhuman primate groups. Berkson (1974, 1993) argues persuasively that

> monkey and ape groups include individuals who have fallen from trees or who have been injured by predators. [They] may survive in natural animal groups when their injury does not actually interfere with foraging or escape from predators. In other words, the injury may not be handicapping.

Injured animals may survive and live in a group because group living itself can provide aid to adaptation. Mother monkeys provide care that compensates for even severe injuries, and other members of the group may "baby sit" injured babies, as they do other young of the group . . . where predation pressure is low and food is plentiful, handicapped animals may live to be adults. (Berkson 1993:5-6)

Citing work by Solecki (1971) and Stewart (1958), Berkson (1993) describes a published description of an adult Neanderthal male with severe arm and head injuries incurred at an early age. He accommodated the injury by using his teeth to hold objects. Berkson also uncovered research documenting the fact that disabling arthritis and other chronic impairments were common in Neanderthals (Goldstein 1969; Straus and Cave 1957). He concludes that individuals with both minor and even highly significant impairments were part of primate societies "even before the evolution of modern Homo sapiens" (p. 6). Thus, the presence of impairments among subsequent prehistoric Homo sapiens should not surprise us.

The Old Testament

Documentation of the treatment and life experiences of people with impairments during the earliest periods of recorded history is extremely limited. Edicts about disability offer some insight into prevailing attitudes, but the messages that they convey are mixed. The Old Testament commanded, "Thou shalt not curse the deaf nor put a stumbling block before the blind, nor maketh the blind to wander out of the path" (Leviticus 19:14). Daniels (1997) argues that this Hebraic command in Leviticus is the first attempt by any nation to legislate for the protection of the deaf. Daniels further asserts that deaf persons without speech were viewed as children under Hebrew law and provided with the same protections as children.

People were also reminded about their responsibilities toward one another with the injunction that "there will always be poor people in the land. Therefore, I command you to be openhanded toward your brothers and toward the poor and needy in your land" (Deuteronomy 15:11).

In contrast, the Old Testament also warned that

if you do not carefully follow His commands and decrees . . . all these curses will come upon you and overtake you: the Lord will afflict you with madness, blindness and confusion of mind. At midday, you will grope around like a blind man in the dark. (Deuteronomy 28:15, 28-29)

These paradoxical statements reflect competing attitudes toward disability. While society seems to have recognized a charitable obligation to people with disabilities, disability was also perceived as a punishment meted out by God. The belief that illness was inflicted by an angry deity or by a supernatural power was widespread among ancient peoples (Rosen 1968). The Old Testament also supports the notion that people with disabilities were classified with prostitutes and menstruating women as unclean and were thereby prohibited from making sacrifices as priests. According to Stiker (1997), people with disabilities were allowed to otherwise participate in religious observances. The early Christian church, however, held that faith came from hearing (Romans 10:17), and therefore the deaf were necessarily without faith in the eyes of the church (Daniels 1997).

In records dating back to 2000 B.C.E., the births of children with congenital impairments were used to predict future events for a community. In the Babylonian region, ancient Semitic Chaldean diviners of the future maintained a list of birth deformities and the specific prophetic meanings each foretold. The manifestation of disability was viewed as a portent of things to come (Warkany 1959).

Ancient Greece and Rome

Average life expectancy in ancient Greece and Rome did not generally exceed 37 and 44 years, respectively, for women and men. Due to the omnipresence of disease, war, poor prenatal care, malnutrition, and injury sustained during the hard work performed by most people, impairments and deformities were doubtless prevalent. Even such minor injuries as broken limbs would have produced disabling impairments in a majority of the population who were too poor to obtain medical care (Garland 1995). As Garland (1995) has noted,

> Life in the ancient world was nasty, brutish, and short. The most privileged were those who happened to be freeborn, well-to-do males in perfect health. But the overwhelming majority did not, of course, belong to that ideal category. (P. 11)

In the midst of this society beset by endemic impairment, the Greeks and Romans had varied interpretations of persons with such conditions. Babies born with congenital deformities were often regarded as signs that their parents had displeased the gods. However, public support was available to individuals whose impairments precluded them from working. In some exceptional situations, having an impairment was not a barrier to attaining power. The Roman Emperor Claudius had significant congenital deformities, and Spartans elected a short-statured man as their king. In any case, care for persons with impairments would have been reserved for those few who were wealthy enough to afford it—disability for the vast majority of Greeks and Romans would have increased the extent to which they were marginalized and excluded from society and living in deprived economic conditions (Garland 1995).

The notion that Greeks practiced infanticide of children with disabilities has been widely accepted (e.g., Mackelprang and Salsgiver 1996; Scheerenberger 1983; Woodill and Velche 1995). However, this practice was not as widespread as has been believed (Garland 1995). In ancient Greece and Rome, infanticide was practiced for economic reasons when there were too many children. In Sparta, however, children born with obvious physical deformities were put to death regardless of a family's means (Stiker 1997; Warkany 1959). Spartan law mandated the practice of killing newborns who had been born with deformities, while there is some limited evidence that Athenians may have been more inclined to raise such children (Garland 1995). Infants with deformities were sometimes perceived to represent the anger of the gods, and murdering such babies was a sacrifice intended to mollify the gods.

> Aberrancy within the species not only threatens the future and continuation of this species, but also announces, threatens, signifies a condemnation by the gods: a condemnation of the group . . . an aberrancy within the corporeal order is an aberrancy in the social order. (Stiker 1997:40)

Stiker (1997) further notes that the subjection of infants with deformities to death by exposure was specifically for infants we would today say have physical disabilities. Infants with hearing impairments, vision impairments, and mental retardation were not categorized as "deformed" and were not put to death, except perhaps for those most profoundly limited intellectually who could have been "diagnosed" early on.

It is likely, however, that many children with physical impairments survived even in Sparta because their impairments would not have been evident until they passed the age at which killing them would have been contemplated (Gaw 1906b). Furthermore, adults with congenital disabilities were a presence in ancient Greece (Stiker 1997). M. L. Edwards's (1996, 1997) reviews of the scant documentary records from ancient Greece indicates that deformity was not perceived as absolutely negative by the Greeks but that this perspective was developed by historians during the nineteenth century, who applied contemporary contempt for people with disabilities to their assessment of the ancient world. She further concludes that the assumption that deformity in a child was automatically associated with economic burden is not appropriate since many people with disabilities had jobs and earned income. It is difficult to determine from these conflicting records the extent to which the infanticide of children with disabilities was practiced; what is clear is that people with congenital disabilities, broadly defined, existed in society, indicating that infants with disabilities were not uniformly put to death.

Given high rates of disease and war, there was likely a higher prevalence of disability in ancient communities. Greeks who sustained injuries on the battlefield would often be expected to continue to fight, as mobility was not always a requisite for combat participation. Existing court records provide compelling evidence that the linkage between disability and entitlement to monetary support from the government was not absolute. Individuals with disabilities in Greece would have had to prove that they truly were economically needy and not just physically disabled to receive a small food grant (Edwards 1997).

Greek records also substantiate a public acknowledgment of providing support for those who were classified as unable to work. Dating from at least the sixth century B.C.E., Athens offered modest public support for those individuals who were unable to work due to their impairments. The *Constitution of Athens* provides information regarding the process of providing this support:

> The Council inspects those who are disabled. For there is a law which bids those who possess less than three minai and who are incapacitated and incapable of work to undergo inspection by the Council, which is to give them two obols per day each at public expense. (Garland 1995:35)

Military medicine was in widespread use in ancient Greece, as was public support of men disabled by war (Stiker 1997). Pensions were granted to soldiers who had been injured in battle, and food was provided to others with disabilities who could prove their economic need. The conclusion that Edwards (1997) draws regarding the status of people with disabilities during ancient Greek times is telling:

> The consequences of physical handicaps varied according to the context and to the individual. Without a codified notion of "able-bodied" on one hand and "disabled" on the other, people were not automatically assigned to one category or the other on the basis of medical diagnosis or appearance.... We see very few instances in which people with physical handicaps were banned a priori from certain roles ... people with disabilities in Greek society were integral to the society. There is no indication that people with physical handicaps in the ancient Greek world identified themselves or were identified as a distinct minority group. (Pp. 43-44)

Surviving historical and literary accounts have indicated that prosthetic devices were used by persons who sustained injuries during battle or had congenital limb malformations (Bliquez 1983). Herodotus recounts a warrior amputating his own foot to free himself and escape his impending execution. In 479 B.C.E., this warrior supported himself fighting on the battlefield by using a wood prosthesis. In a tomb dating to 300 B.C.E., a skeleton was found with an artificial lower right leg. This prosthesis was made of bronze, indicating that its owner was a person of some wealth.

Early Roman law chiefly protected the property rights of people with disabilities. Persons who were designated as intellectually deficient in early Roman times were provided with guardians to assist in the management of their affairs (Winzer 1993). Deaf persons capable of speech were granted authority to discharge legal obligations such as marriage and property ownership. Deaf persons without speech were classified alongside persons with intellectual disabilities, mental illness, and infants and were forbidden to perform any legal acts (Gaw 1906a, 1906b, 1907; Hodgson 1953).

In the Roman Empire, short-statured slaves and slaves with intellectual disabilities were often maintained by wealthy men for entertainment purposes. "Keeping" such individuals was considered good luck. The earliest records of court jesters date from Egyptian pharaohs of the Fifth Dynasty who kept short-statured people (Welsford [1935] 1966). Both ancient China and pre-Colombian American civilizations had short-statured people serve as court jesters as well (Willeford 1969).

Later Roman law enumerated the specific rights of people with disabilities. In the sixth century A.C.E., the Justinian Code classified persons with disabilities in detail and delineated rights pertaining to different types and degrees of disability; for example, people with mental disabilities were not permitted to marry. Drawing on the Jewish discrimination between degrees of deafness (Daniels 1997), the Justinian Code identified five classes of deafness (Gaw 1906a, 1906b, 1907). The code became the basis of law in most European countries from the sixth to the eighteenth centuries.

Writings from the New Testament offer insight into attitudes about disability shortly after the time of Christ. Mark records Jesus' healing of a blind man by spitting and laying hands on the man's eyes (Marcus 1999; Mark 8:22-26). Mark and Matthew also record Jesus' healing of a man with paralysis (Black 1996; Mark 2:1-12; Matthew 8:5-13). The New Testament relates other stories of people with leprosy, epilepsy, mental illness, deafness, and blindness being healed by Christ (Black 1996). These healing tales may be interpreted to mean that people "have disabilities . . . to show the power of God" (Black 1996:29). When asked whether a blind man's sin or his parents' sin had caused the man's blindness, Jesus replied that it was neither but rather a mechanism for "God's work [to be] revealed in him" (John 9:3; Black 1996:29). However, the fact that the disciples believed that the man's blindness was caused by sin may be indicative of prevailing wisdom regarding the supernatural etiology of this condition at the time.

Interpreting disability in antiquity is difficult in that the time span considered is vast, and competing attitudes toward disability are evident at many points. Writings from the Old Testament suggest paradoxical attitudes, which exhorted society to be generous and kind toward individuals with impairments, while also declaring that impairment was a mark of the wrath of God. Ancient Greece and Rome offer similarly complex interpretations of impairment. The killing of newborns with congenital impairments existed in some form throughout Greece and Rome, and society clearly perceived the birth of a child with congenital anomalies as the mark of the anger of the gods. However, the provision of pensions to soldiers injured on the battlefield was also a part of ancient Athenian life, and citizens with impairments were widely known to have worked at different trades. Impairment at the time of Christ was similarly fraught with different meanings, offering both redemption opportunities for kind strangers and signifying superstition. In the ancient world, impairment was accepted, at least in part, as an aspect of the course of life.

MIDDLE AGES

In the fourth to sixth centuries A.C.E., monastically inspired hospices for blind persons were established in what is now Turkey, Syria, and France. These hospices were organized as refuges for people with disabilities within existing religious enclaves (Winzer 1993). Bishop Nicholas cared for persons with intellectual disabilities in a hospice in southern Turkey during the fourth century, and the Belgian village of Gheel initiated the support of persons with mental disabilities in family care settings in the thirteenth century (Roosens 1979; Stevens 1858). The latter community provided vocational opportunities in a community setting that included an infirmary and a church centered around the shrine of St. Dymphna (Kroll 1973; Pollock 1945; Rumbaut 1972). By the sixth century A.C.E., institutions to segregate people with Hansen's disease (leprosy) were developing sporadically. Germany and Italy had hundreds of these facilities by the Early Middle Ages (Howard 1789; Weymouth 1938).

Demonology

Many disabling conditions, including intellectual disability, mental illness, deafness, and epilepsy, were thought to have supernatural or demonological causes during the medieval period.

The devil was believed to cause epilepsy (Alexander and Selesnick 1964). Belief in demonic possession as a primary etiology of mental illness led to attempted cures based on religious ideas about exorcism (Clay 1966; Neaman 1978). Attempts to cure people with disabilities from early medieval times reflect supernatural beliefs in the abilities of magic and religious elements. For instance, Anglo-Saxons offered the following antidote to mental illness:

> A pleasant drink against insanity. Put in ale hassock, lupine, carrot, fennel, radish, betony, water-agrimony, marche, rue, wormwood, cat's mint, elecampane, enchanter's night-shade, wild teazle. Sing twelve Masses over the drink, and let the patient drink it. He will soon be better. (Russell 1980:45)

Interest in persecuting witches developed gradually, culminating in the craze that began in 1450 (Russell 1980). During the Middle Ages, the first heresy executions occurred in France in 1022, and thousands of so-called witches were subsequently executed (Russell 1972). Persecution was frequently led by the Catholic Church, although Protestant European countries also followed papal orders regarding the execution of witches. Pope Innocent IV authorized the seizure of heretics' goods, their imprisonment, torture, and execution (Russell 1980). In 1484, Pope Innocent VIII declared war on witches (Russell 1980). While it is acknowledged that disabled persons were among those who were persecuted, the extent to which this occurred is not known. It seems likely that persons whose impairments were not amenable to contemporary treatment, particularly those with mental illness, would have been disproportionately affected by the witch craze (Winzer 1993).

Some of those individuals later persecuted for witchcraft in colonial New England most likely had mental illness, even given the crude understanding of mental illness at the time. Erikson (1966) recounts instances of clearly mentally disabled colonial women being put to death for their various crimes. American psychiatrists of the mid-nineteenth century described colonial New England's witchcraft as manifestations of mental illness. These psychiatrists interpreted the persecution of people with mental illness as pitiable but not necessarily peculiar. They expressed surprise that physicians misapplied the label "witch" to women who had mental illness ("Witchcraft and Insanity" 1849).

Compassion and Support

Despite the negative impact that widespread superstition had on people with disabilities during medieval times, there is evidence that other attitudes about disabilities, particularly mental illness, were also common (Kroll 1973; Neugebauer 1979; Rosen 1968). Kroll (1973) argues that the absence of demonology in medical texts from the medieval era, the scattered advocates for the natural causes of mental illness, and the town's assumption of responsibility for people with mental disabilities are strong evidence that demonological beliefs were only a part of the picture. However, views toward disability were complex and apparently included "elements of empirical rationality and humane interest" (Rosen 1968:139). Further evidence of positive or at least sympathetic attitudes toward people with disabilities is manifested in the fact that some towns actually funded pilgrimages to distant religious sites for people with epilepsy and mental illness to seek cures (Rosen 1968).

The relationship between poverty and disability during the medieval period is also significant. Malnutrition and infectious diseases were endemic, doubtless contributing to significantly higher rates of impairment, making persons quite visible in their communities. The chances of living to adulthood averaged just 50 percent during the medieval period (Jankauskas and Urbanavicius 1998). In thirteenth-century France, Italy, and England, tax records indicate that as much as 75 percent of the population was too poor to pay taxes and was particularly susceptible to dire consequences if they became disabled (Farmer 1998). This profound poverty meant that adults not capable of working were often a tremendous burden to their families. Even in families where both spouses worked, women often supplemented their low wages with begging (Farmer 1998). In this context, begging by people with disabilities seems more related to their poverty than to their disability. Begging during the Early Middle Ages was not stigmatized as it later would be. The existence of the poor was accepted as part of the natural order, and the poor were perceived to offer opportunities for wealthier citizens to do good by providing alms (Spierenburg 1984). In this context, persons with disabilities doubtless had more widespread acceptance as part of the poor.

Evaluating records from the canonization of St. Louis provides extensive evidence that people with disabilities sought cures for their disabilities at his tomb and that during the medieval period, people with disabilities survived by relying on a variety of supports: family members, neighbors, employers, charitable institutions, and begging (Farmer 1998). Charitable institutions appear to have been the least likely source of support for people with disabilities, often only providing assistance until an individual was sufficiently recovered to leave the hospital and beg for alms. There is also evidence that family, friends, and neighbors, in addition to providing material support as they were able, would assist people with disabilities to beg in the streets even by carrying them if necessary (Farmer 1998). The networks of support that appeared to exist, even for women who were recent immigrants, provide evidence that medieval attitudes toward disability were more complex than is often believed and not entirely negative.

Examining court records between the thirteenth and seventeenth centuries in England, Neugebauer (1978, 1979, 1996) found that demonological beliefs about the origins of brain disorders were not the only etiological beliefs held by society. The Crown's legal incompetency jurisdiction differentiated between intellectual disability (termed *natural fools* and, later, *idiots*) and mental illness (termed *non compos mentis* and, later, *lunacy*) (Neugebauer 1996). The *Prerogativa Regis* in the latter half of the thirteenth century endowed the Crown with specific responsibilities for protecting the person and property of individuals whose mental disabilities rendered them legally incompetent. Differentiation of "idiots" and "lunatics" by the *Prerogativa Regis* enabled the Crown to take custody and profits generated from lands owned by "idiots." In the case of individuals with mental illness, the Crown had the responsibility to ensure the safekeeping of lands held by "lunatics." The Crown, however, was not entitled to profits generated by the "lunatics'" lands that it supervised (Neugebauer 1996).

Perhaps even more significant, verbatim transcripts of custody hearings indicate that the means used to determine the presence of mental disability relied on tests of literacy, numerical ability, reasoning, knowledge as to place and kin, and so on (Neugebauer 1996). The records of these examinations indicate that the essential questions used to determine the presence of mental disability were relatively constant from the thirteenth through the seventeenth centuries, indicating relative stability in the understanding of mental disability during this prolonged period (Neugebauer 1996; Swinburne 1590).

Residential Institutions Emerge

During the Middle Ages, Greek and Roman medical and philosophical traditions were introduced into Europe by the Arabs, who had conquered most of the continent and penetrated Spain and France. Asylums for people with mental disabilities had previously been established by the Arabs in Baghdad, Fez (Morocco), and Cairo in the eighth century and subsequently in Damascus and Aleppo in 1270 (Alexander and Selesnick 1964). Since the Arabs held the general belief that mental disability was divinely inspired and not demonic in origin, care in these facilities was generally benevolent.

In England, the Priory of St. Mary's of Bethlehem was founded in 1247 in London with the explicit purpose of supporting the Order of Bethlehem by gathering alms to provide a base for members of the order visiting from abroad (MacDonald 1981). Although the order may have begun supporting physically ill persons as a hospital as early as 1330, it did not begin caring for mentally disabled persons, except perhaps incidentally and temporarily, until 1403. After this date, mentally disabled persons gradually displaced the physically sick as the primary focus of the facility, but "it was nearly a hundred years later before there is evidence that London's magistrates thought that *only* the mad should be admitted" (Andrews et al. 1997:90). Today, Bethlem Hospital is the longest continually operating mental hospital in Europe.

In Spain, a hospital dedicated exclusively to mental disability was founded by Father Joffre in Valencia in 1409 (Rumbaut 1972). Other asylums also opened in fifteenth-century Spain in Zaragoza (1425), Seville (1436), Valladolid (1436), Palma Majorca (1456), Toledo (1480), and Granada (1527) (Bassoe 1945). A general hospital known to have housed persons with mental disabilities was also opened in Barcelona in 1412. No less an authority than France's great psychiatrist Phillippe Pinel believed Spain's asylums to be the world's most humanely and wisely administered mental hospitals from the fifteenth through the eighteenth centuries. In *Traité Médico-Philosophique sur l'alienation Mentale* (1809), he specifically cited the excellence of the Zaragoza asylum, "the founders of which aimed to construct mental disorder by charm inspired by the cultivating of fields, the instinct which prompts people to render the earth fertile and secure the fruits of their industry" (Pinel 1809:238).

A madhouse was constructed as part of the Georghospital in Elbing in 1326, in what is modern-day Germany. The Grosse Hospital in Erfurt, Germany, included a "mad hut" when it was constructed in 1385. Prior to the building of separate facilities for people with mental illness, general hospitals or infirmaries accepted people with mental disorders (Rosen 1968). However, given the lack of care institutions during the medieval era, people with mental disabilities must have been a relatively common presence in their communities (Digby 1996).

It has become part of the lore that people with mental disabilities were cast out to sea in so-called ships of fools during the Middle Ages (Maher and Maher 1982). The notion of the ship of fools was created in 1494 with the publication in German of a book of the same name by Brant (Swain 1932). There is no evidence that these ships actually existed, however (Maher and Maher 1982). Brant was a preacher who used the fool as a metaphorical device to rebuke his congregation to be pious (Swain 1932).

During the twelfth century, institutions for the quarantine of people with Hansen's disease (leprosy) became prolific (MacArthur 1953). Howard (1789) chronicles the existence of numerous facilities, termed *leprosariums,* throughout Europe, many of which evolved as part of the charitable work done by religious orders (Kipp 1994). This confinement experience with leprosy represents the first time that institutional, segregated facilities were systematically used in Europe to address the issues presented by people with disabilities. Isolation of lepers was a harbinger of the perceived merits of segregation and confinement of other disabled populations, although institutional treatments for people with disabilities other than leprosy were slower to develop. As leprosy virtually disappeared in Europe by the sixteenth century (Weymouth 1938), many converted leprosariums became privately operated madhouses for people with mental illness and, in some cases, for persons with intellectual disabilities (Alexander and Selesnick 1964). Leprosy, however, subsequently spread to the Americas and had a substantial impact. De Souza-Araujo (1937, 1946, 1948) has described in great detail the spread of leprosy from Portugal, Spain, France, Holland, and Africa to Brazil beginning in the fifteenth century. The first Brazilian leprosarium opened in Rio de Janeiro in 1766, followed by the establishment of scores of such facilities nationwide.

During the Middle Ages, begging was a common way for people with disabilities to support themselves when their families were unable or unwilling to do so. Guilds and brotherhoods of blind beggars were organized to address issues of competition and conflict (Covey 1998; French 1932). One of the strongest guilds was developed in 1377 in Padua, Italy. This guild regulated begging and organized pensions for elderly blind beggars (Covey 1998; Gowman 1957). As the active role of the Catholic Church in promoting charity diminished following the Reformation, "little of the medieval fabric of hospices, almshouses and refuges" was left for care of "unfortunates" (Porter 1987a:121). Since monastic institutions were seized by the government during the Reformation and charity concomitantly diminished, the number of beggars increased dramatically. The passage of the Elizabethan Poor Law in England in 1601 was enacted partly in response to the large number of beggars (Covey 1998). And in 1657, Paris outlawed begging within its city limits (Foucault 1965).

In summary, the Middle Ages were notable for the contradictory beliefs held about disability. One common conception of disability was that some disabilities, particularly deafness, epilepsy, and mental disabilities, had demonological origins. This point of view contributed to the persecution of people with disabilities as witches and the use of magic to attempt to cure the disabling condition. A second conception of disability was also widespread—that persons with disabilities were part of the natural order, situated with other poor people and subject to the random havoc occasioned by the plagues in Europe. Stiker (1997) argues that the widespread nature of the plagues actually de-emphasized difference (impairment) more than in any epoch. There is significant evidence that people with disabilities used networks of support in their communities to survive in times that were harsh for nearly everyone. These two competing aspects of disability in medieval society appear to have coexisted, lending credence to the claim that there was no universal definition or interpretation of disability through this period.

EARLY MODERN PERIOD THROUGH THE EIGHTEENTH CENTURY

Renaissance and the Scientific Method

In the fourteenth through sixteenth centuries, beginning primarily in Italy, humanism in art was accompanied by advances in the anatomical and physiological study of hearing, vision, and the human body by Versalius, da Vinci, William Harvey, and others (P. Edwards 1996). In the mid-sixteenth century, Girolamo Cardano pioneered instructional approaches for people with hearing and visual impairments. He also attacked the prevailing practice of witch hunting (Gannon 1981; Wright 1969). While the last witchcraft execution in England took place in 1684, English laws halting the persecution of witches were not repealed until 1736 (Russell 1980).

Despite the advances in human understanding that were secured during the Renaissance, beliefs in the bestial nature of, and possession by, people with mental disabilities continued during the early modern period. During the sixteenth century, Reformation leaders John Calvin and Martin Luther independently preached that persons with mental disabilities were possessed or created by Satan (Colon 1989; Kanner 1964).

During the Renaissance, voluntary beatings of the head were employed to treat people with many mental diseases, including depression, paralysis, and intellectual disability (Bromberg 1975). Physicians would also bore holes in the head or purge persons with mental disabilities to release the "stones" or "black bile" thought to cause illness (Gilman 1982). Treatment for epilepsy included the ingestion of a mountain goat's brain or the still-warm gall of a dog killed at the moment of the seizure (Tuke 1878, [1882] 1968). One treatment of deafness consisted of frying earthworms with goose grease and dropping the solution into the ears (Winzer 1993). While these endeavors to cure illness and disability seem fantastic by today's standards, they focused on biological etiologies and treatments and therefore signified a change in the prevailing beliefs that the causes of disability and illness were supernatural. Cures during this period were related to primitive understandings of anatomical functions and to physicians' abilities to intervene to address bodily difference and dysfunction.

Analysis of an array of legal records in England during the early modern period indicates that society perceived two groups of people with mental disabilities: the "safe" and the "dangerous." The safe would have included most people with intellectual disabilities and many people with mental illness who were not perceived to be violent (Fessler 1956; Rushton 1988; Suzuki 1991). These individuals were cared for largely by their families, with an unclear and diverse amount of assistance from their local communities. The "dangerous" of the mentally ill were either cared for by their relatives, by local constables, or by sending them to a house of correction (Suzuki 1991).

In early modern England, there is further evidence that the general understanding of intellectual disability was understood to arise from birth and to be relatively fixed, whereas people understood that mental illness often had an onset in later life and could be quite transitory. While there were ambiguities in philosophical, medical, and legal interpretations of intellectual disability, fundamental aspects of differentiation clearly existed (Andrews 1998). The perceived need to differentiate between mental illness and intellectual disability seems to be more related to the application of property law than to treatment, which was essentially nonexistent at this time.

An important development of the sixteenth century was the initiation of education of deaf persons, which began in Spain and the Turkish Ottoman court. In Spain, instruction began with deaf aristocratic children who had been hidden in monasteries and convents by their wealthy families. This education was undertaken by the monks with whom they lived (Plann 1997). During the next century, deaf education in Spain was still limited to the wealthy classes, but it moved beyond the monasteries. In 1620, Juan Pablo Bonet of Madrid published the first treatise on the education of the deaf (Gannon 1981; Whitney 1949; Wright 1969). Sixty years later, George Dalgarno published the first finger alphabet designed specifically for deaf persons (Wright 1969).

Miles (2000) found that deaf persons employed in the Turkish Ottoman court were actually training one another in the use of sign language as early as 1500 and for the next two centuries. Their signing system became popular and was used regularly by hearing people, including Sultans and diplomats. Miles observed that

> the use of this language, and the training of deaf people *by* deaf people for responsible employment in a highly privileged but risky environment, was evidently developing from the early sixteenth century at a time when Western Europeans very seldom thought deaf people could be educated or could make any useful contribution to society. (P. 129)

The English statesman and philosopher Francis Bacon ([1605] 1900) believed that the supernatural and speculative philosophies of the Middle Ages and Renaissance had contributed nothing to the advancement of knowledge. He was impressed with the revolutionary discoveries of Copernicus and Galileo, who, for the first time, had proven certain characteristics of the universe. He was impressed with Marco Polo's travels and with the invention of gunpowder. Bacon introduced the notion of science as *systematic study*. He called for experiments to be conducted based on the collection of empirical data (Bacon [1605] 1900; Park and Daston 1981). The secrets of nature could be revealed, he argued, by the systematic observation of its regularities. In 1605, Bacon published *The Advancement of Learning, Divine and Humane*. In it, he refuted the notion of divine punishment as a cause of mental illness. He suggested four lines of inquiry that would guide psychological research for the next 300 years: studies of mental faculties and the interaction of body and mind, individual case studies, anatomical inquiry and postmortem studies, and the interaction between society and the individual (Bacon [1605] 1900).

Poverty and Disability

A profound change in attitudes toward poverty occurred across Europe during the thirteenth through seventeenth centuries that would have an impact on people with disabilities. Poverty traditionally had been associated with followers of Jesus in the Christian European countries, and beggars represented a means for almsgivers to please God (Spierenburg 1984). Ideas about the changing perception of poverty, from a necessary and even blessed state to a curse, began to slowly evolve from the thirteenth century. By the sixteenth century, this transformation was more or less complete, and poor people were deemed suspect. This metamorphosis of attitudes resulted in the eventual development of incarcerating facilities for the poor, particularly for people with mental illness (Spierenburg 1984). As previously noted, begging was outlawed in the streets of Paris in 1657, further marginalizing people with disabilities and separating them from what had been an important source of income for centuries.

England's Poor Law of 1601 was a watershed that specifically designated responsibility for poor and other people unable to provide for themselves. If a person was unable to procure a living for himself or herself, the first line of responsibility was his or her family. Barring the possibility of family provision of support, local communities were charged with providing for such persons in need (Rushton 1988, 1996). "Competent sums of money for and towards the necessary relief of the lame, impotent, old, blind, and such other among them" were to be set aside by the local community (43 Elizabeth 1601, cited in Axinn and Levin 1982:10). These laws became the general model in the American colonies, and local responsibility for people with disabilities who were unable to provide their own care was the common practice (Axinn and Levin 1982).

During the early modern and Renaissance periods, a complex relationship existed between community support, religious and medical institutions, and family resources in coping with mental disability (Adair, Melling, and Forsythe 1997). While the implementation of the English Poor Law was distinguished by the provision of relief in the community, on the Continent, the provision of public welfare "was usually within the context of structures likely to produce a sense of social stigma and alienation. Continental institutions are thus seen as compulsory and segregated from the outside world, and characterized by day-to-day procedures inherently dehumanizing" (Cavallo 1998:91). During the early modern period in Italy, for example, there is evidence that people with disabilities sought admission to hospitals for the poor in large numbers and were thereby subject to stigmatization.

English administrative records of the overseers of the poor indicate that people with intellectual disability were widely supported through the Poor Law, and policies of relief were relatively well organized during the early modern period (Rushton 1996). People with mental illness fared differently from those with intellectual disability. While most people with disabilities remained in the community with their families, there is evidence that people with mental illness were more likely to be incarcerated in gaols and houses of correction than their peers with intellectual disability (Rushton 1996). What is particularly important about the administration of welfare at this time is that it "marked a shift from the predominantly familial system that dominated the medieval period" (Rushton 1988:34). Examining welfare records in England, Rushton found that custodial care was virtually never contemplated for people with intellectual disability or mental illness, but families sought relief when their poverty was related to the impairment of a family member.

The first almshouse in the United States was established in Boston in 1662 and served a heterogeneous population, including persons with physical and mental disabilities, blind persons, deaf persons, the poor, the elderly, and orphans. However, the development of institutions for disabled persons was slow in the United States until the 1820s (Rothman 1990). Privately operated "madhouses" also began to spread across Britain during the Enlightenment period (Parry-Jones 1972). The first English workhouse was established in Bristol in 1697. By the end of the eighteenth century, there were 127 workhouses in England alone. Contagious invalids were turned away from workhouses, but people with mental disabilities were not. Workhouses spread rapidly across Europe by the beginning of the nineteenth century (Foucault 1965). Despite the spread of institutional care for people with mental illness in England between 1650 and 1850, families remained the main source of support during this period for poor people with mental illness (Suzuki 1998).

Philosophical Enlightenment

The *Enlightenment* or *Age of Reason* is a cultural historian's term for revolutionary changes in thinking that began in Europe in the seventeenth century. The Enlightenment represented the intellectual platform for the rise of contemporary Western civilization and drew heavily from the contributions of Francis Bacon, Isaac Newton, and John Locke. Two themes in Enlightenment thinking are related to changes in the care and treatment of people with disabilities. First, a "sensationalist" theory of knowledge laid the foundation for bold new psychological and educational interventions by arguing that experience and reason—rather than innate ideas and divine punishment—were the sources of all knowledge and that social and environmental modification could thus improve humans and society by manipulating society and the environment (de Condillac [1754] 1930; Locke 1690). The second Enlightenment idea of importance to people with disabilities was the growing belief in the merits of natural science to advance the species (P. Edwards 1996).

The Enlightenment's sensationalist school of philosophy spawned changes in attitudes, new institutions, voluntary charitable societies, interest groups, and literary work. In 1656 in Paris, the great "Hôpital General," France's charitable hospital, was formed as a single, semi-judicial administrative entity out of several existing establishments, including the Salpêtriere and the Bicêtre (mental hospitals for women and men, respectively) and several smaller general hospitals (Andrews et al. 1997). The first public charity hospital in France had opened in Lyons in 1612 and functioned in an analogous manner (Foucault 1965). Confinement no doubt accelerated in Paris with the enactment of the aforementioned edict in 1657 that prohibited begging.

Thus, *poverty, disability,* and the *inability to work* came to rank prominently among the major problems of the city. The soon to emerge "sensationalist" philosophies of the Enlightenment, however, provided the moral imperative and the tools for new and constructive interventions with the interconnected problem of disability and poverty (Winzer 1986).

Distinguishing between Intellectual Disability and Mental Illness

While English property law differentiated between intellectual disability and mental illness beginning in the thirteenth century, John Locke's 1690 work, *An Essay Concerning Human Understanding*, presented the most influential distinction to date between "idiots" and "madmen":

> The defect in [idiots] seems to proceed from want of quickness, activity, and motion in the intellectual faculties, whereby they are deprived of reason: whereas mad men seem to suffer by the other extreme. For they do not appear to me to have lost the faculty of reasoning: but having joined together some ideas very wrongly . . . they argue right from wrong principles. . . . But there are degrees of madness as of folly; the disorderly jumbling [of] ideas together, is in some more, and some less. In short, herein seems to lie the difference between idiots and mad men, that mad men put wrong ideas together, and so make wrong propositions, but argue and reason right from them: but idiots make very few or no propositions, but argue and reason scarce at all. (P. 236)

Although Rushton (1996:50) argued that Locke merely "provides a gloss on the pre-existing legal concepts rather than a critical challenge to them," he also acknowledges that Locke had a significant influence on Blackstone's later legal interpretations of intellectual disability. Goodey (1996) credits Locke with establishing the dichotomy between mental illness and intellectual disability that ultimately influenced social policy doctrine for people with intellectual disability. Even before Locke, in 1614, the Portuguese physician Montalto wrote a major medical work in which he distinguished mental illness from intellectual disability and described the diagnosis, prognosis, and treatment for intellectual disability (Woolfson 1984). This work, written while Montalto was personal physician to Italian Grand Duke Ferdinand I, has been largely ignored by historians.

Swinburne's (1590) definition of intellectual disability, published a century earlier, is important as well, in that it points to the importance of basic reasoning ability and suggests the elements of an assessment test to evaluate the provenance of "idiocy":

An idiote or a naturall foole is he who notwithstanding he bee of lawfull age, yet he is so witlesse, that he can not number to twentie, nor can tell what age he is of, nor knoweth who is his father, or mother, nor is able to answer to any such easie question. Whereby it may plainelye appeare that he hath not reason to discerne what is to his profite or damage, though it be notorious, nor is apt to be informed or instructed by anie other. Such an Idiote cannot make any testament nor may dispose either of his lands, or goodes. (P. 39)

Shortly after Locke penned his 1690 essay, Daniel Defoe, journalist and the author of *Robinson Crusoe,* recommended, to no avail, creating government-sponsored residential institutions for persons with intellectual disabilities, to be paid for with an author's tax (Defoe [1694] 1894; Goodey 1996). In 1720, Defoe also made a real deaf-mute person the hero in his book *The History of the Life and Adventures of Mr Duncan Campbell,* and he described sign language and approaches to deaf education in considerable detail.

Institutions for People with Mental Illness Established

In 1700, county asylums for "idiots, blind, and cripples" were proposed in England ("County Asylums Proposed" 1982). Parliament enacted a law in 1714 authorizing confinement, but not treatment, for the "furiously mad" and exempted them from the whippings routinely applied to rogues, beggars, and vagabonds. In 1704, Bethlem Hospital had 130 residents. There were 64 admissions, and 50 persons were cured and discharged that year (Strype 1720). Bethel and St. Luke's Mental Hospitals opened in Norwich in 1724 and in London in 1751, respectively. British Parliament repealed the witchcraft acts in 1736, and pressure mounted to improve conditions in the private madhouses. A statute was enacted regulating madhouses in 1774, and this was followed by a major parliamentary inquiry from 1815 to 1816 covering England, Scotland, and Ireland. According to one noted British authority, glaring deficiencies were noted between the best practices delineated in books about mental disability and actual conditions found in such facilities (Parry-Jones 1972).

In the eighteenth century, madhouses and criminal prisons were combined facilities in what is modern-day Germany. In these facilities, inmates were expected to work to contribute to the upkeep and expenses of the facility, particularly women through spinning (Spierenburg 1984). In Holland and Germany, private confinement was sought by wealthier families for their relatives with mental illness, frequently to avoid dishonor to the family by the person's behavior (Spierenburg 1984).

While the institutionalization of people with mental illness who were violent began during the fifteenth century, by the eighteenth century, facilities accepted people with mental illness who were not violent (Spierenburg 1984). This was the case in England, Germany, Holland, France, and Spain as well as in the New Spain (Mexico).

Developments in the American Colonies and Early United States

In colonial America, the first petition to secure payment for the guardianship of a person with intellectual disability was submitted to England's King Charles I in 1637. Support was sought for custody of Benoni Buck of Virginia (Harris 1971; Hecht and Hecht 1973; Neugebauer 1987). However, Puritans in colonial America still believed that disability was a result of God's divine displeasure (Covey 1998). Increase Mather, president of Harvard and father of witchcraft zealot Cotton Mather, wrote about the birth of children with disabilities as evidence of God's retribution. His son Cotton Mather later preached and wrote the same (Covey 1998; Winship 1994).

The American colonies largely appropriated English laws for their governance, including the Poor Law initially passed in 1601 under Queen Elizabeth. Since towns had ultimate responsibility for the poor under the law, communities took steps to discourage "vagabonds, beggars, or idle persons" (Peterson 1982:109) from settling therein. People who were considered likely to become a public charge would be "warned out" of town, with public whipping—the penalty for not leaving. People with mental illness were particularly susceptible to being warned out; however, there is also evidence that they received public support. The earliest provision for the maintenance of a mentally disabled individual in the Pennsylvania colony, for example, dates to 1676. In that year, the Upland Court in Delaware County, Pennsylvania, ordered that "a small Levy be Laid to pay for the buildings of ye house and the maintaining of ye said madman according to the laws of ye government" (Morton 1897:4).

In 1752, with leadership from the physician Thomas Bond and Benjamin Franklin, the first general hospital was established in the American colonies in Philadelphia. Care for persons with mental illness was a major motive in the founding of this hospital. The principal argument expressed in the petition filed with the Pennsylvania Provincial Assembly and subsequently embodied in the authorizing legislation of May 11, 1751, was to address the growing problem of mental disability in the colony. The petition read as follows:

To the honourable House of Representatives of the Province of Pennsylvania, The Petition of sundry Inhabitants of the said Province, Humbly showeth,

THAT with the Numbers of People, the number of Lunaticks or Persons distempered in Mind and deprived of their rational Faculties, hath greatly encreased in this Province.

That some of them going at large are a Terror to their Neighbours, who are daily apprehensive of the Violences they may commit; And others are continually wasting their Substance, to the great Injury of themselves and Families, ill disposed Persons wickedly taking Advantage of their unhappy Condition, and drawing them into unreasonable Bargains, &c.

That few or none of them are so sensible of their Condition, as to submit voluntarily to the Treatment their respective Cases require, and therefore continue in the same deplorable State during their Lives; whereas it has been found, by the Experience of many Years, that above two Thirds of the Mad People received into Bethlehem Hospital, and there treated properly have been perfectly cured.

Your Petitioners beg Leave farther to represent, that tho' the good Laws of this Province have made many compassionate and charitable Provisions for the Relief of the Poor, yet something farther seems wanting in Favour of such, whose Poverty is made more miserable by the additional Weight of a grievous Disease, from which they might easily be relieved, if they were not situated at too great a Distance from regular Advice and Assistance; whereby many languish out their Lives tortur'd perhaps with the Stone, devour'd by the Cancer, deprived of Sight by Cataracts, or gradually decaying by loathsome Distempers; who, if the Expense in the present manner of Nursing and Attending them separately when they come to Town were not so discouraging, might again, by the judicious Assistance of Physic and Surgery, be enabled to taste the Blessings of Health, and be made in a few Weeks, useful Members of the Community, able to provide for themselves and Families.

The kind Care our Assemblies have heretofore taken for the Relief of sick and distempered Strangers, by providing a Place for their Reception and Accommodation, leaves us no Room to doubt their showing an equal tender Concern for the Inhabitants. And we hope they will be of Opinion with us, that a small Provincial Hospital, erected and put under proper Regulations, in the Care of Persons to be appointed by this House, or otherwise, as they shall think meet, with Power to receive and apply the charitable Benefactions of good People towards enlarging and supporting the same, and some other Provisions in a Law for the Purposes above mentioned, will be a good Word, acceptable to God and to all the good People they represent. (Morton 1897:8)

Initially, cells in the basement of the hospital's temporary quarters were set aside for persons with mental disabilities. Four years later, a special wing in the hospital was used for this purpose, and in 1836, the cornerstone of a separate building was laid for the Pennsylvania Hospital for the Insane ("A Sketch" 1845). In its first years, the treatment of persons with mental disabilities in the Pennsylvania Hospital consisted of an assault on the body and the senses. Morton's (1897) comprehensive history of the hospital describes the treatment of "phrenze" in 1791 as consisting of being

> drenched or played upon, alternately with warm and cold water (which may have accounted for some of the pulmonary fatalities elsewhere mentioned). Their scalps were shaved and blistered; they were bled to the point of snycope; purged until the alimentary canal failed to yield anything but mucous, and, in the intervals, they were chained by the wrist, or the ankle to the cell wall. (P. 125)

The noted American psychiatrist Benjamin Rush may have introduced some improvements in care during his nearly 30 years of continuous service at the hospital between 1783 and 1813, but he is most widely remembered for introducing two mechanical contrivances for treatment (Rush 1812). One, called a gyrator or revolving machine, was used in cases of "torpid madness" to spin the body and raise the heart rate to 120 beats per minute. A second device, the tranquilizing chair, was intended to reduce sensory-motor activity and reduce the pulse. Rush, the only physician signer of the Declaration of Independence, also prescribed bloodletting, a common medical practice he learned in his studies at Edinburgh University, along with low diet, purges, emetics, and cold showers and baths (Morton 1897:164).

Veterans of the Revolutionary War were the first people with disabilities in the new United States to receive a pension, providing compensation for war-related impairments. In 1776, the first national pension law was adopted, and the sentiment of the Continental Congress reveals compassionate and concerned attitudes regarding those men whose impairments were sustained during the war:

> Permit not him, who, in the pride and vigor of youth, wasted his health and shed his blood in freedom's cause, with desponding heart and palsied limbs to totter from door to door, bowing his yet untamed soul, to meet the frozen bosom of reluctant charity. (Glasson, as cited in Obermann 1968:137)

One of the first American states to establish provisions for people with intellectual disability and mental illness was Kentucky. In 1793, the state passed legislation authorizing payment to families too poor to continue caring for members with either mental illness or intellectual disability without assistance (Estabrook 1928). A trial system for determining the person's identity as an "idiot" or "lunatic," as well as their need for such support, was established. This pension system continued throughout the nineteenth century and was still in existence in 1928. Annual payments remained at $75 from 1870 to 1928 (Estabrook 1928). It is noteworthy that professionals felt that the use of this pension encouraged idleness in people with intellectual disabilities and that the only appropriate form of support was institutionalization (Estabrook 1928).

Another American response to meeting the need for care of people with mental disabilities that could not be met by their families was the practice of "bidding out." In this system, a person with mental illness or intellectual disabilities was auctioned off to the lowest bidder, who would receive the bid amount to provide care for a year. This practice of "bidding out" was administered by counties in many states for people with intellectual disability and mental illness until about the 1820s, when it was perceived to become too expensive (Breckinridge 1939). Bidding out was a common form of welfare throughout the nation (Peterson 1982).

Schools for Deaf and Blind Persons Opened in Europe

The eighteenth century saw the gradual proliferation of residential schools for both deaf and blind persons. Schools for the deaf began in Spain and France and gradually spread to other European countries and the United States. The roots of deaf education began in north-central Spain with the birth of Pedro Ponce de León around 1510. de León, a Benedictine monk working in the monastery of San Salvador de Oña in the province of Burgos, is credited with being the first teacher of the deaf in the Western world. The exact date he began his work is not known, but by the mid-sixteenth century, he had initiated a school within the monastery for his students, many of whom were the children of wealthy Spanish families. He apparently used a manual alphabet and conventional signing and instructed about 20 students (Daniels 1997). After de León's death in 1584, Juan Pablo Bonet further disseminated de León's methods, publishing in 1620 in Spanish *The Art of Teaching the Deaf to Speak*. This book is recognized as fully derivative of de León's work; however, no original manuscripts of de León's earlier contributions have been located to date (Daniels 1997).

Ponce de León's methods appeared in mid-eighteenth century France, carried forward by Charles Michael de l'Epée. In 1755 de l'Epée, a Paris priest, established the world's first public residential school for deaf persons in Paris (Gannon 1981; Minski 1957; Wright 1969). By 1783, the school had 68 pupils (Daniels 1997). Signs were the communication technique preferred by de l'Epée (instead of the oral communication championed by his rival Péreire), and the support provided for his school by the king had a lasting influence on deaf communication (Lane 1989; Sacks 1989).

In 1760, Thomas Braidwood established the first British school in Edinburgh, Scotland (Gannon 1981; Minski 1957; Wright 1969). The first school for deaf persons in Germany was opened in 1778 in Leipzig by Samuel Heinicke. Abba Silvestri opened the first Italian school for deaf persons in Rome in 1784 (Gannon 1981). Germany's Heinicke favored "pure oralism," in the belief that articulation was necessary for deaf people to obtain respected status in society (Gannon 1981; Minski 1957; Wright 1969).

Abbé de l'Epée believed that deaf persons were representative of primordial ancestors, not unlike Rousseau's ([1762] 1991) notion of "man in the state of nature," and that their silence made them extremely similar to the first people on earth. He invited the public to visit his school, with the intent that doing so facilitated insight into the "natural path of human mental and linguistic development" (Rosenfeld 1997:157). Scientists and statesmen from Europe and the United States visited his school, and Enlightenment philosophers were intrigued with his educational methods and the unique opportunity represented by studying deaf persons and their sign language.

Although de l'Epée believed that sign language was a primitive form of communication, he believed that it was effective for deaf people. de l'Epée died in 1789 and was succeeded by the Abbé Sicard, who had previously headed a school for the deaf founded in the Bordeaux region of France in 1786. Sicard subsequently hosted Thomas Gallaudet of the United States during the latter's visit to Paris in 1816 and assisted Gallaudet in establishing the first school for the deaf in the United States (in Hartford, Connecticut) the following year.

In 1784, Valentin Haüy opened the first residential school for blind students in Paris (Allen 1899; Farrell 1956; Roberts 1986). He developed the first embossed print and used it to teach reading. The first school for blind students in England was opened in Liverpool in 1791 by Edward Rushton. Between 1804 and 1820, schools for blind children and youth opened in Vienna, Steglitz (Germany), Milan, Amsterdam, Prague, Stockholm, St. Petersburg, Dublin, Copenhagen, Aberdeen, Brussels, Naples, and Barcelona (Farrell 1956). The first U.S. institutions for blind students were opened in Boston (Perkins Institute) and New York City in 1832. Pennsylvania followed one year later, and Ohio opened a public school for blind students in 1837 (Allen 1899, 1914; French 1932).

The early modern period through the eighteenth century was a time of far-reaching change for persons with disabilities. Systematic differentiation between people with mental illness and intellectual disability was established to ensure correct adjudication of property laws. Comprehensive education of deaf and blind children began in Spain and France, respectively. This period saw the first manifestations of criminalizing and regulating idleness and poverty, which had a direct impact on people with disabilities who were usually poor. Institutional solutions to the problems ostensibly posed by poverty and disability—houses of correction, workhouses, asylums, and madhouses—became more common as the eighteenth century ended. The intellectual revolution of the Renaissance and Enlightenment contributed to fundamental changes in the relationships between humans, society, and God. For the first time, people were deemed to be capable of intervening in what had been perceived to be the immutable natural order: a belief that society and human beings could be perfected. This revolution in thinking stimulated extensive efforts to develop treatment interventions for people with disabilities, including the deaf, blind, and people with mental disabilities, and it led to the ascendancy of a professional class of physicians, educators, and caretakers. The medicalization and professionalization of disability reinforced the development and proliferation of institutions and schools across Europe and subsequently in North America. The trend toward institutionalization would gain greater momentum during the nineteenth and twentieth centuries.

THE NINETEENTH CENTURY

Educational Developments

Residential schools for deaf and blind students grew rapidly during the nineteenth century, as did institutionalized segregation of people with mental illness and intellectual disability. Therapeutic advances occurred for people with speech impairments, and controversy developed regarding two competing philosophies for educating deaf persons—oralism and manualism.

Schools for children with physical disabilities opened somewhat later in Europe than did those for deaf and blind students. The first school designed exclusively for children with physical disabilities was opened in 1832 in Bavaria by John Nepinak. Schools subsequently opened in other parts of Germany, France, England, Switzerland, and Italy. Denmark established the first program of industrial training for children with physical disabilities. A program of segregation in workshops became common in European schools by the middle of the nineteenth century (Obermann 1968).

In 1829, Louis Braille published an explanation of his embossed dot code, which was an improvement on a system developed by Barbier in 1808 (French 1932; Roberts 1986). Competing systems of communication would exist until 1932, when American and British committees finally signed an agreement to adopt Standard English Braille as the uniform type (Roberts 1986). In 1858, the American Printing House for the Blind was chartered in Louisville, Kentucky. This organization would become the premier printer of materials for blind persons in the United States, and in 1879, Congress legislated an annual appropriation of $10,000 for the printing of educational materials for blind persons (Allen 1914; American Printing House for the Blind 1999).

An intimate link between the fields of deafness and intellectual disability developed at the dawn of the nineteenth century. In 1800, Jean Itard (1775-1850) joined the medical staff at Sicard's National Institution for Deaf Mutes in Paris to study speech and hearing. The previous summer, a feral child was discovered in southern France, and scholars in Paris were anxious to examine him in the belief that the boy approximated "man in the state of nature." Thus, basic philosophical questions about human learning and development prominent in French Enlightenment thinking of the day could be systematically studied. Since the "wild boy" was mute, he was placed in the school for deaf persons in Paris. Pinel, who first examined the boy at the Bicêtre, was initially convinced that the boy, later named Victor, was unteachable. However, Itard committed the next five years of his life to instructing Victor, using educational approaches pioneered during the mid-eighteenth century by one of the first professional French teachers of deaf persons, Jacob Péreiere. Péreiere's teaching methods drew heavily on Rousseau's interpretation of Locke's "sensationalist" empirical psychology (Winzer 1993). Itard's approach emphasized individualization of instruction in five areas: sensory stimulation, speech, socialization, concept development, and transfer of learning (Itard 1802).

Itard initially believed that Victor suffered from early social and educational deprivation, and he thought his teaching had failed because Victor developed only minimal speech and was not fully restored to a useful life in society. Nevertheless, Itard's work subsequently stimulated highly successful interventions for children with intellectual disabilities by his pupils Edouard Séguin and Maria Montessori. Itard is also known for his early contributions to the oral education of deaf persons, the medical specialty otolaryngology, the use of behavior modification with children with disabilities, and the special education of persons with mental and physical disabilities (Itard 1821a, 1821b; Lane 1989). One of Itard's greatest contributions to his age's understanding of intellectual disability stemmed from his rejection of overly inclusive diagnoses of "idiocy." Also, in an underacknowledged paper he published in 1828 ("Mutism Caused by a Lesion of the Intellectual Functions"), Itard described how to distinguish between children with intellectual disability and those with pervasive developmental disorders such as autism (Carrey 1995).

Seguin expanded Itard's sensory techniques into what he termed the "physiological method," emphasizing sensory-motor training, intellectual training (including academics and speech), and moral training or socialization (Simpson 1999; Talbot 1967). Early in his career, Seguin (1846) acknowledged his debt to Péreiere and noted that intellectual disability, deafness, and congenital blindness shared two key characteristics: early age of onset and permanence of the condition. It followed that there would be similarities in remedial techniques. Seguin's work was embraced by the French Academy of Sciences in 1844 and subsequently became the standard worldwide reference. After heading schools for children with intellectual disabilities at the Bicêtre and in private schools for 20 years, Seguin left Paris for the United States in 1848 to escape political instability (Simpson 1999; Talbot 1967). Elsewhere in Europe, special residential schools for persons with intellectual disabilities were established by Guggenbuhl in Switzerland in 1842, by Saegert in Germany in 1842, and by Connolly and Reid in England in 1846 (Barr 1904; Bucknill 1873; Fernald 1893). It was common during this period for superintendents of facilities in one nation to visit Paris's facilities and report on the methods observed ("A Visit to the Bicêtre" 1847a, 1847b, 1847c).

The nineteenth century also witnessed dynamic changes in the education of other people with disabilities. In 1810, John Thelwall published the first book to be concerned solely with speech disability, *Letter to Henry Cline* (Rockey 1980). Thelwall is regarded as England's first speech therapist, and the nineteenth century marks the beginning of the differential diagnosis, evaluation, and treatment of speech disorders (Rockey 1980). The development of speech correction techniques in continental Europe was largely the province of educators of deaf persons, while in England, orators, clergymen, actors, and singing teachers were principally involved (Rockey 1980).

In Spain, deaf educator Tiburcio Hérnandez at the Royal School decreed a return to oralism following the 1814 opening of the school after Spain's War of Independence. While Hérnandez adopted the subordinate use of signs, borrowed from Frenchmen Abbé de l'Epée and Sicard, he advocated the primacy of oralism (Plann 1997). Hérnandez held derogatory views of deaf students, believing them to be essentially defective and unintelligent. Students were thus encouraged to learn manual trades because of persistent beliefs in their intellectual deficits. The domination of oralism in Spanish education of deaf students did not end with Hérnandez's 1823 execution during a period of political upheaval. Students were subjected to considerable physical abuse, which led to an uprising by some of the pupils against the teachers. For the rest of the nineteenth century in Spain, there was a marked rejection of teachers who were deaf, and education of deaf students became entrenched as the domain of experts who could hear.

In France during the nineteenth century, society continued to perceive deaf people negatively, often as a stereotype of naive, incompetent children. The Deaf Institute in Paris, a state-sponsored facility for deaf persons, served both educational and social welfare purposes. Two professors at the institute, however (Bébian and Paulmier), advocated the use of sign language and fostered a belief in the existence of deaf culture (Quartararo 1995).

First North American Mental Hospitals and Residential Schools

The first mental hospital established on the North and South American continents was opened in Mexico City two centuries before similar initiatives were undertaken in the United States and Canada. San Hipólito Hospital was established in 1566 near San Hipólito Chapel in Mexico City by the Spanish philanthropist Bernadino Alvarez. Alvarez was joined in the effort by several clergymen from an order that subsequently came to be known as "Los Hipólitos." New hospital structures were erected in 1739 and 1777, and the administration of the facility was taken over by the municipal government in 1821. The facility was closed in 1910, when all patients were transferred from this facility and from a second asylum for women that had opened in 1700, to a new institution called La Casteñada Asylum. The women's asylum, "La Canoa Hospital for Mental Disease," also known as the "Divino Salvador Hospital," was a product of the efforts of local carpenter José Sayago and his wife, who provided shelter, food, and care for poor mentally disabled women who were an everyday sight on the streets in the Capitol of the New Spain (Ramirez-Moreno 1937, 1942).

The first American almshouse was constructed in Boston in 1662, and the first mental asylum was constructed in Virginia in 1773. However, such institutions did not become common in the American landscape until the Jacksonian era, beginning in the 1820s. At this time, the nation was faced with increasing urbanization and manufacturing and changing demographics that included the first major influx of immigrants. These changing conditions led to social turmoil, and institutional solutions for social problems were sought for the first time in the United States. There is widespread disagreement among historians and social scientists as to the reasons for the appearance of institutions in the United States beginning in the 1820s (Mora 1992). Rothman (1990) contends that it was absolutely not inevitable for institutions to develop in the United States but that they represented an innovative solution to pressing social problems and profound changes in the economic and social structure of the country. He argues that the concurrent development of orphanages, asylums for people with mental illness, prisons, almshouses, and reformatories was the result of a nation grappling with tremendous social upheaval and a desire to manage the social order by controlling deviant members. Others have argued that the development of institutions followed the European example and was the product of American interest in solving social problems by adhering to the natural course established by Europe (Mora 1992; Grob 1990). Symonds (1995) has argued that mental institutions developed in England during the nineteenth century as a sociological response to perceptions of the threat of deviance, which is consistent with Rothman's (1990) conclusions about the development of such facilities in the United States.

During this period, residential schools in the United States began for deaf persons with the 1817 opening of the American Asylum for the Education of the Deaf and Dumb in Hartford, Connecticut, by Thomas Gallaudet and Laurent Clerc (Fay 1893). Within two years, this first school for deaf students in the United States was accepting students from 11 states (Ely 1893). The national character of the school stemmed in part from the fact that in 1819, the federal government granted the school an endowment of 23,000 acres of land in the Alabama territory (Breckinridge 1927).

The state of New York established the second U.S. school in 1818 in New York City (Gannon 1981). Many of the first schools in the United States were initially begun as day schools and later evolved into residential schools (Gordan 1885). The first separate schools for blind students in the United States began instruction within months of one another in 1832 in New York

City and at the Perkins Institute in Boston (Allen 1899; Farrell 1956; Frampton and Kerney 1953).

The bishop of Québec erected the first building in Canada exclusively dedicated to the confinement of mentally disabled individuals in 1714 (Hurd 1910). The building was located adjacent to the Québec General Hospital. However, people with mental illness and intellectual disability had been cared for in two general hospitals in Québec since at least 1694 (Griffin and Greenland 1981). As previously noted, the colonial government of Virginia opened the first mental hospital in the United States exclusively dedicated to mental disability in 1773 in Williamsburg (Eastern State Hospital). The opening of this facility had virtually no impact as a model on other states. The impulse to establish this facility stemmed from Virginia's English colonial governor, Francis Fauquier, who was motivated through a sense of noblesse oblige to establish similar institutions abroad (Grob 1973). The establishment of this first facility in the United States was not preceded by a public campaign, as would become the common practice for subsequent American facilities. The Virginia facility's capacity was 24 to 36 persons, and the governing authorities "never publicized the work of the hospital, and thereby reinforced its essentially local character" (Grob 1973:29). The facility shut down for 4 years beginning in 1782 due to the American Revolution. The state of Maryland then opened the fledgling nation's second state mental institution in 1798—fully 25 years after the opening of the first facility in Virginia. The third state institution for people with mental illness opened 25 years later, in Kentucky in 1824 (Grob 1973).

Private initiatives in the northeastern United States led to the creation of several mental hospitals modeled after the York Retreat in England. York was a private facility opened by the Quaker William Tuke in 1792. Between 1817 and 1847, private institutions opened in Philadelphia, Boston, New York, Connecticut, Vermont, and Rhode Island (Earle 1845; Hamilton 1944; Kirkbride 1845; Wood 1853). By the time the Butler Hospital opened in Providence in 1847 (Rochefort 1981), however, it had become clear that the exclusiveness and higher costs of private hospitals rendered them inadequate to meet the needs of the poorer classes, particularly the growing populations of urban poor in America's developing cities (Grob 1973; Hamilton 1944).

The development of mental asylums accelerated following Dorothea Dix's advocacy beginning in the 1840s (Brown 1998; Grob 1994; Rothman 1990). Dix traveled across the country, inspecting conditions of people with mental illness kept in prisons, living with their families, and in "bidded-out" contracts. She lobbied individual state legislatures for the construction of asylum facilities for the mentally disabled by writing memorials that described her findings (Brown 1998). In her first memorial, written after canvassing conditions in Massachusetts, Dix (1843) described

the present state of Insane Persons confined within this Commonwealth, in cages, closets, cellars, stalls, pens! Chained, naked, beaten with rods, and lashed into obedience! . . . Irritation of body, produced by utter filth and exposure, incited [one woman] to the horrid process of tearing off her skin by inches; her face, neck, and person, were thus disfigured to hideousness. (P. 7)

Institutions for people with mental illness continued to be constructed, frequently due to Dix's agitation. During the 1840s to 1870s, she was involved in the construction or expansion of more than 30 such facilities across the United States and in Britain (Brown 1998). Mental asylums of the earliest period were generally designed to house fewer than 300 people and were organized under the leadership of psychiatrist-superintendents. These men adhered to the moral treatment method pioneered by Pinel and Tuke (Grob 1966). However, the first institutions were marked by specific divisions in the care and treatment of the poor from the privileged classes (Tuke 1815). This initial segregation within public facilities between the middle class and the poor was the beginning of practices that would eventually become a hallmark of American institutions (Rothman 1990; Trent 1995). During the first half of the nineteenth century, physician-superintendents of the first mental asylums in the United States believed that mental illness was curable (Grob 1966; Kirkbride [1880] 1973). Kirkbride, superintendent of the Pennsylvania asylum, argued that in cases where uncomplicated insanity was "properly and promptly treated, and having this treatment duly persevered in, may be regarded as curable . . . 80%" of the time (Kirkbride [1880] 1973:23).

Overcrowding and the Demise of the Moral Treatment

Beginning almost immediately after they were constructed, mental institutions experienced severe overcrowding as prisons sought to release their most dangerous and disturbed inmates to the newly available facilities (Grob 1966). Overcrowding and expansion soon made the superintendents' attempts at moral treatment impossible as the management of large facilities became paramount. In the later decades of the 1800s, as treatment gave way to confinement and custodial care in larger facilities, cure rates concomitantly dropped, and psychiatrists reported that mental illness was largely incurable (Earle 1877; Grob 1966; Rothman 1990; Scull 1991).

As populations in these asylums swelled, conditions of overcrowding became serious by the end of the nineteenth century. The sheer number of inmates in most facilities, along with growing administrative responsibilities in increasingly complex institutions, translated into less time with patients for the superintendent. The moral treatment subsequently faded, along with beliefs in the curability of mental illness as custodial functions of the asylums became primary (Grob 1966; Rothman 1990).

By the late 1800s, the earlier optimism of rehabilitating patients with mental illness and sending them back to their home communities had been replaced with a rigid pessimism that decried the possibility of cure and demanded the lifelong custody of patients reported as extremely dangerous to their home communities (Earle 1877; Grob 1966; Rothman 1990). Grob (1966) argues that superintendents gave way to the inevitability of poor conditions, given severe overcrowding and limited contact with patients. Rothman (1990) and Scull (1991) contend that superintendents used the opportunities presented by expanding demand for mental asylum space to legitimate their own existence and secure their power. Our review of the *American Journal of Insanity* from its 1844 inception to 1900 reveals extensive discussions of the architecture of asylums and the management of such facilities. However, there were fewer than 10 articles that dealt with patient treatment or care. This lends credence to Rothman's (1990) and Scull's (1991) claims that superintendents were more interested and absorbed in the management of their facilities than in therapeutic issues.

Writing of his experiences of incarceration in the New York Asylum at Utica, a patient with mental illness recounts extraordinary abuse, patient overcrowding, and horrific conditions at the facility during the mid-nineteenth century ("Five Months" 1982). Elizabeth Packard (1868) wrote of being physically abused at the Illinois State Insane Asylum at Jacksonville, and after her eventual release, she campaigned for the civil rights of mental patients in Illinois and other states. Lydia Button (1878) wrote an autobiography recounting abusive conditions she and other inmates endured while institutionalized at the State Asylum in Kalamazoo, Michigan. By all accounts, Packard and Button were not mentally ill but were victimized by a legal system that permitted husbands to institutionalize their wives during the nineteenth century (Peterson 1982). However, the treatment of these individuals is representative of the institutional experiences of many other people with mental illness during the mid-nineteenth century in the United States. Conditions in English mental asylums during the beginning of the nineteenth century were equally severe. Visitors related stories of seeing people with mental illness confined in rooms without heat or clothing, chained, and physically abused (Browne 1837).

Before the first distinct residential institution for persons with intellectual disabilities had opened in the United States in 1848, 31 institutions for persons with mental illness had been established (Hamilton 1944). There were 4,730 residents, a small percentage of whom had intellectual disabilities; 27 of the facilities were public, and 4 were private.

The psychiatrist Phillippe Pinel was a major figure in the care of people with mental illness at the close of the eighteenth century. He is most popularly known for his bold act in 1792 of simultaneously unchaining 50 patients in a Paris mental hospital. The act echoed the "liberty, equality, and fraternity" spirit of the French Revolution popularized by Rousseau ([1762] 1991). Pinel's ([1801] 1977) *Treatise on Insanity* had worldwide influence on the developing field of psychology and psychiatry. Nearly 50 years after its publication, the editors of the *American Journal of Insanity* noted that "we know not of any work on insanity superior to this . . . none more worthy of our daily study" ("The Moral Treatment" 1847:4). In Belgium a generation later, psychiatrist Joseph Guislain similarly unchained mental patients at the asylum in Ghent, earning the nickname of the "Belgian Pinel" (Brierre de Boismont 1867). Despite the efforts of Pinel and Guislain and, in Italy, Chiarugi's notoriety in promulgating the moral treatment (Alexander and Selesnick 1964), there is evidence that it did not originate with them; rather, changing therapeutic philosophies were emerging before Pinel wrote his treatise and even before Chiarugi's works were known in England. English physician William Pargeter wrote *Observations on Maniacal Disorders* in 1792, prior to Pinel's arrival at the Bicêtre (Jackson 1988). Pargeter advocated for humane care of people with mental illness by arguing against the use of restraints, beatings, and forced remedies in advance of Pinel and Tuke (Jackson 1988; Pargeter [1792] 1988). Like Pinel and Chiarugi, he emphasized the importance of the management of insanity in lieu of medicine and punishment:

> The chief reliance in the cure of insanity must be rather on management than medicine. The government of maniacs is an art, not to be acquired without long experience, and frequent and attentive observation. Although it has been of late years much advanced, it is still capable of improvement. (Pargeter [1792] 1988:49)

The emphasis that Pargeter, Pinel, Chiarugi, Guislain, and Tuke placed on management has been interpreted by later analysts as an emphasis on social control and coercion. Thomas Szasz (1973) has argued that involuntary institutionalization of persons with mental illness established a relationship between doctor and patient during the rise of psychiatric power in the seventeenth and eighteenth centuries that is akin to that of master and slave. Szasz further argues that this relationship between doctor and patient still exists in contemporary Western society.

In 1790, only six U.S. cities had more than 8,000 people, and the population of the United States was 3.9 million. By 1850, there were 85 such metropolises, 26 cities had more than 25,000 persons, and the total U.S. population was 23.2 million people (Hamilton 1944). In the period between 1824, when the nation's third state mental institution opened, and 1851, 19 state-operated facilities were established in 15 states, including New York (3), Virginia, South Carolina, Massachusetts (2), Tennessee, Maine, New Hampshire, Georgia, Indiana, New Jersey, Louisiana, Pennsylvania (2), Missouri, Illinois, and California (Hamilton 1944). All of these state facilities, which collectively housed 4,730 persons in 1850, were opened before the first separate and distinct U.S. institution was constructed for people with intellectual disabilities.

Between 1850 and 1890, 55 state psychiatric institutions were opened in the United States, and the census of patients with mental illness in mental hospitals grew dramatically to 40,942 persons (Hamilton 1944:86). It would nearly double by 1890 to 74,028 and double again to 187,791 in 1910. Overcrowding in mental institutions became pronounced during the latter half of the nineteenth century in the United States. During this time, facilities essentially abandoned their therapeutic capacities in favor of custodial arrangements designed to protect society from the perceived threat posed by people with mental illness (Rothman 1990; Scull 1991). However, one innovative response to overcrowding was family care, a program of placing people with mental illness in the homes of unrelated families. In the United States, family care was initiated first in Massachusetts in 1885 (Pollock 1945). A similar program had been in place in Scotland dating back to at least the 1860s (Pollock 1945). The use of family care for people with mental illness represents the first efforts to provide state-sponsored services in community settings. While a few other states followed Massachusetts's lead, family care for people with mental illness never became widespread in the United States (Pollock 1945). Large-scale community-based services would not develop for people with mental illness until late in the twentieth century (Grob 1994).

Growing concern about the number of people with disabilities in the United States resulted in their enumeration by the census. Beginning in 1830, counts were taken of deaf and blind persons, and in 1840, the census began counting people labeled "idiotic" and "insane" (Gorwitz 1974). The 1840 census reflected pervasive racism. All black residents in some towns were classified as insane (Gorwitz 1974). Between 1870 and 1880, the proportion of the population counted as insane rose from 97 to 183 per 100,000, while the proportion of the population counted as intellectually disabled rose from 64 to 153 per 100,000 (Gorwitz 1974). This dramatic increase can be attributed, at least in part, to the fact that census enumerators received extra compensation in 1880 for each person with mental illness or intellectual disability that they counted (Gorwitz 1974). The rapid increase in the mentally disabled population was seen as evidence that society needed to take drastic measures to address mental disability (Knight 1895). These concerns ultimately fueled the agenda of the eugenics movement. The publication and dissemination of the results of such "scientific inquiry" were widely used in propaganda campaigns to catalyze public support for sterilization and marriage restriction laws (Pernick 1996). By 1912, numerous states prohibited the marriage of persons with mental disabilities and epilepsy or allowed such marriages only after age 45 (Smith, Wilkinson, and Wagoner 1914).

Historians and advocates have argued that the professionals involved with the operation of institutions for people with mental illness (Rothman 1990; Scull 1979) and intellectual disability (Blatt 1977; Trent 1995; Tyor 1972; Tyor and Bell 1984) were personally invested in perpetuating the life of these institutions, often at the expense of the residents. Social historians studying leprosy have made similar claims (Navon 1998). Cochrane (1963), Gussow (1989), and MacArthur (1953) argued that Christian missionaries supported the need for segregation and did not criticize the negative images of people with leprosy so that they would continue to receive funding for their missionary efforts.

Deaf Community Organizing

During the mid-nineteenth century, the number of schools for deaf and blind students grew rapidly both in the United States and in Europe. In 1856 in the United States, a donated estate in Washington, D.C., was used to establish a residential school for 12 deaf and 6 blind students, the Columbia Institution for the Instruction of the Deaf and Dumb and the Blind (Gallaudet 1983; Lane 1989). In 1864, President Lincoln signed legislation authorizing Columbia to confer college degrees. Columbia later became Gallaudet University (Gallaudet 1983; Lane 1989).

Suppression of sign language was championed by Alexander Graham Bell in the United States at the end of the nineteenth century. In 1872, he opened a speech-based school for teachers in Boston intending to banish the use of sign language and encouraging deaf persons to "pass" as hearing individuals (Gannon 1981; Lane 1989). In 1880, at the International Congress on Education of the Deaf, which met in Italy, a resolution passed that banned the use of sign language in the education of deaf children (Gannon 1981; Gallaudet 1983). Also in 1880, the National Association of the Deaf was organized by deaf people. This organization would become the leading association fighting the oralists for manual instruction of deaf people in the United States (Baynton 1996).

One of the first self-advocacy organizations by people with disabilities was the British Deaf and Dumb Association (BDDA), now the British Association of the Deaf. The BDDA initially organized in 1890 in direct response to the International Congress's sign language ban and the view that deaf persons did not need to be involved in matters that concerned them. The 1880 International Congress on the Deaf had only two deaf teachers in attendance (British Association of the Deaf 1999).

First U.S. Institution for People
with Intellectual Disability

Superintendents of asylums for the mentally ill were among the first in the United States to call for separate provisions for people with intellectual disabilities. Reflecting on the path-breaking developments in Europe, Samuel Woodward, superintendent of the Worcester State Hospital in Massachusetts, and Amariah Brigham of New York's Bloomingdale facility both recommended in their 1845 annual state hospital reports that their states should make a public educational provision for children and youth with intellectual disabilities (Brigham 1845; Woodward 1845).

In 1846, Samuel Gridley Howe—the noted reformer, leader of the education of blind students, and committed oralist in the education of deaf students—was appointed to chair an epidemiological committee regarding intellectual disabilities appointed by the Massachusetts legislature. Howe carried out the nation's first investigation of the prevalence of intellectual disabilities and presented recommendations to establish an experimental school. Howe's report is replete with purported connections between the etiology of intellectual disability and the immoral behavior of one's parents (Howe 1848). His perspective was no doubt indicative of attitudes of the day that disability was a punishment for violating natural law.

The residential school that Howe recommended opened in October 1848 in south Boston in a wing of the Perkins Institute for the Blind (Howe 1851). A few months earlier, in July 1848, Hervey Wilbur had opened a small private school in his own home for the instruction of children with mental retardation in Barre, Massachusetts (Elm Hill Private School and Home 1911). A few years later, Wilbur left Barre to be superintendent of the new institution at Syracuse, site of the first institution for people with intellectual disabilities constructed specifically for that purpose in the United States. The Syracuse institution opened in 1855 (Fernald 1893; FitzGerald 1900).

It became common for states to initially open experimental schools (Kerlin 1877), and other states followed Massachusetts's and New York's lead. Pennsylvania opened a private school in 1852 that was incorporated in 1853 as the Pennsylvania Training School for Idiotic and Feebleminded Children. In 1855, this school was moved to its present site at Elwyn, Pennsylvania. Ohio, Connecticut, Kentucky, and Illinois established residential schools in 1857, 1858, 1860, and 1865, respectively (Fernald 1917). The Illinois school was administered for its first decade under the auspices of the Illinois School for the Deaf. Twenty-six years after Howe opened the United States' first school for 10 children, seven states had established publicly operated or assisted institutions for 1,041 residents, and there were two private facilities in Massachusetts (Fernald 1917). Although the national census of institutions for people with intellectual disabilities was now growing steadily, almshouses housed more people with intellectual disabilities until 1906 (U.S. Bureau of the Census 1914).

From Training Schools to Custodial Asylums

Institutions for people with intellectual disabilities, similar to those for people with mental illness, grew rapidly both in size and number following their initial construction in the mid-1800s. Early training efforts were quite successful, and many of the children with intellectual disabilities were returned to their communities as "productive workers" (Stewart 1882; Trent 1995). Economic hardship hit the nation following the Civil War, and severe recessions occurred in the 1870s and again in the 1880s. Due to extensive unemployment, it became increasingly difficult for superintendents to discharge trained residents who could not compete for already scarce jobs in their home communities. Superintendents also noted the value of using unpaid resident labor to offset the costs of running the institutions (Fenton 1932; Knight 1891). The exploitation of resident labor, or peonage, prevailed both in institutions for people with mental illness and in ones for those with intellectual disability (Bartlett 1964; Bonsall

1891; Fenton 1932; Johnson 1899; Knight 1891; MacAndrew and Edgerton 1964) until the late 1960s (Scheerenberger 1983).

By 1880, the training schools envisioned by Howe and Seguin had evolved into custodial asylums with reduced emphasis on educating residents and returning them to community life (Trent 1995; Wolfensberger 1976). The optimism of the 1840 to 1870 "amelioration" period confronted two difficult realities, including negative attitudes toward persons with mental retardation held by the general public and the lack of supportive social services, family support, and work opportunities in the community. Wilbur (1888), at the fifteenth annual gathering of the National Conference of Charities and Corrections, observed that institutions would offer lifelong protective custodial care. Other professionals in the field joined Wilbur in calling for lifelong institutionalization of people with intellectual disabilities (Barr 1902; Bicknell 1895; Fish 1892; Fort 1892; Johnson 1896). Samuel Gridley Howe had strongly opposed this trend, arguing in an 1866 speech that people with disabilities "should be kept diffused among sound and normal persons. Separation, and not congregation, should be the law of their treatment." The states, he said, should "gradually dispense with as many [custodial institutions] as possible" (cited in Wolfensberger 1976:26).

But the states did not dispense with custodial institutions. They continued to build them, expand them, and stress self-sufficiency and economical management in all aspects of facility operation. In 1900, the census of mental retardation institutions in the United States was 11,800 persons (Fernald 1917). Many institutions were located in remote areas and farmed extensive lands. Residents worked laundries, farms, and workshops, not so much to develop skills for community out-placement but rather to contribute to the self-sustaining economy of the institution. While most superintendents championed the growth of large institutions during this period (Trent 1995), Seguin (1870) warned against this phenomenon. He wrote, "Let us hope that the State institutions for idiots will escape that evil of excessive growth . . . in which patients are so numerous that the accomplished physicians who have them in charge cannot remember the name of each" (p. 21).

At the dawning of the twentieth century, institutions for persons with intellectual disabilities were firmly established in the developed nations of the world. Barr (1904), who wrote the first U.S. textbook on intellectual disability, completed an international survey and reported that 21 nations were operating 171 institutions for people with intellectual disability. There were 25 institutions in the United States by 1900 (Kuhlmann 1940). Barr also noted that "following the experiments worked out in the continental cities and in England, the special classes for backward children opened first in Providence, Rhode Island and [are] now part of the educational systems of New York, Philadelphia, Chicago, and Boston" (p. 71).

In the United States, the course of the initial development of institutions for people with mental illness and intellectual disabilities had numerous similarities. Superintendents of both types of facilities used existing social and economic issues to develop secondary goals for their facilities after their initial goals of training failed. Both sets of leaders aggressively agitated for the next phase of institutional development—custodial care (Rothman 1990; Scull 1991; Trent 1995).

Freak Shows

Institutions were not the only manifestation of society's attitudes toward people with disabilities during the nineteenth century. So-called freak shows displayed people with physical and mental disabilities throughout the nineteenth century in the United States and Europe (Bogdan 1988; Rothfels 1996; Thomson 1996, 1997). People with intellectual disabilities were among those exhibited, their "abnormal" characteristics exaggerated into caricatures of the grotesque (Bogdan 1988; Thomson 1997). These exhibits were extremely popular at circuses, fairs, and expositions. People with disabilities who were displayed at freak shows were frequently "sold" to the show organizers, who maintained the right to display them for the duration of their lives (Bogdan 1988).

In displaying people with disabilities in these shows, exotic stories of wild and far-flung origins of the exhibited people were fabricated by the show organizers (Bogdan 1988; Thomson 1997). Thomson (1997) argues that the exploitation of people with disabilities in the United States served to reinforce average Americans' notions of their own normality, by emphasizing disability and often race as profound and monstrous differences. Freak shows served to institutionalize notions of disability as the ultimate deviance, thus solidifying Americans' needs to perceive themselves as normal (Thomson 1997). Freak shows reached the height of their popularity at the end of the nineteenth century, at a time when eugenic beliefs in the superiority of the white middle class were crystallizing. In the United States, freak shows continued until the 1940s, when competing forms of entertainment, as well as economic hard times, led to their demise (Bogdan 1986).

While freak shows were at their heyday during the mid- to late-nineteenth century, there is evidence that by their decline in late-eighteenth century England, they had been popular for centuries among all classes (Park and Daston 1981; Semonin 1996). Semonin (1996) describes the "taste for monsters" as "an almost universal craze among English citizens of all ranks" (p. 69). In medieval and modern England, people with disabilities, racial and ethnic minorities, and people with unusual attributes were termed "monsters," and their display in markets for profit was commonplace (Semonin 1996). It was common for people to visit Bethlem during the medieval and later periods for the "entertainment" provided by the inmates (MacDonald 1981).

Threat of the Eugenicists

The period from 1880 to 1925 was a time when persons with intellectual disabilities were viewed as deviant social menaces, and intellectual disability was seen as an incurable disease (Barr 1902; Butler 1907; East 1917; Fernald 1915; Gosney and Popenoe 1929; Kerlin 1887; Scheerenberger 1983; Sloan and Stevens 1976; Switzky et al. 1988; Trent 1995; Watkins 1930; Winspear 1895). The eugenic belief widely held during this period was that intellectual disability was inherited as a Mendelian characteristic that degraded the species (Barr 1902; Fernald 1915; Galton 1883; Rafter 1988; Roberts 1952). Intellectual disability was linked in numerous studies to criminality, immoral behavior, and pauperism (Dugdale [1877] 1910; Evans 1926; Fernald 1915; Goddard 1912; Rafter 1988). Intelligence tests, developed shortly after the turn of the century, were employed widely in the major cities of the United States to identify children with intellectual disabilities and place them in segregated special classes. Intelligence tests were also used to support ethnocentric and class biases against immigrants in the United States (Davenport 1921; Fernald 1915). Subsequent to the implementation of intelligence testing at ports of entry, deportations for mental deficiency increased 350 percent in 1913 and 570 percent in 1914 (Gould 1981). Rampant abuse existed in the classification of both immigrants and poor Americans as mentally deficient. Workers were "trained" to classify people as mentally deficient by sight (Gould 1981).

Economic problems occurred at the same time that Galton's ideas of social Darwinism were beginning to take hold in the United States and abroad. Superintendents' writings reflect changing attitudes toward their charges as their institutional populations soared; the menace and burden of people with intellectual disabilities were frequently discussed (Barr 1895; Bicknell 1895; Fernald 1912; Kerlin 1887). Society needed protection from these menaces, and institutional care became the way to achieve these goals. Trent (1995) argues that the superintendents readily espoused the new social Darwinism and its messages of fear about deviant persons because it offered a way for them to legitimate and consolidate their authority.

The eugenics movement in the United States was accompanied by extensive instances of physicians refusing to treat, thereby facilitating the death of infants born with disabilities and birth defects (Pernick 1996). Newspaper accounts publicized the withholding of lifesaving treatment of babies with disabilities during the decade after 1915, and movies propagating the eugenics agenda became quite common (Pernick 1996).

In England, concern about people termed *mental defective* led to the 1886 passage of the "Idiots Act," which called for further clarification of the distinction between "idiots" and "lunatics" (Gladstone 1996) and preceded the eugenics movement in that country (Carpenter 1996). Passage of the 1899 Education Act led to the growth of institutions for people with intellectual disability and epilepsy in England (Carpenter 1996; Koven 1994).

Social Darwinism had an impact on the deaf community in the United States as well. At the end of the century, the debate between manualists and oralists intensified. Oralists claimed that people who used sign language were less evolved than people who spoke and were like apes or racial minorities (Baynton 1993; Porter 1894). This debate eventually resulted in the near eradication of manual education of deaf students, which was supplanted by oral education, a trend that was strongly opposed by deaf adults but continued well into the mid-twentieth century (Baynton 1996; Semi-Deaf Lady 1908). Zealously opposed to signed instruction, hearing teachers and other oralists used physical abuse of students to suppress sign language (Baynton 1996; Lane 1989; Porter 1894). In 1920, 82 percent of the 13,917 deaf students in school were taught speech ("Statistics of Speech" 1920).

The deaf movement that began in the United States in the late nineteenth century expressed a desire for independence and an evolving commitment to the emergence of deaf culture (de Saint-Loup 1996). The foundation of this movement was the use of sign language, which had been opposed by notable figures such as Alexander Graham Bell. Bell even explicitly rejected marriage among deaf people (Bell [1883] 1969). Deaf culture was further facilitated by the printing and circulation of newspapers among deaf residential schools across the nation. By 1893, at least 29 schools had 35 newspapers (Haller 1993). It is a testament to the strength of the deaf community that sign language survived and thrived during nearly a century of repression, and it is now a primary communication strategy in educating deaf children.

In summary, the nineteenth century is best characterized as the century of institutions and interventions. Schools and institutions for persons with physical disabilities, deafness, blindness, mental illness, and intellectual disability took root throughout Europe and North America. Professionals developed differential diagnosis to particularize disability and devised treatment interventions and educational schemes focused on specific impairments. The medical model of defining and classifying disability became thoroughly accepted in this century. However, the segregation of individuals with similar impairments also afforded people with disabilities opportunities to begin to develop group identities. By the close of the nineteenth century, deaf persons advocating for manual education and control of their own schools had begun to coalesce into the first disability political action groups.

THE TWENTIETH CENTURY

Segregation and Expansion of the Institutional Model

At the opening of the twentieth century, the eugenics era was gaining momentum, and social reformers sought segregation and prohibitions on marriage and procreation by people with disabilities. Conditions in facilities for people with mental disabilities were deteriorating, and deaf persons were fighting to be able to use sign language in their schools.

Despite the rapid expansion of institutions for people with mental disabilities after the turn of the century, poor farms or almshouses were also a significant aspect of state provision for people with intellectual disabilities and mental illness. By the 1920s, poor farms were "dumping grounds" for all undesirables, including people with disabilities and the poor. In 1922, Ohio reported that 70 percent of poor farm inmates had "feeblemindedness," or what is today known as intellectual disability. North Carolina estimated that 85 percent of inmates were "mentally abnormal." Iowa reported that in 1924, 45 percent of its poor farm inmates were mentally ill (Evans 1926:7-8). In a nationwide study of inmates of poorhouses, 36 percent were found to be "feeble-minded, borderline defective, psychopathic, psychoneurotic, epileptic, or suffering from mental disease" (Haines 1925:138).

The sterilization of institutional residents with intellectual disabilities was commonplace in some states (Ferster 1966; Watkins 1930). Between 1907 and 1949, there were more than 47,000 recorded sterilizations of people with mental disabilities in 30 states (Woodside 1950). Of particular interest was the sterilization of people with intellectual disability who would eventually be discharged into the community (Popenoe 1927). Sterilization of women with epilepsy and mental illness was also widely believed by physicians to have therapeutic benefits despite overwhelming empirical evidence to the contrary (Church 1893). In the face of evidence that removal of the ovaries and Fallopian tubes was wholly ineffective, physicians continued to perform such surgery on women with an array of conditions, including hysteria, depression, epilepsy, insanity related to childbirth, and nymphomania. Surgery was also deemed appropriate to "prevent the prospect of illegitimate and defective children" (Church 1893:496).

The U.S. Supreme Court's *Buck v. Bell* (1927) decision affirmed the states' right to sterilize people with intellectual disabilities and propelled the eugenics movement to further lobby for its agenda (Kevles 1985; Radford 1994; Reilly 1991). In 1933, using California's program as a model, Nazi Germany enacted its own eugenic sterilization law (Reilly 1991). This legislation led to the forced sterilization of between 300,000 and 400,000 persons, a majority on the grounds of "feeblemindedness." Most were institutional residents. This unprecedented oppression against disabled persons culminated in the murder by euthanasia of between 200,000 and 275,000 individuals with mental and physical disabilities between 1939 and 1945 in Germany. The eugenics movement had reached its zenith (Friedlander 1997; Gallagher 1995; Reilly 1991; U.S. Holocaust Memorial Museum n.d.; Wolfensberger 1981). Justification for the killing of people with disabilities in Nazi Germany was made on the basis of utilitarian arguments, and German health professionals and psychiatrists were among those who accommodated themselves to these policies (Burleigh 1994). Psychiatrists, particularly, had been responsible for identifying the pool of potential victims and, in some cases, participated in victim selection and murder (Burleigh 1994).

The United States and Germany were not the only nations to sterilize people with disabilities. Denmark had an active program of sterilization between 1930 and 1954, sterilizing at least 8,627 persons over this period. Sweden's program operated throughout the 1930s and 1940s, with 2,278 persons being sterilized in 1948 alone (Trombley 1988).

Contemporaneous with zealous agitation by eugenicists, evidence began to emerge that questioned the assumptions of deviance in people with intellectual disabilities. In Massachusetts, Fernald's (1919) Waverly studies demonstrated that with proper support from their families, individuals with intellectual disabilities could function well in the community. Fernald also concluded that only about 8 percent of a sample of 5,000 schoolchildren with intellectual disabilities in Massachusetts exhibited behavioral problems of any type. In addition, Wallace (1929) presented a compelling paper discrediting the link between intellectual disability and criminality. Also, the "parole plan," which could lead to permanent institutional discharge, was devised in the first decade of the twentieth century as an early release program for institutional residents with milder impairments. Paroled residents were cared for in the community by relatives, employers, or supportive volunteers (Bernstein 1917, 1918, 1921; Davies 1930; Fernald 1902; Hoakley 1922; Mastin 1916; Matthews 1921).

In 1908, with the publication of former mental patient Clifford Beers's *A Mind That Found Itself,* the mental hygiene movement began in the United States (Felix 1957). Beers's autobiographical account of his two-year institutionalization presents chilling details of life for those hospitalized at the turn of the century (Beers 1908; Peterson 1982). Describing constant physical abuse, Beers's narrative resembles those of earlier inmates of the nineteenth century. Like Elizabeth Packard, Beers was interested in reform and established an agenda to promote humane care (Peterson 1982). Influenced by Beers, leaders in psychiatry supported the reform agenda, and psychiatric hospitals began offering clinics in their communities to treat and prevent chronic mental illness (Grob 1983, 1994). In 1909, as a result of Beers's advocacy and leadership, the National Committee for Mental Hygiene was established (Felix 1957).

Shock therapies were developed and implemented in the 1920s, including the use of insulin, metrazol, and malaria to induce shock and, it was hoped, cure patients with mental illness. Electroshock began to be used on people with mental illness in Europe in the 1830s, and a few late-eighteenth-century physicians experimented with electroshock on people with epilepsy, blindness, and mental illness (Harms 1955). However, the widespread acceptance and use of electroshock did not occur until the 1930s, when the Italian Ugo Cerletti invented and publicized modern electroshock therapy. Electroshock involved the application of electricity to induce improvements in psychiatric conditions (Cerletti 1950; Harms 1955).

While psychosurgery had been performed by the Swiss surgeon Gottlieb Burkhardt in 1890, his contemporaries rejected its use (Ramsey 1952; Swayze 1995). The Portuguese neuropsychiatrist Egas Minoz developed modern psychosurgery in 1933, and from its initial use until the 1950s, nearly 20,000 patients were lobotomized (Grob 1994; Ramsey 1952; Swayze 1995; Valenstein 1986). Psychosurgery involved the severing of the frontal lobe from the rest of the brain and frequently left patients with changed personalities, diminished intellectual faculties, and other severe problems (Ramsey 1952; Swayze 1995).

Recent advocates with mental illness have rejected the use of shock therapy and psychosurgery as barbaric attempts to control people with mental illness (Lefley 1996; MadNation 1999; Peterson 1982). Litigation in the United States has resulted in determinations that patients in mental hospitals have the right to refuse electroshock treatment (Levy and Rubenstein 1996; Parry 1995).

The repression and social control of people classified as deviant are an important aspect of discussing the history of disability, particularly the history of mental illness. Historians and social scientists have offered extensive critiques of psychiatry as a social control device. Thomas Szasz (1970), one of the most vocal and articulate critics of psychiatry, has argued that society has scapegoated people with mental illness and severely abused them. Elliot Valenstein (1986) has argued that the uses of psychosurgery and the shock therapies so popular during the first half of the twentieth century were vehicles for ambitious psychiatrists to pursue their own career agendas at the cost of individuals with mental illness.

The census of American psychiatric hospitals continued to increase during the first half of the twentieth century, reaching 461,358 persons in 1940 and peaking at more than 550,000 persons in 1955 (Braddock 1981; Hamilton 1944). The size of many public facilities was truly immense, even by American standards. Hamilton (1944) reported that in 1941, 10 public facilities housed more than 5,000 residents (one had 9,177 residents), 22 had more than 4,000, 40 housed more than 3,000 individuals, and 102 of the nation's 475 mental hospitals on December 31, 1941, contained more than 2,000 patients.

In 1880, there were 1,382 persons with intellectual disability in insane asylums. By 1940, the number of persons with intellectual disabilities living in psychiatric hospitals peaked at nearly 29,000 persons (U.S. Bureau of the Census 1939, 1940). The census of separate state institutions for people with intellectual disabilities swelled to 55,466 persons by 1926 (Lakin 1979). Switzky et al. (1988) described several common practices in institutions of this era. Residents were "patients" who lived on "wards" in a facility, often called a "hospital," which was governed by a hierarchical medical structure. Resident programs were termed *treatments* or *therapy* (e.g., recreational therapy, industrial therapy, and educational therapy). Living units were locked, windows were barred, and the institution became increasingly structured "like a hospital for the care of sick animals rather than as a place for the special education of human children and adults" (Switzky et al. 1988:28). Prolonged institutionalization exacted a price from residents by promoting excessive conformity to the institutional culture at the expense of personal spontaneity, excessive fantasizing, fear of new situations, and excessive dependency on the institution (Sarason and Gladwin 1958).

Because of widespread unemployment and poverty during the Great Depression, families sought institutional care for their relatives with intellectual disabilities in increasing numbers (Noll 1996). Institutional facility censuses continued to swell, and overcrowding became commonplace (Noll 1996; Trent 1995; Tyor and Bell 1984; Watkins 1930). The Depression also brought relief with President Roosevelt's economic recovery programs. Passed in 1935, Title X of the Social Security Act provided specific relief for blind persons but no other disability groups (Axinn and Levin 1982; Braddock 1987; Lende 1941; Scotch and Berkowitz 1990). By 1940, approximately 50,000 blind people across the United States were receiving this aid (Lende 1941). While Title V of the Social Security Act authorized Crippled Children's Services grants of $2.85 million (Braddock 1986a), minutes of the 1936 Crippled Children's Services National Advisory Committee stated that "children with incurable blindness, deafness, or mental defect . . . and those requiring permanent custodial care" were beyond the intended scope of the new program (Social Security Board 1946:1).

The widespread segregation of people with intellectual disabilities in institutions made them targets for medical experiments. At the Wrentham and Fernald facilities in Massachusetts, institutional residents with intellectual disabilities were subjected to tests with foods that had been laced with radioactive elements. Neither the individuals with disabilities who served as subjects in these experiments nor their parents were ever apprised of the nature of the foods that were ingested. This illegal research spanned the period between 1946 and 1973 (Moreno 1999). Residents at the Willowbrook institution in New York were similarly exposed to hepatitis B without their knowledge or informed consent (Rothman and Rothman 1984).

Developments for Persons with Physical Disabilities

Religious charity, as has been previously discussed, had been part of the landscape of support provided to people with disabilities and the poor for centuries. However, numerous secular charitable societies organized in the United States during the period between the 1840s and the 1880s. For example, Clara Barton founded the American Red Cross in 1881, an affiliate of an endeavor already in existence in Europe. The predecessor of the original European Red Cross had been founded to prevent death and disability on an Italian battlefield in 1859 (Obermann 1968).

Secular charitable organizations began to make an impact on persons with disabilities and, in some instances, became forerunners of the vocational rehabilitation movement in the early twentieth century. Among the most important of these was the Red Cross's establishment of the Institute for Crippled and Disabled Men in 1917. This organization was an experimental school for the rehabilitation of veterans, one of the first in the United States. Borrowing on ideas learned from visits to France, Germany, Italy, and England, the institute developed retraining programs for veterans with disabilities that were later used in U.S. Army hospitals as well. The predecessor of the Easter Seal Society, the National Society for Crippled Children and Adults was established in 1907 in Ohio (Obermann 1968).

Legal protections for laboring men were among the first formal provisions enacted for persons with physical disabilities. Germany and Austria legislated compensation for men disabled while working in 1884 and 1887, respectively. In the United States, Maryland enacted the first "workmen's compensation" law in 1902, which specifically provided a stated schedule of benefits to persons who became disabled while they were working (Obermann 1968). During the opening decades of the twentieth century, many other states followed Maryland's lead and established similar laws of their own.

Developments in workers' compensation laws led to discussions about rehabilitating disabled workers, thus providing them with the training necessary to successfully reenter the workforce. The U.S. Congress passed PL 66-236 in 1920, which was the first civilian vocational rehabilitation law in the country (Braddock 1986a; Obermann 1968). Two years earlier, Congress had authorized rehabilitation services for disabled soldiers returning from World War I. While the 1920 law primarily targeted industrially injured persons, services were to be provided to "any person, who, by reason of a physical defect or infirmity, whether congenital or acquired by accident, injury, or disease" (Obermann 1968:161). Persons with mental disabilities were not, however, eligible for rehabilitation services at this time.

Goodwill Industries was established in 1902 in Boston. Goodwill initially collected and distributed clothing and other contributions for the poor. Unemployed persons were subsequently hired to repair and renovate donations before they were sold, with the intention that the income generated would pay the workers. This program was later expanded to provide rehabilitation and sheltered work to persons with disabilities who were perceived as otherwise unable to support themselves (Obermann 1968). Goodwill Industries expanded across the United States and into other countries by the 1940s.

Charitable organizations often involved themselves in the monitoring of physical disability after the turn of the twentieth century. These organizations would conduct surveys to determine the extent of physical disability and then promulgate recommendations to address the needs of those found to have disability. A typical survey was one conducted in New York City in 1919, following a polio epidemic in 1916. The committee sent orthopedic surgeons to the homes of individuals that the survey had identified who had not received treatment and proposed that a system of services be developed that included the following components: education, vocational training, medical treatment, convalescent care, custodial care, social services, home treatment, summer outings, employment placement, braces and appliances, and work in the home (Wright 1920). The result of collaboration among 41 social service agencies in New York, this comprehensive plan for people with physical disabilities reported on nearly every aspect of life with disability and recommended greater access to education and employment opportunities as the central issues of concern.

A similar survey was conducted in Cleveland in 1916 by the Welfare Federation of Cleveland. This survey included numerous interviews with working men with physical disabilities. Their attitudes and advice are insightful. One locksmith stated, "If you have something to offer, you can usually get a job, but you must be sure that what you have to offer is of real value" (cited in Wright and Hamburger 1918:237). This man reported stories of being harassed about his disability by others, but he also told of his ability to persevere and succeed in the working world. Other men with disabilities described similar successes in maintaining employment, albeit in the face of difficult conditions.

Advances in orthopedic treatment and prosthetic devices for people who lost limbs during wartime or in industry were made during World War I. While primitive forms of artificial limbs had been used for centuries, technological advances subsequent to World War I resulted in the development of more comfortable and effective prostheses. These advances enabled greater numbers of men with disabilities to return to work after sustaining impairments. During this period, an understanding of the importance of individually fitting each person, as opposed to mass-producing devices, developed (Martin 1924).

Emergence of Family, Community, and Consumer Models

Although the Depression and World War II inhibited innovation in service delivery for people with intellectual disabilities in the United States (Noll 1996; Trent 1995), some progress was made. New York state, for example, introduced foster family care in the 1930s, authorizing payment for the care of persons with intellectual disabilities in family homes (Vaux 1935). Research subsequently confirmed the beneficial effects of placement in foster or adoptive homes (Skeels and Harms 1948; Speer 1940) and the benefits of preschool intervention programs (Lazar and Darlington 1982; Skeels et al. 1938).

The 1940s witnessed greater public awareness of conditions in mental hospitals brought on by another autobiographical account of institutionalization. Publication of Mary Jane Ward's (1946) *The Snake Pit*, which was subsequently made into an Academy Award–winning movie, heightened awareness of brutal conditions in American mental hospitals (Peterson 1982). The perceived need for enhanced research efforts in mental illness led to the 1946 creation of the National Institute of Mental Health (NIMH), which also led to increased community services for people with mental illness in the United States (Braddock 1986a; Felix 1957). In 1946, when the National Mental Health Act that created the NIMH was enacted, 24 states had community-based mental health programs. By 1957, every state had at least some community-based mental health services stimulated in part by the NIMH (Felix 1957).

In 1940, the National Federation of the Blind was founded, the first consumer advocacy organization for blind persons in the United States. This group opposed the nonblind leadership in the American Foundation for the Blind, which had formed in 1921 (Koestler 1976; Matson 1990). The split between organizations for blind persons and those led by blind people was international as well. In 1964, blind persons decided to separate from the World Council for the Welfare of the Blind and form their own organization (Driedger 1989).

The Social Model of Disability

While some people with disabilities at mid-century wrote about their experiences as a tragedy to be overcome (e.g., Walker 1950), writings of blind Americans in the mid-twentieth century describe not blindness but the social and physical environment as the essential problem of disability. "Not blindness, but the attitude of the seeing to the blind is the hardest burden to bear" (Keller, as cited in Gowman 1957:5). "All too frequently the great tragedy of a blind person's life is not primarily his blindness, but the reactions of the family and social group toward him as a non-typical member" (Maxfield, as cited in Gowman 1957:5). Chevigny (1946) writes,

> The tragic aspect of blindness does not inhere in the condition nor can it do so. In nature it is absent. It is an entirely civilized idea. The world in which a man finds himself creates the tragedy for him and in him. If I found blindness more of a major nuisance than a tragedy, therefore, it was because of the world in which I moved and had my being. (P. ix)

The intellectual basis for these ideas regarding the interaction between disability and society was powerfully advanced in Berger and Luckmann's (1967) sociological treatise on the social nature of knowledge. Their social-constructivist view was a harbinger of the social model of disability that would later emerge in the research of Saad Nagi (1970) and in disability studies and the independent living movement of the 1970s (Bowe 1978; Davis 1997; Linton 1998; Oliver 1983, 1990; Scott 1968). The World Health Organization's (1980) definitions of impairment, disability, and handicap, which proposed a distinction between the socially constructed disadvantages that accrue to persons with impairments and the physical realities of impairment, were grounded in the writings of these early theorists and advocates (Lupton 2000). Explaining the significance of this distinction, Bickenbach (1993) has argued that

> handicaps are thus socially created disadvantages that arise from the social reception of impairments and disabilities. The explicit focus of this dimension of disablement is social valuations of physical states (or perceived physical states); there is no question here of normative neutrality. Moreover, nearly every aspect of the conceptual structure of the notion is shaped by and so relative to social and cultural forces. (P. 48)

Organizational Developments

Beginning in the 1950s, friends and parents of people with disabilities began organizing for more extensive services for people with disabilities in many parts of the world. At that time, schools and activity centers were established, and ultimately international associations were founded, composed of national organizations interested in the prevention of disability.

Parents of people with intellectual disabilities in Washington state had actually organized to advocate for services for their children as early as the 1930s (Jones 1987); however, larger-scale organizing by such groups did not occur until the 1950s. During the 1950s, local groups of parents from many states joined forces and formed the group that became the National Association for Retarded Children (now The Arc). These families organized to advocate for services for their children, including better conditions in institutions and the development of schools and workshops (Goode 1999). A similar nationwide organization of families of people with mental illness would not be developed until the 1979 founding of NAMI, the National Alliance for the Mentally Ill (Grob 1994; Lefley 1996).

In 1953, the Council of World Organizations Interested in the Handicapped (CWOIH, now the International Council on Disability) was formed (Driedger 1989). The constituent organizations of the World Council generally did not include people with disabilities as active leaders, however (Driedger 1989). In the United States, the 1950s and 1960s saw the formation of organizations directed by people with disabilities, a departure from organizations led by the able-bodied for people with disabilities (Roberts 1989). Single-disability-focused international organizations led by consumers with those disabilities were subsequently established, including the World Federation of the Deaf, the International Federation of the Blind, and the Fédération Internationale des Mutilés, des Invalides du Travail et des Invalides Civils (Driedger 1989).

Beginnings of Deinstitutionalization

The introduction of antipsychotic drugs in the 1950s, coupled with public commitments to a community treatment approach, resulted in a rapid decline in the average daily resident population of state- and county-operated psychiatric hospitals (Grob 1994). The aggregate census began declining for two additional reasons. Penicillin, which was used to cure syphilis, led to a decrease in the number of persons with this disease in public mental hospitals. Also, following implementation of the Social Security Act of 1935, many elderly residents were moved to nursing homes (Holstein and Cole 1995; Hughes 1986). Between 1955 and 1975, the census in psychiatric hospitals dropped by 200,000 persons from a high of 559,000 (Braddock 1981; National Association of State Mental Health Program Directors Research Institute 1996). However, the declining overall census of such facilities during this period tells only part of the story. While psychiatric hospitals continued to be exceedingly overcrowded, admissions and discharges operated like a revolving door for many patients. In a typical one-year period, there were more than 147,000 admissions and nearly 188,000 discharges and deaths (Grimes 1964). Homelessness has also been a serious consequence of the deinstitutionalization movement for persons with mental illness (Grob 1994; Lefley 1996). However, the community movement for persons with intellectual disabilities has been considerably more successful in developing services and support programs and avoiding homelessness to the degree experienced by persons with mental illness (Braddock 1992).

The census in public facilities for persons with intellectual disabilities peaked at 194,650 in 1967 (U.S. Department of Health, Education, and Welfare 1972). More than 20,000 additional persons with intellectual disabilities resided in state and county psychiatric hospitals at the time. The average facility population of institutions for people with intellectual disabilities was 1,422 residents in 1962 (Survey and Research Corporation 1965). Several facilities, such as Willowbrook in New York and Lincoln in Illinois, housed 4,000 to 8,000 residents. In the 1960s, despite growing evidence to the contrary, American society still treated persons with intellectual disabilities as a group that needed to be controlled by segregation, sterilization, and isolation.

Political Activism and the Right to Treatment

In light of deplorable conditions in institutions for people with mental illness, discussion began to take shape within the legal community about the right to treatment for people who were incarcerated in these facilities. Morton Birnbaum led this initiative with the 1960 publication of his paper, "The Right to Treatment" (Birnbaum 1965; Levy and Rubenstein 1996). The first case in which an American court recognized the right to treatment was the landmark 1966 case of *Rouse v. Cameron*, which held that if an individual was involuntarily committed to a facility, at a minimum, he or she had the right to receive treatment because the purpose of confinement was treatment and not punishment (Levy and Rubenstein 1996; *Rouse v. Cameron* 1966). Subsequent cases upheld this right, which was extended in the 1970s to include people with intellectual disabilities as well (Levy and Rubenstein 1996; Parry 1995).

The election of John F. Kennedy to the U.S. presidency in 1960 ushered in the modern era of intellectual disability services in the United States and an expanded concern for people with mental illness as well. On October 11, 1961, President Kennedy issued an unprecedented statement regarding the need for a national plan in the field of mental retardation. "We as a nation," he said, "have for too long postponed an intensive search for solutions to the problems of the mentally retarded. That failure should be corrected" (Kennedy 1961:196). Kennedy appointed the President's Panel on Mental Retardation. The panel's 95 recommendations, released in 1962, were broad and far-reaching. They extended from issues of civil rights to the need for scientific research on etiology and prevention. The panel called for a substantial downsizing of institutional facilities and an expansion of community services; most important, it clearly embraced the principle of normalization (Nirje 1976; Wolfensberger 1972) as a guide to future innovation in service delivery.

Many of the 95 recommendations of the President's Panel (1962) were enacted into law by the 88th Congress as Public Laws 88-156 and 88-164. Public Law 88-156, the Maternal and Child Health and Mental Retardation Planning Amendments of 1963, doubled the spending ceiling for the existing Maternal and Child Health State Grant Program and established a new mental retardation planning grant program in the states. The planning effort was unique in the history of the field in that federal legislation required all 50 participating states to produce comprehensive plans for the development of improved residential, community, and preventive services.

President Kennedy also signed into law the Community Mental Health Centers Act of 1963, which stimulated the development of such centers across the country (Grob 1994). While these centers were never funded at a level consistent with the desires of their supporters (Braddock 1987), they did develop into a network of community support for people with mental illness (Grob 1994).

The 1970s was a decade of considerable progress in public policy for people with disabilities in the United States (Silverstein 2000). There were four major catalytic events: (1) the 1971 passage of the ICF/MR (Intermediate Care Facilities/Mental Retardation) program as part of Title XIX (Medicaid) of the Social Security Act, (2) Judge Frank M. Johnson's landmark 1972 right to treatment ruling in the Alabama case of *Wyatt v. Stickney*, (3) the political organizing that led to the 1973 passage of Section 504 of the Rehabilitation Act prohibiting discrimination against disabled individuals in any program receiving federal financial assistance, and (4) the 1975 passage of the Education of All Handicapped Children Act (now known as IDEA) (Braddock 1986b; Scotch 1984).

The passage of the ICF/MR law in 1971 enabled the states to obtain federal funding for institutional services for people with intellectual disabilities if the care provided met minimal federal standards of treatment and space. Insofar as the federal government would reimburse states for 50 to 78 percent of the costs of institutional care, states had great incentives to change their services to conform to federal standards. This led to a tremendous push to deinstitutionalize because the minimum space requirements were well beyond the overcrowded capacities of nearly all the nation's institutions (Rothman and Rothman 1984). Peaking in 1967 at more than 194,000 people, the population of the nation's public institutions for persons with mental retardation and developmental disabilities has declined steadily to 52,801 persons in 1998 (Braddock et al. 2000). Advances in applied behavioral interventions have facilitated community, employment, and social integration (Jacobson, Burchard, and Carling 1992; Koegel, Koegel, and Dunlap 1996; Thompson and Grabowski 1977).

The *Wyatt v. Stickney* decision in regard to people with intellectual disability was built on the principle of right to treatment developed for people with mental illness. Judge Johnson found that people in Alabama's institutions had a constitutional right to treatment (Levy and Rubenstein 1996; Parry 1995; *Wyatt v. Stickney* 1971). This case began a tidal wave of federal class action cases related to conditions in institutions for people with intellectual disabilities, culminating in more than 70 cases in 41 states (Braddock et al. 1998; Hayden 1997; Levy and Rubenstein 1996). Similar litigation was also filed on the right to education (Martin, Martin, and Terman 1996; *Pennsylvania Ass'n. Retarded Child. v. Commonwealth of PA* 1971).

In 1973, the U.S. Congress enacted Section 504 of the Rehabilitation Act, which prohibited discrimination against people with disabilities by any entity that received federal funds (National Council on Disability 1997; Percy 1989; Scotch 1984). The promulgation of regulations that would clarify the operating provisions of Section 504 was delayed by Secretary David Mathews of the U.S. Department of Health, Education, and Welfare (HEW) and then by his successor, Secretary Joseph Califano (National Council on Disability 1997; Scotch 1984). Disabled advocates organized to force promulgation of the regulations, first by suing Secretary Mathews and then by organizing sit-ins and demonstrations in HEW offices in San Francisco, New York, and Washington (Fleischer and Zames 1998). For the first time, American television audiences saw people with disabilities occupying federal buildings to secure their rights (Roberts 1989). These demonstrations resulted in the 1977 promulgation of regulations four years after the law was signed. Judy Heumann, a leader in the fight for release of the regulations, stated, "I don't think the regulations would have been signed without the demonstrations, as they were. I am totally convinced of that. I mean the political pressure was really getting to be heavy. They had to sign those regulations" (as cited in Scotch 1984:116). Highlights of Section 504 included mandating for new construction to be barrier free, mandating accessibility in programs and activities in existing facilities, and supporting reasonable accommodations for the employment of people with disabilities (Scotch 1984).

The coalition building and advocacy by disability groups during the Section 504 political action activities was one of the first times in American history that cross-disability advocacy groups had successfully worked together on a unified disability rights agenda. This cross-disability advocacy helped to establish the foundation for the subsequent passage of the broader advocacy efforts that ultimately led to the passage of the Americans with Disabilities Act in 1990 (Fleischer and Zames 1998; National Council on Disability 1997).

In 1980, after years of seeking equal representation within the professional organization Rehabilitation International (RI), disabled people broke with RI and formed Disabled Peoples' International. Since 1922, RI had been the only international cross-disability organization that addressed the needs of people with a variety of mental, physical, and sensory disabilities (Driedger 1989). In 1980, at a World Congress of RI, a resolution was defeated that would have mandated the equal participation of people with disabilities in each country's RI organization. In response, disabled advocates then established Disabled Peoples' International (DPI), indicating no tolerance for patronizing behavior by professionals. Disabled people would direct their own destiny. DPI worked energetically to establish the presence of people with disabilities on the world stage. By 1983, it had achieved consultative status with several United Nations organizations, and by 1985, organizations of disabled people had been established in nearly every country in the world (Driedger 1989).

The fourth watershed civil rights event in the 1970s in the United States was passage of the Education for All Handicapped Children's Act of 1975, which guaranteed children and youth with disabilities the right to a free, appropriate, public education. For the first time in the history of compulsory education in the United States, parents had a federally enforced right to education for their children with disabilities. Beyond the obviously important changes in education for children with disabilities, this legislation also created a generation of parents who believed that their children were entitled to related community services. Many of these parents would become strong advocates for community services and inclusive education. In the 1995-1996 school year, 46 percent of children with disabilities in the United States were educated in regular classroom settings, while the remainder were educated in a combination of other settings, including resource rooms, separate classrooms, and separate schools (U.S. Department of Education 1998).

The education for deaf and blind students in the United States, however, has traditionally been provided in special residential schools that began in the nineteenth century. Some have objected to the segregated education provided in such schools. For example, research conducted with women with visual impairments in England has demonstrated that the women educated in special schools felt that their experiences had been detrimental to their growth and that dependence was fostered in such settings (French 1996).

Recent analysis of educational data for blind and deaf students indicated that the number of blind students educated in residential schools has declined. Kirchner, Peterson, and Suhr (1988) found that between 1963 and 1978, the percentage of blind students educated in public and private residential schools declined from 45 percent to 24 percent. By 1996, the latest school year for which data are available, 11 percent of deaf children were being educated in residential schools (U.S. Department of Education 1998). In 1998, the number of blind children being educated in residential schools had fallen to 8 percent (American Printing House for the Blind 1999). The total numbers of deaf and blind children being educated in residential schools in 1996 were 7,311 and 2,179, respectively (U.S. Department of Education 1998).

Independent Living and Self-Advocacy

The 1970s was also the decade of the rise of independent living in the United States (DeJong 1979a, 1979b; Stewart, Harris, and Sapey 1999). As previously noted, this movement gathered strength from the advocacy needed to force the promulgation of the Vocational Rehabilitation Act of 1973's Section 504 rules. Such legislation was predicated on the notion that people with disabilities need supports to live independently in their communities, not only because of their impairments but because society is constructed in such a way as to preclude their full participation (Bowe 1978). The initial catalysts for the independent living movement in the United States were drawn from a critical analysis of the processes of medicalization and professionalization in the rehabilitation system (Lysack and Kaufert 1994; Zola 1979). In Canada, the independent living movement emerged in the early 1980s, also driven by the advocacy efforts of people with disabilities (Boschen and Krane 1992).

The independent living movement embraced the notion that the barriers that confront people with disabilities are less related to individual impairment than to social attitudes, interpretations of disability, architectural barriers, legal barriers, and educational barriers (Americans Disabled for Attendant Programs Today 1995; Bowe 1978). The creation in the early 1970s of the nation's first independent living center in Berkeley, California, served as a model for the development of such centers across the country (DeJong 1979a; Roberts 1989). This first center, as well as hundreds of others that followed it, offered an array of services, including peer counseling, advocacy services, van transportation, training in independent living skills, wheelchair repair, housing referral, and attendant care referral, among others (DeJong 1979a; Roberts 1989). Central to the independent living movement is the notion that people with disabilities themselves must set the agenda for research and political action in disability policy (DeJong 1981). Ed Roberts (1989:238-39), one of the founders of the independent living movement, identified the four core principles of independent living as self-determination, self-image and public education, advocacy, and service to all. In the year 2000, there were 336 centers for independent living and 253 subordinate sites operating in the United States. They served 212,000 persons in approximately 60 percent of the nation's 3,141 counties (Innes et al. 2000).

Self-determination in the United States has focused on the independent living center as a primary coordinating organization by which disabled people engage in the advocacy and education activities needed to meet their individual and collective goals. In the Netherlands, the independent living needs of people with disabilities have been embraced by the country's mainstream entitlement programs, wedding a system of residential care and independent living to the country's general health and social welfare systems (DeJong 1984). Denmark and Germany, nations similar to the Netherlands in welfare policy, also have connected programs for people with disabilities to their mainstream entitlement programs (Fröhlich 1982; Jørgensen 1982). In Britain, housing has been a pivotal advocacy and policy concern of the independent living movement (Stewart et al. 1999).

The advocacy organization Disabled in Action was founded in 1970 by Judy Heumann to address barriers faced by people with disabilities, and by 1972 it had 1,500 members. The group engaged in activities ranging from a march on Washington protesting President Nixon's veto of the Vocational Rehabilitation Act Amendments of 1973 to the staging of protests at inaccessible buildings and at Jerry Lewis telethons. The telethons used paternalistic, pity-oriented depictions of people with disabilities to raise funds. These initial political advocacy efforts led to the formation in 1974 of the American Coalition of Citizens with Disabilities, which became an umbrella organization for disability advocacy groups across the nation (Scotch 1989).

In America, states' efforts to "reform" institutions for people with intellectual disabilities in the 1970s gave way to efforts to reallocate institutional resources to community services activities. States began closing institutions in significant numbers for the first time in the early 1980s (Braddock and Heller 1985). In 1991, New Hampshire closed the Laconia Developmental Center and became the first state in the United States to provide all of its services to people with intellectual disabilities in the community (Covert, MacIntosh, and Shumway 1994). By 1998, 36 states had closed 118 state institutions for people with intellectual disabilities, and 4 more closures were scheduled to occur by the year 2000 (Braddock et al. 2000). In addition to New Hampshire, all public institutions for people with intellectual disabilities have also been closed in Alaska, the District of Columbia, Hawaii, New Mexico, Rhode Island, Vermont, and West Virginia (Braddock et al. 2000).

Institutional phase-downs and closures have been accompanied by a growing emphasis on supported community living for individuals with intellectual disabilities. Between 1977 and 1998, the number of persons living in community-based settings for 1 to 6 persons expanded from 20,409 to 237,796 persons, a more than tenfold increase. Much of this tremendous expansion in community services was fueled by the federal-state partnership in the Medicaid Home and Community Based Services (HCBS) Waiver Program (Braddock et al. 1998, 2000).

The reduction in reliance on residential institutions for people with intellectual disabilities occurred in Great Britain and across Western Europe as well (Keith and Schalock 2000). In England, for example, the census of public hospitals for people with intellectual disabilities (those operated by the National Health Service) declined 83 percent, from 44,400 in 1980 to 7,400 persons in 1996. Similarly significant declines were noted in other U.K. countries. In Wales, Scotland, and Northern Ireland, census reductions of 70 percent, 51 percent, and 48 percent, respectively, were noted during the same 1980 to 1996 period (Emerson et al. 2000).

Organized self-advocacy is an important manifestation of the emergence of autonomy and self-determination for people with intellectual disabilities (Dybwad and Bersani 1996; Longhurst 1994). Membership in local and statewide self-advocacy groups such as People First has grown rapidly. Hayden and Senese (1996) identified more than 1,000 self-advocacy groups, some in every state. This represented almost a threefold expansion in the number of groups since 1990 (Longhurst 1994). In 1995, self-advocacy groups established a national organization called Self Advocates Becoming Empowered (SABE). SABE has developed an advocacy agenda calling for the phase-down and closure of all state-operated mental retardation institutions in the United States (Dybwad and Bersani 1996).

Self-advocacy by people with mental illness has included people completely opposed to organized psychiatry, psychotropic medication, and institutional treatment (Lefley 1996). The first group of ex-patients devoted to the "liberation from psychiatry" formed in Portland, Oregon, in 1969. Advocacy by this group has included litigation to combat involuntary, uninformed use of electroconvulsive therapy (ECT), litigation against ECT manufacturers, and pressing for consumer advisory functions at the state level of mental illness service administration (MadNation 1999).

Deaf students at Gallaudet University gained national attention in 1988 by advocating for a deaf president. In addition to initiating the Deaf President Now movement, the students sought a deaf majority on the university's board of directors. The university's first deaf president, I. King Jordan, was subsequently appointed, and the first deaf chair of the board, Philip Bravin, was selected (Gallaudet University 1997).

International Disability Rights Initiatives

The 1990 passage of the Americans with Disabilities Act (ADA) in the United States was a watershed event for disability rights on the international stage. This law recognized that discrimination against people with disabilities in the form of purposeful unequal treatment and historical patterns of segregation and isolation was the major problem confronting people with disabilities and not their individual impairments (National Council on Disability 1997; Parry 1995). The ADA also stated that people with disabilities have been relegated to powerless positions based on stereotypical assumptions about their disabilities. As such, the ADA bars discrimination against people with disabilities in employment, public services, public accommodations, and telecommunications (Parry 1995). The ADA was enacted after a concerted effort by a coalition of mental, physical, and sensory disability rights groups to work together to secure its passage (National Council on Disability 1997). As noted, the cross-disability coalition that advocated for enactment of the ADA was built in part on the foundation initially developed by advocates pushing for the enactment and subsequent promulgation of rules for the Vocational Rehabilitation Act Amendments of 1973 (Scotch 1989).

In Britain, a similar law protecting the rights of people with disabilities, the Disability Discrimination Act, was enacted in 1995 (Doyle 1996; Gooding 1996). This law mandated reasonable adjustments to the policies and physical environments of employers with 20 or more employees, compelling the removal of barriers facing people with disabilities (Gooding 1996). The law also mandated accessibility in public transportation (Doyle 1996; Gooding 1996). While the law has been hailed as an advance in civil rights for people living in Scotland, England, Wales, and Ireland, disability advocates have expressed disappointment that the law did not go as far as it should have in protecting and facilitating enforcement of the rights of people with disabilities (Doyle 1996; Gooding 1996).

At the international level, the United Nations General Assembly unanimously adopted the *Standard Rules on the Equalization of Opportunities for Persons with Disabilities* (United Nations 1994). The *Standard Rules* are not legally enforceable internationally, but they do provide basic international standards for programs, laws, and policy on disability. The *Standard Rules* grew out of earlier pressure from international disability interests to promote greater participation by people with disabilities in society. This philosophy was initially expressed in the 1971 *Declaration of the Rights of Mentally Retarded Persons* (United Nations 1971), the 1975 *Declaration of the Rights of Disabled Persons* (United Nations 1975), and the more comprehensive statement expressed in the 1982 *World Programme of Action Concerning Disabled Persons* (United Nations 1982).

The purpose of the *World Programme of Action* (WPA) is to

promote effective measures for prevention of disability, rehabilitation and the realization of the goals of "full participation" of disabled persons, in social life and development, and of "equality." This means opportunities equal to those of the whole population and an equal share in the improvement in living conditions resulting from social and economic development. These concepts should apply with the same scope and with the same urgency to all countries, regardless of their level of development.

The WPA requires member states to plan, organize and finance activities at each level; create, through legislation, the necessary legal bases and authority for measures to achieve the objectives; ensure opportunities by eliminating barriers to full participation; provide rehabilitation services by giving social, nutritional, medical, educational and vocational assistance and technical aids to disabled persons; establish or mobilize relevant public and private organizations; support the establishment and growth of organizations of disabled persons; and prepare and disseminate information relevant to the issues of the World Programme of Action. (Metts 2000:20)

The United Nation's (1994) *Standard Rules* was predicated on the principles embodied in the *World Programme of Action,* which focuses on the equalization of opportunities for people with disabilities. This commitment to disabled persons goes well beyond traditional international antidiscrimination protections of property, political, and judicial rights by seeking to convey rights to rehabilitation, special education, and access to public and private facilities and programs. The European Union (1996) has also adopted general disability policies similar to the UN's (1982) *World Programme of Action.*

In addition to Great Britain and the United States, a number of nations adopted legislation in the 1990s prohibiting discrimination against persons with disabilities. Australia adopted the Disability Discrimination Act of 1993, outlawing discrimination on the basis of disability, and the constitutions of Germany, Austria, Finland, and Brazil have been similarly amended. Constitutional changes have also been adopted in South Africa, Malawi, Uganda, and the Philippines. These actions are representative of the recent flurry of legislative activity on a worldwide basis to promote the rights of people with disabilities (Metts 2000).

In the United States, the growth of public spending for disability programs during the past 30 years has paralleled the rise of parent and consumer advocacy and of the "disability business" (Albrecht 1992). In fiscal year 1997, an estimated $93.8 billion was allocated for long-term care services and rehabilitation, housing, and veterans activities by federal, state, and local governments in the United States. General health care commanded $50.5 billion, and $36.4 billion was allocated for special education activities. An additional $96.9 billion was spent for disability-related income maintenance in 1997, primarily through the Supplemental Security Income and Social Security Disability Insurance programs (Braddock 2000).

Thus, at the close of the twentieth century, the public sector in the United States was spending $277.6 billion for disability services and income supports for more than 38 million recipients. This spending level is roughly equivalent to 12 percent of the country's total public expenditure for all purposes from combined federal and state sources in 1997.[1] However, a large percentage of the $93.8 billion financial commitment for disability services and long-term care—approximately 46 percent of the funds—supported the placement of hundreds of thousands of persons with disabilities in segregated settings such as nursing homes, sheltered workshops, and mental institutions. Furthermore, a large percentage of the 5.7 million students with disabilities in special education, particularly those with significant disabilities, received services in separate classes, separate educational facilities, or public or private institutions. Sixty-one percent of students with intellectual disabilities ("mental retardation"), for example, were served in segregated educational settings in 1996 (U.S. Department of Education 1998). While it is clear that the United States has made enormous strides in the implementation of disability assistance programs over the past few decades (Silverstein 2000), the basic funding priorities in many programs, such as Medicaid and special education, have not kept pace with contemporary consumer support models based on choice, self-determination, home care, family support, and inclusive education.

CONCLUSION

After the seventeenth century, medical science and the rise of custodial residential institutions undermined the self-determination of people with disabilities during a period of rapid and continuous urbanization and industrialization in the West. It did this by overmedicalizing what was, in large measure, a social, educational, and economic problem, separating many disabled people from their families, communities, and society at large. This socially sanctioned segregation reinforced negative societal attitudes toward human difference. However, the segregation of disabled people in one geographic place—in residential schools for deaf and blind persons, mental institutions for those with emotional problems and intellectual limitations, and, eventually, special public school classes and rehabilitation centers—also facilitated the development of empowered group identities that ultimately led to political activism.

Assertive political activism by people with disabilities and their families emerged primarily in the late twentieth century, and, in the United States, it draws considerable strength from the example of the civil rights movement for people of color (Birnbaum and Taylor 2000). It is, in fact, an often-repeated general truism in the disability field today that prejudicial and exclusionary practices are greater barriers to social participation for disabled people than their particular mental, physical, or sensory impairments (Scotch 1989).

People with disabilities have shared a history that has often been oppressive and included abuse, neglect, sterilization, stigma, euthanasia, segregation, and institutionalization. Disabled people, who have survived by relying on tenacity and resourcefulness and on support provided in different measures by family, friends, and local communities, are currently struggling to claim identity (Anspach 1979; Gill 1997; Linton 1998) and political power (Hahn 1985). While the deaf community has a history of struggling collectively to preserve their culture for more than a century, people with mental and physical disabilities have only emerged to champion their own interests collectively within the past three or four decades.

Advocacy by specific, single-disability groups in the United States began to evolve into cross-disability coalition building in the 1970s, 1980s, and 1990s. Cross-disability advocacy, for example, secured passage of the Americans with Disabilities Act (National Council on Disability 1997). The paternalism of nondisabled nineteenth-century figures such as Howe, Pinel, Gallaudet, and Rushton has been replaced, at least in part, with leadership and self-determination by people with disabilities themselves. Thus, at the close of the twentieth century, the foundation was gradually established in the West for a new era based on civil rights, social participation, and a cross-disability perspective.

Achieving inclusive societies, however, will require persons with mental, physical, and sensory disabilities to learn more about one another and, on common ground, to construct more powerful community, state, national, and international cross-disability coalitions than have been developed in the past. In this chapter, we argued that people across the spectrum of disability have a good deal in common historically and that recognizing and celebrating this shared history are an important step in building stronger and more effective cross-disability coalitions in the future.

The potential strength of cross-disability coalitions should grow as societies age since the prevalence of impairment in a society is directly correlated with aging. Over the course of the next 30 years, the number of persons age 65 and older will double in the United States, triple in Germany and Japan, and advance rapidly in virtually every developed nation of the world (U.S. Bureau of the Census 1997; Janicki and Ansello 2000). As more developing countries make significant economic advances, these nations will experience a concomitant rise in political advocacy by and for people with disabilities. Albrecht and Verbrugge (2000) refer to this growing phenomenon of disability across the developed and developing nations of the world as the global emergence of disability. "With or without anyone's attention," they argue, "global disability will be on the rise for many decades to come, fueled by population aging, environmental degradation, and social violence" (p. 305). The key disability issues for developing societies include controlling infectious diseases that lead to disability; reducing unsafe occupational conditions; managing drought and the environment; limiting ethnic, religious, and regional wars; and launching thoughtful innovations in income support, health promotion, special education, rehabilitation, and the promotion of self-determination (Hoffman and Field 1995). By adopting programs that stress consumer, family, and community values, it is hoped that many developing nations will be able to avoid replicating the developed world's self-destructive preoccupations with segregation, institutionalization, and eugenics.

The principal disability issues currently facing the developed nations in Europe, North America, and Australasia, according to Albrecht and Verbrugge (2000), include fashioning reasonable eligibility standards for income maintenance and service programs for persons with disabilities; advancing civil rights; creating access to employment, public accommodations, and society at large; and minimizing regional, state, and substate differences in public welfare benefits and service programs. To these critically important contemporary issues, we would add that developed nations also must confront (1) ethical and cost-benefit dilemmas accompanying advances in gene therapy, biotechnology, and neuroscience research; (2) the potential for assisted suicide to lead to the widespread euthanasia of persons with disabilities; (3) the continuing segregation of millions of persons with disabilities in nursing homes, institutions, and other segregated settings throughout the world; and (4) the development of productive and reciprocally valued working relationships between consumers with disabilities seeking greater self-determination and political power and the professionals who provide and study services to people with disabilities (Barnes 1996; Humphrey 2000; Oliver 1992; Oliver and Barnes 1999). In particular, the United States must also confront the growing inequality in the distribution of the wealth of its citizenry and the profound health care and educational disparities between rich and poor (Galbraith 1998).

The disability rights struggle of the first half of the twenty-first century will fundamentally be a struggle to delink the enduring and oppressive relationship between poverty and disability. Even in the most economically developed nations of the world today, unemployment rates for disabled persons frequently approach 80 percent, and average personal income is in the bottom decile.

As researchers, we need to mount a series of rigorous, comparative, recurring empirical studies to monitor the growth of public-sector resource and service commitments for disability programs in every country of the world in which it is possible to do so. These recurring studies need to assess the allocation of resources on a nationwide basis for disability programs so that all the nations of the world can be held accountable for their commitments to disabled people and their families. Such studies would permit the priority that a nation assigns to disability to be evaluated over time and to be compared to other nations with similar levels of wealth. The information generated in such studies would be useful in program planning, and, by identifying the leaders and the laggards among the nations of the world, it would be immensely useful to disability advocates seeking to influence public policy on behalf of their constituencies. Several international organizations should be approached to sponsor this research, including the World Bank, the United Nations, the European Union, the Pan American Health Organization, and the World Health Organization. In the United States, the National Institute on Disability and Rehabilitation Research (NIDRR) should also consider launching one or more international rehabilitation research and training centers. These centers would focus on significantly expanding educational and research links on disability between and among the developed and developing nations of the world.

Albrecht and Verbrugge (2000) are right: Disability *is* emerging globally. The number of disabled people in 175 nations of the world today was recently estimated to range between 235 and 549 million people. The lost gross domestic product due to unemployment, underemployment, and services and support costs associated with disability was determined to range between $1.4 and $1.9 trillion per annum in current dollars (Metts 2000). Disability research institutions such as NIDRR and international development organizations such as the World Bank need to acknowledge the global emergence of disability by establishing and funding new strategies for international research leadership and action on disability in the twenty-first century.

One final point is in order. At the outset of this chapter, we noted that the paucity of primary source evidence in most written histories of disability was a significant weakness. It is lamentable indeed that most existing records and publications have inevitably described disability history from the perspective of professionals who controlled the delivery of services. We endeavored in this chapter to use primary sources extensively when possible. However, in evaluating the strengths and weaknesses of this chapter, it is clear that we have barely touched on the potential of one very useful type of primary source material—literary and artistic archives—to complement the institutionally oriented history presented here. Studying the representation of disability in literature and art is an important and relatively unexplored research frontier in disability studies. It is a frontier with the potential to yield a richer understanding of the history of disability, with lived experience and perspective at the center of analysis rather than at the periphery. The work of Allen Thiher (1999), Robert Garland (1995), Rosemarie Garland Thomson (1997), David Mitchell (2000), and Sander Gilman (1988, 1995) exemplifies this approach, and significant growth in research on disability and the humanities can be expected over the next decade. This scholarship will contribute greatly to the developing knowledge base on the history of disability and human diversity.

NOTE

1. Public-sector (federal, state, local) spending for disability programs in fiscal year 1997 was estimated by the authors based on data obtained from the following sources: $36.4 billion on special education (Chambers et al. 1998; U.S. Department of Education 1992, 1998). Federal and state spending for services for individuals with mental illness was estimated based on data collected by the National Association on State Mental Health Program Directors (Lutterman, Hirad, and Poindexter 1999) at $26.7 billion. Spending for individuals receiving housing support through the U.S. Department of Housing and Urban Development (2000) was reported at $9.9 billion. Combined federal and state vocational rehabilitation and independent living services spending totaled $2.9 billion in 1997 (D. Teimouri, Rehabilitation Services Administration, U.S. Department of Education, personal communication, February 16, 2000, and J. Nelson, Rehabilitation Services Administration, U.S. Department of Education, personal communication, March 3, 2000). In addition, federal, state, and locally financed services for persons with developmental disabilities in 1997 totaled $24.2 billion (Braddock et al. 2000). Medicaid health care, Medicare health care, and nursing home spending for persons with disabilities, excluding such funding associated with mental illness and developmental disabilities spending, totaled $51.8 billion (Health Care Financing Administration 1998) and $22.3 billion, respectively (M. Diacogiannis, Health Care Financing Administration, U.S. Department of Health and Human Services, personal communication, March 15, 2000). Payments totaled $6.4 billion for acute health care for veterans with disabilities (M. Pringle, Department of Veterans Affairs, personal communication, March 16, 2000, and W. L. Walsh, Department of Veterans Affairs, personal communication, March 14, 2000).

Income maintenance for persons with disabilities totaled $24.5 billion for Supplemental Security Income, $44.6 billion in Social Security Disability Insurance payments in 1997, $5.2 billion for the Disabled Adult Child Income Maintenance Benefits (Social Security Administration 1998), $12.7 billion for Veterans Compensation (M. Pringle, Department of Veterans Affairs, personal communication, March 16, 2000), $7.6 billion for Housing Rental Subsidy Payments (U.S. Department of Housing and Urban Development 2000), and $2.4 billion for Food Stamps (U.S. Department of Agriculture 1998). Total disability spending of $277.6 billion was then divided by nondefense public (federal, state, and local) expenditures of $2.404 trillion (Office of Management and Budget 1999) to determine the estimated proportion of public spending attributable to disability services and income support in 1997 (11.5 percent).

REFERENCES

Adair, R., J. Melling, and B. Forsythe. 1997. "Migration, Family Structure, and Pauper Lunacy in Victorian England: Admissions to the Devon County Pauper Lunatic Asylum, 1845-1900." *Continuity and Change* 13:373-401.

Albrecht, G. L. 1992. *The Disability Business: Rehabilitation in America.* Newbury Park, CA: Sage.

Albrecht, G. L. and L. M. Verbrugge. 2000. "The Global Emergence of Disability." Pp. 293-307 in *The Handbook of Social Studies in Health and Medicine,* edited by G. L. Albrecht, R. Fitzpatrick, and S. C. Scrimshaw. London: Sage.

Alexander, F. G. and S. T. Selesnick. 1964. *The History of Psychiatry: An Evaluation of Psychiatric Thought and Practice from Prehistoric Times to the Present.* New York: Harper & Row.

Allen, E. E. 1899. "Education of Defectives." Pp. 3-51 in *Monographs on Education in the United States, No. 15*, edited by N. M. Butler. New York: Department of Education for the U.S. Commission for the Paris Exposition of 1900.

————. 1914. *Progress of the Education of the Blind in the United States in the Year 1912-1913: Chapter XXII, Volume I, 1913*. Washington, DC: Government Printing Office.

American Printing House for the Blind. 1999. *Distribution of Eligible Students Based on the Federal Quota Census of January 5, 1998* [Online]. Available: sun1.aph.org/dist98.htm.

Americans Disabled for Attendant Programs Today. 1995. *Long Term Care Policy: It's Good to Have the Facts When You Choose (Statistics, Sources, a Call to Action)*. Rochester, NY: Free Hand.

Andrews, J. 1998. "Begging the Question of Idiocy: The Definition and Socio-Cultural Meaning of Idiocy in Early Modern Britain: Part I." *History of Psychiatry* 9:65-95.

Andrews, J., A. Briggs, R. Porter, P. Tucker, and K. Waddington. 1997. *The History of Bethlem*. New York: Routledge.

Anspach, R. R. 1979. "From Stigma to Identity Politics: Political Activism among the Physically Disabled and Former Mental Patients." *Social Science and Medicine* 13A:765-73.

Axinn, J. and H. Levin. 1982. *Social Welfare: A History of the American Response to Need*. New York: Longman.

Bacon, F. [1605] 1900. *The Advancement of Learning*. Reprint, Oxford, UK: Clarendon.

Barnes, C. 1996. "Disability and the Myth of the Independent Researcher." *Disability & Society* 11:107-10.

Barr, M. W. 1895. "Moral Paranoia." *Proceedings of the Association of Medical Officers of American Institutions for Idiotic and Feeble-Minded Persons* 20:522-31.

————. 1902. "The Imbecile and Epileptic versus the Taxpayer and the Community." *Proceedings of the National Conference of Social Work* 30:161-65.

————. 1904. *Mental Defectives*. Philadelphia, PA: P. Blakiston's Sons & Co.

Bartlett, F. L. 1964. "Institutional Peonage: Our Exploitation of Mental Patients." *The Atlantic Monthly* 214:116-19.

Bassoe, P. 1945. "Spain as the Cradle of Psychiatry." *American Journal of Psychiatry* 102:731-38.

Baynton, D. C. 1993. " 'Savages and Deaf-Mutes': Evolutionary Theory and the Campaign against Sign Language in the Nineteenth Century." Pp. 92-112 in *Deaf History Unveiled: Interpretations from the New Scholarship*, edited by J. V. Van Cleve. Washington, DC: Gallaudet University Press.

————. 1996. *Forbidden Signs: American Culture and the Campaign against Sign Language*. Chicago: University of Chicago Press.

Beers, C. 1908. *A Mind That Found Itself*. New York: Longmans, Green.

Bell, A. G. [1883] 1969. *Upon the Formation of Deaf Variety of the Human Race*. Reprint, Washington, DC: Alexander Graham Bell Association for the Deaf.

Berger, P. and T. Luckmann. 1967. *The Social Construction of Reality: A Treatise in the Sociology of Knowledge*. London: Allen Lane.

Berkson, G. 1974. "Social Responses of Animals to Infants with Defects." Pp. 239-49 in *The Effect of the Infant on Its Caregivers*, edited by M. Lewis and L. E. Rosenblum. New York: John Wiley.

————. 1993. *Children with Handicaps: A Review of Behavioral Research*. Hillsdale, NJ: Lawrence Erlbaum.

Bernstein, C. 1917. "Self-Sustaining Feeble-Minded." *Journal of Psycho-Asthenics* 22:150-61.

————. 1918. "Rehabilitation of the Mentally Defective." *Journal of Psycho-Asthenics* 23:92-103.

————. 1921. "Colony Care for Isolation of Defective and Dependent Cases." *Proceedings of the American Association on Mental Defect* 26:43-59.

Bickenbach, J. E. 1993. *Physical Disability and Social Policy*. Toronto: University of Toronto.

Bicknell, E. 1895. "Custodial Care of the Adult Feeble-Minded." *Charities Review* 5:76-88.

Birnbaum, J. and C. Taylor. 2000. "Introduction: Where Do We Go from Here?" Pp. 1-6 in *Civil Rights since 1787: A Reader on the Black Struggle*, edited by J. Birnbaum and C. Taylor. New York: New York University Press.

Birnbaum, M. 1965. "Some Comments on 'the Right to Treatment.' " *Archives of General Psychiatry* 13:33-45.

Black, K. 1996. *Healing Homiletic: Preaching and Disability*. Nashville, TN: Abingdon.

Blatt, B. 1977. "The Family Album." *Mental Retardation* 15:3-4.

Bliquez, L. J. 1983. "Classical Prosthetics." *Archaeology* 36:25-29.

Bogdan, R. 1986. "Exhibiting Mentally Retarded People for Amusement and Profit, 1850-1940." *American Journal of Mental Deficiency* 91:120-26.

————. 1988. *Freak Show: Presenting Human Oddities for Amusement and Profit.* Chicago: University of Chicago Press.

Bonsall, A. 1891. "Discussion on the Care of Imbeciles." *Proceedings of the National Conference of Social Work* 19:331-32.

Boschen, K. A. and N. Krane. 1992. "A History of Independent Living in Canada." *Canadian Journal of Rehabilitation* 6:79-88.

Bowe, F. G. 1978. *Handicapping America: Barriers to Disabled People.* New York: Harper & Row.

Braddock, D. 1981. "Deinstitutionalization of the Retarded: Trends in Public Policy." *Hospital and Community Psychiatry* 32:607-15.

————. 1986a. "Federal Assistance for Mental Retardation and Developmental Disabilities: Part I.—A Review through 1961." *Mental Retardation* 24:175-82.

————. 1986b. "Federal Assistance for Mental Retardation and Developmental Disabilities: Part II.—The Modern Era." *Mental Retardation* 24:209-18.

————. 1987. *Federal Policy toward Mental Retardation.* Baltimore, MD: Brookes.

————. 1992. "Community Mental Health and Mental Retardation Services in the American States: A Comparative Study of Resource Allocation." *American Journal of Psychiatry* 149:175-83.

————. 2000. *Disability in the United States: A Comparative Analysis of Public Spending.* Chicago: Department of Disability and Human Development, University of Illinois at Chicago.

Braddock, D. and T. Heller. 1985. "The Closure of Mental Retardation Institutions: Part II.—Implications." *Mental Retardation* 23:222-29.

Braddock, D., R. Hemp, S. Parish, and M. C. Rizzolo. 2000. *The State of the States in Developmental Disabilities: 2000 Study Summary.* Chicago: Department of Disability and Human Development, University of Illinois at Chicago.

Braddock, D., R. Hemp, S. Parish, and J. Westrich. 1998. *The State of the States in Developmental Disabilities.* 5th ed. Washington, DC: American Association on Mental Retardation.

Breckinridge, S. P. 1927. *Public Welfare Administration in the United States: Select Documents.* Chicago: University of Chicago Press.

————. 1939. *The Illinois Poor Law and Its Administration.* Chicago: University of Chicago Press.

Bredberg, E. 1999. "Writing Disability History: Problems, Perspectives, and Sources." *Disability & Society* 14:189-201.

Brierre de Boismont, A. J. F. 1867. *Joseph Guislain, sa vie et ses ecrits* (Joseph Guislain, His Life and Writings). Paris: Bailliere.

Brigham, A. 1845. *Annual Report of the Bloomingdale Insane Asylum.* Bloomingdale, NY: Bloomingdale Insane Asylum.

British Association of the Deaf. 1999. *Our History* [Online]. Available: www.bda.org.uk/index1.htm.

Brockley, J. A. 1999. "History of Mental Retardation: An Essay Review." *History of Psychology* 2:25-36.

Bromberg, W. 1975. *From Shaman to Psychotherapist: A History of the Treatment of Mental Illness.* Chicago: Henry Regnery.

Brown, T. J. 1998. *Dorothea Dix: New England Reformer.* Cambridge, MA: Harvard University Press.

Browne, W. A. F. 1837. *What Asylums Were, Are, and Ought to Be: Being the Substance of Five Lectures Delivered before the Managers of the Montrose Royal Lunatic Asylum.* Edinburgh, UK: Adam and Charles Black.

Brundage, A. 1989. *Going to the Sources: A Guide to Historical Research and Writing.* Arlington Heights, IL: Harlan Davidson.

Buck v. Bell, 274 U.S. 200 (1927).

Bucknill, J. C. 1873. "Address on Idiocy." *Journal of Mental Science* 19:167-83.

Burleigh, M. 1994. "Psychiatry, German Society, and the Nazi 'Euthanasia' Programme." *Social History of Medicine* 7:213-28.

Butler, A. W. 1907. "The Burden of Feeble-Mindedness." *Proceedings of the National Conference of Social Work* 35:1-10.

Button, L. A. 1878. *Behind the Scenes; Or, Life in An Insane Asylum.* Chicago: Culver, Page, Hoyne.

Carabello, B. J. and J. F. Siegel. 1996. "Self-Advocacy at the Crossroads." Pp. 237-39 in *New Voices: Self-Advocacy by People with Disabilities,* edited by G. Dybwad and H. Bersani. Cambridge, MA: Brookline.

Carpenter, J. 1996. "Rev Harold Nelson Burden and Katherine Mary Burden: Pioneers of Inebriate Reformatories and Mental Deficiency Institutions." *Journal of the Royal Society of Medicine* 89:205-9.

Carrey, N. J. 1995. "Itard's 1828 Memoire on 'Mutism Caused by a Lesion of the Intellectual Functions': A Historical Analysis." *Journal of the American Academy of Child and Adolescent Psychiatry* 34:1655-61.

Cavallo, S. 1998. "Family Obligations and Inequalities in Access to Care in Northern Italy, Seventeenth to Eighteenth Centuries." Pp. 90-110 in *The Locus of Care: Families, Communities, Institutions, and the Provision of Welfare since Antiquity*, edited by P. Horden and R. Smith. London: Routledge Kegan Paul.

Cerletti, U. 1950. "Old and New Information about Electroshock." *American Journal of Psychiatry* 107:87-94.

Chambers, J. G., T. B. Parrish, J. C. Lieberman, and J. M. Wolman. 1998. *What Are We Spending on Special Education in the US?* CSEF Brief No. 8. Palo Alto, CA: Center for Special Education Finance.

Charlton, J. I. 1998. *Nothing about Us without Us: Disability, Oppression, and Empowerment*. Berkeley: University of California Press.

Chevigny, H. 1946. *My Eyes Have a Cold Nose*. New Haven, CT: Yale University Press.

Church, A. 1893. "Removal of Ovaries and Tubes in the Insane and Neurotic." *American Journal of Obstetrics and Diseases of Women and Children* 28:491-98.

Clay, R. M. 1966. *The Mediaeval Hospitals of England*. London: Frank Cass.

Cochrane, R. G. 1963. *Biblical Leprosy: A Suggested Interpretation*. 2d ed. London: Tyndale Press for The Christian Medical Fellowship.

Colon, D. M. 1989. "Martin Luther, the Devil, and the Teulfelchen: Attitudes toward Mentally Retarded Children in Sixteenth Century Germany." *Proceedings of the PMR (Patristic, Medieval, and Renaissance) Conference* 14:75-84.

"County Asylums Proposed." 1982. P. 277 in *Three Hundred Years of Psychiatry: 1535-1860*, edited by R. Hunter and I. Macalpine. Hartsdale, NY: Carlisle.

Covert, S. B., J. D. MacIntosh, and D. L. Shumway. 1994. "Closing the Laconia State School and Training Center: A Case Study in System Change." Pp. 197-211 in *Creating Individual Supports for People with Developmental Disabilities: A Mandate for Change at Many Levels*, edited by V. J. Bradley, J. W. Ashbaugh, and B. C. Blaney. Baltimore: Brookes.

Covey, H. C. 1998. *Social Perceptions of People with Disabilities in History*. Springfield, IL: Charles C Thomas.

Daniels, M. 1997. *Benedictine Roots in the Development of Deaf Education: Listening with the Heart*. Westport, CT: Bergin & Garvey.

Davenport, A. B. 1921. "Selecting Immigrants." *Proceedings and Addresses of the American Association for the Study of the Feeble-Minded* 25:178-79.

Davies, S. P. 1930. *Social Control of the Mentally Deficient*. New York: Thomas Y. Crowell.

Davis, L. 1997. *The Disability Studies Reader*. New York: Routledge.

———. 2000. "Dr. Johnson, Amelia, and the Discourse of Disability in the Eighteenth Century." Pp. 54-74 in *"Defects": Engendering the Modern Body*, edited by H. Deutsch and F. Nussbaum. Ann Arbor: University of Michigan Press.

de Condillac, E. B. [1754] 1930. *Treatise on the Senses*. Translated by G. Carr. Reprint, Los Angeles: University of Southern California.

Defoe, D.. [1694] 1894. *An Essay upon Projects*. Reprint, London: Cassel.

———. 1720. *The History of the Life and Adventures of Mr Duncan Campbell*. London: E. Curll.

DeJong, G. 1979a. *The Movement for Independent Living: Origins, Ideology, and Implications for Disability Research*. East Lansing: University Center for International Rehabilitation, Michigan State University.

———. 1979b. "Independent Living: From Social Movement to Analytic Paradigm." *Archives of Physical Medicine and Rehabilitation* 60:435-46.

———. 1981. *Environmental Accessibility and Independent Living Outcomes: Directions for Disability Policy Research*. East Lansing: University Center for International Rehabilitation, Michigan State University.

———. 1984. *Independent Living and Disability Policy in the Netherlands: Three Models of Residential Care and Independent Living*. New York: International Exchange of Experts and Information in Rehabilitation, World Rehabilitation Fund.

de Saint-Loup, A. 1996. "A History of Misunderstandings: The History of the Deaf." *Diogenes* 44:1-25.

De Souza-Araujo, H. C. 1937. "The Origin of Leprosy in Brasil and Its Present Situation." *Leprosy Review* 8 (1): 12-16.

———. 1946. *História Da Lepra No Brasil* (History of Leprosy in Brazil). Vol. 1. Rio de Janeiro: Impresa Nacional.

———. 1948. *História Da Lepra No Brasil* (History of Leprosy in Brazil). Vol. 2. Rio de Janeiro: Impresa Nacional.

Digby, A. 1996. "Contexts and Perspectives." Pp. 1-21 in *From Idiocy to Mental Deficiency: Historical Perspectives on People with Learning Disabilities,* edited by D. Wright and A. Digby. London: Routledge Kegan Paul.

Dix, D. 1843. *Memorial: To the Legislature of Massachusetts.* Boston: Munroe & Francis.

Doyle, B. 1996. *Disability Discrimination: The New Law.* Bristol, UK: Jordans.

Driedger, D. 1989. *The Last Civil Rights Movement: Disabled Peoples' International.* London: Hurst & Company.

Dugdale, R. L. [1877] 1910. *The Jukes.* Reprint, New York: Putman.

Dybwad, G., and J. Bersani, Jr., eds. 1996. *New Voices: Self-Advocacy by People with Disabilities.* Cambridge, MA: Brookline.

Earle, P. 1845. "Historical and Descriptive Account of the Bloomingdale Asylum for the Insane." *American Journal of Insanity* 2:1-13.

———. 1877. *The Curability of Insanity.* Bloomingdale, NY: Bloomingdale Asylum for the Insane.

———. 1898. *Memoirs.* Boston: Damrell & Upham.

East, E. M. 1917. "Hidden Feeblemindedness." *Journal of Heredity* 8:215-17.

Edwards, M. L. 1996. "The Cultural Context of Deformity in the Ancient Greek World." *Ancient History Bulletin* 10:79-92.

———. 1997. "Deaf and Dumb in Ancient Greece." Pp. 29-51 in *The Disability Studies Reader,* edited by L. Davis. New York: Routledge.

Edwards, P. 1996. *Encyclopedia of Philosophy.* New York: Macmillan.

Elm Hill Private School and Home. 1911. *Elm Hill: Private School and Home.* Barre, MA: Author.

Ely, C. W. 1893. *History of the Maryland School for the Deaf and Dumb.* Frederick City: Maryland School for the Deaf and Dumb.

Emerson, E., J. Robertson, N. Gregory, C. Hatton, S. Kessissoglou, A. Hallam, M. Knapp, K. Järbrink, P. N. Walsh, and A. Netten. 2000. "Quality and Costs of Community-Based Residential Supports, Village Communities and Residential Campuses in the United Kingdom." *American Journal on Mental Retardation* 105 (2): 81-102.

Erikson, K. I. 1966. *Wayward Puritans: A Study in the Sociology of Deviance.* New York: John Wiley.

Estabrook, A. H. 1928. "The Pauper Idiot Pension in Kentucky." *Journal of Psycho-Asthenics* 33:59-61.

European Union. 1996. *Resolution of the Council and the Representatives of the Governments of the Member States on Equality of Opportunity for People with Disabilities.* Official Journal C 12, 13.01.1997. Brussels: Author.

Evans, H. C. 1926. *The American Poorfarm and Its Inmates.* Mooseheart, IL: Loyal Order of Moose.

Farmer, S. 1998. "Down and Out and Female in Thirteenth-Century Paris." *American Historical Review* 103:344-72.

Farrell, G. 1956. *The Story of Blindness.* Cambridge, MA: Harvard University Press.

Fay, E. A. 1893. *Histories of American Schools for the Deaf, 1817-1893.* Washington, DC: Volta Bureau.

Felix, R. H. 1957. "Evolution of Community Mental Health Concepts." *American Journal of Psychiatry* 113:673-79.

Fenton, R. 1932. "The Pacific Colony Plan." *Journal of Juvenile Research* 16:298-303.

Ferguson, P. M. 1994. *Abandoned to Their Fate: Social Policy and Practice toward Severely Retarded People in America, 1820-1920.* Philadelphia: Temple University Press.

Fernald, W. E. 1893. "The History of the Treatment of the Feeble-Minded." *Proceedings of the National Conference of Social Work* 21:203-21.

———. 1902. "The Massachusetts Farm Colony for the Feeble-Minded." *Proceedings of the National Conference on Charities and Correction* 30:487-91.

———. 1912. "The Burden of Feeble-Mindedness." *Journal of Psycho-Asthenics* 17:87-99.

———. 1915. "State Care of the Insane, Feebleminded, and Epileptic." *Proceedings of the National Conference of Charities and Correction* 42:289-97.

———. 1917. "The Growth of Provision for the Feebleminded in the United States." *Mental Hygiene* 1:34-59.

———. 1919. "A State Program for the Care of the Mentally Defective." *Mental Hygiene* 3:566-74.

Ferster, E. Z. 1966. "Eliminating the Unfit: Is Sterilization the Answer?" *Ohio State Law Journal* 27:591-633.

Fessler, A. 1956. "The Management of Lunacy in Seventeenth Century England: An Investigation of Quarter-Session Records." *Proceedings of the Royal Society of Medicine* 49:901-7.

Fish, W. B. 1892. "Custodial Care of Adult Idiots." *Proceedings of the National Conference of Social Work* 17:203-18.

FitzGerald, J. F. 1900. "The Duty of the State towards Its Idiotic and Feeble-Minded." *Proceedings of the New York State Conference of Charities* 1:172-89.

"Five Months in the New-York State Lunatic Asylum." 1982. Pp. 108-22 in *A Mad People's History of Madness,* edited by D. Peterson. Pittsburgh, PA: University of Pittsburgh Press.

Fleischer, D. Z. and F. Zames. 1998. "Disability Rights." *Social Policy* 28:52-55.

Fort, S. J. 1892. "What Shall Be Done with the Imbecile?" *Maryland Medical Journal* 27:1057-63.

Foucault, M. 1965. *Madness and Civilization.* Translated by R. Howard. London: Tavistock.

Frampton, M. E. and F. Kerney. 1953. *The Residential School: Its History, Contributions and Future.* New York: Edwin Gould Printery, New York Institute for the Education of the Blind.

French, R. S. 1932. *From Homer to Helen Keller: A Social and Educational Study of the Blind.* New York: American Foundation for the Blind.

French, S. 1996. "Out of Sight, Out of Mind: The Experience and Effects of a 'Special' Residential School." Pp. 17-47 in *Encounters with Strangers: Feminism and Disability,* edited by J. Morris. London: The Women's Press.

Friedlander, H. 1997. *The Origins of Nazi Genocide: From Euthanasia to the Final Solution.* Chapel Hill: University of North Carolina Press.

Fröhlich, A. 1982. "Movements toward Greater Independence of the Handicapped in West Germany." Pp. 35-70 in *Independent Living: An Overview of Efforts in Five Countries,* edited by D. G. Tate and L. M. Chadderdon. East Lansing: Center for International Rehabilitation, Michigan State University.

Galbraith, J. K. 1998. *Created Unequal: The Crisis in American Pay.* New York: Free Press.

Gallagher, H. G. 1995. *By Trust Betrayed: Patients, Physicians, and the License to Kill in the Third Reich.* Arlington, VA: Vandamere.

Gallaudet, E. M. 1983. *History of the College for the Deaf, 1857-1907.* Washington, DC: Gallaudet College Press.

Gallaudet University. 1997. *History of Gallaudet* [Online]. Available: www.gallaudet.edu/~pubreweb/visitor/history/page6.html.

Galton, F. 1883. *Inquiry into Human Faculty and Its Development.* London: Macmillan.

Gannon, J. R. 1981. *Deaf Heritage: A Narrative History of Deaf America.* Silver Spring, MD: National Association of the Deaf.

Garland, R. 1995. *The Eye of the Beholder: Deformity and Disability in the Graeco-Roman World.* Ithaca, NY: Cornell University Press.

Gaw, A. C. 1906a. "The Development of the Legal Status of the Deaf: A Comparative Study of the Rights and Responsibilities of Deaf-Mutes in the Laws of Rome, France, England, and America." *American Annals of the Deaf* 51:269-75.

———. 1906b. "The Development of the Legal Status of the Deaf: A Comparative Study of the Rights and Responsibilities of Deaf-Mutes in the Laws of Rome, France, England, and America." *American Annals of the Deaf* 51:401-23.

———. 1907. "The Development of the Legal Status of the Deaf: A Comparative Study of the Rights and Responsibilities of Deaf-Mutes in the Laws of Rome, France, England and America." *American Annals of the Deaf* 52:1-12.

Gill, C. J. 1997. "Four Types of Integration in Disability Identity Development." *Journal of Vocational Rehabilitation* 9:39-46.

Gilman, S. L. 1982. *Seeing the Insane.* New York: John Wiley-Interscience.

———. 1988. *Disease and Representation: Images of Illness from Madness to AIDS.* Ithaca, NY: Cornell University Press.

———. 1995. *Picturing Health and Illness: Images of Identity and Difference.* Baltimore: Johns Hopkins University Press.

Gladstone, D. 1996. "Western Counties Idiot Asylum 1864-1914." Pp. 134-60 in *From Idiocy to Mental Deficiency: Historical Perspectives on People with Learning Disabilities,* edited by D. Wright and A. Digby. London: Routledge Kegan Paul.

Goddard, H. H. 1912. *The Kallikak Family: A Study in the Heredity of Feeble-Mindedness.* New York: Macmillan.

Goldstein, M. S. 1969. "Human Paleopathology and Some Diseases in Living Primitive Societies: A Review of Recent Literature." *American Journal of Physical Anthropology* 31:285-94.

Goode, D. 1999. *History of the Association for the Help of Retarded Children of New York City.* New York: Association for the Help of Retarded Children.

Goodey, C. F. 1996. "The Psychopolitics of Learning and Disability in Seventeenth Century Thought." Pp. 93-117 in *From Idiocy to Mental Deficiency: Historical Perspectives on People with Learning Disabilities,* edited by D. Wright and A. Digby. London: Routledge Kegan Paul.

Gooding, C. 1996. *Blackstone's Guide to the Disability Discrimination Act 1995*. London: Blackstone.

Gordan, J. C. 1885. "Deaf-Mutes and the Public Schools from 1815 to the Present Day." *American Annals of the Deaf* 30:121-43.

Gorwitz, K. 1974. "Census Enumeration of the Mentally Ill and the Mentally Retarded in the Nineteenth Century." *Health Services Reports* 89:180-87.

Gosney, E. S. and P. Popenoe. 1929. *Sterilization for Human Betterment*. New York: Macmillan.

Gould, S. J. 1981. *The Mismeasure of Man*. New York: Norton.

Gowman, A. G. 1957. *The War Blind in American Social Structure*. New York: American Foundation of the Blind.

Griffin, J. D. and C. Greenland. 1981. "Institutional Care of the Mentally Disordered in Canada: A 17th Century Record." *Canadian Journal of Psychiatry* 26:274-78.

Grimes, J. M. 1964. *Institutional Care of Mental Patients in the United States*. Chicago: Author.

Grob, G. N. 1966. *The State and the Mentally Ill: A History of Worcester State Hospital in Massachusetts, 1830-1920*. Chapel Hill: University of North Carolina Press.

———. 1973. *Mental Institutions in America: Social Policy to 1875*. New York: Free Press.

———. 1983. *Mental Illness and American Society, 1875-1940*. Princeton, NJ: Princeton University Press.

———. 1990. "Marxian Analysis and Mental Illness." *History of Psychiatry* 1:223-32.

———. 1994. *The Mad among Us*. New York: Free Press.

Gussow, Z. 1989. *Leprosy, Racism, and Public Health*. Boulder, CO: Westview.

Hahn, H. 1985. "Disability Policy and the Problem of Discrimination." *American Behavioral Scientist* 28:293-318.

Haines, T. H. 1925. "Mental Defect and Poverty." *Proceedings and Addresses of the American Association for the Study of the Feeble-Minded* 30:136-45.

Haller, B. 1993. "The Little Papers: Newspapers at Nineteenth Century Schools for Deaf Persons." *Journalism History* 19:43-50.

Hamilton, S. W. 1944. *One Hundred Years of American Psychiatry*. New York: Columbia University Press.

Harms, E. 1955. "The Origin and Early History of Electrotherapy and Electroshock." *American Journal of Psychiatry* 111:933-34.

Harris, C. C. 1971. "The Treatment of Mental Deficiency in Colonial Virginia." *Virginia Cavalcade* 17:34-41.

Hayden, M. F. 1997. "Class-Action, Civil Rights Litigation for Institutionalized Persons with Mental Retardation and Other Developmental Disabilities." *Mental and Physical Disability Law Reporter* 21:411-23.

Hayden, M. F. and D. Senese. 1996. *Self-Advocacy Groups: 1996 Directory for North America*. Minneapolis: University of Minnesota.

Health Care Financing Administration. 1998. *Health Care Financing Review Medicare and Medicaid Statistical Supplement*. Baltimore: Author.

Hecht, I. W. D. and F. Hecht. 1973. "Mara and Benomi Buck: Familial Mental Retardation in Colonial Jamestown." *Journal of the History of Medicine and Allied Sciences* 28:171-76.

Hirsch, K. 1995. "Culture and Disability: The Role of Oral History." *Oral History Review* 22:1-27.

Hoakley, Z. P. 1922. "Extra-Institutional Care for the Feeble-Minded." *Journal of Psycho-Asthenics* 27:117-37.

Hodgson, K. W. 1953. *The Deaf and Their Problems*. New York: Philosophical Library.

Hoffman, A. and S. Field. 1995. "Promoting Self-Determination through Effective Curriculum Development." *Intervention in School and Clinic* 30:147-56.

Holstein, M. and T. Cole. 1995. "The Evolution of Long-Term Care in America." Pp. 19-47 in *Long-Term Care Decisions: Ethical and Conceptual Dimensions*, edited by L. B. McCullough and N. L. Wilson. Baltimore: Johns Hopkins University Press.

Howard, J. 1789. *An Account of the Principal Lazarettos in Europe*. London: Warrington.

Howe, S. G. 1848. *Report Made to the Legislature of Massachusetts upon Idiocy*. Boston: Coolidge and Wiley.

———. 1851. "On Training and Educating Idiots: Second Annual Report to the Massachusetts Legislature." *American Journal of Insanity* 8:97-118.

Hughes, S. L. 1986. *Long-Term Care: Options in an Expanding Market*. Homewood, IL: Dow Jones–Irwin.

Humphrey, J. C. 2000. "Researching Disability Politics, or, Some Problems with the Social Model in Practice." *Disability & Society* 15 (1): 63-85.

Hurd, H. M. 1910. *A History of Institutional Care of the Insane in the United States and Canada.* Washington, DC: American Medico-Psychological Association.

Innes, B., A. Enders, T. Seekins, D. J. Merritt, A. Kirshenbaum, and N. Arnold. 2000. "Assessing the Geographic Distribution of Centers for Independent Living across Urban and Rural Areas: Toward a Policy of Universal Access." *Journal of Disability Policy Studies* 10 (2): 207-24.

Itard, J. M. 1802. *The Wild Boy of Aveyron.* Paris: Richard Phillips.

———. 1821a. *Traite des Maladies de l'Oreille et de l'Audition.* Vol. 1: Treatment of Hearing and Speech Infirmities. Paris: Chez Mequignon-Marvis.

———. 1821b. *Traite des Maladies de l'Oreille et de l'Audition,* Vol. 2: Treatment of Hearing and Speech Infirmities. Paris: Chez Mequignon-Marvis.

Jackson, M. 1998. " 'It Begins with the Goose and Ends with the Goose': Medical, Legal, and Lay Understandings of Imbecility in Ingram v. Wyatt, 1824-1832." *Social History of Medicine* 11:361-80.

Jackson, S. W. 1988. Introduction. Pp. ix-xl in W. *Pargeter's Observations on Maniacal Disorders,* edited and with an introduction by S. W. Jackson. London: Routledge Kegan Paul.

Jacobson, J. W., S. N. Burchard, and P. J. Carling. 1992. *Community Living for People with Developmental and Psychiatric Disabilities.* Baltimore: Johns Hopkins University Press.

Janicki, M. and E. Ansello. 2000. "Supports for Community Living: Evaluation of an Aging with Lifelong Disabilities Movement." Pp. 519-37 in *Community Supports for Aging Adults with Lifelong Disabilities,* edited by M. Janicki and E. Ansello. Baltimore: Brookes.

Jankauskas, R. and A. Urbanavicius. 1998. "Diseases in European Historical Populations and Their Effects on Individuals and Society." *Collegium Antropologicum* 22:465-76.

Johnson, A. 1896. "Permanent Custodial Care." *Proceedings of the National Conference of Social Work* 24:207-19.

———. 1899. "The Self-Supporting Imbecile." *Journal of Psycho-Asthenics* 4:91-99.

Jones, L. A. 1987. *Doing Justice: A History of the Association of Retarded Citizens of Washington.* Olympia: The Arc of Washington.

Jørgensen, S. 1982. "Independent Living for Handicapped Persons in Denmark." Pp. 11-29 in *Independent Living: An Overview of Efforts in Five Countries,* edited by D. G. Tate and L. M. Chadderdon. East Lansing: University Center for International Rehabilitation, Michigan State University.

Kanner, L. 1964. *A History of the Care and Study of the Mentally Retarded.* Springfield, IL: Charles C Thomas.

Keith, K. and R. Schalock. 2000. *Cross Cultural Perspectives on Quality of Life.* Washington, DC: American Association on Mental Retardation.

Kennedy, J. F. 1961. "Statement by the President Regarding the Need for a National Plan in Mental Retardation." Pp. 196-201 in *National Action to Combat Mental Retardation,* edited by the President's Panel on Mental Retardation. Washington, DC: Government Printing Office.

Kerlin, I. N. 1877. "The Organization of Establishments for the Idiotic and Imbecile Classes." *Proceedings of the Association of Medical Officers of American Institutions for Idiotic and Feeble-Minded Persons* 3:19-24.

———. 1887. "Moral Imbecility." *Proceedings of the Association of Medical Officers of American Institutions for Idiotic and Feeble-Minded Persons* 12:32-37.

Kevles, D. J. 1985. *In the Name of Eugenics: Genetics and the Uses of Human Heredity.* New York: Knopf.

Kipp, R. S. 1994. "The Evangelical Uses of Leprosy." *Social Science and Medicine* 39:165-78.

Kirchner, C., R. Peterson, and C. Suhr. 1988. "Trends in School Enrollment and Reading Methods among Legally Blind School Children, 1963-1978." Pp. 113-21 in *Data on Blindness and Visual Impairment in the US: A Resource Manual on Social Demographic Characteristics, Education, Employment, and Income, and Service Delivery,* 2d ed., edited by C. Kirchner. New York: American Foundation for the Blind.

Kirkbride, T. [1880] 1973. *On the Construction, Organization, and General Arrangements of Hospitals for the Insane.* Reprint, New York: Arno.

Knight, G. H. 1891. "Colony Care for Adult Idiots." *Proceedings of the National Conference of Social Work* 19:107-8.

———. 1895. "The Feeble-Minded." *Proceedings of the Association of Medical Officers of American Institutions for Idiotic and Feeble-Minded Persons,* pp. 559-63.

Koegel, L. K., R. L. Koegel, and G. Dunlap. 1996. *Positive Behavioral Support: Including People with Difficult Behavior in the Community.* Baltimore: Brookes.

Koestler, F. A. 1976. *The Unseen Minority.* New York: David McKay.

Koven, S. 1994. "Remembering and Dismemberment: Crippled Children, Wounded Soldiers, and the Great War in Great Britain." *American Historical Review* 99:1167-1202.

Kroll, J. 1973. "A Reappraisal of Psychiatry in the Middle Ages." *Archives of General Psychiatry* 29:276-83.

Kuhlmann, F. 1940. "One Hundred Years of Special Care and Training." *American Journal of Mental Deficiency* 45:18-24.

Lakin, K. C. 1979. *Demographic Studies of Residential Facilities for the Mentally Retarded: An Historical Review of Methodologies and Findings.* Minneapolis: University of Minnesota.

Lane, H. 1989. *When the Mind Hears: A History of the Deaf.* New York: Random House.

Lazar, I. and R. B. Darlington. 1982. "Lasting Effects of Early Education." *Monographs of the Society for Research in Child Development* 47 (2-3, Serial No. 195).

Lefley, H. 1996. *Family Caregiving in Mental Illness.* Thousand Oaks, CA: Sage.

Lende, H. 1941. *What of the Blind?* New York: American Foundation for the Blind.

Levy, R. M. and L. S. Rubenstein. 1996. *The Rights of People with Mental Disabilities: The Authoritative ACLU Guide to the Rights of People with Mental Illness and Mental Retardation.* Carbondale: Southern Illinois University.

Linton, S. 1998. *Claiming Disability: Knowledge and Identity.* New York: New York University Press.

Locke, J. 1690. *An Essay Concerning Human Understanding.* London: Basset.

Longhurst, N. A. 1994. *The Self-Advocacy Movement: A Demographic Study and Directory.* Washington, DC: American Association on Mental Retardation.

Lupton, D. 2000. "The Social Construction of the Body." Pp. 250-63 in *The Handbook of Social Studies in Health and Medicine,* edited by G. L. Albrecht, R. Fitzpatrick, and S. C. Scrimshaw. London: Sage.

Lutterman, T., A. Hirad, and B. Poindexter. 1999. *Funding Sources and Expenditures of State Mental Health Agencies: Fiscal Year 1997.* Alexandria, VA: National Association of State Mental Health Program Directors Research Institute.

Lysack, C. and J. Kaufert. 1994. "Comparing the Origins and Ideologies of the Independent Living Movement and Community-Based Rehabilitation." *International Journal of Rehabilitation Research* 17:231-40.

MacAndrew, C. and R. Edgerton. 1964. "The Everyday Life of Institutionalized 'Idiots.' " *Human Organization* 23:312-18.

MacArthur, W. 1953. "Mediaeval 'Leprosy' in the British Isles." *Leprosy Review* 24:10-11.

MacDonald, M. 1981. *Mystical Bedlam: Madness, Anxiety, and Healing in Seventeenth-Century England.* Cambridge, UK: Cambridge University Press.

Mackelprang, R. W. and R. O. Salsgiver. 1996. "People with Disabilities and Social Work: Historical and Contemporary Issues." *Social Work* 41:7-14.

MadNation. 1999. *Movement History of the Consumer/Survivor/Ex-Patient/User Community* [Online]. Available: madnation.org/csxuhistory.htm.

Maher, W. B. and B. Maher. 1982. "The Ship of Fools: Stultifera Navis or Ignis Fatuus?" *American Psychologist* 37:756-61.

Marcus, J. 1999. "A Note on Markan Optics." *New Testament Studies* 45:250-56.

Martin, E. W., R. Martin, and D. L. Terman. 1996. "The Legislative and Litigation History of Special Education." *Special Education for Students with Disabilities* 6:25-38.

Martin, F. 1924. *Artifical Limbs: Appliances for the Disabled.* Studies and Reports, Series E (Disabled Men), No. 5. Liége, Belgium: Georges Thone.

Mastin, J. T. 1916. "The New Colony Plan for the Feeble-Minded." *Journal of Psycho-Asthenics* 21:25-35.

Matson, F. 1990. *Walking Alone and Marching Together: A History of the Organized Blind Movement in the United States, 1940-1990.* Baltimore: National Federation of the Blind.

Matthews, M. A. 1921. "One Hundred Institutionally Trained Male Defectives in the Community under Supervision." *Journal of Psycho-Asthenics* 26:60-70.

Metts, R. L. 2000. *Disability Issues, Trends and Recommendations for the World Bank.* Washington, DC: World Bank.

Miles, M. 2000. "Signing in the Seraglio: Mutes, Dwarfs and Jestures at the Ottoman Court 1500-1700." *Disability & Society* 15 (1): 115-34.

Minski, L. 1957. *Deafness, Mutism, and Mental Deficiency in Children.* New York: Philosophical Library.

Mitchell, D. 2000. *Narrative Prosthesis: Disability and the Dependencies of Discourse.* Ann Arbor: University of Michigan Press.

Mora, G. 1992. "The History of Psychiatry in the United States: Historiographic and Theoretical Considerations." *History of Psychiatry* 3:187-201.

"The Moral Treatment of Insanity." 1847. *American Journal of Insanity* 4:1-15.

Moreno, J. 1999. *Undue Risk: Secret State Experiments on Humans.* New York: Freeman.

Morton, T. G. 1897. *The History of Pennsylvania Hospital 1751-1895*. Philadelphia: Times Printing House.

Nagi, S. Z. 1970. *Disability and Rehabilitation: Legal, Clinical, and Self-Concepts and Measurements*. Columbus: The Ohio State University Press.

National Association of State Mental Health Program Directors Research Institute. 1996. *FY'96 SMHA Profiling System* [Online]. Available: www.nasmhpd.org/nri/CLI_T1.htm.

National Council on Disability. 1997. *Equality of Opportunity: The Making of the Americans with Disabilities Act*. Washington, DC: Author.

Navon, L. 1998. "Beggars, Metaphors, and Stigma: A Missing Link in the Social History of Leprosy." *Social History of Medicine* 11:89-105.

Neaman, J. 1978. *Suggestion of the Devil: Insanity in the Middle Ages and the Twentieth Century*. New York: Octagon.

Neugebauer, R. 1978. "Treatment of the Mentally Ill in Medieval and Early Modern England: A Reappraisal." *Journal of the History of the Behavioral Sciences* 14:158-69.

———. 1979. "Medieval and Early Modern Theories of Mental Illness." *Archives of General Psychiatry* 36:477-83.

———. 1987. "Exploitation of the Insane in the New World: Benoni Buck, the First Reported Case of Mental Retardation in the American Colonies." *Archives of General Psychiatry* 44:481-83.

———. 1996. "Mental Handicap in Medieval and Early Modern England: Criteria, Measurement and Care." Pp. 22-43 in *From Idiocy to Mental Deficiency: Historical Perspectives on People with Learning Disabilities*, edited by D. Wright and A. Digby. London: Routledge Kegan Paul.

Nirje, B. 1976. "The Normalization Principle and Its Human Management Implications." Pp. 231-40 in *Changing Patterns in Residential Services for the Mentally Retarded*, edited by R. B. Kugel and A. Shearer. Washington, DC: President's Committee on Mental Retardation.

Noll, S. 1996. *The Feeble-Minded in Our Midst: Institutions for the Mentally Retarded in the South, 1900-1940*. Chapel Hill: University of North Carolina Press.

Obermann, C. E. 1968. *A History of Vocational Rehabilitation in America*. 5th ed. Minneapolis, MN: Dennison.

Office of Management and Budget. 1999. *Budget of the United States Government, Fiscal Year 1999: Budget Information for States*. Washington, DC: Government Printing Office.

Oliver, M. 1983. *Social Work with Disabled People*. Basingstoke, UK: Macmillan.

———. 1990. *The Politics of Disablement*. Basingstoke, UK: Macmillan.

———. 1992. "Changing the Social Relations of Research Production." *Disability, Handicap & Society* 7 (2): 101-14.

Oliver, M. and C. Barnes. 1999. *Disabled People and Social Policy: From Exclusion to Inclusion*. London: Longman.

Packard, E. P. W. 1868. *The Prisoner's Hidden Life, or, Insane Asylums Unveiled: As Demonstrated by the Report of the Investigating Committee of the Legislature of Illinois*. Chicago: J. N. Clarke.

Pargeter, W. [1792] 1988. *Observations on Maniacal Disorders*. Reprint, London: Routledge Kegan Paul.

Park, E. and L. Daston. 1981. "Unnatural Conceptions: The Study of Monsters in Sixteenth and Seventeenth-Century France and England." *Past and Present* 92:20-54.

Parry, J. 1995. *Mental Disability Law: A Primer*. 5th ed. Washington, DC: American Bar Association.

Parry-Jones, W. L. 1972. *The Trade in Lunacy: A Study of Private Madhouses in England in the Eighteenth and Nineteenth Centuries*. London: Routledge Kegan Paul.

Pennsylvania Ass'n., Retarded Child. v. Commonwealth of PA, 334 F.Supp. 1257 (1971).

Percy, S. 1989. *Disability, Civil Rights, and Public Policy: The Politics of Implementation*. Tuscaloosa: University of Alabama Press.

Pernick, M. S. 1996. *The Black Stork: Eugenics and the Death of "Defective" Babies in American Medicine and Motion Pictures since 1915*. New York: Oxford University Press.

Peterson, D. 1982. *A Mad People's History of Madness*. Pittsburgh, PA: University of Pittsburgh Press.

Pinel, P. [1801] 1977. *Treatise on Insanity*. Translated by H. Maudsley. Reprint, Washington, DC: University Publications of America.

———. 1809. *Traité médico-philosophique sur l'aliénation mentale* (Medical-Philosophical Treatise of Mental Illness). 2d ed. Paris: J. A. Brosson.

Plann, S. 1997. *A Silent Minority: Deaf Education in Spain, 1550-1835*. Berkeley: University of California Press.

Pollock, H. M. 1945. "A Brief History of Family Care of Mental Patients in America." *American Journal of Psychiatry* 102:351-61.

Popenoe, P. 1927. "Success on Parole after Sterilization." *Proceedings and Addresses of the American Association for the Study of Feeblemindedness* 32:86-109.

Porter, R. 1987a. *Mind Forg'd Manacles: A History of Madness in England from the Restoration to the Regency.* London: Athlone.

———. 1987b. *A Social History of Madness: The World through the Eyes of the Insane.* New York: Weidenfeld and Nicolson.

Porter, S. 1894. "The Suppression of Signs by Force." *American Annals of the Deaf* 39:169-78.

Quartararo, A. T. 1995. "The Perils of Assimilation in Modern France: The Deaf Community, Social Status, and Educational Opportunity, 1815-1870." *Journal of Social History* 29:5-23.

Radford, J. P. 1994. "Eugenics and the Asylum." *Journal of Historical Sociology* 7:462-73.

Rafter, N. H. 1988. *White Trash: The Eugenic Family Studies, 1877-1919.* Boston: Northeastern University Press.

Ramirez-Moreno, S. 1937. "History of Psychiatry and Mental Hospitals in Mexico." *Journal of Nervous and Mental Disease* 86 (5): 513-24.

———. 1942. "History of the First Psychopathic Institution on the American Continent." *American Journal of Psychiatry* 99 (2): 194-95.

Ramsey, G. V. 1952. "A Short History of Psychosurgery." *American Journal of Psychiatry* 108:813-16.

Reilly, P. R. 1991. *The Surgical Solution: A History of Involuntary Sterilization in the United States.* Baltimore: Johns Hopkins University Press.

Roberts, E. V. 1989. "A History of the Independent Living Movement: A Founder's Perspective." Pp. 231-44 in *Psychosocial Interventions with Physically Disabled Persons,* edited by B. W. Heller, L. M. Flohr, and L. S. Zegans. New Brunswick, NJ: Rutgers University Press.

Roberts, F. K. 1986. "Education of the Visually Handicapped: A Social and Educational History." Pp. 1-18 in *Foundations of Education for Blind and Visually Handicapped Children and Youth: Theory and Practice,* edited by G. T. Scholl. New York City: American Foundation for the Blind.

Roberts, J. A. F. 1952. "The Genetics of Mental Deficiency." *Eugenics Review* 44:71-83.

Rochefort, D. A. 1981. "Three Centuries of Care of the Mentally Disabled in Rhode Island and the Nation, 1650-1950." *Rhode Island History* 40:111-32.

Rockey, D. 1980. *Speech Disorder in Nineteenth Century Britain.* London: Croom Helm.

Roosens, E. 1979. *Mental Patients in Town Life: Gheel-Europe's First Therapeutic Community.* Beverly Hills, CA: Sage.

Rosen, G. 1968. *Madness in Society: Chapters in the Historical Sociology of Mental Illness.* Chicago: University of Chicago Press.

Rosenfeld, S. 1997. "Deaf Men on Trial: Language and Deviancy in Late Eighteenth-Century France." *Eighteenth Century Life* 21:157-75.

Rothfels, N. 1996. "Aztecs, Aborigines, and Ape-People: Science and Freaks in Germany, 1850-1900." Pp. 158-72 in *Freakery: Cultural Spectacles of the Extraordinary Body,* edited by R. G. Thomson. New York: New York University Press.

Rothman, D. J. 1990. *The Discovery of the Asylum: Social Order and Disorder in the New Republic.* Rev. ed. Boston: Little, Brown.

Rothman, D. J. and S. M. Rothman. 1984. *The Willowbrook Wars.* New York: Harper & Row.

Rouse v. Cameron, 373 F.2d 451, 452 (D.C. Cir. 1966).

Rousseau, J.-J. [1762] 1991. *The Social Contract.* Reprint, Norwalk, CT: Easton.

Rumbaut, R. D. 1972. "The First Psychiatric Hospital of the Western World." *American Journal of Psychiatry* 128 (10): 1305-9.

Rush, B. 1812. *Medical Inquiries and Observations, upon the Diseases of the Mind.* Philadelphia: Kimber & Richardson.

Rushton, P. 1988. "Lunatics and Idiots: Mental Disability, the Community, and the Poor Law in North-East England, 1600-1800." *Medical History* 32:34-50.

———. 1996. "Idiocy, the Family, and the Community in Early Modern Northeast England." Pp. 44-64 in *From Idiocy to Mental Deficiency: Historical Perspectives on People with Learning Disabilities,* edited by D. Wright and A. Digby. London: Routledge Kegan Paul.

Russell, J. B. 1972. *Witchcraft in the Middle Ages.* Ithaca, NY: Cornell University Press.

———. 1980. *A History of Witchcraft: Sorcerers, Heretics, and Pagans.* New York: Thames and Hudson.

Sacks, O. 1989. *Seeing Voices: A Journey into the World of the Deaf.* Berkeley: University of California Press.

Sarason, S. B. and T. Gladwin. 1958. "Psychological and Cultural Problems in Mental Subnormality, Part II." Pp. 145-392 in *Mental Subnormality: Biological, Psychological, and Cultural Factors,* edited by R. L. Masland, S. B. Sarason, and T. Gladwin. New York: Basic Books.

Schafer, R. J. 1980. *A Guide to Historical Method*. 3d ed. Chicago: Dorsey.

Scheerenberger, R. C. 1983. *A History of Mental Retardation*. Baltimore: Brookes.

Scotch, R. K. 1984. *From Goodwill to Civil Rights: Transforming Federal Disability Policy*. Philadelphia: Temple University Press.

Scotch, R. K. 1989. "Politics and Policy in the History of the Disability Rights Movement." *The Milbank Quarterly* 67 (Suppl. 2, Pt. 2): 380-400.

Scotch, R. K. and E. Berkowitz. 1990. "One Comprehensive System? A Historical Perspective on Federal Disability Policy." *Journal of Disability Policy Studies* 1:1-19.

Scott, R. 1968. *The Making of Blind Men: A Study of Adult Socialization*. New Brunswick, NJ: Transaction.

Scull, A. 1979. *Museums of Madness: The Social Organization of Insanity in Nineteenth Century England*. London: Allen Lane.

———. 1991. "Psychiatry and Social Control in the Nineteenth and Twentieth Centuries." *History of Psychiatry* 2:149-69.

Seguin, E. 1846. *Traitement Moral Hygiene et Education des Idiots et des Autres Enfants Erroires* (The Moral Treatment and Education of Idiots and Other Handicapped Children). Paris: Bailliere.

———. 1870. *New Facts and Remarks Concerning Idiocy, Being a Lecture before the New York Medical Journal Association, October 15, 1869*. New York: William Wood.

Semi-Deaf Lady. 1908. "The Sign Language and the Human Right to Expression." *American Annals of the Deaf* 53:141-48.

Semonin, P. 1996. "Monsters in the Marketplace: The Exhibition of Human Oddities in Early Modern England." Pp. 69-81 in *Freakery: Cultural Spectacles of the Extraordinary Body*, edited by R. G. Thomson. New York: New York University Press.

Shapiro, J. P. 1993. *No Pity: People with Disabilities Forging New Civil Rights Movement*. New York: Times Books.

Sheldon, E. W. 1921. "Historical Review." Pp. 7-16 in *A Psychiatric Milestone: Bloomingdale Hospital Centenary: 1821-1921*, edited by H. Townsend, B. Winthrop, and R. H. Gallatin. New York: Society of the New York Hospital.

Silverstein, R. 2000. *Disability Policy Framework: A Guidepost for Analyzing Public Policy*. Washington, DC: Center for the Study and Advancement of Disability Policy and the Arc of the United States.

Simpson, M. K. 1999. "The Moral Government of Idiots: Moral Treatment in the Work of Seguin." *History of Psychiatry* 10:227-43.

Skeels, H. M. and I. Harms. 1948. "Children with Inferior Social Histories: Their Mental Development in Adoptive Homes." *Journal of Genetic Psychology* 72:283-94.

Skeels, H. M., R. Updegraff, B. L. Wellman, and H. M. Williams. 1938. "A Study of Environmental Stimulation, an Orphanage Preschool Project." *University of Iowa Studies in Child Welfare* 15 (4).

"A Sketch of the History, Buildings, and Organization of the Pennsylvania Hospital for the Insane, Extracted Principally from the Reports of Thomas S. Kirkbride, M.D., Physician to the Institution." 1845. *American Journal of Insanity* 2:97-114.

Sloan, W. and H. A. Stevens. 1976. *A Century of Concern: A History of the American Association on Mental Deficiency, 1876-1976*. Washington, DC: American Association on Mental Deficiency.

Smith, S., M. W. Wilkinson, and L. C. Wagoner. 1914. "A Summary of the Laws of the Several States Governing: I. Marriage and Divorce of the Feeble-Minded, the Epileptic, and the Insane. II. Asexualization. III. Institutional Commitment and Discharge of the Feeble-Minded and Epileptic." In *Bulletin of the University of Washington*. Seattle, WA: Bailey and Babette Gatzert Foundation for Child Welfare.

Social Security Administration. 1998. *Annual Statistical Supplement*. Washington, DC: Author.

Social Security Board. 1946. *Recommendations of the Children's Bureau Advisory Committee On Services to Crippled Children: December 1935 to April 1946*. Washington, DC: Department of Health and Human Services Archives.

Solecki, R. 1971. *Shanidar: The First Flower People*. New York: Knopf.

Speer, G. S. 1940. "The Intelligence of Foster Children." *Journal of Genetic Psychology* 57:49-55.

Spierenburg, P. 1984. "The Sociogenesis of Confinement and Its Development in Early Modern Europe." Pp. 9-77 in *The Emergence of Carceral Institutions: Prisons, Galleys and Lunatic Asylums, 1550-1900*, edited by P. Spierenburg. Rotterdam: Erasmus Universiteit, Centrum voor Maatschappij Geschiedenenis.

"Statistics of Speech Training in American Schools." 1920. *Volta Review* 22:361-75.

Stevens, H. 1858. "Insane Colony of Gheel." *The Asylum Journal of Mental Science* 4:426-36.

Stewart, J., J. Harris, and B. Sapey. 1999. "Disability and Dependency: Origins and Futures of 'Special Needs' Housing for Disabled People." *Disability and Society* 14:5-20.

Stewart, J. Q. A. 1882. "The Industrial Department of the Kentucky Institution for the Education and Training of Feeble-Minded Children." *Proceedings of the Association of Medical Officers of American Institutions for Idiotic and Feeble-minded Persons,* pp. 236-39.

Stewart, T. D. 1958. "Report of Committee on Research: Anthropology." *Yearbook of the American Philosophical Society,* pp. 274-78.

Stiker, H. 1997. *A History of Disability.* Translated by W. Sayers. Ann Arbor: University of Michigan Press.

Straus, W. L. and A. J. E. Cave. 1957. "Pathology and the Posture of Neanderthal Man." *Quarterly Review of Biology* 32:348-63.

Strype, J. 1720. "Description of Bethlem Hospital Commonly Called Bedlam." Pp. 192-97 in *Three Hundred Years of Psychiatry 1535-1860: A History Presented in Selected English Texts,* edited by R. Hunter and I. Macalpine. Hartsdale, NY: Carlisle.

Survey and Research Corporation. 1965. *Mental Retardation Program Statistics of US—Report to the Department of Health, Education and Welfare Pursuant to Contract PH-86-64-99.* Washington, DC: U.S. Department of Health, Education and Welfare.

Suzuki, A. 1991. "Lunacy in Seventeenth- and Eighteenth-Century England: Analysis of Quarter Sessions Records. Part I." *History of Psychiatry* 2:437-56.

———. 1998. "The Household and the Care of Lunatics in Eighteenth-Century London." Pp. 153-75 in *The Locus of Care: Families, Communities, Institutions, and the Provision of Welfare since Antiquity,* edited by P. Horden and R. Smith. London: Routledge Kegan Paul.

Swain, B. 1932. *Fools and Folly during the Middle Ages and the Renaissance.* New York: Columbia University Press.

Swayze, V. W. 1995. "Frontal Leukotomy and Related Psychosurgical Procedures in the Era before Antipsychotics (1935-1954): A Historical Overview." *American Journal of Psychiatry* 152:505-15.

Swinburne, H. 1590. *A Brief Treatise of Testaments and Last Willes.* London: John Windet.

Switzky, H. N., M. Dudzinski, R. Van Acker, and J. Gambro. 1988. "Historical Foundations of Out-of-Home Residential Alternatives for Mentally Retarded Persons." Pp. 19-25 in *Integration of Developmentally Disabled Individuals into the Community,* 2d ed., edited by L. W. Heal, J. I. Haney, and A. R. Novak Amado. Baltimore: Brookes.

Symonds, B. 1995. "The Origins of Insane Asylums in England during the 19th Century: A Brief Sociological Review." *Journal of Advanced Nursing* 22:94-100.

Szasz, T. 1970. *The Manufacture of Madness: A Comparative Study of the Inquisition and the Mental Health Movement.* Syracuse, NY: Syracuse University Press.

———. 1973. *The Age of Madness: The History of Involuntary Mental Hospitalization.* New York: Jason Aronson.

Talbot, M. 1967. "Edouard Seguin." *American Journal on Mental Deficiency* 72:184-89.

Thiher, A. 1999. *Revels in Madness: Insanity in Medicine and Literature.* Ann Arbor: University of Michigan Press.

Thompson, T. and J. Grabowski, eds. 1977. *Behavior Modification of the Mentally Retarded.* 2d ed. New York: Oxford University Press.

Thomson, R. G. 1996. *Freakery: Cultural Spectacles of the Extraordinary Body.* New York: New York University Press.

———. 1997. *Extraordinary Bodies: Figuring Physical Disability in American Culture and Literature.* New York: Columbia University Press.

Trent, J. W. 1995. *Inventing the Feeble Mind: A History of Mental Retardation in the United States.* Berkeley: University of California Press.

Trombley, S. 1988. *The Right to Reproduce: A History of Coercive Sterilization.* London: Winfield and Nicolson.

Tuke, D. H. 1878. *Insanity in Ancient and Modern Life.* London: Macmillan.

———. [1882] 1968. *Chapters in the History of the Insane in the British Isles.* Reprint, Amsterdam: E. J. Bonset.

Tuke, S. 1815. *A Letter on Pauper Lunatic Asylums.* New York: Samuel Wood.

Tyor, P. L. 1972. "Segregation or Surgery: The Mentally Retarded in America, 1850-1920." Ph.D. dissertation, Northwestern University, Chicago.

Tyor, P. L. and L. V. Bell. 1984. *Caring for the Retarded in America: A History.* Westport, CT: Greenwood.

United Nations. 1971. *On the Declaration on the Rights of Mentally Retarded Persons.* General Assembly Resolution 2856 (XXVI). New York: Author.

————. 1975. *On the Declaration on the Rights of Disabled Persons.* General Assembly Resolution 3447 (XXX). New York: Author.

————. 1982. *World Programme of Action Concerning Disabled Persons.* New York: Author.

————. 1994. *Standard Rules on the Equalization of Opportunities for Persons with Disabilities.* New York: Author.

U.S. Bureau of the Census. 1914. *Insane and Feeble-Minded in Institutions, 1910.* Washington, DC: Author.

————. 1939. *Patients in Mental Institutions.* Washington, DC: Author.

————. 1940. *Patients in Mental Institutions.* Washington, DC: Author.

————. 1997. *International Data Base.* Washington, DC: Bureau of the Census, International Programs Center, Information Resources Branch.

U.S. Department of Agriculture. 1998. *Reaching Those in Need: How Effective Is the Food Stamp Program?* Washington, DC: Author.

U.S. Department of Education. 1992. *Fourteenth Annual Report to Congress on the Implementation of the Individuals with Disabilities Education Act.* Washington, DC: Author.

————. 1998. *Twentieth Annual Report to Congress on the Implementation of the Individuals with Disabilities Education Act.* Washington, DC: Author.

U.S. Department of Health, Education, and Welfare. 1972. *Mental Retardation Sourcebook of the DHEW.* Washington, DC: U.S. Department of Health, Education, and Welfare, Office of the Secretary, Office of Mental Retardation Coordination.

U.S. Department of Housing and Urban Development. 2000. *A Picture of Subsidized Households in 1997: US Summaries.* Washington, DC: Author.

U.S. Holocaust Memorial Museum. n.d. *The Mentally and Physically Handicapped Victims of the Nazi Era.* Washington, DC: Author.

Valenstein, E. S. 1986. *Great and Desperate Cures: The Rise and Decline of Psychosurgery and Other Radical Treatments for Mental Illness.* New York: Basic Books.

Vaux, C. L. 1935. "Family Care of Mental Defectives." *Journal of Psycho-Asthenics* 40:168-89.

"A Visit to the Bicêtre, First Article." 1847a. *Chambers's Edinburgh Journal* 7 (158): 20-22.

"A Visit to the Bicêtre, Second Article." 1847b. *Chambers's Edinburgh Journal* 7 (161): 71-73.

"A Visit to the Bicêtre, Third Article." 1847c. *Chambers's Edinburgh Journal* 7 (163): 105-7.

Walker, T. 1950. *Rise Up and Walk.* New York: Dutton.

Wallace, G. L. 1929. "Are the Feebleminded Criminals?" *Mental Hygiene* 13:93-98.

Ward, M. J. 1946. *The Snake Pit.* New York: Random House.

Ward, N. and B. Schoultz. 1996. "People First of Nebraska: Eight Years of Accomplishment." Pp. 216-36 in *New Voices: Self-Advocacy by People with Disabilities,* edited by G. Dybwad and H. Bersani. Cambridge, MA: Brookline.

Warkany, J. 1959. "Congenital Malformations in the Past." *Journal of Chronic Disabilities* 10:84-96.

Watkins, H. M. 1930. "Selective Sterilization." *Proceedings and Addresses of the American Association for the Study of the Feeble-Minded* 35:51-67.

Welsford, E. [1935] 1966. *The Fool: His Social and Literary History.* Reprint, Gloucester, MA: Peter Smith.

Weymouth, A. 1938. *Through the Leper-Squint: A Study of Leprosy from Pre-Christian Times to the Present Day.* London: Selwyn and Blount.

Whitney, E. A. 1949. "The Historical Approach to the Subject of Mental Retardation." *American Journal of Mental Deficiency* 53:419-24.

Wilbur, C. T. 1888. "Institutions for the Feebleminded." *Proceedings of the Fifteenth National Conference of Charities and Correction* 17:106-13.

Willeford, W. 1969. *The Fool and His Sceptre: A Study in Clowns and Jesters and Their Audience.* London: Edward Arnold.

Winship, M. P. 1994. "Prodigies, Puritanism, and the Perils of Natural Philosophy: The Example of Cotton Mather." *The William and Mary Quarterly* 51:92-105.

Winspear, C. W. 1895. "The Protection and Training of Feeble-Minded Women." *Proceedings of the Association of Medical Officers of American Institutions for Idiotic and Feeble-Minded Persons* 20:160-63.

Winzer, M. A. 1986. "Early Developments in Special Education: Some Aspects of Enlightenment Thought." *Remedial and Special Education (RASE)* 7:42-49.

————. 1993. *The History of Special Education: From Isolation to Integration.* Washington, DC: Gallaudet University Press.

"Witchcraft and Insanity." 1849. *American Journal of Insanity* 5:246-61.

Wolfensberger, W. 1972. *The Principle of Normalization in Human Services*. Toronto, Ontario: National Institute on Mental Retardation.

———. 1976. "On the Origin of Our Institutional Models." Pp. 35-82 in *Changing Patterns in Residential Services for the Mentally Retarded*, rev. ed., edited by R. Kugel and A. Shearer. Washington, DC: President's Committee on Mental Retardation.

———. 1981. "The Extermination of Handicapped People in World War II Germany." *Mental Retardation* 19:1-7.

Wood, G. B. 1853. "History of the Pennsylvania Hospital for the Insane." *American Journal of Insanity* 9:209-13.

Woodill, G. and D. Velche. 1995. "From Charity and Exclusion to Emerging Independence: An Introduction to the History of Disabilities." *Journal on Developmental Disabilities* 4:1-11.

Woodside, M. 1950. *Sterilization in North Carolina: A Sociological and Psychological Study*. Chapel Hill: University of North Carolina Press.

Woodward, S. 1845. *Annual Report of the Worcester State Hospital*. Worcester, MA: Worcester State Hospital.

Woolfson, R. C. 1984. "Historical Perspective on Mental Retardation." *American Journal of Mental Deficiency* 89:231-35.

World Health Organization. 1980. *International Classification of Impairments, Disabilities, and Handicaps*. Geneva, Switzerland: Author.

Wright, D. 1969. *Deafness*. New York: Stein and Day.

Wright, D. and A. Digby. 1996. *From Idiocy to Mental Deficiency: Historical Perspectives on People with Learning Disabilities*. London: Routledge Kegan Paul.

Wright, H. 1920. *Survey of Cripples in New York City*. New York: New York Committee on After Care of Infantile Paralysis.

Wright, L. and A. M. Hamburger. 1918. *Education and Occupation of Cripples Juvenile and Adult: A Survey of All the Cripples of Cleveland, Ohio in 1916*. New York: Red Cross Institute for Crippled and Disabled Men.

Wyatt v. Stickney, 325 F. Supp. 781 (M.D. Ala. 1971), enforced in 334 F. Supp. 1341 (1971); 344 F. Supp. 387 (1972); Wyatt v. Aderholt, 503 F. 2d. 1305 (5th Cir. 1974).

Zola, I. K. 1979. "Helping One Another: Speculative History of the Self-Help Movement." *Archives of Physical Medicine* 60 (10): 452-56.

Counting Disability

2

GLENN T. FUJIURA
VIOLET RUTKOWSKI-KMITTA

OVERVIEW

We are driven to classify and count the human condition. From the Hippocratic division of the Four Humors through contemporary efforts to catalog variations in genome sequences, people (or, more precisely, the society of men and women) have sought to systematize the measurement and subdivision of their own. Such has been the case with disablement.

As we will see in the following sections, disability statistics encompass an enormous range of concepts, method of definition, systems of surveillance, and, indeed, humanity. Those people identified under different approaches are best viewed as overlapping populations, with considerable but not total communality. A central theme of this chapter is that discrepancies among approaches underscore the fluidity of the disability concept and the vagaries of classifying human variability into simple dichotomies. The act of classification and counting is far from a simple matter, often subject to methodological bias and the distortion of the cultural lens. Disability identification is a judgment on the human condition, and its statistical summary represents more than a simple enumeration of those who are disabled and those who are not.

Herein lies the challenge in understanding the numbers—disability is a contested concept, and a critical evaluation of disability data must assume multiple personas. At its most fundamental level, our narrative explores the meaning of classification and numerical representation. Against this backdrop, we overview the basic contemporary conceptual frameworks employed in international surveillance systems and address the basics of disability demographics—population size, the character of international surveillance, and how estimates are profoundly affected by variations in the conception of disability. Finally, and perhaps most important to the intent of this chapter, we reflect on the relationship of a disability studies perspective and statistics on disability. The former is anchored in the relativism of context; the latter favors quantitative certainties in intent if not execution. This chapter challenges the viability or utility of a universally applicable or singular definition of disability. While we do not deny the importance of the details and "rules" of disability measurement, we assert that there are larger messages in the numbers than the numbers themselves.

THE MEASUREMENT OF DISABILITY

I do not plead guilty to taking a shallow view of human nature, when I propose to apply, as it were, a foot-rule to its heights and depths. The powers of man are finite, and if finite they are not too large for measurement. (Galton 1884:4)

British scholar Galton was an early proponent of the statistical analysis of persons and of human nature. While the less metaphysically inclined among us may agree with Galton that the range of the human is "finite," in matters of assessment, we have argued endlessly about the boundaries and dimensions of human measurement. In this vast arena of contention lies considerable ambiguity regarding the meaning of disability and thus its measurement.

Current Approaches

Disability data are typically constructed from assessments of physical or mental anomalies within a population or limitations in the "capacity to perform" or "loss of function"—concepts common to everyday experience. When operationalized, however, layers of nuance are revealed. What if a physical anomaly—sinusitis, for example—has limited impact on basic daily activities? At what threshold of limited capacity or functional loss does one cross and join the ranks of the disabled? Are thresholds and criteria absolute or relative? Which skills or functions should be emphasized in the criteria? Is it just the individual assessed, or do we accommodate the environment in the definition? Or should the environment be the principle unit of analysis? We could go on. These and other related issues reflect the major conceptual definitional frameworks and associated debates in disability statistics. Each are briefly reviewed in the following sections with an emphasis on the meaning and utility of disability data.

Why Measure Disability?

The word *statistics* has its Germanic and Latin roots in the notions of the state and status and political study. It is in the fundamental self-interest of nations to quantify the contours of its population. Although there are notable exceptions, the organized political state exists to promote the well-being of its people. Data inform this process and help inform the planning and organization of state policy. Thus, the surveillance of health status is both an ancient practice and nearly universal among nation-states. More often than not, disability statistics are the by-products of surveillance efforts devoted to a broader public health agenda. The imperative to measure and count disability internationally in large part may reflect the traditional association of disability to disease and illness. In the *World Health Statistics Annual 1990*, for example, disablement is characterized as "a major burden of ill-health in populations" (World Health Organization [WHO] 1990:39).

What is it exactly that we do with the numbers? In 1662, John Graunt published the *Observations upon the Bills of Mortality*, an actuarial effort using the weekly bulletins on plague deaths in the parishes of London (Clark 1972). His analyses led to observations of the impact of migration, poverty, and literacy on health and mortality. Colleagues extended the work of Graunt into what has been termed the *political arithmetic* of demography (Clark 1972:16). The work of these political arithmeticians was reform (Wright 1988). Indeed, Oberschall (1972) notes that the demand for extensive and detailed information by "social reformers, civic groups, and philanthropists" was the foundation of much statistical work in the nineteenth century (p. 6). Contemporary discussions of population statistics suggest that not much has changed in the intervening three centuries. Although applications of demography and popula-

Table 2.1   Published Intent for Disability Surveillance Systems

Surveillance System	Nation	Stated Purpose for Disability Screen
1991 Census	Aruba	To collect systemic information on disability and the social position of disabled persons in Aruba
Central Registry for Rehabilitation	Hong Kong	To facilitate provision of services and to assist in their reaching out to people with a disability[a]
Disability Statistics Database	United Nations	To increase awareness among governments, organizations, and the research community of the limitations and strengths of disability data[b]
Health and Activity Limitation Survey	Canada	To provide information on the living conditions of Canada's disabled population[c]
National Health Interview Survey	United States	To provide information on the distribution of illness and effects in terms of disability and chronic impairments[d]
National Intellectual Disability Database	Ireland	To provide information for decision making in relation to the planning, funding, and management of services[e]
Survey of Disability, Ageing, and Carers	Australia	To provide some indicators of needs for medical, rehabilitation, and welfare services[f]
Survey of Income and Program Participation	United States	To improve measurement of economic status and help manage and evaluate government programs[g]

a. Health and Welfare Bureau (1995).
b. United Nations (1988).
c. Hamilton (1998).
d. National Center for Health Statistics (1992).
e. Health Research Board (1997).
f. Australian Bureau of Health and Welfare (1998).
g. U.S. Bureau of the Census (1991).

tion statistics span many scientific disciplines, the connection to reform as a fundamental purpose remains close to the surface. In a recent debate regarding the proper role of statistical surveillance and epidemiology, Schwartz and Carpenter (1999) argued for research questions that explicitly focus on differences between populations. Through the analysis of group differences (rather than interindividual variations), epidemiologists can directly address social- and cultural-level effects.

These themes of data as a means to inform and reform service are very much infused into contemporary disability surveillance. Table 2.1 lists selected national surveillance systems that incorporate explicit disability screens. The ascribed purpose of the disability screen is listed next to the instrument.

While the mechanics of the systems are very much predicated on traditional public health and medical conceptions of monitoring health outcomes or the distribution of "disease" and impairment, fundamental importance is attached to social and civic participation. There is an underlying social and political dimension to the "science" of measuring disability.

An Overview of the Major Disability Perspectives

A comprehensive critique of the conceptual bases for defining disability is dealt with elsewhere in this volume and will not be addressed in great depth here. Nonetheless, a discussion of disability statistics requires at least a cursory review of disability concepts and their derivative classification schemes. We will anchor our discussion in subsequent sections to the key surveillance systems used to count disability and their conceptual frameworks. Underscored in our overview are the vagaries in the methods of definition and the illusory character of the disability concept as an entity of known and fixed dimensions.

For all the extraordinary technical sophistication required of population-level surveillance, the basic logic of disability data collection is relatively straightforward. A respondent is asked if a specific condition is present, if specific activities can be performed, or if there is a departure from "normal" functions, routines, and rhythms of life. Within this apparently simple procedure, there is extraordinary variability across both surveillance systems and national borders. These variations represent different concepts of what constitutes a disability definition and read like a mysterious language of acronyms: ADLs, DALYs, DFLEs, IADLs, LLIs, and YLDs, among others. At great risk of oversimplification, the central differences across perspectives can be reduced to three variations in emphasis between systems: (1) illness or impairment-based schemes, (2) limited function or restricted life activity schemes, and (3) ecological perspectives that focus on the interaction of person characteristics with the physical and social environment. These are the three pillars on which contemporary disability definitions, in various permutations, are built.

The former is exemplified in what is routinely referred to as the *medical model,* which has long formed the basis of disability identification in education, social welfare, and rehabilitation. Application within statistical systems very much parallels international systems for coding and classifying diseases and injuries (i.e., the International Statistical Classification of Diseases and Related Health Problems). The central feature of an illness- and impairment-based definition is the emphasis on the individual and focus on organ malfunction, anatomical loss, or other physical stigmata. The disability screening questions for the National Morbidity Survey of Bahrain ask, "Do you have any handicapped person(s) in your household? If the answer is yes, then state whether he (she) is blind, deaf, deaf and mute, amputee, paralyzed or mentally handicapped" (Al-Ansari 1989:22). Impairment-based systems are prominently featured in nonmedically oriented systems. Special education service data in the United States are summarized according to eight impairment categories: visual, hearing, speech or language, learning, orthopedic, mental health, autism, and traumatic brain injury. The presumption in this surveillance perspective is that the characteristics of the person are fundamentally important to the purposes of the surveillance; superseded are the consequences of the condition. Implicit in such systems is the identification of deviations from the norm—that is, "defects in the population," a common feature of older statistical efforts. In his introductory remarks to a U.S. census disability statistics report, Special Agent Frederick Howard-Wines (1888) noted,

> The insane, the idiots, the blind, and the deaf are known in the census by the title of defectives, or the defective classes . . . their claim to the protecting care of the government is, therefore, based upon a physical or mental defect. (P. viii)

The second conceptual pillar for disability definition is represented in the *functional limitation model* of disablement proposed by sociologist Saad Nagi (1976). Variously referred to as the Nagi model or functional-limitations approach, the process of disablement was linear, moving from pathology to impairment at the organ systems level, which in turn could result in functional loss. If this decrement in performance or capacity restricts the individual in performing a socially defined role, then disability is present (see Chapter 3, this volume). The significance of Nagi's approach is that it extended disability definition beyond the physical status or mental state of the individual—"an inability or limitation in performing roles and tasks expected within a social environment" (Nagi 1991:315). As we will see in the summary of national surveillance systems, the influence of a functional-limitations perspective resonates throughout contemporary surveillance systems.

The third major conceptual thread in contemporary disability surveillance is represented by the efforts of the WHO in the *International Classification of Impairments, Disabilities, and Handicaps (ICIDH)* (WHO 1980) and its revision, the *ICIDH-2* (WHO 1999). The *ICIDH* was an effort to standardize disability conceptualizations internationally and improve the precision of data collection. A conceptual cousin to the Nagi model, the disablement process in the original *ICIDH* is a similar four-stage sequence of disorder-impairment-activity limitation (referred to as "disability" in the *ICIDH*) and then "handicap," if the limitations put the individual at a disadvantage relative to others. Disadvantage was defined in terms of performing basic *life roles*—orientation, physical independence, mobility, occupation, social integration, or economic self-sufficiency. The concept of *disadvantage* is important here because it incorporates comparisons that are relative rather than absolute, invoking environmental context as well as lack of individual capacity. Nagi (1976) posited disadvantage primarily in the person's impairment. This is a subtle but important distinction between the two approaches.

Yet, the *ICIDH* continued to posit disability primarily in the individual's impairment. As critiqued by Bickenbach et al. (1999), the ambiguity of the language suggested the importance of the linear relationship of impairment to handicap. Though disadvantage was anchored in social context, it occurs *because* of impairment and disability. Largely in response to these and related criticisms, the WHO initiated development of the *ICIDH-2* in 1993. In the *ICIDH-2* revision, there are three components of disablement—impairments, activity limitations, and participation restrictions. Each of these represents *simultaneous dimensions of disablement* rather than different stages on the path to disability status. As in the original handicap concept, participation is anchored in the social context. However, the participation construct is far more expansive and sensitive to specific contextual factors than the six core "survival roles" of handicap in the original *ICIDH* (see Chapter 3, this volume). The parallelism of the forms of disablement—impairment, activity limitations, and participation—yields a less dichotomous, more universal conception of health outcomes. One may have significant impairments that do not limit participation. Each dimension of disablement, in turn, can be considered within an environmental context ranging from the immediate physical surroundings to systems-level policy. This is an oversimplification of the *ICIDH-2* redraft, but it serves to connect concepts to our discussions of the structure of statistical surveillance systems.

A Note on Terminology and Concepts

A statistical review of these concepts is made difficult in that the systems, their conceptual models, and terminology can seem to the uninitiated a "terminological soup" (Kita 1992). There are numerous opportunities for misunderstanding, given the interchangeable and sometimes idiosyncratic use of terminology and meaning, compounded by the ambiguity of the distinction between *disability* and *handicap* (Badley 1987; Campbell-Brown 1991; Chamie 1990; Edwards 1997). We hope not to add to the confusion. Because *ICIDH* concepts underlie (in principle, if not practice) much of the world's disability surveillance, we adhere to *ICIDH* and *ICIDH-2* conventions. Thus, impairments will reflect loss or malfunction at the level of organ or body part, activity limitations to instrumental activities of daily living (IADLs), and activities of daily living (ADLs) as well as more complex clusters of activities such as work, school, self-care, or social interaction behaviors. We invoke the term *handicap* to describe surveillance efforts adhering to the *ICIDH* concepts of disadvantage across multiple dimensions of "survival roles" (WHO 1980).

An Overview of the Major Forms of Disability Data Systems

In addition to variations in the conceptual basis for defining disability, there are variations in the method of data collection. There are three primary sources of population-level data on disability: national censuses, household surveys, and administrative registries. A census is an (attempted) enumeration of every person in a national population. The detail and depth of disability-related queries in a national census are severely limited due to the great cost and substantial data collection demands of comprehensive, national coverage. In the long-form version of the dicennial census of the United States, for example, disability has been defined very simply as limitations in work or use of public transportation (1980 only) or through a few select IADLs, such as going outside the home alone and taking care of personal needs (1990 only).

Household surveys are systematic samplings conducted to estimate some feature of interest (e.g., health status, behavior, and economic well-being) and impute the distribution of its occurrence at the population level. Health surveys are the most common variation. The National Health Interview Survey (NHIS), which forms the core of "disability statistics" for the United States, is an annual multistage stratified survey of the health and health care of American households (National Center for Health Statistics 1998). Disability is imputed from a series of queries on activity limitations within the basic question sets on household and individual demographics, health status, presence of acute or chronic health conditions, and summaries of health care. The 1996 Health Survey of the West Bank is a parallel example on a more modest scale (Palestinian Central Bureau of Statistics 1996). The Palestinian survey was a stratified multistage survey questionnaire composed of three questionnaire components: household questionnaire, women's health, and child health. The general intent was to profile the health of Palestinian society using selected indicators. Within the household questionnaire were questions on the type and cause of disabilities, described in terms of specific functional limitations or limitations in ADLs.

Internationally, household surveys with relevant disability data are implemented annually (U.S. NHIS), intermittently (Australian National Health Survey), or as one-shot special-topic surveys (e.g., the 1986 Spanish Survey on Disabilities, Impairments and Handicaps; the 1994-1995 U.S. NHIS Disability Supplement). Though samples are based on statistically representative sample frames rather than comprehensive canvases of entire populations, the household survey effort remains labor and resource intensive. These demands, in turn, limit the depth of survey detail with implications for how well large-scale surveys will be able to accommodate the newer conceptions of disablement that include environmental or social context in their data codes.

A more specialized variation is the household survey containing disability modules. The Survey of Income and Program Participation (SIPP) is an annual household survey of the U.S. Bureau of the Census designed to gather statistics on the economic status of American households. Interviews are conducted longitudinally at four-month intervals, and in one interview, a supplemental questionnaire set (referred to as a topical module) on functional limitations and disability is administered. The Health Survey for England (Department of Health 1995) is a series of surveys repeated each year containing a "core" of health behavior and demographic questions. Topical modules focus on different chronic conditions. Disability questions, adapted from the WHO, were incorporated into a single-topic module in 1995 and used to identify types of disability found in the private household population.

Disability is not always relegated to an ancillary role in these surveys, though the disability-specific household surveys tend to be infrequently administered or one-time special survey efforts. The Australian Bureau of Statistics conducts the National Survey of Disability, Ageing, and Carers every five years (Australian Bureau of Health and Welfare 1998). China conducted a massive household survey of 1.6 million persons in its 1987 National Sampling Survey of Disability in China (Bureau of Statistics 1990). Data from the survey still represent the core of what is known about disability in China and are widely cited in international analyses of disability (e.g., Liming, Weihua, and Fujie 1997; United Nations 1996). The Health and Activity Limitations Survey (HALS), a national disabilities survey for Statistics Canada, consists of a household component and an institutional component, which were both administered in 1986 and 1991.

The third major subcategory of surveillance system type is the service registry, essentially an administrative tally of individuals who are the recipients of public services or benefits. Children's social and educational services and adult health and employment programs are the most common forms of registries internationally. The Instituto Nacional De Estadistica Geografia e Informatica (INEGI 1998) of Mexico maintains the Registry of Children with a Disability. Children of all education levels, beginning with preschoolers, are identified by type and number of disabilities, along with basic demographic and socioeconomic indicators. In 1995, 2.7 million children were identified in the registry (INEGI 1998). Pension and social welfare programs, designed as income supports, are a second major source of registry data because of their widespread use by persons with a disability. Iceland's Disability Register of the State Social Security Institute tracks pension benefits granted to those with prolonged disability (Ministry of Health and Social Security 1993). Pension eligibility is predicated on earning potential that is one-fourth of what persons with full mental and physical health are able to earn in the same area of work. The U.S. Social Security Administration provides several "disability protection" programs under the Social Security Act—disabled workers' benefits, supplemental security income, and childhood disability benefits.

While an important source of information on access to government programs or extent of service need, registry data have limited utility for population-based demographic analyses. Only a fraction of the total population with a disability is typically a recipient of services or benefits. Studies of the long-term residential care system for persons with mental retardation (MR) in the United States provide exacting annual statistics on the number served (e.g., Braddock et al. 1998); however, the system represents only 11 percent of the total MR population (Fujiura 1998). In nations where formal systems of care and support are less developed, the discrepancy can be even greater. The 1990 census of Mauritius identified nearly 28,000 citizens with a disability, 14,000 of whom were disability pension recipients but only 400 of whom were recipients of services from rehabilitation programs (United Nations 1996:20).

Table 2.2 presents selected data systems classified under the three levels of disablement in the *ICIDH* as well as the participation construct of the *ICIDH-2*, tabulated across the three methods of data collection (census, household survey, or administrative registry).

The distribution of table entries illustrates the emphasis among existing surveillance systems on impairments and restricted activities. While *ICIDH* concepts are nearly universally accepted in international disability surveillance schemes, only limited components of the model are actually implemented. In the developing world, illness and impairment-defined systems dominate. Each of the national data systems in the United States and the major European industrialized nations is predicated in one form or another on restricted activity. Notable exceptions include the Australian National Health Survey (NHS) and the 1986 survey by the Spanish National Institute of Statistics. The Australian Bureau of Statistics survey of disability explicitly assessed each of the survival role domains under the *ICIDH* handicap scheme (Australian Bureau of Health and Welfare 1998). In addition to the usual queries regarding impairments (e.g., loss of sight or hearing) and activity restrictions (e.g., incomplete use of arms or legs), the NHS queries whether a person is limited in the ability to perform tasks in one or more of the survival roles.

Table 2.3 numerically illustrates the impact of definition concept on estimation in the Australian national survey. Shown in the table are estimates of activity limitations versus handicaps associated with selected impairments in the 1993 Survey of Disability, Ageing, and Carers (Australian Bureau of Health and Welfare 1998). The first column includes those Australians citing 1 or more of 15 restrictions or limitations, per the *ICIDH* classification scheme. Estimates are uniformly lower in the second column, which represents those limited in one of the six core survival roles.

As shown in Table 2.3, the more contextually defined "handicap" criterion yields estimates uniformly lower than person-level descriptors based on activity limitations. Similarly, the Spanish survey systematically assessed each of the six survival roles with direct comparisons to the reporting of activity limitations (Rodriguez 1989). The survey found, for example, that among

Table 2.2 Selected International Disability Data Systems by Disability Definition and Form of Data Collection

Disability Concept	Census	Form of Data Collection	
		Household Survey	Administrative Registry
Impairment	Population Census, 1981 (Bahrain) 1980 Census (Comoros, Kuwait, South Africa, Zambia) 1981 Census (Brazil, Hong Kong, Pakistan) 1982 Census of Disabled (Cyprus) Census of Population, 1992 (Cyprus) 1985 Census (Turkey) 1986 Census Bangladesh, Qatar) 1987 Census (Mali)1988 Census (Poland) 1990 Census of Population and Housing Taiwan-Fukien Area (Taiwan) 1990 Census (Panama) 1990 National Census of Population and Housing (Mauritius) 1991 Census (Aruba) 1992 Census (Paraguay) 1994 Census (Jordan) 1996 Census of Population and Dwellings (New Zealand)	1983 Survey (Malawi) 1985 Survey (Singapore) 1989 Health Survey (Cyprus) 1994 Living Condition Survey (Latvia) Accompanying Survey to the General Population and Housing Census of 1994 (Jordan) Household Survey, 1996-1997 (Mozambique) Ministry of Labor Survey (Japan) National Sampling Survey of Disability (CHN) (Thailand) National Survey of Handicapped, 1981 (India) National Survey of Handicapped Adults (Japan) Survey of Disability (Northern Ireland)	1989 registry (Bulgaria) Benefits on Social Insurance Basis (Estonia) Registration system of disabled persons, 1991 (Germany) Registry of Children with a Disability (Mexico)
Activity restriction	Dicennial Census (United States) Health Survey 1989 (Cyprus) Population census, 1981 (Sri Lanka) Population census, 1975 (Turkey)	1984 Survey of the Chronically Ill (Uruguay) 1996 Health Survey in West Bank and Gaza Strip (Palestine) 1996 Household Disability Survey (New Zealand) Health & Activity Limitation Survey (CAN) National Health Interview Survey (United States) National Health and Medical Survey, 1979-1981 (Egypt) National Survey, 1981 (Zimbabwe) Surveys of disability in Great Britain, 1985-1986 (England) Survey of Income and Program Participation (United States) 1995 National Health Survey (Australia) National Disability Survey, 1988 (Australia) Survey of Disability, Ageing, and Carers, 1993, 1998 (Australia)	Disability Register of the State Social (Iceland) National Disability Unit (Barbados) RSA-11 (United States)
Handicap	1996 Census of Population and Housing (Australia)		

Table 2.3   "Disability" versus "Handicap": Australian Survey of Disability, Aging, and Carers

Impairment Category	Population Estimate (thousands)	
	Disability	Handicap
Sensory	571.9	303.8
Arthritis	504.3	439.9
Respiratory diseases	290.4	215.9
Intellectual	283.0	227.3
Head injury/stroke/other brain damage	59.6	53.0

adults ages 44 to 79, the average number of role handicaps across their sample was less than one per person. In short, not all persons described as having an activity limitation (disability) were described as having a "handicap." The Spanish survey also highlighted the dynamism of disablement across age cohorts of the population. The average number of role "handicaps" formed a U-shaped function when plotted across age of respondent. The highest numbers of handicaps were at the younger and older age cohorts (1.4 and 1.7 handicaps, respectively) and trough in the middle-age ranges of 45 to 60 years.

The conceptual demarcation of disability and handicap is a source of considerable debate. Edwards (1997), for example, argued that the distinction was superfluous. His basic premise is that external causes lie at the root of both "disability" (restricted activity) and "handicap" (disadvantage) since one cannot pursue activities if the social context is not in place (Edwards 1997:604). The essence of Edwards's critique lies in the shortcomings of any assessment based only on person-level characteristics—morbidity, impairment, or restricted activity. The relevant unit of analysis must be the external constraints preventing activity.

THE DEMOGRAPHY OF DISABLEMENT

To this point, we have navigated the underlying rationale of basic mechanics of disability surveillance. In this section, we briefly summarize the core demographic features of disability in the world. There are three fundamental questions asked of disability data: (1) How many people have a disability? (2) How is disability distributed within the population? (3) What are the major causes? Other questions are relevant, of course, but these three describe the basic starting point for disability surveillance. There are no simple answers, and we must, at the outset, apologize for what will be a rather generalized overview. Estimates of the magnitude of disability are directly affected by the definition employed and the method of sampling. We proceed, therefore, with a modest agenda—to provide a "big-picture" summary of the magnitude of disablement globally, describe variations in terms of the structure of surveillance, and briefly address general themes regarding the dimensions and etiology of disablement across demographic stratifiers.

Data presented in the following sections were drawn from sources employing a variety of methodologies across multiple definitions and inconsistent consideration of severity in judgments of impairments and activity restrictions. Rather than attempting to portray a single estimate of "disability," we will directly acknowledge in our summaries and syntheses these conceptual and statistical distinctions. A common thread throughout this chapter is the futility of searching for a single better estimate of "disability." We reiterate Zola's (1993) argument that how one chooses to define and thus count disability should largely be driven by the purposes of the count. The linkage of purpose to definition is a key feature of the multiple dimensions of disablement concept in the *ICIDH-2*. Equally critical to a disability studies perspective is a dialogue on the meaning of the numbers we produce. We return to this latter point at the end of the chapter.

The Magnitude of Disablement

Disability is not consistently represented in our global data systems. Unlike those defining moments of birth and death, which are not burdened by conceptual ambiguity, disability data are compiled under different conceptual frameworks, data collection schemes, and sampling frames. Surveillance systems are fragmented, rudimentary, or nonexistent, particularly in developing countries. Chamie (1989) aptly summarizes the current state of affairs with respect to international disability statistics: "a bewildering myriad of detailed impairments and disability codes from surveys, often jumbled together without benefit of a meaningful conceptual framework" (p. 122).

It is difficult to statistically summarize ambiguity. We cannot directly answer the very basic questions of "how much?" or "how often?" without a series of caveats. Such are the nuances of disability statistics and the structure of this section of the chapter—a synthesis of statistical estimates followed by caveats and explanations of the major sources of variance in the estimates. Despite these equivocations, some general statements can be made regarding the size and composition of the population, trends, and underlying demographic dynamics. Most national census and household survey systems employ as their sampling unit some component of the disablement process outlined under the *ICIDH* model discussed above: (1) underlying morbidities or impairments, (2) restriction of activity, or, more rarely, (3) handicap.

International summaries of health status have been compiled by the United Nations Development Programme (UNDP) since 1990 and reported in the annual *Human Development Report* series. Health status indicators include disease exposure, access to physicians and nurses, cigarette consumption, health expenditures, and disability. Data are drawn from national estimates organized primarily by the United Nations (UN) and other international organizations. Figure 2.1 summarizes selected regional tallies of the international prevalence of disability during the years 1985 to 1992 from the 1998 *Human Development Report* (UNDP 1998).

It would appear from the national tabulations that rates of disablement are highest in the developed, industrialized nations and decreased in the less-developed Third World nations. Consider the rates per 1,000 of population reported in the UN's DISTAT for selected countries in Table 2.4.

Although the data represent formal governmental census statistics and ostensibly were collected to represent "disability" within the population, the numbers are remarkable, primarily for their extraordinary range, from 3 in 1,000 in Egypt to 142 per 1,000 population in the United Kingdom. While one may be inclined to attribute the vast differences to some peculiarity of England or the English, the more obvious explanation lies among the issues discussed earlier—namely, the form of disability concept employed in the surveillance. Though the intent of disability surveillance and statistical estimation is the same internationally, the manner of operationalization varies widely.

Impairment definitions are employed among the nations reporting much lower rates of disability (e.g., Egypt). Higher rates are found under restricted activity definitions ("disability" per *ICIDH* terminology). This is a well-established finding in disability statistics. Suris and Blum (1993), in their analysis of DISTAT data and adolescent disability prevalence, reported a *positive* correlation between disability rate and gross national product ($r = 0.65, p < .05$). Disability increased in relatively predictable linear fashion with national wealth. The strength of the linear relationship was based not on the connection of national wealth and disability, but rather

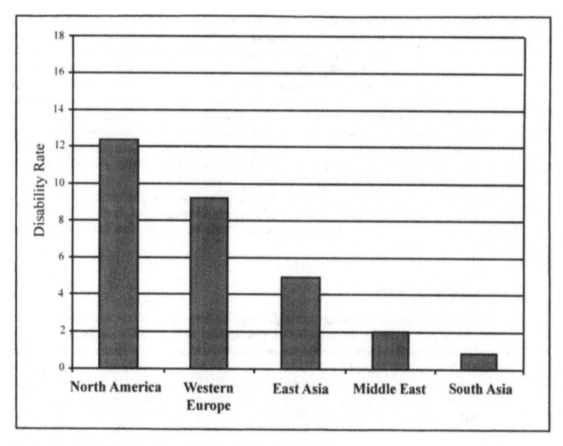

Figure 2.1. Disability Prevalence Rates for Selected World Regions
SOURCE: Data compiled from national statistics during the 1985 to 1992 period.

Table 2.4   Disability Rates Per 1,000 Population Reported in Selected National Statistics

Country	Disability Rate Per 1,000		
	All	Males	Females
Egypt (1976)	3.0	4.4	1.6
Bangladesh (1986)	5.2	6.2	4.1
Zambia (1980)	16.2	16.7	15.6
China (1987)a	49.0	48.5	49.4
United States (1990)a	89.6	93.7	85.6
Poland (1988)	98.6	94.0	103.0
United Kingdom (1986)a	142.0	160.0	152.0

SOURCE: Data from the United Nations (1996).
a. Based on household survey data.

on the inclination of Western nations to employ restricted activity conceptualizations of disability rather than morbidity- and impairment-based definitions. The differences in Table 2.4 represent two manifestations of the differences in impairment and restricted activity definitions of "disability." In her examination of international design strategies, Chamie (1989) found increased rates under activity probes and increased gender differences under impairment probes. Probes focused on the presence of specific impairments yield lower identification rates than queries asking about limited activities. Respondents are more likely to identify activity limitations because the content of the question reflects daily experience. In contrast, an underlying impairment may be of only vague familiarity, or its nomenclature is not recognized. Second, impairment-based identification typically increases the ratio of male-to-female disability due to sex-linked congenital conditions and risks that are associated with gender differences. In their global analysis of disease, injury, and risk, Murray and Lopez (1996) estimated alcohol to be the leading etiology of male morbidity (referred to as "disability" in the original report) worldwide but only the tenth largest cause among women.

Underscored in the cross-national examples is the difficulty in using national disability statistics to draw an unequivocal global portrait of disability demographics. In the following sections, we look separately at impairment, restricted activity, and the few national efforts at evaluations of "handicap."

Demography of Impairment

Despite the clear distinction in our conceptual models between impairment and disablement and our desire not to equate the presence of impairments with disability status, impairment-based surveillance data are a significant source of statistical knowledge of disability. The bias internationally was illustrated earlier in Table 2.2. While a variety of factors account for the skew in emphasis—recency of widespread application of *ICIDH* conceptual standards, for example—clearly, the relative ease in operationalizing impairment-based definitions plays a part. Judgment of the presence or absence of a condition is relatively consistent across cultures. Diagnosis of physical anomalies and organ-level dysfunction come from medical convention, and established standards can be applied to their monitoring. In contrast, the translations of activity, disadvantage, or participation into measurement operations remain works in progress and, by definition, malleable within local culture. Finally, condition-based screening is a form of surveillance very familiar within existing public health infrastructures, with its diagnostic focus on individual pathology.

Table 2.5 lists national estimates of "disability" taken from impairment-based national censuses. Data were reported in the UN's DISTAT (United Nations 1996).

Prevalence rates appear to converge within a relatively narrow range within impairment-based estimates. The apparent variability in reported prevalence within impairment-based systems is largely attributable to the use of severity standards. As summarized by Chamie (1995) in her summary of national data in the UN DISTAT, countries using severe impairments as the criterion for disability tend to yield prevalence rates in the 0.2 percent to 6 percent range, with general impairment estimates falling in the range of 5 percent of the population. Thus, very low impairment rates tend to indicate use of "total loss" definitions. Table 2.6 illustrates the linkage between severity restrictions and derived prevalence estimates with selected national systems.

Underscored in the differences is the fact that disablement is continuously distributed across many different dimensions that are not readily dichotomized. Prevalence will vary widely depending on the cutoff point.

Demography of Activity Limitations

The restricted activity framework dominates surveillance among the industrialized Western nations. The popularity of the perspective lies in its pragmatism—disability is described in terms of function rather than form, with activities familiar to the daily experience of the respondents. Included in this rather broad category are functional limitations in the form of specific ADLs and IADLs, as well as limits in performing the more complex clusters of activities

Table 2.5 Disability Prevalence Estimates Based on Impairment Definitions: National Data from DISTAT (in percentages)

Region	Rate
Africa	
South Africa (1980)	0.6
Zambia (1980)	1.6
Botswana (1991)	2.2
Asia	
Sri Lanka (1981)	0.5
Bangladesh (1986)	0.5
Thailand (1986)[a]	0.7
Hong Kong (1981)	0.8
Japan (1987)[a]	2.7
China (1987)[a]	4.9
Central and South America	
Panama (1990)	1.3
Brazil (1981)	1.7
Europe	
Hungary (1988)[a]	3.4
Middle East–Crescent	
Qatar (1986)	0.2
Egypt (1976)	0.3
Kuwait (1980)	0.4
Pakistan (1981)	0.5
Iraq (1977)	0.9
Syria (1981)	1.0
Turkey (1985)	1.4
Bahrain (1981)	1.7

a. Based on household survey.

such as employment. The range of variations along the continuum of simple-to-complex activity is routinely employed as operational definitions of "disability" among national statistical systems.

An example of the ADL and IADL activity approach is illustrated by an early effort of the Organization for Economic Cooperation and Development (OECD) to facilitate assessment of disability across international borders (see Table 2.7; McWhinnie 1982).

Major national surveys, primarily in the industrialized Western nations, are largely predicated on variations of this approach. Selected surveillance systems, their assessed domains, and respective estimates of activity limitation are listed in Table 2.8. As shown in the Table 2.8, the various activity limitation protocols yield population prevalence rates in the 13 to 19 percent range. The similarity of estimates suggests the relative stability of specific activity assessments.

Table 2.6   Impairment Rates across Severity Definitions

Method	Example/Inclusion Criteria	Rate (percent)
With severity		
Bahrain (1981)[a]	Person is "blind, deaf, deaf and mute, amputee, paralysed or mentally handicapped"	1.0
Jordan (1994)[b]	Person is deaf or dumb, physical, mental, visual, cerebral palsy, other, multiple handicap, chronic, and psychic diseases	1.2
Mozambique (1996-1997)	Person has conditions of "blindness, deafness, paralysis, mute, mental retardation, amputation arms or legs"	1.2
Paraguay (1992)[c]	Person is blind, deaf, mute, mentally retarded, paralyzed, or two or more conditions combined	0.9
Generic impairment		
China (1987)	Screening for the following conditions: hearing, visual and speech disorders, paralysis, mental disorders, epilepsy, amputation, physical stigmata, and cardiopulmonary conditions	4.9
Hong Kong (1994)[d]	Hearing impairment, autism, mental handicap, maladjustment, physical handicap, visual impairment, mental illness, visceral disability, speech impairment	4.3
Japan (1998)[e]	Motional and internal physical disabilities, mental retardation, or mental disorders	4.0

a. Reported in Al-Ansari (1989).
b. Department of Statistics (1996).
c. Direccion General de Estadistica Encuestas y Censos (1992).
d. Health and Welfare Bureau (1995).
e. Ministry of Health and Welfare of Japan (1997).

Table 2.7   Organization for Economic Cooperation and Development (OECD) Disability Questionnaire

1. During the past 2 weeks, did you have to cut down on any of the things you normally do because of illness or injury?
2. Is your eyesight good enough to read ordinary newspaper print (with glasses if usually worn)?
3. Can you hear what is said in a normal conversation with another person (with hearing aid if usually worn)?
4. Can you speak without difficulty?
5. Can you carry an object of 5 kilos for 10 meters?
6. Can you walk 400 meters without resting?
7. Can you move between rooms?
8. Can you get in and out of bed?
9. Can you dress and undress?
10. Can you (when standing) bend down and pick up a shoe from the floor?

SOURCE: McWhinnie (1982).

The ADL-IADL protocol has considerable durability, appearing in various incarnations and applications over the years. McDowell and Newell's (1996) guide to assessment instruments identified more than 50 variations of ADL scales currently in use in health and rehabilitation

Table 2.8 Limitation Prevalence by Nation

Nation	Domains	Limitation Rate (percent)
Australia (1993)[a]	Self-care, mobility, verbal communication, school, employment	14.2
Canada (1986 HALS)	Mobility, agility, seeing, hearing, speaking	13.2
New Zealand (1996 HDS)	Walking, moving, carrying, standing, bending, reaching, dressing, getting in or out of bed, grasping, hearing, seeing, and cognitive impairments	19.0
Spain (1986)	Seeing, hearing, speaking, personal care, walking, climbing, running, out of home, other activities of daily living, behavioral problems	14.9
United Kingdom (1986 HSE)	Seeing, walking, bending, dressing, washing, eating, communication, hearing, personal care, climbing	14.2
United States (1990-91 SIPP)[b]	Seeing, hearing, speaking, walking, climbing, running, out of home, lifting and carrying	17.5

a. Excludes canvas of impairments.
b. Functional limitations definition.

applications. A number of important features are illustrated in the activity-based protocol: (1) reliability and validity (Durkin et al. 1995), (2) ease of use and facilitation of interdisciplinary communication (Shaffer et al. 1983), and (3) cross-cultural and international comparability (Simeonsson, Chen, and Hu 1995). Durkin et al. (1995), for example, evaluated the reliability of the 10-questions screen for the detection of childhood disability. Administered to parents, the 10-questions screen was composed of five queries on cognition, two on movement, and one question each on the presence of seizures, vision, or hearing limits. Samples were drawn from Bangladesh, Jamaica, and Pakistan. The stability (test-retest reliability) of the 10-questions screen, as well as its measurement characteristics (internal consistency, factor structure, and item profiles), was similar across cultures.

Restricted activity encompasses a broad range of phenomena, however, and where measurements are made on the continuum of simple to complex will have a significant impact on derived statistics. The U.S. NHIS defines limits in terms of the more complex clusters of activities (e.g., work, school), while the Canadian HALS system parallels the OECD model with an emphasis on specific ADLs. France employs ADLs but emphasizes severity of limitation in its ADL assessment (Jee and Or 1998).

Intranational examples of the simple-to-complex continuum and use of severity standards can be seen in the activity restriction implementations of the U.S. SIPP, U.S. NHIS, and the Australian Health Interview Survey. Queries range from specific functional IADLs to the more global socially defined role activities. The central NHIS definition focuses on long-term limitations in the performance of a major social role as a consequence of a chronic condition. Respondents could be deemed as having a disability if they were limited by a long-term chronic condition in their primary "role" of working, keeping house, or going to school. The SIPP employs a checklist of functional limitations in ADLs and IADLS as well as selected impairments in its screen for disability (McNeil 1997). If there was evidence of programmatic need (e.g., a developmental disability or receipt of disability benefits) or assistance in basic ADLs or mobility, then the disability was deemed "severe." Similarly, the 1993 Australian Health Interview Survey (Australian Bureau of Health and Welfare 1998) monitors "disability" in terms of specific functional activities (loss of hearing, incomplete use of arms) and restricted activities and sepa-

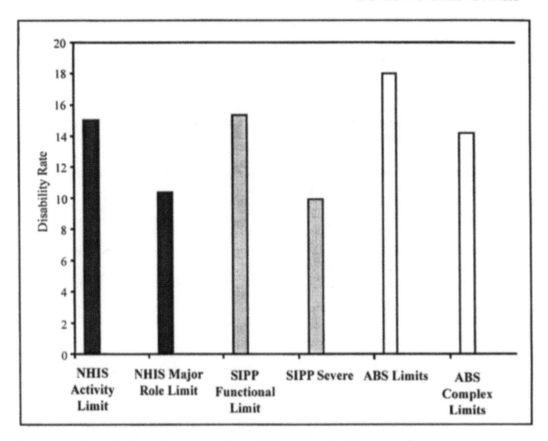

Figure 2.2. Disability Prevalence under Three Different Activity Restriction Screens

rately counts "handicap" as limits in more complex tasks such as self-care, mobility, and communication. Quite apart from the debate regarding the meaningfulness of the "handicap" assessment, the operational measurement is very similar in concept to the "role limits" and "severe disability" of the U.S. NHIS and SIPP, respectively. The key conceptual distinction in each of these examples is that a subset of those reporting discrete functional limits will have difficulty performing the more complex activity. Figure 2.2 graphically illustrates the impact on prevalence estimate using the specific (SIPP, Australian Bureau of Statistics [ABS] disability) and complex definitions (NHIS, ABS handicap).

Estimated prevalence of Americans with an activity limitation in 1994 was 15 percent in the 1994 NHIS (Benson and Marano 1994) and 15.3 percent in the 1994 SIPP under the "inability to perform one or more functional activities" definition (McNeil 1997). Imposing a "severity" standard on the screen (at a minimum, the presence of a limitation in an ADL or IADL, mobility, or work or presence of a developmental impairment) reduced the SIPP estimated prevalence to 9.9 percent. Figure 2.2 illustrates the observation of many regarding the conceptual vagueness of the original *ICIDH* "disability" construct—that, in fact, there are at least two distinct levels at which activity could be assessed, the simple and complex.

The degree to which the distinction poses a problem depends on the use of the data. Preceding discussions underscored how prevalence estimates can be dramatically affected by subtle definitional nuances. The different scalings, however, may not be particularly problematic in other applications. If disablement measures can reliably order individuals and be validated against outcomes such as employment or gross earnings, then multiple conventions may be employed to answer the same form of question. Figure 2.3, for example, illustrates the prevalence of impairment and activity restrictions across the life span, across selected national surveillance systems. Although the overall rates vary substantially across these national statistics systems, the relative ranking of impairment by age grouping is relatively stable.

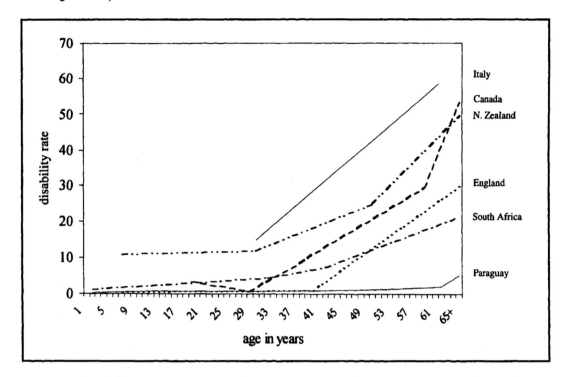

Figure 2.3. Disability Prevalence across Age Cohort: Canada, England, Italy, New Zealand, Paraguay, and South Africa

In Chamie's (1989) review and critique of variations across international classification systems and screening mechanisms, she notes, "Even under these less-than-perfect conditions, it appears that relationships within data sets are relatively stable" (p. 137).

Demography of External Determinants: Environment and Context

If disability as a status of the human condition is not well represented in our international systems of population monitoring, then disablement as a process is largely invisible. Despite the relatively unified surveillance framework provided by the *ICIDH*, the translation of the concepts of person by context interactions into measurement procedures remains at a very exploratory stage of development. There is the methodological challenge of translating what is inherently an interactive and multidimensional concept into measures capable of being incorporated into large-scale statistical systems. The implications of the challenge extend well beyond the domain of data keeping and national surveillance. Some concerns, such as the meaningfulness of any form of disability case definition, reach to the heart of disability studies. We briefly explore these issues from the perspective of statistical systems; we address them more directly later in the chapter. Elsewhere in this volume, the reader will find greater substantive treatment of the conceptual implications of disability definition.

The dominance of impairment and restricted activity approaches worldwide is not surprising. The person is the principle unit of analysis in national surveillance, and it follows that individual characteristics lie at the core of identification methods. The incorporation of measures capturing interactions with social context or environmental setting is relatively unexplored on a large-scale basis. Whether the key-defining element is conceived as social disadvantage (handicap in the *ICIDH*), restricted participation in life situations (*ICIDH-2*), or some other process external to the person, assessment of interactions by definition extends beyond a single domain or function. Multidimensional complexity runs counter to the desire for case definition simplicity in large-scale surveillance (e.g., Teutsch 1994). Complexity confounds both construction of instrumentation and administration of the instrument. In a review of European applications of the *ICIDH* handicap concept, for example, Fougeyrollas (1993) found inconsistencies between the survey's definitional model and actual questionnaire items to be the norm rather than exception in survey operations. Survey items typically assumed "constant environments," effectively focusing the assessment on individual capabilities rather than situational interactions. Instruments and applications were variable in what domains were employed. Abstract classification concepts were not readily operationalized into specific written and oral survey-based questions.

Is the task of incorporating context into surveillance achievable? As the emphasis in disability definition skews toward situational interactions, the complexity of measurement construction is compounded. Local, setting-specific features are the sine qua non of an interaction-focused assessment. The shift in emphasis can be seen indirectly in a comparison of survival domains employed in the *ICIDH* and the much more broadly conceived major life dimensions of the *ICIDH-2*. In the original *ICIDH*, an assessment is made on the six survival domains. In contrast, the *ICIDH-2* (beta draft) participation scheme attempts to represent (by proxy) the full range of human social experience. As context is more explicitly incorporated, the complexity of the taxonomy increases (see Table 2.9).

A parallel can be drawn in the evolution of psychotherapeutic efficacy research after the "uniformity" myths came under challenge in the 1950s (Kiesler 1966). The uniformity perspective treated therapy as a homogeneous process across patients who were presumed to be more alike than dissimilar. In like fashion, outcomes could be measured along uniform dimensions such as behavior or personality change. The causal chain from treatment to outcome operated in a linear and largely deterministic manner. Person and context differences were treated as nuisance variables under the uniformity assumptions, to be controlled via randomization or statistical control. An "interactionist" perspective arose among efficacy researchers (Cronbach 1957) as the appropriate focus of study. Instructive for the present discussion was the challenges of translating the interactionist approach into a measurement methodology. Grand theory and generalizations were in part supplanted by microanalyses that included both context and process variables (Kiesler 1966). Thus, for example, structural features of the dyadic interview were assessed: synchronicity of communication between therapist and client, the reciprocity of verbal influence, and verbal productivity, among others. The character of the research questions changed from dichotomizing therapeutic models into those that were "effective" or "not effective" to identifying the effective components of the process. A similar move away from "disabled" and "not disabled" dichotomies in statistical applications will require an expanded view of disability data and substantially greater measurement challenges if context-based disablement concepts are to be incorporated. As Heller (1971) noted in his evaluation of the new paradigm, "The varied complexity of the therapeutic interaction and the inability to specify and control therapeutic operations make it difficult to obtain reliable information" (p. 127). While the approach constructs a better foundation for understanding disablement, there are extraordinary conceptual and methodological challenges for implementing concept into the coding systems of large-scale assessments. International experience under the more constrained *ICIDH* suggests that we should not expect any simple solutions.

An alternative perspective on disability data is the surveillance of problematic social issues or contexts and specific barriers within a society rather than the counting of "disabled persons." The idea is not new. In concept if not in practice, the *ICIDH* was not conceived as a classification of persons. Chamie (1989), for example, characterized "handicap" as an analytical tool rather than as a screening standard. In Chamie's view, assessment of handicap should focus not on screening of individuals but rather through aggregated statistical reporting on "economic and other opportunity loss . . . that may be explained through the influence of impairments and disabilities in different environments" (p. 137). Under such a perspective, one is not counting persons using a "better" definition. The focus is on explicating the relationship between society, culture, and disablement (Chamie 1995).

Table 2.9   *ICIDH* Handicap and *ICIDH-2* Participation Domains

ICIDH Handicap Domains		ICIDH-2 Participation Domains	
Principle Domain	*Rated on Ability to Do the Following*	*Principle Domain* [a]	*Rated on Extent of Participation across Subdomains of the Following*
Orientation handicap	Orient to surroundings	Personal maintenance	Personal care, health, nourishment, and housing
Physical independence handicap	Sustain independent existence	Mobility	Home, outside of home, transportation, private transport, and public transport
Mobility handicap	Move effectively through surroundings	Exchange of information	Spoken and nonspoken, written, symbols and signs, public symbols, and telecommunication
Occupation handicap	Occupy time in a manner customary to culture	Social relationships	Family relationships, intimate relationships, friends and acquaintances, peers, strangers, other
Social integration handicap	Participate in social relationships	Home life and assistance to others	Housing, management of home, nutrition, health, and mobility for self and others
Economic self-sufficiency handicap	Sustain customary socioeconomic activity	Education	Informal settings, preschool, school, vocational training, and higher education
Other handicaps		Work and employment	Work preparation, self-employment, remunerative work, nonremunerative work, and other types
		Economic life	Transactions, self-sufficiency, public entitlements, other
		Community, social, and civic life	Formal, informal associations, ceremony, recreation and leisure, religion and spirituality, human rights, citizenship

SOURCE: World Health Organization (1999).

a. Interaction with environment can be rated for each domain; three broad classes of environment: immediate, service structure, and systems level.

The Epidemiology of Disablement

Just as the meaning of disability varies, so do the meanings we attach to the concept of causation in disability. In disability statistics, cause is variously defined in traditional terms—as underlying pathologies or as specific, identifiable events such as trauma. Alternatively, underlying chronic conditions are identified as the "cause" of conditions that are an intermediary of some more distal event. Thus, for example, injury may be cited as a cause of an orthopedic impairment, or the orthopedic impairment itself may be cited as a cause of restricted activity, without mention of an earlier determinant in the sequelae of events. The reader of epidemiological data must be aware of the intermingling of impairment as a criterion and cause of disablement, as well as the inconsistent evaluation of injury and other external traumas.

Table 2.10   Top Five Underlying Causes of Disability: SIPP, NHIS, and ABS: Study or Instrument

1990-1991 SIPP[a]		1992 NHIS[b]		1993 ABS[c]	
Conditions	Rate	Conditions	Rate	Conditions	Rate
Arthritis	3.7	Arthritis and other musculoskeletal	4.2	Arthritis and other musculoskeletal	4.3
Heart trouble and high blood pressure	3.5	Circulatory system	4.0	Circulatory system	1.3
Back or spine problem	2.9	Orthopedic impairments	3.4	Intellectual impairment	1.3
Lung or respiratory trouble	1.5	Respiratory conditions	1.9	Respiratory conditions	1.2
Impairment of the limbs	1.0	Nervous systems/sense organs	1.7	Diseases of the ear	1.2

a. Reported as first, second, or third cause of ADL or IADL, age 16 and older (McNeil 1993).
b. Chronic conditions as cause of activity limits, all ages (LaPlante and Carlson 1996).
c. Conditions as cause of limit in self-care, mobility, and communication, all ages.

Relevant to the current discussion are the implications of the causal identification because it goes to the heart of the purposes of the counting. The *World Programme of Action Concerning Disabled Persons* (United Nations 1982) connected specific action goals to the conceptual basis of surveillance. These goals were prevention, rehabilitation, and equalization of opportunity. In accordance with the original *ICIDH* model, monitoring methods were aligned with the three components of disablement: assessment of impairments for the monitoring of prevention programs, disabilities for rehabilitation efforts, and handicaps for opportunity within society.

While the *ICIDH* handicap concept is not well represented in our international surveillance data (and widely criticized, as described earlier in this chapter and elsewhere in this volume), the underlying model introduced significant alterations in the conception of disability causation. Positing handicap in the interaction of person-level factors (impairments and activity limitations) with social and cultural context incorporates external factors (e.g., "opportunity") in the epidemiological framework.

Causes of Restricted Activity

In the national health surveys of the Western industrialized countries, the presence of restricted activity is typically accompanied by queries regarding the condition or conditions causing the restriction. The NHIS in the United States (e.g., NCHS 1998); SIPP (McNeil 1993); Australian Survey of Disability, Ageing, and Carers (Australian Bureau of Health and Welfare 1998); and the Canadian Health and Activity Limitation Survey (Social Trends Analysis Directorate 1986) employ chronic conditions as the unit of analysis rather than "the more distal pathology or trauma event." Comparison of systems and leading causes is shown in Table 2.10.

Despite variations in the coding of conditions and modest differences in the implementation of restricted activity definitions, there is remarkable consistency in identifying conditions underlying ADL and IADL limits. Arthritis and other musculoskeletal conditions, heart and other circulatory system diseases, and respiratory conditions are commonly cited as principal causes.

The WHO framework for the study of causes provides an alternative perspective. An expanded list of external causes was developed on the basis of *International Classification of Disease* codes and proposed as a means for standardizing the surveillance of the determinants of impairments. The taxonomy is shown in Table 2.11 (from the *ICIDH*; WHO 1980).

Table 2.11 Causes of Impairments

Diseases and illness
Congenital anomalies and perinatal conditions
Injury
  Motor vehicle (*ICD-9* codes E810-825)
  Other transport (*ICD-9* codes E800-807, E826-838)
  Accidental poisoning (*ICD-9* codes E850-858, E860-869)
  Injury from falls, fire, and operations of war (*ICD-9* codes E880-888, E890-899, E990-999)
  Other external causes, including natural and environmental factors (*ICD-9* codes E900-909)

SOURCE: World Health Organization (1980).

Table 2.12 Causes of Impairment: Chinese National Survey of the Handicapped, 1987

	Percentage of Total	
	Physical Disabilities	*Reduced Mental Capacity*
Disease and illness	41	12
Congenital anomalies and perinatal conditions	6	20
Injury	26	16
Other	18	12
Unknown	9	40

SOURCE: DISTAT data reported in World Health Organization (1990).

Note that the coding scheme represents broad clusters of underlying pathologies—diseases and illness or congenital conditions or injury. For example, New Zealand's 1996 Household Disability Survey employed chronic conditions (e.g., disease or illness, conditions present at birth), trauma events (e.g., accidents, abuse, environment), and the "natural ageing process" (Statistics New Zealand 1998:41) in their summary of causes. Types of data and the manner of coding are subject to considerable variation across national borders. As stated in the WHO (1990) report on disability causes, national statistics are "not meant to reflect perfectly the proper medical diagnosis . . . rather they summarize the general population's understanding of factors which have caused impairments or disability" (p. 41). Chamie (1995) summarized the UN DISTAT data on causes of restricted activity (Canada, 1986; Spain, 1986; United Kingdom, 1985-1986) and impairment (China, 1987; Germany, 1989; and Japan, 1987). Whether impairments or restricted activity was employed as the unit of analysis, illness and disease conditions were the primary causes, ranging from about 50 percent of all cases in the registry in Japan and Canada to 83 percent in Germany. Congenital and injury-based causes tended to represent a small proportion of cases but varied widely depending on the form of impairment. Injury was a significant cause of physical impairments, while congenital and perinatal causes are most pronounced as causes of intellectual impairments or as causes of childhood activity limitations. These general themes can be seen in Table 2.12, which summarizes external causes data from the 1987 National Survey of the Handicapped in China (Bureau of Statistics 1990; data from WHO 1990).

The Global Burden of Disease Study

An alternative approach to the epidemiology of disability was developed in the WHO- and World Bank–sponsored Global Burden of Disease (GBD) study. The GBD project sought to comprehensively profile worldwide health status using a single index of health—the disability-adjusted life year (DALY). The DALY is a composite measure estimating years lost to premature death as well as years lived with disability (Jamison 1996). The concept of years lived with a disability (YLD) represented the magnitude of impact of a disability. An example helps to illustrate the distinction between the YLD and the "head counts" emphasized to this point in this chapter. A national portrayal of asthma can be quantified using the now-familiar prevalence rate—the number of persons affected divided by the total population. Calculation of impact using the YLD measure requires three numerical inputs: (1) the incidence of untreated asthma, (2) average duration, and (3) a weight representing the "severity" of the condition. (For an in-depth treatment of the methodology, refer to Murray 1996.) The number of untreated cases multiplied by the average years of duration and the severity rate yields the YLD index.

Conceptually, the YLD is a numerical index of the impact of a condition on a nation's health status rather than the rate of occurrence. For example, GBD prevalence estimates of global asthma rates were double those of unipolar depression (.020 vs. .013), but the YLD values for asthma were dwarfed by depression (9.1 vs. 50.8 million YLDs). Although asthma affects more persons, the impact of depression is greater. The GBD methodology is more sensitive to cumulative impact, while cross-sectional surveys better represent their numerical presence.

Altogether, the GBD study estimated a total of 472.7 million YLDs worldwide in 1990. There was divergence in the GBD's estimates of the leading causes of death versus disability. Noncommunicable diseases (heart disease and cancer) were the dominant causes of mortality in the developed world and a close second to infectious diseases in the developing world. In contrast, mental illness, nutritional deficiencies, substance abuse, and injury were critical components of worldwide estimates of YLDs. General conclusions were the following: (1) neuropsychiatric conditions had the greatest impact, estimated to account for 28 percent of all YLDs; (2) alcohol use, motor vehicle accidents, and asthma were important sources of YLDs for males globally, while maternal health and sexually transmitted diseases were primary sources of disability for females; and (3) infectious diseases, health, and nutritional causes had proportionately greater impact in the developing world.

The GBD effort was not without its detractors. In the absence of extant statistical data on the causes of disablement, the study employed a consensus process using experts and research reviews to identify those conditions or injuries most important to disablement. Conditions were equated to disability. Murray (1996) acknowledged the real possibility that the conditions evaluated in the estimation plan were not representative. Briefly, the process involved estimating the impact of 483 causes of death and morbidity from three broad categories: (1) communicable diseases and maternal, perinatal, and nutritional conditions (e.g., parasitic diseases, respiratory infections); (2) noncommunicable diseases (e.g., neuropsychiatric conditions, cardiovascular diseases); and (3) injuries. For example, falls were one form of injury evaluated on four impairment outcomes: long-term skull fracture, spinal cord injury, femur fracture, and intercranial injury. Over the course of a three-year cycle of estimation and revision, epidemiology experts estimated prevalence, fatality rates, and remission rates for each of the sequelae based on review of research. Inconsistencies were identified (e.g., implausible prevalence rates based on known incidence statistics), and the specialists were asked to revisit and revise their estimations.

The procedural detail of the GBD estimation is emphasized in this very brief summary to reinforce to the reader that these are broadly painted portraits rather than exacting statistical summaries. Murray and Lopez (1996) succinctly describe the methodological challenge that is by now familiar to the consumer of disability statistics—"definition and measurement of nonfatal health outcomes are less precise than for mortality" (Murray and Lopez 1996:201). The significance of the present discussion lies less in the methodology than in its effort to systematically profile the epidemiology of disability. Underscored in the study was the relative lack of attention given to disability in the world's public health systems. According to the authors, "For descriptive epidemiology where the objective is to assess the probable or even approximate magnitude of disease or injury so as to inform current policy debates and planning exercises, approximate estimates are better than no estimates" (Murray and Lopez 1996:241).

Unfortunately, the GBD effort is perhaps as pure an example of the linear sequelae of pathology to disability that we (and others in this volume) have rejected as an excessively crude representation of the disablement process. The GBD study employed estimates of specific conditions or injuries that led to impairments, which in turn were equated to disability. Other value-laden decisions undergirded the methodology—principally, that years in old age and childhood are of lesser "value" than years lived during youth, years lived with a chronic condition are years "lost," and the presumption of disablement as a burden.

A Disability Studies Perspective on Epidemiology

Epidemiological analyses are historically anchored to the analysis of the causes of death, diseases, or injury and their distribution. One should expect a disability studies view of epidemiological inquiry to be necessarily harsh, given its focus on underlying pathologies, linear sequelae of causation, and analytic emphasis on dichotomizing populations into those with or without the condition. Implicit as well in epidemiological thinking is prevention strategies. The 1991 Institute of Medicine (IOM) report, for example, argued the need for "cause-oriented disability data" to assist in setting priorities for disability prevention. Yet, there are a number of reasons to believe that standard epidemiological approaches are not wholly inconsistent with emerging paradigms of disability. Epidemiologists realized long ago that conditions and their distributions were only incompletely described by the presence of a causal agent. Agents were necessary but not sufficient as explanations. Multifactorial ecological models were developed to accommodate the influences of person characteristics, causal agents, and their interaction with environmental factors (Mausner and Kramer 1985).

The *ICIDH-2*, with its taxonomy of disablement rather than of people, provides a template for epidemiological surveillance more consistent within a disability studies framework. How causal concepts are characterized will vary depending on what dimensions of disablement are being evaluated—body structures or functions, activities, or participation. Different concepts will have varying utility across the dimensions of disablement. Source of injury, for example, may be an important statistical unit for the study of impairment such as traumatic brain injury but of lesser utility when attempting to evaluate postrehabilitation employment status. The utility of the data is directly related to how well individual variance is accounted for. Pathogenic events are powerful determinants of morbidities but may account for only a fraction of the interperson variability in the manifestation of activity restrictions and even less as an explanation of participation limits. If we accept the perspective of disablement as a process with parallel dimensions rather than as a singular and linear process, then it follows that the determinants of disability must be considered within a multifactorial framework. The study of "cause" can be viewed as a direct window into the analysis of the disablement process, whether the genesis is biological, in the environment, socially constructed, or the manifestation of multiple interacting influences.

THE LIMITS AND PROMISE OF DISABILITY STATISTICS

In its most rudimentary form, the operations of measurement are simple—assignment of a number to represent the presence or the magnitude of an attribute. The most elemental form is arguably the most common, as labels in nominal or ordinal representation of "disability." Thus, one has a disability or does not, or the magnitude of the disability is "mild," "moderate," or "severe." Less frequently implemented but still widely employed are scaled attribute measures on interval (quality of life) or ratio scales (number of functions, years "lost"). The act of quantification refines our manner and method of describing disablement. Numerical associations facilitate independent verification, standardization, and economy of communication. We need not detail the importance of these assignment operations here—these are fundamentals of measurement and empirical inquiry.

As overviewed in this presentation and discussed in greater depth in subsequent chapters, a disability studies perspective shifts the framework from the methodology of classification and measurement to more metaphorical constructions of personal experience and social and cultural context. Disability status is lodged in the interaction of the social and experiential with the physical or psychological. One does not readily operationalize, survey, and classify such phenomena. In fact, the concept of describing, measuring, and counting physical or mental impairment or functional limitation almost by definition lies outside the realm of disability studies (Gill and Longmore 1999).

Which is the truer model? To paraphrase the cartoon character Pogo, Walt Kelly's Okefenokee Swamp opossum philosopher, when you come to a crossroad, take it. In his narrative describing the reanalysis of the Burgess Shale fossils, Stephen Jay Gould (1989) describes the initial misclassification of ancient sea creatures by early twentieth-century paleontologists. Unable to readily classify bizarre 500-million-year-old, Cambrian-era life forms, they pigeonholed the findings into preexisting categories of worms and arthropods. The rediscovery and reanalysis of the fossils decades later revealed the remarkable diversity of early life forms and revised our view of evolution. In his reflections on the nature of description, classification, and science, Gould states, "The beauty of nature lies in detail; the message in generality. Optimal appreciation demands both" (p. 13).

Perhaps the better perspective on counting disability is to interpret measurement operations as imperfect proxies that capture only a fraction of the complex reality that is disablement. The sociologist Irving Zola (1993) challenged the very notion of disability as a condition into which one can be reliably classified. In Zola's analysis, the "fixity" of numbers is undermined by the inherent dynamism of disability status—changing because of temporality of health status, the importance of context in manifesting a limitation, and the vagaries of conflicting classification systems. Above all, Zola argued that disability is not a "thing" possessed by some and not by others but rather "a set of characteristics everyone shares to varying degrees and in varying forms and combinations" (p. 30). In short, the issue is recast from one of measurement methodology to one of the epistemology of the numbers. "It is time to reflect deeply on what they do and do not reveal, what they can tell us as well as what they could" (Zola 1993:31).

Rather than devoting the measurement debate to the search for the definitive or better scale of disability, we should accept the existence of multiple "conventions." A central purpose of this chapter is to disabuse the reader of the notion that disability statistics are the quantification of something singular and "real." By itself, the act of quantification does not impart a greater reality. The full measure of disability supersedes the capabilities of a structured statistical surveillance as currently constructed. Simply put, all the nuances of the disability experience are impossible to capture in a singular numerical index.

"You haven't told me yet," said Lady Nuttal, "what it is your fiancé does for a living."

"He's a statistician," replied Lamia, with an annoying sense of being on the defensive.

Lady Nuttal was obviously taken aback. It had not occurred to her that statisticians entered into normal social relationships. The species, she would have surmised, was perpetuated in some collateral manner, like mules.

"But Aunt Sara, it's a very interesting profession," said Lamia warmly.

"I don't doubt it," said her aunt, who obviously doubted it very much. "To express anything important in mere figures is so plainly impossible that there must be endless scope for well-paid advice on how to do it. But don't you think that life with a statistician would be rather, shall we say, humdrum?"

Lamia was silent. She felt reluctant to discuss the surprising depth of emotional possibility, which she had discovered below Edward's numerical veneer.

"It's not the figures themselves," she said finally. "It's what you do with them that matters." (K. A. C. Manderville, *The Undoing of Lamia Gurdleneck*)[1]

We must continue to continue to count, of course, for that is the nature of the beast, and numbers, however faulty, are necessary. It is equally important that we view these numbers with greater pragmatism. We must cease expecting from them a portrait of a reality they can only partly and imperfectly measure. Required as well is a degree of comfort with the inherent "messiness" of alternative conventions. Different conventions serve different purposes. The task is more appropriately framed as fitting the data to the question with the awareness of what Cook and Campbell (1979) labeled the "presumptive nature" of our observations and measurements.

It is in this spirit of approximation and reconstruction that we approach the challenge of disability statistics and treat statistics as a means rather than as an end—focus determined by function rather than the search for a better, truer count. Above all, counting disability is a "political arithmetic," used to galvanize awareness of the relationship between society and disablement. Therein lies the rapprochement of disability studies and the counting of disability.

NOTE

1. This quote is from Kendall and Stuart (1967), *The Advanced Theory of Statistics.*

REFERENCES

Al-Ansari, A. 1989. "Prevalence Estimates of Physical Disability in Bahrain: A Household Survey." *International Disability Studies* 11:21-24.

Australian Bureau of Health and Welfare. 1998. *Australia's Health: 1998: The 6th Biennial Health Report of the Australian Institute of Health and Welfare.* Canberra: Australian Institute of Health and Welfare.

Badley, E. M. 1987. "The ICIDH: Format, Application in Different Settings, and Distinction between Disability and Handicap." *International Disability Studies* 9:122-25.

Benson, V. and M. A. Marano. 1994. "Current Estimates from the National Health Interview Survey, 1993." *Vital Health Statistics* 10 (190). DHHS Pub. No. (PHS) 95-1518. Hyattsville, MD: National Center for Health Statistics.

Bickenbach, J. E., S. Chatterji, E. M. Badley, and T. B. Ustun. 1999. "Models of Disablement, Universalism and the International Classification of Impairments, Disabilities and Handicaps." *Social Science & Medicine* 48:1173-87.

Braddock, D., R. Hemp, S. Parish, and J. Westrich. 1998. *The State of the States in Developmental Disabilities.* 6th ed. Washington, DC: American Association on Mental Retardation.

Bureau of Statistics. 1990. "National Survey of the Handicapped: 1987." In *World Health Statistics Annual.* Geneva: World Health Organization.

Campbell-Brown, S. 1991. "Conceptualizing and Defining Disability." Pp. 1-14 in *Disability in the United States: A Portrait from National Data,* edited by S. Thompson-Hoffman and I. Fitzgerald Storck. New York: Springer.

Chamie, M. 1989. "Survey Design Strategies for the Study of Disability." *World Health Statistics Quarterly* 42:122-40.

———. 1990. "The Status and Use of the International Classification of Impairments, Disabilities and Handicaps (ICIDH)." *World Health Statistics Quarterly* 43:273-80.

———. 1995. "What Does Morbidity Have to Do with Disability?" *Disability and Rehabilitation* 17:323-37.

Cronbach, L. J. 1957. "The Two Disciplines of Scientific Psychology." *American Psychologist* 12:671-84.

Clark, G. N. 1972. "Social Science in the Age of Newton." Pp. 15-30 in *The Establishment of Empirical Sociology: Studies in Continuity, Discontinuity, and Institutionalization,* edited by A. Oberschall. New York: Harper & Row.

Cook, T. D. and D. T. Campbell. 1979. "Validity." Pp. 37-94 in *Quasi-Experimentation: Design and Analysis Issues for Field Settings,* edited by T. D. Cook and D. T. Campbell. Boston: Houghton Mifflin.

Department of Health. 1995. *Health Survey for England 1995.* London: Department of Health Statistics Division.

Department of Statistics. 1996. *The Accompanying Survey to the General Population and Household Census 1994: Methodology and results.* Amman: Hashemite Kingdom of Jordan, Department of Statistics, Public Relations.

Direccion General de Estadistica Encuestas y Censos. 1992. *Census Nacional de Poblacion y Viviendas* (The National Census of the Populatoion and Dwellings) [Online]. Available: www.dgeec.gov.py/cuadros/censo%201992/P03.xls.

Durkin, M. S., W. Wang, P. E. Shrout, S. S. Zaman, Z. M. Hasan, P. Desai, and L. L. Davidson. 1995. "Evaluating a Ten Questions Screen for Childhood Disability: Reliability and Internal Structure in Different Cultures." *Journal of Clinical Epidemiology* 48:657-66.

Edwards, S. D. 1997. "Dismantling the Disability/Handicap Distinction." *Journal of Medicine and Philosophy* 22:589-606.

Fougeyrollas, P. 1993. *Applications of the Concept of Handicap of the ICIDH and Its Nomenclature.* Strasbourg, France: Council of Europe.

Fujiura, G. T. 1998. "Demography of Family Households." *American Journal on Mental Retardation* 103:225-35.

Galton, Sir Francis. 1884. "Measurement of Character." *Fortnightly Review of London* 42:179-85. (Cited in L. D. Goodstein and R. I. Lanyon, eds., *Readings in Personality Assessment.* New York: John Wiley.)

Gill, C. and P. Longmore. 1999. *Examining the Impact on Postsecondary Students of Three Disability Studies Paradigms.* Chicago: University of Illinois at Chicago.

Gould, S. J. 1989. *Wonderful Life.* New York: Norton.

Hamilton, M. K. 1998. "The Health and Activity Limitation Survey." *Health Reports* 1:175-87.

Health and Welfare Bureau. 1995. "White Paper on Rehabilitation: Equal Opportunities and Full Participation." Hong Kong: Government Secretariat of the Government of the Hong Kong Special Administrative Region (HKSAR).

Health Research Board. 1997. *National Intellectual Disability Database: Annual Report of the National Intellectual Disability Database Committee, 1996.* Dublin, Ireland: Health Research Board.

Heller, K. 1971. "Laboratory Interview Research as Analogue to Treatment." Pp. 126-53 in *Handbook of Psychotherapy and Behavior Change,* edited by A. E. Bergin and S. L. Garfield. New York: John Wiley.

Howard-Wines, F. 1888. *Report on the Defective, Dependent, and Delinquent Classes of the Population of the United States, as Returned at the Tenth Census (June 1, 1880).* Washington, DC: Government Printing Office, Department of the Interior, Census Office.

Institute of Medicine (IOM). 1991. *Disability in America: A National Agenda for Prevention.* Washington, DC: National Academy Press.

Instituto Nacional De Estadistica Geografia e Informatica (INEGI). 1998. *Boletin Del Registro De Menores Con Discapacidad.* Mexico City: Direccion General de Estadistica.

Jamison, D. T. 1996. "Foreword." Pp. xv-xxiii in *The Global Burden of Disease,* Vol. 2, *Global Burden of Disease and Injury Series,* edited by C. J. L. Murray and A. D. Lopez. Cambridge, MA: Harvard University Press.

Jee, M. and Z. Or. 1998. *Health Outcomes in OECD Countries: A Framework of Health Indicators for Outcome-Oriented Policy Making.* Paris: Organization for Economic Cooperation and Development.

Kendall, M. G. and A. Stuart. 1967. *The Advanced Theory of Statistics.* Vol. 2. New York: Hafner.

Kiesler, D. J. 1966. "Experimental Designs in Psychotherapy Research." Pp. 36-74 in *Handbook of Psychotherapy and Behavior Change,* edited by A. E. Bergin and S. L. Garfield. New York: John Wiley.

Kita, M. W. 1992. "Morbidity and Disability." *Journal of Insurance Medicine* 24:268-74.

LaPlante, M. and D. Carlson. 1996. *Disability in the United States: Prevalence and Causes, 1992.* Disability Statistics Report No. 7. Washington, DC: U.S. Department of Education, National Institute on Disability and Rehabilitation Research.

Liming, L., C. Weihua, and X. Fujie. 1997. "Disability among the Elderly in China: Analysis of the National Sampling Survey of Disability in 1987." *Chinese Medical Journal* 110:236-37.

Mausner, J. S. and S. Kramer. 1985. *Epidemiology: An Introductory Text.* Philadelphia: W. B. Saunders.

McDowell, I. and C. Newell. 1996. *Measuring Health: A Guide to Rating Scales and Questionnaires.* New York: Oxford University Press.

McNeil, J. M. 1993. *Americans with Disabilities: 1991-92.* Washington, DC: U.S. Bureau of the Census, Current Population Reports, Government Printing Office.

———. 1997. *Americans with Disabilities: 1994-95.* Washington, DC: Current Population Reports, Government Printing Office.

McWhinnie, J. R. 1982. *Measuring Disability.* Paris: OECD Social Indicator Development Programme.

Ministry of Health and Social Security. 1993. *The Social Security Act.* Reykjavik, Iceland [Online]. Available: brunnur.stjr.is/interpro/htr/htr.nsf/pages/act-socialsecurity.html.

Ministry of Health and Welfare of Japan. 1997. *New Developments in Measures for People with Disabilities in Japan to Ensure the Realization of Normalization in the Community: Extraction from Annual Report on Health and Welfare, 1995-1996* [Online]. Available: www.mhw.go.jp/english/white_p.

Murray, C. J. L. 1996. "Rethinking DALYs." Pp. 1-98 in *The Global Burden of Disease*, Vol. 1, *Global Burden of Disease and Injury Series,* edited by C. J. L. Murray and A. D. Lopez. Cambridge, MA: Harvard University Press.

Murray, C. J. L. and A. D. Lopez. 1996. "Global and Regional Descriptive Epidemiology of Disability: Incidence, Prevalence, Health Expectancies and Years Lived with a Disability." Pp. 201-46 in *The Global Burden of Disease*, Vol. 1, *Global Burden of Disease and Injury Series,* edited by C. J. L. Murray and A. D. Lopez. Cambridge, MA: Harvard University Press.

Nagi, S. 1976. "An Epidemiology of Disability among Adults in the United States." *The Milbank Quarterly* 54:439-67.

———. 1991. "Disability Concepts Revisited: Implications for Prevention." Pp. 309-27 in *Disability in America: A National Agenda for Prevention,* edited by A. M. Pope and A. R. Tarlov. Washington, DC: National Academy Press.

National Center for Health Statistics. 1992. *Field Representative's Manual, HIS-100: National Health Interview Survey.* Hyattsville, MD: Author.

———. 1998. *Data File Documentation, National Health Interview Survey, 1996.* Hyattsville, MD: Author.

Oberschall, A. 1972. "The Sociological Study of the History of Social Research." Pp. 2-14 in *The Establishment of Empirical Sociology: Studies in Continuity, Discontinuity, and Institutionalization,* edited by A. Oberschall. New York: Harper & Row.

Palestinian Central Bureau of Statistics. 1996. *Palestine: The 1996 Health Survey of the West Bank.* Ramallah, Palestine: Health Statistics Department.

Rodriguez, P. G. 1989. "Using the International Classification of Impairments, Disabilities, and Handicaps in Surveys: The Case of Spain." *World Health Statistics Quarterly* 42:161-66.

Schwartz, S. and K. M. Carpenter. 1999. "The Right Answer for the Wrong Question: Consequences of Type III Error for Public Health Research." *American Journal of Public Health* 89:1175-80.

Shaffer, D., M. S. Gould, J. Brasic, P. Ambrosini, H. Bird, and S. Aluwahlia. 1983. "A Children's Global Assessment Scale." *Archives of General Psychiatry* 40:1228-31.

Simeonsson, R. J., J. Chen, and Y. Hu. 1995. "Functional Assessment of Chinese Children with the ABILITIES Index." *Disability and Rehabilitation* 17:400-10.

Social Trends Analysis Directorate. 1986. *Profile of Disabled Persons in Canada: 1983-1984.* Ottawa, Canada: Department of the Secretary of State.

Statistics New Zealand. 1998. *Disability Counts.* Wellington, New Zealand: Publishing and Community Information Division of Statistics New Zealand.

Suris, J. C. and R. W. Blum. 1993. "Disability Rates among Adolescents: An International Comparison." *Journal of Adolescent Health* 14:548-52.

Teutsch, S. M. 1994. "Considerations in Planning a Surveillance System." Pp. 19-30 in *Principles and Practices of Public Health Surveillance,* edited by S. M. Teutsch and R. E. Churchill. New York: Oxford University Press.

United Nations. 1982. *World Programme of Action Concerning Disabled Persons—United Nations Decade of Disabled Persons, 1982-1992.* New York: Author.

———. 1988. *United Nations Disability Statistics Database, 1975-86: Technical Manual.* New York: Author.

———. 1996. *Manual for the Development of Statistical Information for Disability Programmes and Policies.* New York: Statistics Division, Department for Economic and Social Information and Policy Analysis of the United Nations Secretariat.

United Nations Development Programme (UNDP). 1998. "Human Development Indicators." Pp. 125-217 in *Human Development Report 1998.* New York: Oxford University Press.

U.S. Bureau of the Census. 1991. *SIPP Users' Guide.* 2d ed. Washington, DC: Author.

World Health Organization (WHO). 1980. *International Classification of Impairments, Disabilities and Handicaps.* Geneva: Author.

———. 1990. "International Statistics on Causes of Disability." Pp. 39-96 in *World Health Statistics Annual 1990.* Geneva: Author.

———. 1999. *International Classification of Functioning and Disability.* Beta-2 draft. Geneva: Author.

Wright, J. D. 1988. "Survey Research and Social Policy." *Evaluation Review* 12:595-606.

Zola, I. K. 1993. "Disability Statistics, What We Count and What It Tells Us: A Personal and Political Analysis." *Journal of Disability Policy Studies* 4:9-39.

Disability Definitions, Models, Classification Schemes, and Applications

3

BARBARA M. ALTMAN

I t has been observed that there is no neutral language with which to discuss disability (Williams 1996; Zola 1993; Linton 1998), and yet the tainted language itself and the categories used influence the definition of the problem (Williams 1996). For that reason, the objective of this chapter—to define disability—is a daunting one. Thus, while reading this chapter, I ask that readers try to suspend their own preconceived notions of the meaning of the term *disability* to realize the commonalities and differences among and between definitions and the usefulness of this variety.

Part of the difficulty of defining disability has to do with the fact that disability is a complicated, multidimensional concept. Because of the extensive variety in the nature of the problem, a global definition of disability that fits all circumstances, though very desirable, is in reality nearly impossible (Slater et al. 1974). Attempts have been made to define disability with simple statements, theoretical models, classification schemes, and even through different forms of measurement. This has contributed to the confusion and misuse of disability terms and definitions, particularly when operationalized measures of disabilities are interpreted and used as definitions (Altman 1986, 1993). When trying to make sense of this variety of ideas and forms, it is necessary to take into consideration the structure, orientation, and source of the definitions, as well as the difference between simple single-purpose statements of definition, theoretical models that map the relationship of conceptual elements seen as part of the definition, and classifications schemes and other forms of translating the concepts into empirical measures. Identifying the variety of definitions and definitional forms and understanding the strengths and weaknesses of those forms as well as the purposes for which they can be useful are the objectives of this chapter.

This chapter reviews the kinds of intellectual and practical circumstances that create the need for definitions of disability. First it describes the current contexts in which definitions of disability are developed and used. Then it examines the concepts that make up a variety of theoretical definitions of disability, identifying similarities and differences between the various conceptualizations of the components of the definitions. This is followed by an examination of several commonly used models that combine these concepts into definitions of disability. The chapter then discusses the similarities and differences among the chosen models and presents some thoughts on the appropriateness of the various models in the expanding interest and research in this field. It concludes with an example of the definition of disability that results from an application of the various models.

AUTHOR'S NOTE: Work on this chapter was supported by the United States government and is in the public domain.

DEFINITIONS

Disability is an occurrence that has been described from numerous perspectives, including medical, economic, sociopolitical (Hahn 1985), and administrative (Blaxter 1976; Stone 1984). Sixteen years ago, Duckworth (1984) noted that in the context of health care, there is a need for consistent terminology relating to disease consequences or *disablement*, a term used to express the process of becoming disabled. Progress has been made along those lines, but there are still a variety of purposes for which the definition of this phenomenon is necessary and a number of theoretical and research approaches to the problem. The result is conflict, contradiction, and confusion among terms. The need for consistency or at least interpretability between terms persists and is necessary not only within the health context but also across other contexts. Such interpretability would ensure that communications between areas of research, social policy, and social structure are clear and unambiguous. The lack of consistency is most dramatic when a person is defined as disabled in one context and not another, such that she or he receives therapies for serious impairments but does not qualify for certain disability-related benefits provided by his or her employer or by the government. Definitions that have been developed for clinical circumstances and administrative implementation are those most commonly known among the total population and have had the greatest influence on our understanding of this phenomenon until recent years. Research definitions that are used to investigate the process, examine the experience, or identify the incidence and prevalence of disability in a population are a relatively new development compared to those used for purely administrative purposes.

Legal and Administrative Definitions

Programmatic Definitions

Whenever an idea has legal ramifications associated with responsibilities, duties, or benefits, the term is usually defined for the purposes of that particular circumstance by an administrative body. The administrative perspective suggests an emphasis on the individual and the categorization of the individual as a member or nonmember of the disabled class or category (Altman 1986). So we find in the United States, as an example, multiple legal definitions (U.S. Department of Health and Human Services [DHHS] 1990) of the concept of disability enacted by the Congress or by state legislatures. These definitions specify who will receive the benefits provided by the welfare or health policy legislation or who is subject to the civil rights protection that the law provides. The same is true for many other developed countries. While early legal definitions were associated with specific problems such as blindness, increased survival of persons with injuries as the result of wars or accidents and persons affected by serious epidemics such as polio or AIDS has influenced a broadening of definitions to encompass a much larger proportion of conditions and circumstances.

For programmatic administrative purposes, disability is usually defined as situations associated with injury, health, or physical conditions that create specific limitations that have lasted (or are expected to last) for a named period of time. Sometimes, there are additional qualifiers or conditions based on occupation (miners) or circumstances associated with the injury (occurred on the job) or in the performance of hazardous duties (active military, police, other risky occupations). As an example, the U.S. Social Security definition of disability requires that an applicant demonstrate

> the inability to engage in any substantial gainful activity by reason of any medically determinable physical or mental impairment which can be expected to result in death or has lasted or can be expected to last for a continuous period of not less than 12 months. DHHS 1990:5)

Of course, the actual process by which the Social Security Administration determines if an applicant meets this definition is significantly more complicated and, for Social Security disability benefits (Social Security Disability Insurance [SSDI]), includes a requirement that the individual had been employed and paying into the system for a specific period of time prior to the application for benefits.

Other legal definitions of disability vary widely, as dictated by their purpose—from the more narrowly defined definition of developmental disability,[1] which refers to a severe or chronic condition that is acquired before age 22, to the much broader conceptualization in the Americans with Disability Act (ADA).[2] The breadth of the content of the ADA definition is a notable exception to the more narrow definitions found in most of the benefits legislation. However, court cases that test the definitions of disability in ADA legislation continue to involve prominent testimony by physicians, thus emphasizing a medical perspective, and are frequently focused on narrowing that definition. A recent Supreme Court decision related to the ADA has demonstrated that tendency to narrow the definition of disability when it rejected attempts to extend job discrimination protection to persons with conditions that are ameliorated by medication or appliances. In these most recent cases, conditions included hypertension and vision loss (Biskupic 1999).

Public Health

More recently, governments have also been taking an interest in being able to predict the size and nature of the population with disabilities, as well as the epidemiology, to further refine or change benefit programs and understand the disablement process from a public health standpoint. These definitions are similar to those described by Albrecht and Verbrugge (2000) as statistical definitions and are based on survey or census data of the national population. Organizations such as the World Health Organization (WHO) and the World Bank, having recognized the burden of disability in the world—particularly developing countries—and the implications this has on economic development and human rights, have played an active role in developing ways to measure this problem (Albrecht and Verbrugge 2000). As a result of the work commissioned by these two leading international organizations, a composite measure known as disability-adjusted life years (DALYs) was developed for use as a health outcome measure to provide a basis for comparisons across multiple national populations (Murray and Lopez 1996). As an alternative to measures based on mortality, this measure seeks to incorporate nonfatal health outcomes to quantify the effect of what is identified as the "burden" of disease in a way that could be used for cost-effectiveness analysis. Another purpose of the measure is to decouple the epidemiological assessment from advocacy so that estimates are objective and divorced from proposals for policy change.

The measure is calculated by a sum of years of life lost from premature mortality plus years of life with disability that has been adjusted for the severity of disability. A number of versions of calculations for this measure include a weighting process to represent the severity of the disability. The goal is to provide a set of weights for the treated and untreated forms of several hundred outcomes (Murray and Lopez 1996). Definition of disability from this perspective is associated with selected diagnosed chronic conditions or injuries and the accompanying limitations in function based on the conceptualization of disability in the *International Classification of Impairment Disability and Handicap (ICIDH,* discussed below). However, the definition of disability is only a starting point since the measure is time based (years lived with disability) and incorporates judgments about the value of time spent in different health states.

Clinical Definitions

Clinical definitions have their basis in the authority that is attached to medicine and carried out by medical specialists. As such, the clinical category, as named and documented by the medical provider, becomes the label and legitimization required to qualify a patient for rehabilitation, education, or welfare programs. Clinical definitions are associated with the pathology that medical practitioners identify within the individual and the prognosis that the practitioner expects relative to the type of condition and the characteristics of the patient.

The Committee on the Rating of Mental and Physical Impairment of the American Medical Association authorized the publication of a series of guides to evaluate permanent impairment and disability beginning in 1958. These guides make the point of differentiating between permanent impairment and permanent disability and are also very concerned with the scope of responsibility of the medical professional for that evaluation, although no specification of that responsibility is described in the guides. A patient's *permanent disability*, which is how the term is presented in these guides, is defined as "not a purely medical condition . . . but when his [the patient] actual or presumed ability to engage in gainful activity is reduced or absent because of 'impairment' which in turn may or may not be combined with other factors" (Engelbert 1988:104). These guidelines provide evaluation ratings of permanent *impairment* that are interpreted within the purview of physicians alone since they are seen as uniquely competent to perform such a judgment of function. The guidelines point out that evaluation of permanent disability, in the last analysis, is an administrative as well as a medical function, and since the evaluation of permanent disability is an appraisal of the patient's present and future ability to engage in gainful activity (probably referring to employment), the emphasis is put on evaluating permanent impairment. The guidelines are provided in publications of the American Medical Association and are based on specific body systems such as the digestive system or the urinary system. While physicians are discouraged from making evaluations of permanent disabilities, these guidelines provide a method of evaluation of permanent impairment on which most administrative definitions rely extensively.

Scholarly Research Definitions

Scholarly academic and research definitions attempt to provide a conceptual framework with which to approach the complete phenomena of disability regardless of age, gender, race, and other social characteristics. While there is still the impetus to create a dichotomy between persons identified as having a disability and those who do not, the scholarly research approach is not predicated on the need to identify persons for either clinical or administrative purposes as either-or. Within the research perspective, there is recognition of the idea of disability as a continuum rather than an absolute, as first proposed by Zola (1989). The nature of that continuum is currently being developed through some of the conceptualization, modeling, and operationalization of disability measures currently taking place (Bickenbach et al. 1999; Altman and Barnartt 2000).

Unlike administrative definitions of disability, research approaches to the definition of disability are much more cognizant of the multiple factors involved in the relationship between health, functioning, context, and the dynamics of conditions that go into the process that is ultimately labeled as disability. As with the definition of health, which Kelman (1975) has pointed out is the "most perplexing and ambiguous issue in the study of health," this is equally true for the definition of disability, which bridges the space between "health" and the context of health. "Disability," if envisioned as Kelman (1975) envisions "health," is no less a social construct than "health" and is not an intrinsic condition of the individual. The remainder of this chapter will examine the research approaches to this conceptualization of "disability" and the structure of those conceptualizations along with their uses, strengths, and limitations.

CONCEPTS, MODELS, AND MEASURES

Most of the definitions of disability frequently found in scholarly research are actually models made up of several concepts that have either directed or reciprocal relationships with one another. Concepts serve as components or building blocks of definitions, models, and theories and are therefore critical elements of explanation and prediction. Concepts can serve a number of important functions. They are the foundations of communication or symbols of the phenomena under investigation (Frankfort-Nachmias and Nachmias 1992), which introduce the perspective or way of looking at some aspect of reality. Of particular interest in understanding the variety of different ways to explain the meaning of disability is the definition of the concepts used in creating those meanings and the subtleties of differences in those definitions. It should be noted that conceptual definitions are neither true nor false (Frankfort-Nachmias and Nachmias 1992) but are the explanations of the symbols or communications of the researcher, scientist, or person creating them. Concepts, as reflected in their definitions, are either understandable or not, useful or not, or used consistently or not. As a first step in understanding the various approaches to disability definitions, I will compare the meanings of the various conceptual components associated with the definitions of disability found in models currently used for research.

As a second step, I will examine the similarities and differences among several models used to explain the multidimensional aspects of disability. I will discuss the definition of disability that these models convey, and, using a specific empirical example, I will describe the usefulness of the various models to understand the example. Though there have been many conceptual models of disability put forth, space restraints require that I concentrate on just a few. Those I have chosen to include are Nagi's (1965, 1969, 1991) model; Verbrugge and Jette's (1993) model; the two versions of the World Health Organization model associated with the *International Classification of Impairment, Disability and Handicap* (WHO 1980, 1999); the two models produced by the Institute of Medicine at the National Institute of Medicine (Brandt and Pope 1997; Pope and Tarlov 1991), known as the IOM models; and the social model proposed by disability theorists in Great Britain (Abberley 1987; Oliver 1990, 1993, 1996). If space allowed, other thoughtful models would have been interesting to examine as well, including another contemporary general model, the Quebec model (see Fougeyrollas and Beauregard's chapter, this volume), and more limited earlier models proposed by Suchman (1965), Wan (1974), Altman (1984), the National Center for Medical Rehabilitation Research (1993), and Johnson and Wolinsky (1993), among others.

The usefulness of concepts and conceptual models or frameworks is ultimately to be found in their translation into empirical observation. To accomplish that translation, one needs to convert the concept through a procedure, either observational or through inquiry, which establishes the empirical existence of the concept in question. Such a set of procedures is known as an operational definition and creates the link between the concept and the real world. They tell "what to do" and "what to observe" to identify a circumstance that has been a priori decided; this would represent an example of the concrete indication of the abstract meaning of the concept (Frankfort-Nachmias and Nachmias 1992). So, for example, if wheelchair use were accepted as an indicator of the concept of disability, then a question asking about the use of a wheelchair would become a measure of disability in this instance. Though space does not allow the full exploration of this process of converting the conceptual definitions into measurable qualities, in the subsequent section on application, I will examine how the concepts and models of disability relate to an actual example. To understand the relationships to be explored in this chapter, I indicate in Figure 3.1 the transition from the conceptual to observational level.

BASIC CONCEPTUAL COMPONENTS

Frequently, models use the same terminology but ascribe a different meaning to the terms. To understand the different shades of meaning that various models develop, one must start at the concept level to see how the ideas are similar or different across conceptualizations regardless of terminology. To follow the discussion of the various uses of the terms, I have provided Tables

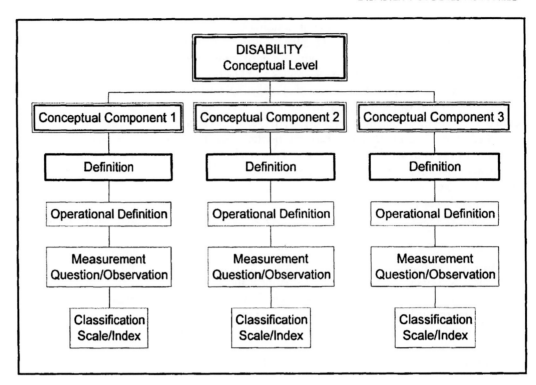

Figure 3.1.   Transition from the Conceptual to the Observational Level

3.1 and 3.2 to serve as a guide to the discussion. When definitions of terms are different enough to affect the meaning of the concept, a unique identifier has been attached to the term, so that the reader can identify with which conceptual model that term is associated. Therefore, the term *disability* has five separate identifiers in the tables and in the following discussion. For example, the first mention of disability is identified as *disability (A)* and represents the meaning of the term as used in the second component of the social model.

First Components

Pathology or some concept close to it is the starting point for most, but not all, of the conceptual models of disability included here. Nagi (1965) begins his model of disability[3] with a discussion of active pathology, which refers to the state of mobilization of the body's defenses against a condition associated with infection, traumatic injury, or some other etiology. In all his discussions (Nagi 1965, 1977, 1991), pathology represents an interruption in normal body processes while the body attempts to restore that normal state. Its association with disease as well as traumatic injury and other etiologies is discussed as part of the definition, but its relationship to diagnoses is not spelled out.

Pathology in the Verbrugge and Jette (1993) model of disability refers very specifically to biochemical and physiological abnormalities that are detected *and* medically labeled as disease, injury, or congenital or developmental conditions. These authors note that many of the bodily changes represented by pathology are not always directly measurable in medical practice where detection relies on evaluation of manifest signs and symptoms. Their perspective requires a diagnosis since it represents a pathology that has satisfied clinical significance and can therefore be considered public. Undiagnosed pathologies would not be included in this version of the concept.

The Institute of Medicine (IOM) models are prefaced on the Nagi model and include a similar definition of the meaning of pathology as proposed by Nagi. However, the first IOM group

Table 3.1 Names of Conceptual Components of Theoretical Definitions of Disability Included in This Analysis

	First Component	Second Component	Third Component	Fourth Component	Fifth Component
Nagi model	Pathology	Impairment	Functional limitation	Disability (C)	—
Verbrugge and Jette model	Pathology/disease	Impairment	Functional limitation	Disability (D)	—
IOM-1 model	Pathology	Impairment	Functional limitation	Disability (E)	—
IOM-2 model	Pathology	Impairment	Functional limitation	Disability (E)	—
ICIDH-1 model	Disease and disorders	Impairment	Disability (B)	Handicap	—
ICIDH-2 model	Health context	Body function/body structures/impairment	Activity/activity limitation	Participation/participation limitation	Context: environmental and personal
Social model	Impairment	Disability (A)	—	—	—

Table 3.2 Variety of Meanings Given the Term *Disability* in Five Theoretical Models

	Disability (A)	Disability (B)	Disability (C)	Disability (D)	Disability (E)
Model	Social model	ICIDH-1 model	Nagi model	Verbrugge and Jette model	IOM-1 and IOM-2 models
Definition	Limit or loss of opportunities to take part in community life because of physical and social barriers	In the context of health experience, any restriction or lack (resulting from an impairment) of ability to perform an activity in the manner or within the range considered normal for a human being	Pattern of behavior that evolves in situations of long-term or continued impairments that are associated with functional limitations	Disability is experiencing difficulty doing activities in any domain of life due to a health or physical problem	The expression of a physical or mental limitation in a social context —the gap between a person's capabilities and the demands of the environment

to work on defining disability was empaneled to address issues of preventing potentially disabling conditions from developing into disability and on minimizing the effects of such conditions on a person's productivity and quality of life (Pope and Tarlov 1991). With such a mandate, their perspective included an approach that also examined and discussed risk factors that can lead to pathology. These have not been included in this examination.

The original WHO model used a slightly different concept, *disease,* to represent the medical model that is depicted as etiology, pathology, and manifestation. Noting that the medical model is incomplete because it does not include the consequences of disease, the WHO (1980) proposed as the precondition of a model of disability a pathological state that is "exteriorized" —that is, the pathology is evident to the individual or to those around him or her. This "exteriorized" (but not necessarily diagnosed) pathology or awareness of illness leads to the recognition of the impairments or abnormalities of body structure or appearance that serve as the basis for most models of disability.

In the second WHO model, *ICIDH-2*, the concept of disorder and disease has been included in the model as subsumed under the context of health. It has been redefined to avoid misinterpretations that were induced by the 1980 WHO model. No definition of disorder and disease is included in the elaboration of the components or concepts that make up the new model (WHO 1998, 1999). A recent version of this model is framed "in the context of a health condition," although health condition is not defined as a concept either (WHO 1998, 1999). However, in examples provided in one publication (WHO 1998), diagnosed health conditions, along with their considered impairment, activity limitation, and participation restriction, are provided (health condition—leprosy; impairment—loss of sensation of extremities; activity limitation—grasping difficulties; participation restriction—denied employment because of stigma).

The social model of disability is oriented to societal oppression as the source of the experience of disability (Abberley 1987; Bury 1996; Oliver 1990). While disease or pathology is seen as the causal precedent for disability in the other models, the authors of the social model interpret the cause of disability as residing within the social structure and its treatment and control of the individual; neither the concept of pathology nor disease is seen to have a place in this model (Abberley 1987; Oliver 1990, 1996). Instead, the first identified component of this model is *impairment*. Impairments, as defined by the Disabled People's International, "is the functional limitation within the individual caused by physical, mental or sensory impairment" (Oliver 1996:41). The tautology of such a definition is immediately recognizable in the fact that the definition includes the term being defined. Probably, the earlier definition—"lacking part of or all of a limb or having a defective limb, organism or mechanism of the body"—also put forth by Oliver (1990) should also be included, although the exact meaning of *organism* in this context is not clear.

Second Components

Impairment is defined as anatomical or physiological abnormalities and losses in the initial Nagi (1965) formulation. While he acknowledged that such abnormalities can also be reflections of an active pathology, he made a distinction by also including abnormalities and losses associated with residuals of pathology, that is, abnormalities and losses that remain after an active pathology has been arrested or eliminated. In this way, he accounted for paralysis remaining after a disease such as polio has been neutralized or organ deficiencies that remain after multiple flare-ups of lupus have damaged such organs. In further elaboration of his model, Nagi (1977, 1991) specifically included abnormalities, such as congenital deformities, which are not necessarily associated with a pathology. He noted that impairments can vary among a number of dimensions that can influence the nature and degree of disability observed (Nagi 1977, 1991). These dimensions include

> degree of visibility and disfigurement, stigma, the predictability of the underlying pathology, the prognosis and prospects for recovery or stabilization, threat to life, types and severity of limitations in function they impose and the point of onset in the life cycle. (Nagi 1991:314)

It should be pointed out that except for references to severity, these are very important characteristics of impairment that are not included in descriptions of this term in other models.

For Verbrugge and Jette (1993), "*impairments* are dysfunctions and significant structural abnormalities in specific body systems" (p. 3). "Significant" is used to indicate that the abnormality can have consequences for physical, mental, or social functioning. The authors also specify that the impairment can occur not only in the primary locale of the pathology but also in secondary locales, immediately or on a delayed basis. So, for example, a hip injury can impair a person's ability to walk, but continued walking on such a damaged hip can also have an effect on the functioning of the person's lower back muscles. Impairments are identified via medical procedures, including exams, laboratory tests, imaging, and the patient's medical histories and reports of symptoms. This latter method is an extension of their original concept of the necessity of diagnosis as a precondition for pathology. As in the first WHO model, this emphasis on diagnosis or "exteriorization" implies a need for legitimation from the medical profession, which is a central element of the administrative definition discussed earlier. From this perspective, self-reports are questionable and effects from new conditions, such as chronic fatigue syndrome, fibromyalgia, or Gulf War syndrome, are invalid until such conditions are identified and accepted by the medical system.

In the first IOM model, *impairment* is defined as a discrete loss or abnormality of mental, physical, or biochemical function, including losses caused by all forms of pathology (Pope and Tarlov 1991). Specific impairments may have different etiologies and different types of pathologies. Impairments include anomalies, defects, or losses that relate to the specific functioning of an organ or organ system but not the organism or person as a whole. The severity of impairment is seen to vary by the condition, by the tissues and organs affected, and by the extent to which they have been damaged. The definition of impairment is not changed between the two IOM models (Brandt and Pope 1997).

In the introduction to the first *ICIDH* system, WHO (1980) defined *impairment* as "any loss or abnormality of psychological, physiological or anatomical structure or function" (p. 27). This was qualified as within the context of a health experience. Two points are made in relation to this definition. First, the term *impairment* is interpreted to be more inclusive than disorder, and, second, to resolve boundary distinctions that lacked clarity in earlier versions, *functional limitations* were included with impairments. This means that something like an arthritic shoulder joint with restricted range of motion would be considered as an impairment, along with the inability to reach overhead caused by the impaired joint. Impairment, which could be permanent or temporary, was seen as representing deviation from some norm in the person's biomedical status.[4] It was not contingent on etiology (i.e., how it was caused) but included an anomaly, defect, or loss in a limb, organ, tissue, or other body structure or the defect in a functional system or body mechanism, including systems of mental functioning. Use of the term *impairment* did not necessarily indicate that a disease is present or that the person should be regarded as sick.

The concept of *impairments* from the first WHO model is identified as "body function and structure" in the second WHO model, *ICIDH-2,* and described as "problems in body function or structure as a significant deviation or loss" (WHO 1999:16). The emphasis in the definition is that this dimension refers to the body, although the indication is that *body* refers to the whole human organism, including the brain and its functions. Limitations in certain functions such as the inability to carry out a basic function of the body or body part, a concept that was included in 1980 within impairments, is still included in the new version. Reference to the impairment as a deviation from "generally accepted population standards" in the biomedical status of the body and its functions is more clearly expressed in this version. Definition of those "standards" is to be arbitrated by "those qualified to judge physical and mental functioning according to generally accepted standard" (WHO 1999:16). The implication is that such judgments are carried out by professionals, are outside the person's own experience with the impairment, and are based on a group standard rather than the person's capabilities prior to the impairment.

The second component of the social model is identified as *disability (A).* The definition of *disability (A)* is based on the Disabled Peoples' International definition, which interprets it as "the loss or limitation of opportunities to take part in the normal life of the community on an equal level with others due to physical and social barriers" (Oliver 1996:56). It is not clear if *disability (A)* is a singular, primary role resulting from the oppression that ultimately curtails any other role opportunities, or if multiple roles are considered available and all or most are circumscribed by the oppressive reaction of the society. Clearly, the emphasis is almost totally on the society as the regulator of the individual's access and, in that way, has a similarity to the original WHO conception of handicap, which will be discussed below. The earlier definition of *disability (A)*, offered by Oliver (1990), conceptualized it as "the disadvantage or restriction of activity caused by a contemporary social organization which takes little or no account of people who have physical impairments and thus excludes them from the mainstream of social activities" (p. 80). The change in definition within this model demonstrates the evolution of the conceptualization of *disability (A)* as being separate from impairment since the newer definition does not refer to any type of impairment or limitation as was done in the earlier one.

Third Components

The concept of *functional limitations* as a separate element is not common to all conceptual models of disability. Nagi (1965) initially identified functional limitations as the restrictions that impairments set on the individual's ability to perform the tasks and obligations of his or her usual roles and normal daily activities. These include tasks associated with family roles, such as taking care of a child; work roles, such as holding down a job; community roles, such as participation in church or club activities; and roles in other interactional settings as well as activities or tasks associated with self-care. The degree of limitation is seen not only as a function of the impairment but also involves the requirements of the specific roles and activities. Though Nagi does not say it specifically, the implication is that the functional limitation is observable when an individual is involved in purposeful activity associated with roles rather than in the situation when a function is being tested. An example of the latter is an orthopedic surgeon flexing a patient's knee or hip to observe the rotation or movement to ascertain the joint "range of function" associated with an impairment of the joint, whereas an example of the former is the actual distance that a person is able to walk or run within her or his responsibilities of caring for a child. If the person did not have to care for the child, the functional limitation may not be obvious. It was further recognized that not every impairment results in a functional limitation, and functional limitations may result for reasons other than impairments. In the latter case, an example is technological unemployment, which is caused by changes that occur in the work role requirements and are associated with lack of training or changes in expectations rather than lack of ability.

Nagi (1977) clarified this concept of the nature of limitation in other papers. He referred to functional limitations as the most direct way impairments contribute to disability and noted that functional limitations might be grouped into four categories: physical, emotional, intellectual, and sensory. Another way of understanding this conceptualization would be to consider functioning that is common across roles, so that purposeful mobility and communication are functions that involve the whole person and are necessary to carry on many roles. Examples used in all the Nagi papers also clarify the interpretation of this concept. They included being unable to reach overhead or an inability to lift a heavy weight (Melvin and Nagi 1970; Nagi 1965, 1991).

While Verbrugge and Jette (1993) introduced a definition of *functional limitations* very similar to Nagi—"restrictions in performing fundamental physical and mental actions used in daily life by one's age-sex group"—their elaborations were more extensive. They made the point that these are "generic actions [required] in many specific circumstances" (Verbrugge and Jette 1993:3). In all, they defined functional limitations in terms of the physical and mental actions that are required for an individual to interact with their social and physical environment, including overall mobility; discrete motions and strengths; trouble seeing, hearing, or communicating; and more general examples. They were more specific about the mental functions to be considered than was Nagi and include such things as short-term memory, intelligible speech, orientation in time and space, and positive affect. In addition, Verbrugge and Jette identified ways of getting these data from self or proxy reports to observer- or equipment-based evaluations, which include indications of whether the activity is accomplished with or without assistive devices. They were more concerned with a *task* orientation toward the limitation than to a *role* orientation.

The definition in the IOM original model was very brief. It defined *functional limitation* as "the term proposed by Nagi to describe effects manifested in the performance or performance capacity of the person as a whole" (Pope and Tarlov 1991:80). It also reminded the reader that the same type of functional limitation, such as the example of the inability to lift a 25-pound box and carry it 25 feet, can be caused by multiple forms of impairment but that not all impairments result in a functional limitation. The second version of the IOM model made no adjustments to the definition of functional limitation used in the first version (Brandt and Pope 1997).

The WHO model did not incorporate functional limitations as one of its defined concepts, but the actions referred to in examples of functional limitations in the models discussed above are present in the WHO model as the concept of *disability (B)*. Specifically, as noted above, the WHO (1980:27) model makes reference to including functional limitations with impairments. It appears that the use of the idea "of anatomical structure *or function*" and the reference to "*functional system or mechanism*" in the discussion of impairment is meant to encompass functional limitations at the system level rather than at the person level. As an example of this perspective, the *ICIDH-1* classification of "impairment category, language impairments" includes two entries under the category "severe impairment of communication": (1) severe functional impairment of communication and (2) impairment of higher centers for speech with inability to communicate (WHO 1980:68). However, other types of functioning at the individual level, which Nagi emphasizes (1965, 1991), are included in the *disability (B)* segment of the *ICIDH* classification scheme in 1980.[5]

Activity/activity limitations are the terms used as the third component in the second WHO model, *ICIDH-2*. This new model component, which was previously referred to as disabilities, is now focused on *activities* or the "performance of a task or action by an individual" (WHO 1999).

In the original WHO model, the conceptualization of the exact limits in functioning appeared to be split between the "impairment" section and what was identified as the "disability (B)" section of the classification scheme. What was once the impairment section, now identified as body function and structure, contains two segments—the impairment of function and the impairment of structure—which are representative of impairment at the mechanism level as opposed to the whole persons. The changes have gone a long way toward removing the overlap between the two conceptualizations, substantially improving the classification scheme. For example, in Chapter 7, "Neuromusculoskeletal and Movement Related Functions," there is a category under "functions of joints and bones," identified as "mobility of a single joint" (WHO 1999:80). This can be elaborated on by referring to the structure section, which would allow the researcher to identify the essential limb or part thereof associated with the mobility pattern. If the mobility problem is located in a leg, for example, then under the renamed activity section, the previously identified impairment in function or structure can or cannot be indicated to be associated with the activity of walking at the level of the person.

This new term that has been introduced to replace *disability (B)* in the WHO model, *ICIDH-2*, is defined as "the performance of a task or action by an individual" (WHO 1999:18). Specifically, the activity dimension is seen to represent the integrated use of body functions in a purposeful way to perform the individual's life tasks. The A code, which represents the classification of activity, is depicted as a neutral list of activities that deals with actual performance or execution of a task or activity. The emphasis is on the objectification or actual limitation or performance that can be observed in everyday life. These activities can include simple or basic physical functions of the person as a whole or more complex functions that require coordination of physical and mental capacities. The complexity of some of the activities, as illustrated in the classification scheme, appear to move beyond Nagi's meaning and begins to overlap with role activities such as the section of the *ICIDH-2* that applies to "moving around using transportation" (WHO 1999:116). An activity limitation, then, is a difficulty in driving a motorized vehicle in *all* the ways that engaging in that activity might be affected (i.e., not in the manner expected) (WHO 1999:18). The discussion indicates that activity is concerned with the performance of the task, while the participation dimension addresses involvement of the individual in a life area, particularly whether involvement is restricted or facilitated (WHO 1999:19). This approach organizes the concept of role and role behavior used in the Nagi and IOM perspectives into two parts: the tasks involved in the role and inclusion or exclusion in the role environment, assuming that the parts can be separated.

The social model does not contain a third, fourth, or fifth component.

Fourth Components

Except for one model, the fourth components are the outcome terms and the crux of the models that are developed from these concepts. They are also the conceptual components on which there is the most contention. In his original conceptualization of the meaning of the term, Nagi (1965) saw *disability (C)* as a "pattern of behavior that evolves in situations of long-term or continued impairments that are associated with functional limitations" (p. 103). The conception of behavior differs from performance in that behavior connotes a particular manner in which one conducts or manages himself or herself, while performance refers to the actual execution or accomplishment of a task and possibly the effectiveness with which the action is done. Nagi differentiates *disability (C)* from illness in the case when the impairment that limits the person's functioning is not associated with the presence of a disease, but he also notes that *disability (C)* and illness can overlap.

The patterns of behavior associated with *disability (C)* are influenced by the characteristics of the impairments, which include the degree of limitations imposed and the potential for rehabilitation, as well as individual's definition of the situation and his or her reactions, which are also largely influenced by the definition of the situation by others' reactions and expectations (Nagi 1965). This definition of the influences on behavior patterns is elaborated in Nagi's (1965) presentation in a discussion of roles and role behavior. Referring to Gross, Mason, and McEachern (1958), he discusses role definitions that are normative and others that are interactive and differentiates between systems that include a status or position for the ill or disabled and systems that do not. Systems that include a status or position for the ill or disabled are hospitals and rehabilitation organizations that have a specific role and role behavior expectations for the patient or client. When a role system does not have a status or position for a person who is ill or disabled,[6] such as the role of mother, the nature of the behavior that occurs would result from the reciprocal nature of interactions in the role and would evolve on the basis of ongoing interactions. So, a mother with mobility limitations would adapt her behavior to accommodate both functional limitations and role expectations in various ways, depending on the number of children, their ages, and their specific needs; the types of assistance the mother has available; and the mother's understanding of what aspects are important about the role. Disability conceptualized in terms of behavior is not a stagnant, singular action but a dynamic process that evolves in the context of role interactions.

In one revisit to these concepts, Nagi (1981) clarifies the social nature of *disability (C)* and reinforces the essential interpretation in terms of *roles*, identifying them as organized spheres of life activities and noting that they include self-care, education, family relations, other interpersonal relations, recreation, economic life, and employment or vocational concerns. In another revisit to the topic, he elaborates on the earlier definition, explaining that disability is "an inability or limitation in performing socially defined roles and tasks expected of an individual within a sociocultural and physical environment" (Nagi 1991:315). He also places more emphasis on environmental factors by replacing the first characteristic of the behavior noted in 1965 with the following: "characteristics of the environment and the degree to which it is free from, or encumbered with physical and sociocultural barriers" (Nagi 1991:315). *Disability (C)*, as its conceptualization by Nagi has evolved, is the behavior developed within the physical and social context interaction by the individual, based on personality and functional limitation, and it is associated with role opportunities.

The definition of *disability (D)* in Verbrugge and Jette's (1993) model is somewhat simpler: "Disability is experienced difficulty doing activities in any domain of life due to a health or physical problem" (p. 4). Though the Nagi perspective on the interactive or dynamic quality of *disability (C)* is not mentioned, it is also not precluded by this definition. An interesting addition to this conceptualization is the specification of a comprehensive view of individual activity that is taken from earlier work by Verbrugge (1990), which includes all domains of human activity from self-care to leisure activities. Domains organize tasks and actions in a somewhat different manner than roles. They do not allow for the fact that the same task may be performed differently based on which role the individual is playing when doing that task. So, for example, the process of cooking dinner as carried out within the family role can be different from the process of cooking dinner when one is participating in a group function and the individual is performing as a group member or when one is cooking in the role of chef as part of a job.

The original IOM model defined *disability (E)* as "the expression of a physical or mental limitation in a social context—the gap between a person's capabilities and the demands of the environment" (Pope and Tarlov 1991:81). While that sounds restrictive in that a person has only certain capabilities but the environment has specific (unamenable) demands, the discussion goes on to indicate the interactive nature of the physical or mental limitations with social and environmental factors that determines whether there is a disability. The concepts of role and task are introduced as well, with the indication that roles are made up of many tasks that are specific physical and mental actions through which the individual interacts with the social and physical world (Pope and Tarlov 1991:82). While the second IOM model does not specifically change the conceptual definition of disability, it does revise its positioning and interpretation in the model itself (Brandt and Pope 1997:69). This change will be discussed below in the explanation of the total model.

Handicap is the fourth component in the first WHO model. This component attempted to classify the outcomes of disease and impairment and, in so doing, moved away from the interactive nature of a role perspective to focus on the "disadvantage experienced by the individual as a result of impairments and *disabilities (B)*" (WHO 1980:14). The exact definition of this concept is recorded as the following:

> In the context of health experiences, a handicap is a disadvantage for a given individual, resulting from an impairment or a disability, that limits or prevents the fulfillment of a role that is normal (depending on age, sex, and social and cultural factors) for that individual. (WHO 1980:14)

While this definition acknowledged that handicap is a social phenomenon and is moderated by the expectations of the particular group of which the individual is a member, the focus was on the *"disadvantage to the individual* that stems from the impairment or *disability (B)*" (WHO 1980:29). This disadvantage was seen as a discordance between an individual's performance and the expectations of the group, imposed by the group and arising despite the individual's intentions. As a departure from a group norm, it was also seen to have a value either by the individual or the group. The value is dependent on cultural norms and so may change from group to group, over time and by type of role. The understanding of the deviation from a norm can be based on several approaches, including a purely statistical conception of normal; some ideal, such as body height or weight; an arbitrary criterion specified for nonquantifiable characteristics, such as the necessity to produce human speech rather than using a synthesized voice; or norms determined by social reactions that indicate either the individual or the group perceives that there is a problem.

The emphasis in the categorization of *handicap,* as it was proposed in the original WHO model, is limited to disadvantages associated with activities that are related to existence and survival, and the classification scheme identifies six dimensions (WHO 1980:39). The modelers recognized that survival roles do not exhaust the dimensions of handicap but found that higher needs are more difficult to measure and categorize in any mutually exclusive and hierarchical way. Since survival is the most important in any hierarchical scheme, they chose to limit the third classification to the basic need for orientation, independence, mobility, occupation, social integration, and economic sufficiency.

The fourth component is reconceptualized as *participation* in the second WHO model, *ICIDH-2. Participation* in the *ICIDH-2* is defined as "an individual's involvement in life situations in relation to health conditions, body functions and structures, activities and contextual factors" (WHO 1999:19). The *participation* classification does not focus on disadvantage but allows the individual to be rated on a point scale that ranges from 0 (*not restricted*) to 5 (*complete restriction*) (WHO 1999:141). An examination of the classification elements of participation indicates the complexity of this component and includes a discussion of how to avoid confusion between items in the classification of participation and in the classification of activities. Participation involves judgment about the extent to which a person with an activity limitation is involved in some area of human life as compared with the involvement of a person without an activity limitation. Rather than interpret this participation in terms of roles, role interaction, and other features of role-playing, participation is seen as involvement that can mean being included or engaged in an area or being accepted or having access to needed resources. The mechanism of this "involvement," via role socialization and interpersonal interaction or some other mechanism, is not seen as part of the elaboration of the relationships between the concepts necessary to understand the model. However, capacity to interact in relationships is seen as one part of the dimension of activity, and the dimension of participation includes both involvement in the exchange of information and participation in social relationships as separate components.

Fifth Component

Only one of the models contains a fifth component, the second WHO model, *ICIDH-2*. That component is identified as *contextual factors* that represent the complete background of an individual's life. Contextual factors are made up of personal factors, reflecting an individual's background, and environmental factors represented by the physical and material features of the person's environment, the available formal and informal social structures and services in the community, and the overarching systems established in a culture. Personal factors are not classified in the *ICIDH-2*, but environmental factors are organized in the classification and include individual environments (including home, workplace, and school), service systems available in the community, and cultural systems (including laws as well as attitudes).

Discussion of Concepts

An identification of the most pronounced differences in these conceptualizations is noticeable in three areas:

> In some instances, the same term is used to represent several different concepts (see the use of disability A, B, C, D, and E).
> Models vary in the number of conceptual elements and in the unit of analysis.
> The conceptualization involves how difficulties in functioning are perceived and the use of positive language.

The greatest difference is noted between the individually oriented models and the social model, which examines disability from a macro level, beginning with disabled people as a group rather than a collection of individuals. More subtle differences can also be observed among those conceptualizations that profess to be based on the Nagi model. While there are notable similarities, particularly in definitions of pathology, impairment, and functional limitations, the definitions of disability outcomes show some variety. The Verbrugge and Jette (1993) model moves away from the conception of roles to domains that are more generalized and occasionally cut across roles. The second IOM model also pays less attention to behavior and introduces new nuances with the interaction of individual and environment, which particularly captures the enabling or disabling qualities that environments impose.

The basic differences between the definitions of the Nagi-type models and those associated with the World Health Organization have been widely noted (Badley, 1995; de Kleijn de Vrankrijker, Heerkens, and van Ravensberg 1998; Nagi 1991). A particular difference is the conceptualization of the term *disability* and the location of the concept of disability as the outcome of the Nagi model, while the term is conceptualized in the first WHO model as associated with the limits in physical and mental functioning and is included as the component that leads to the outcome. Also in comparison with the first WHO model, both the Nagi model and the IOM model interpret the outcome, disability (C), as a *relational* concept, while in the first WHO model, the outcome is conceptualized as a *handicap,* interpreted as a *disadvantage* for the individual relative to other people.

Differences between some of the definitions associated with the two World Health Organization models are notable as well. Participation, which has replaced handicap in the current model, is conceptualized more broadly and has taken on a more positive connotation of involvement and represents inclusion as well as exclusion. However, the participation is seen in terms of individual domains that can be common across roles rather than an organized set of tasks or activities that make up a single role.

Finally, although all the models refer to the larger social context as being very important in the development of disability, this is the least well-specified aspect of the models. Even the social model, which proposes that disability begins with the social structure, has not yet specified the mechanisms or relationships originating in the social structure that generates a disability outcome other than to propose that it takes the form of oppression (Abberley 1987; Oliver 1990). The most recent WHO model attempts to include the contextual elements but in a limited way, and the second IOM model portrays the environment in a somewhat trampoline effect but without further specificity.

CONCEPTUAL FRAMEWORKS AND MODELS

Models, as systematic organizations of conceptual elements, represent the relationships between or among concepts using symbols representing the component concepts, along with relevant connecting lines or arrows to denote the connection and possible direction of those relationships. The model, then, "delineates certain aspects of the real world as being relevant to the problem under investigation, it makes explicit the significant relationships among the aspects, and it enables the formulation of empirically testable propositions regarding the nature of these relationships" (Frankfort-Nachmias and Nachmias 1992:44). In the remainder of this section, I will discuss the relationship frameworks of four of the models whose conceptional components were discussed earlier and will examine the purpose for which these models were developed. To preserve the historical origins and show the changing thought processes of the two models currently in the forefront of disability studies, I will first examine the Nagi conceptual framework and the first WHO model. Second, I will examine the most recent IOM model and the current WHO model, *ICIDH-2.* As a way of understanding the similarities and differences between the models, I will discuss the congruence of the models with their purposes, the types of answers the models give us as to the definition of disability, and the value and problems of multiple models.

Purposes of Models

The original Nagi article that served as a basis for the Nagi model was written for a conference co-sponsored by the American Sociological Association and the Vocational Rehabilitation Administration. According to the editor of the volume, which was a product of that conference, the "overriding consideration in developing the conference and in selecting participants was *the usefulness and applicability of current sociological theory and research* (beyond just medical sociology) to the field of rehabilitation" (Sussman 1965:iii, emphasis added). In additional remarks, Mary Switzer, the commissioner of the Vocational Rehabilitation Administration at that time, reinforced the need for new and creative thinking about the problem of dependency (Switzer 1965:vii). She noted the "generations of prejudice against the provision of proper opportunity" and looked to "mobilize sociological findings in such a manner that we call attention to those things that must be recognized before anything can be done about a problem" (Switzer 1965:vii-viii).

The other formulations of a disability model that follow from the Nagi model are those put forth by the two IOM panels. The second IOM panel was established at the request of the U.S. Congress.[7] In response to that request, they produced a report that assesses the current knowledge base in rehabilitation science, evaluates current rehabilitation models, recommends ways to transfer scientific findings to promote health and health care for persons with disabling conditions, and evaluates the federal programmatic efforts in these areas (Brandt and Pope 1997:1). As a part of describing priorities and strengthening the fields of rehabilitation science and engineering, this panel included an elaboration of the original IOM model of disability, or the enabling-disabling process, to include "clear reference to the *importance of the environment in causing, preventing, and reducing disability*" (Brandt and Pope 1997:1, emphasis added).

The introduction to the first WHO model and *ICIDH* manual indicates that the classification schemes within the manual are offered as *frameworks to facilitate the provision of information* that was seen as essential to decisions that need to be made for those concerned with health and welfare. The purpose of the development of the *ICIDH* is "to provide a classification scheme similar to the *International Classification of Disease* (ICD) with the intent to facilitate study of the consequences of disease" (WHO 1980:35). The classifications were designed as coding schemes to allow information from an individual's case records to be interpreted into numerical form for counting and other numerical analysis forms to evaluate health care processes.

The second WHO model is similar to the first, with the aim "to provide a scientific basis for understanding and studying the functional states associated with health conditions" (WHO 1999:9). In addition, its purposes are to establish a common language for describing functional states to assist in communication about those functional states, permit comparisons, and provide a systematic coding scheme for health information (WHO 1999:9). The *ICIDH-2* is seen as belonging to a "family" of WHO classifications that encompass a wide range of health care information and are seen as essential to communication about health and health care across nations, disciplines, and sciences. The *ICIDH-2* specifically is intended to provide a synthesis of the different dimensions of health at both a biological and social level. It is represented as a tool for many users, including people with disabilities, people responsible for social programs, and policymakers and clinical providers. Its envisioned use to promote more comprehensive assessment of individual problems at the clinical level, to facilitate the evaluation of health service use at the population level to identify social priorities and evaluate policy issues, and to generate statistics for use in surveillance, planning, and epidemiological research represents the high expectations of the model and taxonomy held by its developers (WHO 1997, 1999).

Nagi Symbolic Model

Although many have interpreted Nagi's formulation of the concepts of disability into a symbolic relationship form (Albrecht 1997; Verbrugge and Jette 1993), Nagi himself did not originally present his ideas in that manner (Nagi 1965, 1969). Directional relationships between the concepts were implicit in some instances in the examples that were given but were not proposed outright. For example, in the discussion of functional limitations, Nagi uses the classic example of the loss of a finger, "which could be severely limiting to a pianist, may not be limiting at all, to a teacher" (Nagi 1965:102). In this example, he implies that impairment is associated with functional limitation but also indicates that it is not a one-to-one relationship. In addition, his example suggests that a pianist will be disabled (i.e., his or her role behavior will be affected by

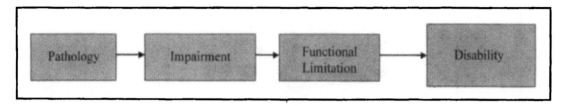

Figure 3.2. Nagi Model as Generally Portrayed in Literature

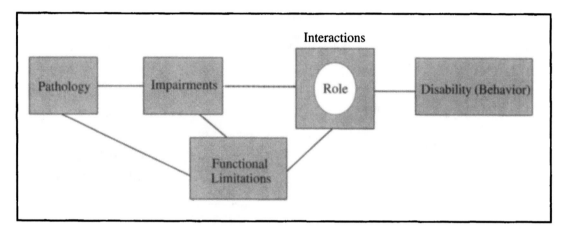

Figure 3.3. Nagi Model: Symbolic Representation
SOURCE: Adapted from Nagi (1965) by Altman.

the impairment), but this same effect will not hold for the teacher, the implication being that the impairment does not create a functional limitation that affects the teacher's enactment of his or her teaching role. In his discussion of the concept of disability, Nagi (1965) indicates that "while disability indicates the existence of an impairment which limits the individual's functioning, it may not be associated with the presence of disease as in the case of healed amputations and residual polio" (p. 103). This implies that while in some instances, a causal relationship is evident—starting with pathology and then moving from impairment to functional limitation and finally to disability—this also is not always the case. Figure 3.2 indicates the Nagi model as it has been represented symbolically by others. Figure 3.3 represents a possible symbolic representation of the Nagi model when the ideas about role interactions and behavior are incorporated.

In the same discussion about the concept of disability, Nagi (1965) indicated that disability behavior is influenced by things outside the individual as well—specifically, the "definition of the situation by others, their reactions and expectations" (p. 103). His emphasis on this was more explicit in his follow-up work, where he included "characteristics of the environment" as one of the three factors that contribute to or shape the dimensions of disability (Nagi 1991:315). Where these components are placed in the model is not specified.

IOM Symbolic Model

The IOM models (Brandt and Pope 1997; Pope and Tarlov 1991) are much more explicit than the Nagi model about the relationships, the direction of the relationships, and where the environmental effects take place. The second IOM model begins with the complete first portion of the earlier IOM model and revises the final or disability element. This element is expressed three-dimensionally, rather than two-dimensionally as in the other models, and identifies the person with impairment or functional limitation as having a *potentially* disabling

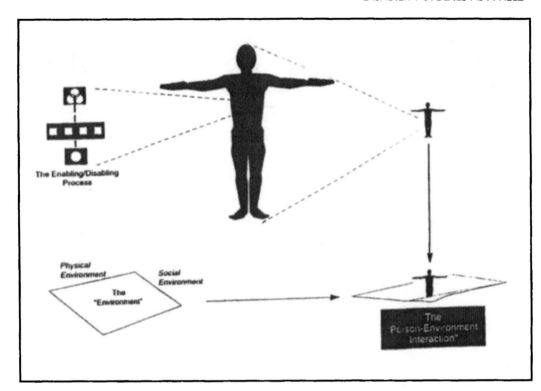

Figure 3.4. Current Institutes of Medicine Model
SOURCE: Brandt and Pope (1997). Copyright 1965 by the National Academy of Sciences. Used courtesy of the National Academy Press, Washington, DC.

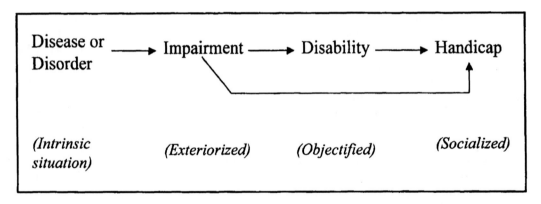

Figure 3.5. World Health Organization Model—Original
SOURCE: World Health Organization (1980).

condition (Brandt and Pope 1997:70). The person is projected onto a square mat that depicts the physical and social environment. The amount of displacement made by the person within that mat is identified as proportional to the amount of disability the individual experiences. Although the IOM model does not emphasize the interactive mechanisms, this visual device implies some of the interactive quality of the intersection of functional limitation and environment. While this visual device is intuitively useful, the IOM model does not provide any indication of how this displacement in the mat of physical and social environment would be

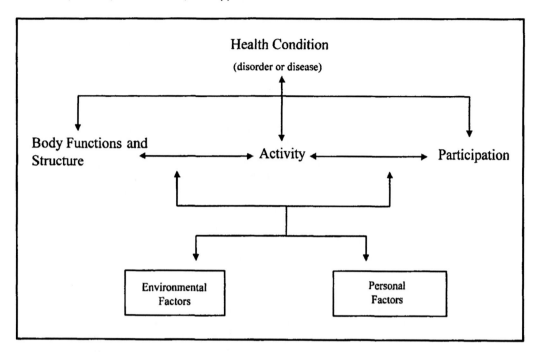

Figure 3.6. World Health Organization Model—*ICIDH-2*
SOURCE: World Health Organization (1999).

operationalized and measured, nor does it give examples of what would constitute a small displacement or a large one (see Figure 3.4).

WHO Symbolic Models

The original WHO model indicated four concepts linked together, with arrows moving in one direction from disease or disorder, which was identified as an *intrinsic situation,* to the outcome handicap, identified as *socialized* (WHO 1980:30). The model also indicated a second directional arrow between impairment and handicap, implying that impairment can lead directly to handicap without associated disability. The text indicated that this sequence can be interrupted at any stage, so that an individual can be impaired without being disabled or disabled without being handicapped, but such interruptions are not part of the symbolic representation (WHO 1980:30). While the text also indicated that the direction of the relationships could in some instances be in the opposite direction, the arrows indicated a unidirectional movement from impairment to handicap.

The current symbolic model proposed by the WHO (1999) as a basis for the classification scheme includes the concepts of health condition (disease/disorder), which is seen as directly related to the three elements of impairment, activity, and participation (Figure 3.5). The model does not indicate a unidirectional flow as in the earlier model. Impairment is depicted as part of a reciprocal relationship with activity, and activity is also represented in a reciprocal relationship with participation (see Figure 3.6). Contextual factors, which refer to both environmental and personal factors, are incorporated into the model between impairment and activity and imply an interventional interpretation between activity and participation. The authors of this model, however, clearly point out that other depictions are possible, and "any diagram would be insufficient and could be prone to misrepresentation because of the complexities of interactions in a multidimensional model" (WHO 1997:12).

APPLICATIONS

Defining Disability from the Models

To understand the differences and similarities of what these models tell us about the definition of disability, I have chosen to use a single example and examine it in light of each of the four models elaborated above as well as the social model, which has not been represented in symbolic form. The example is a 27-year-old man with cerebral palsy and extensive physical limitations from the condition. Jim uses a reclining motorized wheelchair, which he manipulates with his right hand. His speech is not affected by his condition, but most if not all of his body functioning is, and he uses a personal assistant for his physical needs and has a job coach at his place of employment to help with the physical lifting and other physical activities associated with his employment that he cannot manage. Jim is an actual person who works in a local hardware store.

From the perspective of the Nagi model, we can identify that Jim has a condition (pathology) that has resulted in impairments in his musculature that has created a set of functional limitations (restricted use of his arms and legs; inability to walk, lift, finger, or grasp). This has resulted in adaptations to his social performance of things such as self-care behavior and work behavior. He directs his personal assistant in how to do most of his self-care, rather than doing it himself, and he directs his job coach in moving items off shelves and ringing up charges for the customers he assists in the sales job he holds. From the perspective of the Nagi model, an examination of Jim's disability would be one that is concerned with social performance or Jim's self-care behavior and work role behavior and how it is similar to or different from some comparison group. The fact that Jim lives independently and has a job would be an indication of lessor levels of "disability (C)," as interpreted by behavior than the level of impairment or functional limitation may imply.

Using an IOM model perspective to understand disability as it is explained by that recent model, the first elements would be similar or identical to those identified in the Nagi model. In the IOM model, disability is a relational outcome that is dependent not only on the person and his characteristics but also on the physical and social environment. On the basis of the visual model, which shows deflection in the mat that represents the environment, Jim's disability can be reflected by how much his environmental support score compensates for his potential disability score that would be based on some measure of his functional limitation. In this case, where the support system is available, at least in terms of a personal assistant and a job coach, Jim's disability could be interpreted as less than if he were not able to function in those self-help and work roles because of the lack of support. Comparisons could also be made with others with different impairments and levels of functional limitation, as well as with those with no impairments.

The first WHO model would identify Jim's impairment, cerebral palsy, and disability or lack of ability to perform self-care or certain aspects of his job. His outcome would be interpreted in terms of his disadvantage that limited the fulfillment of the self-help role and the work role in a way that was "normal" for his age, sex, and other characteristics. It is not clear how Jim's access to the personal assistance help and job coach help would affect an evaluation of his level of handicapness. The outcome here (not identified as disability, but rather as handicap) is relative to other people.

In the current WHO model, *ICIDH-2*, Jim's body function and structure would be more specifically identified than previously. The level of activity could be identified, so the parts he is capable of doing relative to his job, for example, would indicate communication with the customers but would also indicate the inability to lift the items off shelves or manipulate the cash register. A measure of his participation, however, would indicate his involvement in a work role and in his self-help role. The use of the context level of measurement would elaborate how that participation is accomplished. *Disability*, which in the *ICIDH-2* is used as an umbrella term for all the dimensions of the model, could be interpreted as the interrelational aspects of all these elements.

The Models as Tools for Research

These models represent a very exciting evolution of thought about the circumstances associated with impairment, functional limitations, disability, and participation in society. The differences in purposes and objectives associated with the development of the models, as well as the differences in disciplines, very clearly have influenced the definition of concepts and the relationship of concepts to outcome that are proposed in these models. However, all are useful to the promotion of research on the topic of disability.

These models reflect both the purposes that brought them into existence and the disciplinary orientation of their originators or sponsors. The Nagi model was developed by a sociologist for the purpose of applying sociological theory and knowledge to the problems of disability, particularly in a rehabilitation context. It demonstrates a strong affinity for a sociological perspective on how an individual functions in the social group and for the use of a large body of social theory known as role theory. If the developers of the IOM model, which builds on the Nagi model, continue to pursue the mechanisms that will provide an understanding of the way to change the role participation of an individual through the rehabilitation process, then further elaboration of the model will continue along the same lines.

The second WHO model, *ICIDH-2*, reflects the orientation to develop classification schemes—in this case, to extend the classification of disease to the characteristics of the outcomes or consequences of disease as is stated in its purpose. The classification scheme in this instance is the central concern, and its evolution over a period of 20 years has gone hand in hand with the changes in the model itself. Even the movement away from conceptualizing the outcomes in terms of roles as in the Nagi and IOM models or disadvantages as detailed in the first WHO model is dictated by the need to separate the overlapping aspects of role and domain. Multiple definitions of different actions cannot be tolerated if a mutually exclusive categorization is the goal. The action of cooking could not be viewed in terms of its form in the family role as different from its form in an occupational role without undermining the purpose of the classification development.

A second very important difference between the models discussed is that one comes with a measurement coding scheme, *ICIDH-2*, and the others do not. The Nagi model and the IOM models are generalized conceptual definitions and patterns of relationships that leave the operational interpretation and empirical measurement of the components very much in the hands of those who would use them. The *ICIDH-2* gives the illusion of uniformity in the definition of disability through the use of a very detailed set of mutually exclusive categories, subcategories with the additional levels of severity, while the other models provide nothing other than the conceptual definitions as a guide to the user for measuring the phenomena at the individual or group level. Operationalizing the general concepts, on one hand, will be very difficult because of the lack of uniformity of measures that are currently available in survey data or even in clinical data. The exaggerated specificity of the classification scheme offered by the *ICIDH-2*, while impressive in its completeness, is also misleading. There is no assurance that professionals will identify the activity ability or participation in a uniform way or that the subject will demonstrate uniform ability or participation over time, depending on the trajectory of the condition associated with the body function and structure deficits. Self-reporting of body function and structure, activities, and participation is equally at risk for subjective interpretation, and self-reporting would also suffer from the burden of questions necessary to identify the detailed aspects of the classification scheme. So, while the *ICIDH* classification scheme is a useful comprehensive complement to the *ICD*, its usefulness as a measurement tool in the study of disability in an individual or population is very dependent on the development of successful measurement tools.

The value of any model lies in the way that it is related to the empirical world and thus its usefulness to investigate real problems that exist in that empirical world. Many times, the events or attributes that are represented by the concepts of a theory or model are not directly observable empirically. Or, as in the case of disability, a concept is a complex one with multiple empirical interpretations for which no one empirical measure is adequate. In that instance, the translation of the concept into an empirical measure requires a set of procedures that describe the activities to perform in order to establish the existence of the phenomenon described by the concept. This is an operational definition, and it helps bridge the conceptual-observational levels. Operational definitions tell what to do and observe, bringing the concept to a measurable level. Once this operationalization is accomplished, the relationships proposed in the models can be examined. This is the missing element in developing a conceptual understanding of disability and linking it to the empirical world.

In the hard sciences, these operational definitions can involve the use of instruments to weigh or measure a sample specimen or various other manipulations to test the hardness or porousness of the object. In social science, where the subject of research is human rather than inanimate objects, physical manipulation of individuals or events is difficult and often unethical. The methods of simulation of the underlying concepts are more restricted to interaction with or observation of the individuals who are to be studied. This is partially possible at the clinical level, but if the concept cannot be directly observed, it must be inferred. In social science, this is most often done by constructing questionnaires that attempt to get at the underlying components of the conceptual construction.

A very important problem arises in the transition from the conceptual level to the empirical observational level. It is associated with the level of congruency between conceptual and operational definitions (Frankfort-Nachamias and Nachamias 1992). If disability is defined conceptually as "experienced difficulty doing activities in any domain of life due to a health or physical problem" (Verbrugge and Jette 1993:4) or as "an inability or limitation in performing socially defined roles and tasks expected of an individual within a sociocultural and physical environment" (Nagi 1991:315), and if it is operationally defined as the inability or limitation in the ability to work, go to school, or do housework,[8] what is the degree of congruence between the definition and the measure? In addition, is any one operational definition necessarily appropriate for all the different definitions of disability indicated above, or are there multiple ways to operationalize and measure the concepts?

The more complex the social phenomenon being defined, the greater the possible *variety* in operationalization. Blalock (1968, 1979) discussed the concept of prejudice and showed that one definition will not suffice for all circumstances. In the same way, disability is a complex social phenomenon, and we have just demonstrated multiple components of disability, as described in the various models discussed above. Disability, then, is undefinable empirically unless one reduces the focus of the definition to a specific aspect of experience. Northrop (1947) referred to theoretical definitions as "concepts by postulation" and to operational definitions as "concepts by intuition." He denied that there was a way of connecting these except by common agreement. Blalock (1968, 1979), on the other hand, offered the possibility that a theoretical concept could have a number of different operational definitions and associated indices, "provided it does not lead to endless bickering about which of the procedures is really measuring prejudice (the essence of which is presumed understood)" (Blalock 1968:36). The gist of Blalock's point was that the research process can be used to *clarify* theoretical concepts.

The operational process has the purpose of making the concept, taken from the theory or model, more concrete and creates a way to measure the phenomenon. However, once an operational definition is accepted, it also creates a gap between the conceptual and operational definition that narrows the meaning of the theoretical concept to that represented by the operational tool or question used in measurement. So using the two definitions given above and the operational example, we note that the measure of disability has been reduced from the conceptualization of its occurrence in all domains (Verbrugge and Jette 1993) or all social roles (Nagi 1991) to one specific set of roles or one domain: work, school, or housework. Using the WHO definition of an outcome of body function and structure and activity, as identified as participation, the concept can also be operationalized in terms of involvement in work or school. Selecting only one of those areas of participation is just as limiting of the WHO concept as is the limiting of the operationalization of the other definitions of disability to one type of role. This points to the next step in understanding and defining disability—the process of translating the conceptual elements of the models into valid and reliable empirical measures that economically represent the complexity of the problem.

NOTES

1. The Developmental Disabilities Assistance and Bill of Rights Act Amendments of 1987 specified that such a severe or chronic condition was attributable to a mental or physical impairment; manifested before age 22; is likely to continue indefinitely; results in substantial functional limitations in *three* or more areas of major life activity, such as self-care, receptive and expressive language, learning, mobility, self-direction, capacity for independent living, and economic self-sufficiency; and reflects the need for a combination and sequence of special, interdisciplinary, or generic care and treatment or other services that are of lifelong or extended duration and are individually planned or coordinated (Amado, Lakin, and Menke 1990).

2. The Americans with Disabilities Act (ADA) defines disability with respect to an individual as the following: (1) a physical or mental impairment that substantially limits one or more of the major life activities of such individual, (2) a record of such impairment, or (3) being regarded as having such an impairment (Sec. 3(2), 42 U.S.C. 12102, 1990).

3. The term *disability* will be used several different ways in this discussion. When referencing the general idea of disability, as defined by the various models to be discussed, it will be written simply as "disability." When reference is made to a specific definition of the term *disability* by the authors of the models, the term will be italicized and will be followed by a letter in parentheses that will identify which model is the source for the specific definition. In that way, I will attempt to discuss *disability (A), disability (B),* and *disability (C)* and keep the subtle differences of meaning separated.

4. It is not clear how the term *norm* is used in this context, whether it refers to the "prior norm" for the individual before the onset of the pathology or a "norm" of a population with whom the individual is being compared.

5. For example, locomotion disabilities are indicated to refer to "an individual's ability to execute distinctive activities associated with moving, both himself and objects, from place to place" (WHO 1980:161).

6. Nagi specified that in some systems, there is a role for persons with an illness or disability, such as in a hospital where a person is a patient or in rehabilitation where a person is a client. This differs from the family context or the work context where there is not a special role for someone who is ill or disabled but where adaptations or changes may be made to accommodate the effects of role behavior caused by the functional limitations involved.

7. Although the two panels that authored the Institute of Medicine (IOM) models were closely related and sponsored by the same organization, they were brought together for two different purposes. The first panel report focuses on "preventing potentially disabling conditions from developing into disability and on minimizing the effects of such conditions on a person's productivity and quality of life" (Pope and Tarlov 1991:v). This prevention is seen as occurring not only before a pathology begins but before a pathology can lead to an impairment, before an impairment becomes a functional limitation, before a functional limitation develops into a disability, or before any stage creates secondary conditions.

8. This question, or ones similar to it, is an operationalization of the concept of disability that has widespread use in numerous national surveys around the world.

REFERENCES

Abberley, P. 1987. "The Concept of Oppression and the Development of a Social Theory of Disability." *Disability, Handicap and Society* 2 (1): 5-19.

Albrecht, G. L. 1997. "The Health Politics of Disability." Pp. 367-83 in *Health Politics and Policy*, 3d ed., edited by T. J. Litman and L. S. Robins. Albany, NY: Delmar.

Albrecht, G. L. and L. M. Verbrugge. 2000. "The Global Emergence of Disability." Pp. 293-307 in *Handbook of Social Studies in Health and Medicine*, edited by G. L. Albrecht. London: Sage.

Altman, B. M. 1984. "Examination of the Effects of Individual, Primary and Secondary Resources on the Outcomes of Impairment." Ph.D. dissertation, University of Maryland, College Park.

———. 1986. "Definitions of Disability in Empirical Research: Is the Use of an Administrative Definition Co-opting the Results of Disability Research?" Paper presented at the annual meetings of the American Sociological Association, August, Washington, DC.

———. 1993. "Definitions of Disability and Their Measurement and Operationalization in Survey Data." In *Proceedings of the Public Health Conference on Records and Statistics*, pp. 1-12. Hyattsville, MD: National Center for Health Statistics.

Altman, B. M. and S. N. Barnartt. 2000. "Introducing Research in Social Science and Disability: An Invitation to Social Science to 'Get It.' " Pp. 1-30 in *Expanding the Scope of Social Science Research on Disability*, edited by B. M. Altman and S. N. Barnartt. Stamford, CT: JAI.

Amado, A. N., K. C. Lakin, and J. M. Menke. 1990. *Services for People with Developmental Disabilities*. Minneapolis: University of Minnesota, Center for Residential and Community Services, Institute on Community Integration.

Badley, E. M. 1995. "The Genesis of Handicap: Definition, Models of Disablement, and Role of External Factors." *Disability and Rehabilitation* 17 (2): 53-62.

Bickenbach, J. E., S. Chatterji, E. M. Badley, and T. B. Üstün. 1999. "Models of Disablement, Universalism and the International Classification of Impairments, Disabilities and Handicaps." *Social Science and Medicine* 48:1173-87.

Biskupic, J. 1999. "Supreme Court Limits Meaning of Disability." *Washington Post*, June 23, pp. 1, 10.

Blalock, H. 1968. "The Measurement Problem: A Gap between the Languages of Theory and Research." Pp. 5-27 in *Methodology in Social Science*, edited by H. Blalock and A. Blalock. New York: McGraw-Hill.

———. 1979. *Social Statistics*. 2d ed. New York: McGraw-Hill.

Blaxter, M. 1976. *The Meaning of Disability*. London: Heinemann.

Brandt, E. N. and A. M. Pope, eds. 1997. *Enabling America: Assessing the Role of Rehabilitation Science and Engineering*. Washington, DC: National Academy Press.

Bury, M. 1996. "Defining and Researching Disability: Challenges and Responses." Pp. 17-38 in *Exploring the Divide: Illness and Disability*, edited by C. Barnes and G. Mercer. Leeds, UK: The Disability Press.

de Kleijn de Vrankrijker, M. W., Y. F. Heerkens, and C. D. van Ravensberg. 1998. "Defining Disability." Pp. 34-47 in *Introduction to Disability*, edited by M. A. McColl and J. E. Bickenbach. Toronto, Canada: W. B. Saunders.

Duckworth, D. 1984. "The Need for a Standard Terminology and Classification of Disablement." Pp. 1-13 in *Functional Assessment in Rehabilitation Medicine*, edited by C. V. Granger and G. E. Gresham. Baltimore: Williams & Wilkins.

Engelbert, A., ed. 1988. *American Medical Association Guides to the Evaluation of Permanent Impairment*. 3d ed. Chicago: American Medical Association.

Frankfort-Nachmias, C. and D. Nachmias. 1992. *Research Methods in the Social Sciences*. 4th ed. New York: St. Martin's.

Gross, W. S. Mason, and W. McEachern. 1958. *Explorations in Role Analysis*. New York: John Wiley.

Hahn, H. 1985. "Toward a Politics of Disability: Definitions, Disciplines, and Policies." *The Social Science Journal* 22 (4): 87-105.

Johnson, R. J. and F. D. Wolinsky. 1993. "The Structure of Health Status among Older Adults: Disease, Disability, Functional Limitation, and Perceived Health." *Journal of Health and Social Behavior* 34:105-21.

Kelman, S. 1975. "The Social Nature of the Definition Problem in Health." *International Journal of Health Services* 5:625-42.

Linton, S. 1998. *Claiming Disability: Knowledge and Identity.* New York: New York University Press.

Melvin, J. L. and S. Z. Nagi. 1970. "Factors in Behavioral Responses to Impairments." *Archives of Physical Medical Rehabilitation* 51 (9): 552-57.

Murray, C. J. and A. M. Lopez. 1996. *The Global Burden of Disease.* Boston: Harvard University Press.

Nagi, S. Z. 1965. "Some Conceptual Issues in Disability and Rehabilitation." Pp. 100-13 in *Sociology and Rehabilitation,* edited by M. Sussman. Washington, DC: American Sociological Association.

———. 1969. *Disability and Rehabilitation: Legal, Clinical, and Self-Concepts and Measurement.* Columbus: The Ohio State University Press.

———. 1977. "The Disabled and Rehabilitation Services: A National Overview." *American Rehabilitation* 2 (5): 26-33.

———. 1981. "Disability Concepts and Implications for Programs." Pp. 33-48 in *Cross National Rehabilitation Policies: A Sociological Perspective,* edited by G. Albrecht. Beverly Hills, CA: Sage.

———. 1991. "Disability Concepts Revisited: Implications for Prevention." Pp. 309-27 in *Disability in America: Toward a National Agenda for Prevention,* edited by A. M. Pope and A. R. Tarlov. Washington, DC: National Academy Press.

National Center for Medical Rehabilitation Research. 1993. *Research Plan for the National Center for Medical Rehabilitation Research.* Washington, DC: National Institutes of Health.

Northrop, F. S. C. 1947. *The Logic of the Sciences and the Humanities.* New York: Macmillan.

Oliver, M. 1990. *The Politics of Disablement: A Sociological Approach.* New York: St. Martin's.

———. 1993. "Disability and Dependency: A Creation of Industrial Societies?" Pp. 49-60 in *Disabling Barriers—Enabling Environments,* edited by J. Swain, V. Finkelstein, S. French, and M. Oliver. London: Sage.

———. 1996. "Defining Impairment and Disability: Issues at Stake." Pp. 39-53 in *Exploring the Divide: Illness and Disability,* edited by C. Barnes and G. Mercer. Leeds, UK: The Disability Press.

Pope, A. M. and A. R. Tarlov, eds. 1991. *Disability in America: Toward a National Agenda for Prevention.* Washington, DC: National Academy Press.

Slater, S. B., P. Vukmanovic, T. Macukanic, T. Prvulovic, and J. L. Cutler. 1974. "The Definition and Measurement of Disability." *Social Science and Medicine* 8:305-8.

Stone, D. A. 1984. *The Disabled State.* Philadelphia: Temple University Press.

Suchman, E. A. 1965. "A Model for Research and Evaluation on Rehabilitation." Pp. 52-70 in *Sociology and Rehabilitation,* edited by M. Sussman. Washington, DC: American Sociological Association.

Sussman, M. 1965. "Preface." Pp. iii-vi in *Sociology and Rehabilitation,* edited by M. Sussman. Washington, DC: American Sociological Association.

Switzer, M. E. 1965. "Remarks." Pp. vii-xii in *Sociology and Rehabilitation,* edited by M. Sussman. Washington, DC: American Sociological Association.

U.S. Department of Health and Human Services (DHHS). 1990. *Federal Programs for Persons with Disabilities.* Washington, DC: Office of the Assistant Secretary for Planning and Evaluation, Department of Health and Human Services.

Verbrugge, L. M. 1990. "The Iceberg of Disability." Pp. 55-75 in *Longevity: Health and Health Care in Later Life,* edited by S. M. Stahl. Newbury Park, CA: Sage.

Verbrugge, L. M. and A. M. Jette. 1993. "The Disablement Process." *Social Science and Medicine* 6 (1): 1-14.

Wan, T. T. 1974. "Correlates and Consequences of Severe Disabilities." *Journal of Occupational Medicine* 16 (4): 234-44.

Williams, G. 1996. "Representing Disability: Some Questions of Phenomenology and Politics." Pp. 194-212 in *Exploring the Divide: Illness and Disability,* edited by C. Barnes and G. Mercer. Leeds, UK: The Disability Press.

World Health Organization (WHO). 1980. *International Classification of Impairments, Disabilities, and Handicaps: A Manual of Classification Relating to the Consequences of Disease.* Geneva: Author.

———. 1997. *International Classification of Impairments, Activities and Participation: A Manual of Dimensions of Disablement and Health.* Beta-1 draft for field trials. Geneva: Author.

———. 1998. *Towards a Common Language for Functioning and Disablement: ICIDH-2.* Geneva: Author.

————. 1999. *ICIDH-2: International Classification of Functioning and Disability.* Beta-2 draft, full version. Geneva: Author.

Zola, I. K. 1989. "Toward the Necessary Universalizing of a Disability Policy." *The Milbank Quarterly* 67:401-26.

————. 1993. "Self, Identity and the Naming Question: Reflections on the Language of Disability." *Social Science and Medicine* 36:167-73.

Theorizing Disability

4

GARETH WILLIAMS

> And there stirs in me a little of the same anger as the Negro writer James Baldwin reveals
> in *The Fire Next Time* when I remember the countless times I have seen disabled people
> hurt, treated as less than people, told what to do and how to behave by those whose only
> claim to do this came from prejudice and their power over them.
>
> —Hunt (1998:14)

The most persuasive sociological writing emerges from a personal feeling. Whether it be of anger or delight, it forms into a conviction about something good or bad in society. It unfolds into a story of loss and change, protest or revolution, and then develops into something more abstract, ecumenical, and systematic but recognizably spoken nonetheless, by a voice still breaking with the emotion that first fired it into the world. Such writing is often driven by a desire to proclaim the truth in situations in which power demands "lies, secrets, and silence" (Rich 1995). The first step is the recognition of something unjust, and while people may not always be in a position to articulate common concerns, let alone develop political strategies, they may nonetheless be profoundly "sensitive to inhibitions, prohibitions, and threats to their freedom" (Kaye 1996:198).

Although the disability movement and studies of disability have traveled a long way since Paul Hunt's anger stirred in him—and new languages and theories have proliferated in response to economic, social, and cultural change—the ability to think about disability as both a "personal trouble" and a "public issue," as hurt and prejudice, and to write about it with a vivid sociological imagination marks out the most interesting work in the field, by both medical sociologists and disability theorists. The trick is to see the thing nondualistically, to recognize impairment/disability not as something that is either-or but as simultaneously and ontologically both personal and public—to see it, therefore, as something that requires methodological lenses to help us change focus easily, without feeling that talking about one excludes or even betrays the other. Much of the literature on disability is angry literature, and it is also replete with guilt, shame, betrayal, and a well-intended desire to say the right thing.

"Theorizing disability" is no longer a dry intellectual or technical task. Long gone are the days when an interest in something called "disability" signaled only a concern with the clinical

AUTHOR'S NOTE: I am grateful to Helen Busby for her contribution to many of the ideas contained in this chapter. Responsibility remains with the author alone.

effectiveness of particular prosthetic interventions or drug therapies or a passion for the changing rules for accessing welfare benefits. Although in the view of some scholars working in the burgeoning field of disability studies, "disability has continued to be relegated to hospital hallways, physical therapy tables, and remedial classrooms" (Davis 1997:1), the existence in Britain and the United States, in particular, of 30 years of movement in disability politics has ensured a strong platform from which the academic discipline of disability studies was able to take off in the 1990s (Shakespeare 1998:1). Moreover, if disability studies has opened up a space for reconceptualizing disability in more social terms (Thomas 1999), it is important to recognize that it has done this dialectically with those working within medical sociology and elsewhere. Between medical sociology and disability studies in Britain, years of frosty silence and occasional abuse have evolved into something more like a constructive argument.

The growing field of disability studies has many facets and numerous styles, including Marxist, feminist postmodern, and poststructuralist. Some of these styles emphasize the social oppression of disabled people; others focus on the cultural and ideological construction of impaired bodies (Barton and Oliver 1997; Davis 1997; Shakespeare 1998). However, all this work has as its common root a rejection of the medical model as the foundation for any effective understanding of impairment or disability. As disability has become politicized and the body has become a domain of theorization, the challenge for sociological writing has become one of how to embrace structuralist and poststructuralist work in disability studies while continuing to remain alert to the shape-shifting powers of orthodox biomedicine.

Nearly all work in disability studies explicitly rejects conventional medical, administrative, welfare, or other "property definitions" of disability (definitions in which disability is seen as the property of the person with an impairment) (Thomas 1999). Insofar as epidemiologists and policymakers emphasize social aspects only while continuing to elaborate their positions in language, which makes disability the property of individual people (see, e.g., Chatterji, Üstün, and Bickenbach 1999), they will remain profoundly antagonistic to people working within the field of disability studies. However, it remains the case that developments in rehabilitation medicine, state social security systems, and the entire "disability business" in Western societies can have a profound impact, not only on the lives of disabled people but also on what disability in society is taken to be (Albrecht 1992; Stone 1985).

Insofar as the social reality of disability is in part constructed by the activities and discourses of powerful professional and political interests, without engagement with them (as well as resistance to them), it is not possible to take any effective part in discussions about how many "disabled people" there are, what "problems" they face, or how (as they say in the United Kingdom nowadays) "joined up policies for a national disability strategy" might be developed (Howard 1999). While "relational" definitions of disability might be more powerful components of sociological and political theories of disability (Thomas 1999), the property definitions found in both welfare and medical categorizations are part of the "historical materialism" of disability, without which neither personal nor collective experiences of disability can be understood.

Medical sociological writing on both chronic illness/impairment and disability has generally been less antagonistic to the medical model but has emphasized the importance of seeing the experience of impairment and disability from the disabled person's point of view. The theoretical perspectives used in this work derive from symbolic interactionism and phenomenology (Williams 1996a, 1998). While much of this work developed is in opposition to medical dominance, it has recently found itself in the curious position of being lambasted for covertly supporting the biomedical model (Williams 1996a). What such work often produces are complex lay accounts or narratives of experiences of impairment and disability (Booth 1996; Frank 1995; Williams 1984), not dissimilar from those self-authored autobiographical accounts that are also increasingly visible on the intellectual landscape of disability studies (Couser 1997). These narratives or stories—often personal, sometimes political, occasionally religious or spiritual—offer their own definitions of disability of which professionals in the "disability business" need to take into account. Such narratives of experience are dealt with more fully elsewhere in this volume, but they are touched on here as important contributions to the continuing theoretical exploration of disability.

One consequence of this Babel of discourses is that the study of disability lacks any unifying theory or perspective. However, this absence of theoretical coherence is not necessarily a bad thing. A unifying theory of disability constructed out of the different terms of diverse disciplines would depend on the resolution of enormous problems of translation, and any claim to success would quite rightly give rise to considerable suspicion. Moreover, in the wake of the postmodern turn in sociological theory and social philosophy, not having a unifying theory may, paradoxically, be regarded as evidence of theoretical sophistication. Perhaps this greater pluralism will also make people more relaxed about terminology that has been the focus of intense discussions about words and their meanings (Oliver 1993; Zola 1993a). Although Abberley (1998) is right to suggest that "the most fundamental issue in the sociology of disability is a conceptual one" (p. 79), it is important not to allow the history of words as bearers of ideology to prevent us from thinking creatively about the use of words in the contemporary situation, however limited our control over language may actually be.

This chapter makes the argument that both medical sociology and disability studies have had a critique of the medical model at their core. It looks at the different ways in which something called "disability" has been defined and theorized, and it considers the way in which the medical model of disability has developed from one that looks solely at biological impairment to one that recognizes the multidimensionality of the consequences of disease. Alongside this movement of medical thinking from the body to society—which some see as a welcome sign of medical progress and liberalization, while others see it as imperialistic medicalization—activists and theorists from within the "disability movement" have forged their own definitions that are rooted in their self-defined struggles and conflicts in what is regarded as an able-bodied world. What is called the "social model" in the United Kingdom and the "minority group model" in the United States has been the guiding framework of disability theorists since the 1970s, pushing with increasing strength for disability to be seen as a form of social oppression, and the appropriate response is one of civil rights rather than medical or social care. In recent years, a number of theorists within sociology and disability studies have tried to develop more systematically pluralistic approaches to disability and break away from what I would argue is a theoretically sterile and rather contrived distinction between a social model and a medical model. This chapter concludes with a discussion of some of this work and the possibilities for future development.

BIOMEDICAL DEFINITIONS

The medical model that informs traditional approaches to disability takes the presumed biological reality of impairment as its fundamental starting point. This biological reality is taken to be the foundation of all forms of illness and impairment, whether "mental" or "physical." Although ill health may arise from sources in the environment surrounding the individual person, it is the individual body within which illness is situated. In relation to the rehabilitation of disabled people, the focus of the analysis and the intervention is on the functional limitations that an individual has, the effect of these on activities of daily living, and attempts "to find ways of preventing, curing, or (failing these) caring for disabled people" (Marks 1997:86). This property definition of disability has been the foundation of all developments in rehabilitation, the epidemiology of disability, and much of the social science–orientated work on the consequences of chronic disease and the quality of life of disabled people. Examples of such work can be found in the medically defined fields of rheumatology, neurology, and elsewhere where a number of medically orientated social scientists have found a comfortable home developing various kinds of measures of outcome and health status (Yelin 1992).

In the period immediately following World War II, health and social welfare for disabled people were characterized by a mixture of formal, institutional neglect and charitable, humanitarian concern, related to national attitudes to those who had been maimed in war (Bury 1996). In this context, assessments of function were oriented toward simple arithmetic calculations regarding the effect of damage and deficit in particular limbs. In this work, the assumption was that measuring the impairment was a sufficient basis to assess the needs of a disabled person. However, as chronic disease emerged as a major public health problem, a variety of different medical specialties emerged to deal with impairments, and assessments of medical and social need became more complex. Much of the initial sociological interest in disability emerged from this context and involved social scientists working alongside rehabilitation specialists and public health physicians.

In response to the changing nature of disability in individuals, rehabilitation models and assessment techniques became more complex, with an emphasis on the multidimensionality of the whole person and the person in his or her "environment" (Gritzer and Arluke 1985). Since the early 1970s, those who were professionally engaged in rehabilitation recognized the need to move away from the highly reductive conceptions of functional limitations focusing on deficits in limbs and organs, which had traditionally characterized physical medicine and physical therapy. This holism was enshrined in official reports, with the promulgation of broader definitions of rehabilitation as the restoration of patients to their fullest physical, mental, and social capability (Tunbridge 1972).

Increasingly, broader definitions of health status in patients with chronic illness and disability were used for two main reasons (G. H. Williams 1987): first, to assess needs for treatment, therapy, services, or benefits and, second, to provide a baseline from which to perform more realistic evaluations of change in the health and functional status of patients, both informally and as part of research and evaluation. The focus of these evaluations was still very much on the individual but with a recognition that it was the person who could or could not perform certain kinds of activities rather than the organ, the limb, or the body conceived abstractly as a bundle of capacities and incapacities. The idea of individual deficit continued to have a profound influence on policies, notwithstanding the influence of some other models of disability and associated reforms.

New types of descriptor (developed by sociologists, among others) consisted of assessments of performances in daily living stressing those activities that are purportedly carried out habitually and universally (G. H. Williams 1987); thus, their measuring of a range of daily activities does extend the conventional clinical measures of "functional capacity." However, the fact that they are deemed to be universal rather than context bound implies that they can be used across multiple settings without any substantial reconsideration of their validity and without consideration being given to the meaning of the items for the person with the impairment. The Barthel Index, for example, asks only whether a person can walk 50 yards on level ground regardless of whether he or she wants to, needs to, or has anywhere to walk to (Granger, Albrecht, and Hamilton 1979). Although rehabilitation practitioners have increasingly made reference to the way in which disability affects the "whole person" or "all aspects of an individual's life," the nature of this wider context is rarely built systematically into analysis or recommendations for intervention (College Committee on Disability 1986; Gloag 1985).

More recently, disability policy has changed, and definitions have had to alter too. To some extent, these policy changes have incorporated new definitions, but they are also a response to wider changes in economy and society, and they in turn inform conceptual thinking about the nature of disability. However, whether in medicine or social security, there is a continuing emphasis on defining "the problem" as within the individual, albeit as something amenable to change by interventions outside the individual in the wider environment. As far as some disabled commentators are concerned, therefore, fundamental premises have remained unaltered (Dalley 1991), and changes in social and economic policy as they affect disabled people are still imprisoned by their exclusive emphasis on some form of "property definition" (Thomas 1999). In the words of one critic, head counts of numbers of disabled people as the basis for policy have failed because "they have focused on the wrong thing; that is they have tried to measure the numbers of disabled people rather than the effects of disabling environments" (Oliver 1998:13).

In line with the positivistic underpinnings of medical science, the emphasis of traditional assessments is on some universal definition and measure that can be applied by appropriately qualified people without reference to disabled people's own perspectives, the roles they occupy, the relationships in which they are embedded, the circumstances of their milieux, or the wider political context of barriers, attitudes, and power. However broad their frames of reference, measures of health, disability, well-being, and quality of life continue to be driven by classical positivist concerns with universality and generalizability. In other words, such assessments provide a picture of "activities of daily living" devoid of any phenomenological grasp of the individual's own experience or any political analysis of the structures and contexts within which the activity takes place.

Reframing Disability

As Michael Bury (1996), one of the leading medical sociologists in the United Kingdom, has argued, the field of disability research and policy in the immediate postwar period was conspicuous largely by its absence. Social scientists working within the growing fields of social medicine, social policy, and rehabilitation in this period began to make a contribution to researching the social aspects of chronic illness and disability relating to injury. Most of this work was concerned with the prevalence of disability, but it was hampered by a lack of any clearly agreed definition or approach to measurement. Since the mid-1970s, there have been a number of attempts to clarify the meaning of disability and associated concepts. The pressure to clarify comes from a number of different sources representing very different interests. In Britain, following the government reports of Amelia Harris (Harris, Cox, and Smith 1971), which documented for the first time the numbers of people with impairments, it was recognized that the use of terms such as *impairment, disability,* and *handicap* was very confused. On behalf of the World Health Organization (WHO), Philip Wood and his colleagues attempted to develop a set of definitions that was clear and acceptable to different groups (WHO 1980). In the United States, the work of Saad Nagi was driven by the system imperative of reconciling contradictions between definitions of *medical impairment* and *ability to work* as a way of rationalizing the allocation of Social Security benefits. He came up with definitions that were similar but not identical to those produced by Wood (Nagi 1979).

Over the same period, various movements of disabled people in Britain and the United States had been adding their own voices to arguments that had previously been conducted in the studious calm of seminars and rehabilitation clinics. In the United States, as early as 1973, the independent living and disability rights movements have made an important contribution to the framing of the Rehabilitation Act, but the problem of definition was circumvented, if not wholly resolved, by an emphasis on people with disabilities. It was in Britain that the Union of the Physically Impaired against Segregation published its own definitions of disability (UPIAS 1976). At the same time, Wood produced the first version of his definitions (Wood 1975), which were picked up and used by others who were concerned with the wider economic and social costs of disability (Taylor 1976).

It is not my intention to recapitulate the history of these different definitions and their conceptual characteristics. The point is that disability can be placed within a number of different frames. These frames can be seen as methodological: tools for helping us to understand what is there in the world. They can also be seen as ontological: mechanisms or practices whereby things that we cannot see because they are taken for granted, or things that are too blurred to see are brought into being, created, or constructed. This ontogenetic capacity of the frames we employ also makes those frames political because they have the power to make us see disability in one way rather than another. Disability is something—if it actually is anything at all—that is framed in a number of different ways with very different implications for our knowledge, policies, and practices. For most of the twentieth century, disability has been understood to be the property of individuals who are "different from normal," whether cultural "anomalies" or institutionalized "chronic patients" (Arney and Bergen 1983). Biomedicine has been at the heart of defining and managing the meaning and implications of this on behalf of governments and societies.

Definitions and Classifications

At the time that the *International Classification of Impairments, Disabilities, and Handicaps (ICIDH)* was published, many sociologists worked happily alongside medical and other scientists working within this scientific orthodoxy. It was this Enlightenment-style concern with clearer, sharper definitions that drove the work that culminated in the development of the *ICIDH* published by the World Health Organization in 1980. A number of features of this model have made it attractive to some clinicians and repellant to many within the disability movement: its continuing use of bodily impairment as the apparent "first cause" in a causal chain, its emphasis on things lacking or restricted in an individual's abilities, and its dependence, for all the sociological relativism of the concept of *handicap,* on assumptions about the normal human being. Nonetheless, it is certainly the case that in relation to the history of rehabilitation and epidemiological surveys of disability, the *ICIDH,* particularly the concept of *handicap,* was an attempt to break away from an obsessive focus on impaired bodies and limited human beings to a perspective that emphasized the emergence of disadvantage from the individuals' interaction with the social world. In the context of independently developing sociological work on the experience of chronic illness and disability, this kind of definition made a lot of sense.

Arcane as some of the discussions about definition may seem, they provided the basis for a much more realistic assessment of the prevalence of disability and an argument for increases and shifts in forms of provision. Until 1979, disability was part of the wider discussions about the strengths and weaknesses of the welfare state. This was very much a reformist program, informed by some input from disabled people themselves, situated within either a medical or welfarist framework. While beginning to develop a larger picture of the social ontology and consequences of disability, disability itself was ultimately situated within individual lives and experiences.

For a whole range of epidemiological, economic, and policy reasons, the attempt to find a satisfactory "socio-medical model of disabling illness" (Bury 1997:138) underpinned this enterprise. Against the dominant biomedical model, it was argued that the differences between the impairments arising out of clinically different diseases or accidents were less important than what they shared in terms of their psychological, social, and economic consequences. In part, this was a recognition of the limited impact that much disease-based rehabilitation had on the lives of those people going through long periods of treatment. What was important for someone with multiple sclerosis, it was argued, was not so much the nuanced variation of the unfolding of disease in different cases but the broad impact of living with such symptoms on global areas of social life: work, education, family, sex, identity, self-esteem, and so on.

The growing involvement of social scientists in this area also began to open up different ways of looking at disability. Although many of the social scientists working in the area shared the dominant interests and assumptions of the experts in rehabilitation and public health with whom they worked, they also brought with them a set of theoretical and empirical approaches to thinking about social phenomena that were radically different. The work of Goffman (1968) on stigma, in particular, had a significant impact not just on what social scientists thought mental and physical illness were but also on the legitimacy of different ways of researching and writing about them. The "symbolic interactionist" approach in which Goffman can be located included a notion of individual roles and identities that was seen to be highly relevant to the way in which sociological research on disability might be conducted (S. J. Williams 1987).

These debates between various lay and professional experts all take place in the context of global economic and social change. While theorizing disability develops its own logic, it is necessary for those who engage in it to move back and forth between their experience and concepts to the realities of power and interest in the modern world (Stone 1985; Williams 1991). In most Western societies, politicians are increasingly scrutinizing the claims made on their welfare states and moving away from notions of universal entitlement toward various forms of targeted help underpinned by an emphasis on individual self-reliance. In view of these developments inside and outside disability studies, this debate is not one that can be finally resolved at the conceptual level because the intellectual terrain in which the debate takes place is contested by an increasingly wide range of intellectual and political stakeholders. The terrain is multiparadigmatic, and the development of and relationships between different paradigms need to be seen in a historical context (Oliver 1996) if the analysis is to avoid the kind of standoff across a divide that badly needs bridging (Barnes and Mercer 1996).

In this fecund theoretical environment, Marx, Foucault, and Goffman, at the very least, are required to explain why disabled people "have been isolated, incarcerated, observed, written about, operated on, instructed, implanted, regulated, treated, institutionalized, and controlled to a degree probably unequal to that experienced by any other minority group" (Davis 1997:1). Disabled people and their bodies have been framed, intellectually and politically, in a wide variety of ways. Indeed, one important component of our understanding of the way in which disability is to be understood is through an appreciation of the history of disabled people themselves, a complex subject that is covered elsewhere in this volume. These histories themselves are, of course, written within particular theoretical frameworks, but they also help to reveal to us the way in which the categories we use for making sense of human differences have changed over time.

Theorizing disability, therefore, involves the analysis of a number of dimensions of experience and the relationships between them. These dimensions include theorizing the bodily or mental processes that someone experiences; theorizing the relationship and context in which they are placed; theorizing the meanings that emerge, for the person, from the relationship between the two; and theorizing the oppression or disadvantage that arises out of this, particularly social and historical circumstances. In other words, there are multiple ontologies of disability. These ontologies exist in the biomedically constructed body, in the person's relationship to the "lived body," between the person and the people with whom he or she comes into contact, and between the historically formed society (encompassing political economy, social welfare, culture, and ideology) and the person as a member of that society.

MEANING AND INTERACTION

As the pseudonymous W. N. P. Barbellion illustrates in an entry in his journal of a disappointed man, the experience of symptoms, or what Thomas (1999) suggests we refer to as "impairment effects," is de facto a social experience:

> The numbness in my hand is getting very trying. . . . The Baby puts the lid on it all. Can't you see the sordid picture? I can and it haunts me. To be paralysed with a wife and child and no money—ugh! (Barbellion 1984:253)

The development of sociological research on chronic illness, impairment, and disability since the mid-1970s has been characterized by an attempt to understand the relationship between experiences of symptoms or impairment, the social situations in which people live, and the combined effect of these on the kind of life someone has. Concepts such as *representation, trajectory,* and *career* have been developed to make sense of the experience of illness and impairments and the way in which they are shaped (or even "constructed") by social interaction and organization. It is this quality of human experiences of symptoms, illness, impairments, suffering, and how they are formed by things outside personal experience that characterizes the main thrust of sociological theorizing about disability.

This work focuses on meaning in one or other of two senses of meaning identified by Bury (1991). Bury argues that the meaning of an illness can be defined in terms of its "consequences," which refers to the impact it has on practical aspects of the person's roles and relationships in everyday life or in terms of its "significance," which relates to the cultural connotations, symbols, and significations surrounding different sorts of illness and disability. Both these forms of analysis of the meaning of chronic illness and disability have the notion of embodied experience at their center, but rather than attempting to define functional incapacity or activity restriction in biomedical terms, they explore the ramifications of the experience from the point of view of the person affected. In other words, while the biomedical model has disease or dysfunction at the center of its picture, sociological approaches focus on illness as something whose meaning and reality vary depending on the biography of particular individuals and the circumstances in which they find themselves. Stigma and deviance are the processes of societal definition and framing in social interaction.

The quote from Barbellion's (1984) journal illustrates very well how important both senses of meaning are in theorizing chronic illness and impairment and how the two kinds of meaning merge within an individual's experience. The numbness in his hand is upsetting for him because of what it might signify about him, and what it might signify about him is dependent on his circumstances—a new father with financial responsibilities in the context of British society prior to the development of a health service and a welfare state. Taken together, these represent a "sordid picture" in his mind. Regardless of the fact that his symptoms at the time he was writing were limited in the sense that he was not restricted in most activities of daily living, from his point of view and situation, the symptoms were highly significant and consequential.

The attempt to understand the meaning of experience by looking at it in its context lies at the heart of the medical sociological project. The focus on chronic illness and the experience of disability associated with it can be seen as an attempt to move away from the rehabilitation models that were rather static, reductive, and focused on the mechanics of functional limitations and activity restriction. While the experience of "adaptation" to a limb amputation or some other trauma-induced impairment clearly has its own dynamics, influenced by personal, situational, and treatment factors, chronic illness introduces new problems of enormous variability and unpredictability (Bury 1982; Strauss and Glaser 1975). While disability might have certain unifying features, sociologists have been interested in both subjective variation in response to the "same" illness and impairment and variation in the meaning (in the second of Bury's senses) of different kinds of symptoms in society. Explorations of breathlessness, itching and weeping skin, painful joints, heart problems, end-stage renal failure, and many others have allowed sociologists and anthropologists to explore the seemingly infinite permutations of the experience of being physically different in a highly normalizing society (Anderson and Bury 1988; Strauss and Glaser 1975).

Some of these sociological analyses are phenomenologically "deep" or "thick"; others are more inclined to skate over the surfaces of meaning but nevertheless deal with the interaction between symptoms and situations. The hallmarks of this kind of work are, therefore, its focus on the symbolic and material interaction between the individual and society and the interpretive processes whereby individuals construct meaning from their experiences. The environment focused on is that which emerges in the meaning-giving processes of interaction between the individual, the individual's milieux, and the wider society. It therefore follows from this that disability (or "handicap"), in the World Health Organization's (1980) definition, is the product of complex processes of interaction between an individual with an impairment and the discriminating, disadvantaging, stigmatizing, and prejudiced wider society. It is neither in the individual nor outside the individual in society:

> The extent to which functional limitations and activity restrictions constitute a problem, or are otherwise handicapping, is not only variable historically and culturally but is also somewhat dependent upon more immediate contexts; their meaning is not the same across different social and environmental settings. (Locker 1983:5)

The point for Locker (1983), therefore, is that "disability" or "handicap" (he makes use of the WHO schema) as a social reality of people's experiences is caused neither by the externalities of the environment nor by any "facts" of biological trauma or deterioration. This kind of analysis is primarily concerned with meaning as consequences rather than meaning as significance, though it may, as Locker does, explore at some level the "significance" of symptoms to individuals in terms of some notion of "felt stigma" (Scambler 1989). The traditions of sociological theorizing about "disability," therefore, have tended to focus on two of the ontologies to which I referred earlier: the lived body and the everyday relationships between the person with impairment and family, friends, and professionals.

THEORIZING BODILY EXPERIENCE

Much of the early work theorized the disabling consequences of impairments by way of a very specific empirical focus on the management of symptoms, the organization of medical regimens, and the handling of interactions with people known and unknown. In that sense, it was work that provided a complement to, rather than direct criticism of, the biomedical model. More recently, however, with the growing interest in relationships between the body and identity, analysis of the experience of illness or impairment has turned more and more toward the meaning of embodied experience. These analyses may also concentrate on the interactions within the mundane world, but there is a sense in which the purpose of these interactions can be interpreted as having rather more transmundane qualities. Such a path leads us away from the empirical features of the impaired individual's interaction with the material world back into the "self" and "body." The focus of the problem shifts from interactionism to the exploration of the lived body, the body incarnate in which the meaning of illness is revealed.

There are some skilful examples of this mode of analysis, such as the work of Kathy Charmaz, who has written of the process of "immersion in illness," which "means experiencing the vulnerability of one's body" (Charmaz 1991:80). It is possible to see how this kind of work is attempting to do more than descriptively report on the empirical dimensions of the consequences of illness and impairment. It is somehow trying to touch that place in which loss, suffering, pain, degradation, and humiliation are actually felt and offer witness to the truth of the human condition. It is at this point that the dividing lines between sociology, phenomenology, and a kind of nonspecific religiosity become very difficult to find. The "existential-ontological language" of theology and the more theological forms of philosophy and literature (Macquarrie 1967) are powerful resources for meaning, and some sociologists have drawn on these in trying to interpret the experience of illness and impairment.

Some of the more powerful phenomenological analyses come from individuals, usually middle class and often academics or writers themselves, who have tried to explore autobiographically the depths of their own experiences of cancer, neurological disease, heart attack, or whatever else (Couser 1997; Frank 1991; Murphy 1987). The best of this work gives preeminence to the ill person's perspective, emphasizing the "illness" (the social experience) above the "disease" (the physiological processes). However, the aim within this project "to consider illness stories as embodied also deconstructs the distinction: the illness experience is an experience in and of a diseased body" (Frank 1995:187). In much of this work, the storied or narrative nature of illness and disability is emphasized (Hyden 1997). Although most of the sociological work on this theme would not admit to what is criticized from within the disability movement as a "personal tragedy" view of disability, it does take as axiomatic the importance of bringing the tragic dimensions of human experience to the forefront of discussion and debate. The exploration of the experience of illness becomes a vehicle or location for exploring basic questions about the nature of the self in the world and the fundamental meaning structures in a person's life. The concept of a narrative is a powerful framework for analyzing "tragic" experiences of illness for a number of reasons. It provides a temporal framework for thinking about illness, it describes a life both as a sequence of events and as unified around some purpose or purposes, and it moves back and forth between the subjective experience and the world in which the experience is lived out.

THEORIES IN NARRATIVES

Narratives are epistemic concentrates of experience in place and time. If impairment and disability can be seen as disrupting "biography," making problematic the relationship between the individual and the environment, it makes sense to regard the experience of having a chronic illness or disability as part of a process of "narrative reconstruction" (Bury 1982; Williams 1984). Some of this work is explored in other chapters. The point for our purposes is to recognize that theorizing disability is not merely about abstractly conceptualizing the relationships between impairment and situations—it is about how those relationships work for people in dynamic and complex personal and social processes. It is a body of work that has many origins. It partly originates in a growing interest in narratives or other first-person accounts, across a range of disciplines and beyond the specific issues of illness and disability (see Hinchman and Hinchman 1997 for examples). It is also a form of discourse about illness that has been given a high public profile by the history of HIV/AIDS, in which the intersections of personal identity and the history of a societal response to disease, disability, and death have, of course, been particularly sharply defined (Couser 1997). While some of this work emphasizes the materiality and the historicity of such narratives—the political economy of illness (Radley 1993)—other research engages more and more deeply with the subjectivity of the experience—the negotiation and renegotiation of identity through talk, the rediscovery of self in the chaos of illness, and so on (Sacks 1985). Some have explored with great skill and empathy the different kinds of narratives that can be constructed about the experience of chronic—often terminal—illnesses (Frank 1995; Mathieson and Stam 1995).

In much of this narrative-based work, what started as a sociological analysis becomes part of a quasi-religious or spiritual quest for the truth, which illness is supposed to reveal. So profound is the truth of illness that even the person experiencing the illness is merely a vehicle for allowing the body to speak of its suffering. This is truly the body incarnate:

> The body is not mute, but it is inarticulate; it does not use speech yet begets it. The speech that the body begets includes illness stories; the problem of hearing these stories is to hear the body speaking in them. (Frank 1995:27)

Some (but by no means all) of this work can shed a bright light on "human" conditions. However, there is a danger that the process of living with chronic illness becomes represented as so idiosyncratically idiographic that it leads us further and further away from any sense of the society in which the anguish of experience is embedded and, indeed, shaped. As a consequence, the processes through which the response to chronic illness and disability emerges become less and less social and collective and more and more rooted in the psychological, cognitive, and existential world of the individual. There is less exploration of the interaction between the person and the "environment" in the presence of the disruptive effects of chronic illness and more searching the constitution of the self in the presence of a disordered body.

While Christian theology and the learning of other world religions certainly provide rich languages for exploring questions of ultimate concern (life and death, suffering, guilt, and redemption), they can also—if we are not very careful—reduce the individual to a body and limit the experience of illness and disability to a personal quest for meaning and truth. The politics and history of illness and disability become marginalized, and medical sociologists begin to "reproduce the disablism that sociology exhibits everywhere else" (Barnes 1996:19), and the realities of health and social care become forgotten. All that is left is the individual engaged in some abstract process of overcoming bodily "failure" and "coming back" to normality. Even when there is no specific reference to a religious or spiritual interpretation, the language suggests suffering, redemption, and resurrection.

> Coming back is the process of returning to a satisfactory way of life, within the physical/mental limitations imposed by a disabling condition. . . . To come back is a very personal experience. Although others can provide assistance, only the individual can come back. (Corbin and Strauss 1991:138-39)

I have tried to show in this section how sociologists have responded to the limitations of traditional rehabilitation perspectives and theorize disability in a more holistic way. They have done this by emphasizing the need to move away from professional definitions of impairment and disability to explore the ways in which people with chronic illness and disability defined the relationship between their symptoms and situations. Using various forms of qualitative methods, they have attempted to reconstruct from people's own accounts of their experiences the reality of chronic illness and disability as something that emerges out of the relationship between the person and the environment. The World Health Organization's (1980) classification illustrates at a conceptual level what most of these studies attempt to accomplish at an empirical level.

However, I have also indicated how the relational can at times slip into a phenomenological analysis in which the individual or even the body returns to the center of attention, albeit constructed in a discourse somewhat different from that employed within rehabilitation medicine. While explorations of the lived body can illuminate experiences of extreme situations, once detached from the political economy and history of disability and its relationship to state and society, they can become an unhelpful form of self-analysis. The coming back or overcoming is not seen in relation to a collective response to societal barriers but rather in terms of some kind of individual self-transformation.

In the end, so seduced is such theorizing by the voyeuristic delight and horror of looking in on the dark secrets of the self that it loses sight altogether of the structures—of society, policy, and organization—that provide the inescapable framework of experience. History and even biography are dissolved in ever-deeper phenomenological penetration into the interstices of self and world. The politics of the life writing Couser (1997) describes are cultural: a politics of representation and discourse rather than a politics of resources and structures. An AIDS narrative is interpreted as counterhegemonic in that the "sickroom" becomes "a battlefield, a scene of struggle, rather than a site of isolation and invalidity, passivity and despair" (Couser 1997:166). And although Couser (1997) acknowledges the increasing politicization of disabled people and the existence of the "social model," his definition of disability seems caught between seeing it as "a physical and existential condition" and as something created by the "cultural site" in which it is located.

It is certainly not the intention of this sociological analysis to produce a prescription for what is to be done that denudes the situation of its politics and material basis. Indeed, the point of taking a "sociological perspective" for most practicing sociologists is precisely that "it provides an alternative perspective in which individualized, homogenized, and disablist conceptions of policy and practice are subject to critical analysis" (Barton 1998:54). Nonetheless, the consequence of this has been that what began as an attempt to see chronic illness and disability as the product of the complex relationships between individuals, milieux, and social structures becomes a picture in which the illness is portrayed as something that causes certain social consequences.

The central criticism from within disability studies of sociological approaches is that they fail to retain a sharp enough understanding of the politics of both the experience of disability and the construction of the categories we use to speak about it. In short, the sociological imagination has not been exercised sufficiently robustly by sociologists, and it is argued that it is more evident in those engaged in praxis at the heart of the disability movement (Oliver 1996). In addition, what passes for the "sociology of disability" is unreservedly condemned for being "both theoretically backward and a hindrance rather than a help for disabled people" (Abberley 1987:5).

SOCIAL OPPRESSION

In these terms, it is not surprising that those working from within the disability movement should want to distance themselves from sociological contributions to the study of chronic illness and impairment. Insofar as medical sociological work retained a key interest in clinical conditions, even if seen from the point of view of the person with the condition rather than the doctor, it is "destined to lead to a partial and inhibiting view of the disabled individual" (Brisenden 1998:20). In contrast, within much work in disability studies, the prime mover, in causal terms, is most certainly not the "clinical condition" or the individual in a state of tragic adaptive "failure" but the oppressive society in which disabled people live. If disability is seen as a personal tragedy, disabled people are treated as the victims of circumstance. If disability is defined as social oppression, disabled people can be seen as the collective victims of an uncaring, discriminatory society (Oliver 1990).

The object on which many of the conceptual knives of the disability movement have been sharpened is the WHO's *ICIDH,* partly because this classification was developed outside the disability movement (albeit, *pace* Barnes 1995 in consultation with disabled people), but mostly because it is seen to place impairment at the center of its taxonomic efforts. It has been rejected by people involved in the disability movement in Britain and the United States. It has continued to be less objectionable in Europe, perhaps because non-English-speaking people recognize the enormous philosophical and linguistic difficulties that the authors of the *ICIDH* grappled with in coming to a settled view on the definitions of impairment, disability, and handicap that also made sense in other languages. It is unfortunate that the debate over terms got rather mired in etymological issues. For example, much has been made of the origin of *handicap* in the nineteenth-century Poor Laws in England, even though the historical evidence for such a claim is not clear (Devlieger 1999).

However, the rejection of the *ICIDH* is an important historical moment, marking the divide between those who see disability as an emergent property of the interaction between person and society and those who see it as an expression of social oppression. For these latter, medicine, social security, charity, social work, occupational therapy, and so on are all engaged in an ideological practice that defines disability in ways in which it becomes—in the final analysis—a property of the individual rather than a feature of the society. So profound is the assumption of individual property and properties within the Western ideology of "possessive individualism" (Macpherson 1962) that it is difficult to hold conceptually to this, even when it is supported politically. Individualism, as Steven Lukes (1973) argued, has political, economic, religious, ethical, epistemological, and methodological manifestations.

There are different versions of the social model of disability. In the United States, it is more commonly referred to as the "minority group" model of disability, the basic thrust of which is that

> disabled men and women have been subjected to the same forms of prejudice, discrimination and segregation imposed upon other oppressed groups which are differentiated from the remainder of the population on the basis of characteristics such as race or ethnicity, gender and aging. (Hahn 1997:174)

This fundamental position is that which underpins most of the writing by disability theorists in Britain too. However, while in Britain the theoretical driver of the early statements of principle (UPIAS 1976) was a neo-Marxism that defined itself in opposition to welfare-Fabianism and well-meaning liberal-functionalist sociology, in the United States, much of the work has combined a subtle Marxist analysis with a political perspective derived from concepts of civil and constitutional rights. In the United States and in the United Kingdom, however, the arguments developed by people who saw themselves as activist-academics sought to "turn the world upside down" in a tradition of popular revolt that would upset structures of both power and knowledge. It is a position that leads to a very different picture of, for example, the nature of dependency when compared with sociological perspectives. Let me contrast two quotations to highlight this difference between medical sociology (or one example of it) and the work of one very influential disability theorist:

> Certainly physical dependency, if not also social and economic dependency, can result from illness. (Charmaz 1991:80)

> Dependency is created amongst disabled people, not because of the effects of functional limitations on their capacities for self-care, but because their lives are shaped by a variety of economic, political and social forces which produce it. (Oliver 1990:94)

The problem to be overcome is not anything within the individual's body, mind, or soul. There is no personal road to redemption and salvation. It is, as some of the sociological work indicates (Locker 1983), to do with resources in society. However, in this case, the relationship between the individual and society is much more clearly stated. Disability and dependency are caused by society. On this analysis, "hostile environments and disabling barriers—institutional discrimination" are seen as the "primary cause of the problem" (Barnes 1992:20). Proponents of this "social model" turn the conventional models of those working in rehabilitation on their heads, arguing that if you change society, disability will disappear.

The causal relation is reversed, and, as a consequence, the traditional theories and practices of those engaged in rehabilitation come to be seen as part of the problem. If the dominant ideology of the medical model informing rehabilitation defines the focus as what has happened to an individual and what can be done "for the patient," attention is distracted from the primary structural causes, and the medical profession and those working next to them become key figures in the perpetuation of oppression. In view of the overwhelmingly political impulse in much of this work, sociologists who concede any primary role to the bodily disorder or impairment can be criticized for participating in an oppressive ideological practice, and the WHO classification that, in my judgment, was put forward to socialize and collectivize our understanding of "disablement" becomes transformed into an extension of the medical model. Sociological analysis of what disability is like, from the point of view of someone with an impairment or disability—the phenomenological or interactionist exploration of the construction of reality—becomes another ideological justification for the oppression of disabled people.

I have developed my arguments against this position in a number of publications (Williams 1983, 1988, 1991, 1996a). It seems to me that the oppressive quality of everyday life for many disabled people is indubitable, and the origins of much of this oppression lie in the hostile environments and disabling barriers that society (politicians, architects, social workers, doctors, and others) erects. However, to theorize disability wholly in terms of "social oppression" seems to me to be profoundly limited for three reasons. First, most disability in modern societies emerges from chronic illness, and illness, unlike ethnicity or gender, emerges slowly over time. Second, someone who is able-bodied is only temporarily so. Disability is therefore a category theoretically open to everyone and, as populations age, one that becomes a more likely end point for any given individual. Third, notwithstanding the socially constructed nature of embodied experiences, phenomenologically, disability has undeniably to do at some level with the pain or discomfort of bodies, and this is a dimension of the oppressive quality of chronic illness and disability for large numbers of people. To say that disability is social oppression and that the body has nothing to do with it is curiously solipsistic and clearly not the whole story, and among those who otherwise support the broad viewpoint, there has been an attempt to bring impairment back into the picture (Crow 1996; Thomas 1999).

Nonetheless, the social model or the minority group perspective is a powerful story, supporting a theoretical perspective that needs to be argued and justified because on a number of grounds—empirical, political, cultural, epistemological—the dominance of medical knowledge in this area has to be challenged and turned upside down. But having turned the world upside down, it is then necessary to rearrange the pieces. It can be seen, therefore, that while both medical sociology and disability studies stand in contrast to the biomedical model of disability, the interest of medical sociologists in subjective experiences of symptoms and impairments places them in a complementary position in relation to the medical model. Disability studies, on the other hand, rejects the medical model on the grounds that it defines disability primarily in terms of things that have gone wrong with an individual's body. As Davis (1997) points out, "We live in a world of norms," and both medical and welfare definitions of disability define people in their relation to "the norm." Yet, as he goes on to point out, "the idea of a norm is less a condition of human nature than it is a feature of a certain kind of society" (p. 9).

Moreover, the perpetuation of the norm, as well as the cultural dichotomization of normal and abnormal, is inscribed in photographic and cinematic representations of disability (Darke 1998; Hevey 1997) and in architectural assumptions about the normal human body (Imrie 1998). If norms are a product of society, and disability is defined as a departure from the norm, then disability is a social construct. If disability is a social construct, changing the dominant construct, biomedicine, and the practices undertaken in its name will transform or eliminate disability. While many sociologists writing about disability would agree with this, they stop short of a full revolution of the epistemological sphere. The conflict that emerged between the "medical model" and the "social model" during the 1970s and 1980s has become, to this author at least, less clear-cut in recent times. While the medical model has become more social in response to sociological criticism, political protest, and the limits of medical interventions, the social model has become less unitary as it has been exposed to debate inside and outside disability studies. The politics of the social model are as fragmentary as the cultural politics in which they are embedded. In recent times, the post-Foucauldian focus on the nature of the body has made a number of adherents of the social model search for new ways of theorizing impaired bodies without losing the political edge of the social model. Most people writing within the tradition of the disability movement have treated disability as if it had nothing to do with illness.

More recently, however, disabled writers and others have written of impairment as an inescapable part of the politics of disability, and this provides a place of common ground with much of the sociological writing on chronic illness and disability. There are now signs of hope that the rather sterile divide between disability studies and medical sociology can be bridged or at least acknowledged with greater openness than has been the case in the past (Barnes and Mercer 1996). The sources of this new enthusiasm for collaboration and partnership have many sources. Some of these sources include the following:

the increasing diversity and differentiation within the disability movement itself and the need to bring impairment and the body back in (Crow 1996; Williams 1996b);

the recognition of the similarities and differences of experience among those with physical impairments, learning difficulties, and mental health problems (Barton and Oliver 1997);

the continuing need in government for some kind of "individual" head count of people eligible for benefit, whatever the social definitions of *disability* may be;

within sociology and cultural studies, the growing interest in the body and new forms of political resistance that lie outside or across the conventional dividers of gender, race, and class.

In the next section, I will examine the implications of this new pluralism for theorizing disability.

POLYPHONY OR CACOPHONY?

To recapitulate, sociological perspectives on disability have been criticized by disability theorists on a number of different (and sometimes seemingly contradictory) grounds: for not paying attention to disability, for enhancing rather than rejecting the medical model, and for becoming obsessed with the details of illnesses and impairments. All these concerns contain some truth: Disability has not excited the same interest in mainstream sociology as class, gender, or race. Early work on disability by social scientists was undertaken in collaboration with rehabilitation specialists and epidemiologists who took the reality of individual impairments as a starting point (Bury 1996). Some of the more phenomenologically orientated work on chronic illness has attempted to reach the deepest interiors of people's subjective experiences to a point where the connection between those experiences and the outside world is not easy to see.

However, these criticisms contain a truth that depends to a large extent on the setting up and knocking down of straw men and women and on a tendency to theorize anachronistically. Mainstream sociology may have neglected disability, as Barton (1996) and others have argued, but the sociology of health and illness—a large and growing constituency—has not, even if the conceptualization of its interest has not been to everyone's taste. Social scientists' work on the conceptualization and measurement of need among disabled people was, to some extent, individualistic, medically orientated, and "paternalistic." Yet much of this work was important politically in drawing attention to large numbers of people whose needs were not being met by the health service or the welfare state more generally.

Moreover, the work of sociologists such as Blaxter (1976) in the United Kingdom and Strauss and Glaser (1975) in the United States did start an important process of using laypeople's own accounts of life with symptoms and the difficulties they experienced with professionals as the basis for developing an understanding of chronic illness and disability and making recommendations for how doctors, health services, and society should be educated, organized, or constituted. While such studies may be criticized from the viewpoint of the social or minority group model for having looked at social aspects of chronic illness and disability with the individual, who uses illness or disability as his or her starting point (Oliver 1996), when individuals with chronic illness or disability are allowed to speak, they will start with themselves, autobiographically, and the virtue of this kind of work is that it allows that to be possible.

Increasingly, knowledge and frameworks developed by sociologists are interrogated, interpreted, and made use of by groups who were formerly its objects. More recent critiques of sociology by disability theorists point to the assumptions that have framed much of the research agenda, with the methods that are used producing answers that reinforce predominant models of disability (Barnes and Mercer 1997). Taking as his example some of the questions used in the U.K.'s Office for Population Censuses and Surveys (OPCS) to ascertain "levels" of disability, Oliver (1990) suggests how questions that ask about an individual's "difficulty in holding, gripping, or turning things" could be reframed as a question about defects in the design of everyday equipment that limit a person's activities, or how a question about an individual's "scar or blemish" could be reframed to ask about difficulties caused by other people's reactions to any such blemish.

While the extent to which these questions offer any practical alternative to current survey items is debatable (Bury 1996) and is being exposed to some empirical examination (Zarb 1997), they do turn the world upside down in a manner that requires us to question our framing of the relationship between individual experiences and social circumstances. Oliver's (1990) satire also raises questions about the relationship between lay and professional expertise within the processes whereby knowledge about "disability" is produced. However, we need to be sensitive to the way in which methods and research questions are embedded in the political economy and culture of a certain time and place—be it postwar collectivism, the individualism and consumerism of the 1960s, 1970s corporatism, or Thatcherite and Reaganite monetarism—

and are the outcome of particular decisions by politicians, civil servants, and, to some extent, researchers to ask questions in one way rather than another (Abberley 1996a).

The critique of the dominant methods used in the social sciences for understanding disability goes beyond a replacement of one set of survey questions by another. It seeks to contextualize the concept of disability within "knowledge which arises from the position of the oppressed and seeks to understand that oppression. Such sociology requires an intimate involvement with the real historical movement of disabled people if it is to be of use" (Abberley 1996b:77; see also Barnes and Mercer 1997). However, to imply that the position of disabled people is uniquely oppressive replaces one kind of exclusivity with another. It defines disabled people as an undifferentiated class in itself without the differences of body and identity, which clearly have cultural significance for disabled and able-bodied people (Hughes and Paterson 1997). This strategy leaves disabled women, for example, "perennial outsiders" in both disability studies and feminism (Begum 1992:73; see also Meekosha 1998; Morris 1996; Thomas 1999).

Recent poststructuralist, neo-Foucauldian analysis attempts to bring the body back in by conceptualizing it as the object of knowledge and the target of power. In Hughes and Paterson's (1997) terms, "Post-structuralism can be useful in theorising impairment out with a medical frame or reference" (p. 333). In this way, it is argued, the embodied experience of different impairments and their relationship to identity can be part of a more inclusive disability politics. Theorizing disability as fluid and continuous rather than permanent and dichotomous would help to open things up epistemologically and politically (Zola 1993b). If this were to be developed, some of the current difficulties involved in including people with learning disabilities, mental health problems, and other less visible forms of impairment into theoretical frameworks and policy discussions might be reduced, thus allowing an understanding of politics that is as much about aesthetics as economics (Hughes and Paterson 1997). It would also allow for "the near universality of disability" and the diverse "chorus of voices" that disability represents to be part of the movement in the manner advocated by Zola (1989, 1994).

Marginalization of debate about the body has been characteristic of the disability movement, perhaps for good reasons. As Benoist and Cathebras (1993) point out, closure of "the body" is characteristic of most systems of thinking underpinning utopian projects and visions. Pinder's (1995) work about how fixed definitions of disability may have obscured the experiences of some disabled people at work draws attention to some of the consequences of excluding the dimension of lived experience. Pinder argues that many fall into "no-man's land" between definitions of able and disabled and that these have done some disservice to the task of promoting the interests of disabled and differently abled people at work. Similarly, Zola has argued that the exclusivist leaning of some of the writing about disability has led to the marginalization of the growing numbers of older people whose bodies will slowly, but surely, let them down (Zola 1991).

Increasingly, poststructuralist, postmodernist, and feminist analyses have argued that all encompassing theories of disability and oppression can never encompass the diversity of lived experiences (Crow 1996; Hughes and Paterson 1997). As Radley (1995) argues, being disabled involves distinctive bodily experiences, but such experiences cannot be seen as unique inasmuch as they "symbolize and are symptomatic of social contradictions and struggles sited on the body" (p. 19). Peters (1996) draws on the postmodern perspective for what she calls critical pedagogy—working toward a critical understanding of the world and one's relation to the world—with disabled people and others. In Peters's interpretation of postmodernity, one implication is that different insider voices can be articulated and heard and can challenge those of the academy (in this case, professional sociologists). For her, as for other feminists, making private experience speak to public policies is a radical act.

For those who hold firmly to the "social model," however, it is argued that these revisionists do not seem to realize that experience was what drove the disability movement in the first place, as I indicated by reference to Hunt (1998) at the start of this chapter. Also, much of the apparently new work, which tries to bring impaired bodies back in, is really going over old ground rather than building on what has gone before. The consequence of too much emphasis on diversity and difference in impairment, it is argued, is that the boundaries between impairment and disability as social oppression become blurred. In addition, much of the new wave of work in disability studies stands in danger of replicating the sentimental autobiography or disease-based analyses found in medical sociology (Barnes 1998).

Cutting across sociology and disability studies, the work of Irving Zola, a sociologist and disability activist, represents an important attempt to link the material, social, and cultural dimensions of disability (Thomas 1999; Williams 1996b). During the early 1980s, Zola recognized that while his politics had to be unwavering in the articulation of demands for independence and an end to discrimination, there was more to a sociological analysis of disabled people's oppression than an empirical identification of environmental barriers conjoined with a conspiracy theory regarding the interests of professionals engaged in rehabilitation. In line with many other activists in both Britain and the United States, Zola recognized the undermining power of the dominant ideology of disability that regarded "it"—that is, the thing from which the individual "suffers"—as a personal tragedy. It is, perhaps, his ability and willingness to combine the personal and the political, subjectivity and materialism, that makes adherents of the orthodoxy of the social model, with their denial of the structured silence of subjective bodily experiences (Meekosha 1998; Zola 1991), uncomfortable with him.

Zola resisted the temptation to allow his sociology to be reduced to political ideology. This allowed him to avoid a rigid "us and them" theorization of disability and helped him recognize, for example, the enormous implications of aging societies peppered with chronic illnesses for the development of the disability movement (Zola 1991). Zola pointed out that the processes of aging linked the interests of "the able-bodied" to those of "the disabled." However imperative it may be politically to define people with disabilities as a minority group, it is a curious minority that includes us all—if not today, then tomorrow, or the day after—and that

> only when we acknowledge the near universality of disability and that all its dimensions (including the biomedical) are part of the social process by which the meanings of disability are negotiated, will it be possible fully to appreciate how general public policy can affect this issue. (Zola 1989:420)

In addressing the debate on the words used about disability, Zola preferred to talk about "people with disabilities," putting people first. He emphasized that in choosing certain terms, he was "not arguing for any 'politically correct' usage but rather examining the political advantages and disadvantages of each" (Zola 1993a:171). In Zola's view, there was no single, unequivocal authentic voice of disabled people (Zola 1988), nor is there any set of definitions of the universe of disability that can or should be adopted as a standard. A similar argument has been developed in Britain by Corker (1998) and Shakespeare (1996), who see in postmodern and poststructuralist analysis a way of remaining critical in relation to biomedicine while also challenging the tendency to essentialism in the "metanarrative" of the social model.

In place of the monochrome languages of the "medical model," on one hand, and the "social model," on the other, we find in Zola a willingness to examine disability from many points of view and a desire to understand the contribution the growing polyphony has to make to our discussions about disability. Zola's work was a bold attempt to hold firm to the politics of disability while remaining free to explore its darker phenomenological waters. He wanted to place at the forefront of any discussion of disability the bleak realities of economic deprivation, disenfranchisement, and marginalization while insisting on the continuing need to find a place for research in clinical rehabilitation and an interpretive phenomenology of the personal worlds of people with disability and chronic illness. Within this context, the ontological reality of the impaired body was central to the development of any social theory of disability. It could be argued that when some of the more recent writing in disability studies is examined, Zola was an avant-garde poststructuralist. As Corker (1998) argues,

> Post-structuralist discourse on disability does not "reject" the social model. Rather it suggests that, since disability is now located in a postmodern world, it is appropriate to begin to look at the relationship between the individual and society rather than to focus on the individual or society. (P. 232)

This brings us back to some of the central problems currently facing social theory and the social sciences as we attempt to develop better ways of understanding the relationships between agency and structure. While much of the attempt to bring the body back into the sociology of disability can overemphasize self-authorship of possibilities, work on the lived body has the potential to respond to some of these challenges. Thinking about the lived body forces recognition of the constraints as well as the possibilities of interpretation. As Nussbaum (1995) argues, "We all live our lives in bodies of a certain sort, whose possibilities and vulnerabilities do not as such belong to one human society rather than another" (p. 76). There are, of course, other ways of situating knowledge and praxis in relation to disability that cut across this poststructuralist conceptualization. For example, it has recently been argued that a more productive way to think of the oppression of disabled people is to see it as part of the history of disabled people across the world, one that is grounded in a materialist analysis of oppression that exists outside disability per se (Charlton 1998). Charlton (1998) argues that we need to see the oppression experienced by disabled people as a global phenomenon—80 percent of the world's 500 million disabled people live in "developing countries." This oppression, argues Charlton, results from structures of domination and subordination and ideologies of superiority and inferiority. The oppression—exploitation, marginalization, and powerlessness—of disabled people cannot be understood within a poststructuralist framework. While there are cross-cutting identities and relationships of disability, gender, race, age, and class, these cannot be understood in a nonstructural way. As Charlton puts it, "The oppression of individual disabled bodies is not the basis for the oppression of people with disabilities, it is the oppression of people collectively that is the basis for the oppression of their bodies" (p. 57).

Such an analysis allows impairment and disability to be situated within a framework that encompasses disabled people and others whose relationship to the means of production, distribution, and exchange is disadvantaging. In this context, challenging "disablist oppression is a necessary step in the struggle to eradicate all forms of oppression" (Barton 1996:10). Both Marx and Foucault, at the very least, are required to explain why disabled people "have been isolated, incarcerated, observed, written about, operated on, instructed, implanted, regulated, treated, institutionalized, and controlled to a degree probably unequal to that experienced by any other minority group" (Davis 1997:1). Charlton recognizes the importance of acknowledging the oppression of the body within sickrooms dominated by professional experts and developing points of resistance to it, but it is impossible to do this effectively without understanding it in the context of the distribution of power and status in the broader society.

CONCLUSION

Placing too much emphasis on the politics of exclusion may be regarded as a way of underplaying the real effects of different impairments and the complex, "negotiated" aspects of everyday life, thereby creating a spurious homogeneity. Crow (1996) has written with feeling about the discounting of the experience of impairment resulting from "keeping our experiences of impairment private, and failing to incorporate them into our public analysis" (p. 66). Others have begun to point out the need to explore the nature and status of impairments, without being restricted by seeing them as purely biological or purely social (S. J. Williams 1996). However, as we have indicated, focusing too much on impairment is seen to deflect attention from the systematic way in which the social and material environment excludes people from participation in civil society.

Any theory, whether expounded by sociologists or by disability theorists and activists, that overdetermines social control risks paralyzing the possibilities for change. The anger that originally fired Hunt and others gets doused with an overdose of theorizing—structuralist or poststructuralist. Within sociology, we see the turn toward "the body" as representing a longing for community, for connection, and for meaningful participation (Kirkmayer 1992)—a turn away from some of the more sterile territories of critical theory. However, if theory is not to incapacitate meaningful politics altogether (Hallsworth 1996), then it must use the insight of lived experience as grist for its development, and closure of the subject of the body is no longer possible. As Smart (1992) reminds us, "Postmodernism signifies incredulity towards meta-narratives in general, and towards the grand narrative of emancipation in particular" (pp. 176-77), with the attendant dangers of slipping into a politics of hopelessness. However, a focus on the politics of identity alongside the politics of structures might provide the basis for the development of the liberative theory of disability called for by Abberley (1998), which would assert "the rights of the human 'being' against the universalization of the human 'doing' " (p. 92). Without a continuing incorporation of subjective experience into structuralist theories, they become impoverished and meaningless for the lives of those who they are supposed to explain (Thompson 1978).

Where next for theorizing disability? This has been a long but necessarily partial tour through what I see as some of the key issues emerging from the fields of disability studies and medical sociology and the effects of the growing willingness to exchange ideas and perspectives between them. My own perspective is one that I would characterize as "materialist phenomen-ology": a commitment to understanding other people's experiences in the context of what used to be called the objective conditions in which they find themselves. It could be argued that con-siderable political mileage has been clocked up by holding to a fairly tough and uncompromis-ing definition of the "social model" or the "minority group" approach. However, the social reality of disability is one of considerable variation in the experience of impairment by large numbers of people who nonetheless share common conditions of exclusion, marginalization, and disadvantage.

Like Zola, we need to resist the temptation to allow our sociology to be reduced to political ideology. Zola (1991) avoided an "us and them" theorization of disability, and this helped him recognize the enormous implications of aging societies peppered with chronic illnesses for the development of the disability movement. He pointed out that the processes of aging link the in-terests of "the able-bodied" to those of "the disabled." However imperative it may be politically to define people with disabilities as a minority group, it is a curious minority that will include us all—if not today, then tomorrow, or the day after that.

While it is clearly possible to theorize disability with medical categorization, poststruc-turalist theorizing about disability will reproduce the methodological and political individual-ism of the medical model unless it retains in its analysis a connection of the material forces that produce poverty, powerlessness, and discrimination. It is clear how work in both sociology and disability studies attempts in different ways to retain that connection.

REFERENCES

Abberley, P. 1987. "The Concept of Oppression and the Development or a Social Theory of Disability." *Disability, Handicap and Society* 2:5-19.

———. 1996a. "Disabled by Numbers." Pp. 166-84 in *Interpreting Official Statistics,* edited by R. Levitas and W. Guy. London: Routledge Kegan Paul.

———. 1996b. "Work, Utopia and Impairment." Pp. 61-79 in *Disability and Society: Emerging Issues and Insights,* edited by L. Barton. London: Longman.

———. 1998. "The Spectre at the Feast: Disabled People and Social Theory." Pp. 79-93 in *The Disability Reader: Social Science Perspectives,* edited by T. Shakespeare. London: Cassell.

Albrecht, G. 1992. *The Disability Business.* London: Sage.

Anderson, R. and M. Bury, eds. 1988. *Living with Chronic Illness: The Experience of Patients and Their Families.* London: Unwin Hyman.

Arney, W. R. and B. J. Bergen. 1983. "The Anomaly, the Chronic Patient, and the Play of Medical Power." *Sociology of Health and Illness* 5:1-24.

Barbellion, W. N. P. 1984. *Journal of a Disappointed Man and a Last Diary.* London: Hogarth.

Barnes, C. 1992. "Institutional Discrimination against Disabled People and the Campaign for Anti-Discrimination Legislation." *Critical Social Policy* 34:5-22.

———. 1995. "Disability, Cultural Representation and Language." *Critical Public Health* 6:9-20.

———. 1996. "Theories of Disability and the Origins of the Oppression of Disabled People in Western Society." Pp. 43-60 in *Disability in Society: Emerging Issues and Insights,* edited by L. Barton. London: Longman.

———. 1998. "The Social Model of Disability: A Sociological Phenomenon Ignored by Sociologists?" Pp. 65-78 in *The Disability Reader: Social Science Perspectives,* edited by T. Shakespeare. London: Cassell.

Barnes, C. and G. Mercer. 1996. *Exploring the Divide: Illness and Disability.* Leeds, UK: The Disability Press.

———. 1997. *Doing Disability Research.* Leeds, UK: The Disability Press.

Barton, L. 1996. "Sociology and Disability: Some Emerging Issues." Pp. 3-17 in *Disability and Society: Emerging Issues and Insights,* edited by L. Barton. London: Longman.

———. 1998. "Sociology, Disability Studies and Education." Pp. 53-64 in *The Disability Reader: Social Science Perspectives,* edited by T. Shakespeare. London: Cassell.

Barton, L. and M. Oliver. 1997. *Disability Studies: Past, Present and Future.* Leeds, UK: The Disability Press.

Begum, N. 1992. "Disabled Women and the Feminist Agenda." *Feminist Review* 40:70-84.

Benoist, J. and P. Cathebras. 1993. "The Body: From One Immateriality to Another." *Social Science and Medicine* 7 (36): 857-65.

Blaxter, M. 1976. *The Meaning of Disability.* London: Heinemann.

Booth, T. 1996. "Sounds of Still Voices: Issues in the Use of Narrative Methods with People Who Have Learning Difficulties." Pp. 237-55 in *Disability and Society: Emerging Issues and Insights,* edited by L. Barton. London: Longman.

Brisenden, S. 1998. "Independent Living and the Medical Model of Disability." Pp. 20-27 in *The Disability Reader: Social Science Perspectives,* edited by T. Shakespeare. London: Cassell.

Bury, M. 1982. "Chronic Illness as Biographical Disruption." *Sociology of Health and Illness* 4:167-92.

———. 1991. "The Sociology of Chronic Illness: A Review of Research and Prospects." *Sociology of Health and Illness* 14:451-68.

———. 1996. "Defining and Researching Disability: Challenges and Responses." Pp. 17-27 in *Exploring the Divide: Illness and Disability,* edited by C. Barnes and G. Mercer. Leeds, UK: The Disability Press.

———. 1997. *Health and Illness in a Changing Society.* London: Routledge Kegan Paul.

Charlton, J. I. 1998. *Nothing about Us without Us: Disability, Oppression, and Empowerment.* Berkeley: University of California Press.

Charmaz, K. 1991. *Good Days, Bad Days: The Self in Chronic Illness and Time.* New Brunswick, NJ: Rutgers University Press.

Chatterji, S., B. Üstün, and J. Bickenbach. 1999. "What Is Disability After All?" *Disability and Rehabilitation* 21:396-98.

College Committee on Disability. 1986. "Physical Disability in 1986 and Beyond: A Report of the Royal College of Physicians." *Journal of the Royal College of Physicians* 20:160-94.

Corbin, J. and A. Strauss. 1991. "Comeback: The Process of Overcoming Disability." In *Advances in Medical Sociology,* vol. 2, edited by G. Albrecht and J. Levy. Greenwich, CT: JAI.

Corker, M. 1998. "Disability Discourse in a Postmodern World." Pp. 221-33 in *The Disability Reader: Social Science Perspectives,* edited by T. Shakespeare. London: Cassell.

Couser, G. T. 1997. *Recovering Bodies: Illness, Disability and Life Writing.* Madison: University of Wisconsin Press.

Crow, L. 1996. "Including All of Our Lives: Renewing the Social Model of Disability." Pp. 55-73 in *Exploring the Divide: Illness and Disability,* edited by C. Barnes and G. Mercer. Leeds, UK: The Disability Press.

Dalley, G. 1991. *Disability and Social Policy.* London: Policy Studies Institute.

Darke, P. 1998. "Understanding Cinematic Representations of Disability." Pp. 181-97 in *The Disability Reader: Social Science Perspectives,* edited by T. Shakespeare. London: Cassell.

Davis, L., ed. 1997. *The Disability Studies Reader.* London: Routledge Kegan Paul.

Devlieger, P. J. 1999. "From Handicap to Disability: Language Use and Cultural Meaning in the United States." *Disability and Rehabilitation* 21:346-54.

Frank, A. 1991. *At the Will of the Body: Reflections on Illness.* Boston: Houghton Mifflin.

———. 1995. *The Wounded Storyteller: Body, Illness and Ethics.* Chicago: University of Chicago Press.

Gloag, D. 1985. "Severe Disability: Tasks of Rehabilitation." *British Medical Journal* 290:301-3.

Goffman, E. 1968. *Stigma.* Harmondsworth, UK: Penguin.

Granger, C. V., G. L. Albrecht, and B. B. Hamilton. 1979. "Outcome of Comprehensive Medical Rehabilitation: Measurement by PULSES Profile and the Barthel Index." *Archives of Physical Medicine and Rehabilitation* 60:145-54.

Gritzer, G. and A. Arluke. 1985. *The Making of Rehabilitation: A Political Economy of Medical Specialization, 1890-1980*. Berkeley: University of California Press.

Hahn, H. 1997. "Advertising the Acceptably Employable Image: Disability and Capitalism." Pp. 172-86 in *The Disability Studies Reader*, edited by L. J. Davis. London: Routledge Kegan Paul.

Hallsworth, S. 1996. "Confronting Control: Finding a Space for Resistance in Theory." Aldgate Papers in Social and Cultural Theory, No. 1, 1996-97, Department of Sociology and Applied Social Studies, London Guildhall University.

Harris, A., E. Cox, and C. Smith. 1971. *Handicapped and Impaired in Great Britain*. 2 vols. London: Her Majesty's Stationery Office.

Hevey, D. 1997. "The Enfreakment of Photography." Pp. 332-47 in *The Disability Studies Reader*, edited by L. Davis. London: Routledge Kegan Paul.

Hinchman, L. P. and S. K. Hinchman, eds. 1997. *Memory, Identity, Community: The Idea of Narrative in the Human Sciences*. New York: State University of New York Press.

Howard, M. 1999. *Enabling Government: Joined Up Policies for a National Disability Strategy*. London: Fabian Society.

Hughes, B. and K. Paterson. 1997. "The Social Model of Disability and the Disappearing Body: Towards a Sociology of Impairment." *Disability and Society* 12:325-40.

Hunt, P. 1998. "Condition Critical." Pp. 7-19 in *The Disability Reader: Social Science Perspectives*, edited by T. Shakespeare. London: Cassell.

Hyden, L.-C. 1997. "Illness and Narrative." *Sociology of Health and Illness* 19:48-69.

Imrie, R. 1998. "Oppression, Disability and Access in the Built Environment." Pp. 129-46 in *The Disability Reader: Social Science Perspectives*, edited by T. Shakespeare. London: Cassell.

Kaye, H. J. 1996. *"Why Do Ruling Classes Fear History?" and Other Questions*. London: Macmillan.

Kirkmayer, J. 1992. "The Body's Insistence on Meaning: Metaphor as Presentation and Representation in Illness Experience." *Medical Anthropology Quarterly* 6 (5): 323-46.

Locker, D. 1983. *Disability and Disadvantage*. London: Tavistock.

Lukes, S. 1973. *Individualism*. Oxford, UK: Blackwell.

Macpherson, C. B. 1962. *The Political Theory of Possessive Individualism*. Oxford, UK: Oxford University Press.

Macquarrie, J. 1967. *God-Talk: An Examination of the Language and Logic of Theology*. London: SCM Press.

Marks, D. 1997. "Models of Disability." *Disability and Rehabilitation* 19:85-91.

Mathieson, C. M. and H. J. Stam. 1995. "Renegotiating Identity: Cancer Narratives." *Sociology of Health and Illness* 17:283-306.

Meekosha, H. 1998. "Body Battles: Bodies, Gender and Disability." Pp. 163-80 in *The Disability Reader: Social Science Perspectives*, edited by T. Shakespeare. London: Cassell.

Morris, J., ed. 1996. *Encounters with Strangers: Feminism and Disability*. London: The Women's Press.

Murphy, R. 1987. *The Body Silent*. New York: Holt, Rinehart & Winston.

Nagi, S. Z. 1979. "The Concept and Measurement of Disability." In *Disability Policies and Government Programmes*, edited by E. Berkowitz. New York: Praeger.

Nussbaum, M. C. 1995. "Human Capabilities, Female Human Beings." Pp. 61-104 in *Women, Culture and Development: A Study of Human Capabilities*, edited by M. C. Nussbaum and J. Glover. Oxford, UK: Clarendon.

Oliver, M. 1990. *The Politics of Disablement*. Basingstoke, UK: Macmillan.

———. 1993. "Re-Defining Disability: A Challenge to Research." Pp. 61-67 in *Disabling Barriers—Enabling Environments*, edited by J. Swain, V. Finkelstein, S. French, and M. Oliver. London: Sage.

———. 1996. "A Sociology of Disability or a Disablist Sociology." Pp. 18-42 in *Disability and Society: Emerging Issues and Insights*, edited by L. Barton. London: Longman.

———. 1998. *Disabled People and Social Policy: From Exclusion to Inclusion*. London: Longman.

Peters, S. 1996. "The Politics of Disability Identity." Pp. 215-34 in *Disability and Society: Emerging Issues and Insights*, edited by L. Barton. London: Longman.

Pinder, R. 1995. "Bringing Back the Body without the Blame? The Experience of Ill and Disabled People at Work." *Sociology of Health and Illness* (17) 5: 605-31.

Radley, A., ed. 1993. *Worlds of Illness: Biographical and Cultural Perspectives on Health and Disease*. London: Routledge Kegan Paul.

———. 1995. "The Elusory Body and Social Constructionist Theory." *Body and Society* 1:3-23.

Rich, A. 1995. *On Lies, Secrets and Silence*. London: Norton Wiley.

Sacks, O. W. 1985. *The Man Who Mistook His Wife for a Hat*. London: Duckworth.

Scambler, G. 1989. *Epilepsy*. London: Tavistock.

Shakespeare, T. 1996. "Disability, Identity, Difference." Pp. 94-113 in *Exploring the Divide: Illness and Disability*, edited by C. Barnes and G. Mercer. Leeds, UK: The Disability Press.

———, ed. 1998. *The Disability Reader: Social Science Perspectives*. London: Cassell.

Smart, B. 1992. *Modern Conditions, Postmodern Controversies*. London: Routledge Kegan Paul.

Stone, D. 1985. *The Disabled State*. Basingstoke, UK: Macmillan.

Strauss, A. and B. Glaser. 1975. *Chronic Illness and the Quality of Life*. St. Louis, MO: C. V. Mosby.

Taylor, D. 1976. *Physical Impairment: Social Handicap*. London: Office of Health Economics.

Thomas, C. 1999. *Female Forms: Experiencing and Understanding Disability*. Buckingham, UK: Open University Press.

Thompson, E. P. 1978. *The Poverty of Theory*. London: Merlin.

Tunbridge, R. 1972. *Rehabilitation: Report of a Sub-Committee of the Standing Medical Advisory Committee*. London: Her Majesty's Stationery Office.

Union of the Physically Impaired against Segregation (UPIAS). 1976. *Fundamental Principles of Disability*. London: Author.

Williams, G. H. 1983. "The Movement for Independent Living: An Evaluation and Critique." *Social Science and Medicine* 17:1003-10.

———. 1984. "The Genesis of Chronic Illness: Narrative Reconstruction." *Sociology of Health and Illness* 6:175-200.

———. 1987. "Disablement and the Social Context of Daily Activity." *International Disability Studies* 9:97-102.

———. 1988. "Independent Living: Rolling Back the Frontiers of the State?" *Disability Studies Quarterly* 8:50-54.

———. 1991. "Disablement and the Ideological Crisis in Health Care." *Social Science and Medicine* 32:517-24.

———. 1996a. "Representing Disability: Some Questions of Phenomenology and Politics." Pp. 194-212 in *Exploring the Divide: Illness and Disability*, edited by C. Barnes and G. Mercer. Leeds, UK: The Disability Press.

———. 1996b. "Irving Kenneth Zola (1935-1994): An Appreciation." *Sociology of Health and Illness* 18:107-25.

———. 1998. "The Sociology of Disability: Towards a Materialist Phenomenology." Pp. 234-44 in *The Disability Reader: Social Science Perspectives*, edited by T. Shakespeare. London: Cassell.

Williams, S. J. 1987. "Goffman, Interactionism, and the Management of Stigma in Everyday Life." In *Sociological Theory and Medical Sociology*, edited by G. Scambler. London: Tavistock.

———. 1996. "The Vicissitudes of Embodiment across the Chronic Illness Trajectory." *Body and Society* 2:23-47.

Wood, P. H. N. 1975. *Classification of Impairments and Han   dicaps*. Geneva: World Health Organization.

World Health Organization. 1980. *International Classification of Impairments, Disabilities and Handicaps*. Geneva: Author.

Yelin, E. 1992. "The Cumulative Impact of a Common Chronic Condition." *Arthritis and Rheumatism* 35:489-97.

Zarb, G. 1997. "Researching Disabling Barriers." Pp. 49-66 in *Doing Disability Research*, edited by C. Barnes and G. Mercer. Leeds, UK: The Disability Press.

Zola, I. K. 1988. "Whose Voice Is This Anyway? A Commentary on Recent Recollections about the Experience of Disability." *Medical Humanities Review* 2:6-15.

———. 1989. "Toward the Necessary Universalizing of Disability Policy." *The Milbank Memorial Fund Quarterly* 67 (Suppl. 2): 401-28.

———. 1991. "Bringing Our Bodies and Ourselves Back In: Reflections on the Past, Present and Future Medical Sociology." *Journal of Health and Social Behaviour* 32:1-16.

———. 1993a. "Self, Identity and the Naming Question: Reflections on the Language of Disability." *Social Science and Medicine* 36:167-73.

———. 1993b. "Disability Statistics, What We Count and What It Tells Us: A Personal and Political Analysis." *Journal of Disability Policy Studies* 4:9-39.

———. 1994. "Toward Inclusion: The Role of People with Disabilities in Policy and Research in the United States: A Historical and Political Analysis." Pp. 49-66 in *Disability Is Not Measles: New Research Paradigms in Disability*, edited by M. Rioux and M. Bach. Toronto, Ontario: Roeher.

Methodological Paradigms That Shape Disability Research

5

SCOTT CAMPBELL BROWN

The best available methods of sociological research are at present so liable to inaccuracies that the careful student discloses the results of individual research with diffidence; he knows that they are liable to error from the seeming ineradicable faults of the statistical method, to even greater error from the methods of general observation, and, above all, he must ever tremble lest some personal bias, some moral conviction or some unconscious trend of thought due to previous training, has to a degree distorted the picture in his view. Convictions on all great matters of human interest one must have to a greater or less degree, and they will enter to some extent into the most cold-blooded scientific research as a disturbing factor.

—DuBois (1899:2-3)

Previous chapters in this volume have made the case that theories, definitions, and classifications of disability play an important role in how persons with disabilities are viewed in various contexts and in how results for persons with disabilities are interpreted. These chapters have discussed *disability paradigms,* which reference the theoretical, definitional, and taxonomic view toward the disability experience.

Rather than focusing primarily on disability paradigms, this chapter shifts the scope to the paradigms for the conduct of research, referred to as *methodological paradigms.* In discussing methodological paradigms, this chapter mostly references social research. Engineering and medicine are important disciplines within the disability and rehabilitation science field. These disciplines have often been associated with particular research constructs and methods. In the area of social research, however, the choice of a particular research method to study disability has been increasingly recognized as critical beyond methodological appropriateness because that choice in itself may predetermine the results. Guba and Lincoln (1989) elaborate the rationale behind such comments, by noting that "values permeate every paradigm that has been proposed or might be proposed, for paradigms are human constructions, and hence cannot be impervious to human values" (p. 65). Hence, following that logic, the choice of a particular research method may influence study results just as much as the disability paradigm employed.

It may be useful to state specifically the goal of this chapter. First, this chapter does not seek to settle the question of whether one type of paradigm is better than another. Indeed, as researchers who employ different methodologies are forming dialogues, such a quest would be counterproductive. Second, in some parallel to the first issue, this chapter will not attempt to settle the question of whether the choice of a particular methodology will drive a result, as opposed to whether the methodology is properly applied. As different methodologies "borrow" techniques from other paradigms, such a distinction would be difficult and would probably require a major research study in itself. Third, in a more pedestrian vein, this chapter will not attempt to provide a rigorous review of all aspects of all methodologies. This clearly would require a book in itself.

This chapter does explore the underlying values of particular modes of inquiry and how these values might interact with the various disability paradigms to shape conclusions drawn from studies. Indeed, just as some disability advocates have argued that disability cannot be viewed outside of an environmental context, the environmental context of research may also influence how underlying research value paradigms and corresponding methodological paradigms affect conclusions.

The argument is that the underlying value behind a qualitative research technique—triangulation—needs to be adopted by the disability field as a key criterion for the conversion of research conclusions into policy and practice. As noted by Marshall and Rossman (1995),

> Triangulation is the act of bringing more than one source of data to bear on a single point. . . . Designing a study in which multiple cases, multiple informants, or more than one data gathering method are used can greatly strengthen the study's usefulness for other settings. (P. 144)

This notion has been criticized by some who argue that consistency itself is a positivist value similar to reliability. The argument made here is not for the value of consistency but for the application of heterogeneous modes of inquiry to answer particular research questions. To support this argument, the chapter first briefly describes some basic terms—the two value paradigms (positivist and constructivist) in social research and the two methodological paradigms (quantitative and qualitative) often associated with each of the value paradigms. Then, I argue that social research studies of minority groups in the nineteenth century did integrate a variety of research methodologies. However, for at least the first half of the twentieth century, while social disciplines developed and coalesced, public health research shifted from stressing the study of the environment to emphasizing the study of individuals. At the same time, disability policy and research also stressed the study of the individual. More recently, emphases on community-based approaches to public health and rehabilitation have placed greater emphasis on the role of the environment in these fields. These shifts in the disability paradigm at times correlate well with a challenge to the value paradigm of positivism by a constructivist view in social research on disability but not as much in engineering and medical research. This raises the question of whether new disability paradigms demand constructivist value paradigms. In response to this question, this chapter calls for a synthesis or triangulation of the value and methodological paradigms but raises three points to consider for the reader. First, if paradigms are synthesized, different criteria for evaluation from each paradigm need to be blended. Second, if persons with disabilities are to be empowered in research studies through participatory action research (PAR), issues for incorporation of PAR into quantitative research need to be addressed. Third, ethical considerations need to be considered. Finally, this chapter argues for the application of triangulation principles to assess the important concept of access of persons with disabilities to the environment as well as other issues. Some demonstrations of how triangulation concepts can be employed to study this important issue of access to the environment by shifting the unit of analysis, the reporting source, and the methodological paradigm are provided. By the end, one hopes that the reader will be convinced that the merging of different methodological paradigms is not only a desirable goal but also a practical consideration for the conduct of research.

SOME BASIC TERMS

Social Research Paradigms as Compared to Other Fields

In some sense, the division of methodological paradigms into quantitative and qualitative is, itself, a value. One could classify research paradigms into any number using any particular concept. For instance, a significant distinction often made in biomedical research is between basic and applied research. *Basic research* generates knowledge without necessarily pursuing an application or good. *Applied research* seeks to produce knowledge that will have tangible benefits. The roles of both are valued. Indeed, basic research results often lay the foundation for applied research results in later studies.

The quantitative *methodological paradigm* is associated with research problems in the hard sciences. For instance, product safety and procedure reliability are core values in many fields, and reliability almost demands a quantitative methodology. However, quantitative and qualitative paradigms appear to be broadly recognizable in social science. Right or wrong, they have been viewed as somewhat competitive with each other (Cizek 1995). Increasingly, this distinction may influence other fields—if not in product development, then in product application. Thus, it is important to understand that the methodological paradigms of quantitative and qualitative research have underlying value paradigms, and it is important to explore precisely what these value paradigms are.

The *value paradigm* of most kinds of quantitative research is based on the ideas of either positivism or postpositivism. Mertens and McLaughlin (1995) have noted this longstanding value in educational research:

> The dominant orientation in educational research history has been derived from the philosophical orientation of positivism. Epistemologically, positivism is represented by the rationalistic paradigm, which employs a quantitative research design. Alternative perspectives have emerged (i.e., the constructivist paradigm) that typically have been associated with qualitative research designs and are described as contextual, inclusive, experimental, involved, socially relevant, multimethodological, and inclusive of emotions and events as experienced. (P. 5)

As shown in Table 5.1, contrasts between these value paradigms occur along three dimensions of basic beliefs—how reality is viewed, the interaction between those who seek knowledge and the phenomena about which knowledge is sought, and the methodology employed. More detail on the two major methodological paradigms follows.

Quantitative Methodological Paradigms

The values underlying quantitative research consist of the following:

> the notion of one reality,
> the objectivity in the exploration of that reality, and
> the estimation of some probability that the reality has been found.

In other words, a truth can be discerned if the researcher removes as much bias as possible from the study and estimates some likelihood that the truth has been found. According to Cook and Campbell (1979), postpositivists recognize that the investigator's ideas can strongly influence the observed phenomena or his or her observation of those phenomena.

Table 5.1   Basic Beliefs Associated with the Major Value Paradigms

Basic Beliefs	Positivism/ Postpositivism	Interpretive/ Constructivist	Critical Theory
Ontology (nature of reality)	One reality; knowable within probability	Multiple, socially constructed realities	Multiple realities shaped by social, political, cultural, economic, ethnic, gender, and disability values
Epistemology (nature of knowledge; relation between knower and would-be known)	Objectivity	Interactive link between researcher and participants	
		Values are made explicit; created findings	Knowledge is socially and historically situated
Methodology	Quantitative	Qualitative; contextual factors described	
			Construct of oppression

SOURCE: Derived from Guba and Lincoln (1994:105-17).

These assumptions contain the value of linearity from design to study to conclusion. For example, the researcher should design his or her research question and then gather materials to explore this question. As the researcher begins the work, a critical point then is the conversion from the research question to the methodology. Then, a methodology is applied to answer the question in some way, results are obtained, and conclusions are drawn. Many quantitative research articles are organized around this linearity.

Qualitative Methodological Paradigms

According to Marshall and Rossman (1995),

Qualitative research is evolving, through intellectual, political, and even technological struggles and advances. Critical theorists and feminists demonstrate that openly ideological or value-explicit stances in research are essential for identifying the political assumptions embedded in our social institutions. (P. ix)

In contrast to quantitative research, the underlying value paradigms for the qualitative methodological paradigm are quite different (Denzin and Lincoln 2000). According to Mertens and McLaughlin (1995), assumptions are the following: (1) reality is created as a part of social construction, and there is no reality waiting to be "discovered"; (2) both the inquirer and inquiree are interlocked, each affecting the other; and (3) facts are products of social construction; hence, values surrounding statements of "fact" must be explored and made explicit. Thus, qualitative research has a different set of beliefs and values. For instance, context is extremely important in qualitative research.

Patton (1990) gives four characteristics in which the use of qualitative research is warranted. First, the research program emphasizes individual outcomes. Second, detailed, in-depth information about the phenomena under study is needed. Third, the study's focus is on diversity and unique qualities of individuals. Finally, there is no available standardized, valid, and reliable instrument.

Whereas quantitative research values linearity, qualitative research has a valued fluid nature with a lack of linearity. According to Marshall and Rossman (1995),

> The researcher should demonstrate to the reader that she reserves the right to design the research as it evolves: Building flexibility into the design is crucial. The researcher does this by (1) demonstrating the appropriateness and the logic of qualitative methods for the particular research question; and (2) devising a research plan that includes many of the elements of traditional plans but reserves the right to modify and change that initial plan. (P. 39)

These include the interactive linkages between observers and participants.

Whereas quantitative research de-emphasizes the personality of the researcher, quantitative analysis stresses that the role of the researcher cannot be controlled. Issues to be addressed include technical, interpersonal, and data collection considerations. For example, Harding (1993) argues that results are less likely to be biased toward racism or sexism if the design is politically guided rather than value neutral. From this viewpoint, knowledge is limited by one's original standpoint. The researcher has both technical and interpersonal roles (Marshall and Rossman 1995). Spradley (1980) describes five different levels for participant observation as they relate to the role of the researcher. In nonparticipation, the researcher is virtually removed from an activity (i.e., watching a videotape of subjects engaged in an activity). In passive participation, the researcher observes but does not interact with those engaged in the activity. For moderate participation, the researcher participates in some but not all of the activities. Active participation comprises participation in all but a few activities. Finally, there can be complete participation. This assessment for participation is important not only to identify the role of the researcher but can also come into play when the role of persons with disabilities in research is assessed.

Interpretive/constructivist approaches to this research acknowledge multiple realities. Within qualitative research, some distinguish between interpretive/constructivist and critical theory/emancipatory value paradigms. Emancipatory approaches support the notion that reality and knowledge are shaped by situation, particularly in terms of the power relationship between the researcher and those being studied. It differs from the interpretive/constructivist approaches by describing historical factors that create oppression.

Mertens (1998) rejects the label of critical theory because of its close association with Marxist theory. She calls it the emancipatory paradigm, which is characterized by (1) focusing on the marginalization and oppression of diverse groups, (2) explaining inequalities, (3) linking results to political and social action, and (4) developing emancipatory theory. This paradigm relies heavily on values and methodologies from feminist research, including strands acknowledging the standpoint or social and historical context of the knowers, the centrality of the lived experiences of those being studied, and the role of text in sustaining the integration of power and oppression (Olesen 1994).

Blending the Paradigms

It is important to note that the association of particular value and methodological paradigms is not rigid. As will be seen in the next section, it is possible to use qualitative methodologies with a positivist search for truth. By contrast, some quantitative survey designs could operate under constructivist and critical theory/emancipatory paradigms. Indeed, two historical researchers mixed elements of the value and methodological paradigms and applied concepts of triangulation well before these concepts were defined.

Table 5.2   Estimates on the Proportion of Deaf Students Who Could Acquire Articulation, Selected Schools in Europe, 1867

Institution, Country, and Level	Percentage	Reporting Source
Milan, Italy	30	Signor Tarra
Paris, France		Professor Vaisse
Converse some	90	
Converse with teachers	70 to 80	
Converse readily	50 to 60	
Converse on all subjects with ease	10 to 20	
Vienna, Austria		Mr. Venus
Converse readily	80	
Converse with strangers	50	
Weissenfels, Germany		Mr. Hill
Converse some	85	
Converse readily	62	
Converse with strangers	11	

SOURCE: Derived from text in Fischer and de Lorenzo (1983:246-47).

TWO HISTORICAL STUDIES THAT INTEGRATED METHODOLOGIES

Edward Miner Gallaudet's Study of Teaching Methods

In 1867, Edward Miner Gallaudet toured Europe to examine all methods for teaching deaf students (Fischer and de Lorenzo 1983). For this research, he visited institutions in Great Britain, France, Germany, Belgium, Switzerland, and Italy and gathered materials from those countries, as well as from Russia (including Finland at the time), Sweden, Denmark, Holland, and Ireland (Fischer and de Lorenzo 1983). Gallaudet attempted to discern the proportion of deaf students who could acquire articulation. He engaged in personal observations of practices, yet he noted, "Not satisfied to form my opinions solely from the observations I might be able to make in a single tour of inspection, I have taken pains to gather the views of many teachers on this point" (Fischer and de Lorenzo 1983:246). Thus, he gathered data summarized in Table 5.2 from a variety of reporting sources on this question. One can observe from such sources that the reported percentages of students who could acquire articulation varied and, on the surface, appear difficult to synthesize.

Gallaudet combined his own observations with these data and concluded that between 10 and 20 percent of deaf students could gain the ability to communicate with strangers. However, he also noted that "with reference to the additional 40 to 60 per cent who may aspire to converse on commonplace subjects with their teachers, family and intimate friends, my mind is not so clear" (Fischer and de Lorenzo 1983:247).

In combination with this data gathering and personal observation, Gallaudet reviewed many books and pamphlets collected in Europe (Fischer and de Lorenzo 1983). Based on these and his observations, he classified methodologies for teaching deaf students into the natural method (signing), the artificial method (developing speech), and the combined method. He subclassified schools teaching the combined method into types that stressed articulation and those that did not. He learned the historical origins of the methods and observed them personally.

From this effort, Gallaudet concluded,

> Thus it would seem that attempts at articulation should be made with all deaf-mutes, lest, unhappily, some possessing ability to acquire it, by neglect fail to do so. I am inclined to seriously question the desirableness of continuing instruction in speech during a series of years, when no higher result can be expected than to enable the pupil to converse on common place subjects with his teachers, family and intimate friends [because those groups could use sign language]. (Fischer and de Lorenzo 1983:248)

Given his background as the son of Thomas H. Gallaudet, the person largely responsible for introducing the use of sign language as a mechanism for teaching deaf people, Edward Gallaudet could hardly have been a dispassionate observer. Indeed, he had a strong record as an advocate for the sign approach. However, more than 130 years ago, Edward Miner Gallaudet employed both quantitative and qualitative paradigms and triangulated data sources to research a particular issue.

The Philadelphia Negro

A similar integration of methodologies was conducted a little more than 100 years ago by Dr. W. E. B. DuBois in his landmark study, *The Philadelphia Negro*. In an introduction to the book, Samuel McCune Lindsay reported,

> He devoted all of his time to systematic field-work among the Negroes, especially in the Seventh Ward, attending their meetings, their churches, their business, social and political gatherings, visiting their schools and institutions, and, most important of all, conducting a house-to-house visitation in their families, through which he came into personal contact with over ten thousand Negro inhabitants of the city. (DuBois 1899:vii)

DuBois used both descriptive and statistical techniques to explore the conditions for a minority group. Indeed, one chapter in the book is devoted to the environment of the minority group (DuBois 1899).

DuBois may seem to have been in favor of a view of absolute truth in the quotation that begins this chapter. Indeed, the tables in his book are quite extensive for a work of that time. He also notes,

> We must study, we must investigate, we must attempt to solve; and the utmost that the world can demand is, not lack of human interest and moral conviction, but rather the heart-quality of fairness, and an earnest desire for the truth despite its possible unpleasantness. (DuBois 1899:3)

Nevertheless, he stands for moral conviction, indicating a sense of advocacy on the part of the researcher. In his case, it was to yield an improvement in the lives for African Americans in Philadelphia at the time.

Summary

It would appear that the research conducted by Edward Miner Gallaudet and W. E. B. DuBois in the nineteenth century did have an underlying value paradigm of a search for truth consistent with positivist thinking. However, these two were scholar-advocates who saw their work not simply as a quest for truth but also as work that would inform and, in so doing, improve the conditions for the groups being investigated. To achieve their research, they triangulated a variety of perspectives and research methods that today would be recognized as coming from different methodological paradigms.

THE SHIFT TOWARD COMPARTMENTALIZATION OF PARADIGMS

The Emergence of Field Specialization

During the first half of the twentieth century, social research appeared to become more compartmentalized. These paradigms not only related to how people with disabilities were viewed but also appeared to promote the quantitative methodological paradigms in the fields of public health and disability.

Public Health Paradigm Changes

In the case of public health, as noted by Susser and Susser (1996a), modern epidemiology took shape with the demonstration of statistical clustering of mortality and morbidity to pinpoint poisoning by foul emanations from air, soil, and water. The authors state,

> An irony of the history of public health is that, while the sanitarians were mistaken in their causal theory of foul emanations, they nonetheless demonstrated how and where to conduct the search for causes in terms of the clustering of morbidity and mortality. The reforms they helped to achieve in drainage, sewage, water supplies, and sanitation generally brought major improvements in health. Their mistake lay in the specifics of biology rather than in the broad attribution of cause to environment. (P. 669)

Statistics were replaced by infectious disease epidemiology based on germ theory. Instead of altering the environment, the new emphasis was on interrupting the transmission through vaccines, quarantine, and ultimately antibiotics (Susser and Susser 1996a). McKeown (1976) argued that this emphasis on interruption did not cause the decline in infectious diseases; rather, the decline was caused by nutrition and improved living standards. Susser and Susser (1996a) note, "While closer analysis does not sustain the arguments against the role of science, the primary role of economic development and social change is not in doubt" (p. 670).

The period during World War II saw the beginnings of a positive holistic community-based paradigm toward public health. The Gluckman Report (Union of South Africa 1945) emphasized

> the practical expression of two of the most important, and universally accepted, conclusions of modern medical thinkers. The first is that the day of individual isolationism in medical practice is past, and that medical practitioners and their auxiliaries can make their most effective contribution to the needs of the people through group or team practice. The second is that the primary aim of medical practice should be the promotion and preservation of health. (Phillips 1993:1038)

As part of the team involved in implementing the report's recommendations in South Africa, Sidney Kark made three innovations: (1) establishing a national system of community-based health centers, (2) recruiting and training community health teams who would care for families as a whole, and (3) establishing an underlying model of an integrated view of medicine in a societal context, encompassing the biological, psychological, and social sciences (Susser 1993:1040-41). Perhaps the ultimate expression of these perspectives was the World Health Organization's 1948 definition of *health* as not merely the absence of disease but physical, psychological, and social well-being (World Health Organization 1964).

Despite these promising efforts at an environmental perspective, the perspective of chronic disease epidemiology took root at the end of World War II. Referred to as the black box (Susser and Susser 1996a), the emphasis became focused on risk factors of exposure to outcome at the individual level. In the context of history, this paradigm is quite different, with its focus on the individual as opposed to the environment. However, the rise of HIV and the fact that other diseases have never been eradicated in developing countries have undermined confidence in the universal applicability of the black box paradigm (Susser and Susser 1996a).

Susser and Susser (1996b) also argue that in the 1990s, "an exclusive focus on risk factors at the individual level within populations—even given the largest numbers—will not serve. We need to be equally concerned with causal pathways at the societal level" (p. 674). The authors argue for a system emphasizing relations within and between localized structures at a variety of levels. The analysis of determinants and outcomes must occur at different levels of organization, within and across contexts.

The previous discussion may strike the reader as a digression. However, the key points are the following: (1) the consideration of the environment in major aspects of public health has long-term precedent; (2) from a public health perspective, the emphasis on the individual has been criticized; and (3) holistic family and community-based positive approaches to health have been practiced since the 1940s.

Disability Paradigm Concept of "Normal"

It is ironic that even with the public health's focus on the environment, the emerging disability paradigms in the first half of the twentieth century focused on trying to measure an "objective" phenomenon from the standpoint of deviation from the normal. Kuhn's (1996) classic work on paradigm change discusses conceptual shifts in the hard sciences within particular scientific networks. For example, Kuhn notes that interest in investigation can occur when data highlight departure from expected results. This is broadly applicable to disability, in which the concept of "normal" has often driven disability research. More recently, Kirchner (2000) has commented that Kuhn's work lacks broadly applicable insights on how social movements associated with changes in paradigms influence research. One reason for this is the increased emphasis on the role of the environment that, in itself, affects the subject matter under study—persons with disabilities.

Much of the early thinking related to disability emerged after World War I. Technical breakthroughs in science, such as the developments of antibiotics, artificial limbs, and assistive devices, allowed for the formulation of a philosophy of restoring function, without necessarily having to "cure" the individual through restoration of the limb. This represented a breakthrough in establishing a new philosophy for rehabilitation, but the disability paradigm shift still relied on a concept of normality. Instead of concerning the "normal" presence of functioning limbs, the shift concerned the "normal" ability to engage in an activity and somehow substitute something for the limb to enhance "normal" functioning. In terms of the World Health Organization's (1980) *International Classification of Impairments, Disabilities, and Handicaps (ICIDH)*, discussed in detail in this volume, the focus shifted from impairment to disability, but the concept of "normal" remained. These two concepts of normal were reflected historically in disability policy.

For example, taking the example of hearing, from an impairment concept, the "problem" of disability related to hearing might be viewed as the prevention of loss of "normal" aural function in the ear or restoration of that loss to "normal." "Normal" would be defined as the ability to hear at a particular decibel level for particular frequencies measured in hertz. From a disability concept, "normal" would be defined as, recognizing the failure of organ function, returning the individual's ability to communicate to "normal," probably through hearing amplification. These concepts would then force the measurement of deviation from "normal" to measures within the person, as opposed to measures within the environment. Indeed, the first *ICIDH* did not provide for a classification of the environment.

THE SHIFT TOWARD A NEW DISABILITY PARADIGM

Disability Paradigm Changes and Policy

Historically, the value of "normal" relating to the person was mirrored in international disability policy. Prior to 1970, the United Nations (UN) approached disability issues from a social welfare model perspective. In the period from 1955 to 1970, an emphasis on prevention and rehabilitation was established (United Nations Secretariat 1997). Little attention was paid to obstacles created by social institutions and society in general (United Nations Secretariat 1997). The 1960s, particularly the late 1960s, became a time for reevaluation.

Three early resolutions that moved the United Nations toward a human rights approach were the following: (1) the *Declaration on Social Progress and Development* (United Nations 1969), (2) the *Declaration on the Rights of Mentally Retarded Persons* (United Nations 1971), and (3) the *Declaration on the Rights of Disabled Persons* (United Nations 1975). The first declaration advocated the provision of measures to rehabilitate the mentally and physically disabled and to facilitate their integration into society. The second stated that people with mental retardation have the same rights as other human beings and should live with their families and participate in the community. The final resolution clearly stated that all persons with disabilities have the same rights as persons without disabilities.

These initiatives culminated in passage of the *World Programme of Action Concerning Disabled Persons* (United Nations 1983). In addition to promoting the prevention of disability and rehabilitation, the program promoted equalization of opportunities for disabled persons. This represented a disability paradigm shift toward a human rights model. Although not abandoning the more traditional efforts regarding disability, the human rights approach is clearly placed on an equal par with the more traditional concerns. In the resolution, care is taken to define equality as a parity of opportunities with those of the whole population. This parity is viewed not as a static phenomenon but as one that would be fostered and maintained as countries engaged in economic and social development (United Nations 1983).

Equalization of opportunity means the process of enhancing accessibility to the general system of society. Note here how the concept of "normal" is expanded. Moving to the *ICIDH* handicap level, the concept of "normal" is moved outside the person into the environment. To return to the example of hearing, "normal" may now be measured in terms of access of people to sign language interpreters or other societal mechanisms to enhance communication.

In the United States, passage of the Individuals with Disabilities Education Act (IDEA) in 1975 and the Americans with Disabilities Act (ADA) in 1990 ran parallel with these international human rights approaches. These initiatives put a legal emphasis on altering the environment to improve opportunity. In some sense, the concept of "normal" was still in place, but the stress now was placed on altering the environment, as opposed to the individual.

Perhaps because IDEA came first and because IDEA authorized federally funded support for research in special education, a large body of research has been generated within that field. For example, the concept of the Individualized Education Plan (IEP) helped to shift a focus to altering the educational environment to provide free appropriate public education (FAPE) to all students with disabilities. Research on persons with disabilities in general has been expanding too. These changes have expanded the diversity of paradigms for viewing disability and the shifting view of the "problem" of disability toward one of ableism.

Implications of Changes for Research

Three points need to be elaborated on for their impact on disability research, as well as on the choice of methodological paradigms. First, a view has emerged that argues that there is no objective concept as disability; hence, disability is a subjective, socially derived concept. Second, disability must be viewed as a function of historical attitudes and political structures. Finally, disability research cannot be viewed as valid without the empowerment in persons with disabilities in that research. Notice how these three concepts blend fairly well with the critical theory/emancipatory value paradigm previously discussed. Scholars viewing issues of race and those studying disability incorporate many of these three points having emancipatory elements, although not all of these researchers would label themselves critical theorists.

Turning first to the notion that there is no objective concept of disability, the comparison to race is warranted. For instance, Fullilove (1998) has asked two questions related to the use of race as a variable in health research:

> First, if racism is a principal factor organizing social life, why not study racism rather than race? Second, why use an unscientific system of classification in scientific research? For racial classification systems are developed only when "race" is accepted as a legitimate variable. (P. 1297)

From this, Fullilove (1998) concludes, "I believe the time has come to abandon race as a variable in public health research. Following the illusion of race cannot provide the information we need to resolve the health problems of populations" (p. 1298).

One can take a parallel argument for disability. For example, McBryde-Johnson (1981) has argued, "There is no need to measure who is handicapped except when discrimination occurs. The concept of handicap as a product of behavior is appropriate to a statute which seeks only to eliminate the behavior of discrimination" (p. 53). Here, as Fine and Asch (1988) argue, people with disabilities comprise a minority group. Under this viewpoint, past attitudes create certain political and social structures that continue to this day even as some reforms have occurred.

Taking race as an example, the legal analyses of Judge A. Leon Higginbotham are instructive. In his book, *In the Matter of Color: Race and the American Legal Process, the Colonial Period,* Higginbotham (1978) noted the variety of mechanisms by which discrimination historically occurred against only one group:

> The mechanisms of control through judicial decisions and statutes span the sanctioning of slavery and the special limitations imposed on free blacks, to the prohibitions against interracial marriage and sexual activity, to the eliminating of the legal significance of blacks' "conversions to Christianity," to generally restricting any activities or aspirations of blacks that might threaten the groups in control. The law is usually perceived as a normative system, founded on a society's custom and convention. (P. 14)

This is viewed not merely as a past occurrence but also as one that he believed continued into the current period. In a later book, *Shades of Freedom: Racial Politics and Presumptions of the American Legal Process,* Higginbotham (1996:5) poses the "Ten Precepts of American Slavery Jurisprudence." "These precepts summarize the operational perceptions that underlay the maintenance of the slave system to 1865." The first precept is the "Precept of Inferiority":

It posed as an article of faith that African Americans were not quite altogether human. What's more, "inferiority" did not owe its existence to the legal process. Although the law came to enforce the precept, it did not create it. From the time the Africans first disembarked here in America, the colonists were prepared to regard them as inferior. When the Thirteenth Amendment abolished slavery and, presumably, all its attendant conditions, it did not eliminate the precept of inferiority. Even much later, when the law abolished state-enforced racial segregation, it still did not eliminate the precept. (Higginbotham 1996:9)

Higginbotham (1996) argued that this precept continues, thus continuing the long-term and ongoing impact of past discrimination:

I submit that the centuries-old precept of inferiority in American slavery jurisprudence and the contemporary events I have cited are part of a continuum that still has an unfair impact on African Americans, even at the present time. The perception of inferiority that motivated these false accusations against blacks in the 1990s is not unrelated to the perception of inferiority that legitimized slavery. (P. xxvii)

The precept of perceived inferiority can be inferred to persons with disabilities. In his work, Harlan Hahn (1993) makes similar points by noting the historical origins of discrimination in creating the majority group, persons with disabilities. Hahn states, "People with disabilities are a minority group because they have been the objects of prejudice and discrimination" (p. 47). This past discrimination reinforces attitudes that are the primary cause of conditions facing persons with disabilities. Hahn thus places

the focus on public attitudes rather than physical limitations as the primary source of difficulties facing disabled people. Other postulates of the minority-group model specify that all facets of the environment are molded by public policy and that government policies reflect widespread societal attitudes or values; as a result, existing features of architectural design, job requirements, and daily life that have a discriminatory impact on disabled citizens cannot be viewed merely as happenstance or coincidence. (P. 46)

One effect of this is that the research on disability would then have to focus on either society as a whole or persons without disabilities because they are the source of the disability, not the disabled individual. As Hahn (1993) notes,

Whereas the effects of a disabling environment are the penultimate origins of the restrictions encountered by persons with disabilities, an even more fundamental source of their difficulties can be located; it is the societal attitudes of the nondisabled majority that may finally be responsible for all types of environmental restraints. (P. 47)

If this is so, then the search for the norm may not necessarily be the person without disability but rather a universally designed society. For example, Hahn (1993) proposes that "the appropriate standard of assessment is the-as-yet-unrealized ideal of a totally nondiscriminatory habitat adapted to the needs of everybody" (p. 46).

Rioux (1997) actually subdivides elements of the "new" paradigm into environmental and human rights approaches. In the environmental approach, the research focus would be placed on the arrangements of the environment and their impact on persons with disabilities (Bercovici 1983). The human rights approach would analyze how society marginalized people with disabilities and how the social environment could be changed (Oliver 1992). Elements of both approaches can be observed in Hahn's (1993) formulations.

The effect on research is powerful. Not only is the phenomenon under study no longer objective, but the phenomenon under study is also completely shifted. Moreover, the standard for

Table 5.3   Contrast of Disability Paradigms for Research, 1999

Characteristic	Old Paradigm	New Paradigm
Definition of disability	An individual is limited by his or her impairment or condition	An individual with an impairment requires an accommodation to perform functions required to carry out life activities
Strategy to address disability	Fix the individual, correct the deficit	Remove barriers, create access through accommodation and universal design, promote wellness and health
Method to address disability	Provision of medical, psychological, or vocational rehabilitation services	Provision of supports (e.g., assistive technology, personal assistance services, job coach)
Source of intervention	Professionals, clinicians, and other rehabilitation service providers	Peers, mainstream service providers, consumer information services
Entitlements	Eligibility for benefits based on severity of impairment	Eligibility for accommodation seen as a civil right
Role of disabled individual	Object of intervention, patient, beneficiary, research subject	Consumer or customer, empowered peer, research participant, decision maker
Domain of disability	A medical "problem" involving accessibility, accommodations, and equity	A socioenvironmental issue

SOURCE: Derived from materials prepared by DeJong and O'Day (1999).

measurement is an ideal, as opposed to an observable construct of "normal." However, a third piece moves the argument even further—the notion of empowering the recipients of discrimination. A good example of this notion of empowerment can be observed in the National Institute on Disability and Rehabilitation Research's (1999) long-range plan, which proposes a "new" paradigm for disability research, as summarized in Table 5.3.

In Table 5.3, one can observe a shift in a number of characteristics. Elements of the new paradigm can be observed as empowering the person with a disability and shifting the emphasis to changing the environment, as opposed to the individual. Some of the changes appear to link well with the underlying value paradigms of constructivism and critical theory/emancipatory paradigms. This raises the question of whether the new paradigm has a better fit with any particular methodological paradigm.

Association of Research and Disability Paradigms

Although one can argue that there need not be any correlation between research paradigms and any discipline or topic, this may not be true in practice. To take an extreme case, are there many examples of interpretive or constructivist studies in physics? If not, is there any reason why? With few exceptions, researchers tend to be divided more by methodology than by area of interest. For example, a researcher may be interested in implementation of the ADA. It is rare that one sees a researcher making a distinction between topics and then choosing quantitative research for one problem because it is most appropriate and qualitative research for another. Rather, a more likely scenario is that two researchers, one quantitative and one qualitative, may be addressing the same problem. This creates a danger that the training drives the research rather than the problem. For example, Marshall and Rossman (1995) state, "We recommend most strongly that the researcher not decide to do a qualitative study and then search for a research problem. The methods should be linked epistemologically with the problem and the research questions" (p. 36). The same would apply to quantitative research. Yet, if people are well trained in a particular methodology, they may be drawn to problems appropriate for that methodology.

This is important because, rightly or wrongly, the emergence of the new paradigm is often associated with constructivst thinking, as noted earlier. For instance, if disability is not a truly "knowable" phenomenon, one could argue that this demands constructivist assumptions and qualitative methodologies to investigate the issue adequately. Indeed, Cizek (1995) gives his opinion "that qualitative research has become inextricably linked with sociopolitical causes" (p. 27).

However, Cizek (1995) also argues that this need not be the case and that there is a growing recognition that disability research needs to encompass different underlying assumptions and methodologies. He calls for "an inclusive perspective that integrates evaluative concerns across methodologies." He states that "there must be a renewed awareness that qualitative and quantitative methodologists are often investigating the same things, or at least different facets of the phenomena of interest. The problem is how to synthesize these observations" (p. 28).

THREE IMPORTANT CONSIDERATIONS
FOR PARADIGM SELECTION AND SYNTHESIS

General Research Principles

The notion of synthesizing may appear to be a daunting task due to differences in the methodological paradigms. However, basic research principles cut across paradigms. For example, Mertens and McLaughlin (1995) argue,

> In both quantitative and qualitative studies, the researcher should tie the results back to the purpose of the study, and to the literature in the discussion section of the report. Further, findings should be based on data, and caution should be exercised in recommendations for practice. (P. 112)

Three critical issues do emerge, however, related to the choice of paradigm or the synthesis of paradigms. First, in this era when translating disability research to policy and practice is quite important, how research results are evaluated is a critical consideration. Second, if under the new paradigm, the role for a person with a disability changes from a research subject to a research participant, an understanding of participatory action research (PAR) and how it might be applied to quantitative research is necessary. Finally, ethical issues need to be raised. All of these are discussed in the following section.

Criteria for Evaluation

The differences in the basic values underlying quantitative and qualitative methodological paradigms are important because of the emphasis of research on the measurement question—does the research actually measure the concept under study? A shift away from a "true" notion of disability could have implications on the kind of social research methodological paradigm employed to study the issue or attempts to blend the paradigms. These distinctions notwithstanding, there appear to be some parallels between some of the criteria for evaluation, according to Guba and Lincoln (1989), as follows:

Qualitative	Quantitative
Credibility	Internal validity
Transferability	External validity
Dependability	Reliability
Confirmability	Objectivity
Authenticity	???

These parallels indicate that both kinds of research submit to the test of rigor in evaluation. Also, both have rigorous methods for subject identification and selection, information collection, and data analysis. Although each type of research may favor certain methodologies in these areas, there can be overlap.

Quantitative research stresses the importance of variable construct to describing reality and achieving objectivity. This introduces the important objectives of validity and reliability (Williams 1991). Validity is the degree to which researchers measure what they claim to measure. Reliability is the external and internal consistency of measurement. For example, if another researcher measures what you measure, will the result be the same? Validity implies reliability. Hence, results may be reliable but not valid. If results are valid, however, they will always be reliable.

Of the two concepts, validity is the more problematic. Reliability can be assessed through a variety of repeated measurements. Validity offers a problem to the researcher—that of certainty that the goal has been achieved. Although validity is an issue in a variety of quantitative studies, much of the thinking underlying the concept relates to studies derived from traditional scientific experimental methods.

One can observe an important value paradigm for disability research here. As the research is conducted over time, the researcher is trying to limit the effect of the research on the persons being studied to the "response to the treatment." Any changes due simply to the fact that research is being conducted would be avoided.

Considerations for validity honor the principle of linearity—that the research moves from design to execution, without the research methodology itself being influenced by events that occur while the project is under way. In moving linearly from definition to a valid research operationalization, the particular form of measurement becomes crucial. In general, there are four different kinds of scales for measurement.

1. Nominal—classifies or categorizes but does not order (i.e., male/female)
2. Ordinal—ordered but unspecified intervals (i.e., neutral/agree/agree strongly)
3. Interval—ordered and specified intervals but an arbitrarily assigned zero point (i.e., temperature scales)
4. Ratio—ordered and specified intervals with an absolute zero point (i.e., age)

These precise and other values raise the important question—do the values of this measurement construct drive findings? For example, whatever the choice of scale, each value within that scale is presumed to be mutually exclusive. For example, if you are classified as a male, you cannot be a female, and vice versa. This has had a particular interaction with disability, where persons with disabilities tend to be classified according to a primary disability.

For example, under IDEA, students have been classified according to 13 disability categories (U.S. Department of Education 2000). In this system, a student is classified under only one category. If a student is hearing impaired with a learning disability, he or she could be classified as learning disabled, hearing impaired, or multiply disabled. The point here is not to criticize this system but rather to note that such categories attempt to meet the criteria of mutually exclusive categories. However, some might argue that disability might not lend itself to such a classification system because the phenomena may be more fluid.

In recent years, new techniques based on "fuzzy logic," such as grade of membership (GOM) analysis, have attempted to cluster people according to a variety of characteristics. Persons may belong to more than one cluster. These techniques have been used in studies of elderly populations. Such techniques, if applied to disability issues, may meet rigorous scaling criteria but provide a little more flexibility in quantitative analysis.

The principles of validity and reliability are not necessarily duplicated in qualitative research. This does not mean, however, that qualitative research does not have its own set of evaluative criteria. Examples of such criteria are credibility, transferability, dependability, confirmability, and authenticity (Mertens and McLaughlin 1995). *Credibility* assesses whether the subject was accurately described and identified. *Transferability* means that the researcher must describe the research so that results can be transferred appropriately. However, although there may be applicability in other contexts, ultimate responsibility rests with the person doing the transfer, not the original researcher. Triangulation may help determine transferability. *Dependability* refers to change over time that can be tracked. Under *confirmability*, the influence of the researcher's judgment is minimized by openly acknowledging the viewpoints and activities of the researcher vis-à-vis the persons being studied. *Authenticity* requires the presentation of a balanced view of all perspectives, values, and beliefs.

Seeing these evaluation criteria set side by side, one can argue that the research need not be rigidly identified as either quantitative or qualitative. For instance, quantitative research issues have traditionally included consideration of replication issues and competing explanations, as well as recognizing the limitations of data. By contrast, Tesch (1990) has outlined a variety of qualitative issues for analysis. Researchers can borrow techniques from each or use both at the same time. This may raise the following question, however: How can differing results be reconciled, particularly in the field of disability?

One could argue for a universalistic approach to research to integrate all of the paradigms. Indeed, Reswick (1994) argues that all types of research can be scientific if they are valid and reliable. However, others might argue that the concepts of validity and reliability are a function of a particular value paradigm of positivism and that the application of these values to qualitative research might undermine the essential value paradigm of the qualitative methodological paradigm of constructivism. As noted earlier, still others can argue that qualitative research has parallel criteria to validity and reliability, but they are not applied in the same way as in quantitative research.

Meta-analysis can be employed to summarize research because it is a quantitative synthesis of existing research (Glass, McGraw, and Smith 1981). If employed, however, qualitative researchers would need to review the results so that the quantitative methodology does not bias the summary against the qualitative results.

Participatory Action Research

Empowering the person with a disability as a research participant is the key element of PAR. However, just as the new paradigm for disability and qualitative research are separate entities, it is also important to distinguish between these two elements and PAR. According to its prime originator, William Foote Whyte (1991), the goal of PAR is to increase the relevance of research by placing individuals being studied at the center of the decision-making process and ultimately to empower people. It is a method in which the research subjects participate throughout the entire process, from the initial design to the completion of the study (Whyte 1991). As noted by Tewey (1997),

> Participatory Action Research recognizes the need for persons being studied to participate in the design and conduct of all phases (e.g., design, execution, and dissemination) of the research that affects them. PAR is an approach or strategy for research not a methodology. (P. 1)

Table 5.4 Contrast of Emphasis between Traditional and Participatory Action Research (PAR) Paradigms

Characteristic	Traditional	PAR
Learning . . .	"About"	"About" and "from"
Value	Objectivity	Subjectivity
Researcher acts as . . .	Professional	Consultant or educator
Research conducted by . . .	Outsiders	At least some insiders
Role of subjects	Subjects	Subjects and researchers
Subject mode	Passive	Active
Type of study	Controlled	Qualitative, disability
Subject role at end	Completed	Act as "change agent"
Research agenda	Professional/sociopolitical	Set by many constituents, including end users

SOURCE: Derived from Rogers and Palmer-Erbs (1994).

According to Corbet (1995), related trends to PAR are the advances in innovations such as consumerism self-help, civil rights, and total quality management (TQM). Danley and Ellison (1999) note that the concept of action is important too. The goal of the research is to improve a situation and to make concrete changes. "It will typically result in 'action steps' that are context bound rather than in developing or testing theory that can be generalized" (Danley and Ellison 1999:1). These actions are then owned by the stakeholders (Walton and Gaffney 1991).

Just as the issue was raised as to the correlation between certain disability paradigms and qualitative research, the issue can be raised as to whether PAR is simply another form of qualitative research or merely an operationalization of the critical theory/emancipatory value paradigm. For instance, if traditional research tends to be linear (from theory to data to results to use), PAR tends to be reflexive and cyclic. Danley and Ellison (1999) state,

> PAR has developed out of the challenges made by qualitative research to the traditional scientific paradigm; however it can be employed with quantitative research. . . . Subject participation challenges traditional research philosophy but does not make PAR incompatible with traditional research. (P. 2)

While the fit with qualitative research appears more natural, incorporation with quantitative research requires careful planning.

McTaggert (1991) provides four basic values to PAR, defining the relation between the researchers and the subjects—power sharing, mutual respect for experience and expertise, informed decision making, and maximum involvement. These values change the emphasis from a traditional research program to PAR, as given in Table 5.4. Note how these values alter a variety of characteristics, such as the basic value of the research and the roles of the researcher vis-à-vis the subjects of the research employed.

Important issues in participant selection are determining who is the customer, determining the qualifications of PAR participants, and achieving representativeness in the study. Of these, the customer issue is critical because this issue is of high importance in disability research. The Institute on Rehabilitation Issues (1992) defines its customers as "individuals with disabilities and persons significantly involved in improving the quality of life of such individuals outside the 'systems of care' such as family members, friends and employers" (p. 16). This definition is clearly determining that the service provider is not the customer.

It is possible to use a definition that includes service providers and others as the users of the research. Menz (1995) defines constituencies as "people and organizations that have a perspective about what needs to be accomplished in rehabilitation, through sound rehabilitation research" and beneficiaries as "individuals, organizations, and/or processes that will make use of research findings" (p. 10). Note here that groups are defined not in terms of the ultimate beneficiary of the research but rather in terms of the kind of use they would make of the research.

Doe and Whyte (1995) take a scale approach to definitions identifying groups in reference to the persons receiving services. Primary customers are individuals with disabilities receiving services, and secondary customers are service providers, parents, and consumer groups. This splits the groups included as customers by the Institute on Rehabilitation Issues (1992) (i.e., persons with disabilities from their families). Tertiary customers are composed of agencies, policymakers, and leaders.

Because participants are to be involved in all aspects of the research, an expansive view of their role is necessary. According to Seekens (1992), participants can provide resources for information, functions (such as linking to the community and advocating for research), operation, application and research utilization, dissemination and marketing, and advocacy for the use of findings.

Not only must the customers' roles be defined, but the intensity of participation must also be determined. Note that in the qualitative research described earlier, the participation level of the researcher could be classified at five levels, from nonparticipation to complete participation (Spradley 1980). Likewise, continuums of PAR implementation can be determined based on the degree of consumer control, the extent of collaborative decision making, and the levels of input from consumers, as well as the commitment of the researchers to consumers (Tewey 1997).

Children with disabilities and persons with mental disabilities or mental retardation historically have been viewed as not being able to articulate their concerns. Researchers must now be sensitive to mechanisms whereby people can participate meaningfully in the research in ways not previously thought possible. While family members are important participants, if persons with disabilities can participate meaningfully, researchers may want to consider that a first choice.

Ethical Issues

Of course, books can be written on the issue of ethics and disability research. In this section, ethics are discussed in terms of issues related to the choice of research paradigm and the application of PAR. Three basic issues are the tension between research objectivity and full disclosure, the role of people with disabilities as it relates to privacy, and the potential impacts of research on persons with disabilities.

As noted earlier, quantitative research methods seek to obtain objectivity. Qualitative methods may operate under the assumption that objectivity may be unattainable, but full disclosure allows the reader to assess the context of the research accurately. The move toward full disclosure may put pressure on quantitative researchers to describe the contexts of their research studies more accurately. Likewise, pressures for replicability, if not objectivity, particularly in policy-related studies, may put pressure on qualitative researchers to "control" for context in some ways. As noted, the tendency to synthesize research methodologies may be a welcome development. However, ethical issues may be raised that actually could produce some serious problems for each kind of research.

Turning first to objectivity and quantitative research, the pressure to describe contexts may have an impact on the privacy rights of participants in the study. Even if some rules are rigorously enforced (i.e., no reporting of data in which a sample is less than five), does the description of context provide information sufficient to identify the particular situation of people in the study that could have adverse consequences for persons in the study? In qualitative research, there is some expectation that a description of adverse environments takes place to bring about positive change. In quantitative research, there is no such expectation. Thus, detailed description is good for evaluating the study but may adversely affect study participants. Moreover, if researchers find truly adverse situations for people with disabilities, what is their obligation to try to correct them? This may be of particular concern in longitudinal studies in which quantitative researchers want the study to have as little impact on the participants as possible.

Now turning to the issue of replicability and qualitative research, the drive to "objectify" qualitative research in some way may not only undermine its underlying paradigm but also have adverse consequences for persons with disabilities. One reason is that without a control group, it is difficult for a researcher to assert which pieces could be replicated and to identify all the environmental contexts. A particular context may be unimportant in one situation but the driving factor in another. In this sense, the determination of a "fact" becomes an ethical question. If the drive for replicability pressures the researcher to "overpromise," this could have serious implications as results are translated to policy. In this sense, it is important to develop methods to truly identify cultural and historical contexts and values.

It should be noted that PAR, while not a solution to all these problems, at least brings people with disabilities into the decision-making process. As such, their involvement can help to safeguard issues related to privacy, to determine what to do when adverse contexts are discerned, and to guard against overpromising results related to replicability.

As noted earlier, under PAR, the role of people with disabilities needs to be addressed. This must also be done from the ethical perspective. For instance, does a distinction need to be made between a "professional" person with a disability versus persons with disabilities who are actually in the situation being studied? Going further, the issue of who actually conducts the research is considered an ethical question. Some have argued that nondisabled people should not conduct disability research. However, if disability is a relative experience, does this imply that only a person who has experienced social discrimination on the base of disability should direct research? Moreover, if disability studies are really to focus on what society as a whole does to isolate people into the disabled population, would not PAR require nondisabled participants?

These questions bring us back to the issue of privacy. If people with disabilities find themselves saturated with participating in research studies, are they then forced to identify in a way that some of them may not wish? In situations where those who have some control over the context desire change, this may not pose a problem, but in adverse situations, the problem may be very real.

Finally, there is a useful distinction between long-term and short-term outcomes of research. If the choice of a methodology affects the direct lives of persons in some ways, what is the influence of that choice over the long run? Given that most studies do not follow persons for the long term, what are the ethical issues related to the fact that there could be long-run impacts of any kind of research on people that cannot be known?

As can be observed from this brief discussion, no answers have been provided to these complex research questions. The most important is to note that the choice of a particular disability paradigm, a particular methodological paradigm, or PAR may have ethical consequences. At the minimum, the researcher must consider the impact of these choices related to ethical issues and record the decisions made and why those decisions were made. Again, the involvement of people with disabilities in the study may go a long way to addressing some of these issues.

ACCESSING AND IMPLEMENTING THE VALUE OF TRIANGULATION

Understanding the Interactive Issue of Access

As noted earlier, the new paradigm stresses the role of the environment in disability. One could argue that constructivist and participatory paradigms also stress this issue. To operationalize these paradigms, one must understand that the nature of the interaction with the environment is critical because interaction is a difficult concept to measure. If the purpose of research is to evaluate access to the environment, the distinction between the environment, participation, and access must be understood. By its nature, participation refers either to an *act* of taking part or to a *state of being related to a large whole*. Access is not an act or a state but a *liberty* to enter, approach, communicate with, pass to and from, or make use of a situation. The environment is either that large whole or parts thereof or that situation that is accessed. From these distinctions, it is clear then that the elements of accessibility are characteristics of environmental availability (in this case, educational availability) but are not characteristics of the environment.

Whiteneck, Fougeyrollas, and Gerhart (1997) argue that there are three approaches toward viewing the environment. First, different types of environments can be examined (i.e., economic, social, legal). Then, the environment can be ranked from the immediate personal to the broad social (micro, meso, macro) (Fougeyrollas 1995). Finally, five characteristics of the environment may be examined as follows:

1. Accessibility—can you get to *where* you want to go?
2. Accommodation—can you do *what* you want to do?
3. Resource availability—are your special *needs* met?
4. Social support—are you accepted by *those around you*?
5. Equality—are you treated *equally* with others?

The five characteristics do not constitute a classification of the environment or a ranking of the environment, as noted earlier, but rather a classification of different kinds of *interactions* that the environment has with individuals from the point of view of the environment. Despite the use of the term *accessibility* for one of the interactions, this taxonomy of interactions can be viewed as an attempt to describe the dimensions in which environments can be made accessible to people. Note that the systematic description of the dimensions of access proposed by Whiteneck et al. (1997) is somewhat similar to the elaboration of the dimensions of access to health care outlined earlier by Pechansky and Thomas (1981)—availability, accessibility, accommodation, affordability, and acceptability. They define access as "a concept representing the degree of 'fit' between the clients and the system" (Pechansky and Thomas 1981:128). Thus, in both models, the unit of analysis is the environment, and how it interacts with people is what is discerned.

While the use of different units of analysis to discern access may seem complicated, the notion is rooted in the qualitative research technique of triangulation of data. Here, the single point referenced would be access. The reasons for having more than one unit of analysis are consistent with the new paradigm, constructivist theory, and PAR. If, as noted earlier, the new paradigm's strategy to address disability is to remove barriers and create access through accommodation and universal design, the environment must comprise a unit of analysis to understand how environments can be altered to best serve the needs of all people. However, because the role of the disabled individual is as customer, consumer, empowered peer, or decision maker, the actual experiences of individuals with their environments must be taken into account.

For example, in 1983, the Ethiopian National Children's Commission conducted a study of children with disabilities who were younger than age 15. The commission collected data not only on children but also about family issues and community issues. As shown in Table 5.5, community leaders were asked questions about their perceptions of family and community attitudes. These measures show how the social environment responds to people with disabilities. Here, the reporting source is held constant (community leaders), but the unit of analysis changes from community (measuring those attitudes) to families (measuring their attitudes). Note that the overwhelming majority of community leaders felt that the community was sympathetic and ready to assist but that they also felt that families had negative attitudes toward disability, including feeling ashamed or depressed and failing to offer parental care (see Table 5.5).

Table 5.5   Percentage Distribution of Opinions of Community Leaders of Family and Community Attitudes toward Children with Disabilities, 1983

Group with Attitudes	Attitudes toward Disability	Percentage Distribution
Total		
Number		4,891
Percent		100.0
Family	Tend to hide/feel ashamed	22.6
	Feel depressed	56.8
	Fail to offer parental care	7.2
	Others	10.0
	No response	3.4
Community	Sympathy/ready to assist	92.6
	Neglect	7.4

SOURCE: Ethiopia National Children's Commission (1983).

So far, the notion of different units of analysis has been stressed. As noted earlier, however, different reporting sources should also be considered. Mertens and McLaughlin (1995) state, "Triangulation involves checking information that has been collected from different sources or methods for consistency of evidence across sources of data" (p. 54). The distinction between units of analysis and reporting sources is important. Like community leaders, families can report data on *both* children with disabilities *and* the environments they encounter. The children and the environments are the units of analysis, and the parents and providers are the reporting sources.

Turning back once more to the Ethiopian example, in Table 5.5, the community leaders' perceptions of family attitudes were measured. For example, the community leaders may feel that families have negative attitudes, but how do the families feel? In Table 5.6, parental attitudes are measured. This change represents a shift in the reporting source (from community leaders to parents), but the unit of analysis is constant (parental attitudes). Here we see that almost three-quarters of families felt that the disabilities of their children had created problems. This may lend some support to the views of community leaders, although it should be stressed that the same questions were not asked of the families and community leaders. Moreover, the family's opinion of the community was not solicited.

Some qualitative researchers have criticized the search for consistency as inconsistent with the recognition of alternative realities in qualitative research. Thus, it should be stressed that the emphasis on triangulation for studying access is not so much on consistency as on whether customers believe that programs are delivering the needed services and, if not, what circumstances would need to change for that to happen. Thus, if a program provider describes an environment as A and a customer describes it as B, the focus is not on who is correct but rather on how service delivery can be improved.

Note, too, that there is a third potential aspect of using triangulation—the use of different methodologies to study the same problem. As noted earlier, one might anticipate that the integration of quantitative and qualitative approaches to study the issue of access would yield improved information and would be consistent with the new paradigm. For example, qualitative probes of family opinions might reveal concerns about the environment, as opposed to merely believing that the disability had created problems.

Table 5.6   Percentage Distribution of Opinions of Families on the Problems of
Their Children with Disabilities, 1983

Family Opinion on Handling Child	Percentage Distribution
Total	
Number	29,631
Percent	100.0
Have created problems	73.5
Have created no problems	14.0
Irrelevant response	0.0
No response	12.5

SOURCE: Ethiopia National Children's Commission (1983).

Although the World Health Organization's (1980) handicap taxonomy from the *International Classification of Impairments, Disabilities, and Handicaps* does not purport to be a classification of accessibility, the dimensions offered provide a framework to discern the essential elements of accessibility. As shown in Table 5.7, these dimensions have some correspondence with the different kinds of interactions that the environment has with individuals, from the point of view of the environment proposed by Whiteneck et al. (1997). Four elements, as shown in Table 5.7, are virtually the same. These are independence/accommodation, mobility/accessibility, social integration/social support, and economic self-sufficiency/social support. The Whiteneck et al. grouping does not include orientation, occupation of time, and transition, while the handicap classification does not include equality.

A question then arises, in the case of the nonoverlaps, whether the exclusion of any of them from the domains of access hinders the description of access. It is interesting to note that orientation, occupation, and transition refer to extrinsic and nonphysical characteristics that people possess—information, time, and preparation. Some might argue that these three pieces might constitute prerequisites for people doing what they wish to do, going where they wish to go, and the like. However, they clearly are different characteristics not included in the model proposed by Whiteneck et al. (1997).

Equality poses a different problem. While clearly a desirable attribute, one could argue that it is a valued measure that could be applied to the other four elements proposed by Whiteneck et al. (1997), as well as the other elements (orientation, occupation, and transition). For instance, if the environment is not accessible to persons with disabilities, or it does not accommodate them but is accessible to and accommodates others, then equality would not have occurred.

Clearly, then, equality is important and should be measured. However, it is so important that it cannot stand alone as a characteristic of the environment but rather as a measure that can be applied to all environmental interactions with human beings. Thus, the seven handicap groupings can be employed to ascertain whether environmental access has occurred, and equality would constitute one of the desired measures to discern access.

Transition, an element not included in the original handicap dimensions, deserves some special mention. While these dimensions constitute important aspects of access, how the environment interacts with individuals changes over the course of their lives. Thus, individuals may have good access at one age but not at other ages, or they may have good access in a rural environment but not in an urban environment. The concept of transition refers to access to quality preparation prior to major situational changes in life phases. Thus, one would have access to environmental resources to enhance readiness.

Table 5.7   Contrast of Handicap Dimensions with Environmental Attributes Describing How Environments Interact with Human Beings

Construct	World Health Organization Handicap	Whiteneck et al.
Who—do you have the information you wish?	1. Orientation	(Nothing)
What—do you choose what you wish to do?	2. Independence	2. Accommodation
Where—do you go where you wish?	3. Mobility	1. Accessibility
When—do you engage when you wish?	4. Occupation	(Nothing)
With whom—are you accepted by others?	5. Social integration	4. Social support
With what—do you have the resources you need?	6. Economic self-sufficiency	3. Resource availability
Change—are you prepared for change?	7. Transition (new)	(Nothing)
Equal—are you treated equally with others?	(Nothing)	5. Equality

SOURCE: For handicap categories, World Health Organization (1980); for environmental elements, Whiteneck, Fougeyrollas, and Gerhart (1997).

Restrictions in access to transition are not just simply determined by changes occurring in two points in time. Rather, transition is a classification of active engagement in any process designed to prepare for changes in one's life situation. There are many dimensions to transition access. Aside from age-related transitions, there are other demographic transitions for which preparation may be of concern. Family migration status is also related to age-related transitions but raises its own issues that are different from the view of play and school as major activities. Moreover, there are also health transitions of concern for access, including transitions related to anticipated changes due to or associated with genetic conditions (Usher's syndrome), disease (AIDS), or rehabilitation. Some health-related transitions might be age related, as Usher's syndrome appears to be.

With these seven concepts in place, the extent of access to a situation can be explored. If nothing else, the dimensions serve as a checklist for access. Programs serving children can ask themselves in any situation the following questions: Do clients have access to (1) critical information, (2) choices, (3) travel, (4) time, (5) social relationships, (6) economic resources, and (7) preparation for change? If these questions are addressed positively by disabled persons, their families, and all people, then progress toward accessibility has probably occurred. Triangulation can be employed to assess these dimensions from a variety of perspectives.

Diversity

Similarly, triangulation related to diversity can be employed. Two critical issues here are disability diversity and sociocultural diversity. Examples of triangulation given above were shifts in the reporting source, the units of analysis, or the research paradigm employed. However, disability diversity and sociocultural diversity are also two dimensions for triangulation.

Disability diversity accounts for the heterogeneous experiences of people with disabilities. Even if one grants that disability is not an objective phenomenon and is a function of discrimination, societal discriminations against a sign language user may be quite different from those encountered by a person who uses a wheelchair. By checking sources across the range of disability experiences, researchers can more effectively determine the particular influence of context.

Sociocultural diversity is also very important. One clear example is in the development of language and how that interplays with a learning disability. Again, by checking diverse viewpoints, the researcher can determine the sensitivity of a research methodology to different cultural contexts. Broad applicability may not be determined, but the particular influence of the environment can be more clearly elaborated.

Again, the use of triangulation approaches relating to diversity need not establish a knowable truth. Rather, the tool is employed to assess the full range of perspectives that may be applicable to the study. If employed with PAR, triangulation for diversity can then assist in bringing about change in a way that will respect differences by disability or by sociocultural variables.

SUMMARY AND CONCLUSION

Today, Edward Miner Gallaudet's research concerns and opportunities might include cochlear implants, speech recognition, and the nuances of American Sign Language (ASL). When he conducted his study, he did not know he was engaging in the practice of triangulation. At that time, perhaps because research methodology was not so well articulated, he used all the tools at his disposal to obtain the information he needed. However, he was shifting the units of analysis, the reporting sources, and the techniques of analysis to gather information to draw his conclusions. W. E. B. DuBois engaged in a similar process.

Ironically, today's research concerns make the value of triangulation more, not less, necessary. For example, what has been called the "new universe of disability" reflects an increasing heterogeneity in how disability is viewed. This shift requires the incorporation of many more diverse perspectives.

As paradigms shift, grow, and develop, debates about the proper way to study disability are not likely to diminish. With a focus on access, however, the interactive nature of the phenomena can be properly assessed through the syntheses of a variety of paradigms as well as by greater use of research techniques that employ multiple reporting sources and units of analyses. These changes make the researcher's task harder but in the end could represent a great advancement for the field.

REFERENCES

Bercovici, S. 1983. *Barriers to Normalization: The Restrictive Management of Retarded Persons*. Baltimore: University Park Press.

Cizek, G. C. 1995. "Crunchy Granola and the Hegemony of the Narrative." *Educational Researcher* 24 (2): 26-28.

Cook, T. D. and D. T. Campbell. 1979. *Quasi-Experimentation: Design and Analysis Issues for Field Settings*. Chicago: Rand McNally.

Corbet, B. 1995. "Consumer Involvement in Research: Inclusion and Impact." Pp. 213-33 in *Clinical Outcomes from the Model Spinal Cord Injury Systems*, edited by S. L. Stover, J. A. Delisa, and G. G. Whiteneck. Gaithersburg, MD: Aspen.

Danley, K. and M. L. Ellison. 1999. *A Handbook for Participatory Action Researchers*. Boston: Boston University, Sargent College of Health and Rehabilitation Sciences, Center for Psychiatric Rehabilitation.

Denzin, N. K. and Y. S. Lincoln, eds. 2000. *The Handbook of Qualitative Research*. 2d ed. Thousand Oaks, CA: Sage.

Doe, T. and J. Whyte. 1995. "Participatory Action Research." Paper presented at Forging Collaborative Partnerships in the Study of Disability: A NIDRR Conference on Participatory Action Research, April, Washington, DC.

DuBois, W. E. B. 1899. *The Philadelphia Negro*. New York: Benjamin Bloom.

Ethiopia National Children's Commission. 1983. *Report of Survey of Disabled Children in Ethiopia*. Addis Ababa: Government of Ethiopia.

Fine, M. and A. Asch. 1988. "Disability beyond Stigma: Social Interaction, Discrimination and Activism." *Journal of Social Issues* 44 (1): 3-21.

Fischer, L. J. and D. L. de Lorenzo, eds. 1983. *History of the College for the Deaf 1857—1907 by Edward Miner Gallaudet.* Washington, DC: Gallaudet College Press.

Fourgeyrollas, P. 1995. "Documenting Environmental Factors for Preventing the Handicap Creation Process: Quebec Contributions Relating to ICIDH and Social Participation of People with Functional Differences." *Disability and Rehabilitation* 17 (3/4): 145-53.

Fullilove, M. T. 1998. "Comment: Abandoning 'Race' as a Variable in Public Health Research—An Idea Whose Time Has Come." *American Journal of Public Health* 88 (9): 1297-98.

Glass, G. V., G. McGraw, and M. Smith. 1981. *Meta-Analysis in Social Research.* Beverly Hills, CA: Sage.

Guba, E. G. and Y. S. Lincoln. 1989. *Fourth Generation Evaluation.* Newbury Park, CA: Sage.

———. 1994. "Competing Paradigms in Qualitative Research." Pp. 105-17 in *The Handbook of Qualitative Research,* edited by N. K. Denzin and Y. S. Lincoln. Thousand Oaks, CA: Sage.

Hahn, H. 1993. "The Political Implications of Disability Definitions and Data." *Disability Policy Studies* 4 (3): 41-52.

Harding, S. 1993. "Rethinking Standpoint Epistemology: What Is Strong 'Objectivity?' " Pp. 49-82 in *Feminist Epistemologies,* edited by L. Alcoff and E. Porter. New York: Routledge.

Higginbotham, A. L., Jr. 1978. *In the Matter of Color: Race and the American Legal Process, the Colonial Period.* New York: Oxford University Press.

———. 1996. *Shades of Freedom: Racial Politics and Presumptions of the American Legal Process.* New York: Oxford University Press.

Institute on Rehabilitation Issues. 1992. *Consumer Involvement in Rehabilitation Research and Practice.* Little Rock: University of Arkansas at Fayetteville, Arkansas Rehabilitation Research and Training Center.

Kirchner, C. 2000. "Commentary: Disability Policy, Social Research and the Social Movement." Paper presented at the National Institute on Disability and Rehabilitation Research's Conference on the New Paradigm on Disability, January, Bethesda, MD.

Kuhn, T. S. 1996. *The Structure of Scientific Revolution.* 3d ed. Chicago: University of Chicago Press.

Marshall, C. and G. B. Rossman. 1995. *Designing Qualitative Research.* Thousand Oaks, CA: Sage.

McBryde-Johnson, H. 1981. "Who Is Handicapped? Defining the Protected Class under the Employment Provisions of Title V of the Rehabilitation Act of 1973." *Review of Public Personnel Administration* 29:49-61.

McKeown, T. 1976. *The Modern Rise of Population.* New York: Academic Press.

McTaggart, R. 1991. "Principles for Participatory Action Research." *Adult Education Quarterly* 41 (3): 168-87.

Menz, F. E. 1995. *Constituents Make the Difference: Improving the Value of Rehabilitation Research.* Menomonie: University of Wisconsin–Stout, Rehabilitation Research and Training Center on Improving Community-Based Rehabilitation Programs.

Mertens, D. M. 1998. *Research Methods in Education and Psychology.* Thousand Oaks, CA: Sage.

Mertens, D. M. and J. A. McLaughlin. 1995. *Research Methods in Special Education.* Thousand Oaks, CA: Sage.

National Institute on Disability and Rehabilitation Research. 1999. *Long Range Plan.* Washington, DC: Government Printing Office.

Olesen, V. 1994. "Feminisms and Models of Qualitative Research." Pp. 158-74 in *The Handbook of Qualitative Research,* edited by N. K. Denzin and Y. S. Lincoln. Thousand Oaks, CA: Sage.

Oliver, M. 1992. "Changing the Social Relations of Research Production." *Disability, Handicap and Society* 7 (2): 101-14.

Patton, M. Q. 1990. *Qualitative Evaluation and Research Methods.* Newbury Park, CA: Sage.

Pechansky, R. and C. Thomas. 1981. "The Concept of Access: Definition and Relation to Customer Satisfaction." *Medical Care* 19 (2): 127-40.

Phillips, H. T. 1993. "The 1945 Gluckman Report and the Establishment of South Africa's Health Centers." *American Journal of Public Health* 83 (7): 1037-39.

Reswick, J. B. 1994. "What Constitutes Valid Research? Qualitative vs. Quantitative Research." *Journal of Rehabilitation Research and Development* 31:7-9.

Rioux, M. H. 1997. "Disability: The Place of Judgement in a World of Fact." *Journal of Intellectual Disability Research* 41 (2): 102-11.

Rogers, E. and V. Palmer-Erbs. 1994. "Participatory Action Research: Implications for Research and Evaluation in Psychiatric Rehabilitation." *Psychosocial Rehabilitation Journal* 18 (2): 3-12.

Seekens, T. 1992. "Report from the NARRTC Subcommittee on Consumer Involvement." Preliminary report to the annual meeting of the National Association of Rehabilitation Research and Training Centers, May, Washington, DC.

Spradley, J. S. (1980). Participant observation. New York: Holt, Rinehart, & Winston.

Susser, M. 1993. "A South African Odyssey in Community Health: A Memoir of the Impact of the Teachings of Sidney Kark." *American Journal of Public Health* 83 (7): 1039-42.

Susser, M. and E. Susser. 1996a. "Choosing a Future for Epidemiology. Part I—Eras and Paradigms." *American Journal of Public Health* 86 (5): 668-73.

———. 1996b. "Choosing a Future for Epidemiology. Part II—From Black Box to Chinese Boxes and Eco-Epidemiology." *American Journal of Public Health* 86 (5): 674-77.

Tesch, R. 1990. *Qualitative Research: Analysis Types and Software Tools.* New York: Falmer.

Tewey, B. P. 1997. *Building Participatory Action Research Partnerships.* Washington, DC: National Institute on Disability and Rehabilitation Research.

Union of South Africa. 1945. *Report of the National Health Services Commission on the Provision of an Organised Health Service for All Sections of the People of the Union of South Africa 1942-1944 [The Gluckman Report].* Cape Town: South African Government Printer.

United Nations. 1969. *Declaration on Social Progress and Development.* Supplement Number 30 at 47, U.N. Doc. A/7630. New York: Author.

———. 1971. *Declaration on the Rights of Mentally Retarded Persons.* Supplement Number 30 at 93, U.N. Doc. A/8429. New York: Author.

———. 1975. *Declaration on the Rights of Disabled Persons.* Supplement Number 34 at 88, U.N. Doc. A/10034. New York: Author.

———. 1983. *World Programme of Action Concerning Disabled Persons.* New York: Author.

United Nations Secretariat, Division for Social Policy and Development. 1997. *The United Nations and Disabled Persons—An Historical Overview: First Fifty Years.* New York: United Nations.

U.S. Department of Education. 2000. *Twenty-First Annual Report to Congress on the Implementation of the Individuals with Disabilities Education Act.* Washington, DC: Government Printing Office.

Walton, R. and M. E. Gaffney. 1991. "Research, Action, and Participation: The Merchant Shipping Case." Pp. 99-126 in *Participatory Action Research,* edited by W. F. Whyte. Newbury Park, CA: Sage.

Whiteneck, G. G., P. Fougeyrollas, and K. A. Gerhart. 1997. "Elaborating the Model of Disablement." Pp. 91-102 in *Assessing Medical Rehabilitation Practices: The Promise of Outcomes Research,* edited by M. J. Fuhrer. Baltimore: Brookes.

Whyte, W. F., ed. 1991. *Participatory Action Research.* Newbury Park, CA: Sage.

Williams, F. 1991. *Reasoning with Statistics: How to Read Quantitative Research.* Orlando, FL: Harcourt Brace.

World Health Organization. 1964. *Constitution of the World Health Organization.* Geneva: Author.

———. 1980. *International Classification of Impairments, Disabilities, and Handicaps: A Manual of Classification Relating to the Consequences of Disease.* Geneva: Author.

Disability

6

An Interactive Person-Environment Social Creation

PATRICK FOUGEYROLLAS
LINE BEAUREGARD

Not such a long time ago, disability was systematically identified as characteristic of the person. The presence of body or functional differences was considered to automatically provoke personal tragedy, exclusion, or stigmatization. Any person with a significant impairment was labeled handicapped or disabled. Even though this perspective is still widespread, this conception of disability has progressively changed since the 1960s. In fact, several people began to question this reductionist representation of disability and emphasized the role of environmental factors in the disability process, notably through the emergence of the disability rights movement.

Despite much advancement, it remains today that there is no true consensus as to these determinant factors of disability, notably with regards to the environment. In fact, it would be more accurate to say that there is consensus on the importance of the environment but disagreement on the exact role this factor plays. On one hand, there is the social model that attributes the disability entirely to the environment, ignoring factors relevant to the person. On the other hand, there is the biomedical model that mainly focuses on the person and resists consideration of environmental factors. This resistance is especially manifested within the scope of the revision process of the *International Classification of Impairments, Disabilities, and Handicaps* (*ICIDH*) by the World Health Organization (WHO 1980).

This chapter aims to explain and analyze how the social and physical environment has become an essential concept in understanding the disability creation process. It is made up of two main parts. The first part illustrates that within several disciplines, as well as theoretical or intervention domains, environmental factors are taken into consideration as explanatory or constituent factors of diverse phenomena. We will explore some generic approaches to human development and within the health domain. This part demonstrates, among other things, the unavoidable nature of considering the environment in health domains and the generalization of this consideration to several disciplines and domains of intervention. As such, the resistance manifested by WHO with regards to the revision of *ICIDH* will be even further questioned.

The second part of this chapter documents the evolution of explanatory conceptual models of the consequences of disease and trauma. We will present the factors that are at the basis of a better understanding of the variables involved in the disability process. The *ICIDH* being one of these factors, a brief presentation of the *ICIDH* will follow, along with reactions that it provoked within the international community. Several reactions centered on the role the environment played as a determinant of disablement. The reaction of Disabled Peoples' International (DPI), in particular, will be seen along with those of certain conceptual models, elaborated on with the aim to better understand the factors involved in the disability process. All of these emergent sociopolitical models explicitly integrate environmental factors. Next, a brief description of the revision process of the *ICIDH* will be presented, a process that led to the proposal of the *ICIDH-2* Beta-2 draft in 1999. Because of its contribution to the conceptual debates of the revision and its international influence on the role of the environment, the Quebec Classification, known as the disability creation process (DCP), will be introduced. A synthesis and critique of the evolution of debates concerning the conceptual domains, segmentation, and relationships, as well as the environment and its role in the systemic biopsychosocial model of the *ICIDH-2*, will be presented. Finally, the text will plead the following:

- the necessity of a balanced interactive process between personal intrinsic characteristics and environmental factors in the creation of disability that is not compatible with the present *ICIDH-2* conceptual approach;
- the consideration of environment as the essential key to an adequate understanding of the long-term social consequences of disease and trauma.

Now, it is important to define what we mean by environment. The generic definition provided by Law (1991) describes environments as being "those contexts (situations) which occur outside the individual and elicit responses in them" (p. 175). In this chapter, environment's meaning is taken broadly—not only physical characteristics, such as buildings, landscapes, climatic conditions, and others, but also social, political, economic, institutional, and cultural dimensions. We will designate all of these characteristics with the term *environmental factors*, whose taxonomy is in the process of being defined at an international level.

PART I: EVOLUTION OF THE CONCEPT OF ENVIRONMENT WITHIN DIVERSE GENERIC APPROACHES OF HUMAN DEVELOPMENT AND WITHIN THE CONCEPT OF HEALTH

Numerous theoretical models have put into relationship the person and his or her environment within diverse disciplines. This increased interest for person-environment theoretical models has developed as the Cartesian vision of the world has disintegrated since the end of the nineteenth century. In fact, before the twentieth century, in the Occident, the world was perceived according to a mechanistic perspective. The human being was seen as separate from his or her environment. Controlled and objective empirical knowledge that is inherent to a mechanistic vision of the world was accepted within natural, human, and social sciences.

Toward the end of the nineteenth century, notably with the work of Darwin and Haeckel, awareness of the impact of the environment on human beings began. Over the course of the twentieth century, two scientific revolutions shook the representation of the world as perfectly ordered and predictable (Ramsay 1991). The first revolution was quantum physics, which introduced concepts such as *organic, holistic,* and *ecological.* The second revolution was the theory of chaos, which refers to irregularity in nature.

Within the domain of social and human sciences, authors from different disciplines have developed theories that call on the necessity of taking the environment into consideration. Park, Burgess, and McKenzie from the University of Chicago founded human ecology during the 1920s. The basic idea of human ecology was that urban social problems are influenced and even determined by urban space. Social ecology stems from human ecology and was mostly developed in psychology during the early 1940s with the work of Kurt Lewin. The work of Lewin, as well as that of von Bertalanffy, also sensitized psychology as to the importance to life environment. Lewin brought an important contribution to Gestaltism with his work on the interdependency between the person and his or her surrounding environment. Biologist Ludwig von Bertalanffy is at the origins of the general systems theory (GST). The goal of the GST is to form valid principles for "systems" in general, independently of the nature of the elements that compose them and the forces that link them (von Bertalanffy 1968). Systems are defined as groups of elements in interaction. Systems may be of different natures, such as physical, biological, or sociological. von Bertalanffy opposes a mechanistic conception of human beings and prefers a holistic vision of the organism.

Bronfenbrenner (1977), whose work was influenced by Lewin, elaborated on the ecology of the human development model. The ecology of human development is

> the scientific study of the progressive, mutual accommodation, throughout the life span, between a growing human organism and the changing immediate environments in which it lives, as this process is affected by relations obtaining within and between these immediate settings, as well as the larger social contexts, both formal and informal, in which the settings are embedded. (Bronfenbrenner 1977:514)

The notion of environment "is conceived topologically as a nested arrangement of structures, each contained within the next" (Bronfenbrenner 1977:514). Four levels are defined: the micro-system, the meso-system, the exo-system, and the macro-system. In the 1990s, Bronfenbrenner elaborated a "Process-Person-Context-Time" model that operationalizes the ecological conception of human development (Bronfenbrenner 1990). His work has had a significant impact on the development of environmental factors' taxonomies and systemic understanding of simultaneous proximal, community, and societal environmental levels influencing the disability process (Fougeyrollas et al. 1996; Whiteneck et al. 1997; WHO 1999).

Gregory Bateson also played an important role in the development of ecosystemic thought. After his work in anthropology and psychiatry, Bateson became interested in the relation that people foster with their ecosystem and the ecology of ideas (Bateson 1972). His major contribution to communication theory was concretized by the remarkable innovations of the Palo Alto school. Within an interdisciplinary perspective, the following perfectly illustrates the change from an analytical process to a systemic process in his elaboration of a methodology of change. In contrast with the linear search for causes in Freudian psychoanalysis, Milton Erickson (1967) and Paul Watzlawick's (1978) brief therapies are based on a circular causality that attempts to clarify the objective to be attained, rather than the causes of a problem. It is a projection toward the future that influences the present and the construction of reality. The fundamental character of the "subjective viewpoint" as the key to change is of great utility for understanding human functioning and the disability process (Kourilsky-Belliard 1995).

Other authors from diverse disciplines have also developed ecological models. For example, within architecture, Weisman (1981) proposed a systemic environment/behavior model. Lawton and Nahemow (1973) developed an ecological model that they applied to the aging process. Moos (1980) elaborated a model that demonstrates the relationship between environmental factors and personal factors, as applied to the evaluation of elderly people's living environment. The influence of ecological theories and GST was also felt by the social work profession, which adopted an ecosystemic perspective (Kemp 1994).

Other disciplines, such as ergonomics and occupational therapy, consider the environment to be an essential component of human behavior. Thus, ergonomics considers the importance of including environment in the explanation of human performance at work. Important among the models issued from this discipline are the man-machine systems (Grandjean 1980; Oborne 1982) and the person-process-environment model of Webb et al. (1988).

The more generic models related to human occupation in occupational therapy include the work of Dunn, Brown, and McGuigan (1994), who elaborated the ecology of human performance (EHP) model; Kielhofner's (1993) human occupation model; and Law et al.'s (1996) person-environment-occupational model. Theory in occupational therapy has had an important influence on paradigm change in the rehabilitation sciences by its insistence on a holistic and ecological approach and its impacts on the development of interdisciplinarity. In the domain of vocational rehabilitation, ecological models, such as those developed by Dobren (1994) and Vondracek, Lerner, and Shulenberg (1986), also reflect the dynamic relationship between the person and his or her environment.

These brief descriptions of models illustrate the increased consideration of environment in diverse domains. The concept of health was also subject to this tendency. In the nineteenth century and in the beginning of the twentieth century, health was considered to be the absence of disease (Minaire 1992). Moreover, because of the increasing popularity of scientism at the beginning of the twentieth century, the dominating health model was mechanistic (Butrym 1989). Within this perspective, the human body is considered to be a machine. Disease is thus viewed as a break that occurred within the human machine, a break that only doctors can repair (Ramsay 1991). Thus, the malfunctioning part of the body must be repaired or replaced (Evans and Stoddart 1990), and little attention is paid to the subjective experience of the "patient." This mechanistic vision of the human body is at the origin of the biomedical model.

After World War II, health and disease began to be viewed as the product of complex and interactive factors that touch on the biological, psychological, spiritual, and environmental aspects of the person (Butrym 1989). Within the domain of public health and epidemiology, the emergence of models that integrate environmental factors as health determinants appeared and were adopted in the field of primary and secondary prevention, which aims to identify and control risk factors for the appearance of disease and trauma. Today, it is recognized that the determinants of health extend beyond the simple framework of health care services, and it is important to consider the genetic inheritance of individuals, hygienic conditions, quality of diet and lodging, social support, socioeconomic conditions, and others (Evans and Stoddart 1990; Ottawa Charter for Health Promotion 1986).

It is surprising, however, to note the slowness with which this new vision is applied in practice in the curative approach and in interventions on chronic consequences of disease. The physician has the tendency to concentrate on the physiological aspects and to overspecialize, to the detriment of a more holistic vision of the human being. There is thus a large discrepancy between what is recognized at a theoretical level and what is actually put into practice.

The ever-increasing scientific and administrative powers given to physicians for assessing disease and their consequences seem to mean that disability statuses and eligibility to compensation programs are captured by the organic perspective situating the problem in the individual. Health policies, particularly for tertiary prevention, take little notice of the environmental and social determinants of health, social participation, and quality of life despite their recognized importance.

In short, *health* is currently defined by the WHO as a state of physical, mental, and social well-being. Health is also considered to be the capacity of the individual to function optimally within his or her environment or the adaptation of the person to his or her environment or setting (Minaire 1992; WHO 1989). This positive definition of health supposes a larger approach to the factors that influence health, an approach within which the role of social and physical environmental factors must be taken into account. This synthesis shows that contemporary models of human development, as well as those that apply to health, all take into account environmental variables. Thus, there is a strong convergence regarding theoretical development. The mechanistic vision, which existed at the beginning of the twentieth century, is rejected along with linear explanations of phenomena. It is now a question of holistic vision and of interaction between elements; we are within the era of complexity (Morin 1990). Unfortunately, this convergence of ideas has not always been translated into practice in a way that intervenes with the goal of improving the life situations of people.

A parallel can now be made with the concept of disability. This evolution of the mechanistic vision toward a systemic perspective that takes into account the factors of the environment in understanding the long-term consequences of disease and trauma has also manifested. The concept of disability has evolved in such a way that it is now possible to speak of a paradigm change (Kuhn 1970). The next part of this chapter documents the evolution of the conceptual models of disability by focusing on the question of environment.

PART II: MODELS OF THE CONCEPT OF DISABILITY

Toward a Better Understanding of the Variables Involved in the Disability Process

Chronic disease, or the persistent consequences of disease or trauma limiting people in functionality and social independence, has become the subject of increasing concern in health and socioeconomic systems of developed countries, particularly since World War II. This tendency, which is related to the success of medicine, hygiene, and socioeconomic conditions of the population, is currently accelerating due to an increase in the rate of disability within the population, particularly because of the aging of the population.

Noticing the disturbing increase of the phenomena of chronicity, the WHO, in the late 1960s, became aware of the inadequacy of the *International Classification of Disease (ICD)* to take it into account. In fact, it classifies medical diagnoses and specifically responds to the needs of a curative approach. The *ICD* is based on the biomedical model whose aim is to cure, without considering eventual after-effects. Because the necessity of estimating the cost of injuries and providing compensations for them implies assessment of the consequences after the acute phase of trauma or disease has ended, disability insurance programs for veterans and persons injured in work or traffic accidents were the first to push the development of concepts related to functional consequences (Bickenbach 1993; Stiker 1982).

Furthermore, the curative medical model is incomplete when it comes to intervening or providing information on the realities experienced by people with durable, functional limitations once the acute phase has ended (WHO 1980). Models of disability are thus orienting toward defining a direct causal link between corporal injury and its consequences on the accomplishment of a person's activities. Types of definitions of disability, such as that of Jazairi, were elaborated: "all limitations of the individual's activities due to illness and injury" (cited in Duckworth 1983:12).

Since 1965, American sociologist Saad Nagi proposed conceptual works intended to clarify the concepts surrounding the phenomenon of disablement (Nagi 1965). His conceptual framework distinguished between (1) pathology, (2) impairment, (3) functional limitation, and (4) disability. His work identified rehabilitation as focusing primarily on functional limitations and disabilities. This contrasts with the traditional biomedical model that focused on pathology and cure. The Nagi concepts are widely used in English-speaking North America. It is important to note that his disability concept is related to the social consequences and not to the personal attributes, which are impairments and functional limitations. It is very clear, in Nagi's explanations, that there are no linear causal relationships between functional limitations and social impact on activities and roles.

During this period, the deviance and stigma theories developed by Freidson (1965) and Goffman (1963) introduced the ideas that physical limitations influence the attitudes of others because of values related to social expectations and cultural definitions of what constitutes a "normal" and acceptable range of performance. Their work contributed to our understanding of social obstacles that restrict the participation of individuals in social roles. These ideas have helped change the views of disability from those focused on problems within the person to those that recognize "disability" as a societal problem with important social consequences. Thus, models orient themselves toward an understanding of social obstacles to the participation or carrying out of social roles that are not only related to the nature of the person but also related to normative cultural factors or "social representations."

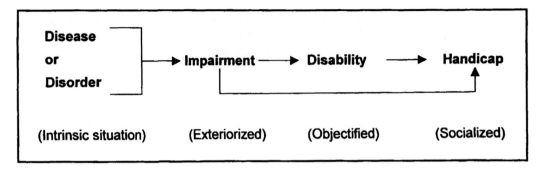

Figure 6.1. Conceptual Schema of the *ICIDH-1*

Other models influenced by the systemic approach were developed, including Wan's (1974) epidemiological model of invalidity and Warren's (1977) interactive model of disability. These models put much emphasis on the importance of environmental factors and socioeconomic status as determinants of a person's loss of functioning. In the early 1980s, the WHO published a classification related to the consequences of disease for experimental purposes: the *International Classification of Impairments, Disabilities, and Handicaps* (*ICIDH*) (WHO 1980). The conceptual framework of this classification had a significant impact throughout the 1980s on the development of public interventions among the population with disabilities (Fougeyrollas 1990).

The ICIDH Conceptual Framework and Its Reception at an International Level

The *ICIDH-1* conceptual framework is based on the following trilogy: body, person, and society (WHO 1980). As illustrated in Figure 6.1, the *ICIDH-1* model presents a cause-and-effect relationship between impairment, disability, and handicap. Thus, an injury leads to the impairment of an organ's functions and structures, which then leads to a disability in the person's behavior and activities, which generates one or many handicaps or disadvantages concerning social or survival roles. Because Nagi did not produce a full classification but only a conceptual framework, the *ICIDH* introduced, for the first time, taxonomies of the different dimensions of experiences related to the organic, personal, and, above all, social consequences of disease and trauma.

Since the diffusion of the *ICIDH* and its experimentation within diverse fields of application, the problems identified, the critiques, and the adaptations to the conceptual model and classification manual have been rich and stimulating for the development of knowledge. The most passionate debate is related to the critique of the linearity of the *ICIDH* model and the work that attempted to explicitly introduce the systemic approach and environmental dimension into the conceptual model. The modifications brought forth by these emergent conceptual models aim to illustrate the person-environment relationship in the construction or prevention of "handicap."

Thus, in 1983, Minaire proposed his concept of "situational handicap," defined as the result of the confrontation between the functional disability presented by an individual and the situations encountered in daily life (Minaire 1983). In 1992, he published an improved version of the conceptual model, explicitly integrating diverse categories of environmental factors (Minaire 1992). The process of disablement, therefore, includes environmental aspects analyzed in terms of situation. Minaire specified that one is handicapped (or disabled in Nagi's terminology, used in North America) not in the absolute but with reference to something. In his opinion, the situational handicap model completes the dimensions of the WHO model by integrating the person within the environment (Minaire 1992). Thus, a "handicap" is a characteristic not of the person but of the interaction between the person and his or her environment. In that way, Minaire refutes the linearity of the WHO classification.

Afterwards, several authors—notably Badley (1987), Chamie (1989), and Hamonet (1990)—elaborated conceptual models that integrate the concept of environment as a determining factor in the disablement process.

The *ICIDH* was published during a period that also witnessed the International Year of Disabled Persons, proclaimed in 1981 by the United Nations, and the Decade of Disabled Persons, which ended in 1992. This period was characterized by the preparation, adoption, and application of policies and legislative measures aiming to promote and ensure the exercise of the rights of disabled people (Office des personnes handicapées du Québec [OPHQ] 1984; United Nations [UN] 1983). Despite its innovative conception at the beginning of the 1970s, with the introduction of the social concept of handicap to the very biomedical universe of the WHO, the *ICIDH* and its conceptual framework failed to become the international reference tool for persons with disabilities (Barry 1989).

A worldwide disability movement, Disabled Peoples' International (DPI), did reject the *ICIDH* definitions in 1981 and adopted definitions that are now known as those of the "social model of disability" (Enns 1989; Oliver 1996). According to this model, disability is exclusively caused by the presence of barriers within the environment and occurs because the environment does not succeed in adapting to the needs of people who have impairment. To improve the life situations of people with disabilities, one must remove the environmental factors that create obstacles to their integration, and little interest is paid to their organic or functional differences (Enns 1989; Hurst 1993).

The DPI defines *impairment* and *disability* as follows:

> Impairment is the functional limitation with the individual caused by physical, mental, or sensory impairment.
> Disability is the loss or limitation of opportunities to take part in the normal life of the community on an equal level with others due to physical and social barriers (DPI 1982).

Within a political perspective, the social model has insisted that there is no causal relationship between impairment and disability. The achievement of the disability movement has been to break the link between bodies and social situation and to focus on the real cause of disability: discrimination and prejudice (Shakespeare and Watson 1997).

The concept of equalization of opportunities, meaning the process by which society is modified to become accessible for people with disabilities, is putting the social model into action. It was first used in a United Nations document, *Decade of Disabled Persons 1983-1992: World Program of Action Concerning Disabled Persons* (UN 1983).

> These radical changes in the early 1980s were largely the result of partnerships between the disability movement and various governments, like Canada and Sweden, who adopted the new principle of participation. This new perception of disability has influenced the development of disability legislation like The Charter of Rights and Freedoms in Canada and The Americans with disabilities Act. (Enns 1998:xii)

In this perspective, disability is a political issue. Disability rights activists (Driedger 1989; Hahn 1985) consider that the social environment structurally creates social disadvantages and discrimination situations experienced by people with disabilities. Disability is socially constructed by environmental barriers, and causality is no longer placed within the body and functional limitations but in the systemic inadequacy to adapt to their specific needs and oppression (Oliver 1990).

It is important to point out that the adoption and application of social policies and legislation ensuring the rights of the person and equal opportunities constitute modification of the environment that has an obvious impact on the disability process. The impossibility to monitor the evolution and impact of these factors through biomedical and compensation models centered on an inside-the-individual model of disability. This led numerous government planners and decision makers to support the movement for the defense of rights in the critique of the *ICIDH* and the inclusion of environmental variables for monitoring and measuring the impact of socio-economic policies in the field of rehabilitation, deinstitutionalization, and social participation. This is well exemplified with the UN standard rules for equalization of persons with disabilities (Barry 1995).

Another major criticism of the *ICIDH-1* was its lack of conceptual clarity and overlap between the concepts of impairments, disabilities, and handicaps (Nagi 1991). This is mentioned by the Committee on a National Agenda for the Prevention of Disabilities in its report, "Disability in America," to explain the rejection of the *ICIDH* as a conceptual framework. The committee preferred the concepts used by Nagi and presented a disabling process made up of four elements: pathology, impairment, functional limitation, and disability (Pope and Tarlov 1991). Another model developed was that of the Advisory Board of the National Center for Medical Rehabilitation Research (NCMRR) within the U.S. National Institutes of Health. The board decided to expand the classification approach presented in "Disability in America" to include "societal limitation" (NCMRR 1992). Furthermore, other explanatory models for the consequences of disease and trauma developed over the course of the 1990s; consider that "handicap" or "disability" is not a characteristic of the person but rather the result of the relationship between the person and the environment (Robine, Ravaud, and Cambois 1997; Verbrugge and Jette 1994).

As can be noted, recent theoretic reflections on the disability process integrate environmental factors. Despite this developing consensus, also among scholars, service providers, public officers, and disability community advocates, the importance of an ecological perspective was not recognized by the WHO for a long time within the framework of the *ICIDH* revision.

In Quebec, the first major application of the *ICIDH* model was in connection with development of the "On Equal Terms" policy, adopted as governmental policy in 1985 in the area of prevention, rehabilitation, and social integration of persons with disabilities (OPHQ 1984). The Quebec Committee on the *ICIDH* (QCICIDH)[1] played an important role in the recog-n ition of environmental factors in the revision process of the *ICIDH*. In fact, following an international meeting, which took place in 1987 and brought together expert users of the *ICIDH*,[2] the QCICIDH received the mandate to propose improvements to the third conceptual domain of the *ICIDH*: the handicap. In 1988, research began, and it continues within the QCICIDH. This work led to the integration of the dimension of environmental factors into a conceptual model that illustrates the interactive relationships between impairments, disabilities, and environmental obstacles and defines handicap situations as the result of this interaction (Fougeyrollas et al. 1991).

Revision of the 1980 ICIDH-1

Despite the constant increase of criticism brought to the *ICIDH* of 1980, the WHO delayed triggering the revision process. Thus, it was not until 1992 that the revision process began. The first result was the update of the *ICIDH* introduction (WHO 1993) in which the Quebec work[3] is well identified and several of the characteristics of their proposals are recognized.

An important task in the revision of the *ICIDH* will be to clarify the role and interrelationships of environmental factors in the definition and development of the different aspects addressed by the *ICIDH*, most notably—but not exclusively—handicap. . . . The current model of the consequences of disease and its graphic representation are effective in distinguishing between impairments, disabilities, and handicaps as separate concepts, but do not provide adequate information on the relationship between them. . . . Furthermore, the graphic representation of the *ICIDH* framework does not adequately reflect the role of the social and physical environment in the handicap process. (WHO 1993:4-5)

These statements, published in 1993 in the new foreword of the reprint of the *ICIDH* by the WHO, were very encouraging as recognition of more than 10 years of struggles and politico-scientific development in the field.

At this time, the United States joined the revision work, creating the North American Collaborating Center on the *ICIDH* at the U.S. National Center for Health Statistics, in partnership with Statistics Canada. The planning of the *ICIDH* revision was expected to last six years, until 1999. From a period in 1993 to the summer of 1996, responsibilities were divided between the various WHO collaborating centers. The French center was responsible for impairments, the Dutch center for disabilities, and the North American center for handicaps. During 1994 and after much pressure, an official North American Environmental Factors Task Force was created.

At the 1994 international meeting on the revision of *ICIDH*, no real debate or modifications were made on the boundaries of the concepts, and the trilogy of body, person, and society was confirmed, despite implications of overlapping problems between "disabilities" and "handicaps." There was a growing consensus for defining *handicap* as the result of the interaction between impairments and disabilities, on one hand, and environmental factors, on the other hand, as proposed in the reprint. The term *handicap* was strongly attacked by English-speaking consumers. During this meeting, the first proposal for a positive alternative concept of *social participation* was made but was not agreed on at that time. There was a lot of discussion for opting toward positive or neutral concepts, a position defended by the North American center and Scandinavian countries, yet still no agreement. The biomedical perspective defending the maintenance of negative concepts was still dominant, particularly by the WHO and the French collaborating center. The issue of recognizing environmental factors as a fourth conceptual domain was again discussed as social model advocates promoted it at each international meeting. A good consensus was reached as to its importance, but the WHO team's orientation to place it in an appendix as a list and not as a full conceptual domain and taxonomy in the classification of dimensions of disablement was consolidated. In September 1995, the Canadian Society for the *ICIDH* (CSICIDH) and QCICIDH organized in Quebec City, the third North American meeting of experts on *ICIDH* revision. Representatives from the sociopolitical disability movement participated in this meeting. It marked a decisive turning point, with the debates aimed at clarifying the distinction between the conceptual-level "handicap," also now called "social participation," and environmental factors. Major confusion between handicap and environmental barriers was stressed at the arrival of the United States and English Canada because of differences between their understanding of the disability concept, which partly covered the social consequences dimension (as proposed by Nagi) and was thus an equivalent of handicap in the *ICIDH* terminology. This tendency to confuse handicap and environmental obstacles is the source of recurrent conceptual ambiguities. Proposals related to environmental factors were presented by the Environmental Factors Task Force (Whiteneck et al. 1997; Whiteneck and Fougeyrollas 1996). Quebec classification proposals clarify the role of environmental factors in the disablement process. To appreciate the contribution of the Quebec classification, it is necessary to present it now.

Presentation of the Disability Creation Process (DCP)

The Quebec proposal is the fruit of several consultations and the reflections of numerous experts, including people with disabilities.[4] One major difficulty of explanatory models of the consequences of disease and trauma, such as those of the *ICIDH-1* or of Nagi, is related to the disease context from where they originate. Although understandable and legitimate, this tends to affect all of the classification processes by a sectarian vision of health problems. These models are not based on a universal model of human development that applies to every human being. Such a model allows the QCICIDH's team to illustrate the dynamics of the interactive process between personal factors (intrinsic) and environmental factors (extrinsic) determining

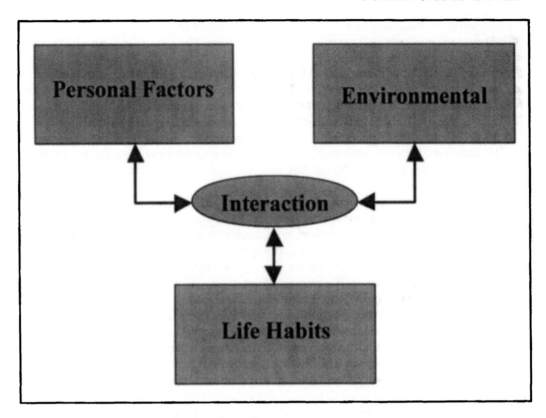

Figure 6.2. Simple Human Development Model

the situational result of accomplishing social activities and roles corresponding to the person's age, sex, and sociocultural identity. For this reason, it appears essential to first illustrate a fundamental model that is simple (see Figure 6.2) and applicable to everyone before introducing the determinants of differences, initiated by traumatic or pathological phenomena.

Thus, the disability creation process is not an independent reality that is separate from the universal model of human development. It is only a variation of possibilities in relation with the biological, functional, and social. This position agrees with the ecological, systemic, and destigmatizing perspective aimed at constructing a classification applicable to all, but it is compatible with the presence of the phenomenon of creating unique differences belonging to the explanation of the causes and consequences of disease and trauma. This theoretical perspective seems to be consistent with human rights ideology and with the movement promoting optimal social participation and the equalization of opportunities for people with functional and organic differences (Zola 1989). On the basis of this ideological choice, Figure 6.3 distinguishes two major conceptual dimensions intrinsic to every human being: organic systems and personal capabilities.

Furthermore, the "personal factors" box is larger and more comprehensive than the "organic systems" and "capabilities" subgroups. This means that other personal identity variables (age, gender, and sociocultural identity) must also be considered in the person-environment interaction, as well as in the explanation of the quality-of-life habits accomplishment. These other personal variables have tended to be omitted in applications centered on organic and functional abnormality taxonomies, identifying the person in terms of the direct manifestations of the pathology.

In Figure 6.3, the interactive process dynamic is symbolized by arrows in bold type. The point of central convergence, symbolized by the word *interaction,* solely aims at naming the continual relationship and interinfluence of the three large domains: personal factors, environmental factors, and life habits. The model's objective is to clarify the determinant variables of

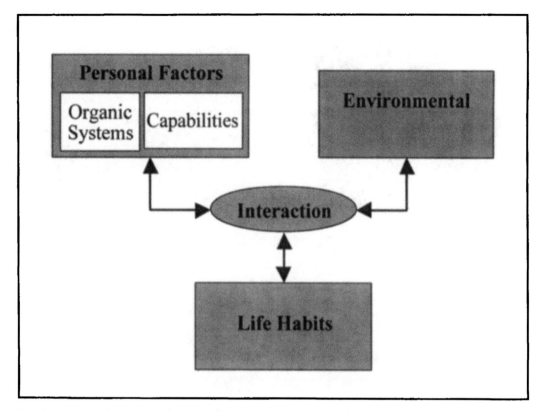

Figure 6.3. Human Development Model (organic systems and personal capabilities)

the interactive process and to consider the interaction as in a continual flux. It is now possible to illustrate the DCP explanatory model more precisely (see Figure 6.4) by specifying its components.

A *risk factor* is an element that belongs to an individual or the environment and is likely to cause a disease, trauma, or any other disruption to a person's integrity or development. These risk factors can become the effective causes that lead to a disease, trauma, or any other disruption to a person's integrity or development as intellectual developmental restrictions related to a lack of social stimulation (Fougeyrollas et al. 1996). Risk factors are an essential component for understanding and explaining the DCP. They were not included in the *ICIDH-1*. The Quebec classification developed a distinct conceptual dimension because it covers both personal and environmental variables requiring a taxonomy whose organization is different from that proposed for environmental determinants of social participation or handicap situations.

Personal factors correspond to a person's intrinsic characteristics, such as age, gender, sociocultural identity, organic systems, capabilities, and others (Fougeyrollas et al. 1996). Contemporary literature brings out the importance of acknowledging all of these variables to explain the disability process (Robine et al. 1997; Verbrugge and Jette 1994).

An *organic system* is a group of corporal components sharing a common function (Fougeyrollas et al. 1996). The taxonomy identifies all components of the human body. Integrity is the quality of an unaltered organic system according to the human biological norm. Impairment is an organic system's degree of anatomical, histological, or physiological anomaly or alteration. This conceptual segmentation is different from the one made in the WHO's *ICIDH-1* and in the *ICIDH-2*'s 1999 Beta-2 draft. It excludes any functional abilities and any externalized functional limitations considered as the result of the internal physiological and structural quality of organs and of their physical components. As a consequence of this change, the Quebec classification excludes the intellectual and psychological functions from the organic system dimension and is consistent in replacing them with functional capabilities whereby we

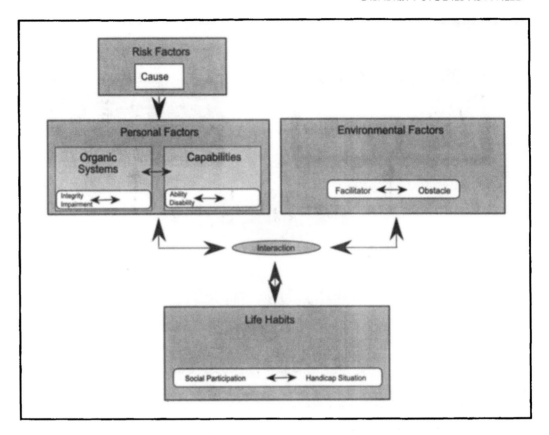

Figure 6.4. The Disability Creation Process

NOTE: This is an explanatory model of the causes and consequences of disease, trauma, and other disruptions to the integrity and development of a person (Fougeyrollas et al. 1996).

can objectively observe their manifestations without necessarily having to identify their etiology. This leads to operationally distinguishing two levels of very different realities that can be independently qualified and does not imply a mechanistic linear causal relationship. It is an organic consequences profile, clearly distinguished from a functional capability profile.

Capability is a person's potential to accomplish a mental or physical activity (Fougeyrollas et al. 1996). Capability has been retained as a classificatory concept, given the clear-cut support from the positive conceptual perspective. This choice also agrees with scientific references distinguishing between the potential for accomplishment and its accomplishment as the result expected according to a norm (Verbrugge and Jette 1994). Therefore, a taxonomy of human capability, applicable to everyone, is proposed. A capability's quality is measured on a scale ranging from optimal ability to total disability.

Within this point of view, we have an operational conceptual dimension. It corresponds to the intrinsic dimension of the person's ability profile, classified with regards to carrying out basic physical or mental activities such as walking, breathing, hearing, understanding, and behavior (some authors, such as Verbrugge and Jette [1994], suggested that one should refer to "actions" instead of "activities"). The real-life environment is not taken into account here; instead, a standardized context is used, as defined in the functional assessment protocols of rehabilitation specialists, for instance. The strength of this conceptual segmentation, besides its positive perspective contrasting with *ICIDH-1,* is translated through its assertion of the necessity of distinguishing complex social activities requiring consideration of social and physical environmental variables specific to the person's real-life situation.

Environmental factors are physical or social dimensions that determine a society's organization and context (Fougeyrollas et al. 1996). We must have a positive classification group that

Table 6.1   Major Environmental Factor Categories

1. Social factors
   1.1. Political economic factors
      1.1.1. Political system and governmental structures
      1.1.2. Judicial system
      1.1.3. Economic system
      1.1.4. Sociohealth system
      1.1.5. Education system
      1.1.6. Public infrastructures
      1.1.7. Community organizations
   1.2. Sociocultural factors
      1.2.1. Social network
      1.2.2. Social rules
2. Physical factors
   2.1. Nature
      2.1.1. Physical geography
      2.1.2. Climate
      2.1.3. Time
      2.1.4. Sound
      2.1.5. Electricity and magnetism
      2.1.6. Lighting
   2.2. Development
      2.2.1. Architecture
      2.2.2. National and regional development
      2.2.3. Technology

SOURCE: Fougeyrollas et al. (1996).

applies to everyone, not only to people with disabilities (see Table 6.1). An Environmental Quality Assessment Scale ranging from optimal facilitators to total obstacles is introduced. Assessing environmental quality only makes sense within the dynamic interaction between an expected social participation result and consideration of personal variables (organic systems, capabilities, and personal identity). Severity assessment is conducted by adding a positive dimension, that of facilitators. A facilitator is an environmental factor that contributes to the accomplishment of life habits when interacting with personal factors. Similarly, an obstacle hinders the accomplishment of life habits or social participation.

A *life habit* is a daily activity or social role valued by the person or his or her sociocultural context according to his or her characteristics (age, gender, sociocultural identity, and others) (Fougeyrollas et al. 1996). Life habit accomplishment quality is measured on a scale ranging from full social participation to a total handicap situation. Clarification of the life habits concept, as defined in the Quebec classification, requires inclusion of all that we designate as "activities of daily living" in rehabilitation into the level of social consequences, within the same conceptual domain as social roles. Therefore, activities such as dressing, personal hygiene, and preparing meals are not intrinsic characteristics of the person. It is rather a question of degree of performance in a social activity within an actual life context. It is that person's encounter with his or her environment, in keeping with a socially determined expected result (Bolduc 1996; Fougeyrollas 1995; Robine et al. 1997; Verbrugge and Jette 1994).

We assert that the conceptual clarification between capabilities in mental and physical activities (e.g., being able to maintain balance, perceive colors, hear in a noisy environment, understand abstract ideas, and remember) and performance in the accomplishment of socially determined life habits is the fundamental operational issue in response to the demands of people with disabilities. As previously mentioned, it is essential to have a conceptual dimension that is intrinsic to the person at the capabilities level being translated into abilities and functional disabilities. It is also essential to distinguish them from the performance result, which requires that we consider the result of using capabilities according to the tasks specific to a social activity or role conditioned by contextual variables. These conceptual dimensions must be related, but it is impossible to deduce handicap situations on the basis of functional ability assessment without taking into account environmental variables in real-life situations. Therefore, within this perspective, the environmental factors dimension constitutes the crucial variable that enables one to distinguish between personal capabilities and quality of social participation.

Toward the ICIDH-2 Draft

On the basis of a growing consensus on the definition of handicap as a domain distinct from environmental factors and the acceptability of a positive concept, a social participation taxonomy proposal, greatly influenced by the Quebec life habits taxonomy, was discussed and adopted by the North American Task Force. As for environmental factors, the QCICIDH's proposal had been almost entirely validated. However, the impairment and disability proposals remained conceptually very similar to those of the original ICIDH.

An Alpha draft of the ICIDH-2 was developed in May 1996, incorporating the work of all collaborating centers. Until 1997, the collaborating centers and task forces provided comments. Basic questions were discussed, but major concerns about conceptual framework and boundaries between concepts were somewhat fixed by the WHO team, which made new modifications in the proposed drafts on its own. Social participation and environmental factors drafts were amended and reorganized.

The Beta-2 draft of the ICIDH-2 was available during the summer of 1999 for a new round of field trials, and the final version for adoption by the World Assembly was planned for May 2001.

Beta-2 Draft of the ICIDH-2

The introduction states that "the overall aim of the ICIDH-2 classification is to provide a unified and standard language and framework for the description of human functioning and disability as an important component of health" (WHO 1999:7). The classification covers "any disturbance in terms of functional states associated with health conditions at body, individual, and society levels" (WHO 1999:7). The new draft of the ICIDH-2 proposes three dimensions—body functions and structure, activities at the individual level, and participation in society—and a list of environmental factors. The title of the classification has been changed to ICIDH-2: International Classification of Functioning and Disability. Functioning and disability are defined as umbrella terms. Thus, disability was preferred over disablement, which was used in the Beta-1 draft.

The current scheme, shown in Figure 6.5,

demonstrates the potential role that contextual factors play in the process. These factors interact with an individual with a health condition and determine the level and extent of the individual's functioning. Environmental factors are extrinsic to the individual (e.g., the attitudes of the society, architectural characteristics, the legal system) and are classified in the classification. Personal factors, on the other hand, are not classified in the current version of ICIDH-2. Their assessment is left to the user, if needed. They may include: gender, age, other health conditions, fitness, lifestyle, . . . all or any of which may play a role in disability at any level. (WHO 1999:26)

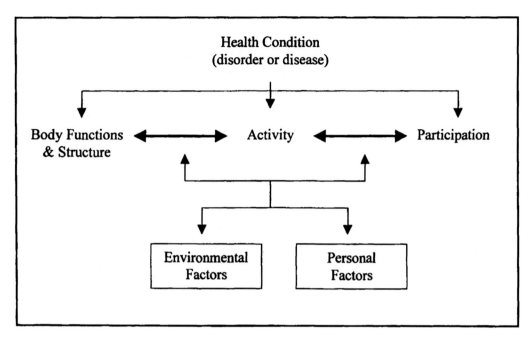

Figure 6.5. Conceptual Schema of the *ICIDH-2*

Critical Analysis of the Beta-2 Draft of the ICIDH-2

The Beta-2 draft is the result of various influences. It indicates positive change because it recognizes the disability, sociopolitical, and environmental models as essential for counterbalancing the biomedical and economic models based on the individual (Bickenbach 1993).

Changes seem to be under way because options previously viewed as impossible have been accepted, such as the adoption of a neutral and positive terminology. Even the biomedical resistance concerning the dimension of impairment, which was present in the Beta-1 draft, has been overcome. The importance of environmental factors is recognized, but there is resistance to making this a separate and full fourth conceptual dimension. The systemic nature of the disability phenomenon is acknowledged, but the explanation is made even more confusing by the proposal of a complex conceptual framework that fails to clearly identify the interaction between the individual and the environment as a central factor. The importance of personal factors is recognized, but their roles are not clear as they are presented as contextual factors, thereby creating some confusion with environmental factors. Finally, there has been no improvement of the conceptual overlapping in the 1980 *ICIDH*, and the famous trilogy—body, person, and society—has been maintained. Yet it perpetuates confusion about what really pertains to the individual and what pertains to the environment. In addition, the Beta-2 draft version reinforces the perception that performance in human activities within one's life context is an intrinsic personal characteristic. "The Activities covers the complete range of activities performed by an individual" (from simple to complex activities) (WHO 1999:12). It severely undermines the adoption of the participation dimension proposed by the North Americans, which is correctly defined as the result of the interaction between a person and external factors but is, in fact, operationalized as an attempt to assess environmental influence. "The Participation dimension classifies areas of life in which an individual is involved, has access to, has societal opportunities or barriers" (WHO 1999:12). We understand that this is a political decision by the WHO that is designed to satisfy the social model. However, it is a cosmetic choice, as we end up with taxonomies that allow each dominant group to maintain its ideological position: An individual's disability is viewed in terms of impairments of body functions, structures, and activity restrictions of the person as a whole. The immediate effect is to put the weight of the responsibility on the individual, satisfying the biomedical gatekeepers and their mandates to attribute disability status and eligibility to compensations.

ICIDH-2 recognizes the importance of a list of environmental factors in the classification. "Environmental factors have an impact on all three dimensions and are organized from the individual's most immediate environment to the general environment" (WHO 1999:12). However, in the facts, these crucial relations with the three conceptual domains are only operationalized with the concept of participation. The relationship between activities and participation is yet to be clarified. "Activities are what an individual does" (WHO 1999:18). It deals with the actual performance and does not refer to an aptitude, potential, capacity, or what an individual might do.

> "[The] activity dimension differs from the Participation (P) dimension in that participation addresses involvement of the individual in a life area and in particular whether or not that involvement is restricted or facilitated by environmental factors. . . . For example, attending school is something a child does, so it is an activity; being allowed to attend and being included in all school activities, however, is a matter of participation. (WHO 1999:19)

WHO's explanations are very ambiguous, and one must state that despite all the positive modifications that link the *ICIDH-2* and DCP, the conceptual disagreement still exists. The *ICIDH-2* measures the same conceptual domain twice, leaving one to believe that human activities are personal characteristics and making participation a disguised measure of the environment. It is better to understand why the WHO resists recognizing environmental factors as a fourth conceptual domain so much and why it persists in relegating them to a list. Within the DCP, a clear segmentation between capabilities that are intrinsic to a person (such as understanding, remembering, keeping one's balance, and walking) and the concept of *life habits,* defined as the result of the interaction between personal factors and factors within the life context of the person, is fundamental. The quality of the accomplishment of life habits is in fact a measure of the person's involvement in society. It is not possible and, in our opinion, is even dangerous to believe that complex social activities, such as achieving at school, preparing meals, and engaging in physical intimacy, can be separated into either a personal performance or a societal involvement! The dramatic consequence of this is that conceptual overlap and incoherency of the *ICIDH-1* trilogy still exist in *ICIDH-2.* Far from being integrated, the three domains can be used independently, and the body and activity ones will be well accepted by biomedical, compensation, and program eligibility gatekeepers. Omitting the necessity to use all conceptual domains together to document human functioning and disability process, *ICIDH-2* makes room for continued consideration of the individual unfitness for work, the inability to be educated, or the inability to use certain means of transportation as intrinsic characteristics. This perspective seems unacceptable to the independent living and equalization of opportunities movements. Historically, all of these categories were attributed to the individual to assign a status justifying his or her social exclusion and failure to consider the relative and dynamic character of the accomplishment of daily activities and social roles as the result of the interaction between the individual and the environment. No individual is intrinsically unfit for work or unable to prepare a meal. The limitations affecting the achievement of these activities are equal to the restrictions affecting participation and only have meaning within a specific real-life context in which the objective outcome can be assessed. Also, this outcome is always relative and changing, as it depends on the evolution (time improvement or deterioration) of the individual's functional abilities and variations in the environment as facilitators or obstacles. To this must be added the meaning and value that the individual assigns to this outcome or that his or her family or social relationships assign to this social situation (Albrecht and Devlieger 1999; Robine et al. 1997).

To illustrate why the outcome of the interactive process is always relative, one must choose a social life or participation situation. At work, for example, the level and quality of an individual's participation are the result of the interaction between functional abilities and limitations, personal identity (education, work experience, personal values), and environmental obstacles or facilitators related to the components of a specific work situation.

In terms of one's personal micro-environment, we can talk about the level of adjustment of the specific tasks required by the job. This will determine the individual's ability to do the job and perform the specific productive tasks. In terms of the community (meso-environment), we take into account the quality of attitudes displayed by the employer and colleagues at work, the quality of physical accessibility or communication aids in the workplace, the availability of adapted transportation resources, and physical assistance at home. All of these are prerequisite social participation situations conditional to job participation. These community variables are positive or negative determinants of an individual's ability to work and are dependent on needs related to functional abilities and limitations and other contexts, such as the home, family network, and urban or rural environment. In terms of the societal macro-environment, the following must be taken into consideration: socioeconomic context, legislation related to employment, and social policies, which are also obstacles or facilitators determining an individual's possibility to participate in the workforce or to "find and hold a job" that is currently classified under activities in the Beta-2 draft version.

From this concrete example, then, it is very clear that the interactive process determining performance in the achievement of social activities, handicap situations, or restrictions to participation, which is a single dimension, is always relative and dynamic. It is necessary to define the following as components of the analytical methodology or application of the disability process models (Bronfenbrenner 1990; Robine et al. 1997; Verbrugge and Jette 1994):

> expected achievement of social life activities, life habits, or spheres of participation;
>
> personal characteristics: personal identity, organic systems' structural and internal functions quality, and functional abilities profile;
>
> the influence of environmental factors on a personal (micro), community (meso), and societal (macro) level.

There can be no shortcuts, and any simplification (administrative, professional prognosis, and common prejudices) designed to shorten this complex systemic process is destined to result in an impasse, which will stigmatize individuals with significant differences. This reinforces the still prevailing tendency to attribute to the individual responsibility for social consequences, for his or her performance in the activities of daily life, and the social roles that constitute social participation situations. One of the most harmful and violent consequences of this process occurs when the individual who is different adopts this label and bases his or her identity on all of the disabilities and oppression situations attributed to him or her. It was precisely to denounce this social violence—widely propagated by health care, rehabilitation, and social support service providers—that radical movements focusing on social change developed.

Environmental Relationships with Three Conceptual Dimensions

Although there was never any explanation of these relationships, the WHO made an ongoing assumption that environmental factors interact with body structures and functions, activities, and participation.

> Environmental Factors make up the physical, social, and attitudinal environment, in which people live and conduct their lives. The factors are external to individuals and can have a positive or negative influence on the individual's participation as a member of society, on performance of activities of the individual, or on the individual's body function or structure. (WHO 1999:22)

It is correct to say that the environment is always present in the evaluation of each conceptual dimension. However, we hold that the utility of the analysis does not truly become operational and essential unless it is in relation to the real-life context of the person (i.e., the life habits or social participation dimension).

Regarding impairments, it is relevant to emphasize that an evaluation of the integrity of the organic structure or its internal functioning must be carried out while taking into account clearly defined and controlled environmental variables (asepsis, air pressure, atmosphere, quality of matters, and others). In doing so, we enter into the universe of biomedical clinical assessment instruments for diagnostic and treatment purposes. It is an ultra-specialized and technical field, and it does not seem at all desirable to complicate the classification system with this field of professional diagnosis. In the activities dimension, the conceptual segmentation of the *ICIDH-2* (with its very large concept of human activities) poses, from our point of view, a major problem for its relationship with the environment. In fact, this dimension integrates, at the same time, functional capabilities and performance in home, daily, or social life. These latter activities are always complex and relative because they require consideration of all the real-life contextual variables of people, if we claim to be carrying out a measure in vivo. As illustrated in the literature (Alexander and Fuhrer 1984), this clarification becomes difficult because of currently available clinical functional assessment instruments. In fact, these tools confuse basic or elementary functional capabilities, such as seeing, talking, holding an object, understanding, and remembering, with performance in the accomplishment of complex activities such as eating a meal, making one's bed, or driving a car. The problem resides within the formulation of the instrument's questions. Assessment of the functional capability of taking an object, holding it, moving it toward the mouth, and directing it right or left requires the formulation of a question that needs to be applied to a concrete context such as eating soup. Thus, we call on a higher conceptual level—social life habit. Actually, we could define a general principle that distinguishes a classification of elements belonging to a conceptual dimension from evaluative questions necessary for measuring the quality of these elements that obligatorily call on a superior conceptual level. Ignorance of the fundamental distinctive principle between the classification and assessment instrument is at the basis of profound confusion, currently within the revision process of the *ICIDH-2*. Thus, with regards to the capabilities dimension, we propose an agreement whereby evaluation is functional and in vitro. The objective here is to make a profile of the person's functional abilities and not a profile of the person's accomplishment of daily and social activities in his or her usual life environment.

We thus note a tendency to confuse "classification" and "evaluation instrument" when we envisage the relationship of the environment with the organic dimension and with the physical and mental capability dimension. In our opinion, environmental variables that are useful at these levels are related to technology, human assistance, and the accommodation of the tasks. Yet these environmental dimensions should be considered in severity scales, measuring impairments and disabilities. These are founded on a presumption of availability and aim to describe or identify with which type and quality of external support the capability to accomplish physical or mental action is possible on a theoretical or clinical, standardized, or controlled basis: in vitro. It is the field of functional rehabilitation.

Thus, as explained by Alexander and Fuhrer (1984), the ability to perform is a phenomenon that is very different from real performance in a situation. It seems essential to avoid any confusion about this and to propose that the criteria of environment (in vitro/in vivo) be considered as the fundamental distinction between the dimension of capabilities and the dimension of situational results of the person-environment interaction: social situations or life habits or even social handicap or participation situations.

Thus, these considerations lead us to assert that the environmental determinants of social participation situations should first be defined and identified to respond adequately to the expectations of people with disabilities, as well as to the requirements of a structured analysis of the social consequences of impairments and functional restrictions within the context of the *ICIDH* revision. Within a perspective of social change and equal opportunities favoring social participation, one must focus attention on the interaction between personal characteristics and the environment's characteristics in the creation of social participation or the prevention of handicap situations, defined as results (Fougeyrollas 1997).

The environment concerns everyone, and its elements are not specific to people with disabilities. Here is another precision that is often misunderstood in the conceptualization of external factors in the revision process of the *ICIDH*.

A Balanced Model Compatible with Personal and Sociopolitical Change

ICIDH-2 (Beta-2 draft) and the DCP Quebec classification are compatible with the disability sociopolitical model. They emphasize in different ways the consideration of environmental variables and support the collective project to modify them within a perspective to ensure the exercise of human rights and equalization of opportunities. They are also compatible with the practical and real demands of taking into consideration the organic and functional consequences of disease, trauma, and other disruptions. These practical requirements interest clinicians at the biomedical and rehabilitation levels and are also needed for defining eligibility for support and benefits programs. This double compatibility is adequate because if there were no functional- or organic-level gaps, there would be no reason to think about the problems of people with impairments or disabilities and the explanation of their consequences on the social participation dimension. The existence of organic and functional differences is a fact. The issue is not to deny them or to minimize their importance since they constitute differences in the identity of those concerned. The central idea is to have a user-friendly explanatory conceptual model and a classificatory system that enable consideration of the group of variables at stake—a model that does not identify people as responsible for the social consequences of their differences. The conceptual segmentation of the *ICIDH-2* presents this risk again, even if it was not the intention expressed by the WHO. We need an explanatory framework in which a dynamic of change will be made possible by deconstructing the social exclusion creation process—not by exclusively concentrating on personal components, as the classic biomedical model has done, as well as the rehabilitation model, which centers on the individual's modification. The challenge, then, is to modify the socioeconomic organization, act on the attitudes and social representations, develop the implementation of perspectives of a universal design, make resources and compensatory and adapted services for functional differences available, and adapt the ways of life habit accomplishment.

These universal models are built on a progressive dynamic perspective centered on the respect of identities and on the necessary acknowledgment of the context to reach the sociopolitical challenge of equalizing opportunities in relation to fields of social participation entrenched in human rights charters. The social norm is not to attend to the rights of people with disabilities but to ensure that people's rights are exercised despite differences, including those related to organic and functional differences. It is also to see that the necessary sociopolitical foundations are laid down to ensure that human rights are exercised. This right to equity can be evaluated by comparing the degree of accomplishment of life habits of people with disabilities to people without disabilities (which is in our view equivalent to the measure of involvement proposed in the *ICIDH-2* participation concept), within a given physical and sociocultural environment. The gaps make up the sociopolitical agenda of social change, as well as the assessment of oppression or social exclusion to be corrected at the societal level.

Is the Environment the Key?

Whether we recognize it or not, the environment constitutes the driving force of change. It is fundamentally historical and anchored in reality. Without the definition of an expected result and the attribution of meaning by the normative cultural context, differences have no predetermined effect. Without the observer's point of view, there is nothing to observe. This is why the interpretation of the significance of corporal and functional differences and of their consequences is a subject or a project that is largely anthropological and interdisciplinary. Variation of human development and the disability creation process is closely linked to its cultural construction (Albrecht and Devlieger 1999; Bickenbach et al. 1999; Robine et al. 1997).

Demonstrating that environment is the key, one must assert that nothing can be said in advance. With regards to human development and the disability creation process, the environment cannot be considered as an accessory. Everything should be put into context, along with the difficulties and complications that result from this, particularly from the administrative and mechanistic logic points of view. Nothing can be deducted from linear cause-and-effect relationships. The inherent opening of the conceptual model of the disability creation process is definitely revolutionary, innovative, and oriented toward social change. The "disability creation process" model does not claim to say what is correct to do or think. Rather, it is an instrument to facilitate the identification and situation of different variables involved in the interaction, without predefining the conclusions. These conclusions are being linked to "judgment," to the point of view of the producer of meaning, and to the context defining the expected sociocultural norm. The challenge is thus to render possible the expression of this expectation without it being set within linear reasoning. The stake of adopting an international frame of reference for the *ICIDH* has made possible this opening to social change and has recognized the systemic and ecological conception of the necessity for the documentation of the environment, personal factors, and their interactions. Anything is possible, but nothing is determined on the basis of any diagnosis, type of organic impairment, profile of abilities, or intrinsic activities. No one can say what a person with organic or functional differences is or what he or she can accomplish. This is not possible, except according to a specific environment and a subjective point of view, whether it be that of the person and his or her family, professionals evaluating eligibility to a service or compensation, or general public opinion. Finally, this model must put into evidence organic and functional differences, the intrinsic personal variables without which it would be useless to evaluate the quality of environmental variables to become facilitators or obstacles according to the accomplishment of life habits or specific social participation situations.

CONCLUSION

The review of the literature demonstrates the generalization of the systemic and person-environment interaction in understanding human development. This approach highlights the erroneous and mechanistic nature of one of the biomedical model's premises and its expansions in rehabilitation and compensation, which considered disease, impairment, or functional limitation as anchorage points. This premise of the biomedical model overshadows the whole person and his or her unique identity and experience. It isolates features, distinctions, or anomalies to explain social situations, life conditions, and the realities experienced by the people who own these signifiers.

Founded on a logic of intervention, treatment, repair or correction of pathology, or deviation from the physiological, anatomical, behavioral, or functional norm, these normalization models that situate the cause of the problem as being intrinsic to the person are erroneous and dangerous—especially when they isolate specific differences and make them explanatory determinants of their consequences at the social level. One may thus note normative processes of naturalization, oppression, social disadvantage, and inferiority as being inherent to the corporal, behavioral, or functional condition. In this way, the principle of creating the social being, which is the basis of the ecological, systemic, and social anthropological approach, is ignored for all human beings.

The sociopolitical model of disability stems from this denunciation of the historical process of social exclusion and oppression based on corporal, behavioral, or functional distinctions. This model situates the source of this problem within the environment. Rather than concentrating on the "responsible" individual, the collective intervention target becomes the modification of environmental factors. Constructed on the reasoning of a sociopolitical struggle, the radical environmentalist movement's approach appears to be coherent and justified. It lies within the relationship of societal forces and within a simplifying argumentation aiming to rally, under a collective identity of social outcasts, a group of the population that is stigmatized and partitioned by diagnoses and administrative statuses, based on the cause of disabilities. It clearly identifies a change of paradigm founded on the transformation of the rules of the social production of inequality. It is exactly this phenomenon that motivated social movement struggles against racism, male domination, or intolerance of minority sexual orientations.

In itself, it emphasizes the social and physical environment as a creator of disability. As with other movements, the struggle against disability is also based on claiming the valorization of corporal and functional difference, a source of unique experience, pride, and a specific knowledge that is ally to a culture belonging to the bearers of these differences.

What is justified and coherent of a political point of view, which defines the global principles of belonging and is staked on a common situation of experience and exclusion, also creates paradoxes and abusive generalizations when it bases its identity on a extremist conceptualization. This results in minimizing and sometimes denying the diversity of differences related to the consequences of disease and trauma, as well as multiple experiences that are of individual expression. Thus, to say that socioeconomic organization, social rules, and the physical environment are determinants of the disability creation process that cannot be bypassed is fundamental. However, asserting that social change is likely to resolve and correct all social "handicap" or "disability" situations experienced by people, while denying the importance of impairments, functional limitations, and the conditions in which they appeared, may lead to new sources of oppression and unrealistic expectations. The courageous position of Sally French (1993) with regard to this subject illustrates the limits of the radical discourse of certain leaders of social models of disability and warns us of the danger of generic solutions applied for the people's "good," leaving little space for experience and individual choice. In fact, it must be recognized that the realities experienced and the personal factors of each different body are just as fundamental as environmental solutions with their own limits.

It is toward this delicate balance that a systemic conceptual perspective, which situates all of the variables involved, must maintain. It consists of a continually changing open game, within which personal factors are as essential as the environmental factors.

NOTES

1. The QCICIDH is a nonprofit organization, founded in 1986, with the mission to promote knowledge, application, validation, and, above all, the improvement of the *ICIDH*. To accomplish this mission, the QCICIDH favored research and the development of relationships between experts and Quebec, Canadian, and international organizations concerned with the development of a common language and a better understanding of the consequences of disease and trauma.

2. Those present were representatives of the movement for the defense of rights of people with disabilities, such as Disabled Peoples' International, and representatives of international organizations such as the World Health Organization (WHO), United Nations, and the Council of Europe.

3. We will see later the results of this work with the presentation of the disability creation process (DCP) model.

4. For more details on the history of the DCP, see Fougeyrollas (1988).

REFERENCES

Albrecht, G. L. and P. J. Devlieger. 1999. "The Disability Paradox: High Quality of Life against All Odds." *Social Science and Medicine* 48:977-88.

Alexander, J. L. and M. J. Fuhrer. 1984. "Functional Assessment of Individuals with Physical Impairments." Pp. 45-60 in *Functional Assessment in Rehabilitation,* edited by Andrew S. Halpern and Marcus J. Fuhrer. Baltimore: Brookes.

Badley, E. M. 1987. "The ICIDH Format: Application in Different Settings and Distinction between Disability and Handicap." *International Disability Studies* 9 (3): 122-25.

Barry, M. 1989. "Disability Concept." *ICIDH International Network* 2 (2-3): 6-8.

———. 1995. "Rules for Equalization of Opportunities for Persons with Disabilities." *ICIDH and Environmental Factors International Network* 7 (3): 10-13.

Bateson, G. 1972. *Steps to an Ecology of Mind.* New York: Ballantine.

Bickenbach, J. E. 1993. *Physical Disability and Social Policy.* Toronto, Canada: University of Toronto Press.

Bickenbach, J. E., S. Chatterji, E. M. Badley, and T. B. Üstün. 1999. "Models of Disablement, Universalism and International Classification of Impairments, Disabilities and Handicaps." *Social Science and Medicine* 48:1173-87.

Bolduc, M. 1996. "Social and Political Issues of an ICIDH: In Depth Revision and the Introduction of Environmental Factors." *ICIDH and Environmental Factors International Network* 8 (3): 49-54.

Bronfenbrenner, U. 1977. "Toward an Experimental Ecology of Human Development." *American Psychologist* 32:513-30.

———. 1990. "Le modèle Processus-Personne-Contexte-Temps dans la recherche en psychologie: Principes, applications et implications." Pp. 9-59 in *Le modèle écologique dans l'étude du développement de l'enfant,* edited by Réjean Tessier. Sainte-Foy, Québec: Presses de l'Université du Québec.

Butrym, Z. 1989. "Health Care and Social Work: What Kind of Relationship?" Pp. 21-31 in *Social Work and Health Care,* edited by Rex Taylor and Jill Ford. London: Jessica Kingsley.

Chamie, M. 1989. "Survey Design Strategies for the Study of Disability." *World Health Statistics Quarterly* 42 (3): 122-40.

Disabled Peoples' International (DPI). 1982. *Proceedings of the First World Congress.* Singapore: Author.

Dobren, A. A. 1994. "An Ecological Oriented Conceptual Model of Vocational Rehabilitation of People with Acquired Midcareer Disabilities." *Rehabilitation Counseling Bulletin* 37 (3): 215-26.

Driedger, D. 1989. *The Last Civil Rights Movement.* London: Hurst.

Duckworth, D. 1983. *The Classification and Measurement of Disablement.* London: Her Majesty's Stationery Office.

Dunn, W., C. Brown, and A. McGuigan. 1994. "The Ecology of Human Performance: A Framework for Considering the Effects of Context." *American Journal of Occupational Therapy* 48 (7): 595-607.

Enns, H. 1989. "Disabled People International (DPI) Statement on the WHO's." *ICIDH International Network* 2 (2-3): 27-29.

———. 1998. "Foreword." Pp. xi-xii in *Introduction to Disability,* edited by Mary Ann McColl and Jerome B. Bickenbach. London: W. B. Saunders.

Erickson, M. H. 1967. *Advanced Techniques of Hypnosis and Therapy.* New York: Grune & Stratton.

Evans, R. G. and G. L. Stoddart. 1990. "Producing Health, Consuming Health Care." *Social Science and Medicine* 31 (12): 1347-63.

Fougeyrollas, P. 1988. "Canadian and International Changes to Conceptual Definition and Classification Concerning Persons with Disabilities: Critical Analysis Issues and Perspective." *ICIDH and Environmental Factors International Network* 9 (2-3): 4-44.

———. 1990. "Les implications de la diffusion de la CIH sur les politiques concernant les personnes handicapées." *Rapport Trimestriel de Statistiques Sanitaires Mondiales* 43 (4): 281-85.

———. 1995. "Documenting Environmental Factors for Preventing the Handicap Creation Process: Quebec Contributions Relating to ICIDH and Social Participation of People with Functional Differences." *Disability and Rehabilitation* 17 (3-4): 145-53.

———. 1997. "Les déterminants environnementaux de la participation sociale des personnes ayant des incapacités: le défi sociopolitique de la révision de la CIDIH." *Canadian Journal of Rehabilitation* 10 (2): 147-60.

Fougeyrollas, P., H. Bergeron, R. Cloutier, and G. St-Michel. 1991. "The Handicap Creation Process: Analysis of the Consultation. New Full Proposals." *ICIDH International Network* 4 (1-2): 5-37.

Fougeyrollas, P., R. Cloutier, H. Bergeron, J. Càté, and G. St-Michel. 1996. *Quebec Classification "Disability Creation Process."* Québec: International Network on the Disability Creation Process.

Freidson, E. 1965. "Disability as Social Deviance." Pp. 71-99 in *Sociology and Rehabilitation,* edited by Marvin B. Sussman. Washington, DC: American Sociological Association.

French, S. 1993. "What's So Great about Independance?" Pp. 44-48 in *Disabling Barriers—Enabling Environments,* edited by John Swain, Vic Finkelstein, Sally French, and Mike Oliver. London: Sage.

Goffman, E. 1963. *Stigma: Notes on the Management of Spoiled Identity.* Englewood Cliffs, NJ: Prentice Hall.

Grandjean, E. 1980. *Man-Machine Systems: Fitting the Task to the Man: An Ergonomic Approach.* London: Taylor & Francis.

Hahn, H. 1985. "Towards a Politics of Disability: Definitions, Disciplines and Policies." *The Social Science Journal* 22 (4): 87-105.

Hamonet, C. 1990. *Les personnes handicapées.* Paris: Presses Universitaires de France.

Hurst, R. 1993. "The Definition of Disability, Our Right to Define Ourselves." *ICDIH International Network* 6 (2): 7-8.

Kemp, S. P. 1994. "Social Work Systems of Knowledge: The Concept of Environment in Social Casework Theory, 1990-1983." Ph.D. dissertation, University of Colombia.

Kielhofner, G. 1993. "Functional Assessment: Toward a Dialectical View of Person-Environment Relations." *American Journal of Occupational Therapy* 47 (3): 248-51.

Kourilsky-Belliard, F. 1995. *Du désir au plaisir de changer.* Paris: Interéditions.

Kuhn, T. S. 1970. *The Structure of Scientific Revolutions.* Chicago: University of Chicago Press.

Law, M. 1991. "The Environment: A Focus for Occupational Therapy." *Canadian Journal of Occupational Therapy* 58 (4): 171-80.

Law, M., B. Cooper, S. Strong, D. Stewart, P. Rigby, and L. Letts. 1996. "The Person-Environment-Occupation Model: A Transactive Approach to Occupational Performance." *Canadian Journal of Occupational Therapy* 63 (1): 9-23.

Lawton, M. P. and L. Nahemow. 1973. "Ecology and the Aging Process." Pp. 610-74 in *The Psychology of Adult Development and Aging,* edited by Carl Eisdorfer and M. P. Lawton. Washington, DC: American Psychological Association.

Minaire, P. 1983. "Le handicap en porte-à-faux." *Prospective et Santé* 26:39-46.

———. 1992. "Disease, Illness and Health: The Critical Models of the Disablement Process." *Bulletin of the World Health Organization* 70 (3): 373-79.

Moos, R. H. 1980. "Specialized Living Environment for Older People: A Conceptual Framework for Valuation." *Journal of Social Issues* 36 (2): 75-94.

Morin, E. 1990. *Introduction à la pensée complexe.* Paris: ESF éditeurs.

Nagi, S. Z. 1965. "Some Conceptual Issues in Disability and Rehabilitation." Pp. 100-13 in *Sociology and Rehabilitation,* edited by Marvin B. Sussman. Washington, DC: American Sociological Association.

———. 1991. "Disability Concepts Revisited: Implications for Prevention." Pp. 309-27 in *Disability in America: Toward a National Agenda for Prevention,* edited by Andrew M. Pope and Alvin R. Tarlov. Washington, DC: National Academy Press.

National Center for Medical Rehabilitation Research (NCMRR). 1992. *NCMRR Research Plan* [Online]. Available: silk.nih.gov/silk/ncmrr/archive/rplan/PIFor.htm.

Oborne, D. J. 1982. *Ergonomics at Work.* New York: John Wiley.

Office des personnes handicapées du Québec (OPHQ). 1984. *A part égale, l'"intégration sociale des personnes handicapées: un défi pour tous.* Québec: Gouvernement du Québec.

Oliver, M. 1990. *The Politics of Disablement.* London: Macmillan.

———. 1996. "Defining Impairment and Disability: Issues at Stake." Pp. 39-54 in *Exploring the Divide: Illness and Disability,* edited by C. Barnes and G. Mercer. Leeds, UK: The Disability Press.

Ottawa Charter for Health Promotion. 1986. *An International Conference on Health Promotion.* Ottawa, Canada: World Health Organization, Health and Welfare Canada, Canadian Public Health Association.

Pope, A. M. and A. R. Tarlov, eds. 1991. *Disability in America: Toward a National Agenda for Prevention.* Washington, DC: National Academy Press.

Ramsay, R. 1991. "Preparing to Influence Paradigm Shifts in Health Care Strategies." Pp. 29-44 in *Social Work Administrative Practice in Health Care Setting,* edited by Patricia Taylor and Janet Devereux. Toronto: Canadian Scholars' Press.

Robine, J. -M., J.-F. Ravaud, and E. Cambois. 1997. "General Concepts of Disablement." Pp. 63-83 in *Osteoarthritis: Public Health Implications for an Aging Population,* edited by David Hamerman. Baltimore: John Hopkins University Press.

Shakespeare, T. and N. Watson. 1997. "Defending the Social Model." *Disability and Society* 12 (2): 293-300.

Stiker, H. J. 1982. *Corps infirmes et sociétés*. Paris: Dunod.

United Nations (UN). 1983. *Decade of Disabled Persons 1983-1992: World Program of Action Concerning Disabled Persons*. New York: Author.

Verbrugge, L. M. and A. M. Jette. 1994. "The Disablement Process." *Social Science and Medicine* 38 (1): 1-14.

von Bertalanffy, L. 1968. *General System Theory*. New York: Braziller.

Vondracek, F. W., R. M. Lerner, and J. E. Shulenberg. 1986. *Career Development: A Life-Span Developmental Approach*. Hillsdale, NJ: Lawrence Erlbaum.

Wan, T. T. H. 1974. "Correlates and Consequences of Severe Disabilities." *Journal of Occupational Medicine* 16 (4): 234-44.

Warren, M. D. 1977. "The Need for Rehabilitation." Pp. 6-10 in *Rehabilitation Today*, edited by Stephen Mattingly. London: Update.

Watzlawick, P. 1978. *The Language of Change: Elements of Therapeutic Communication*. New York: Basic Books.

Webb, R. D. G., P. Lamanna, G. Kovacs, P. Hall, and S. Dickson. 1988. "Ergonomics and Job Placement of Workers Disabled through Occupational Injury." Pp. 99-114 in *Ergonomics in Rehabilitation*, edited by Anil Mital and Waldemar Karwowski. New York: Taylor & Francis.

Weisman, G. D. 1981. "Modeling Environment-Behavior Systems: A Brief Note." *Journal of Man-Environment Relations* 1 (2): 32-41.

Whiteneck, G. G. and P. Fougeyrollas. 1996. "Environmental Factors Task Force Position Paper: Environmental Factors and ICIDH." *ICIDH and Environmental Factors International Network* 8 (3): 14-18.

Whiteneck, G. G., P. Fougeyrollas, and K. A. Gerhart. 1997. "Elaborating the Model of Disablement." Pp. 91-102 in *Assessing Medical Rehabilitation Practices: The Promise of Outcomes Research*, edited by Marcus J. Fuhrer. Baltimore: Brookes.

World Health Organization (WHO). 1980. *International Classification of Impairments, Disabilities and Handicaps: A Manual of Classification Relating to the Consequences of Disease*. Geneva: Author.

————. 1989. *Recherches prioritaires liées à la santé pour tous*, no. 3, Série Européenne de la santé pour tous, Copenhagen: Author.

————. 1993. *International Classification of Impairments, Disabilities and Handicaps: A Manual of Classification Relating to the Consequences of Disease*. Rev. version. Geneva: Author.

————. 1999. *ICIDH-2 International Classification of Functioning and Disabilities*. Beta-2 draft, short version. Geneva: Author.

Zola, I. K. 1989. "Toward the Necessary Universalizing of a Disability Policy." *The Milbank Quarterly* 67:401-28.

Representation and Its Discontents

7

The Uneasy Home of Disability in Literature and Film

DAVID T. MITCHELL
SHARON L. SNYDER

INTRODUCTION: THE UNEASY HOME OF REPRESENTATION

Because a brief exchange can often capture the core of a conflict, let us begin this chapter with an anecdote. Following a Society for Disability Studies meeting address by Henri-Jacques Stiker on the history of disability in European painting, noted disability scholar Paul Longmore ended the evening by asking, "Does disability *ever* represent anything other than a negative image?"[1] Stiker had presented a lengthy history of teratological images during his talk—disabled people projected from slides and transparencies as the embodiments of every period's cripples, lunatics, mendicants, drunkards, misfits, fools, court dwarves, maimed veterans, and cheating card players. A painted catalogue of grotesques.[2]

Members of the audience openly wondered how worldly ruin could be symbolized without resorting to the spectacle of disabled bodies. And, conversely, could disability represent anything other than ruined bodies? Stiker argued that his interpretations demonstrated three important points: the transhistorical nature of artistic interest in disability, the ability of art to serve as an archive for recapturing historical attitudes that would otherwise be lost, and the capacity of artists for creating disability images that continued to resonate (negatively or otherwise) with viewers across history and cultures. None of these responses directly addressed the issue of negative symbolism. Instead, Stiker implied that recognizing the nuances in characterizations of disability from one period to another could sufficiently complicate our historical understanding of its cultural properties. As the evening's participants walked away, we overheard musings on Stiker's responses as only partially satisfactory. The event threatened to go down in the collective history of the Society for Disability Studies as more evidence of the problem with disability studies in the humanities.

As that year's program coordinators, we wondered how humanities scholars could better respond to this most basic query. Similar questions had come up following presentations on disability in literary narratives. Where could one locate more affirming depictions of people with disabilities? Weren't literary and artistic archives perverse in their representational distortions of the disabled body? Didn't one become disheartened over time with the unbearable symbolic weight of literary characterizations? This is, not to mention, the central issue of how study in the humanities could contribute to the pragmatic needs of disabled communities and the contemporary political rights movement!

Beginning nearly 30 years ago, a resurgence of concern over the consequences of dehumanizing representations (i.e., monster, freak, madman, suffering innocent, hysteric, beggar) of the disabled has resulted in suspicion over the ultimate utility of representational studies about disability. Truly, literary and historical texts have rarely appeared to offer disabled characters in developed, "positive" portraits.[3] But the belief that literary study has little to offer our more politicized understandings of disability experience rests uncomfortably with us.

Previously, proponents of the universality in art had sought to salvage the significance of disabled literary characterizations by viewing them as evidence for inherent frailties in what used to be called "the human condition." For example, Herbert Blau (1981) defends literary portraits of disability by explaining that they cause us to "concede that we are all, at some warped level of the essentially human, impaired" (p. 10). A catalogue of disabled representations in literature includes some of the most influential figurations of "suffering humanity" across periods and cultures: the crippled Greek god, Hephaistos; Montaigne's sexually potent limping women; Shakespeare's hunchbacked king, Richard III; Frankenstein's deformed monster; Brontë's madwoman in the attic; Melville's one-legged, monomaniacal Captain Ahab; Nietzsche's philosophical grotesques; Hemingway's wounded war veterans; Morrison's truncated and scarred ex-slaves; Borges's blind librarians; and Oe's brain-damaged son. Astonishingly, this catalogue of "warped" humanity proves as international as it does biologically varied. Why does disability characterization so often result in indelible, albeit overwrought, literary portraits? With this in mind, the exchange between Stiker and Longmore takes on the contours of a disciplinary crisis that needs to be theorized directly.

We suggest that the "problem" of disability representation is the result of two predominating modes of historical address: overheated symbolic imagery and disability as a pervasive tool of artistic characterization. Yet while scholars in literary and cultural studies have produced important readings of individual disabled characters and the centrality of disabled types to specific genres, we have largely neglected to theorize the utility of humanities work for disability studies in particular and disabled populations in general. This chapter seeks to survey developments in the study of disability across the humanities in an effort to provide a governing logic for the necessity of the humanities to the evolution of disability studies in general.

We also seek to explain the myriad ways that scholars have complicated the question of "negativity" without surrendering usable politics. Recent studies of disability in the archives provide a manifestly multifaceted base on which to build our own period's address of disability representations. Consistent throughout will be our own efforts to assess both the pervasive and the hypersymbolic nature of disability. Somewhere between these difficulties, humanities scholars make their uneasy home in disability studies.

NEGATIVE IMAGERY

From the outset, most critical approaches to disability representation sought to theorize negative imagery as the impetus of their scholarship.[4] Like many areas of humanities' investigation into questions of the social construction of identity, disability scholars first interrogated common stereotypes that pervaded the literary and filmic archives. Disability was viewed as a restrictive pattern of characterization that usually sacrificed the humanity of protagonists and villains alike. A few key characters continually surfaced as evidence of this tendency: Shakespeare's murderous hunchbacked king, Richard III; Melville's obsessive one-legged Captain Ahab; and Dickens's sentimental hobbling urchin, Tiny Tim. The repeated citation of these three figures as central to disability characterization initially demonstrated, at the most basic level, that disability existed in canonical literary works. Unlike the marginal presence of racial and homosexual characters, for example, literary scholars promoted the idea that disability played a visible role in several of the most important works in European and American literature.[5] Although the recourse to these three examples gave the impression that this presence proved hardly overwhelming, interpretations of negative images nonetheless secured the argument that disability had been neglected in the critical tradition. The early scholarship also demonstrated a complicity of the literary in the historical devaluation of people with disabilities.

For instance, one of the first disability studies collections to devote space to questions of literary and media images—Gartner and Joe's (1987) *Images of the Disabled, Disabling Images*—emphasized the pernicious nature of stereotypes. Disability writers and scholars, such as Leonard Kriegel, Deborah Kent, and Paul Longmore, exposed representation as a devious device of mainstream and artistic mediums. Kriegel's (1987) essay, "Disability as Metaphor in Literature," took on the entire literary tradition by boldly declaring that depictions of disability fell far short of realistic portrayals of human complexity. In his analysis of the coronation scene in Shakespeare's *Richard III*, he located what he believed to be the two most pervasive and insidious images in the literary tradition:

> In the ascent, the red-caped figure crawls up the steps [to the throne], like some gigantic insect, to take that which he has cheated others of. Imposing its limitations to rob legitimacy, the broken body begs for compassion. In the history of Western literature, both before and after Shakespeare, there is little to be added to these two images, although there are a significant number of variations upon them. The cripple is threat and recipient of compassion, both to be damned and to be pitied—and frequently to be damned as he is pitied. (Kriegel 1987:32)

Importantly, Kriegel's sense of outrage parallels many disability critics who see the metaphoric opportunism of literature as a form of public slander. In establishing the two poles of disability characterization—threat and pity—Kriegel (1987) provided a shorthand method for disability scholars to gain control of a limiting literary archive. Richard III represented an early example of stigmatizing cultural dictates to which even Shakespeare capitulated. The writer's world, according to Kriegel, evidenced the "vantage point of the normals" (p. 32), and in doing so, characters with disabilities would evidence a scapegoating attitude rife in culture and history writ large. Even if, as Shari Thurber (1980) pointed out, "the disabled have a bad literary press" (p. 12), the literary archive would at least serve as a reliable repository for documenting demeaning attitudes toward people with disabilities.

Kriegel's (1987) commentary proved emblematic of what we refer to as the negative image school of disability criticism that sought to diagnose literature as another social repository of stereotypical depictions. Unlike other minority studies of literary representation (such as race and sexuality) that found a desired counter to demeaning cultural attitudes in their own literary traditions, literary scholars of disability found little refuge in creative discourses. The negative image school found literary depictions to be, at best, wanting and, at worst, humiliating: "While metaphoric use of disability may seem innocuous enough, it is in fact a most blatant and pernicious form of stereotyping" (Thurber 1980:12). The core of this argument centered on disabled characters as one and the same with disabled people. There was a direct correlation, argued these scholars, between debasing character portraits and demeaning cultural attitudes toward people with disabilities.

In this way, the argument of the negative imagery school set out to establish a continuum between limiting literary depictions and dehumanizing social attitudes toward disabled people. In his seminal essay, "Screening Stereotypes: Images of Disabled People in Television and Motion Pictures," Paul Longmore (1997a) helped to diagnose film and television as influential reinforcers of cultural prejudice toward disabled people. Rather than Kriegel's (1987) two-pronged analysis of disability types in literature, Longmore found three common stereotypes perpetuated by electronic media representations: "Disability is a punishment for evil; disabled people are embittered by their 'fate'; disabled people resent the nondisabled and would, if they could, destroy them" (Gartner and Joe 1987:67). Longmore's analysis of popular mediums created a neat parallel with Kriegel's arguments in that they both saw contemporary attitudes about people with disabilities informed by these repeated paradigms and plots.

The restrictive elements of stories about disability created a portrait of an uncompromising public belief in the limited options for people with disabilities. "Disabled characters abound, but the ways in which they are portrayed and the development of narrative around them is relentlessly negative" (Pointon and Davies 1997:1). From the outside, the meager nature of the lives of disabled characters was depicted as inevitably leading toward bitterness and anger that made them objects of suspicion. In fact, Kriegel and Longmore argued in tandem that disability portrayals could be understood best as a form of cathartic revenge in which the stigmatizers punish the stigmatized to alleviate their own worries and fears about bodily vulnerability and inhumane social conditions.

What stands out in the analyses of the negative image school is the importance of plots that emphasize individual isolation as the overriding component of a disabled life. The angst surrounding the status of people with disabilities surfaced in expressive discourses as a desire to seclude the offending party within a drama of his or her own making. Longmore (1997a) first identified this element as the most pervasive and debilitating aspect of disability representation. By depicting disability as an isolated and individual affair, storytellers artificially extracted the experience of disability from its necessary social contexts. The portraiture of disability in literature and electronic media became a matter of "psychologizing" the cultural understanding of disability. Disabled characters were either extolled or defeated as a result of their ability to personally adjust to or overcome their tragic situation. Longmore pointed out that "[social] prejudice and discrimination rarely enter into either fictional or nonfictional stories, and then only as a secondary issue" (Gartner and Joe 1987:74). Because representations of disability tend to reflect the medicalized view, which restricts disability to a static impairment entombed within an individual, the social navigation of debilitating attitudes fails to attain the status of a worthy element of plot or literary contemplation.

The failure of a politicized interest in the disability plot could be evidenced in any number of ways within a variety of genres. For instance, Hafferty and Foster (1994) argue that the defining feature of disabled experience comes as a result of "an awareness that issues when disabilities and handicaps are created through interactions between people with physical impairments and an unyielding and antagonistic environment" (p. 189). Yet, in their analysis of disabled detectives in crime novels, Hafferty and Foster discover that the reading public is encouraged to "view matters that are rightly located within social settings as residing in individual achievements and/or failures" (p. 189). The collusion of literary techniques, such as passive dialogue and readerly identifications with individual protagonists in the detective genre, serves as stylistic conventions that help "shape the messages being delivered" (p. 193). This almost exclusive focus on negative representations functioned as a means of humanities-based "proof" that discrimination against disabled people not only existed but also was fostered by the images consumed by readers and viewers alike.

While the analysis of the negative image was carefully supported by a largely structuralist model that slotted disability types into generic classifications and representational modes, the unearthing of discriminatory images tended to collapse all representations into a sterile model of false consciousness. In *The Cinema of Isolation*, Martin Norden (1994) extended and exaggerated Longmore's argument of isolating disability media portraits by drawing up all of film history into a net of conspiracy. The Hollywood filmmaker, according to Norden, participates in an exploitative scheme that seeks to capitalize on the visual spectacle that disabilities offer to the camera eye. Film has taken the place of the nineteenth-century freak show "in the name of maintaining patriarchal order" (p. 6). Despite the historical prevalence of disabled people in film, Norden condemned nearly every image as the product of filmic castration anxiety and discriminatory beliefs. As the editors of *Framed: Interrogating Disability in the Media,* point out, "It is too simplistic to talk about 'negative' compared with 'positive' images because although disabled people are in general fairly clear about what might constitute the former, the identification of 'positive' is fraught with difficulty" (Pointon and Davies 1997:1). The scholarship on the negative image strained beneath the weight of such wholesale condemnations of representational portraits.

Yet despite research that saw most artistic and popular representations of disability as debilitating to reigning cultural attitudes, the analysis of negative images helped to support the idea that disability was socially produced. Identifying common characterizations that reinforced audiences' sense of alienation and distance from disability began an important process of scholarly attempts to rehabilitate public beliefs. Literature and film provided a needed archive of historical attitudes from which to assess ideologies pertaining to people with disabilities. While social scientists sought to understand contemporary beliefs about disabled populations, humanities scholars began to sift through expansive representational preserves. These materials solidified arguments in disability studies about disabled people's position as historical scapegoats. In many ways, this impulse still undergirds humanities-based politics of critiquing the trite and superficial portraits churned out on a daily basis by the mainstream media. To change negative portrayals, a powerful commentary was needed to make authors more self-conscious of the conventions at work in their own media.

In addition, humanities scholars of the negative image looked for the opportunity to identify against the grain of disability's presumed malignancy or excessive fragility. For example, Leonard Kriegel (1987) found himself declaring identification with Richard III's personal antipathy toward the incomprehension of an able-bodied world, even as he condemned Shakespeare's too-easy bid for dramatic pathos. If Kriegel's affectation proved somewhat perverse, he nonetheless anticipated later efforts to embrace the definitive humanity (or alienness) of disabled characters as a move of transgressive identification. In this manner, disability studies scholars in the humanities began to seek out the lines of convergence and divergence from their own experiences in literature and film.

SOCIAL REALIST DISABILITY

One important insight that consistently surfaced in the scholarship on negative imagery was the charge that most disability portraits proved inaccurate and misleading. A new social realism[6] was needed to counter misguided attitudes about people with disabilities. As Deborah Kent (1987) argued in "Disabled Women: Portraits in Fiction and Drama," one could posit a direct correlation between the lives of fictional disabled females and social attitudes toward women with disabilities in general. "An assessment of the disabled woman's place in literature may serve as a barometer to measure how she is perceived by society. Conversely, the literary image of the disabled woman may influence the way disabled women are seen and judged in real life" (Kent 1987:48). The equation between fictional images and lived experiences of a disabled person was viewed by the social realist perspective as a way of elevating the analysis of literature to a pragmatic necessity.

Like many materialist literary movements before—Georges Lukacs for Marxism, Virginia Woolf for feminism, and W. E. B. DuBois for African American studies—disability critics rushed to explain the inadequacy of historical images by posing that which was left out of the picture or distorted for the sake of a dramatic portrayal. Social realism called for the solution of more realistic representations. The social realists' primary criteria centered on whether literary depictions served as correctives to social misapprehensions about the specifics of disability experiences. We can sum up this line of approach in the humorous point made by Irving Zola (1987) in his survey of popular detective fiction. Out of hundreds of novels that forward disabled detective "heroes," never once did Zola find a wheelchair user commenting, "God dammit, how I hate stairs" (p. 505). Realism promoted a more direct depiction of the political reality of disabled characters, from architecture to attitudes. Realistic depictions, argued social realism, will offer familiarity with an experience that has been understood as thoroughly alien.

Social realist scholarship sought to decrease the kinds of alienation that pervade social views of disabled people. If the negative image resulted from associations of disability with personal failure, tragic loss, and excessive dependency, then social realists searched for more accurate images that could effectively counterbalance this detrimental history. For example, one positive exception to the cinema of isolation was found in *Waterdance*, a 1980s film drama that documents the medical, romantic, and social life of a recently paralyzed man. The realism of *Waterdance* could be located, for some, in its depiction of the punishing technology of modern medicine or by the camaraderie that develops between disabled men on a hospital ward. The call for social realism also helped to boost critical interest in autobiography as a counter-representational reality to artistic metaphors and opportunistic spectacle. G. Thomas Couser's (1997) *Recovering Bodies* analyzes the restorative properties of recent disability memoirs not only to the writers but also to the literary tradition itself. In each of these examples, humanities scholars sought reparation in the idea that a more adequate representation could be found in films, autobiographies, or fictions that attended directly to the embodied experience of disabled characters. In attempts to offset a negative portrait of the disabled, realist images would offer up a more substantive, fleshy substitute.

Following Zola's (1987) lead, several disability commentators tried to stress the issue of inaccurate portraiture by striking at the literal level of representation itself—disabled characters, they argued, failed to measure up to the "reality" of disabled lives. In his discussion of the award-winning film *Passion Fish*, the paraplegic writer, Andre Dubus (1996), amusingly explained the limitations of Hollywood film productions about disability:

> I remember one scene in Louisiana, they're [the paraplegic protagonist and her aide] on a wharf and there's this little skiff, and she tells the nurse, "Get me in the boat." Now these are things I live with all the time. Next scene, she's in the boat, and I said, How the fuck did she lower this woman from the chair into the boat in the water? Show me that and you've got some story. (P. 5)

Others, such as Hafferty and Foster's (1994) discussion of deaf detectives in crime novels, argued that despite the characteristic feature of "deafness," the protagonist rarely experienced the dilemmas of life as a hearing-impaired person negotiating a hearing world. Deaf or hearing-impaired detectives were rarely depicted as having to supply themselves with "a steady stream of sign language interpreters to facilitate [their] daily communication with others," nor were they subject to the routine or disastrous misinterpretations of daily life. Their summation of this lack of fictional realism evidences that "[fictional detectives] may be deaf, but [their] lack of hearing seems to have no impact on, or even relationship to, [their] work as . . . detectives" (Hafferty and Foster 1994:195).

In identifying examples of inaccurate characterizations, social realism did not resort to a superficial call for "positive images" that would celebrate the lives of people with disabilities in a romanticized light. Rather, scholars approached even the production of self-styled "positive" portraits with skepticism and saved some of their most severe critiques for notions of disabled "heroism." In his essay on David Lynch's *The Elephant Man*, Paul Darke (1994) ended with the following admonition to readers: "[Lynch's film] is not the liberal, tolerant, and pro-difference film it, and its supporters, suppose it to be . . . often the positive image of disability is really very negative, so, beware of bearers of positive images!" (p. 341). For Darke, not only did the film of Merrick's life distort the facts of his experience within an incarcerating medicalized view of monstrous oddity, but the production also objectified his image in a freak show–like spectacle of difference for the titillation of its viewers.

Within the social realist perspective, the problem of inadequate representation was attributed to two predominating issues: either the complete paucity of "positive" examples in narrative traditions or to the undertheorized nature of what constitutes a negative image. In other words, the call for more realistic depictions of disability provided another side of the negative imagery coin because to critique inadequate, dehumanizing, or false representations is to simultaneously call for more acceptable representations. Yet the distinction between negative and positive proved a difficult one to define. As Darke (1994) points out, that which parades itself as "fixing" the historical record often ends up in the pathos of an individual life or in the falsely superhuman portrait of the overcompensating crip.

Most important, the social realist perspective developed arguments that demonstrated the narrative penchant for extracting the social conditions of disability from the act of characterization itself. British scholars, such as Tom Shakespeare (1994), argued this point most succinctly by noting that fictional portraits often ignore "the way in which disability is a relationship between people with impairment and a disabling society" (p. 287). Unlike other identity movements that called for a politics based on a more individualized representational approach to their lives, social realism argued that depictions of disability had suffered from a history of excessive individuation. Isolation and excessive idiosyncrasy were the bane of disabled people's representational lives, and social realism would push for the necessity of a relational or social model.

As David Hevey (1992) argues in *The Creatures That Time Forgot,* "The reformation of oppressive imagery is only important (or, at least, more than superficially) if it is linked to wider social issues, such as access" (p. 102). "Positive images" would not be determined by their ability to portray disabled people in a good light. Instead, Hevey argued that acceptable portrayals primarily entailed the refusal to deny, disavow, or suppress the site of struggle and oppression that characterizes a contemporary understanding of disability. Hevey and other social realist perspectives insisted on politicizing disability by portraying it as the result of the interaction between impairment and physical and attitudinal environments. Limitation needed to be represented in a visceral way, but it should not be relegated to the level of an individual predicament or a purely embodied phenomenon.

The call for action in social realism ultimately centered on a belief that disability would continue to be misconstrued and relegated to the "dustbins" of history if the able-bodied were left to construct disability images from their own prejudices (Shakespeare 1994:283). The issue came down to a matter of controlling the means of production. If disabled people took responsibility for the production of their own images, then, the social realists reasoned, the image would effectively "evolve" into more acceptable forms. On one hand, a literal representation of disability would capture the myriad negotiations of a fraught social environment; obstacles would prove themselves of societal making rather than individual limitation. Also, technology, previously hidden in the corners of homes and institutions, would take center stage in the drama of disability as a lived experience. In this vein, the recent remake of Alfred Hitchcock's 1955 film *Rear Window,* with Christopher Reeve, would be revolutionary in its tracking shots of respirator tubing and high-tech sets sporting gurneys and elevators.

On the other hand, the social realist perspective would supply an openly politicized image of disability. As Hevey (1992) puts it, the issue of positive representation would be "tied to the general movement for rights . . . whereby image-politics become[s] a part of the struggle for access, not an excuse for it" (p. 103). The acceptable image legislated by the social realists would be based first and foremost on a representational advocacy in which images function as a weapon of political action and as one site of redress to social incomprehension.

NEW HISTORICISM

The significance of the social realist model has continued to dominate recent theories of disability in the humanities. The political objectives that informed this perspective helped to fuel some of the innovations of recent work in the development of a nuanced historical revisionism. Yet, while the influence of social realism continues, recent work has fueled its own investigations by diverging from some of the foundational assumptions of the social realists. Critiques or revisions of social realism have been based on four key principles relating to issues of aesthetics and historical retrieval.

1. Social realism assumed that disability tended to be concealed rather than pervasive in the literary and filmic traditions.
2. The practitioners of social realism created a largely ahistorical paradigm that overlooked the specificity of disability representation as an ideological effect of particular periods.
3. Social realism presumed that no disability perspective had ever informed the "inaccurate" images that pervaded the social realist's critique.
4. Social realism projected its own contemporary desires onto the images that it sought to rehabilitate.

Both the scholarship on negative images and the paradigms promoted by social realism adopted a relatively static structuralist bent to their shared methodology. Interpreters quickly channeled all images into a few representational possibilities, and the results became rather monolithic. There was the passively suffering angel of the house, the overcompensating supercrip, the tragically innocent disabled child, the malignant disabled avenger, and the angry war veteran. Yet, while these shorthand categorizations would show up in a variety of popular texts and genre formulas, they nonetheless preempted a more engaged historical scholarship. The generic classification of disabled types produces an ahistorical interpretation that tends to see disability representations as slanderously consistent across cultures and periods.

How could disability scholars complicate the issue of negative representation by placing disability within a more specific historical context? Could disability scholars develop a theory capable of explaining the seemingly paradoxical idea that dehumanizing portraits of disabled characters could also buttress a previous generation's critique of debilitating institutions such as medicine? Would disability studies in the humanities rest its contribution on the depreciation of its own archival material in the name of stereotypical creations and suspect politics?

To begin with, a new historicism of disability representations in the humanities sought to perform an anthropological unearthing of images that could help to reconstruct a period's point of view on human variation. Stories provided more than cultural escapism. They situated themselves as explanatory paradigms for revealing the supernatural and social origins of disability's appearance in the world. An early example came in Susan Schoon Eberly's (1988) discussion of the figure of the changeling in European folklore. Like the shifting and faerie-like changeling himself (these figures are usually male), Eberly argued that cultural uncertainly about the origins of physical disabilities such as dwarfism, cretinism, cerebral palsy, Down syndrome, and so on often engendered tales of fantastical children. "Specific examples of changelings, solitary fairies—both domesticated and reclusive—and the offspring of fairy-human matings . . . seem to offer identifiable portraits of children who were born, or who became, different as a result of identifiable congenital disorders" (Eberly 1988:58). The "special nature" of changelings, who often did not walk, talk, or run unless they were not being watched, suggests a literary effort to explain a mysterious physical phenomenon. The changeling tales sat on the cusp of a historical shift between medieval superstition and medical diagnoses of congenital disabilities.

In a parallel vein to Eberly's (1988) arguments about disability as an explanatory mystery of literary interest, Davidson, Woodill, and Bredberg (1994) argued that the rampant representations of disability in nineteenth-century children's literature served a similar function. Borrowing from a primarily religious discourse of social instruction for the middle classes, Victorian tracts on disability forwarded physical variation as a divine mystery that could not be comprehended by empirical discourses. "Disability cannot be understood in human terms. Like all forms of human suffering, it needs to be placed within God's mysterious scheme of things" (Davidson et al. 1994:43). As instructional tales, Victorian children's literature reveals a penchant for discussing disability in terms of individual responsibility and the need for charity toward the infirm. Nineteenth-century authors sought to mitigate social readings of malignancy by enfolding disabled children within a paternalistic cultural logic of financial and moral benevolence.

Unlike social realist methodology, historical revisionists focused most of their attention on the function of disability in "high art." The importance of efforts to historicize disability representations demonstrated that artistic narratives played a key role in forwarding a logic or system of explanation for birth anomalies and environmental accidents. Even after the professionalization of modern medicine, literature continued to serve an important explanatory function in the cultural understanding of disability. The changeling figure offered up by Eberly (1988) and Davidson et al. (1994) proffered disability as a product of mainstream beliefs, and literature participated in the process of trying to pierce its mystery by offering up tales of other-worldly creatures or social "unfortunates." The historical analysis of disability helped identify the shifting investments of cultures when confronted with the variability of human biology and psychology.

Within the studies developed by the new historicists, disability was recognized as a product of specific cultural ideologies that did not simply reveal reductive or stigmatizing attitudes. As Diane Price Herndl (1993) theorizes in her work on the female invalid in Victorian literature, the disabled subject should neither be interpreted as an "entirely passive construct nor as an entirely active agent" (p. 12). Instead, the writer and disability as the representational object of the writer's discourse situate themselves more dynamically with respect to the culture within which they are produced. "Neither the woman experiencing an illness nor the author writing a story about a woman's illness is free of the ways that illness has been represented before, but neither one is entirely constrained either" (Herndl 1993:12). Herndl's turn helped to complicate the terrain of previous approaches by arguing that disability portraits provided a window into a more dynamic interchange between culture, author, text, and audience. Disability was a product of an interchange between all of these positions that create and re-create the disabled body as a potent product of literary investment.

Thus, while the prototypical image of the leisurely Victorian woman may fit comfortably with the image of suffering femininity because each is stripped of her agency within a patriarchal and ablist order, nineteenth-century women writers also sought to challenge that image. Consequently, while Charlotte Perkins Gilman's portrait of a woman's descent into madness in *The Yellow Wallpaper* could be interpreted as an unflattering portrait of cognitive disability, the storyteller's strategy seeks to upend the controlling medical model of femininity's excessive frailty and emotional instability. Or, while the infamous hunchbacked doctor, Chillingworth, in *The Scarlet Letter* grows increasingly decrepit as his immoral motivations deepen, Hawthorne's characterization strategy evolved out of nineteenth-century literary efforts to condemn medical practitioners to the deterministic dictates of their own pathologizing discourse on the body. Both of these stories evidence a "negative" outcome with respect to the disabled character, but their object of critique parallels the political objectives of the contemporary disability movement.

The resistance to dismissing disability images as merely detrimental proved evident in an array of essays included in our anthology, *The Body and Physical Difference* (Mitchell and Snyder 1997a). Historical revisionist efforts produced interpretations that situated disability as both a perpetual societal obsession in the West and as the object of complex cultural beliefs. Many of these efforts unearthed examples of cultures that integrated, rather than scapegoated, people with disabilities in surprising ways. Martha Edwards (1997) argues that rather than holding a static, denigrating belief about disability as had been previously argued, ancient Greek texts evidence that disabled people were often integrated into the fold of ancient communal life. Felicity Nussbaum (1997) locates a utopian political alliance between marginalized disabled and feminist communities depicted in Sarah Scott's eighteenth-century novel, *Millenium Hall.* Maria Frawley (1997) analyzes Harriet Martineau's Victorian autobiographical explorations of invalid subjectivity that revised the traditionally passive medical patient into an active negotiator of her own corporeal experience. Cindy LaCom (1997) argues that nineteenth-century women writers countered the monstrous sexuality of female disability in male novels with more empowering images of disabled women who escaped the patriarchal discourse of feminine objectification. In her discussion of twentieth-century German literary representations of disability, Elizabeth Hamilton (1997) documents a movement from the grotesque to the political in the works of disability autobiographers. Rosemarie Garland Thomson (1997) argues that disability in the works of African American women writers serves to destabilize the dominant binary codes of abnormal/normal, male/female, and desired/undesired by openly exploring marginal identities in political, rather than stigmatizing, terms. Finally, Caroline Molina's (1997) reading of the film *The Piano* argues that the female protagonist's "disabling" muteness is resignified by the end of the story into a sign of female refusal to participate in masculinist discourses.

What connected these alternative interpretations of disability was a twofold interest in using an expansive literary archive to solidify the variability of human physiology and reactions to biological mutability. Disability had begun to be recognized as a potent vehicle of political critique at various moments in the literary tradition. By and large, these alternative representational modes had been ignored or overlooked by literary and disability critics alike because of insufficient paradigms for analyzing disability as a site of literary investment. What changed in these analyses was not the disabled object of representation itself but rather the goals of the methodology brought to bear on those objects. This archival resurrection of disability helped to demonstrate that disability, like all representational objects, could be mobilized in a variety of directions. In demonstrating the existence of alternative disability discourses within literature and film, disability scholars provided evidence that challenged the assumption that our moment occupied the only "forward-looking" cultural perspective on disability in history.

Other disability scholars in *The Body and Physical Difference* anthology interpreted historical reactions to disability as the site of conflicting ideological agendas. Scholars applying this approach deflected attention away from disability representation and toward a critique of social institutions that authored disability as "Other." Lennard Davis (1997) assesses the paradox of the art historian's ability to interpret the armless body of the Venus de Milo as a vision of aesthetic perfection, while cultures continued to devalue human "armless" figures as less than ideal. Following the American Civil War, David Yuan (1997) finds that the rise of a modern prosthetics industry sought to "rehabilitate" not only wounded war veterans but also the national wound that disrupted North-South relations. Jan Gordon (1997) interprets the potent symbolism of male disability in D. H. Lawrence's *Lady Chatterley's Lover* and other modernist works as an effort to symbolize the decline of privilege and power in the British aristocracy. Martin Pernick (1997) demonstrates that eugenics, as exemplified in propaganda films that rationalize the medical murder of disabled infants, ultimately premise the determination of expendability on an aesthetic criterion. David Gerber (1997) compares competing ideological interests between the political right and left in the patriotic "repair" of war hero Al Schmid's blindness in *The Pride of the Marines* and in his relation to the Blind Veterans Association. Paul Longmore (1997b) reads the telethon industry's sentimental display of childhood disability as a product of nineteenth-century American discourses on paternalistic philanthropy. In a critical look at contemporary U.S. disability autobiography, Madonne Miner (1997) contrasts the stories of disabled men and women to assess their purchase on traditional narrative schemas of male emasculation and female victimization.

At work in these approaches has been a developing conception of what Lennard Davis (1995) set out to define in *Enforcing Normalcy* as the "construction of the normal world" (p. 22). Within this schema, Davis and the essayists mentioned above invert the historical imperative to designate, define, and diagnose disabilities by turning the "normal" into the producer of pathology. Rather than authorize cultural institutions as the arbiters of deviance, the study of normalcy would expose disability as "not a discrete object but a set of social relations" (p. 11). The production of disability as human oddity or exceptional limitation in science, as in art, would be founded on the norm's ability to disguise itself as transparently average. In this way, the corporeal norm poses as universally desirable—the barometer against which all biologies are assessed and compared. Normalcy studies seek to debunk the norm as an ideological abstraction that is based on a faulty empiricism.

Medical anthropologist George Canguilhem (1991) had argued that medicine's decision to use a bodily ideal to assess an inherently dynamic and adaptive biology effectively surrendered any claim to scientific objectivity in the nineteenth century. Much recent literary criticism rests on the following inversion: Rather than simply serve as deviations from widely expressed biological traits, disabilities exemplify that the ideal of the norm cannot exist without its "deviant" contrast. By using literary and filmic archives to demonstrate that norms shift throughout history and across cultures and thus are definitively unstable, normalcy scholars effectively theorize concepts of the norm as not only flawed and artificial but also feeding a eugenicist mind-set in society. In doing so, the humanities continue to wage a pivotal battle against the objectification of disability in medical science and its popular offshoots.

All of these studies speak to the primacy of disability in representational discourses. Yet, while disability has proven one of the most commonly applied features of narrative characterization, readers and viewers have consistently received disabled characters as isolated cases. Building on the narrative theories of Susan Stewart, we have argued that "disability studies seeks to understand the ways in which we produce the 'private room' of disability in our most public discourses" (Mitchell and Snyder 1997a:17). The historical revisionist turn in the humanistic study of disability sought to dismantle this "private room" by consolidating a body of scholarship that demonstrates what the French disability historian, Henri-Jacques Stiker, argues was the necessity of recognizing disability as not only *integrable* but also *integral* to human communities and biologies across time (Stiker 1999). In other words, the historical revisionists argued that physical and cognitive difference was the rule rather than the exception of historical experience.

BIOGRAPHICAL CRITICISM

One result of this historical revisionism has been to seek out authors and artists in history who are disabled—or who experienced serious involvement with disabled people. With disability saturating narrative discourses in the literary and filmic archives, one may also presume that some of the works were produced by disabled people or by writers with disability-identified perspectives. Within the approach of biographical criticism to the disability contexts of authorship, three tendencies have predominated:

1. the analysis of critical readings on disability by able-bodied and disabled scholars alike,
2. the analysis of the relationship between literature and medicine, and
3. the interpretations by disabled writers of other disability characterizations in history.

Biographical archival work on notoriously "deformed" storytellers, such as Aesop and Socrates, and disabled and chronically ill authors such as John Milton, Alexander Pope, George Byron, Samuel Johnson, John Keats, Stephen Crane, Katherine Mansfield, Virginia Woolf, and Marcel Proust (to name a few) have sought to discern a "disability logic" in their individual artistic works and personas. This undertaking has resulted in serious corrections and complications of the literary historical record while also challenging the idea that disability images have been exclusively the product of able-bodied authors. Since disability offers its own routing of an author's experience in the world, biographical scholarship on disabled authorship properly assumes that revisiting texts from this disability studies orientation will yield important insights into the influence of disability identities on creative efforts. Whereas "successful disabled people . . . have their disability erased by their success" (Davis 1995:9), this scholarly work seeks out the inevitable impact of disability on the creator's worldview.

In our essay, "Infinities of Forms" (Mitchell and Snyder forthcoming), we claimed scholarly works for disability studies such as Eleanor Gertrude Brown's *Milton's Blindness*. Originally published in 1934 and recently reissued by Columbia University Press as a landmark in Milton studies, Brown grounds her interpretation of Milton's poetry on her own experience as a blind person. Taking on an openly essentialist claim to her understanding of Milton's verse, Brown acknowledges the power that disabled experience can lend to disability interpretation:

To the interpretation of Milton's life and writing after the loss of sight, I add my knowledge of blindness. And on account of this bond of union, I bring to the task an interest
such as Milton must have given to the writing of *Samson Agonistes*. Thus, by similarity of
experience alone, I am rendered a more able critic. (Brown 1934: preface)

From a disability vantage, with a decidedly "contemporary" inversion of "able" rhetoric,
Brown (1934) asks disability questions of Milton's poetics—a method that results in fresh and
compelling interpretations.

The importance of the critic's commitment to locating the contexts of disability experience
in history cannot be understated. For instance, Alexander Pope's influential standard
biographer, Maynard Mack, placed Pope's scoliosis in a separate sphere from that of his
poetics—a move that results in fairly abstract pronouncements about Pope's oft-quoted line,
"This long disease my life." However, disability scholar Helen Deutsch (1996) overlaps
Pope's "deformed" body and his classical poetics to insightful results. In *Resemblance & Disgrace: Alexander Pope and the Deformation of Culture,* Deutsch contends that "deformity enables Pope's particular brand of imitation to go originality one better: his poetry marks itself not
as original but as impossible to duplicate" (p. 27). In her recent work, "The Exemplary Case of
Dr. Johnson," Deutsch (forthcoming) also explores the implications of disabled authorship for
eighteenth-century poetics. Her research

considers the history of the authorial body in eighteenth-century Britain, beginning with
the visible deformity of Alexander Pope's curved spine and closing with the indecipher-
able inwardness figured by Samuel Johnson's unruly body. . . . Disability has in fact distinguished the English literary canon—itself a product of the eighteenth century—as a
catalog of authorial monsters and paradoxically representative oddities. (Deutsch forthcoming)

The discovery and "outing" of disabled authors in literary history have followed archival
work undertaken by practitioners in the field of literature and medicine. As borne out by its
name, the field of literature and medicine partakes of an affinity with the disposition of medical
practice. Hence, scholars have undertaken research to label authors in history with contemporary medical diagnoses and assess their attitudes toward their doctors (never very good)! One
finds, in this branch of literary study, a focus primarily on literary depictions of doctors and
their treatment of diseased patients. This allows literary and medical critics, for example, to focus on a birth scene in Toni Morrison's *The Bluest Eye* to critique Polly's insulting treatment
from white doctors while overlooking her "crippled gait" as a key component of her character
and her relationship to her husband.

Pivotal in the literature and medical arena, Philip Sandblom's (1982) *Creativity and Disease*
usefully discerns examples whereby artists and writers throughout history have found creative
potential in the experience of a physical or cognitive impairment. Sandblom's research serves as
a useful casebook of disabled writers; he even claims an identification with disabled people by
recalling his own victimization at the hands of medical error. At the same time, like many medical professionals, his assessments rest on psychologizing the attitudes of disabled artists with all
the distance, prejudice, and misconstruence engendered by an objective posturing. Indeed, he
also seeks to rehabilitate the good intentions of literary history's doctors against the insults of
their writer-patients. Among many examples of ill-founded literary diagnosis, Sandblom
quotes Sir Francis Bacon's equation between deformity and vengeful personality as a means for
understanding the psyches of Lord Byron and Daniel Defoe. "These unfortunates [people with
congenital malformations], then, sometimes react with quiet resignation but more often with
revolt and extreme efforts to compensate, now and then with artistic creation" (Sandblom
1982:107). In Sir Francis Bacon's words, "Whosoever hath anything fixed in his person that
doth induce contempt, hath also a perpetual spur in himself to rescue and deliver himself from
scorn, therefore all deformed persons are extreme bold" (Sandblom 1982:107).

Whereas Sandblom (1982) interprets Byron's artistic work as an overwrought revenge on the universe, the new disability biographical criticism would reread Byron's poetics with an eye toward his artistic vantage on social attitudes. In other words, just as sociological disability studies assesses the social, as opposed to the personal, origination of disability issues, so does the new disability literary study look to the social and aesthetic grounds for the artist's revisionary efforts. Disability biographical critics would more likely argue that Byron's embrace of Shakespeare's villainous hunchback, Richard III, and his refiguring of the play in his drama, *The Deformed Transformed,* follow Alexander Pope's own penchant for claiming as personal monikers all the slings and arrows ("bottlenecked spider," "hunchback'd toad") tossed in the direction of "monstrous" humans. This transformative impulse in literary work, undertaken by disabled literary artists, figures prominently in our own moment's effort to find evidence of disability perspectives—even disability as a social role and subjectivity—in history.

This biographical line of disability interpretation has led literary scholars to analyze the disability involvement of able-bodied writers in history as well. Scholarship is currently immersed in interpreting the effects of disability households and experiences on writers such as Walt Whitman, Mark Twain, and Mary Austin. How does Walt Whitman's nursing of wounded and disabled Civil War veterans inform his poetical claims about fostering perfect national health? How do Mark Twain's significant relationships with deaf friends affect his depictions of deaf characters and American Sign Language? Does Mary Austin's institutional incarceration of her cognitively disabled daughter find expression in her art and writing? Many literary scholars have assessed Virginia Woolf's sickbed seclusion as key to her creative life. How might we also interpret her repeated complicity in squabbles over the invalid pronouncements of men with disabilities on women's writing?

While one might expect to find a natural sympathy toward disabled communities and other socially marginalized identities based on gender, ethnicity, sexuality, and race, often the opposite is true. For example, throughout *A Room of One's Own,* Woolf complains that society rates women's abilities even below those of crippled men in the great ladder of existence. Critiquing the superfluous nature of male discourse on female mystery, Woolf asserts that "whether they were old or young, married or unmarried, red-nosed or humpbacked—anyhow, it was flattering, vaguely, to feel oneself the object of such attention, provided that it was not entirely bestowed by the crippled and the infirm" (Woolf [1929] 1981:28). Other examples abound in the tradition, for minority commentators tend to place disability as a social grouping from which they must escape to assert the positivity of their own culturally devalued identity. For instance, film scholar Judith Halberstam has argued that imposing stigmatized physical traits on minority bodies reveals an ideological devaluation of the dominant culture toward sexual and racial minorities (Halberstam 1995:3). In other words, the "real" stigma of a disability deforms the otherwise evident value of gender and race as cultural differences.

Counter to the participation of authors in the historical devaluation of disability identity, many writers have sought alternative models in the archive to balance against their own experience as disabled people. The Japanese writer Kenzaburo Oe (1996), who fathered an autistic son, reclaims the work of Flannery O'Connor as an example of a disabled author who wrote eloquently out of her own experience of lupus. In rereading O'Connor's posthumously published letters, Oe argues that the very basis of her originality sprang from her navigation of a debilitating condition. "I am sure it is the same accumulated practice that comes into play when the obstacles encountered by all those who labor in the fields of art are somehow—by trial and error—cleared to reveal a landscape no one has seen before" (Oe 1996:57).

Likewise, the nineteenth-century German philosopher Friedrich Nietzsche, who suffered severe migraines and stomach ulcers and, later in his life, underwent a stroke and became aphasic, spent much of his life's work ironically championing social outsiders such as "cripples" and "grotesques." Because the physically unsightly are cordoned off from the stultifying clichés of mainstream thought, Nietzsche (1969, 1990) reasoned, their value would find ironic location in their originality and lack of conformity. His work on Socrates' well-known deformities claims that the philosopher's body disrupted the Athenian faith in the correlation between bodily beauty and moral goodness. Yet, despite Socrates' physical nonconformity, Nietzsche criticizes him for championing the supremacy of rationality and ignoring the power of his own aberrant corporeality. According to Nietzsche, much of the Greek philosopher's appeal for the ancient Athenians was based on a freak show–like spectacle of a thinker who champions rationality as beauty despite the physical evidence to the contrary. While arguing that Socrates' visible presence introduced the destabilizing power of physical difference into philosophical discourse, Nietzsche nonetheless berates Socrates and his followers for sacrificing the power of "the ugliest man" to the more banal superiority of abstract reason.

Just as disability scholars in the humanities now search the archive for evidence of a countertradition of disability representation, so have researchers and writers before them searched in a similar vein. This championing or critique of one disabled writer by another demonstrates that a disability consciousness has been available during prior ages. If one is cut off or isolated from a community of like-minded individuals, the archive can operate not only as a repository of dehumanizing values but also as an imaginative refuge for alternative ways of seeing. Disability, like other devalued social groupings, is first imposed from the outside as a source of stigma and then navigated from the inside as a mode of social redress. The inversionary tactics at work in Nietzsche and Oe involve an open embrace—even a stalwart declaration—of those who are most debased by cultures of the normal.

Future work will continue to review literary archives to counterpose artistic lives and the literary corpus. These textual studies inevitably complicate a socially progressive model of disability history, if only because many disabled people have made names for themselves as literary artists. This notoriety has often occurred despite an open grappling with the meaning of disability. Rather than negativity, disability has provided the spur that allowed writers to unveil new landscapes of contemplation. Much work is currently under way in this new and fruitful line of inquiry—one that dovetails with efforts to show the foundational nature of disability to social and aesthetic work.

TRANSGRESSIVE RESIGNIFICATIONS

Whereas much disability studies work in the humanities has focused on interpretations of disability as a social process or a minority experience, Nietzsche's embrace of outsiderness (those whom he ironically termed "the higher men") points to the possibility of a transgressive narrative space for disability. Rather than rail against or bemoan the unjust social exclusion of cripples, scholars have begun to attend to the subversive potential of the hyperbolic meanings invested in disabled figures. Much of the early work in disability studies centered on the extreme emotions, such as fascination and repulsion, that disability conjures up in the cultural imaginary. The potency of these visceral reactions suggests that there is something significant at stake in the suppression of disability from public view. In a recent introduction to a special issue of *Disability Studies Quarterly*, we argue that while other minority identities have been allowed a space in liberal discourse for reclaiming their cultural meanings as a form of empowerment, disability has been viewed as revealing the ludicrous extremes of identity politics (Mitchell and Snyder 1997b). Whereas "Black is beautiful" or "Gay Pride" will redress the social derision heaped on one minority community by a dominant culture, disabilities have been precluded from access to a similar political status. The category of disability, according to many of the most "liberal" advocates, represents an undesirable state of being that no political triage can repair. Disability has been portrayed within many circles as the straw that breaks the camel's back of identity politics.

Yet, like these other social movements, disability rights advocates, artists, and scholars have recognized the power available in resignifying formerly demeaning terms such as *cripple* and *gimp*. Rather than trying to simply substitute more palatable terms for previously slanderous ones, the ironic embrace of derogatory terminology has provided the leverage of force that belongs to openly transgressive displays. The power of transgression always originates at the moment when the derided object uncharacteristically embraces its deviance as a value. In perversely championing the terms of their own stigmatization, marginal peoples alarm the dominant culture with a seeming canniness over the terms of their own subjugation. The embrace of denigrating terminology by the minority forces the dominant culture to face its own violence head-on because the authority of devaluation has been openly claimed in an ironic fashion. Thus, the minority culture effectively deflects the stigmatizing definition back to the offenders by openly advertising them in public discourse. The effect shames the dominant culture into recognition of its own dehumanizing precepts. What was most devalued is now discovered to have been stood on its head by an act of self-naming that detracts from the original power of the condescending terms.

In a parallel fashion, disability scholars have also attempted to identify and reclaim the power of formerly stigmatized representations in literature. Influential literary critic Leslie Fiedler's (1981) early essay, "Pity and Fear: Myths and Images of the Disabled in Literature and the Popular Arts," explains the potential power of literary transgression most pointedly:

> We will have to exorcize our ambivalences toward the afflicted . . . by turning not to ersatz paeans of the heroism of the crippled, but to disturbing mythic literature; including *Richard III,* over which (let me confess in closing) I still shudder, and *A Christmas Carol,* over which I have wept more than once—and will, I suspect, weep again. (P. 13)

For Fiedler, the literature of disability poses the problem of feeling drawn to that which seems most reprehensible (fear) or sentimental (pity). Yet, in doing so, he does not bemoan or celebrate literary portraits but rather situates them within the realm of human psychology. For Fiedler, literary representations of disability do not resolve as much as tap into visceral emotions.

Fiedler's (1981) argument rests on a complication of the idea of unsatisfactory imagery by framing the question of literary representation within a psychoanalytical framework. The ambivalence sensed by readers in literary presentations of disabled characters is akin to a vicarious experience of a culture's uncertainty about their disabled populations. While literature does not pose an antidote to this ambivalence, it does provide a window into the complex nature of attitudes and their origins. Rather than explain away the visceral nature of responses to physical and cognitive differences, Fiedler seizes the experience of ambivalence as a universal response to the mystery of human variation. The upshot of this position is not that negative imagery reveals dehumanizing attitudes but rather that disability representation explicitly evokes powerful sentiments within the safe space of textual interactions. These "powerful sentiments" can be designated as emanating from the transgressive power signified by physical and cognitive difference. Readers are seduced into an encounter with their most extreme reactions as a way of facing up to the imagined threat that they pose.

It is this visceral potential in the disruption caused by the disabled body that makes it both a primary tool of disruption for writers and an important vein to tap for scholarly investigation. In Fiedler's (1978) book-length study, titled *Freaks,* he explains that the viewer of the freak show spectacle involves an encounter between the self and the other:

> The true Freak, however, stirs both supernatural terror and natural sympathy, since, unlike the fabulous monsters, he is one of us, the human child of human parents, however altered by forces we do not quite understand into something mythic and mysterious, as no mere cripple ever is. . . . Only the true Freak challenges the conventional boundaries between male and female, sexed and sexless, animal and human, large and small, self and other, and consequently between reality and illusion, experience and fantasy, fact and myth. (P. 24)

There are two issues of importance in Fiedler's (1978) effort to define the power of the freak's physical spectacle. First, the terror of the self's boundaries being challenged, boundaries that are believed to be more or less absolute, suggests that the spectacle of extraordinary bodily difference upsets the viewer's faith in his or her own biological integrity. The viewer of the freakish spectacle does not experience a feeling of superiority in his or her proximity to the normal ideal but rather senses his or her own body to be at risk. The power is in the challenge of the self's stability rather than in its security. Second, the division that Fiedler attempts to maintain between the ordinary "cripple" and the spectacular freak is less absolute than he claims. While freak show displays, as Robert Bogdan (1990) has shown, artificially exaggerated physical differences to enhance the encounter with difference, there is a continuum from the freak to the routine encounter with disability. The display of disability discomforts the viewer's identification with bodily ability or normalcy by destabilizing (albeit in a less spectacular manner) that which she or he takes to be biologically "typical." The freak show enhances rather than singularly produces a reaction that already exists within the viewer.

Whereas Fiedler would argue for a lack of correspondence between the freak and the disabled person, disability scholars such as Rosemarie Garland Thomson have argued for the identification of a continuum between two constructed social positions. In her anthology, *Freakery: Cultural Spectacles of the Extraordinary Body,* Thomson (1996) designates the arrival of freak shows in the United States as anything but a fleeting historical anomaly. Tethered to a period of rapid industrialization in America's "golden age" that "put bodies on arbitrary schedules instead of allowing natural rhythms to govern activity" (p. 11), the freak show promised the spectacle of a glimpse into the taboo underworld of human oddity. The appeal of such an amusement was to "assuage viewers' uneasiness either by functioning as a touchstone of anxious identification or as an assurance of their [own] regularized normalcy" (Thomson 1996:11). Such an approach to the "distasteful" freak of negative imagery or social realism not only helps to investigate the overwrought symbolism of physical differences but also identifies the transgressive power invested in the social encounter with aberrancy.

Rather than view the freak as a rarified deviation, the essays in *Freakery* supply portraits of a widespread cultural phenomenon that speaks to the cultural fascination with spectacles of difference. As Thomson (1996) argues, the late nineteenth-century and early twentieth-century phenomenon of the freak show did not end but rather dispersed into "the entertainment discourses of vaudeville, circuses, beauty pageants, zoos, horror films, rock celebrity culture, and Epcot Center" (p. 13). In charting out this proliferation of discourses around figures of human difference, *Freakery* identifies the political undercurrents of disability as a centerpiece of contemporary American popular culture. Yet what these studies also demonstrate is a model of political power available to those who tap into the transgressive reservoirs of fascination and repulsion. Even the scholarship of its discomforting borders breaks down the assumed distance between spectator and object by violating the cultural dictum of silence that surrounds bodily deviation.

As a corollary to Thomson's (1996) overall critical project, which seeks to explore "a critical gap between disabled figures as fashioned corporeal others whose bodies carry social meaning and actual people with atypical bodies in real-world social relations" (p. 15), Felicity Nussbaum and Helen Deutsch (2000) pursue a related project in their book on eighteenth-century disability, titled *DEFECT! Engendering the Modern Body.* Tracing out the implications of a host of objectifying social and medical categories from "monstrosity" to "aesthetic ugliness" to the "exotic deformed," the collection focuses on the dovetailing of physical differences with categories of otherness such as femininity and impoverishment. As many of the essayists in the collection demonstrate, the eighteenth century became one of the most active centuries for carrying on open public discussions about what "marks the boundaries between the increasingly significant categories of the typical and atypical human being, the 'normal' and the 'abnormal' " (Nussbaum and Deutsch 2000:5). In the process of conversing about these issues, nonetheless, many eighteenth-century writers (including some with disabilities) seized the opportunity to harness the transgressive power of physical otherness and shake the foundations of aesthetic and cultural value:

Swift's Lemuel Gulliver in his giant incarnation and as a pigmy exhibited for money is among the most obvious examples [of the physical and mentally "defective"] from literature. The lesser-known *Memoirs of Martin Scribblerus* includes discussions of Siamese twins joined at the back, the little Black Prince, and the "Man-mimicking Manteger." Alexander Pope's own diminished height, humpback, and general frailty made him a curiosity, and his *Dunciad* (1728) teems with monstrosities. In addition, the deaf-mute Duncan Campbell attracted Eliza Haywood's attention and that of several other commentators because of his second sight and his ability to use sign language. Sarah Scott's colony of the maimed served the women of *Millenium Hall* (1762), and she linked ugliness to virtue in her midcentury translation of a French novel, *Agreeable Ugliness: Or, the Triumph of the Graces* (1766). . . . Damaged literary heroines include Henry Fielding's *Amelia* (1751) who met with an accident that injured her nose, and the learned but lame and pock-marked Eugenia in Frances Burney's *Camilla* (1796). (Nussbaum and Deutsch 2000:5)

Importantly, these examples evidence not only the centrality of disability to the period but also an emerging recognition of ways in which difference can be harnessed to the alternative ends of minority and literary cultures. The critical connection between disability and femininity as monstrous deviances allows the editors to create a representational continuum between two surveyed and devalued biologies. Each emphasizes not the parallel category's alien qualities but rather that the body itself contests restrictive social ideals and controls. As both Fiedler and Thomson point out, the literary encounter with deviance at first heightens alienation and then ultimately seeks to collapse the distance between disability and the inherently social processes that mark bodies as falling outside acceptable norms.

While most of the work in the humanities to date has centered on physical disability as its grounding object of study, one of the major new areas of research in disability studies will need to be that of cognitive disabilities. Although cognitive disabilities have surfaced in the current research, only a few studies privilege the representation of psychological difference as their primary concern. For instance, Otto F. Wahls's (1995) *Media Madness: Public Images of Mental Illness* begins by pointing out that images of madness pervade popular discourses such as mainstream television and film. Yet, while Wahls's study largely pursues the negative connotations of these images via the social realist school by arguing that "harmful images" exert a divisive pull on audiences, other scholarship has begun to share an interest in the transgressive potential of "madness" as a shared fascination for literature and medicine alike. For instance, Allen Thiher's (1999) monumental study, *Revels in Madness: Insanity in Medicine and Literature,* seeks to analyze a surprising history of concordance between these two seemingly disparate (even antithetical) fields of study. According to Thiher, literature has historically provided the "applied" basis for "articulating the ways that madness can be experienced, lived as it were, in its alterity . . . [for b]oth medicine and literature have had constant recourse to theater and to theatrical metaphors to describe, in various ways, the dynamics of madness" (p. 24). The import of this approach has been to place literature and medicine (particularly psychology and psychiatry) as much more intimate bedfellows than has been previously recognized.

Beginning with ancient Greece, Thiher's (1999) study demonstrates in great detail how literary stories of mental discordance have provided the foundation for scientific explanations of cognitive deviance. Rather than view this historical material as superficial and primitive, Thiher argues for a historical vision of madness as that which could productively give voice to the existence of disparate and even antithetical "realities." For instance, the autobiographies of the French Romantic, Rousseau, sought to validate "madness" as essential to the acquisition of insight, for "the power of madness to effect disclosure and bring about vision" brought writers "beyond the collectivity to an unmediated relation with the Word" (Thiher 1999:216-17). This exclusive access of those designated mad in their own time to a direct encounter with truth proved both a longstanding association of madness with divine revelation and also an example of the transgressive possibilities offered by an individual's claim to various kinds of insanity. For Thiher, the power to claim the transgressive alterity of madness proved so alluring that even during periods that openly sought to eradicate people with mental disabilities, such as the Salem witch trials, individuals would don the mantle of insanity to articulate their experience of an alternative cognitive reality. Within this perspective, individuals (artistic and otherwise) have openly claimed psychological difference rather than dissimulate its power over their own lives. This disruption of a reader's identification with fictional ideals of normalcy through encounters with "transgressive disabilities" provides an unusual opportunity to rechart a period's fashioning of the meaning of disability. Disability interrogation of received beliefs and values situates the power of stigmatized bodies and minds as profoundly disconcerting rejoinders to biological absolutism. Since literature so often imagines its project as one of social questioning and radical critique, an important continuity can begin to be formulated between contemporary disability politics and artistic production. While disability humanities scholars have been careful to avoid romanticizing the possibilities implicit in disability's transgressive "outings" of a culturally closeted phenomenon, disability studies has begun to revise more simplistic assumptions about disability characterization. If the display of radical physical and cognitive deviance in narrative proves ultimately ambiguous to the values of our own disability movement, it nonetheless reveals that even the most "derisive" portrait harbors within it the antithesis of its own disruptive potential. At the least, disability studies scholars have provided a means for contemplating the ways in which earlier periods may have recognized and deployed the transgressive possibilities that aberrancy proffered.

CONCLUSION: THE NECESSITY OF REPRESENTATION (AND ITS DISCONTENTS)

Representation inevitably spawns discontent. All acts of portrayal (artistic or documentary) prove potentially allegorical in the sense that the act of characterization encourages readers and viewers to search for a larger concept, experience, or population. Thus, the effort to represent is an inevitably fraught and inherently political activity. Like the exchange between Longmore and Stiker, with which we began, the question of disability's service to "negative" portrayals is profoundly complex. Any response proves riddled with difficulty because the question is, first and foremost, social in its making. What one generation of interpreters view as "humane" can be challenged by the next, and so on and so forth. This is particularly true of the representation of disability because even "well-meaning" representations so often result in violent justifications.

Let us provide just a brief example to underscore this point. Recently, we were contacted by a journalist who wanted to write a story about a new wave of children's books that place characters with disabilities in the central role of protagonist. His hypothesis was that these were new identity-affirming portraits (this was spoken with a tinge of sarcasm for political correctness) that sought to instruct readers that "people with disabilities were just like everyone else." He wanted to know if previous stories about children with disabilities usually represented disability as a cautionary tale about bad things that can happen to you. We offered examples of disability studies research that argued medieval stories about children with disabilities as visitors from fairy kingdoms who sought to explain the appearance of congenital disabilities to premedical cultures. Or that early twentieth-century children's stories tended to use disabilities as evidence that one had entered a fantastical world of imagination where the impossible could come true. Our point was that other generations in history had produced ways of thinking about disability that were not solely in the form of warnings. Then we added that, of course, such stories also provided a rationale for many parents to leave their disabled children to die on beaches because the fairies would be returning them to their fantastical place of origin.

The issue of representation and what it produces in readers proves exceedingly complex. The ironic championing of the segregation of disabled people in the writings of Nietzsche was later used by the Nazis as an ideological manual to support the murder of disabled people, gypsies, and Jews during the Holocaust. The first Shinto myth records the birth of a "deformed" child to First Man and First Woman, who then ship their offspring out into the ocean in a makeshift boat to erase the evidence of their failure. Disability is both origin and end—its desired eradication in each generation is countered only with the ferocity of an ultimate recalcitrance to such violent "utopian" programs.

This is the very real and dangerous terrain of representation that humanities scholarship attempts to navigate. It is the heart of our own politics that cannot be strictly channeled into straightforward catalogues of "acceptable" and "unacceptable" representations. Because the seemingly abstract and textual world affects the psychology of individuals (and thus the cultural imaginary), the interpretation of these figures and their reception prove paramount to the contribution of the humanities to disability studies. One cannot assess the merits or demerits of a literary portrait, for example, without understanding the historical context within which it was constructed and imbibed. Nor can one ignore the often-disastrous consequences of even the most inspired tales.

What has proven most striking in the humanities study of disability is the way in which literary and filmic archives provide an overview of the prevalence of disability throughout history and across cultures. While one can charge discrimination and the lack of civil rights for people with disabilities in our own moment, the contention cannot be adequately demonstrated as systemic until a historical record of treatment has been reconstructed. In addition, disabled people inevitably navigate the representational types of an era as coordinates operative in their own psyches. Imaginative works are integral to the alternatives produced for imagining disability by those "contained" within the rubric itself. Readers and viewers find their own personal interpretations of disability inevitably influenced by their imaginative encounters with disabled people in the fictional works they encounter. For instance, Martha Stoddard Holmes's (forthcoming) work, *Fictions of Affliction,* argues that while Victorian culture produced two predominating definitions of disability—that of the innocent afflicted child and that of the disabled beggar as an enemy of the state—writers with disabilities and authors who wrote about disability necessarily navigated these polar oppositions. In turn, the repetitious referencing of these discursive tropes provided a field of options for interpreting disability in the Victorian period, which profoundly influenced the subjective experience of disability and the evolution of disabled subjectivity. Because literary archives provide a repository for historical reactions along these lines, the humanities have begun the important task of bequeathing a more in-depth and sophisticated history of disability to disability studies and people with disabilities as a whole.

Whereas the survey of policies, incarcerating institutions, legislation, and so on helps to provide an overview of state-authored responses to quandaries posed by disabled populations, fictive representations provide access to less legalistic or "official" contexts for understanding disability. Whereas the ancient Athenians' belief in the perfectability of the physical body produced a mythology that proffered only one disabled god (Hephaistos), disability scholar Lois Bragg (1997) has argued that the pantheon of gods with disabilities in ancient Norse myths demonstrates a popular emphasis on the value of personal sacrifice for one's community. In this sense, the analysis of imaginative works allows humanities scholars to record a history of people with disabilities that comes closer to recapturing the "popular" values of everyday lives. If disability is the product of an interaction between individual differences and social environments (architectural, legislative, familial, attitudinal, etc.), then the contrast of perspectives between discourses of disability places art and literature as necessary to further complicate and reconstruct the dynamics of this interaction in history.

This history is by no means complete, but recent work has proven that attitudes and programs toward disabled people prove less static or exclusively detrimental than most humanities scholars originally anticipated. The history of disability, like the history of any socially produced constituency, proves surprisingly uneven and multifaceted. Our work is to understand this multiplicity in its richness. After all, how do we adequately assess our own era's reactions and representations without a thorough knowledge of other cultures and generations? What does it say about our own culture's penchant for designating disability if previous cultures did not see the need for doing so? How do we address the significant differences that exist between disability and other minority methodologies without the linguistic and identity-based interpretative methodologies that have been largely pioneered in the humanities?

As a linguistic "signifier," disability also incites discontent, for the rubric proves as slippery as any minority category imposed from without. Singular designations attempting to contain a diverse people with widely variable histories represented by categories—such as "demoniacs," "the halt and lame," "cripples," "the handicapped," or even our own contemporary rubric of "disabled people"—inevitably result in those who are labeled chaffing against the imprecision and monolithic representational characteristics assigned to the category.

Yet importantly, this inevitable discontent that representation incites serves as one of the primary catalysts to culture formation. Many of us have wondered if disability cultures exist; if so, in what forms? Because cultural groupings always occur in reaction to prior exclusionary definitions that obscure the human multiplicity of the designated population, the critique of representation consolidates a process of identification itself among those who forward the critique. In our video, *Vital Signs: Crip Culture Talks Back* (Mitchell and Snyder 1996), we platform the political critiques of artists and academics with disabilities to identify that disability culture exists within the space of shared critique. This does not suggest that the critique is monolithically formulated across the community but rather that the necessity of talking back to an uncomprehending and ablist parent culture proved to be the shared component of a bona fide, even impudent, minority culture. As one identifies the voices that seek to redress the inadequacy of dominant representations of experiences, one also delineates the contours of a rapidly consolidating community.

Thus, the productivity of discontent is more than purely academic or negative in nature. The humanities study of disability, even through its various repudiations of representational models, serves to construct a more formidable disability "identity." This identity proves to be most resilient because it does not consist of a "positive" content. It does not simply replace a poorer or less acceptable representation with another equally fictive but alluring one. Rather, disability culture remains largely reactionary because no adequate representational antidote exists. As John Frow (1995) has argued,

> The diversity of language games is a prerequisite for the openness of the social system; conversely, the achievement of a "concensus"—and therefore of an end to discussion—would represent a form of violence (or "terror") done to the dynamic of social argument. (P. 139)

Instead, disability culture continues to levy its critiques of contemporary and historical representations while playing the trickster's game of being everywhere and nowhere at once.

However, even a communal identity cannot spring up wholesale and unprecedented without being accompanied by the work of historical retrieval. If one of the main projects of disability studies is to assert, once and for all, that disability is an integral part of the human condition, then there is great advantage in demonstrating the persistence of disabled people and their contributions in history. Henri-Jacques Stiker (1999) makes a similar point in *A History of Disability* when he argues that integration will prove inadequate if it must be on the terms of the dominant culture's "normalizing" criteria. Instead, one must argue for the integral nature of disability as a category of human difference that cannot be usurped into a more homogenizing scheme of a people's shared attributes. If one seeks to argue that the current predicament of and social attitudes toward people with disabilities are inadequate, then demonstrating the kaleidoscopic nature of historical responses to disability can prove an important tool for interrogating the "naturalized" ideology hiding behind current beliefs.

Yet how do we make the historical presence of disabled people visible when they were so often erased from the human record? One answer to this perplexing social question is through the analysis of preserved discursive and visual mediums such as literature, art, and film. Rather than merely privileging the representational modes of texts that come under the purview of humanities scholars, our scholarship seeks to recognize a more complex constellation of relationships made available in these domains. Writers, painters, historians, and filmmakers, like all of us, are subject to the limiting beliefs of their own historical moments, but whereas people with disabilities are often peripheral to other domains outside of medicine, art persists in returning to portrayals of disability as a sustained preoccupation. Thus, while these representational portraits often prove unsatisfactory, they allow us viscerally to encounter disability in a way that we could not otherwise. The very discontent produced by representation provides a fulcrum for identifying the culture that *should be* rather than that which *is*.

NOTES

1. Stiker's presentation occurred during the annual meeting of the Society for Disability Studies in 1998. The address provided a powerful example of the ways in which artistic representations of disability provided a contrastive site of social investments from one period to another. The import of Stiker's analysis was that disability either could provide cultures with examples of corrupt humanity or serve as transgressive commentary on the base instincts of cultures themselves. In either instance, disability provides a window to the source and nature of historical attitudes toward disabled populations.

2. Stiker's (1999) book on disability in Western history and literature provides an insightful overview of shifting investments in disabled individuals and communities. Instead of pushing for a purely civil rights program of inclusion, Stiker argues that disability movements must also argue for the inherent variability of human bodies and psychologies. In doing so, his argument demonstrates that what has maintained people with disabilities in a historically subordinate position to able-bodied populations is a desire to repress the naturalness of human difference. Stiker's book is now published in a new English translation from the University of Michigan Press under the title *A History of Disability* (1999).

3. Our collective and individual work on disability literary figures has included interpretations of a range of biological "crises" such as Socrates' limping Oedipus, Michel de Montaigne's "Of Cripples," Shakespeare's humpbacked king (Richard III), Francis Bacon's "Of Deformity," Puritan physiognomy, Emerson's metaphors of truncated humanity, Hawthorne's hunchbacked Chillingworth, Melville's one-legged Captain Ahab, Nietzsche's cripples at the bridge, Anderson's small-town grotesques, Salinger's institutionalized Holden Caulfield, Robert Lowell's ill narrators, Pynchon's deaf mutes, Didion's multiple sclerosis, Morrison's club-footed Polly Breedlove, and Richard Powers's ward of disabled children.

4. The earliest interpretations of disability in literature involved sociological research that tended to use films and stories as briefly exemplary of contemporary concerns with cultural attitudes. The sociological approach to literature provided some of the earliest categories of disability types, such as the supercrip, tragic innocence, beggarly imposters, and limping villains. The paradigm tended to reduce literary and filmic texts to the purely exemplary by rendering representation as merely indicative of public responses.

5. We discuss this important distinction between disability and other areas of minority studies in literature in our introduction to *The Body and Physical Difference* (Mithcell and Snyder 1997a). In particular, see our comments on pages 4-9.

6. We use the phrase *social realism* in this chapter to identify a group of critical essays that demonstrated the measurable gap existing between the reality of contemporary lives lived with disabilities and the images of those lives in film and literature. We borrow the term from Marxist criticism, which forwards artistic efforts as valuable insofar as they attempt to correct the historical record by representing the lives and material conditions of the "real" working classes. While the phrase has been used somewhat pejoratively in some critical circles, we mean to employ it here as descriptive of an influential approach to disability studies in the humanities.

REFERENCES

Blau, H. 1981. "Responses to Leslie Fiedler." Paper presented at a literary symposium on "Pity and Fear: Myths and Images of the Disabled in Literature, Old and New," International Center for the Disabled, in collaboration with the United Nations (sponsors), October, New York.

Bogdan, R. 1990. *Freak Show: Presenting Human Oddities for Amusement and Profit.* Chicago: University of Chicago Press.

Bragg, L. 1997. "From the Mute God to the Lesser God: Disability in Medieval Celtic and Old Norse Literature." *Disability & Society* 12 (2): 165-77.

Brown, E. G. 1934. *Milton's Blindness.* New York: Columbia University Press.

Canguilhem, G. 1991. *The Normal and the Pathological.* New York: Zone.

Couser, G. T. 1997. *Recovering Bodies: Illness, Disability, and Life Writing.* Madison: University of Wisconsin Press.

Darke, P. A. 1994. *The Elephant Man* (David Lynch, EMI Films, 1980): An Analysis from a Disabled Perspective." *Disability & Society* 9 (3): 327-42.

Davidson, I. F. W. K., G. Woodill, and E. Bredberg. 1994. "Images of Disability in 19th Century Children's Literature." *Disability & Society* 9 (1): 33-46.

Davis, L. 1995. *Enforcing Normalcy: Disability, Deafness, and the Body.* New York: Verso.

———. 1997. "Nude Venuses, Medusa's Body and Phantom Limbs: Disability and Visuality." Pp. 51-70 in *The Body and Physical Difference: Discourses of Disability,* edited by D. T. Mitchell and S. L. Snyder. Ann Arbor: University of Michigan Press.

Deutsch, H. 1996. *Resemblance & Disgrace: Alexander Pope and the Deformation of Culture.* Cambridge, MA: Harvard University Press.

———. Forthcoming. " The Exemplary Case of Dr. Johnson." In *Enabling the Humanities: A Disability Studies Sourcebook,* edited by B. Brueggemann, R. Garland-Thomson, and S. Snyder. New York: Modern Languages Association.

Dubus, A. 1996. "An Interview with Andre Dubus." *AWP Chronicle* 29 (1): 1-6.

Eberly, S. S. 1988. "Fairies and the Folklore of Disability: Changelings, Hybrids and the Solitary Fairy." *Folklore* 99 (1): 58-77.

Edwards, M. 1997. "Constructions of Physical Disability in the Ancient Greek World: The Community Concept." Pp. 35-50 in *The Body and Physical Difference: Discourses of Disability,* edited by D. T. Mitchell and S. L. Snyder. Ann Arbor: University of Michigan Press.

Fiedler, L. A. 1978. *Freaks: Myths and Images of the Secret Self.* New York: Simon & Schuster.

———. 1981. "Pity and Fear: Myths and Images of the Disabled in Literature and the Popular Arts." Paper presented at a literary symposium on "Pity and Fear: Myths and Images of the Disabled in Literature, Old and New," International Center for the Disabled, in collaboration with the United Nations (sponsors), October, New York.

Frawley, M. 1997. " 'A Prisoner to a Couch': Harriet Martineau, Invalidism, and Self Representation." Pp. 174-88 in *The Body and Physical Difference: Discourses of Disability,* edited by D. T. Mitchell and S. L. Snyder. Ann Arbor: University of Michigan Press.

Frow, J. 1995. *Cultural Studies & Cultural Values.* Oxford, UK: Clarendon.

Gartner, A. and T. Joe, eds. 1987. *Images of the Disabled, Disabling Images.* New York: Praeger.

Gerber, D. 1997. "In Search of Al Schmid: War Hero, Blinded Veteran, Everyman." Pp. 111-33 in *The Body and Physical Difference: Discourses of Disability,* edited by D. T. Mitchell and S. L. Snyder. Ann Arbor: University of Michigan Press.

Gordon, J. 1997. "The 'Talking Cure' (Again): Gossip and the Paralyzed Patriarchy." Pp. 202-22 in *The Body and Physical Difference: Discourses of Disability,* edited by D. T. Mitchell and S. L. Snyder. Ann Arbor: University of Michigan Press.

Hafferty, F. W. and S. Foster. 1994. "Decontextualizing Disability in the Crime Mystery Genre: The Case of the Invisible Handicap." *Disability & Society* 9 (2): 185-206.

Halberstam, J. 1995. *Skin Shows: Gothic Horror and the Technology of Monsters.* Durham, NC: Duke University Press.

Hamilton, E. 1997. "From Social Welfare to Civil Rights: The Representation of Disability in Twentieth-Century German Literature." Pp. 223-39 in *The Body and Physical Difference: Discourses of Disability,* edited by D. T. Mitchell and S. L. Snyder. Ann Arbor: University of Michigan Press.

Herndl, D. P. 1993. *Invalid Women: Figuring Feminine Illness in American Fiction and Culture, 1840-1940.* Chapel Hill: University of North Carolina Press.

Hevey, D. 1992. *The Creatures That Time Forgot: Photography and Disability Imagery.* New York: Routledge.

Holmes, M. S. Forthcoming. *Fictions of Affliction: Physical Disabilities in Victorian Culture.* Ann Arbor: University of Michigan Press.

Kent, D. 1987. "Disabled Women: Portraits in Fiction and Drama." Pp. 47-63 in *Images of the Disabled, Disabling Images,* edited by A. Gartner and T. Joe. New York: Praeger.

Kriegel, L. 1987. "Disability as Metaphor in Literature." Pp. 31-46 in *Images of the Disabled, Disabling Images,* edited by A. Gartner and T. Joe. New York: Praeger.

LaCom, C. 1997. " 'It Is More Than Lame': Female Disability, Sexuality, and the Maternal in the Nineteenth-Century Novel." Pp. 189-201 in *The Body and Physical Difference: Discourses of Disability,* edited by D. T. Mitchell and S. L. Snyder. Ann Arbor: University of Michigan Press.

Longmore, P. 1997a. "Screening Stereotypes: Images of Disabled People in Television and Motion Pictures." Pp. 65-78 in *Images of the Disabled, Disabling Images,* edited by A. Gartner and T. Joe. New York: Praeger.

———. 1997b. "Conspicuous Contribution and American Cultural Dilemmas: Telethon Rituals of Cleansing and Renewal." Pp. 134-60 in *The Body and Physical Difference: Discourses of Disability,* edited by D. T. Mitchell and S. L. Snyder. Ann Arbor: University of Michigan Press.

Miner, M. 1997. " 'Making Up Stories as We Go Along': Men, Women, and Narratives of Disability." Pp. 283-96 in *The Body and Physical Difference: Discourses of Disability,* edited by D. T. Mitchell and S. L. Snyder. Ann Arbor: University of Michigan Press.

Mitchell, D. T. and S. L. Snyder, producers. 1996. *Vital Signs: Crip Culture Talks Back* [Video]. 48 min. Beta SP. Marquette, MI: Brace Yourselves Productions.

———, eds. 1997a. *The Body and Physical Difference: Discourses of Disability.* Ann Arbor: University of Michigan Press.

———. 1997b. "Exploring Foundations: Languages of Disability, Identity, and Culture." *Disability Studies Quarterly* 17 (4): 241-47.

———. Forthcoming. "Infinities of Forms: Figuring Disability in Artistic Traditions." In *Enabling the Humanities: A Disability Studies Sourcebook,* edited by B. Brueggemann, R. Garland-Thomson, and S. Snyder. New York: Modern Languages Association.

Molina, C. 1997. "Muteness and Multilation: The Aesthetics of Disability in Jane Campion's *The Piano.*" Pp. 267-82 in *The Body and Physical Difference: Discourses of Disability,* edited by D. T. Mitchell and S. L. Snyder. Ann Arbor: University of Michigan Press.

Nietzsche, F. 1969. *Thus Spoke Zarathustra.* Translated by R. J. Hollingdale. New York: Penguin.

———. 1990. *Twilight of the Idols/The Anti-Christ.* Translated by R. J. Hollingdale. New York: Penguin.

Norden, M. 1994. *The Cinema of Isolation: A History of Physical Disability in the Movies.* New Brunswick, NJ: Rutgers University Press.

Nussbaum, F. 1997. "Feminotopias: The Pleasure of 'Deformity' in Mid-Eighteenth-Century England." Pp. 161-73 in *The Body and Physical Difference: Discourses of Disability,* edited by D. T. Mitchell and S. L. Snyder. Ann Arbor: University of Michigan Press.

Nussbaum, F. and H. Deutsch, eds. 2000. *DEFECT! Engendering the Modern Body.* Ann Arbor: University of Michigan Press.

Oe, K. 1996. *A Healing Family: A Candid Account of Life with a Handicapped Son.* New York: Kodansha International.

Pernick, M. 1997. "Defining the Defective: Eugenics, Aesthetics, and Mass Culture in Early-Twentieth-Century America." Pp. 89-110 in *The Body and Physical Difference: Discourses of Disability,* edited by D. T. Mitchell and S. L. Snyder. Ann Arbor: University of Michigan Press.

Pointon, A. and C. Davies, eds. 1997. *Framed: Interrogating Disability in the Media.* London: British Film Institute.

Sandblom, P. 1982. *Creativity and Disease: How Illness Affects Literature, Art and Music.* Philadelphia: George Stickley.

Shakespeare, T. 1994. "Cultural Representations of Disabled People: Dustbins for Disavowal." *Disability & Society* 9 (3): 283-99.

Stiker, H.-J. 1999. *A History of Disability.* Ann Arbor: University of Michigan Press.

Thiher, A. 1999. *Revels in Madness: Insanity in Medicine and Literature.* Ann Arbor: University of Michigan Press.

Thomson, R. 1996. *Freakery: Cultural Spectacles of the Extraordinary Body.* New York: New York University Press.

———. 1997. "Disabled Women as Powerful Women in Petry, Morrison, and Lorde: Revising Black Subjectivity." Pp. 240-66 in *The Body and Physical Difference: Discourses of Disability,* edited by D. T. Mitchell and S. L. Snyder. Ann Arbor: University of Michigan Press.

Thurber, S. 1980. "Disability and Monstrosity: A Look at Literary Distortions of Handicapping Conditions." *Rehabilitation Literature* 41 (1-2): 12-15.

Wahl, O. F. 1995. *Media Madness: Public Images of Mental Illness.* New Brunswick, NJ: Rutgers University Press.

Woolf, V. [1929] 1981. *A Room of One's Own.* Reprint, New York: Harcourt, Brace.

Yuan, D. 1997. "Disfigurement and Reconstruction in Oliver Wendell Holmes's 'The Human Wheel, Its Spokes and Felloes.' " Pp. 71-88 in *The Body and Physical Difference: Discourses of Disability,* edited by D. T. Mitchell and S. L. Snyder. Ann Arbor: University of Michigan Press.

Zola, I. 1987. "Any Distinguishing Features? The Portrayal of Disability in the Crime-Mystery Genre." *Policy Studies Journal* 15 (3): 487-513.

Philosophical Issues in the Definition and Social Response to Disability

8

DAVID WASSERMAN

Disability should be of interest to philosophers because it raises fundamental issues about the significance of variations in physical and mental functioning for human performance and well-being, for personal and social identity, and for justice in the allocation of resources and the design of the physical and social environment. Recent Anglo-American philosophy, in turn, should be of interest to disability scholars because of its close analysis of concepts critical to the conceptualization and social response to disability, such as health, normality, and disease; human action and well-being; and discrimination, justice, and equality.

Yet there is tension in the relationship between philosophy and disability. To the extent that philosophers turn to disability in addressing more general questions about well-being or justice, they may be inclined to misrepresent or oversimplify disabilities for the sake of argument. The distortion need not be intentional; philosophers are hardly immune to the "myths, fears, and stereotypes" about disabilities that prevail in contemporary society. Disability advocates, for their part, may be inclined to treat philosophy as the handmaiden of policy and may be unduly suspicious of or impatient with any philosophical analysis not in the service of a reform agenda. Despite these cross-purposes, however, philosophers can bring much-needed clarification to many debates about disability classification and policy. Disability advocates, in turn, can help to educate philosophers about the functional and social significance of human variation and to disabuse them of familiar myths and stereotypes about impairment.

In this chapter, I will begin by outlining several areas of philosophy that are relevant to the conceptualization and social response to disability. In some of these areas, the potential contribution of philosophy to disability policy has been widely recognized; in others, it has been largely ignored. I will focus on a subset of issues that highlights the tensions between two aspects of disability: as functional limitation or deficiency and as stigma or social marker. I will examine the meaning and the implications of the impairment classification, the causal role of impairments in personal and social limitations, and the significance of impairments for well-being. I will not attempt to resolve these issues but merely outline the debate over them and suggest that their resolution does not have the implications for social policy that some disability advocates fear.

AUTHOR'S NOTE: I am grateful to Ron Amundson, Jerome Bickenbach, Robert Wachbroit, and Gary Albrecht for their comments on earlier drafts of this chapter.

I will then turn to political philosophy, where the tension between the two aspects of disability has been most explicit and most acute. Distributive-justice approaches to disability focus on deficits in capacity and performance. Antidiscrimination approaches to disability focus on stigmatization and exclusion. I will examine the potential of each approach standing alone to provide an adequate foundation for disability policy and the prospects for integrating the two.

Three terminological matters: I will follow the *International Classification of Impairments, Disabilities, and Handicaps (ICIDH)* (World Health Organization 1980) in speaking of "impairments" as biomedically defined conditions, but I will depart from it in using "disabilities" to cover both the activity limitations and participation restrictions associated with impairments. I will have little to say about the necessity or utility of drawing a line between activity and participation, except to discuss one way of drawing that line that is not embodied in the *ICIDH*: between basic and nonbasic actions. I may also depart from the *ICIDH* on occasion in speaking of the limitations of "basic" actions, such as the inability to raise one's arm or wiggle one's ears, as impairments rather then activity limitations, blurring the tripartite classification scheme on the other end as well.

My theoretical commitments are less ambiguous on another matter. I generally use the term *people with impairments* rather than *people with disabilities,* which is the term that prevails in the American legal context. While the latter term may be perfectly appropriate in that context, I want to use a term that identifies people with biomedically defined conditions without making any assumptions about their degree of limitation, well-being, or fair treatment. For some who adopt a social or minority group model of disability or who see the impairment classification as form of stigmatization, my usage may seem naive or question begging. On their view, disability is either conceptually prior to or entirely separate from impairment. I disagree and believe that it is analytically appropriate and useful to start with impairments.

Finally, I will frequently contrast "mainstream philosophers" and "disability advocates." There is a small, growing, and welcomed overlap between the two groups: philosophers trained in the mainstream analytic tradition who also engage in disability research and advocacy, such as Ron Amundsen, Anita Silvers, Susan Wendell, and Jerome Bickenbach. In contrasting mainstream philosophers and disability advocates, then, I will often be contrasting not different individuals but (what I take to be) different perspectives or allegiances of the same individuals. My reason for referring to distinct groups is simply convenience, which I want to make clear from the outset.

OVERVIEW: HOW IS PHILOSOPHY RELEVANT TO DISABILITY POLICY?

Several areas of philosophy have shared interests with and implications for disability studies. The philosophy of science analyzes the concepts of causation and explanation, concepts with broad relevance to claims about the contribution of biological, environmental, and social factors to disability. Philosophical accounts of the distinction between causes and conditions and of the relationship and ordering of different causal factors may be useful in evaluating medical, interactive, and social models of disability, with their apparently conflicting claims about the primary cause, or locus, of disability. Is it ever appropriate to attribute particular activity limitations or participation restrictions exclusively to physical or mental impairment or to the physical or social environment? Is it meaningful to assign proportions of an individual's limitation or restriction to his or her impairments and environment? Is it meaningful to even compare the contributions of his or her impairments and environment and judge one greater than the other?

Within the philosophy of science, the philosophy of biology and medicine examines concepts such as health, disease, normality, fitness, and functioning, addressing issues about the meaning, significance, and normative content of biological classifications and medical diagnoses. Is the underlying notion of normality in terms of which impairments are identified biological, statistical, or normative? Is there a difference in this respect between physical and mental impairments? Are "universal" processes or states such as pain (perception), tooth decay, and aging to be understood as impairments? Is the distinction between normal and abnormal conditions a matter of degree or kind; is it arbitrary or conventional or grounded in scientific theory?

The philosophy of action is concerned with the relationship between human agents and the external world. It examines the widespread tendency to see human actions as hierarchical, with more complex and contingent interventions in the world resting on a bedrock of "basic actions" that the agent can perform more or less independently of the world. Theories of basic action tend to treat impairments as having a presumptively negative impact on agents' efficacy and to underwrite a distinction between disability and handicap (or between activities and participation, to use the language of the *ICIDH-2* [World Health Organization 1997]). Critics of basic action tend to treat the agents' efficacy as more contingently related to their physical endowments.

Epistemology, or the philosophy of knowledge and belief, bears on disability in its concern for the importance and reliability of sense perception and the relationship of different sensory modalities. Perennial philosophical questions about the extent to which our understanding of the world must be obtained from sensory experience or from the operation of various senses have obvious and important implications for the assessment of disabilities. For example, do people who can see have access to knowledge and understanding that people who cannot see cannot acquire or can acquire only derivatively? Do the senses of touch and sight necessarily yield consistent information about the world? Could an external world be perceived or constituted solely through sound? The philosophy of language examines the completeness and comparability of different systems of communication, an examination relevant to the appraisal of the sign languages and tactile communication employed by deaf and blind people.

Aesthetic and moral philosophy examine questions of value that bear on the appraisal of differences in function and structure. Can we make meaningful comparisons about the beauty, richness, or complexity of the experience yielded by different senses or combinations of senses? Are various sensory and motor functions or combinations of functions necessary for or only contingently related to well-being? Do limitations in cognitive function have a more direct or less contingent relationship to well-being than differences in sensory and motor function? Is some minimal level of sensory or cognitive function necessary for humanity or personhood, for enjoying moral rights against various harms or for various goods, or for exercising certain moral powers, that is, to make promises?

Finally, recent social and political philosophy has taken two different and potentially conflicting approaches to justice that focus on different aspects of disability. The dominant approach understands justice primarily in distributive terms, in terms of the pattern of individual resources, opportunities, or welfare across society. This approach tends to treat impairments as functional limitations that may generate various distributive claims. A second approach understands justice primarily in terms of social structures and processes, in terms of relationships of power, privilege, and status among social groups. This approach tends to treat impairments as the markers of oppressed social groups and sees justice for impairments in terms of the elimination of oppressive and discriminatory attitudes and practices.

These competing approaches to justice and disability highlight a tension existing in several areas of philosophical inquiry outlined above—between approaching disabilities as functional limitations and as social markers. This difference in orientation yields a familiar but by no means necessary alignment of positions on questions related to disability. Thus, philosophers who approach impairments as functional limitations tend to see the impairment classification as, at least in theory, value neutral and objective. While denying that that classification is based on value judgments, they also tend to regard normal functions as presumptively desirable and many, though not all, impairments as disadvantageous in causing various limitations and in denying or restricting valuable experiences or opportunities. They tend to see these disadvantages as exacerbated, but not created, by neglect and exclusion. They tend to favor medical correction or monetary compensation as the presumptive social response to disability.

In contrast, philosophers who focus on impairment as stigma tend to regard the impairment classification as value laden and subjective. Moreover, they tend to reject the values they see as informing that classification. They deny that the conditions classified as impairments cause disadvantage or limit human flourishing and that people with those conditions have lives that are any less rich, complex, or satisfying than those classified as normal. They tend to regard the appropriate social response to disability as the transformation of the basic cultural, political, and economic structures of society or, more modestly, as the elimination of discriminatory attitudes and practices and their pervasive structural manifestations. They acknowledge that these changes may well affect the distribution of resources and the comparative advantage of individuals with impairments, but they do not have that as their primary purpose.

This alignment of positions, however, is unnecessary. It oversimplifies the complex relationship between the conceptualization of and social response to disability. As I will argue in the following sections, the understanding of impairments as sources of functional limitation is fully compatible with the recognition of impairment as stigma and with the endorsement of environmental reconstruction and social reform as the primary responses to disability. The claim that the impairment classification is value neutral may be adduced to argue that biological normality has only a contingent relationship to human flourishing and that the disadvantages associated with disability arise largely because social practices are tailored to normal human functioning. The claim that certain impairments preclude valuable experiences does not mean that they thereby make life any less rich or valuable overall; it may rather support the conclusion that there is an indefinite variety of ways in which human lives can flourish. A focus on the functional significance of impairments is compatible with understanding disability as a poor fit between the individual and his or her environment, such as an obsolete skill or membership in a very small linguistic or cultural minority. This view lends support to environmental modification over medical correction or monetary compensation as the presumptive response to disability.

WHAT DOES IT MEAN TO CLASSIFY A PHYSICAL OR MENTAL CONDITION AS AN IMPAIRMENT?

It is widely agreed that "physical or mental impairment" is a biomedical classification—one made by doctors or other health professionals. Yet there is considerable disagreement about what that classification means. This disagreement is part of a wider debate about the meaning of health—whether it simply is the absence of disease, injury, or impairment and whether disease, injury, and impairment are distinct categories, appropriately grouped together as adverse health states.[1] I will focus on the question of whether the classification of a physical or mental condition as an "impairment" is value free or value laden. Is one claiming or assuming that a condition is at least presumptively undesirable by classifying it, or is one making a scientific judgment that, standing alone, has no normative implications? I will not discuss the questions of how "thick" a notion health is or how to distinguish disease from injury from impairment, although both questions are closely related to the one on which I focus. If the notions of impairment and disease are value neutral, it may be tempting to deny that health consists of nothing but their absence. If health is merely the absence of disease or impairment, it may be tempting to deny that those notions are value neutral.

As I mentioned earlier, some philosophers and disability advocates have tended to assume that the impairment classification is value laden and to question the values they see as underlying it. Their claim is not merely that the actual classification of impairments at any given time and place will reflect the influence of prevailing social norms and values but that those norms and values are integral to the classification, not sources of error or bias. Some who attack the medical model of disability suggest that conditions classified as impairments are mere differences, akin to skin and hair color, stigmatized because they are uncommon or unfamiliar. A more modest and perhaps more widespread claim is that to judge a structure or function "impaired" is to hold it up against some moral or aesthetic ideal. About health and related concepts, Tristram Engelhardt (1986), one of the leading "normativists," said,

> To see a phenomenon as a disease, deformity, or disability is to see something wrong with it. Diseases, illnesses, and disfigurements are experienced as failures to achieve an expected state, a state held to be proper to the person afflicted. (P. 165)

The normativist need not endorse or reject the values underlying the impairment classification; his or her claim is merely that that classification is not a strictly scientific matter and that it involves the fallible and controversial applications of moral and aesthetic ideals to human variation.

The principal alternative to this view maintains that the classification of disease and impairment is descriptive and scientific, that it is not based on, even though it may be distorted by, moral or aesthetic values. Thus, Christopher Boorse (1977), the leading exponent of this view, argues that the diagnosis of disease or impairment is a strictly biological judgment: that some part or system of the organism is not performing its normal or species-typical function with at least statistically typical efficiency. Boorse understands the species-typical function of a part or system to be

> its ultimate contribution to certain goals at the apex of the [biological] hierarchy. . . . The function of the heart is to pump blood rather than produce heart sounds, and the function of the kidney is to eliminate wastes rather than to keep the bladder full. It is the former effects, not the latter, that contribute to the organism's highest-level goals. . . . I suggest that those functions are, specifically, contributions to individual survival and reproduction. (P. 556)[2]

Other philosophers of science have disputed Boorse's assumption that species-typical levels can be identified for most functions. According to Alexander Rosenberg (1986), for example,

> Modern biology suggests that variation of many endowment is not a matter of normality and disturbances from it, but of the random distribution of relatively discrete traits . . . contemporary biological theory does not identify the average as the normal or natural level. There is no such thing. (Pp. 5-6)

Somewhat more cautiously, Ron Amundson (2000) maintains that "it is an open empirical question whether evolution results in the kind of functional uniformity that would license normality definitions" (p. 7). He finds grounds for skepticism in a variety of case studies from developmental biology and disability research, which suggests that

> functional adults can develop in an indefinitely large number of ways. . . . Development yields adults that *function,* but not adults that *function identically.* Functional diversity is a product of developmental plasticity. (P. 9)[3]

These case studies certainly illustrate the loose connection between typical and successful functioning. The question is whether they can be generalized to challenge the very notion of biostatistical normality. Even if they can, it is unclear how they are relevant to other value-neutral accounts of biological normality that do not identify with the central tendency of a statistical distribution of functioning (e.g., Wachbroit 1994). I will not attempt to judge the merits of this dispute. My interest is rather in what it means for an account of biological normality to be value neutral and what, if anything, such neutrality implies about the appraisal of and social response to impairments.

Boorse (1987) claims that his definition of disease or impairment, in terms of departures from species-typical functioning, "is value-neutral, or as value-neutral as biology itself" (p. 372).

The determination that a condition is an impairment does not imply that it is undesirable or disadvantageous. As he observes,

> At least in some circumstances, a disease state may be preferable to normality: it is advantageous to have cowpox in a smallpox epidemic, rubella prior to pregnancy, myopia or flat feet during a military draft, or oviduct blockage if one wishes no more children. . . . [Moreover,] some normal conditions are far worse than some pathological conditions. For example, short stature, low intelligence and moderate ugliness are by most standards greater handicaps than athlete's foot or myopia, even if the latter last a lifetime. (Boorse 1987:369)

In highlighting the extent to which environmental conditions and personal goals mediate the impact of impairment, Boorse's (1987) account appears fully compatible with an interactive model of disability. The extent to which a departure from species-typical functioning is disadvantageous to an individual depends on her or his environment and goals. Boorse's account makes no judgment about the moral importance of individual survival and reproduction, as opposed to other goals and projects. Rather, it invites an explicit resolution of the issues of value that, according to normative accounts, are implicitly resolved by the very act of classification.[4]

Thus, for example, a Boorsean would probably uphold the classification of deafness as an impairment simply because the auditory systems of deaf people did not make a statistically average contribution to their individual survival and reproduction. Yet he would not thereby be committed to the proposition that deaf activists emphatically deny that it is undesirable or disadvantageous to lack hearing (see Lane 1992; Wasserman 1996). In places where sign language was widely used (or interpreters plentiful), where Deaf culture flourished, or where cacophonous sounds abounded, it might be desirable or advantageous to lack hearing.

The resistance to value-neutral accounts by disability advocates may have less to do with their actual implications than with a concern that they lend scientific credibility to social bias. Even if doctors and other health professionals believe that they are making a value-neutral judgment in classifying physical and mental conditions as impairments, their aversion to or disapproval of those conditions may often influence their judgments. The sway of social norms is now obvious with respect to some conditions long classified as diseases or impairments, such as masturbation; it may be as great, though less obvious, for many conditions still classified as diseases or impairments. It does not follow, however, that the need to justify that classification in scientific, value-neutral terms serves to protect, rather than expose, those social biases.

A related concern is that doctors are notorious for their embrace of individual survival (if not reproduction) as the overriding goal of medical practice. Even if the priority of that goal is not inherent to the impairment classification, those making the diagnosis often assume it. However, a nonnormative account does not support that assumption. Rather, by treating individual survival as only one goal among many, it requires that that assumption be independently justified.

A final concern, however, closely related to the previous two is more difficult to dismiss. On a value-neutral account, a person correctly classified as impaired does have something objectively wrong, defective, or lacking, even if it is something she or her might be indifferent toward or, in some circumstances, welcome. For some disability advocates, this provides a strong foothold for erroneous attributions of responsibility: Thus, Amundson (2000) argues,

> Philosophers and medical practitioners have used the category [biological normality] to conclude that the disadvantages of disabled people result from their own abnormality; they have only themselves (and nature) to blame. . . . When an inaccessible environment causes the confinement of a wheelchair user, the abnormality of the wheelchair is identified as the cause of the confinement. The doctrine of biological normality . . . the linkage of normality to opportunity . . . and hence to quality of life . . . rationalizes the assessment. The opportunity losses of abnormal people are theorized to be not only natural and obvious, but morally innocuous. (P. 29)

Amundson may be correct that the doctrine of biological normality has been used to rationalize neglectful (or intrusive and demeaning) social responses to disability. But none of the linkages he describes are compelled by the acceptance of a value-neutral account of biological normality. That doctrine does not support the claim that the wheelchair user's abnormality is the cause of his confinement, let alone that he is responsible for his confinement or that his confinement is "morally innocuous." In the next section, I will discuss the difficulty of finding a principled basis for designating any factor as *the* cause of a limitation or disadvantage and suggest that causal attribution is more plausibly seen as grounded in, rather than as grounding, judgments of moral responsibility and political obligation.

WHAT DOES IT MEAN TO CLAIM THAT AN IMPAIRMENT IS THE CAUSE OR A CAUSE OF THE PERSONAL AND SOCIAL LIMITATIONS WITH WHICH IT IS ASSOCIATED?

There is a broad consensus among scholars writing about disabilities that the limitations associated with impairment are a joint product of biological features, environmental factors, and personal goals. As Amundson (1992) explains in a representative passage,

> A person with a disability [impairment] is handicapped only with respect to a particular environment and a particular goal. This is because the structure of the environment determines which goals are accessible to people with certain disabilities. Blind people are handicapped with respect to access to information because so much information in the present social environment is stored only in visually accessible form. Wheelchair users are handicapped with respect to travel because so little public transportation is accessible to wheelchairs. (P. 110)

The recognition that impairment alone does not cause limitations in personal activity and social participation is central to the tripartite classification scheme of the *International Classification of Impairments, Disabilities, and Handicaps (ICIDH)*. The revised version (*ICIDH-2*) explicitly assigns a causal role to environmental and social factors in producing both disabilities (referred to in the *ICIDH-2* as personal activity limitations) and handicaps (referred to in the *ICIDH-2* as social participation restrictions). Although there are several competing schemes for classifying the effects associated with impairments of biological function, they all take an interactive approach to disability, recognizing environmental and social as well as biological contributions.

The existence of a plurality of causal factors for any personal or social limitation raises the question of what it means to claim that a particular factor is *the* cause of an outcome or is a cause rather than a mere condition of its occurrence. As Robert Wachbroit (2001) notes, philosophers have made various proposals for distinguishing causes from mere conditions:

> Some have claimed that causes are factors that we can control or manipulate, whereas conditions are factors beyond our control. Thus, the blow from the bat swing caused the baseball to land in the bleachers; gravity was a (background) condition. Others have identified causes as the unusual or salient factors. Thus, the driver being drunk caused the accident last night; that the road was also dark was a (background) condition. Still others have identified causes as those factors that address the interests we may have in the inquiry. Thus, what the road engineer regards as the cause of a car accident (the banking of the turn) might be different from what the automotive engineer regards as the cause of the accident (the way the power is distributed on each of the car wheels). (Pp. 69-70)

Wachbroit (2001) argues that the distinction between causes and conditions can be regarded as subjective, "in the sense of [depending] upon what we find salient or what interests motivate the inquiry rather than objective features of the world" (p. 70). Whether the impairment classification is subjective or value laden, the attribution of personal or social limitations to impairments is likely to be.

One reason why impairments are often seen as the causes of the limitations associated with them is their salience. If a wheelchair user cannot get up a flight of stairs, we tend to attribute his or her failure to lack of leg movement rather than to the stairs. If a person with standard limb function cannot get up a sheer concrete wall, we tend to attribute his or her failure to the wall rather than to his or her lack of suction-cupped feet. The absence of standard leg movement is salient; the absence of suction-cupped feet is not, but there is no scientific or neutral basis for making an exclusive causal attribution in either case.

Similarly, the background features of the environment are unlikely to figure in a causal account because they are, as Harlan Hahn (1999) observes, taken for granted. Although gravity contributes to the limitations experienced by would-be stair and wall climbers alike, it would rarely be cited as the cause of their limitations, just because of its pervasiveness. Again, however, there is no scientific warrant for its omission, just a pragmatic or psychological explanation.

In light of the general recognition that disability results from the interaction of a variety of factors and that the selection of a given factor as *the cause* is subjective or context dependent, why should there be controversy over the causal role of biological and social factors in disability? In part, the controversy reflects conflicting intuitions about *how much* each type of factor contributes. The claim that disabilities are naturally or socially caused may be taken to express (somewhat hyperbolically) the claim that one kind of factor predominates. If the lack of standard limb function is more likely to be regarded as the cause of a mobility limitation than the lack of suction-cupped feet, it is not only because the former is more salient but also because, in a wider range of environments, the former is believed to be associated with greater mobility limitations. Such intuitions, however, are notoriously difficult to make more precise. This is illustrated by the somewhat analogous attempt to apportion the causal contributions of genetic and environmental factors to various mental and behavioral traits in an analysis of variance (Sober 2001; Wachbroit 2001). Without a generally accepted way of enumerating environments or of measuring the distance between them, assigning causal shares to biological and social causes is virtually meaningless.

Yet the stubborn conviction that biological or social factors predominate in the creation of disability is rarely based on a canvass of all possible environments, even an incomplete or selective one. Rather, the judgment that one type of factor is the real or predominant one reflects the tacit choice of a baseline environment for making causal attributions. For many mainstream political philosophers, that baseline is a "state of nature" in which no one has the advantages of technology or social cooperation; for some disability advocates, it is a state in which people with impairments have unlimited access to existing and emerging technology. Those who adopt the first baseline regard any limitation that would arise in a state of nature as caused (predominantly) by natural or biological factors; those who adopt the second baseline regard any technologically surmountable limitation as caused (predominantly) by social factors.

The selection of either baseline is clearly value laden, and the resulting divergence in causal attributions is more likely to reflect moral than empirical disagreement. Thus, the adoption of the second baseline is likely to reflect the conviction that people with impairments should enjoy unlimited access to adaptive technology, a conviction that singles out limitations in access to such technology as the cause of disability. The adoption of the first, state-of-nature baseline is based on a view of organized society as a contract among self-interested people who bargain or deliberate in light of their default position—how they would fare in the absence of a cooperative scheme. There are a variety of contractarian theories, but almost all share the assumption that a society has a greater obligation to avoid creating or exacerbating differences among its members than to eliminate differences that exist in a precontractual setting. A society's most stringent obligation is to leave its members no worse off, in comparative or absolute terms, than they would be in a state of nature; its obligation to make them better off is more qualified or contingent.

The moral convictions that underlie these opposing baselines can be criticized on moral grounds—that they demand too much or too little of us and that they embrace a conception of society that is too encompassing or too atomistic. I will turn to these concerns in the final section, on disability and justice. Here, I want to consider a threshold difficulty: that both these baselines provide a shaky foundation for causal attribution because they are ambiguous or indeterminate. I will focus on the state-of-nature baseline because it is adopted more widely and uncritically in making causal attributions.[5]

The interactive nature of disability makes it difficult, if not impossible, to assess how individuals would fare in the absence of a scheme of social cooperation. Human beings are social animals and relentless artificers; a state in which people lived without frequent contact and cooperation, or in which they did not modify their environment to accommodate their needs and limitations, would be a highly unnatural one. An indefinite variety of informal arrangements might exist or develop in the absence of organized civil and political society. People with impairments might fare very differently under those different arrangements, and there is no obvious basis for deciding which to regard as "the state of nature."

The problem with a state-of-nature baseline is not merely that there is an indefinite number of alternatives to the present society or to any organized society. It is also that many of the disadvantages people experience in a given society must be understood in terms of the framework of advantages that society creates. It may not make sense to ask if they would have experienced those disadvantages outside of that framework, in a state of nature.

The difficulties of abstracting away from a specific social order, or any social order, in making causal attributions are readily apparent in Thomas Pogge's (1989) attempt to distinguish natural and social disadvantages in the service of a theory of justice that regards society as having stronger obligations to the latter than to the former. Pogge asserts that "human life is exposed to a wide range of natural contingencies, such as genetic handicaps, illnesses, accidents, and other misfortunes not socially induced" (p. 45). He views the distribution of social goods as "superimposed upon [the distribution] of natural goods and ills" (p. 46). Although a person's genome can, at least until the advent of routine genetic therapy, be reasonably regarded as a natural contingency (although social policies and practices pervasively affect what genetic features get reproduced), the extent to which a given genetic feature is a "handicap" or "misfortune" may be due, to a considerable extent, to environmental factors that are "socially induced."

Pogge (1989) recognizes that diseases and impairments themselves will sometimes be "socially produced, that is, due to the interactions among participants in the social system." He includes pollution, crimes, and traffic accidents as conditions whose incidence is affected by political decisions (Pogge 1989:190-91). He appears to regard these cases of social causation as marginal, rather than central, threats to the distinction that he wants to draw. In fact, as recent studies of influenza, hepatitis, and AIDS suggest, virtually all contagious diseases owe their epidemic character, and many owe their particular biological form, to various features of organized social life, especially agriculture and trade. The contribution of organized social life is even more obvious with respect to most types of adventitious injury.

Social arrangements contribute not only to the incidence of various types of biological impairments but, more pervasively and more important for our purposes, to the impact of those impairments on the lives of those who possess them—from the impact of literacy on dyslexia to the impact of the telephone on deafness.[6] If it is difficult to attribute the production of the underlying impairment to a natural or social cause, it will be even more difficult to make such an attribution with respect to the personal and social limitations associated with impairments.

The difficulty with a state-of-nature baseline is not just a matter of uncertainty or indeterminacy about the conditions that would prevail in such a state. Even if we could, for example, extrapolate from the mortality statistics of less developed nations, showing dramatically lower life expectancies for people who are blind or paraplegic in an attempt to conclude that people with those conditions would generally have fared poorly in certain parts of the world in the absence of civil and political society, this gives us a very tenuous basis for attributing their present disadvantages to "nature." Thus, imagine a technologically sophisticated society built in an inhospitable environment, where precivil life for blind or paraplegic people can be presumed to have been nasty, brutish, and short. Assume that this society made no provision for sightless communication or legless mobility but kept its blind and paraplegic members in physically comfortable institutions. Apart from the obvious injustice of this state of affairs, it would seem odd to attribute the disadvantages of those blind and paraplegic individuals to "nature" or to their natural endowment. What they lacked could only be characterized in terms of the activities and opportunities available to other members of the society and in terms of the social and political decisions that made those activities and opportunities unavailable to them.

This is not to deny that the past can sometimes be a benchmark for making causal attributions. We may not be able to compare our present social arrangements with a hypothetical state of nature, but we can compare them to the state of society before the introduction of a new social practice or a new technology to assess whether those changes have exacerbated or alleviated various types of disadvantage. The introduction of the telephone caused much business and social communication to shift to a medium to which deaf people had no access. In addition, icon-based computer software poses a similar threat to the blind, for whom it is considerably harder to access than the DOS software it replaced. Such ante/post comparisons provide a basis for attributing the increased exclusion of people with impairments to changes in technology and social practice, but not for attributing their disadvantages generally to natural or social causes.

One alternative to the state of nature as a baseline for causal attribution would be a state of "maximum feasible adaptation." Such a state would allow people with impairments to enjoy the benefit of all technologically possible measures to adapt the environment to their needs and goals. This baseline has not, to my knowledge, been clearly articulated, but it appears to be implied by the claims of some disability advocates to the effect that any barrier that could be removed by human technology, at any cost, is socially constructed rather than natural. Thus, the Union of the Physically Impaired against Segregation (UPIAS) declares that "in our view, it is society which disables physically impaired people" (quoted in Oliver 1996:22). The apparent denial of any causal role to biological factors seems to reflect both a very strong view of entitlement and a very strong technological optimism. Whether it is a morally more appropriate baseline than a "state of nature" is not the issue. In a world of infinite need and limited resources, it is an equally ambiguous or indeterminate one. It is notoriously difficult to assess the limits of technological possibility. Investment in technology yields unpredictable results, and a greater investment at an earlier time might have made possible enhancements in mobility and sensation that now seem fanciful.[7]

It is not clear, however, that the claims of exclusive social causation made by some disability advocates should be taken at face value. Unlike some political philosophers, these advocates appear to recognize the morally and politically contentious character of causal attributions. Thus, the claim that disability is socially caused is seen by some proponents as a reaction against the opposing tendency to treat the disadvantages associated with disability as solely biological. As Tom Shakespeare explains,

> The achievement of the disability movement has been to break the link between our bodies and our social situation, and to focus on the real cause of disability, i.e., discrimination and prejudice. To mention biology, to admit pain, to confront our impairments, has been to risk the oppressors' seizing on evidence that disability is "really" about physical limitation after all. (Quoted in Oliver 1996:39)

This passage suggests that the claim of exclusive social causation is a calculated overstatement, a corrective for the opposing and more damaging misrepresentation, but the analysis of causation also really involves the attribution of moral and political responsibility. These suggestions are made more explicit by Amundson (2000):

> Causation is a complicated thing. We pick out one antecedent event or condition and baptize it as *the cause* of a phenomenon. Different perspectives, different theoretically orien-

tations, of different prejudices can lead to the baptism of different events as *the cause*. The Social model of disability never identifies the biomedical condition as *the cause* of that person's disadvantages. The causes are always identified in the environment and the social context. A critic might dismiss this approach as politically motivated and therefore not scientifically objective. But consider the alternative. . . . Philosophers and medical practitioners have used the category [biological normality] to conclude that the disadvantages of disabled people result from their own abnormality. They have only themselves (and nature) to blame. Is *this* assessment scientifically objective? (P. 29)

The answer to Amundson's question, of course, is that neither assessment is scientifically objective. Instead of choosing the politically more congenial oversimplification, it would be preferable to reject the false dichotomy between biology and society as *the cause* of disability and to break the link between causation and responsibility—to hold society responsible for the alleviation of disadvantage, whether it can be said to have caused it or not.[8]

Even if we had some basis for attributing the disadvantages associated with impairments to natural causes, it would hardly mean that the individuals were to blame or that their alleviation was not society's responsibility. As long as those disadvantages were not voluntarily chosen or risked, their source or locus will have no direct relevance on most plausible accounts of distributive justice. What will matter on those accounts is the cost to others of alleviating those disadvantages and the possible intrusiveness or indignity of particular forms of alleviation. Yet those considerations will have only a tenuous relationship with the attribution of those disadvantages to natural or social causes. There may be good reasons for favoring one kind of intervention over the other, particularly for modifying the environment rather than the individual (although the distinction between the two will not always be clear). It may be more respectful, dignified, or effective. But the fact that a disadvantage can be attributed to natural causes hardly means that it is not amenable to environmental modification.

WHAT, IF ANYTHING, IS BAD ABOUT IMPAIRMENTS? DO IMPAIRMENTS DETRACT FROM WELL-BEING?

Philosophers, as we have seen, disagree about whether the classification of a physical or mental condition as an impairment implies a judgment that it is undesirable and about the extent to which impairments can be said to cause the disadvantages associated with them. In discussing these issues, I have deferred, or sidestepped, the obvious and important issues of what makes a physical or mental feature undesirable and what counts as a disadvantage.

The two sets of issues are connected in the following way: the more general or abstract the description of a desirable state or condition, the more tenuous or limited the causal role of impairment appears to be.[9] Thus, various neuromuscular impairments appear to affect the ability to move one's limbs more directly than they affect the ability to get around. Yet even the ability to move one's limbs is environmentally mediated. On Jupiter, none of us could move our legs very well or far without assistive devices; on Earth, a person with a neuromuscular impairment could move his or her legs with the right assistive device. As I argued in the last section, it is difficult to be more precise about the intuition that the causal role of impairments is more direct in the case of some actions or states than in others. Certain impairments may contribute definitionally to the absence of certain activities (e.g., the absence of limbs to voluntary arm or leg movements). But even if the connection is not a matter of definition, there may be no known or achievable environment in which a person with a given anatomical or physiological impairment could engage in particular action. It is certainly worth asking what loss of value he or she would thereby experience. And even when the connection is more contingent than this, it makes sense to ask what, if anything, is desirable or valuable about the various personal and social activities that impairments play some role in limiting.

Philosophers have addressed such questions at length, though rarely under the rubric of disability. They have typically debated the more general questions about what makes a life go well, how or whether we can measure well-being and compare the well-being of different individuals, and whether certain forms of well-being matter more for certain purposes, such as political justice (Pogge 1999). These questions have been of special interest to philosophers who embrace some form of utilitarianism because they base the moral appraisal of actions on the evaluation of their (expected) outcomes. Yet many nonutilitarian philosophers have addressed these questions as well, especially those who adopt what Robert Nozick (1974) has called "end-state" conceptions of justice, in which the justice of a society or cooperative scheme depends to some extent on who ends up with what or in what condition.

Historically, utilitarians understood well-being in terms of pleasure or happiness, without regard to the ways in which individuals achieved those states. Contemporary welfare economists have tended to adopt the less psychological, even more general, metric of preference-satisfaction, without regard to the specific preferences chosen or the ways they are satisfied. Recent utilitarian philosophers have been drawn to constrained preference and desire-satisfaction accounts, which count only the preferences or desires that an individual would have with full or adequate information. Despite considerable differences among them, these accounts of well-being are all subjective in two senses. First, they define well-being in terms of psychological states, such as pleasure and desire, or psychological constructs, such as preferences. Second, they involve no judgment about the objective worth or value of different sources of pleasure or happiness or different objects of (informed) preference or desire. (Preference or desire accounts may be objective in another sense, in treating the satisfaction of preferences as a matter of fact, about which the preference holder can be mistaken. Informed preference and desire accounts may also be objective in imposing a high standard of knowledge or rationality on the preference formation process.)[10]

More objective conceptions understand human well-being in terms of states or activities that are valuable "in themselves," whether or not anyone values them and whether or not they yield pleasure or happiness (although pleasure or happiness may be among the objectively valuable states, and well-being may require or even consist of taking pleasure in objectively valuable activities). What counts as valuable may be determined by ideals of human perfection; by the telos of humanity, revealed in theology, biology, or history; or by critical generalizations about what people have found valuable across times, places, and cultures. Objective accounts vary in the specificity with which they describe what is valuable for people and in the extent to which they emphasize valuable experiences or activities or the opportunity or capacity for such experiences or activities. Distinguishing subjective and objective accounts can be difficult since the constraints imposed on informed desire and belief accounts may bring them into rough correspondence with some objective ones, while objective accounts may rely heavily on what people actually desire or have desired in determining what is desirable or worthy. Moreover, some metrics of well-being appear to have an irreducibly hybrid character, such as opportunity for welfare (where "opportunity" is not based on the individual's own unconstrained probability judgments).

On subjective conceptions of well-being, the impact of impairments is largely contingent. With the exception of impairments that are defined in terms of pain, unhappiness, or frustration or that involve limitations in the capacity to form coherent and stable preferences or desires, people with impairments can have as much pleasure, happiness, or satisfaction as people without them, and research on subjective well-being suggests that they often do. Indeed, some philosophers regard this as a reason for rejecting subjective accounts. They see the "happy cripple" as a *reductio ad absurdum* of any view that regards subjective states as the primary constituents of well-being (see Crocker 1995; Sen 1980). Not surprisingly, some disability scholars have been drawn to subjective metrics out of a concern that more objective accounts of well-being place it beyond the reach of people with impairments. It is not clear, however, that objective accounts must render the adverse judgments about impairments that are often made in specific arguments for those accounts.

In examining how impairments fare on objective accounts of well-being, it will be useful to consider two influential but problematic distinctions: between intrinsic and instrumental value and between basic and nonbasic action. The first distinction is integral to the commonsense explanation of motivation and behavior. An activity may be valued instrumentally because of what it brings about, contributes to, or facilitates, or it may be valued intrinsically in itself. As intuitive as the distinction is, it can be hard to make—in part because there is deep disagreement about what is of ultimate value, in part because it is possible to parse many activities and states almost indefinitely into instrumentally valued means and intrinsically valued ends. For example, making money or friends can be seen as an end in itself or as a means to obtaining comfort and security.

The interactive approach to disability encourages the parsing of activities in this manner. Thus, for example, much of what we value in talking, seeing, and walking is instrumental. We value them as ways of achieving communication with other people, reading, and moving from place to place—activities we regard as valuable in themselves. (Of course, we also recognize that these activities have instrumental value as well, e.g., for finding social partners and business opportunities.) None of these intrinsically valuable activities is precluded by deafness, blindness, or paraplegia; each can be achieved in alternative ways, by signing, reading Braille, or operating a wheelchair.

This parsing of activities into instrumentally valued means and intrinsically valued ends is often informed by a hierarchical conception of action, in which simpler actions, more fully under our control, generate more complex actions, whose successful completion is more dependant on environmental factors. A general characterization of this hierarchy can be made with reference to a distinction philosophers have debated for decades. This is the distinction between basic actions, which a person does not do by doing anything else but "just does," and nonbasic or generated actions, which a person does by doing other actions, ultimately—on pain of regress—basic ones. Nonbasic actions can be generated causally. I make a breeze by waving my hand. Or they can be generated conventionally. I say goodbye by waving my hand, but I do not, or need not, do anything else to wave my hand (Danto 1965; Goldman 1970). This is an intuitively appealing notion that seems helpful in clarifying how impairments are associated with the loss or absence of intrinsic value. As I suggested earlier, impairments may preclude basic actions definitionally; that is, whatever distinctive value there is in moving one's legs and eyes is precluded by impairments that involve the absence of the anatomical structure necessary for walking or seeing. Contingently, a neuromuscular impairment may prevent limb movement in all known environments. In either case, impairments can be said to deny the value that inheres in the basic actions they preclude.[11] Blindness does not preclude reading, but it does preclude seeing; deafness does not preclude communication, but it does preclude hearing; leg paralysis does not preclude mobility, but it does preclude walking and running.[12] Impairments may also be thought to be disadvantageous instrumentally, in limiting the stock of basic actions with which the individual can generate other, more valuable or advantageous actions.

Some philosophers, however, doubt that we can give an adequate account of basic actions (e.g., Candlish 1984); others have argued that the actions, which are truly basic, are mental events such as volitions (e.g., Hornsby 1980), which seem relatively immune from or less directly vulnerable to (physical) impairments. And even those philosophers who accept a notion of basic action, under which many such actions are precluded by particular impairments, differ about the extent to which the precluded actions are a source of instrumental or intrinsic value. Several philosophers have argued that, at least in technologically advanced societies, most of the actions we value intrinsically are nonbasic and can be generated with widely varying sets of basic actions. Thus, Steven Edwards (1997) argues that

> basic actions are not interesting in their own right, but only in so far as they have an effect at the level of persons.... [But] a person may still be able to perform an extensive range of types of actions whether or not it is possible to perform a particular range of basic actions. (Pp. 602-3)

Similarly, John Dupre (1998) maintains that

> most of the significant capacities of even fully able people are contextually determined.
> . . . Indeed, as far as mobility goes, it is surely the case that the financial resources neces-
> sary for access to cars, train tickets, or plane fares are far more determinative than are con-
> trol over one's limbs. Similar remarks apply to sensory limitations of sight or hearing. In
> summary, though it is no doubt uncommon to lack the use of one's legs or the evidence of
> one's eyes, and although such deficits are hugely inconvenient to those who suffer from
> them, such deficits should not be seen as more than some among a range of characteristics
> that determine the vastly diverse range of capacities of different people in different societ-
> ies. (Pp. 230-31)

Other philosophers regard these claims as too extreme. They do not deny the availability of
alternate means of generating the kinds of activity people value; they merely claim that the instrumental importance of the standard set of basic actions can be underestimated. Even if there
are alternative ways of generating less basic activities, they may be less effective, more expensive, or costlier in less tangible ways. Thus, Nordenfelt (1997) argues,

> There may be one type of basic action which is the dominant means for realizing a certain
> endstate, and where we cannot see a good replacement. It is, admittedly, rarely the case
> that the favored basic action is absolutely necessary for achieving the desired end. The ac-
> tion may in practice, however, be necessary, given the way society works; or it may be the
> only way that can lead to the desired state in an expedient and efficient manner, given the
> way society works. (P. 617)

Nordenfelt (1997) gives the example of the hand and finger movement involved in signing a
wide range of documents. The comparative difficulty of executing a document without manu-
ally signing depends, of course, on existing social practices and technology, and a reduction in
comparative difficulty may be claimed as a matter of justice. However, in assessing this claim of
justice, it is also necessary to weigh the cost to others in modifying existing social practices and
technology. It would surely count as instrumentally disadvantageous if those costs were very
high "given the way society works."
    There is disagreement about the intrinsic and instrumental value of many standard sensory
and motor functions and the actions closely associated with them—seeing, hearing, and walking. One threshold issue is whether the value in such functions and actions inheres in their exercise or performance or in the "internal" experience they yield. If the latter, then the value of
those functions and actions themselves would be instrumental, and the loss of value from their
impairment would be contingent. Examples such as Nozick's (1974) "experience machine,"
which faithfully simulates the experience of climbing a mountain and reaching its summit, suggest that what matters is not just the experience but attaining it *through* certain actions. This intuition, however, may be stronger for experiences that are also achievements, such as mountain
climbing, for which simulation seems to be a form of cheating. It is not clear that we would find
a similar loss of intrinsic value in the simulation of more a passive experience, such as experiencing the programmed arousal of the acoustical centers of the brain to produce the sensations
of listening to a symphony versus listening to a digital recording of that symphony—at least if
the simulation were shaped by the actual symphony performance to the same extent as the digital recording. Yet it may not be clear whether a symphony could be simulated or how it could be
judged to be successfully simulated for someone who was congenitally deaf. Also, it may not
make sense to talk about the simulation of cognitive functions and activities, such as imaging,
imagining, and reasoning, since it may be impossible to distinguish their simulation from their
occurrence.
    Setting aside the issue of simulated experience, it is hard to deny that many standard sensory
and motor functions or the activities closely associated with them have intrinsic value. But it is
almost as hard to assess how the absence of that value affects overall well-being. One obvious

source of intrinsic value for standard sensory functions and activities, for example, is aesthetic—their beauty, richness, and complexity. But we do not regard color blindness, tone deafness, or impairments of smell or taste as inimical to well-being, although they preclude vast ranges of rich aesthetic experience. We generally assume that people who have never had those sensory functions (as opposed to, say, an artist or food critic dependent on his or her daily exercise) can lead perfectly good lives without such admittedly valuable experiences. This suggests that we cannot infer from the fact that there is great intrinsic value in a basic action that those who cannot perform that action have lives with significantly less intrinsic value. As Silvers, Wasserman, and Mahowald (1998) argue,

> Things have intrinsic value when we esteem them for themselves or, more precisely, for the character of the direct experience of them. It might seem to follow, then, that the absence of intrinsically valuable experience might be deleterious, injurious, or disadvantageous. But this inference is incorrect. Indeed, missing one kind of experience can enhance the quality of the remaining kinds. (P. 89)

Silvers et al. (1998) claim that once we distinguish the absence from the loss of valuable sensory and motor experiences, there is no reason to believe that the absence of intrinsically good experiences is intrinsically bad. They note that the value of sensory and motor experiences increases with the attention we are able to devote to them and that a smaller range of experience may permit greater concentration. Silvers et al. also observe that we do not make the assumption that unimpaired people who can, but do not, have particular sensory or motor experiences necessarily lead impoverished lives.

It may be that arguments such as Silvers et al.'s (1998) take an overly narrow view of the intrinsic value to be found in certain sensory and motor functions. As Magee and Milligan (1995) argue,

> The practical usefulness of seeing plus its power to provide aesthetic pleasure come nowhere near to accounting for the awed value that sighted people place on it. There are several other large ingredients. One, of course, is the sheer avidity of the desire to see. . . . This has no parallel with the senses of hearing, taste, or smell; we are under no slavish compulsion to be hearing sounds all the time, or tasting tastes, or smelling smells. However, there might be a similarity with the fifth remaining sense, that of touch. (P. 105)

Magee and Milligan (1995) go on to suggest a second "ingredient"—that seeing and touch link us to the world more directly and closely than do the other senses and that their loss involves a profound isolation from physical and social reality (Magee and Milligan 1995:105-6). It is not clear, however, that we need *both* seeing and touch to avoid such isolation[13] or that any of the other senses has comparable importance.

A more general claim about the relevance of impairment to well-being has been made by several recent philosophers. Martha Nussbaum (1990), for example, maintains that having some form of sense perception and mobility is necessary for humanity and that "being able to move from place to place" and "being able to use the five senses" are essential to human flourishing (Crocker 1995:170-80; Nussbaum 1990:219, 225). Nussbaum, however, does little to justify these claims. She views them as generalizations derived from and supported by "a wide variety of self-understandings of people in many times and places" (Crocker 1995:171; Nussbaum 1992). Our conception of human flourishing, she maintains, has evolved around the standard complement of human functions, and we cannot step outside of our collective experience to demand a freestanding justification.

Yet without more specific argument about the role of specific functions in our relationship to the physical world or to other people, we have no way of resolving conflict about the importance of those functions or of addressing the charge that the consensus "of people in many times and places" reflects nothing more than widespread prejudice or error. To respond, for example, to the claim of deaf activists that people's lives can go as well without hearing as with it,

Nussbaum could not merely assert what no one would deny—that there is great aesthetic value in hearing. Without claiming that hearing is essential for some broader social or intellectual good, a claim that would almost certainly be false, it is unclear what Nussbaum could argue. More broadly, as Jerome Segal (1998) points out, we can hardly deny that some people flourish without many of the capabilities Nussbaum seems to regard as essential. The most successful lives of people lacking those capabilities appear to go as well as the most successful lives of people with a standard complement of sensory and motor functions. While a life could hardly go well without at least some of the capacities Nussbaum enumerates, we have no clear basis for establishing a minimum set.

An alternative to the dogmatic enumeration of essential human goods is suggested by Sen's (1993, 1980) approach to capabilities as a metric of positive freedom. Instead of insisting that any particular function is necessary for well-being, Sen places a more abstract emphasis on positive freedom as a good in itself. This emphasis suggests that the greater the number of valuable functionings we have the capability to engage in, the better off we are, even if we do and can engage in only a limited number of them. If there is intrinsic value in the opportunity or positive freedom to do as many activities as possible, in as many different ways as possible, then impairments may be intrinsically undesirable in reducing our range of opportunity. But it is unclear why there should be greater intrinsic value in larger "capability sets," beyond some minimum needed to ensure a meaningful choice among different options. It may be wrong for the government to limit people's options on the basis of a parochial or contested view of human flourishing, but it is not necessarily bad for a person to face life with a narrower than average but still capacious set of options. An emphasis on positive freedom, like an emphasis on material goods, can become obsessive or fetishistic.

The difficulties in finding an appropriate metric of well-being suggest that no single metric may be appropriate for all purposes. Several philosophers (e.g., Griffin 1993, 1986) have suggested that different conceptions of well-being are appropriate in different contexts. For example, it may be more appropriate to adopt a comprehensive, value-laden conception in assessing how one's own life is going, or would go, than to allocate resources based on relative disadvantage. Thomas Scanlon (1998) has contended that well-being is not the "master value" it is assumed to be by some philosophers who are primarily, but not exclusively, consequentialists. He argues that from the first-person point of view, "the things that contribute to (one's own) well-being are obviously important, but the concept of well-being plays very little role in explaining why they are important" (p. 142). It is simply an "inclusive" concept encompassing many or most of the person's specific aims and concerns. From a third-person point of view, some but not all aspects of well-being matter. For instance, a parent or guardian will be concerned about specific ways in which things go well or badly for his or her charges, while a political society or cooperative scheme may be obliged to promote or equalize some aspects of well-being but not others.

So perhaps we do not need a general answer to the question of how impairments affect well-being. What matters to the individual are his or her aims and special concerns; what matters to the society to which he or she belongs are those aspects of well-being that are a source of political obligation, and that may be quite distinct from what matters to the individual and his or her family or friends. In the next section, I will focus on the question of how impairments affect what we owe each other as a matter of justice.

HOW ARE IMPAIRMENTS RELEVANT TO SOCIAL AND POLITICAL JUSTICE?

The question of whether or how much impairments reduce well-being has often been conducted in the shadow of the more general debate about how well-being is relevant to the allocation of resources and to the design of society. In denying that impairments reduce well-being, some disability advocates may be responding to the perceived consequences of conceding that they do reduce well-being. This is seen in the assignment of low priority to the lives of impaired people in choices among lives and the assignment of high priority to the often unwelcomed medical "correction" of impairments. Disagreements about the impact of impairments on various aspects well-being might be more tractable if they were not seen as having such questionable distributive implications.

Nowhere are the implications of impairment for resource allocation starker or more controversial than in utilitarian accounts of health care decision making. In its classical form, utilitarianism assesses the value of lives by the pleasure, happiness, or satisfaction they contain and produce and judges decisions among lives by their impact on the sum of pleasure, happiness, or satisfaction in the world. Individuals matter only as bearers and producers of utility: The more utility they gain or produce from a resource, the stronger their claim to it. To the extent that impairments reduce utility, the preservation of the lives of people with disabilities has lower priority; to the extent that the correction of impairments increases utility, the medical treatment of people with impairments has higher priority.

The classical utilitarian calculus provides apparently straightforward, if often unpalatable, answers to questions about creating and extending lives. If the birth of an impaired child increases overall utility, the child should be born, unless its "replacement" by a child without an impairment would increase utility even more (see, e.g., Kuhse and Singer 1985). If a hospital can save the life of two disabled people or one nondisabled person, but not both, it should save the nondisabled person if his or her life would be sufficiently longer, happier, or more productive (see Brock 1995, 1997; Daniels 1997; Murray 1996).

Some utilitarians attempt to deny these implications by insisting that it is necessary to consider the full range of consequences—not only the length and quality of the lives immediately at stake but also the possibility of mistaken judgments about length and quality, as well as the distrust and demoralization that would result from the use of a utilitarian decision criterion. Other utilitarians, while not denying that all such consequences must be taken into account, are more inclined to challenge than accommodate popular sentiment. Among the latter, by far the most prominent and controversial is Peter Singer (1993), who has proposed that parents be allowed to let severely impaired newborns die. Singer's (1999) conviction is that "philosophy ought to question the basic assumptions of age" (p. 466), whether the assumption that *only* humans matter morally or the assumption that *all* humans matter to the same extent. Singer's challenge to the former has made him a champion to many in the animal rights movement, while his challenge to the latter has made him a nemesis to many in the disability rights movement. The consistency Singer claims for these positions may be superficial or foolish, but his vigorous advocacy has challenged opponents to articulate their own conceptions of equality more clearly.

Utilitarianism is often thought to demean the lives of people with disabilities. Yet it gives equal weight to the utility of all persons and favors the interests of people with disabilities in any context where their relative disadvantage promises high marginal utility for interventions on their behalf. Unlike some of the egalitarian and "prioritarian" theories of justice I will discuss below, it does not treat people with impairment as special cases. It takes an equally calculating and instrumental view of all lives. Moreover, the interpersonal comparison and aggregation mandated by utilitarianism seem difficult to banish altogether from theories of justice since considerations of aggregate well-being exercise a powerful intuitive constraint on the reduction of inequality and the improvement of the position of the worst off.

For political philosophers committed to equalizing rather than maximizing well-being, people with lower well-being generally have stronger claims to resources. To the extent that impairments reduce well-being, people with impairments have priority for both life-extending and life-enhancing resources. Philosophers with such egalitarian commitments have often assumed that physical impairments such as paraplegia and blindness dramatically reduce well-being because functions such as seeing and walking are critical for a wide variety of life plans. They have proposed a variety of special provisions to compensate for the absence of those functions, from a cash allowance approximating the insurance that people with impairments would have purchased against their deficits in hypothetical circumstances (Dworkin 1981) to an unlimited allowance to restore them to normal functioning (Daniels 1986, 1990).[14]

Disability advocates have not been much happier with the high priority accorded by egalitarian approaches to people with impairments on the basis of their presumed disadvantage than with the low priority accorded them by utilitarian approaches on the basis of their presumed misery. The inappropriateness of standard egalitarian provisions for disability has led some disability advocates to regard egalitarian justice as part of the problem, not the solution. They have concluded that any theory of political justice that sees its mission as equalizing people or reducing inequality on some metric of well-being or advantage will inevitably demean those it regards as disadvantaged.

In the remainder of this section, I will discuss three responses to these misgivings, suggested by three critiques of egalitarian theories of distributive justice. While these critiques have not, for the most part, been informed by the complaints of disability advocates, they reflect similar concerns. The first, friendliest critique is that egalitarian theories have set about equalizing the wrong thing, either external resources or subjective welfare. An individual's share of material resources is not the appropriate metric of advantage for purposes of political justice, nor is her or his happiness or satisfaction. People with impairments are poorly served by both metrics: Equality in individual resources takes no account of the disabling effect of the physical and social environment and tends to exaggerate the limitations of people with impairments, while equality in welfare ignores those limitations altogether. What is needed is a metric that takes into account differences in functioning by recognizing claims to environmental adaptation.

The second, most hostile critique calls into question the very idea of justice as principally concerned with the distribution of resources or the well-being of individuals. Some philosophers have argued that distributive accounts make inappropriate provisions for disability because they fail to recognize the locus of injustice for people with impairments. In focusing on the symptoms of material disadvantage, distributive justice ignores the underlying structural causes: oppressive and exploitative economic, social, and political relations among groups. Disparities in material resources across social groups may be important evidence of oppression and exploitation, but they have no independent significance. In addition, heroic efforts to extend distributive justice beyond material resources to intangible, participatory, and collective goods are futile; they merely "reify" concerns that are properly understood as relational and procedural, in terms of oppression and domination, not maldistribution (Young 1990).[15]

In its application to impairments, this approach focuses on their character as stigma rather than as causes of functional limitation. Impairments are of concern to justice not because of any direct or proximate effect they have on the performance or well-being of the impaired but because they are, like skin color or ancestry, the markers of an oppressed and subordinated social group. Justice for people with impairments requires the transformation of these relationships. Any change in the share of resources assigned to people in an oppressed group would be a by-product of that more fundamental change.

A third critique attempts to steer a middle course between justice as equality in resources, welfare, opportunities, or capabilities and justice as the absence of oppression and domination in social structures and relationships. Justice must be understood primarily in social and political terms, as a matter of equal citizenship. On this approach, impairments are relevant to justice only to the extent that people with impairments are not treated as equal citizens, not in the more pervasive way they are to utilitarian and some egalitarian accounts. The philosophers who argue for a distinct notion of political equality claim or assume that such equality imposes a threshold that can be reached or exceeded by almost everyone in modern postindustrial societies. They claim that equality is not an elusive goal whose partial achievement must be balanced against other values and whose pursuit requires intrusive and insulting assessments of individual well-being.

The next three subsections examine the adequacy of these competing approaches for disability policy. They consider

1. whether distributive justice is broad or flexible enough to encompass environmental adaptation;
2. whether nondistributive approaches to justice have the resources to prescribe appropriate modifications in the physical and social environment, without recourse to distributive considerations; and
3. whether an account of justice, in terms of political equality, can successfully combine distributive and nondistributive considerations relevant to disability.

Can Distributive Justice Encompass Claims for Environmental Adaptation?

In debates over the appropriate conception of well-being or comparative advantage for distributive justice, impairments are often presented as hard cases. Both the profound misery of the blind and the crippled and their unaccountable euphoria are invoked to criticize various metrics as demanding too much or too little for the disabled or of the able-bodied (Cohen 1989; Dworkin 1981; Sen 1980). The caricatured picture of impairments that informs these debates has led some philosophers and disability advocates to conclude that merely framing the issue of justice for people with impairments in distributive terms is to present them as defective and helpless (e.g., Silvers 1994).

While this conclusion is understandable, it is too sweeping. The treatment of impairments as a problem of deficient natural endowment is not dictated by a distributive conception of justice; it arises in part from a failure to appreciate the interactive character of disability. An awareness of the myriad ways that individuals' environment and goals mediate the impact of their impairment on their well-being would surely reduce the temptation to assume that their misery was inconsolable, their euphoria unreasonable, or their needs inexhaustible (see, e.g., Albrecht and Devlieger 1999). Thus, the assumption that people with impairments invariably require a significantly larger bundle of resources to pursue their (reasonable) life plans reflects a failure to take into account the disabling effects of what Hahn (1999) has aptly described as the "taken-for-granted" environment and of the enabling effects of environmental adaptations.

The question, however, is whether claims to greater environmental adaptation can be captured by a theory of distributive justice. Typically, such theories have sought to equalize or reduce inequalities in the resources possessed or controlled by individuals or their welfare, that is, their pleasure, happiness, or satisfaction.[16] It is difficult to express claims for environmental reconstruction in terms of either a resource or a welfare metric.

Theories of justice that take resources as the metric of comparative advantage tend to take the environment for granted. The (hypothetical) division of resources into individual bundles takes place either within the present scheme of social cooperation and economic production or else in a state of nature that is assumed to evolve into a scheme such as the present one through transactions among the equally endowed participants. Giving people with impairments equal economic shares in a society constructed as our own, with a physical environment and social practices designed for people with standard endowments, might improve their material circumstances, but it would be likely to leave them at the margins of society.

It is doubtful that any approach to justice based on the partition and allocation of external or material resources could give people with impairments an adequate say in the design of the physical and social environment to bring them into the mainstream of social activity and political decision making. In failing to provide an accommodating environment, a scheme of resource equality might, as disability advocates fear, legitimize the inferior status of people with impairments, as individuals disadvantaged by deficits in natural endowment, not in external resources.[17] A resource metric can only respond to these concerns with more of the same, giving people with impairments larger bundles of goods or special compensation for their inefficiency in converting those goods to their own purposes by a cash allowance or medical correction.

Theories of justice that take welfare as the metric of comparative advantage do not require or encourage such special treatment for people with impairments. They either defer to the individual's own assessment of how she or he is doing or else base her or his status on some independent measure of her or his pleasure, happiness, or preference satisfaction. However, welfare approaches seem manifestly unsatisfactory as a basis for determining political obligations or what we owe each other as members of the same political community. It seems intuitively unfair that we should owe more to those who, because of extravagance or self-importance, would be miserable with less, or less to those who, because of self-denial or self-denigration, would be happy with very little. While the euphoria of a blind or paraplegic person should hardly be taken as a *reductio ad absurdum* of a welfare approach (that euphoria may be entirely warranted), it does suggest a stronger, more general objection to welfare metrics. Even if extreme misery or frustration is a concern of justice, what we owe each other is not some level of happiness or satisfaction but a reasonable means to lead a happy and satisfying life. Moreover, the assessment of individual welfare for distributive purposes would seem likely to be a particularly intrusive, demeaning, and unreliable process. An adequate theory of political obligation requires a more objective metric of human flourishing.

Recent political philosophers have been keenly aware of the inadequacy of both resource and welfare metrics. They have proposed a variety of alternative metrics that assess well-being for purposes of distributive justice not, or not only, in terms of what the individual has or feels but also in terms of his or her opportunities, capacities, or activities in terms of opportunity for welfare (Arneson 1989, 1990), access to various kinds of advantage (Cohen 1989), or range of capabilities (Sen 1980; Nussbaum 1990).[18] These "midfare" metrics (Cohen's 1993 term) are more objective than welfare metrics in looking beyond the individual's feelings or preferences to assess her or his comparative advantage, but they are more individualized than resource metrics in looking at what a person can do with the resources at his or her disposal. Although they regard impairments as undesirable to the extent that they limit opportunity or access or preclude valuable activities, they also treat the physical and social environment as a source of disadvantage and underwrite claims to environmental modification.

Perhaps the most comprehensive metric for assessing comparative advantage for purposes of political justice is offered by the capabilities approach of Sen and Nussbaum, discussed in the last section. Their approach does treat impairments as inherently undesirable in precluding valuable functions or capacities, such as seeing, hearing, or walking. But most of the capabilities regarded as essential or important bear a highly contingent, environmentally mediated relationship to impairments. Thus, for example, the capabilities approach abstracts from the physical differences between people with limb impairments and normal limb function to find a common claim to the means of moving about from place to place. Those means will often but not always be the same for both; they may be architectural, vehicular, mechanical, or prosthetic, or they may involve making places more accessible or making the individual more mobile. In some circumstances, it may well be more difficult or costly for people with limb impairments to achieve or maintain that capability, but the difference will not be a categorical one. In general, the capabilities approach and other midfare metrics allow the disadvantages of people with impairments to be seen as problems of environmental fit rather than deficient endowment.

A recognition of the critical role played by the environment in creating and alleviating disability is found not only in the development of more flexible or comprehensive metrics of well-being but also in the analysis of social and technological changes that affect the participation of people with impairments. Several philosophers have observed that social decisions and policies about the deployment of new technology and the design of social rules and practices make impairments more or less disabling (Buchanan 1996; see also Silvers and Wasserman 1998; Wikler 1979). The introduction of the telephone and Windows software, the raising and lowering of competence standards for legal responsibilities and social activities, and the modification of requirements for earning a college degree or playing in a golf tournament have all had profound effects on the access and participation of people with various impairments. In each case, there appears to be a conflict between the inclusion of some and the satisfaction of others—a quintessential problem of distributive justice. A society could develop an indefinite number of cooperative schemes and social practices that would be more or less inclusionary, rewarding, and productive. No doubt some of the alleged trade-offs are avoidable, and others are exaggerated. However, there will inevitably be trade-offs, and an adequate theory of distributive justice is needed to resolve them on a principled basis.

To provide such guidance, one must enlarge that subject matter of a theory of distributive justice without losing focus on individual outcomes. Although such a theory must be comparative, concerned with how the members of a society are faring relative to each other, it need not and often cannot be achieved through individual allocations; it may require changes in the structure and organization of society.[19] Such changes are required not only for people with impairments but also for people who belong to minority cultures, for people who possess obsolete skills, and, more broadly, for people who value goods that can be realized only in social institutions and practices. Thus, for example, similar issues of environmental modification arise in deciding how to accommodate atypical functions and minority languages; they arise for users of American Sign Language as well as for speakers of Spanish or Chinese. The fact that Spanish- and Chinese-speaking children learn Standard English more easily than deaf children may be relevant to the way the issues are resolved, but it does not change their fundamental character. Assimilation may be possible for deaf as well as for Spanish and Chinese children through oralism or cochlear implants, and, to the extent that it is possible, it raises similar concerns about cultural survival and intergenerational estrangement. Impairments are merely some of the more significant and conspicuous variations that a just society must accommodate.

The rejection of a distinction between natural/internal and social/external causes of disadvantage will, if anything, sharpen the conflicts over environmental accommodation because the claims of people with impairments cannot be accorded lower priority on the grounds that they concern naturally occurring disadvantages.[20] Yet if such claims cannot be treated as less urgent than those of able-bodied people, they will not necessarily prevail against conflicting claims. Environmental modifications can be very expensive, and modifications that serve people with one type of impairment may be useless or inconvenient for those with other impairments or for nonimpaired people.

Thus, consider the issue of how to educate and support people with severe cognitive and developmental impairments. It is, of course, important to recognize that the classification of cognitive limitation may be driven by the economic demands of modern industrial and postindustrial societies and that the disadvantages associated with the levels and styles of mental functioning, classified as impairments, are largely due to the failure to accommodate atypical functioning in the design of educational institutions, the provision of caregiving services, and the structuring of jobs. However, we still need to decide how to redesign our educational, caregiving, and employment institutions to fairly accommodate people classified as cognitively and developmentally impaired. It would be naive to assume that the designs that best serve those individuals will best serve individuals with normal or superior cognitive functioning or will have no adverse impact on productivity, safety, wealth, or other values and concerns.

More broadly, it is likely that we will have to choose between cooperative schemes that have higher average or total well-being on any metric, not based exclusively on material goods, and schemes that have smaller disparities in well-being. People with impairments have often been unfairly typecast to illustrate this conundrum, but a less distorted view of impairment would hardly eliminate it. Some philosophers have responded to the obvious difficulty of achieving equality on any adequate metric of well-being by arguing that equality needs to be balanced against other values, such as beneficence. Others have argued for giving priority to the worst off rather than attempting a general reduction in inequality (Parfit 1997). Just as egalitarian accounts must decide how much inequality to tolerate for the sake of other values, "prioritarian" accounts must decide how much priority to accord the worst off at the expense of such values. The moral uncertainty of these trade-offs is as daunting as the individualized assessment of well-being they require.

Can Justice for People with Impairments Be Achieved
by Eliminating Discrimination against Them or, More
Broadly, by Eliminating Oppression and Subordination?

The complexities of more comprehensive theories of distributive justice have a moral cost. They appear to diminish the urgency of the pursuit of justice by shifting its focus away from the elimination of great social evils—slavery, caste, political repression, child labor—to the pursuit of an elusive goal with debatable criteria. Much of the appeal of procedural or relational accounts of justice,[21] which focus on such specific evils, is that they seem to capture the moral importance of justice better than the abstract assessment of outcome disparities.

The strengths and limitations of a relational account of justice for disability policy, based on the elimination of oppressive attitudes, practices, and structures, are suggested by the antidiscrimination approach taken by the Americans with Disabilities Act of 1990. While that approach does not embody a complete relational theory of justice for people with impairments, it treats the locus of injustice as the underlying attitudes of contempt and devaluation, as well as their pervasive structural and institutional manifestations. It relies on and extends the broad notion of discrimination that has evolved in American civil rights law over the past generation, treating impairments as the markers of an oppressed social group. The antidiscrimination approach identifies a core evil in the treatment of people with impairments and provides effective means of responding to it. Yet as a social policy for disability, it is, as I will conclude, radically incomplete.[22]

Several philosophers and legal scholars have argued that the core notion of discrimination that informs recent American civil rights law involves contempt or devaluation of individuals based on their membership in a social group (Wasserman 1998). For more than 30 years since the passage of the 1964 Civil Rights Act, this notion has been enlarged by legislation, judicial decisions, and legal commentary to cover not only deliberately unfavorable treatment based on hatred or contempt but also the long-term and institutional effects of intentional discrimination and the "facially neutral" practices that embody or perpetuate it.[23]

The analysis of discrimination, as embedded in ostensibly neutral norms and standards, owes much to the feminist critique of earlier civil rights law, with its narrow focus on the direct and indirect effects of intentional discrimination (see Rebell 1986). Feminists have argued that the design of physical structures and social practices for one group—able-bodied males—constitutes a significant form of discrimination against the rest.

If the structures and practices of our society embody a norm of male functioning, they also embody a norm of healthy functioning. As Susan Wendell (1989) argues,

> Life and work have been structured as though no one of any importance in the public world . . . has to breast feed a baby or look after a sick child. . . . Much of the world is structured as though everyone is physically strong . . . as though everyone can walk, hear and see well. (P. 111)

This position was anticipated a generation ago by Jacobus tenBroek (1966), who argued that the right of the disabled "to live in the world" required comprehensive changes in our physical and social order, not just in the design of buildings and public spaces but also in the duties of care owed by "abled" pedestrians, drivers, common carriers, and property owners to disabled people traveling in public places. The refusal to make these changes denied the disabled their right to live in the world as much as the exclusion of blacks and women from public facilities.

The ADA famously embodies this notion of structural discrimination. It treats the failure to make "reasonable accommodation" for people with disabilities, in the design of buildings and facilities and in the structuring of jobs, as a form of discrimination. It provides exemptions only for undue burdens and for changes that would alter the fundamental nature of the activity.

Some commentators maintain that an antidiscrimination approach is not appropriate for disability because of vast differences in the prevailing attitudes and practices toward different impairments and in the experiences of people with those impairments. Thus, Bickenbach (1996) argues, "Not only are the social responses to different forms of mental and physical difference vastly different, there is almost no commonality of experience, or feelings of solidarity, between people with diverse disabilities" (p. 6).

Because I wish to consider a different question, I will assume, for the sake of argument, that people with impairments face the kind of prejudice necessary to claim discrimination and that many or most of the environmental barriers they face are attributable directly or indirectly to that prejudice.[24] The issue I will address is not whether people with disabilities can be regarded as victims of structural discrimination but whether we can eliminate structural discrimination without the guidance of a substantive theory of justice.

Clearly, the elimination of structural discrimination involves more extensive reconstruction for disabled people than for women. As one judge commented about an early disability discrimination statute,

> What must be done to provide handicapped persons with the same right to utilize mass-transportation facilities as other persons? Does each bus have to have special capacity? Must each seat on each bus be removable? Must the bus routes be changed to provide stops at all hospitals, therapy centers, and nursing homes? Is it required that buses be able to accommodate bedridden persons? (Quoted in Wegner 1984:404)

Even tenBroek (1966) conceded that "the policy of integration has its limitations: it cannot be pushed beyond the physical capacity of the disabled" (p. 914). The limitations are not physical so much as technological and economic. The "physical capacity of the disabled" depends on available technology, and that, in turn, depends on the resources invested in research and implementation. For example, opening doors is "beyond the physical capacity" of many disabled people, but that limitation can be overcome by electric door openers. Securing the right of people with disabilities to "live in the world" involves an indefinite commitment of resources.

An injunction against discrimination does not, by itself, tell us the extent to which we must modify our physical and social environment to accommodate people with disabilities. It is one thing to agree that physical structures and social practices have been designed for those who fall within a very narrow range of physical and mental variation, that this results in part from the devaluation of those outside the range, and that this constitutes a powerful, if unwitting, form of discrimination. It is quite another matter to decide how we should redesign those structures and practices to end discrimination against people who fall outside the range. What norm should we adopt? A requirement that structures and practices be designed to strictly equalize burdens or benefits (e.g., the time to get by public transit from point A to point B) for all people in every conceivable mental or physical condition is obviously problematic, as the judge's comments suggest. A standard based on the structures and practices that we would obtain if we did not devalue people with disabilities would require that we suspend the attitudes we have every reason to regard as entrenched and pervasive.

Even if we could imagine a society in which people with impairments were not devalued, however, that exercise would not yield a determinate standard for structuring the physical and social environment to accommodate the full range of human physical and mental variation. While the members of such a society, free of the prejudices that taint our own judgment, would doubtless condemn many social practices and arrangements to which we are indifferent or inured, they would still need a theory of justice to decide on the practices and arrangements they should adopt for themselves. How would they, for example, design their educational systems and structure their jobs to accommodate people with very limited cognitive functioning? Doubtless, they would find solutions through the rough-and-tumble of their untainted political processes. But it would still make sense to ask if those solutions were just.

This reflects a more general problem with procedural or relational approaches to justice. We can acknowledge that some procedures have criteria for fairness that are independent of the outcomes they produce and that in some contexts, justice may be purely procedural, such that any outcome produced by a fair procedure is ipso facto fair. However, when we are assessing not discrete, context-specific procedures such as lotteries but whole social systems, it is doubtful that we could find procedural or relational criteria—that is, of nondiscrimination, nonoppression, and nonsubordination—adequate to assess the justice of the society and of the outcomes experienced by its members. Even if we could establish and apply such procedural criteria independently of distributive considerations, we could not assume that their satisfaction would always yield just outcomes or that any outcome that seemed intuitively unjust could be traced to an infirmity in social relationships. It is a sociological question whether oppressive and exploitative social relationships must produce great disparities in various kinds of advantage, but it is a conceptual or moral question whether we can judge disparities in advantage as unjust without having traced them to such a relationship. Some philosophers suggest that we cannot. Thus, Richard Norman (1999) argues,

> What is unjust is not the bare fact that some are better off than others, but the facts of *domination* and *exploitation*. These terms are central to the vocabulary of injustice, and they serve to pick out the facts that power is unequally distributed, and that this enables some members of a community to make use of others and to prosper at their expense. (P. 191)

But this seems mistaken if domination and exploitation mean anything more than participation in a social scheme that gives one unjustified advantages. The use of force or deception to create or maintain such advantages (or even an improper reliance on psychological or physical vulnerability) surely makes them more objectionable. Yet they are objectionable even if they are acquired without force or deception (or exploitation, if it means more than participation in a scheme that produces such advantages). There are circumstances in which better-off people will be guilty of tolerating injustice but not of dominating or exploiting worse-off people.

Thus, consider a society earnestly striving for justice, in which better-off people have relinquished many of their perquisites and their claims to them. There may well be reasonable disagreement within that society about what justice requires on issues ranging from the fairness of academic tracking, the acceptability of significant income disparities between managers and workers, and the appropriate level of investment in geriatric medicine. It should be possible to argue that the society had made the wrong decision in any of these areas and was to that extent unjust, without condemning it for domination and exploitation. To deny this possibility is either to make the implausible empirical claim that domination and exploitation are present whenever unjustifiable disparities in outcome are found or else to strip those terms of their opprobrium by *defining* them to be present whenever such disparities are found.

Is an Account of Equality as Equal Citizenship Adequate for Disability Policy?

Several recent political theorists have argued that justice is concerned with equality only in a limited social and political sense. While justice imposes constraints on distribution and on disparities in certain forms of advantage, it does not require equality of resources or welfare, let alone equality on some more comprehensive metric of well-being (Anderson 1999; Miller 1997, 1999). This general point, reminiscent of Scanlon's (1988) suggestion that different conceptions of well-being are appropriate in different contexts, is well made by Richard Norman (1997):

> Egalitarian distribution cannot plausibly be comprehensive, and the idea that it should be is an idea which has standardly incurred the derision of anti-egalitarians. Some people are incurably shy and find it difficult to form deep emotional relationships with others. Some people are emotionally volatile, forming relationships only to destroy them and move on. Some people strike a balance between these extremes. The third group are likely to have

more satisfying lives than those in the first or second group. Is this inequality "a bad thing"? ... The commonsense answer is "That's life." The idea that we ought to redistribute emotional sensitivity (by genetic engineering?) so that everyone has an equally fulfilling emotional life would be a caricature of egalitarianism. (P. 246)

A more modest and appropriate egalitarianism would treat disparities in well-being as relevant to justice only to the extent that they undermined equality in basic social or political roles, in status and participation. Proponents of this narrow notion of political equality see its principle virtue as identifying the core injustice in various social and economic disparities—the denial of equal citizenship—and as avoiding the intrusiveness of more comprehensive egalitarian theories.

I will focus on the recent account of "democratic equality" offered by Elizabeth Anderson (1999) because it draws from both the distributive and the procedural or social relationship approaches discussed above and because it is informed by disability scholarship and has explicit implications for disability policy. Her account suggests that equality, in the sense relevant to justice, can be secured for people of varying physical and mental endowments without quixotic and demeaning attempts to achieve a more comprehensive equality.

Democratic equality, as Anderson (1999) presents it, is an interesting hybrid of distributive and procedural approaches. Like many philosophers who reject comprehensive equality as a social or political imperative (Miller 1997, 1999; Norman 1997, 1999; Young 1990), she sees injustice as something quite distinct from and more egregious than mere unjustified disparities in well-being. She identifies as the core of social and political injustice what others have identified as the core evil of discrimination—the treatment of some people or groups of people as moral inferiors:

> Inegalitarians asserted the justice or necessity of basing social order on a hierarchy of human beings, ranked according to intrinsic worth. Inequality referred not so much to distributions of goods as relations between superior and inferior persons. ... Such unequal social relations generate, and were thought to justify, inequalities in the distributions of freedom, resources, and welfare. (Anderson 1999:312)

Anderson recognizes, however, that the elimination of such hierarchy requires a certain kind of equality among the members of a society, and she attempts to offer a positive account of that equality. She builds on Sen's (1980, 1993) capabilities metric and endorses its emphasis on activity and participation. But she regards only a small set of capabilities as critical for the kind of equality a just society should pursue:

> Negatively, people are entitled to whatever capabilities are necessary to enable them to avoid or escape entanglement in oppressive social relationships. Positively, they are entitled to the capabilities necessary for functioning as equal citizens in a democratic society. (Anderson 1999:317)

The set of capabilities Anderson finds necessary for these purposes is fairly extensive, however:

> To be capable of functioning as an equal citizen involves not just the ability to effectively exercise specifically political rights, but to participate in the various activities of civil society more broadly. ... And functioning in these ways presupposes functioning as a human being. ... To be capable of functioning as a human being requires effective access to the means of sustaining one's biological existence—food, clothing, medical care—and access to the basic conditions of human agency—knowledge of one's circumstances and options, the ability to deliberate about means and ends. (Anderson 1999:317-18)

While this might seem like a tall order, Anderson emphasizes that it does not require equality in many things that people dearly value, such as sensual pleasure, romantic fulfillment, or intellectual stimulation. She argues that her functional democratic orientation to equality avoids the objectionable implications for disability of welfare or resource metrics. It does not seek to compensate people with impairments for their alleged unhappiness or inefficiencies in consumption but to ensure their standing as full citizens:

> Democratic equality . . . demands, for instance, that the disabled have good enough access to public accommodations that they can function as equals in civil society. To be capable as functioning as an equal does not require that access be equally fast, comfortable, or convenient, or that one get equal subjective utility from using public accommodations. There may be no way to achieve this. But the fact that, with current technology, it may take an extra minute or two to get into city hall does not compromise one's standing as an equal citizen. (Anderson 1999:334)

Anderson appears to be claiming that the important thresholds for democratic equality can be met and that any more precise, exacting, or comprehensive equality is not necessary. Both these claims are questionable. On its face, Anderson's conception of equal citizenship requires the indefinite expenditure of resources to achieve partial reductions in inequality, while her placement of certain capabilities outside the purview of democratic equality may not satisfy a robust notion of equal concern and respect.

The suggestion that democratic equality imposes thresholds that can be met by all or nearly all citizens is belied by Anderson's list of relevant capabilities. Thus, for example, "effective access . . . to medical care" would require indefinite expenditures for citizens with chronic and degenerative health conditions, unless *effective* is understood to mean only formal or logistical access to perfunctory care. However, such a spare understanding would hardly serve the purposes of democratic equality because it would not secure (to the limited extent that current or emergent medical technology permitted) the freedom from debility and pain necessary to take part in civic life. Such freedom cannot be guaranteed; it can only be achieved to a greater or lesser extent, by a greater or lesser number of people, through the use of scarce resources. There is no universally achievable threshold for the capability of "functioning as a human being," only a goal that competes with the enhancement of other capabilities.

A similar point could be made about competence in deliberation, which Anderson (1999) regards as an element of "access to the basic conditions of human agency." We could spend an indefinite amount on education, training, and support for people with cognitive disabilities without achieving such competence (Veatch 1986). As protracted litigation over the requirement of a "free and appropriate education" under the Individuals with Disabilities Education Act has made painfully clear, there are sharp trade-offs involved in even marginally enhancing this capability (Howe 1996). Such trade-offs arise regardless of whether we treat cognitive disability as a problem of internal function or environmental accommodation. Although mental incompetence is socially constructed, in the sense that society determines the cognitive complexity of many tasks and sets the minimum standards for proficiency (Buchanan 1996; Wikler 1979), decreasing the complexity of those tasks or lowering the standard for proficiency may have considerable social costs. Again, there is no universally achievable threshold for the capability of "functioning as a human being," only a goal that competes with the enhancement of other capabilities.

If Anderson (1999) underestimates the difficulty of achieving "sufficient"—as opposed to equal—levels of functioning, she also underestimates the harshness of excluding a wide range of capabilities from the scope of democratic equality. She offers examples of relatively trivial pursuits, such as playing cards expertly, enjoying luxury vacations, and competing in beauty pageants, as capabilities that democratic equality can safely ignore. However, to extend G. A. Cohen's (1989) criticism of Sen's capabilities approach, an impaired individual might be able to function quite well "as a human being, as a participant in a system of cooperative production, and as a citizen of a democratic state" (pp. 918-21) while in constant low-grade pain, bereft of friends, lovers, and family and devoid of aesthetic and cultural stimulation. It seems uncomfortably instrumental to regard a person's pain, loneliness, and drudgery as matters of collective or public concern only to the extent that they affect his or her capacity to work or vote. The refusal to view the alleviation of severe and protracted pain or loneliness as a general obligation seems inconsistent with an equal concern for those who experience such pain or loneliness. We may have to accept comprehensive measures of well-being and considerable intrusion into our private lives as the price of a robust commitment to equal concern and respect.

In focusing on the weaknesses of Anderson's (1999) account, I do not want to overlook one of its most significant achievements. It represents one of the first sustained efforts of a mainstream political philosopher to take disability scholarship seriously.[25] Even if Anderson underestimates the extent to which democratic equality requires harsh trade-offs and intrusive interventions, she has made great strides in elevating people with impairments from caricatures and cameo appearances to equal partnership in a challenging intellectual and moral inquiry.

CONCLUSION: THE PROSPECTS FOR CONVERGENCE

There is an intriguing symmetry in the challenges facing distributive and relational accounts of justice as they apply to disability. Distributive accounts must recognize the centrality to justice of equal social and political participation and develop metrics of individual well-being in which the capacity and opportunity for such participation figure prominently. Relational accounts, in turn, must make the notions of nondiscrimination and nonoppression sufficiently determinate to guide the reconstruction of the physical and social environment. Hybrid approaches such as Anderson's (1999) raise hopes for a convergence between distributive and relational accounts of justice.

Those hopes, however, may be illusory. Justice, as Walzer (1983), Miller (1999), and others argue, may be irreducibly plural. Although both distributive and relational accounts of justice appear to be guided by a principle of equal concern and respect, the former emphasize concern, the latter respect. The two kinds of accounts focus on inequalities that, however closely correlated, may be morally distinct. The failure to take adequate account of atypical functioning in the design of the physical and social environment may be a fundamentally different kind of wrong than the treatment of people with atypical functions as inferior beings. These wrongs may require different remedies: the former, redistribution; the latter, recognition (Fraser 1995). Perhaps, then, a single theory of justice cannot do justice to both aspects of impairments, as sources of functional limitation and as stigmatized differences. We may require both distributive and relational accounts to guide disability policy.

Whether justice for people with impairments is singular or plural, it will be better understood and perhaps more fully realized if philosophers and disability scholars take each other seriously. That requires philosophers to become more attentive to the perspectives and research of disability scholars and disability scholars to become less skeptical and dismissive of philosophical inquiry. The prospects for dialogue are improving, as philosophers become more restless with armchair analysis and disability scholars expand their disciplinary frontiers beyond social science.

NOTES

1. Useful overviews of this debate are found in Caplan (1998) and Wachbroit (1998).

2. While Boorse (1977) defines the goal of functions as *individual* survival and reproduction, he also asserts that "function statements are about a trait's *standard* contribution in some population or reference class" (p. 556), so that a single life-saving contribution by a trait does not make it a function. "One squirrel might catch its tail in a crack *en route* to being run over by a car, but that would not make defense against cars a function of the squirrel tail" (p. 557). In taking the species as the reference class for functions, Boorse implicitly restricts the settings in which functions are

claimed to contribute to individual survival and flourishing to the standard environments where the trait was established in the species.

3. An interesting example of postgestational plasticity was presented in the recent U.S. Supreme Court case of *Albertson's, Inc. v. Kirkinburg* (1999), in which the plaintiff's subconscious adjustment for monocular vision apparently prevented that condition from "substantially limiting" his work as a truck driver.

4. Boorse (1975) himself offers two reasons why species-typical functioning may be generally desirable. First, typical functions such as heart pumping and digestion "tend to contribute to all manner of activities neutrally; second, people enjoy engaging in many of these functions, like eating and sex, quite apart from their contribution to other goals and activities" (p. 60). The first reason, which Boorse regards as "surely the main [one]," may suggest no more than that physical survival is a prerequisite to the pursuit of many goals and activities. Or it may suggest that species-typical functions owe their utility to their typicality and to the fact that the social environment is tailored to people with normal functions, a claim often made by disability advocates. The second reason is more an empirical than an evaluative claim—that species-typical functions are desired, not that they are desirable.

5. The appeal of a state-of-nature baseline, as well as the associated view that a society is more responsible for the misfortunes it causes than those it merely allows (see note 6), arises, I suspect, from an unwarranted extension of the deontological principle that agents are more responsible for what they cause than for what they allow. However valid this principle may be for individuals, it is untenable for society. Our commonsense understanding of human agency allows us to draw a reasonably clear distinction between action and omission. To the extent that the distinction between causing and allowing diverges from the distinction between action and omission (since, for example, we can cause by strategic omission), we can have recourse to a counterfactual world where the individual agent never existed. Even if that counterfactual poses conceptual difficulties in certain cases (e.g., the mother's existence in the case of abortion) or yields surprising results (e.g., *It's a Wonderful Life*), it seems adequate for routine cases.

In contrast, we have no clear idea of what it means for a society or other collective entity to act (except in narrow domains such as corporate law), and the counterfactual comparison, to a world without this particular society or organized society in general, is far harder to make. Moreover, a primary motivation for drawing the causing/allowing distinction for individuals—to recognize a sphere of special responsibility and preserve discretion elsewhere—hardly applies to a collectivity, which does not need personal space, pursue ground-level projects, or enjoy prerogatives. Even more clearly than individuals, societies can be judged to have caused those disadvantages they are responsible for, rather than as being responsible for those disadvantages they have caused.

This is not to deny that a society or state may incur special obligations to certain members as a result of specific actions or policies. It may owe compensation for neglect or mistreatment (e.g., to Japanese internees or the subjects of the Tuskegee study) or for special services rendered or risks assumed (e.g., to combat veterans).

6. At some points, Pogge (1989) suggests that the relevant distinction is not between socially caused and naturally occurring disadvantages but between those a society causes and merely allows. The latter would include disadvantages that were socially caused but not attributable to the present social order (e.g., that were caused by other societies or by social developments that antedate the present society). But the caused/allowed distinction is difficult enough to draw for individual agents; it may be untenable for collective or social agents. The distinction is particularly difficult for Pogge to draw because he cannot rely on the kindred distinction between the effects that a cooperative scheme intends and those that it merely foresees. The latter distinction does not make a moral difference on the Rawlsian theory of justice that Pogge is elaborating.

The difficulty in teasing apart natural and social causes for various limitations on activity poses a challenge for Amundson's (1992) distinction between "those features of the handicapping environment that are socially constructed [and] those which are independent of human choice" (p. 116). Amundson is well aware, of course, that the "handicaps" associated with biological impairments arise from their interaction with the physical and social environment. Yet he fails to consider the problem this interaction raises for attributing a handicapping feature of the environment to either natural or social causes. Increasingly few handicapping features remain "independent of human choice" as technology expands the potential for human control of the physical environment, and even those features still beyond human control, such as earth's gravity, can be exploited by humans to exclude people with various impairments.

7. A somewhat more modest, but no more determinate, baseline is advanced by Harlan Hahn, the leading proponent of the minority group model of disability. Hahn (1999) endorses Michael Oliver's suggestion that justice for people with disabilities be assessed by principle of "equal environmental adaptation." He argues that "few judges or lawyers seem willing to acknowledge the heavy burdens imposed on disabled citizens by the demands of the existing environment . . . most appear to be in a state of denial about the massive advantages bequeathed to the non-disabled majority by the present 'taken-for-granted' environment" (p. 39). Hahn is careful enough to recognize that the acknowledgment of those advantages would not preclude the attribution of some disadvantages to the impairments of the nondisabled minority. But the very notion of "equal environmental adaptation" is misleading, in part because of the asymmetrical character of disability. "Equal adaptation" for people who speak two different languages might be

bilingual instruction or equal classroom time in both languages; an equal adaptation for people of two vastly different sizes, Lilliputians and Brobdagnagians, might consist of facilities and equipment in both sizes or in some intermediate size. However, despite the familiar examples of stairs versus ramps and spoken language versus signing, the very idea of equal adaptation to standard and impaired functions is obscure, in part because many adaptations for the latter would also serve the former. This is partially because it is unclear how equality in adaptation is to be assessed in a way that would distinguish it from equality in result.

8. A final claim about social causation would be based on the intentional character of the disadvantages faced by people with disabilities. The claim would be that those in positions of power keep people with impairments marginalized and oppressed to serve their own interests (e.g., to keep "able-bodied" workers docile and inexpensive by maintaining a large reserve of unemployed individuals). On this view, the biological impairments of disabled individuals would be seen as causally inert and pretextual, playing much the same role as differences in skin color and ethnicity. This would provide a clear sense in which the "real cause" of disability was social. Yet it is simply not plausible to attribute most of the disadvantage of people with disabilities to such calculated policy, as opposed to pervasive neglect.

9. The *ICIDH-2* recognizes that the environment plays a causal role at the level of impairments as well as activity limitations and participation restrictions. Proponents of some alternative classification schemes insist that the impairment category must be free of environmental influence, but this seems clearly misguided since even physiological states are mediated by environmental factors. However, there is certainly a strong intuitive sense that the environment plays a greater role in less basic activities than in more basic ones and in impairments than in activity limitations.

10. Griffin (1986) discusses a range of utilitarian and nonutilitarian positions on well-being.

11. One philosopher (Nordenfelt 1997) has argued that the *ICIDH* distinction between disability versus handicap should be refined or replaced with a distinction between basic and nonbasic action. On this account, disabilities would be a subclass of impairments—impairments of basic actions or the most proximate effects of impairments—on the capacity to perform basic actions.

12. Some of these functions or actions straddle the categories of disability classification schemes. Thus, the Americans with Disabilities Act lists seeing, hearing, and walking as major life activities, along with working and caring for oneself, activities that obviously have a more contingent relationship to impairment. The drafters of the *ICIDH-2* continue to struggle over whether to treat seeing and hearing as bodily functions, activities, or both.

13. The relationship between touch and sight is raised by "Molyneux's problem." Would a person acquiring vision for the first time as an adult immediately recognize the shapes he saw as the same ones he knew by touch? Recent philosophical writing on the problem suggests that the connection between visual and tactile experiences of the world is especially close (Grice 1962; Thomson 1974).

14. For a more detailed account of how egalitarian theories of justice treat disability, see Wasserman in Silvers et al. (1998).

15. The contrast between these first two approaches reflects a broader division among theories of justice. Those theories, which have proliferated since the publication of John Rawls's (1971) *A Theory of Justice,* differ in their basic orientation—to the procedures or processes by which resources are generated, appropriated, and exchanged or to the distribution or end state resulting from those processes (Nozick 1974). A purely procedural theory would have no need for a metric of well-being with which to assess end states since it would endorse any outcome reached by fair procedures. Libertarian accounts, for example, treat any distribution as fair that results from the exchange of legitimately acquired resources by voluntary transactions devoid of fraud or force (Nozick 1974). But libertarian accounts require some criteria of justice in acquisitions or holdings, and it has been argued that distributive standards are already built into those criteria, such as the "Lockean proviso," which requires that any appropriation of initially unclaimed resources leave "as much, and as good, in common." (Many distributive accounts also have procedural elements. For example, in Rawls's theory, any distribution will be just that arises from the political and economic processes occurring under a just "basic structure"—one that embodies the two (substantive) principles of justice for which Rawls argues.) Other procedural accounts focus on political processes, such as democratic voting. Again, it has been argued that distributive constraints are required to make such mechanisms fair. Still, other procedural accounts, more familiar in the disability context, assess fairness in terms of the relationships between social groups, particularly the presence or absence of oppression, domination, and hierarchy (e.g., Young 1990), or in terms of the attitudes informing those relationships, such as the presence or absence of hatred, contempt, and devaluation.

16. To some extent, the distinction between resources and welfare tracks that between objective and subjective conceptions of well-being discussed in the last section. However, the overlap is only partial. First, most objective accounts of well-being treat the possession of material resources as having mainly instrumental value. Second, many philosophers believe, with Scanlon, that not all aspects of well-being, important to the individual or to her or his loved ones, are the proper concern of political justice. They believe that even if what we regard pleasure or satisfaction as part of what makes our own lives, or those of our family and friends, goes well, it may not be something we owe each other as fellow citizens.

17. Some proponents of resource equality have attempted to encompass internal and external resources, usually by giving everyone a claim on each other's skills and talents. Such schemes seem oppressive, however, in creating a "slavery of the talented." No one has a special say over his or her own time and energy, and the talented must pay dearly for leisure because their labor is in so much demand.

18. Other philosophers (e.g., Kymlicka 1991) have expanded Rawls's list of primary social goods to include more participatory goods such as membership in a culture or community.

19. Several other political philosophers have suggested ways of expanding the subject matter of distributive justice beyond the ownership or control of material resources. Thus, some of the claims of linguistic and cultural minorities can be framed in distributive terms by recognizing "the social bases of self-respect" (Rawls 1971) or cultural membership (Kymlicka 1991) as goods, subject to distributive goals or constraints, because they provide the context for the selection and enjoyment of other goods. Iris Young (1990) expresses a widespread skepticism about these prospects for extending the subject matter of distributive justice to such intangible goods. She asks, for example,

> What can it mean to distribute self-respect? Self-respect is not an entity or measurable aggregate, it cannot be parceled out of some stash, and above all, it cannot be detached from persons as a separable attribute adhering to some unchanged substance. . . . It is certainly true that in many circumstances the possession of distributable material goods may be a condition of self-respect. Self-respect, however, also involves many nonmaterial conditions and cannot be reduced to distributive arrangements. . . . None of the forms and not all of the conditions of self-respect can be meaningfully conceived as goods that individuals possess; they are rather relations and processes in which the actions of individuals are embedded. (P. 27)

Yet a theory of distributive justice does not require that self-respect or cultural membership itself be subject to distribution or that it be based entirely or even primarily on the possession of goods that can be distributed. Rather, it merely requires that we be able to assess, however crudely and fallibly, individuals' self-respect or cultural affiliation and that we be able to alter social arrangements to reduce the disparities we find in those social goods or aspects of well-being.

20. Justice will also require expensive medical intervention for some impairments, particularly those acquired adventitiously by adults. While the restoration of normal functioning should not have the lexical priority it is accorded by some accounts of justice in health care (e.g., Daniels 1986), it will often be an urgent and weighty interest.

21. As I explain in note 15, I am treating relational accounts of justice as a subclass of procedural account.

22. A relational theorist such as Iris Young might reach the same conclusion for different reasons because discriminatory attitudes and practices are so entrenched that "they are beyond the reach of law and policy to remedy" (Young 1990:124). As Young argues,

> The behavior, comportments, images, and stereotypes that contribute to the oppression of bodily marked groups are pervasive, systematic, mutually generating and mutually reinforcing. They are elements of the dominant cultural practices that lie as the normal background of our liberal democratic society. Only changing the cultural habits themselves will change the oppression they produce and reinforce. (P. 152)

Young may underestimate the capacity of law and policy to alter such habits, but this is a distinct issue from the one I address in the text, which concerns the ends rather than the means of antidiscrimination policy.

23. There is an ongoing debate, which several philosophers have recently joined, about the adequacy of such an antidiscrimination rubric for disability policy. For a more detailed discussion of this issue, see Bickenbach (1993), Bickenbach et al. (1999), Kelman and Lester (1997), and Silvers et al. (1998).

24. This is not to assume that conscious attitudes of aversion are the main causes of structural bias—merely that they are an integral part of the complex web of attitudes, behaviors, and practices that constitute what Young (1990:122-48) calls oppression and subordination. See note 15.

25. In this effort at interdisciplinary dialogue, Anderson is assisted by the fact that one of her "informants," Anita Silvers, is herself an experienced professional philosopher who has written influentially on disability.

REFERENCES

Albertson's v. Kirkinburg, 527 U.S. 555 (1999).

Albrecht, G. and P. Devlieger. 1999. "The Disability Paradox: High Quality of Life against All Odds." *Social Science and Medicine* 48:477-88.

Amundson, R. 1992. "Disability, Handicap, and the Environment." *Journal of Social Philosophy* 23 (1): 105-19.

———. 2000. "Against Normal Functions." *Studies in the History and Philosophy of Biological and Biomedical Sciences* 31 (1): 33-53.

Anderson, E. 1999. "What Is the Point of Equality?" *Ethics* 109:287-337.

Arneson, R. 1989. "Equality and Equal Opportunity for Welfare." *Philosophical Studies* 56:77-93.

———. 1990. "Liberalism, Distributive Subjectivism, and Equal Opportunity for Welfare." *Philosophy and Public Affairs* 19:158-94.

Bickenbach, J. 1993. *Physical Disability and Social Policy*. Toronto: University of Toronto Press.

———. 1996. "Equality, Rights, and the Disablement Process." Paper presented at the annual meeting of the American Philosophical Association, Central Division, April, Chicago.

Bickenbach, J., S. Chatterji, E. M. Badley, and T. B. Üstün. 1999. "Models of Disablement, Universalism, and the International Classification of Impairments, Disabilities, and Handicaps." *Social Science and Medicine* 48:1-15.

Boorse, C. 1975. "On the Distinction between Disease and Illness." *Philosophy and Public Affairs* 5:49-68.

———. 1977. "Health as a Theoretical Concept." *Philosophy of Science* 44 (4): 542-73.

———. 1987. "Concepts of Health." Pp. 359-93 in *Health Care Ethics: An Introduction*, edited by Donald VanDeveer and Tom Regan. Philadelphia: Temple University Press.

Brock, D. 1995. "Justice and the ADA: Does Prioritizing and Rationing Health Care Discriminate against the Disabled?" *Social Philosophy and Policy* 12 (2): 159-85.

———. 1997. "Ethical Issues in the Development of Summary Measures of Population Health Status." Paper presented at the Institute of Medicine, National Academy of Sciences, Workshop on Summary Measures of Population Health Status, December, Washington, DC.

Buchanan, A. 1996. "Choosing Who Will Be Disabled: Genetic Intervention and the Morality of Inclusion." *Social Philosophy and Policy* 13 (2): 18-46.

Candlish, S. 1984. "Inner and Outer Basic Action." *Proceedings of the Aristotelian Society* 84:83-102.

Caplan, A. L. 1998. "The Concepts of Health, Disease, and Illness." Pp. 57-73 in *Medical Ethics*, edited by Robert Veatch. Boston: Jones & Bartlett.

Cohen, G. A. 1989. "On the Currency of Egalitarian Justice." *Ethics* 99:906-44.

———. 1993. *Equality of What? On Welfare, Goods, and Capabilities: The Quality of Life*. New York: Oxford University Press.

Crocker, D. 1995. "Functioning and Capability: The Foundations of Sen's and Nussbaum's Development Ethic: Part II." Pp. 153-98 in *Women, Culture, and Development*, edited by Martha Nussbaum and Jonathan Glover. New York: Oxford University Press/Clarendon.

Daniels, N. 1986. "Justice and Health Care." Pp. 290-325 in *Health Care Ethics: An Introduction*, edited by Donald Van DeVeer and Tom Regan. Philadelphia: Temple University Press.

———. 1990. "Equality of What: Welfare, Resources, or Capabilities?" *Philosophy and Phenomenological Research* 50 (Suppl.): 273-97.

———. 1997. "Distributive Justice and the Use of Summary Measures of Population Health Status." Paper presented at the Institute of Medicine, National Academy of Sciences, Workshop on Summary Measures of Population Health Status, December, Washington, DC.

Danto, A. 1965. "Basic Actions." *American Philosophical Quarterly* 2:108-25.

Dupre, J. 1998. "Normal People." *Social Research* 65 (2): 221-48.

Dworkin, R. 1981. "What Is Equality? Part II—Equality of Resources." *Philosophy and Public Affairs* 10:283-345.

Edwards, S. D. 1997. "Dismantling the Disability/Handicap Distinction." *Journal of Medicine and Philosophy* 22:589-606.

Engelhardt, H. T., Jr. 1986. *The Foundations of Bioethics*. New York: Oxford University Press.

Fraser, N. 1995. "From Redistribution to Recognition: Dilemmas of Justice in a 'Post-Socialist' Age." *New Left Review* 212:68-93.

Goldman, A. 1970. *A Theory of Human Action*. Englewood Cliffs, NJ: Prentice Hall.

Grice, W. P. 1962. "Some Remarks about the Senses." In *Analytical Philosophy*, edited by R. J. Butler. Oxford, UK: Oxford University Press.

Griffin, J. 1986. *Well-Being Its Meaning, Measure, and Moral Importance*. Oxford, UK: Oxford University Press.

———. 1993. "Commentary on Dan Brock: Quality of Life Measures in Health Care and Medical Ethics." Pp. 133-39 in *The Quality of Life*, edited by Martha Nussbaum and Amartya Sen. Oxford, UK: Clarendon.

Hahn, H. 1999. "A New Approach to Developmental Disabilities: From Perspective to Proposals." Unpublished paper, Disability Forum, Santa Monica, CA.

Hornsby, J. 1980. *Actions.* London: Routledge Kegan Paul.

Howe, K. R. 1996. "Educational Ethics, Social Justice and Children with Disabilities." Pp. 46-64 in *Disability and the Dilemmas of Education and Justice,* edited by Carol Christensen and Fazal Rizvi. Buckingham, UK: Open University Press.

Kelman, M. and G. Lester. 1997. *Jumping the Queen: An Inquiry into the Legal Treatment of Students with Learning Disabilities.* Cambridge, MA: Harvard University Press.

Kuhse, H. and P. Singer. 1985. *Should the Baby Live? The Problem of Handicapped Infants.* Oxford, UK: Oxford University Press.

Kymlicka, W. 1991. *Liberalism Community and Culture.* Oxford, UK: Clarendon.

Lane, H. 1992. *The Mask of Benevolence: Disabling the Deaf Community.* New York: Knopf.

Magee, B. and M. Milligan. 1995. *On Blindness.* Oxford, UK: Oxford University Press.

Miller, D. 1997. "Equality and Justice." *Ratio* 10 (3): 222-37.

———. 1999. *Principles of Social Justice.* Cambridge, MA: Harvard University Press.

Murray, C. 1996. "Rethinking DALYs." Pp. 1-98 in *The Global Burden of Disease: A Comprehensive Assessment of Mortality and Disability from Diseases, Injuries, and Risk Factors in 1990 and Projected to 2020,* edited by C. Murray and A. Lopez. Geneva: World Health Organization.

Nordenfelt, L. 1997. "The Importance of a Disability/Handicap Distinction." *Journal of Medicine and Philosophy* 22:607-22.

Norman, R. 1997. "The Social Basis of Equality." *Ratio* 10 (3): 238-52.

———. 1999. "Equality, Priority, and Social Justice." *Ratio* 12 (2): 178-94.

Nozick, R. 1974. *Anarchy, State, and Utopia.* Cambridge, MA: Harvard University Press.

Nussbaum, M. 1990. "Aristotelian Social Democracy." Pp. 203-52 in *Liberalism and the Human Good,* edited by R. B. Douglass, G. Mara, and H. Richardson. London: Routledge Kegan Paul.

———. 1992. "Human Functioning and Social Justice: A Defense of Aristotelian Essentialism." *Political Theory* 20:202-46.

Oliver, M. 1996. *Understanding Disability: From Theory to Practice.* London: Macmillan.

Parfit, D. 1997. "Equality and Priority." *Ratio* 10 (3): 202-21.

Pogge, T. 1989. *Realizing Rawls.* Ithaca, NY: Cornell University Press.

———. 1999. "Human Flourishing and Universal Justice." *Social Philosophy and Policy* 16:332-61.

Rawls, J. 1971. *A Theory of Justice.* Cambridge, MA: Harvard University Press.

Rebell, M. 1986. "Structural Discrimination and the Disabled." *Georgetown Law Journal* 74:1435-89.

Rosenberg, A. 1986. "The Political Philosophy of Biological Endowments." *Social Philosophy and Policy* 5 (1): 2-31.

Scanlon, T. 1988. "The Significance of Choice." Pp. 177-85 in *Tanner Lectures on Human Values VIII,* edited by S. McMurrin. Salt Lake City: University of Utah Press.

———. 1998. *What We Owe to Each Other.* Cambridge, MA: Harvard University Press.

Segal, J. M. 1998. "Living at a High Economics Standard: A Functionings Analysis." Pp. 342-65 in *Ethics of Consumption: The Good Life Justice, and Global Stewardship,* edited by David Crocker and Toby Linden. Lanham, MD: Rowman & Littlefield.

Sen, A. 1980. "Equality of What?" Pp. 195-220 in *Tanner Lectures on Human Values I,* edited by S. McMurrin. Salt Lake City: University of Utah Press.

———. 1993. "Capability and Well-Being." Pp. 30-54 in *The Quality of Life,* edited by Martha Nussbaum and Amartya Sen. Oxford, UK: Clarendon.

Silvers, A. 1994. "'Defective' Agents: Equality, Difference and the Tyranny of the Normal." *Journal of Social Philosophy* 25:154-75.

Silvers, A. and D. Wasserman. 1998. "Competence and Convention: Disability Rights in Sports and Education." *Report from the Institute for Philosophy & Public Policy* 18 (4): 1-7.

Silvers, A., D. Wasserman, and M. Mahowald. 1998. *Disability, Difference, Discrimination.* Lanham, MD: Rowman & Littlefield.

Singer, P. 1993. *Practical Ethics.* 2d ed. Cambridge, UK: Cambridge University Press.

———. 1999. "All Animals Are Equal." Pp. 461-70 in *Bioethics: An Anthology,* edited by Helga Kuhse and Peter Singer. Oxford, UK: Blackwell.

Sober, E. 2001. "Separating Nature from Nurture." Pp. 47-78 in *Genetics and Criminal Behavior: Methods, Meanings, and Morals,* edited by David Wasserman and Robert Wachbroit. New York: Cambridge University Press.

tenBroek, J. 1966. "The Right to Live in the World: The Disabled in the Law of Torts." *California Law Review* 54:841-919.

Thomson, J. 1974. "Molyneux's Problem." *Journal of Philosophy* 71:637.

Veatch, R. 1986. *The Foundation of Justice: Why the Retarded and the Rest of Us Have Claims to Equality.* Oxford, UK: Oxford University Press.

Wachbroit, R. 1994. "Normality as a Biological Concept." *Philosophy of Science* 61:579-91.

———. 1998. "Health and Disease, Concepts of." *Encyclopedia of Applied Ethics* 2:533-38.

———. 2001. "Understanding the Genetics of Violence Controversy." Pp. 25-46 in *Genetics and Criminal Behavior: Meanings, Methods, and Moral.* New York: Cambridge University Press.

Walzer, M. 1983. *Spheres of Justice.* New York: Basic Books.

Wasserman, D. 1996. "Some Moral Issues in the Correction of Impairments." *Journal of Social Philosophy* 27 (2): 128-45.

———. 1998. "Discrimination, Concept of." *Encyclopedia of Applied Ethics* 1:805-13.

Wegner, J. 1984. "The Antidiscrimination Model Reconsidered: Ensuring Equal Opportunity without Respect to Handicap under Section 504 of the Rehabilitation Act of 1973." *Cornell Law Review* 69:401-516.

Wendell, S. 1989. "Toward a Feminist Theory of Disability." *Hypatia* 4 (2): 104-24.

Wikler, D. 1979. "Paternalism and the Mildly Retarded." *Philosophy and Public Affairs* 8 (4): 63-87.

World Health Organization. 1980. *International Classification of Impairments, Disabilities, and Handicaps.* Geneva: Author.

———. 1997. *ICIDH-2 Beta-1 Draft: International Classification of Impairments, Activities, and Participation.* Geneva: Author.

Young, I. M. 1990. *Justice and the Politics of Difference.* Princeton, NJ: Princeton University Press.

Disability and the Sociology of the Body

BRYAN S. TURNER

INTRODUCTION: TWO SOCIOLOGICAL TRADITIONS

The issue of disability had been until recently somewhat neglected within both mainstream sociology (Ingstad and White 1995) and the humanities (Mitchell and Snyder 1997). In addition, classical studies of the cultural meanings of the body and disability, such as Henri-Jacques Stiker's *Corps infirmes et societes* (1982), have not received the attention that they deserve in the conventional sociology of health and illness. Apart from influential works by Erving Goffman (1959, 1964) and Irving Zola (1982, 1988), sociology has contributed surprisingly little in terms of systematic theory and research to the study of disability. With respect to the study of mental health and social deviance, the tradition of symbolic interactionism has produced an influential literature that gave rise to radical criticism of taken-for-granted notions of normality and questioned the conventional division between norm, normal, and deviance (Williams 1987). Grounded theory has of course addressed important issues in the analysis of chronic illness (Strauss and Glaser 1975). In these studies, there is a common assumption that the human body can be read as a text that can disclose important facts about the person, and these corporeal texts provide significant information about the inner life of the individual (Skultans 1977).

Against conventional criminology, which accepted a narrow legal definition of crime and deviance, deviancy studies argued that deviance is "in the eye of the beholder," and as a consequence, sociological research concentrated on the processes of stigmatization and institutionalization. If sociologists had an interest in the sociology of disability, it was somewhat submerged in studies of stigma and stigmatization (Goffman 1964). Symbolic interactionism developed an array of useful concepts around the idea of "discredited" and "discreditable" identities and studied the management of interaction between "normals" and the chronically sick and disabled (Davis 1963). In a similar fashion, disability in medical sociology has not been a major research interest. Studies of disability typically appeared in research on aging, where it was represented under the heading of "dependency" (Hocking and James 1993). In this setting, disability became associated with negative "images of ageing" (Featherstone and Wernick 1995).

However, this situation of relative scientific neglect changed in the 1980s with the growth of the disability movement and the political quest for social rights. As a result, there is greater public awareness that the prejudicial assumptions of the media and the deployment of a "disabling language" have the consequence of reinforcing negative stereotypes (Auslander and Gold 1999). It is now recognized that there is an ideology of "able-ism" that has exclusionary social functions. As a result, writers such as Wendy Seymour (1989, 1998) have more systematically analyzed the negative consequences of the medicalization of patients and the medical model in rehabilitation in medical sociology. This emphasis on ability as an assumption of the dominant culture may be particularly true of American society, where, in the twentieth century, the "youth complex" (Parsons 1999) gave a salient position to individualism, achievement, and success. Youthfulness became the principal criterion for aesthetic judgments of the body. As a result, "able-ism" underpins more general values about the cultural importance of sport, athleticism, and masculinity; that is, the notion of physical dexterity becomes an index of more general distinction. In contemporary consumer societies, the youthful and powerful body has increasingly become a sign of social worth; the body has become a principal theme in the notion of the self as a project (Giddens 1991). Against a background of relative neglect, there has been an emerging critical literature on disability that has had an effect on the social sciences for which the notions of disability, handicap, and impairment are now thoroughly contested (Barnes, Mercer, and Shakespeare 1999). These intellectual changes were indicated, to some extent, in disability studies by Zola's (1991) critical lecture on "bringing bodies back in." In this chapter, I attempt to show that, both politically and analytically, there is a growing appreciation of the body and embodiment in modern sociology and that the sociology of the body can make important contributions to the study of impairment and disability.

This chapter has three specific aims. The first is to develop a sociology of the body that combines both an appreciation of the phenomenology of the body in the everyday world and an awareness that the body is constructed as an object of professional concern. The chapter examines both the subjectivity of the "lived body" in the phenomenological tradition (O'Neill 1972) and the external social and political structures that regulate, produce, and govern bodies and populations in the tradition of Michel Foucault (Burchell, Gordon, and Miller 1991; Jones and Porter 1994). The term *embodiment* attempts to describe the subjectivity of the lived body in the life-world in the phenomenological tradition, whereas the term *governmentality* attempts to describe the production of the body as an object of professional practice in the poststructural tradition. The second aim is to examine the notions of vulnerability and contingency in relation to the idea of the embodied self to further disrupt the idea of "natural" disability. Finally, the chapter considers how a sociology of the body can provide an analysis of human and social rights that is grounded in an understanding of the social ontology of human beings as both frail and vulnerable. These three objects can be regarded as in fact one: to undertake a critique of the Cartesian dualism of mind and body to situate the sociology of the body at the center of disability debates.

In exploring the relevance of sociology to an understanding of disability, we should therefore examine two versions of the sociology of the body in contemporary social thought. The first is the debate opened up by the critical writings of Michel Foucault (1926-1984) about the social production of the human body that leads into an analysis of how disability is socially constructed. Such an approach is radical in the sense that it treats, for example, the rehabilitation process as normalization, which is how the "disabled body" is discursively produced, governed, and regulated. This Foucauldian approach has in recent years been increasingly summarized as the study of "governmentality" (Rose 1989:5). This concept refers to the development of micro-systems of social regulation that exercise normative control over individuals and populations. In this sense, rehabilitation is a form of governmentality that orchestrates various medical and welfare practices that aim to create the rehabilitated person. Another illustration is the spread of dietary practices in which "diet" as a "government of the body" brings about a detailed self-regulation of the body to exercise more control over the self (Turner 1982). More broadly, this "social constructionist" approach avoids the difficulties of "essentialism." There are many versions of the constructionist argument, some of which converge with philosophical pragmatism in which scientific facts are produced rather than discovered. As Richard Rorty (1999:xvi) has argued, relativists are people who believe that truths about the world are produced for pragmatic reasons and not discovered. For example, social constructionist approaches to the body argue that the ways in which we categorize and classify bodies are characteristically products of political struggles within the field of the medical professions. For example, Foucault (1980) has shown that the absolute binary division between the sexes emerged from bureaucratic and political conflicts between professionals, where individuals of indeterminate sex nevertheless have to be unambiguously ascribed to a specific category, either male or female. The history of gender classification shows that the allocation of individuals to positions within the gender map is arbitrary and that the map itself changes and evolves over time (Laqueur 1990). In a similar fashion, social constructionism challenges the assumption that there is a fixed and unchanging essence of human disability and asserts, by contrast, that disability is a not a phenomenon with shared characteristics across cultures and across time but is a product or consequence of medical classification. The paradox of the social constructionist position is that the specific character of embodiment in the everyday lives of people who are regarded as disabled disappears because the "body" appears as only a phantasm that is produced by the discourses and practices of "ablement."

The second possibility is the elaboration of the phenomenology of the body through the study of embodiment in everyday life. This perspective has its intellectual origins in the philosophical tradition of Maurice Merleau-Ponty (1907-1961). The phenomenology of the body keeps the body in focus as an object of intellectual inquiry, but it treats as problematic the relationship between the official objective body of rehabilitation and the subjective body of personal experience. It recognizes the complex interplay between the objectified body of medical discourse, the phenomenal body of everyday experience, and the body image that, as it were, negotiates the social spaces between identity, experience, and social relationships. Chronic illness presents specific interactional problems in which the individual must negotiate a new set of everyday practices that can manage the tensions between the self, the experience of embodiment, the biological changes, and the medical appropriation of the body. These issues have been subtly explored by Monks and Frankenberg (1995) in terms of the experience of multiple sclerosis in which the expectations of time for the self have to be adjusted to the temporal demands that are imposed by the biological body. Erving Goffman's (1964) study of stigma might be a useful additional illustration of this line of argument. A stigmatized and stigmatizing body has to be managed in everyday life in terms of managing a body image in an interactional context, in which a negative body image gives off information that may be damaging to the self. The presentation of the self in everyday life (Goffman 1959) requires successful management of the body and, more critically, management of the body image if the self is to avoid the existential damage that follows from embarrassment. The interactional problems that arise with stigma are carefully explored by Goffman, who recognized that individuals may or may not invest in action; there are always opportunities of "role distance" that involve subjective withdrawal from interaction.

There has been much debate as to whether Goffman's approach involved a cynical assumption that there is no true or continuous self, only an endless and playful presentation of masks. The phenomenology of the body assumes that the continuity of the self across space and time requires the continuity of embodiment. Without this continuity of embodiment, how could we be effectively recognized over time? For phenomenologists, the notion of a continuous self is thus predicated on the idea of embodiment, and therefore it argues that any sharp differentiation of mind and body is inadequate as a basis for understanding the self in society. Who I am cannot be separated from how I am embodied, and thus any traumatic disruption of my body through accident or disease brings about disruptions to the self. Parkinson's disease threatens to disrupt the self in everyday life because the victim of the disease may be inadvertently classified as an alcoholic.

The phenomenological approach is a crucial challenge to the assumptions of the medical model, which assumes a clear division between mind and body, rejects the subjective experience of the patient as irrelevant to treatment, and approaches the body as simply a collection of parts. One crucial problem with the medical model is that in the case of amputation, for example, it treats limbs as merely parts of the physical organism rather than as components of the embodied self. In response to patients who suffer from phantom limb experiences, the medical model provides a criticism of the patient's "failure" to adjust in terms of the dominant values of American society—namely, individualism and pragmatism (Deegan 1978). Contemporary philosophers, inspired by the work of Martin Heidegger, have argued that to transcend existing dualities and develop a more adequate understanding of the embodied self, we need "a conception of a single entity that is at once a self and a body" (Olafson 1995:199). In this chapter, I propose that the idea of "embodiment" is such a conception.

These two traditions (poststructuralism and phenomenology) are normally regarded as mutually exclusive. Foucault rejected both phenomenology and existentialism to develop an understanding of social and cultural relationships as products of discourses. The result was to expunge an interest in the actual phenomena of the experience of everyday life. Foucauldian poststructuralism has examined the enormous variety of discourses by which "bodies" have been produced, categorized, and regulated (Foucault 1981, 1987, 1988). At the same time, it denies the sensuous materiality of the body in favor of an "antihumanist" analysis of the discursive ordering of bodily regimes. Such an approach rejects the commonsense assumption that the body (in the singular) can have any unitary coherence or uniform significance. Foucault's work is briefly summarized in his own words from *Technologies of the Self* (Martin, Gutman, and Hutton 1988:11)—"All of my analyses are against the idea of universal necessities in human existence. They show the arbitrariness of institutions." His legacy has produced a range of historical inquiries into the government of the body resulting from institutionalization. By contrast, the phenomenology of the body examines the ways in which the everyday world is organized from the perspective of the embodiment of human beings. Merleau-Ponty's (1962) approach to perception and understanding argued against any separation of mind and body; our perceptions of the world are always grounded in the relationship between our embodiment and the world.

Although these two traditions are typically regarded as incommensurable, this chapter develops an interpretation of the body that seeks a theoretical rapprochement between Foucault's poststructuralism and Merleau-Ponty's phenomenology to bring out the positive political and theoretical benefits of combining both positions for an analysis of disability (Turner 1992, 1995a, 1996). An adequate sociology of the body in disability studies must examine different levels of disability—namely, how individuals experience disability, the social organization of disability in terms of sociocultural categories, and the macro or societal level of welfare provision and the politics of disability (Barnes et al. 1999:35). On one hand, Foucault's idea of normalization is useful in understanding how medical interventions standardize human experience. On the other hand, a phenomenology of the body provides a basis for a better appreciation of the actual experiences and subjectivities of embodiment. This chapter is consistent with the position taken by Susan Reynolds Whyte (1995), who has criticized the tradition of Foucault and Stiker as frameworks for analysis of individuals' experiences of misfortune, disease, disability, and so forth because "discourse analysis does not leave much room for their subjectivity and agency" (p. 276). She makes the important point that the ethnographic tradition of anthropology has therefore much to offer to the exploration of an issue (the subjective experiences of the everyday world) about which discourse analysis is wholly silent.

The argument here claims that it is possible to combine (what we can call) ontological foundationalism with cultural constructionism, and such a combination, particularly in medical sociology, can have a number of theoretical benefits. It is important to distinguish between epistemological questions that relate obviously to questions about knowledge and understanding and ontological questions that relate to problems about the nature of the existence of things. By combining these two questions—namely, foundationalism and constructionism—we can recognize a number of logical possibilities. The two extreme positions assert either that the body is socially produced (radical constructionism) or that it is biologically given (positivism). In contemporary social theory, the most commonly held position is that of radical constructionism. This tradition has been significantly influenced by the writings of Foucault, postmodernists, feminists, and epistemological relativists. It has also been attractive to political activists in the disability movement, precisely because it recognizes the contingencies of social responses to disability—namely, the arbitrariness of institutions.

It is possible, however, to identify some traditions in social theory when social construction is combined with ontology. For example, in sociology, the work of Peter Berger and Thomas

Luckmann was particularly important in the development of the theory that the social world is constructed by the endless activities of social agents. Indeed, their book, *The Social Construction of Reality* (Berger and Luckmann 1966), was a major development in the modern sociology of knowledge and was welcomed as a particularly radical turn in the history of sociology. Their sociological position was actually based on the work of Arnold Gehlen, who attempted to integrate biology and sociology. Gehlen (1980, 1988) argued that human beings are "not yet finished animals"; that is, human beings are biologically ill equipped to deal with the world because they have no specific instinctual basis and depend on a long period of socialization to adapt themselves to the world. Gehlen argued that to cope with this "world openness," human beings had to create a cultural world to replace their instinctual world or at least to supplement their instinctual world. Berger and Luckman developed this perspective to argue that because human beings are biologically underdeveloped, they have to construct a social canopy around themselves to supplement their biology. Because human beings are "unfinished," they are vulnerable and require the support and protection of institutions to cope with the exigencies of life.

It is important to note, therefore, that one of the most useful contributions to the debate about social constructionism was in fact based on a foundationalism ontology. This theoretical combination may explain why the reception of Berger and Luckman's (1966) approach was characterized by a profound ambiguity. Ontological foundationalism often appeared to point to a rather conservative theory of institutions, while the social constructionist position in the sociology of knowledge implied a profound criticism of the taken-for-granted nature of social institutions. This ambiguity in the work of Berger and Luckman should help us identify the political nature of constructionist theories. They arise in contexts within which certain categories of behavior, such as homosexuality, have become highly politicized. They make the somewhat obvious point that while individuals may not fully accept the application of a stigmatized identity, such individual discrepancies only become politically important once a group of individuals presents a counterdefinition of social reality. This is evident in the historical case of the emergence of leper colonies (Berger and Luckmann 1966:184-90). Through such collective redefinition of deviance, individual cases of abnormality are transformed by acts of collective reorganization of social definitions of normality. Similarly, the idea that anorexia is socially constructed typically arises when feminists want to deny the importance of physiology in social behavior. The same issue is at stake in the political debate around disability, in which the social construction of disability is emphasized (in the words of Foucault) to show the arbitrary nature of the institutions that surround, produce, and maintain disability as an exclusionary device. "Disability" is, in terms of the sociology of knowledge, not unlike "gender" in that its very existence has been questioned by the politics of constructionism. It is for this reason that the UPIAS (Union of the Physically Impaired against Segregation) model, which defines disability in terms of citizenship (as a loss of opportunities), is appropriate for advocacy purposes. In this perspective, it is society that "disables people with impairments; disability is imposed on people" (Bickenbach et al. 1999:1176).

Social constructionism is probably best regarded as a historical and sociological account of how certain conditions (disease, sickness, impairment, or disability) become accepted over time by the medical profession and the wider society and how that historical process is shaped by political struggles and economic interests. The historical reception of repetitious strain injury is probably a particularly good illustration of the idea that a nonspecific discomfort or condition can be transformed over time into a distinctive medical condition (tenosynovitis) as a result of a successful political lobby by the victims of the condition against employers and insurance companies (Turner 1995a:14-15). Phenomenological studies offer a rich tradition of research that can provide a detailed understanding of the everyday experiences of disability (Nettleson and Watson 1998; Toombs 1995; Williams 1984). As I have suggested, the main problem with constructionism is that it is either unable or unwilling to give an account of the experience of the condition, which is socially constructed, and the subjective consequences of disabling labels. Finally, an understanding of this shared phenomenology of human embodiment can transcend the trap of cultural relativism and suggest how a human and social rights discourse can overcome the able-disable dichotomy.

These examples from the work of Berger and Luckmann (1966) are intended to demonstrate two (possibly obvious) issues: (1) that a concern for the phenomenology of individual experiences of illness does not preclude the development of a political agenda for collective responses to inequality, and (2) as a result, it is a short step between the phenomenological description of chronic illness to an account of social rights. My concern for a sociology of ethics and politics is connected with a desire that sociology might make a contribution to the study of human rights through the concept of embodiment (Turner 1993, 1997a, 1997b, 1997c). The ontological theory that lies behind this discussion of embodiment attempts to develop a general sociology that has three components—the frailty (of human beings), the precariousness (of institutions), and the interconnectedness (of social life). In this respect, my approach has been influenced by the existentialist reflections of Oliver Sacks (1986) in *A Leg to Stand On* and by the notion of "the pain of vulnerability" in the social philosophy of Arthur Kleinman (Kleinman 1988; Kleinman and Kleinman 1996). The analytical goal is to produce an ethics of embodiment through an understanding of the debates on chronic illness, impairment, and disability.

IMPAIRMENT AND DISABILITY

Many of the philosophical issues discussed above have been effectively identified by Hughes and Paterson (1997) in a valuable article titled "The Social Model of Disability and the Disappearing Body." Their argument is that the disability movement has been based on the creation of a "social model" of disability, which is a direct challenge to the medical model. A medical model regards both disease and sickness as medical conditions that are produced by specific entities (such as a virus) and assumes that the role of medical intervention is to control the symptoms of a disease and, where possible, remove their causes. It does not attend, therefore, to the subjective worldview of patients as constitutive of the condition and does not recognize the role of politics and culture in shaping human suffering (Turner 1995b). Hughes and Paterson note that by "focusing on the ways in which disability is socially produced, the social model has succeeded in shifting debate about disability from biomedically dominated agendas to discourses about politics and citizenship" (p. 325). However, this displacement is made possible by a division between the concepts of impairment and disability that is not satisfactory. By defining disability as a social and political condition of exclusion and impairment as a medical category to describe an absent or defective limb, organism, or mechanism of the body, the social construction of the disabled body confines impairment to a medical framework. While a constructionist interpretation of the body liberates disability, the medical model still dominates the field of impairment.

The result of postmodern and poststructuralist theories is that the palpable, living body disappears because postmodern perspectives preclude the possibility of an "ethnography of physicality" (Shakespeare and Watson 1995:16) that would be highly valuable to the disability movement. Indeed, one can argue that it would be difficult to imagine what, in general, a postmodern ethnographic methodology would look like. At best, it would be concerned to decode the images of disability in modern societies, and in that respect it is simply a branch of cultural studies. By contrast, one illustration of an ethnographic approach to the physicality of the impaired body can be found in Wendy Seymour's moving account of the experience and consequences of spinal cord injury. Her research represents an intellectually creative approach to the injured body that transcends the separation of the objective and subjective body in the clash between the legacy of Foucault and Merleau-Ponty. *Remaking the Body* (Seymour 1998) and *Bodily Alterations* (Seymour 1989) are two studies of trauma that open up creative directions in the study of disability. Her analysis of disability closely follows the distinction between the experience of embodiment, the physical body, and the medical or objective body (Frankenberg

1990). Employing qualitative data from interviews, Seymour examined the social construction of the body in a literal sense—namely, how bodies are remade following trauma, whether by accident or disease. The posttraumatic rebuilding of the body also involves, in the language of Anthony Giddens (1992), a "second chance" at refashioning the self. This remaking is not merely a discursive process; it involves, following Merleau-Ponty, the reconstruction of the lived, sensual body. This remaking of the body also takes place within the professional "gaze" of rehabilitation, which holds out the typically false promise of normalization, that is, the production of a socially "normal" body—young, athletic, and sexual. It is not enough to return to society via rehabilitation; the rehabilitated body has to be discursively normal. Seymour's ethnographic study shows how, through endless medical encounters in the everyday world, these individuals are coached and coaxed into the vestiges of normal and routine social roles.

One solution to these conceptual difficulties with both the medical and the social model of disability has been to propose a synthesis of the medical and social processes—namely, a biopsychosocial model. Such a model has been incorporated into the *ICIDH-2* (*International Classification of Impairments, Disabilities, and Handicaps*) proposals of the World Health Organization (1997), in which every dimension of disablement is analyzed in terms of an interaction between the individual and his or her social and physical environment. The model assumes that different types of intervention are appropriate at different levels. While medical intervention may be appropriate in relation to the specific features of impairment, sociopolitical action is appropriate at the level of the disability. Although the model has been criticized by movement activists because it labels individuals in terms of an official and professional system of classification, it is claimed that the model transcends the limitations of both the social and the medical models and holds out the promise of a more universalistic approach (Bickenbach et al. 1999). Although the idea of a synthesis is attractive, to argue that the biological should not be dismissed is quite separate from an account of human embodiment. From the perspective of sociology, "the body" is not in some elementary framework "the biological." The point of the sociology of embodiment is to go beyond a Cartesian medical framework in which mind-body dualism is replaced; there is little advantage in substituting a psychology-biology dualism for the traditional mind-body dualism.

Embodiment, Self, and Society in Western Cultures

Contemporary studies of the phenomenology of impairment and disability serve to further question the legacy of Cartesian dualism. The sociology of disability demonstrates the limitations of a simple mind-body dualism and takes us into a discussion of the embodied self and the disruptions of everyday life. The nature of corporeality and embodiment leads directly into the question of the self and the social actor (Charmaz 1994; Deegan 1978; Oberg 1996). The characterization of the social actor has been an issue that has dominated the entire development of the social sciences. It involves questions about the rationality of social action, the importance of affective and emotional elements, and the role of symbol and culture in the constitution of the social self. Disability, while socially produced by systems of classification and professional labels, also has profound significance for the self because who we are is necessarily constituted by our embodiment. Because our biographical narratives are carried in our embodiment, disability has to be mediated by its meaning for the self. The day-to-day difficulties of mobility and autonomy are not, as it were, merely accidental features of everyday life of the chronically ill, the disabled, or the elderly; they actually constitute selfhood by transforming the complex relationships between the self, body image, and environment. These disabilities, for instance, impinge on the everyday capacity of individuals to make and sustain intimate partnerships; in this respect, the problems of sexual intimacy in old age and in chronic illness are not dissimilar (Riggs and Turner 1999).

This issue of the embodiment of the social actor has also to be cast in a distinctively historical context; we are obliged to explore the historical setting of the corporeality of the social self. Sociologists are not only concerned with the phenomenology of the embodied self but also must be aware that in certain historical periods, the relationship between body and society is very different. Therefore, the debate about the relationship between selfhood and disability can take very different forms in different cultural and historical settings. In contemporary Western societies, there is, within the context of an individualistic and hedonistic culture, an emphasis on youth, youthfulness, and activity. For example, in critical gerontology, there is an important emphasis on activity and engagement against the idea that successful aging requires disengagement (Phillipson 1998:15-16). This emphasis on the youthful, active, and slim body is connected with the importance of reflexivity as a component of modernity. Recent writing on the body has indeed associated the emergence of the debate about the body with the growing importance of the postmodern or reflexive self in high modernity. For example, Anthony Synnott (1993) has asserted that "the body is also, and primarily, the self. We are all embodied" (p. 1). In a similar fashion, Chris Shilling (1993), following the approach of Anthony Giddens (1991, 1992) to contemporary forms of intimacy, also argues that the project of the self in modern society is in fact the project of the body; "there is a tendency for the body to become increasingly central to the modern person's sense of self-identity" (p. 1).

The transformation of medical technology has made possible the construction of the human body as a personal project through cosmetic surgery, organ transplants, and transsexual surgery. In addition, there is the whole panoply of dieting regimes, health farms, sports science, and nutritional science that are focused on the development of the aesthetic, thin body. Both Synnott (1993) and Shilling (1993) have noted that modern sensibility and subjectivity are focused on the body as a representation of the self, such that the body is a mirror of the soul in contemporary society. This involves a profound process of secularization whereby diet is transformed from a discipline of the soul into a mechanism for the expression of sexuality, which is in turn the focus of modern selfhood (Turner 1996). Whereas traditional forms of diet subordinated desire in the interests of the salvation of the soul, in contemporary consumer society, the diet assumes an entirely different meaning and focus—namely, as an elaboration or amplification of sexuality. The project of the self is intimately bound up with these historical transformations of the nature of the body, its role in culture, and its location in the public sphere. Although sociologists have invested much effort into understanding cosmetic surgery as a technique for refashioning the self through body transformations, there is, as we have noted in the work of Wendy Seymour (1989, 1998), an important system of rehabilitation in contemporary medicine and social work that contributes both to rebuilding the self and to normalizing the body. Given this emphasis on the body beautiful in the commercial culture of contemporary capitalism, there is an important "aestheticization of everyday life" that puts considerable social pressure on conformity with these health norms. Both old bodies and impaired bodies need rehabilitation to conform to the values of youthfulness, beauty, and athleticism (Featherstone 1991:15). In contemporary America, even smallness has become a medical condition, thereby preventing the election of small men to the presidency; the size of the presidential role requires the presence of a large and handsome body. The word *ailment* is derived from the Old English *egl(i)an,* indicating "troublesome" (*egle*) and, in its Gothic form, "disgraceful" (*agls*); an ailing body is therefore without grace (charisma). A charismatic leader should be, whenever possible, equipped with a graceful body that as a result indicates the existence of a charismatic power.

To clarify these debates, we need to develop an adequate definition of embodiment or at least to list its necessary components. It is interesting that despite the enthusiasm for the development of the sociology of the body, we do not as yet possess any adequate definition. First, following Norbert Elias's (1978) notion of the social as process, it is important not to reify the term but to treat embodiment as a process—namely, the social processes of embodying. Embodiment is the effect or consequence of ongoing practices of what we might call "corporealization." In this respect, it requires the learning or mastery of body techniques (Mauss 1973)—walking, sitting, dancing, eating, and so forth. Embodiment is the ensemble of corporeal practices, which produce and give "a body" its place in everyday life. Embodiment locates or places particular bodies within a social habitus. In this respect, embodiment could be readily described in terms of Pierre Bourdieu's (1990) notions of practice, disposition, and habitus. Embodiment is an accomplishment by which a social actor embraces a set of dispositions, practices, and strategies and, as a result, comfortably occupies a unique habitus. Second, embodiment is about the production of a sensuous and practical presence in the life-world. Embodiment is the lived experience of the sensual or subjective body, and it is, in this sense, very close to the notion of practice (praxis) in the early philosophical anthropology (Csordas 1994). The sensual, lived body is a practical accomplishment in the context of everyday social relations, but it is also the active shaping of the lived world by embodied practices. Third, embodiment is a social project in the sense that it takes place in a life-world that is already social. Embodiment is not an isolated or individual project; it is located within a social and historical world of interconnected social actors, within a social network. The phenomenology of the lived body is not grounded in any individualistic assumptions; on the contrary, it treats the body as necessarily a social product. Finally, while it is the process of making and becoming a body, it is also the project of making a self. Embodiment and enselfment are mutually dependent, interdependent, and reinforcing projects. The self involves a corporeal project within a specific social nexus where the continuous but constantly disrupted self requires successful embodiment, a social habitus, and memory.

BODY AND TIME

Although embodiment is a social project that is routinely accomplished (with comfort or ease), it also has its own specificity (Turner 1998a). My embodiment is uniquely accomplished within wholly routine and predictable contexts. We can express this paradox of particularity and uniformity in terms of the relationship between sociology and ontology in a formulation taken from Martin Heidegger's (1958) *The Question of Being*. On the social or horizontal plane, an individual is routinely defined by a series of social roles that specify a standardized position in the public world of the economy and society. There is also an ontological plane, which forms a vertical axis, that is defined by the finite and unique embodiment of a person. The horizontal social plane is the precarious world of the social system; the vertical plane is the world of embodied frailty. In this sense, we might argue that sociological (horizontal) analysis is concerned to understand the contingent and arbitrary characteristics of social being, while philosophical (vertical) analysis attempts to grasp the necessities of our human being. This formulation can be adopted as a further perspective on Foucault's notion of the arbitrariness of institutions. The horizontal planes of social relations are indeed arbitrary; they are also precarious. The institutions of disability and rehabilitation have been radically transformed in the late twentieth century, and the traditional systems of rehabilitation no longer hold sway. However, on the vertical plane of human existence, certain necessities are concerned with aging, disability, and dependency.

In many respects, Gay Becker's (1997) *Disrupted Lives* perfectly captures the relationship between these vertical and horizontal relationships; it addresses a carefully formulated theoretical problem, which concerns the relationship between the body, metaphor, and personal identity. The notion of "disruption" leads us toward a reflexive uncovering of the frailty of our lives and the precarious character of the institutions that underpin them. Becker's book is composed of five separate but interconnected studies of infertility, midlife crisis, strokes, old age, and chronic illness. *Disrupted Lives* can be understood as a further reflection on the problems of the Cartesian legacy of the mind-body dichotomy. Both sociology and anthropology have demonstrated that identity is fundamentally embodied because subjective and objective identity cannot be easily separated from embodiment. It follows that "self" is not an enduring or stable fact but changes with aging, the life course, and the disruptions of illness. Hence, radical disruptions to self occur as a result of traumatic illness, which often breaks our relationship with significant others, reorganizes our life-world, and threatens to destroy the comfortable relationship between self, body, and others. In North America, where there is an important emphasis on youthfulness, activism, and independence, disruptions to everyday life from accident, chronic illness, and aging represent a profound challenge to the sense of self-identity. Talcott Parsons's (1951) sick role defined sickness in terms of inactivity; to be sick was essentially not to be at work. In a society that values activism, chronic illness and impairment are in this sense deviant. Parsons's model of the sick role was implicitly about the occurrence of acute illness and does not easily fit the experience of chronicity. As such, the Parsonian model implies that disability is a form of more or less permanent sickness and thus of permanent stigmatization. When the disruptions of life from sickness and disability transform the body image, then other social actors experience disruptions to the social routines of interaction. According to Goffman's (1964) analysis of stigma, impairments create systematic representational ambiguities.

Becker (1997) argues that metaphors of illness and impairment play an important part in helping people to make sense of these unwanted discontinuities. Metaphors help us to understand, but they also have therapeutic qualities; as a result, narratives of disruption constitute moral accounts of people's lives. Metaphors are the cultural vehicles that express the values that make life meaningful and coherent. Thus, narratives of healing are part of the process of healing. Given the importance of activism and individualism in American culture, healing narratives are typically structured around themes of disruption and the assumption of personal responsibility. Power relationships are crucial to the negotiation of these narratives. The interaction between therapist and patient in the rehabilitation process also involves power. The hierarchical structure of power in relation to medical knowledge is fundamental to questions such as the following: What metaphors are available to patients, and how are they legitimized? Can deviant narratives of illness subvert medical power? Because meanings and metaphors are negotiated in medical settings where resources are unequal, the critique of the medical model has been central to the disability movement.

There is a submerged theme to Becker's (1997) study that requires special attention and suggests a radical alternative to the conventional perspective on the body-self relationship. The stability of everyday life requires the presumption of a continuous and reliable self, and hence we assume that disruptions are exceptional interventions within this normality. For interaction to take place at all, one must be able to make assumptions about the continuity of an embodied self through time and space. Toward the end of her study, Becker came to the conclusion that "continuity is an illusion. Disruption to life is a constant human experience. The only continuity that has staying power is the continuity of the body, and even that is vulnerable" (p. 190). Hence, the everyday world involves a constant struggle to sustain the illusions of order and continuity against a backdrop of persistent and ineluctable disorder. Metaphors, which mediate between the self and chaos, provide the building blocks of cultural meaning. The social world has to be constantly socially constructed against the disruptions that threaten the continuities of the identities of social actors.

Any account of disruption has to take into account the biography of the individual in terms of whether trauma occurred to a person previously regarded as whole and healthy or whether impairment has its origins in the fetus—namely, whether a person is born with an impairment. In the medical history described by Geyla Frank (1984, 1986), Diane DeVries was born without fully developed limbs and therefore had no memory of the "missing limbs." This fact explains why she responded to the notion of being an amputee with amazement. In fact, she came to think of herself as an image of beauty—an embodiment of the limbless Venus de Milo. Similar experiences of the phenomenology of the body would characterize people who are thalidomide victims because they have no experience of a different type of body. We need to make an important distinction in studies of disruption to life involving impairment at birth, accident, and processes such as aging. These three contrasting situations have an importance for any sociological understanding of disruptions to the self.

In conclusion, the diseases and discomforts of human beings have their own peculiar temporalities and rhythms—onset, duration, crises, and terminations are different for different diseases in relation to different patients. Some are slow and insidious, others confronting and quick. Oliver Sacks (1976) has given us poetically inspired accounts of the rhythms of chronic sickness and the capacity of drugs to bring about personal awakenings. The temporal dimensions of disease have different implications for the self. The same is true for different impairments and disabilities. We need to distinguish between people who are born with impairment and who have no pre-impairment experience of the embodied self. Second, we can identify a range of disabilities that are consequences of a traumatic event, such as a traffic or sporting accident. In this case, the assault on the integrity of the embodied self is massive. An individual with spinal injury has a clear phenomenological experience of a pre- and posttraumatic personality. The rhythm of disruption is total and abrupt. In Seymour's (1989, 1998) terms, such accidents require a reconstruction of self and body. Third, we may distinguish a slow and crippling ailment such as rheumatism, in which the transformations of embodiment are painful but uneven and unpredictable; however, the long-term outcome may be immobility and marginalization. Finally, forms of disability and impairment accompany the aging process in which the loss of mobility, independence, and status is profound and inevitable. However, with aging, the loss of mobility and autonomy is an expected, anticipated, and possibly normal outcome of aging (Schieman and Turner 1998).

CONCLUSION: VULNERABILITY AND RIGHTS

My discussion has involved an account of how the notion of embodiment can contribute to the phenomenology of disability to provide a sociology of rights that is grounded in the notion of a shared frailty. To pursue this line of argumentation, I need to provide an elaboration of the idea of ontological insecurity, which has the following components. First, there is the assertion that we are biologically frail. Both impairment and aging are important illustrations of this position. While of course age and aging are culturally defined, it is also the case that we are subject necessarily to an aging process. This process is individually variable, but our immune systems tend to decline with age, and we are more exposed to physical dangers as we grow older. Most people will experience some form of disability in old age, and there is a definite experience of a loss of mastery after 60 years (Mirowsky 1995). Because there is a scarcity of resources, there is a social conflict over the allocation of resources to the elderly and the impaired, which, in a state of nature, means that life is "nasty, brutish, and short." In this Hobbesian world, the state is the product of a contract between rational actors to protect their collective security. In my sociology version of social contract theory, embodiment for human beings creates insecurity because we are all prone to illness, aging, and disability. We can derive the need for (protective) human rights from this Hobbesian notion that human beings are biologically frail, they are socially vulnerable, and their lives are politically precarious. Human beings as embodied creatures are subject to illness and disease, aging and disability, and suffering and mental decay (through dementia, Alzheimer's disease, Parkinson's disease, etc.). Human beings have to manage the problem of their "ontological security" (Giddens 1991:44) through the development of everyday routines, but in my argument, these routines are prone to fail because our social and political world is precarious. Daily routines and norms are constantly disrupted because our embodiment means that we are exposed to physical risks that cannot be easily predicted.

In addition to being biologically frail, we are also vulnerable at a social level. Once more, the aging process provides a clear illustration of the issue. As we age, in biological terms, we are exposed to social vulnerability because old age is, particularly in modern society, a period of increasing isolation and loneliness. We cannot provide easily for our own wants and needs, and we become dependent on the family and kinship networks. With growing longevity in societies where traditional family systems have broken down, the elderly become increasingly dependent and exposed to marginalization and social abuse. Biological frailty and social vulnerability tend to reinforce the problems of marginality and isolation that the sick, disabled, and elderly experience.

In addition to the human body being fragile and frail, we live in a societal environment that is essentially precarious, and this precariousness is an inevitable consequence of the nature of power and its investment in the state. Powerful institutions such as the state, which are set up according to social contract theory to protect the interests of rational actors, can of course function to terrorize and dominate civil society. While strong states may protect society from civil wars, they can, for that very reason, be a danger to the very existence of citizens. By precariousness, I also mean that institutions, which are rationally designed to serve certain specific purposes, may evolve in ways that contradict these original charters. Social life is essentially contingent and risky; individuals, even when they collect together for concerted action, cannot necessarily protect themselves against the vagaries of social reality. Following through with the theme of aging, we are precarious at the societal level because we cannot effectively control macro-policy decisions about issues such as compulsory retirement, mandatory superannuation contributions, inheritance taxation, health coverage, and so forth.

While social theorists might grant that social reality is precarious, the argument that human beings are universally frail may appear to be controversial and contentious. There are a number of problems here. If human beings are frail by definition, then frailty is variable, and my argument could easily be converted into a Darwinistic theory of the survival of the fittest. Those who are least frail may combine to dominate and subordinate the vulnerable and fragile. The disposition of the strong to support and protect the weak must be based consequently on some collectively shared sympathy or empathy for human beings in their collective frailty and weakness. Following Richard Rorty (1998), one can derive a theory of human rights from certain aspects of feminist theory, from a critical view of the limitations of utilitarian accounts of reason, and from an interest in notions of sympathy, sentiment, and emotionality. Insofar as the strong protect the weak, it is through recognition of likeness, which is itself a product of affective attachment and sentiment. People will want their rights to be recognized because they see in the plight of other human beings their own (potential or actual) unhappiness and misery (Turner 1994, 1998b). Because individual aging is an inevitable biological process, we can all anticipate, in principle, our own vulnerability and frailty. We can anticipate our own impairment. More important, sympathy is crucial in deciding to whom our moral concern might be directed. Sympathy derives from the fundamental experiences of reciprocity in everyday life, particularly from the relationship between mother and child.

However, if this argument is to prevail, we need a more elaborate notion of human frailty. For example, the argument could be made more sophisticated by developing a distinction between pain and suffering. Human beings can suffer without an experience of pain; conversely, they can have an experience of pain without suffering. Suffering is essentially a situation in which the self is threatened or destroyed from outside, for example, through humiliation. We can suffer the loss of a loved one without physical pain, whereas a toothache may give us extreme physical pain without a sense of loss of self or the humiliation of self. While suffering is variable, pain might be regarded as universal. This is closely related to a position adopted by Richard Rorty (1989) in *Contingency, Irony and Solidarity,* where he argues that

> the idea that we have an overriding obligation to diminish cruelty, to make human beings equal in respect of their liability to suffering, seems to take for granted that there is something within human beings which deserves respect and protection quite independently of the language they speak. It suggests that a non-linguistic ability, the ability to feel pain, is what is important, and the differences in the vocabulary are much less important. (P. 88)

There is an additional claim that can be made here, namely that while pleasures are variable, human misery is universal. Although we find it difficult to agree about a common definition of happiness, there is little disagreement as to the nature of human suffering (Moore 1970).

This claim about the unity of suffering can provide a universalistic foundation for human rights: Frailty is a universal condition of the human species because pain is a fundamental experience of all organic life. Such an argument runs counter to the conventional anthropological view of cultural relativism, but the notion that there is an organic foundation to pain and suffering could be compatible with the idea of cultural diversity. Such a position finds strong support in Irving Zola's (1989) defense of universalism with respect to disability and impairment. Zola was acutely aware of the paradox or "dilemma of difference" (Goffman 1964) that political demands to end various forms of discrimination require a social analyst to identify those who are experiencing discrimination. This identification of a minority requires a special focus on their difference, but to ignore the difference delays the development of positive policies against discrimination. Against a "special needs approach," Zola argued that, in the long term, we need to support universal policies that recognize that the entire population is in some sense "at risk" in terms of chronic illness and disability. He took this universalistic stance because

> only when we acknowledge the near universality of disability and that its dimensions (including the biomedical) are part of the social process by which the meanings of disability are negotiated will it be possible fully to appreciate how general public policy can affect this issue. (P. 406)

The aging of the populations of Western society, the growing prevalence of chronicity, and the globalization of health risks are important demographic and sociological aspects of Zola's (1989) view of the universality of disability. The basis of his view (the need to universalize policy responses to disability) rested on the claim that only by "bringing bodies back in" could an adequate sociology of disability be finally created. The challenge of Zola's view of embodiment for the social sciences should remain a permanent feature of both disability studies and policy formation.

REFERENCES

Auslander, G. K. and N. Gold. 1999. "Disability Terminology in the Media: A Comparison of Newspaper Reports in Canada and Israel." *Social Science & Medicine* 48 (10): 1395-1405.

Barnes, C., G. Mercer, and T. Shakespeare. 1999. *Exploring Disability: A Sociological Introduction.* Cambridge, UK: Polity.

Becker, G. 1997. *Disrupted Lives: How People Create Meaning in a Chaotic World.* Berkeley: University of California Press.

Berger, P. L. and T. Luckmann. 1966. *The Social Construction of Reality.* Garden City, NY: Doubleday.

Bickenbach, J. E., S. Chatterji, E. M. Bailey, and T. B. Ustun. 1999. "Models of Disablement, Universalism and the International Classification of Impairments, Disabilities and Handicaps." *Social Science & Medicine* 48 (9): 1173-88.

Bourdieu, P. 1990. *The Logic of Practice.* Cambridge, UK: Polity.

Burchell, G., C. Gordon, and P. Miller, eds. 1991. *The Foucault Effect: Studies in Governmentality.* Hemel Hempstead, UK: Harvester Wheatsheaf.

Charmaz, K. 1994. "Identity Dilemmas of Chronically Ill Men." *The Sociological Quarterly* 35 (2): 269-88.

Csordas, T. J. 1994. *Embodiment and Experience: The Existential Ground of Culture and Self.* Cambridge, UK: Cambridge University Press.

Davis, F. 1963. *Passage through Crisis: Polio Victims and Their Families.* Indianapolis, IN: Bobbs-Merrill.

Deegan, M. J. 1978. "Living and Acting in an Altered Body: A Phenomenological Description of Amputation." *Journal of Sociology and Social Welfare* 5 (3): 342-55.

Elias, N. 1978. *The Civilising Process.* Vol. 1. Oxford, UK: Basil Blackwell.

Featherstone, M. 1991. *Consumer Culture and Postmodernism.* London: Sage.

Featherstone, M. and A. Wernick, eds. 1995. *Images of Aging: Cultural Representations of Later Life.* London: Routledge Kegan Paul.

Foucault, M. 1980. *Herculine Barbin.* Brighton, UK: Harvester.

———. 1981. *The History of Sexuality.* Vol. 1, *An Introduction.* Harmondsworth, UK: Penguin.

———. 1987. *The History of Sexuality.* Vol. 2, *The Use of Pleasure.* Harmondsworth, UK: Penguin.

———. 1988. *The History of Sexuality.* Vol. 3, *The Care of the Self.* Harmondsworth, UK: Penguin.

Frank, G. 1984. "Life History Model of Adaptation to Disability: The Case of a 'Congenital Amputee.' " *Social Science & Medicine* 19 (6): 639-45.

———. 1986. "On Embodiment: A Case of Congenital Limb Deficiency in American Culture." *Culture, Medicine and Psychiatry* 10:189-219.

Frankenberg, R. 1990. "Disease, Literature and the Body in the Era of AIDS: A Preliminary Exploration." *Journal of Health and Illness* 12 (3): 351-60.

Gehlen, A. 1980. *Man in the Age of Technology.* New York: Columbia University Press.

———. 1988. *Man, His Nature and Place in the World.* New York: Columbia University Press.

Giddens, A. 1991. *Modernity and Self-Identity: Self and Society in the Late Modern Age.* Cambridge, UK: Polity.

———. 1992. *The Transformation of Intimacy: Sexuality, Love and Eroticism in Modern Societies.* Cambridge, UK: Polity.

Goffman, E. 1959. *The Presentation of Self in Everyday Life.* New York: Doubleday Anchor.

———. 1964. *Stigma: Notes on the Management of Spoiled Identity.* Englewood Cliffs, NJ: Prentice Hall.

Heidegger, M. 1958. *The Question of Being.* New York: Twayne.

Hocking, J. and A. James. 1993. *Growing Up and Growing Old: Ageing and Dependency in the Life Course.* London: Sage.

Hughes, B. and K. Paterson. 1997. "The Social Model of Disability and the Disappearing Body: Towards a Sociology of Impairment." *Disability & Society* 12 (3): 325-40.

Ingstad, B. and S. R. Whyte, eds. 1995. *Disability and Culture.* Berkeley: University of California Press.

Jones, C. and R. Porter, eds. 1994. *Reassessing Foucault: Power, Medicine and the Body.* London: Routledge Kegan Paul.

Kleinman, A. 1988. *The Illness Narratives: Suffering, Healing and the Human Condition.* New York: Basic Books.

Kleinman, A. and J. Kleinman. 1996. "Social Suffering." *Daedalus* 125 (1): 1-24.

Laqueur, T. 1990. *Making Sex: Body and Gender from Greeks to Freud.* Cambridge, MA: Harvard University Press.

Martin, L. H., H. Gutman, and P. H. Hutton, eds. 1988. *Technologies of the Self: A Seminar with Michel Foucault.* London: Tavistock.

Mauss, M. 1973. "Techniques of the Body." *Economy & Society* 2:70-88.

Merleau-Ponty, M. 1962. *Phenomenology of Perception.* London: Routledge Kegan Paul.

Mirowsky, J. 1995. "Age and the Sense of Control." *Social Psychology Quarterly* 58:31-43.

Mitchell, D. T. and S. L. Snyder, eds. 1997. *The Body and Physical Difference: Discourses of Disability.* Ann Arbor: University of Michigan Press.

Monks, J. and R. Frankenberg. 1995. "Being Ill and Being Me: Self, Body, and Time in Multiple Sclerosis Narratives." Pp. 107-34 in *Disability and Culture,* edited by B. Ingstad and S. R. Whyte. Berkeley: University of California Press.

Moore, B. 1970. *Reflections on the Causes of Human Misery and upon Certain Proposals to Eliminate Them.* Boston: Beacon.

Nettleson, S. and J. Watson, eds. 1998. *The Body in Everyday Life.* London: Routledge Kegan Paul.

Oberg, P. 1996. "The Absent Body: A Social Gerontological Paradox." *Ageing and Society* 16:701-19.

Olafson, F. A. 1995. *What Is a Human Being? A Heideggerian View.* Cambridge, UK: Cambridge University Press.

O'Neill, J. 1972. *Sociology as a Skin Trade.* London: Heinemann.

Parsons, T. 1951. *The Social System.* London: Routledge Kegan Paul.

———. 1999. "Youth in the Context of American Society." Pp. 271-91 in *The Talcott Parsons Reader,* edited by B. S. Turner. Oxford, UK: Blackwell.

Phillipson, C. 1998. *Reconstructing Old Age: New Agendas in Social Theory and Practice.* London: Sage.

Riggs, A. and B. S. Turner. 1999. "The Expectation of Love in Older Age: Towards a Sociology of Intimacy." Pp. 193-208 in *A Certain Age: Women Growing Older,* edited by M. Poole and S. Feldman. St. Leonards, UK: Allen & Unwin.

Rorty, R. 1989. *Contingency, Irony and Solidarity.* Cambridge, UK: Cambridge University Press.

———. 1998. *Truth and Progress.* Cambridge, UK: Cambridge University Press.

———. 1999. *Philosophy and Social Hope.* Harmondsworth, UK: Penguin.

Rose, N. 1989. *Governing the Soul: The Shaping of the Private Self.* London: Routledge Kegan Paul.

Sacks, O. 1976. *Awakenings.* Harmondsworth, UK: Penguin.

———. 1986. *A Leg to Stand On.* London: Pan.

Schieman, S. and H. A. Turner. 1998. "Age, Disability and the Sense of Mastery." *Journal of Health and Social Behavior* 39 (3): 169-86.

Seymour, W. 1989. *Bodily Alterations: An Introduction to a Sociology of the Body for Health Workers.* Sydney, Australia: Allen & Unwin.

————. 1998. *Remaking the Body: Rehabilitation and Change*. St. Leonards, UK: Allen & Unwin.

Shakespeare, T. and N. Watson. 1995. "Defending the Social Model." *Disability and Society* 12 (2): 293-300.

Shilling, C. 1993. *The Body and Social Theory*. London: Sage.

Skultans, V. 1977. "Bodily Madness and the Spread of the Blush." Pp. 145-60 in *The Anthropology of the Body*, edited by J. Blacking. London: Academic Press.

Stiker, H.-J. 1982. *Corps infirmes et societes*. Paris: Aubier Montaigne.

Strauss, A. L. and B. Glaser. 1975. *Chronic Illness and the Quality of Life*. St. Louis, MO: C. V. Mosby.

Synnott, A. 1993. *The Body Social: Symbolism, Sex and Society*. London: Routledge Kegan Paul.

Toombs, K. S. 1995. "The Lived Experience of Disability." *Human Studies* 18:9-23.

Turner, B. S. 1982. "The Government of the Body: Medical Regimens and the Rationalization of Diet." *British Journal of Sociology* 33:254-69.

————. 1992. *Regulating Bodies: Essays in Medical Sociology*. London: Routledge Kegan Paul.

————. 1993. "Outline of a Theory of Human Rights." *Sociology* 27 (3): 489-512.

————. 1994. "Preface." Pp. vii-xvii in *The Consuming Body*, edited by Pasi Falk. London: Sage.

————. 1995a. *Medical Power and Social Knowledge*. 2d ed. London: Sage.

————. 1995b. "Aging and Identity: Some Reflections on the Somatization of the Self." Pp. 245-62 in *Images of Aging: Cultural Representations of Later Life*, edited by M. Featherstone and A. Wernick. London: Routledge Kegan Paul.

————. 1996. *The Body and Society: Explorations in Social Theory*. Oxford, UK: Basil Blackwell.

————. 1997a. "A Neo-Hobbesian Theory of Human Rights: A Reply to Malcolm Waters." *Sociology* 31 (3): 565-71.

————. 1997b. "What Is the Sociology of the Body?" *Body & Society* 3 (1): 103-7.

————. 1997c. "From Governmentality to Risk: Some Reflections on Foucault's Contribution to Medical Sociology." Pp. ix-xxi in *Foucault, Health and Medicine*, edited by A. Petersen and R. Bunton. London: Routledge Kegan Paul.

————. 1998a. "Foreword." Pp. v-viii in *Remaking the Body*, edited by Wendy Seymour. St. Leonards, UK: Allen & Unwin.

————. 1998b. "Forgetfulness and Frailty: Otherness and Rights in Contemporary Social Theory." Pp. 25-42 in *The Politics of Jean-Francois Lyotard: Justice and Political Theory*, edited by C. Rojek and B. S. Turner. London: Routledge Kegan Paul.

Whyte, S. R. 1995. "Disability between Discourse and Experience." Pp. 267-92 in *Disability and Culture*, edited by B. Ingstad and S. R. Whyte. Berkeley: University of California Press.

Williams, R. S. 1984. "Ability, Disability and Rehabilitation: A Phenomenological Description." *Journal of Medicine and Philosophy* 9:93-112.

Williams, S. 1987. "Goffman, Interactionism and Stigma." Pp. 134-64 in *Sociological Theory and Medical Sociology*, edited by G. Scrambler. London: Tavistock.

World Health Organization. 1997. *ICIDH-2 Beta-1 Draft: International Classification of Impairments, Activities, and Participation*. Geneva: Author.

Zola, I. 1982. *Missing Pieces: A Chronicle of Living with a Disability*. Philadelphia: Temple University Press.

————. 1988. "Aging and Disability: Toward a Unifying Agenda." *Educational Gerontology* 14:365.

————. 1989. "Toward the Necessary Universalizing of Disability Policy." *The Milbank Quarterly* 67:401-26.

————. 1991. "Bringing Our Bodies and Ourselves Back In: Reflections on a Past, Present and Future Medical Sociology." *Journal of Health and Social Behavior* 32 (1): 1-16.

Intellectual Disabilities— *Quo Vadis?*

10

TREVOR R. PARMENTER

. . . while we live, while we are among human beings, let us cultivate our humanity.

—Seneca, "On Anger"

It is probably difficult for anyone newly approaching the study of Mental Deficiency to appreciate the great advances which have taken place in the past thirty or forty years. At the beginning of the Century it was regarded as a comparatively unimportant subject, and interest in it was mainly confined to a few mental specialists and social workers. Today it is realised to be a serious social problem; a large number of medical practitioners and officials of public bodies are actively engaged in it; and it is recognized as an important branch of psychological medicine.

—Tredgold (1937:vii)

P lus ça change! Tredgold's preface to the sixth edition of *Mental Deficiency (Amentia)* is as evocative today as it was more than 60 years ago. While the language of the 1930s, in contemporary terms, is archaic and to many offensive, the book's chapter titles are topics that are still being vigorously explored in the millennium. Issues such as the concept and nature of mental deficiency, incidence, etiology, classification and definition, pathology, psychology, educational defect, clinical varieties of primary and secondary amentia, diagnosis and prognosis, treatment and training, the law, and sociology have remained major themes throughout the latter half of the twentieth century.

While Tredgold, one of the pioneers in the study of intellectual disability,[1] applauded the advances made in this field in the early twentieth century, there would be differences of opinion as to whether the first half of the twentieth century, in fact, made significant advances that led to positive outcomes in the lives of persons with intellectual disability. A key difference between the way Tredgold and his contemporaries viewed intellectual disability and the way it is viewed by most present-day commentators rests in the interpretation of the term *serious social problem.* The former group, people diagnosed with "primary or secondary amentia," presented a range of social problems, including a lack of moral sense somewhat akin to that of "primitive man." The psychological basis for "misconduct" was ascribed to faulty upbringing, inherent peculiarity, inherent incapacity for development, or a delay of inhibiting mechanisms (Tredgold 1937). The predominant contemporary view is that the social issues of intellectual disability, to-

267

gether with those of other disability groups, rests as much with the nature of society as it does with the person with the disability. There are, of course, current commentators whose views would range from those more akin to Tredgold's position to those who would see disability to be entirely a manifestation of a society unwilling or unable to cater for people with impairments (Stainton 1998).

This chapter will first explore, from a historical perspective, the place in society of persons with an intellectual disability. This analysis will establish that these people have been consistently denied personhood; they have been seen as objects of pity, fear, or both; they have been oppressed; and, with the rise of the eugenics movement, they have been seen as a threat to the very quality of the human race. The second section will analyze a number of the forces that spearheaded changes in the attitudes toward this group of people and the subsequent provision of more enlightened supports that enabled them to participate more fully in the general community. The pivotal role played by the normalization principle, together with scientific and technological advances, will be critically explored. Finally, it will be proposed that the full realization of personhood for these people may be found in the development of an "ethical community," rooted in the philosophy of a mutuality of need and responsiveness to the needs of all individuals in our society.

THE PLACE OF A PERSON WITH AN INTELLECTUAL DISABILITY IN SOCIETY

Philosopher Martha Nussbaum (1997) has identified three capacities that are essential to the cultivation of humanity in today's world. The first is an ability to examine oneself and one's traditions critically. The second is an ability to see beyond some local region, group, or country. As Nussbaum suggested, "The world around us is inescapably international" (p. 10). To cultivate our humanity, we must try to understand the variety of ways different groups realize our common needs and aims. Finally, she suggested that the development of a "narrative imagination" or "the ability to think what it might be like to be in the shoes of a person different from oneself, to be an intelligent reader of that person's story, and to understand the emotions and wishes and desires that someone so placed might have" (pp. 10-11) is the quintessential quality for the purposes of this discussion. It is only in recent years that we have come to recognize that to appreciate the essence of an intellectual disability, we must try to identify with the lives as they are lived by people with an intellectual disability.

Historically, society's continued denial of humanity toward persons with intellectual disability, as well as society's seeing such persons as a disposable commodity, challenges us. We move from a century that started with pride in scientific rationality and the triumph of logic over superstition to a century in which we should, in Nussbaum's (1997) terms, "make all human beings part of our community of dialogue and concern, showing respect for the human wherever it occurs" (pp. 60-61).

While not gainsaying Clegg's (1998) argument that in looking at past events in present time, one should not simply organize a set of ideas into chronological order, it is useful to examine the way society has almost consistently demeaned the place of persons with an intellectual disability in society. There are, of course, a number of positive signs that may be a harbinger for the future emancipation of this group. However, as will be indicated, significant though these signs may be, they were still quite tenuous within the overall social, cultural, political, and economic milieu at the beginning of the twenty-first century.

A categorization of historical eras suggested by Cliff Judge (1987), an early Australian leader in the field of intellectual disabilities, provides a useful framework in which to trace the evolution of community practices and attitudes toward this population. Judge has appropriately warned, however, that it is difficult to distinguish categorically one particular period in history from any other as a complex set of customs, social attitudes, and political imperatives define the character of an era. For example, infanticidal practices that were once found acceptable in an earlier period of history are still practiced in some communities today. Although we currently believe that community attitudes toward people with significant disabilities are more accommodating of diversity, religious prejudices, ethnic persecution, and discriminatory practices against minority groups are still manifested in all continents of the world. People with disabilities are more often than not a part of these minority groups.

A Prescientific Era

Infanticide, a practice that dates back to antiquity, typifies the fact that it is only in recent times that children have been seen to have a distinct place in society. The outlawing of child slavery and abuse and the principle that children are not mere chattels of their parents are relatively recent phenomena that are still not being applied in all countries. For instance, in many countries, including India and China, male babies are preferred for a variety of reasons. One example is that in some countries, males are seen as better agricultural workers. The practice of providing dowries for females, which can impoverish a family, is suggested as a reason for the preference for males.[2]

In the case of children with intellectual disability, however, there is an added and more insidious reason that Stainton (1998) has described as the oppression of people labeled as having an intellectual disability. Stainton has argued that

the central idea in their oppression lies at the heart of the idea of modernity, that is, the association of reason and value and this accounts for the pervasiveness and consistency of oppression . . . in modern societies. (P. 115)

Unlike other disabilities, especially physical and sensory, Stainton has posited that a distinctive and consistent characteristic of intellectual disability is the phenomenon of *otherness*,[3] which led to the practice of infanticide in classical Greece and the keeping of intellectually disabled people as slaves and fools by the nobility in ancient Rome (Stainton 1994).

In answering the question as to what lies at the heart of this *otherness* and its consistent and potent source of oppression for this population, Stainton's (1998) thesis is that

intellectual disability strikes at the very heart of classical and modern ideas of value and humanness. Shakespeare at his most Aristotelian sums up this central plank in the modernist project: "What a piece of work is man! How noble in reason! How infinite in faculty! . . . the paragon of animals" [*Hamlet*, II.ii]. (P. 115)

The notion that a defect of the human mind can be equated with subhuman species is found in the natural philosophy and the social and ethical writings of both Plato and Aristotle. For Plato, low intelligence was something to do with the nature of slave mentality (Goodey 1992), and Aristotle maintained that

the deliberative faculty is not present at all in the slave; in a female it is present but ineffective, in a child present but underdeveloped. (*Politics*, lxii, cited in Stainton 1998:116)

The eugenics movement, so often typified as a phenomenon of the late nineteenth and early twentieth centuries, can be seen to have had its foundations in the classical era. For instance, there is a road sign near Sparta that reads, "The law giver of Sparta threw deformed and invalid children for the good development of the human race" (Judge 1987:4).

The principle that persons with an intellectual disability were considered less than human and, more important, were ascribed as being possessed by the devil had strong foundations in religious beliefs of the Christian era. For instance, Martin Luther saw demonic forces underlying mental disorders:

> Idiots[4] are men in whom devils have established themselves, and all the physicians who heal these infirmities as though they proceeded from natural causes are ignorant blockheads, who know nothing about the power of the demon. (Cited in Judge 1987:4)

Superstitions concerning the origins of mental disorders became entwined with the origins of medicine. The writings of Hippocrates (460-359 B.C.) and Galen (131-200 A.D.) had profound effects on medical thinking for centuries. For instance, Galen is reported as saying that idiotic patients had large and outstanding ears (Judge 1987:7). In the sixteenth century, the pseudoscience of palmistry gained popularity. Palmists maintained that the shape, size, and marking of a person's hand and palm provided indications of a person's intellectual ability and character. Phrenology, another pseudoscience, gained popularity in the eighteenth century through the work of Franz Joseph Gall (1758-1828).

The movement went from a long period of superstition and the belief that intellectual disability had its origins in demonic and satanic forces (somewhat akin to witchcraft, with "treatments" such as exorcism and ritual burning) to the pseudoscientific era, which resulted in a search for a cure. Remedies such as purification with water treatment, bloodletting, the ingestion of "bitters" (quinine), multivitamin and cell therapy, movement training, and faith healing have been prescribed and are still being prescribed in parts of the world. It is this search for curative treatments that gave rise to the "medical model" of intervention for people with an intellectual disability.

"Moral training," which became advocated for "moral imbeciles," can be seen as related to exorcism, as mental disorders after the Middle Ages were seen as something quite distinct from the body. The thesis that the mind is basically distinct from the body can be traced to Cartesian philosophy. Descartes's view, suggested by Edwards (1998), was that "the self can be identified with the mind or soul, and is only contingently related to the body" (p. 47). In this view, "the self is encased, housed or trapped within a body; the mental and physical realms, are clearly demarcated; and the body is an object different from inanimate objects only by virtue of the degree of complexity and its organization" (Edwards 1998:49).

The Age of Enlightenment

In the seventeenth century, John Locke (1623-1704) set the philosophical groundwork for the "Age of Enlightenment" and heralded the then radical belief in the value of education, which countered the deeply held religious view of "man" having to bear the ineradicable stain of original sin. The prevailing view was that education could do very little to ameliorate the human condition without "the previous impression of God's saving grace" (Spellman 1988:2). Despite this new optimism, Locke's writings still reflected the widely held view that persons with intellectual disability do not attain the same level of personhood as those of higher intelligence. For instance, in his analysis of what constitutes "personal identity," Locke emphasized the role that "continuity of consciousness" plays in the identity of self and the identity of a person (Gibson 1968). Locke, too, drew comparisons between animal and "idiot" intellect (cf. Locke [1690] 1959:II.11.12-13 and II.9.14). For Locke, "a 'person' was a 'thinking' intelligent Being, that has reason and reflection, and can consider itself as itself, the same thinking thing in different terms and places" (cited in Lowe 1995:103). Thus, the defining characteristics of personhood, for Locke, were rationality and consciousness, including self-consciousness.

Goodey (1992) has cited contemporary writers whose views also highlight the permanence of the concept that persons with intellectual disabilities are less than human. For example, Gilbert Ryle's (1949) *The Concept of Mind* gives as its definition of *specifically human behavior* "behaviour which is unachieved by animals, idiots and infants" (Goodey 1992:28). From antiquity, then, there has been a pervasiveness of the concept of the separateness of those labeled "intellectually disabled" from full personhood. The optimism that the Age of Enlightenment brought for many did not include those with intellectual disability.

An Abandonment Era

Just as the practice of infanticide typified the denial of personhood for children, especially those who were deemed never likely to attain this status because of their disability, the practice of abandonment became more common with the advent of the Industrial Revolution. For children with an intellectual disability, this era saw the emergence of a number of sensationalized cases of "feral children"[5]—children who, when abandoned, did not die from exposure but were either cared for by animals or were able to care for themselves. Malson (1972) documented 53 such cases between 1344 and 1961. While the authenticity of many of these reports is open to question, the immense publicity surrounding such events spawned the morbid curiosity of the public that was always eager to observe "deviant" examples of humanity, typified by displays of such people in sideshow alleys.

The most celebrated case, however, was Victor, the so-called Wild Boy of Aveyron or, in French, *l'enfant sauvage.* Victor was found in the woods of Aveyron and subsequently became the protégé of the French physician Jean Itard. Itard's attempts to educate Victor were to have a significant impact on another French physician, Edouard Seguin, who worked under Itard's supervision. The sensationalism of the feral child phenomenon gave impetus to the ongoing nature-nurture debate or the heredity versus environment question, which was to have a profound impact on the way people with intellectual disabilities were viewed in the first half of the twentieth century. Itard's work, and later that of Seguin, produced a spirit of optimism concerning the educability of persons presumed to have intellectual disability.

An Institutionalization Era

The phase of institutionalizing persons with intellectual disability, the effects of which still permeate disability policies worldwide, can, in a sense, be traced to the development of homes for foundlings—children often born out of wedlock. One of the earliest reports of such a facility was a home founded by Archbishop Datheus in Milan in 787 A.D. The founder of the celebrated Catholic welfare society, St. Vincent de Paul (1581-1680) is credited as being one of the first to take in not only foundlings but also people with leprosy, mental illness, and intellectual disability in the Paris home that was to become the Hospice Bicêtre. This, together with the Hospice of the Salpêtrière, was the site where the great French reformers Pinel, Esquirol, Itard, Morel, Bourneville, and Seguin led the world in drawing attention to the special needs of people with intellectual disabilities.

Institutions exclusively for intellectually handicapped people, as we have come to know them more recently, however, grew out of the "back wards" of hospitals for people with mental illness. In many cases, the needs of people with intellectual disabilities in these facilities were not met with the same vigor as those needs of people with mental illness. For instance, it was not until recent times that it has become generally accepted that intellectually disabled people can also experience mental illnesses.[6] Two major factors that contributed to the scandals exposed in the latter half of the twentieth century by figures such as Bank-Mikkelsen, Nirje, Blatt, and Wolfensberger were the "therapeutic" practices applied to either cure or contain behavior and the gross overcrowding that occurred as a result of the pressures of industrialization and urbanization and, more recently, the increased life span of the inmates.

Emerging Educational Influences

Seguin's influence on the role of education to ameliorate the effects of intellectual impairments cannot be underestimated (Talbot 1964). His belief in the efficacy of intensive sensory-motor activities as an aid to learning and his exposition of detailed step-by-step instructional procedures reflected the intense optimism that flourished in the 1850s and 1860s around new ideas about the educability of "idiots." While the Age of Enlightenment provided the basis for the modern-day educational systems, influenced by figures such as Johann Heinrich Pestalozzi (1746-1827), the apparent incurability of "mental deficiency" challenged the very foundations of the Enlightenment ethos. Radford (1994) clearly summed up the position as follows:

> In an age that celebrated intelligence as much as beauty, perfection and rationality, the "idiot" was dull, flawed, defaced with stigmata and above all incurable. In the blunt terms of the philosopher John Locke: "where the 'lunatic' has lost his mind, the 'idiot' never had one." (P. 12)

However, in 1844, the Paris Academy of Science proclaimed that Seguin had solved the problem of "idiot education" (Baumeister 1970). In 1848, he moved to North America, where he was instrumental in the foundation of several institutions for people with intellectual disabilities. Together with five medical colleagues, in 1876 he established the Association of Medical Officers of American Institutions for Idiots and Feeble Minded Persons, renamed the American Association for the Study of the Feeble Minded in 1907 and then, in 1933, the American Association on Mental Deficiency. The influence of the medico-psychologists of the nineteenth century, including Seguin, Guggenbühl, and Howe, extended throughout much of the then Western world and continued into the early twentieth century.

Assessment and Classification

Educational approaches to training persons with an intellectual disability were influenced by the rising discipline of psychology, which was to eventually usurp the power role formerly held by the medical profession (Crocker 1999). Theories propounded by Francis Galton (1922-1911), William James (1842-1910), Arnold Gessell (1880-1961), Charles Spearman (1863-1945), Cyril Burt (1883-1971), and Jean Piaget (1896-1979) had a profound effect on the way people with intellectual disabilities were assessed and classified.

Frenchman Alfred Binet (1857-1911), however, is credited with being the founder of psychometrics, the measurement of intelligence. As discussed above, there had been earlier "scientific" attempts to diagnose or explain the phenomena of low intelligence—from Galen's reference to the association between idiocy and large ears to palmistry and phrenology. Other movements included polygenism, which emphasized that among the human races, there were separate biological species; craniometry, or the measurement of the skulls and its context; and the measurement of bodies to search for signs of apish morphology in groups that were deemed undesirable.

Binet, director of the psychology laboratory at the Sorbonne, eschewed his early attachment to craniometry and the work of his countryman, Paul Broca, in his development of a scale to identify those children whose lack of success in normal classrooms suggested their need for some form of special education. His first scale, published in 1905, consisted of a number of everyday problems of life involving processes of reasoning. The tasks were arranged in an ascending order of difficulty, with an age level assigned to each task, giving rise to the concept of mental age and, subsequently, the intelligence quotient (IQ).

Despite Binet's deep interest in the theoretical aspects of intelligence, his scale had a practical, empirical focus. He explicitly avoided imposing any theoretical interpretation to his scale and denied that it was a measure of "intelligence" (Gould 1981). Contrary to the later misuses of his and later scales as a means to label and limit, in the belief that measures of intelligence are markers of permanent inborn limits, Binet devised his scale to identify those children whose poor performance identified them as needing special education. He had definite pedagogical suggestions as to how these children might be instructed. For instance, he suggested that prior to being taught the basic subjects, they needed "mental orthopedics." These included exercises to develop motivation, attention, and cognition discipline. Like Seguin, Binet's pedagogy was a harbinger for instructional techniques developed by learning theorists in the latter part of the twentieth century. He certainly believed that intelligence could be augmented by good education and was not necessarily an immutable and inborn quantity.

The Menace of the Feebleminded

The publication in 1859 of Charles Darwin's *Origin of Species* and its interpretation by his cousin Francis Galton, the attribution of the causes of intellectual disability to the sinful behavior of parents (promiscuity and or alcoholism—usually of the mother), the documentation of mongolism and cretinism, and the genetic discoveries of Gregor Mendel (1822-1884) gave rise to the science of eugenics. Interestingly, eugenics did not have its original roots in the study of the epidemiology of intellectual disability but in the study of the epidemiology of genius. However, Mendel's formulation of inheritance laws concerning dominant and recessive conditions gave rise to oversimplified interpretations. For instance, the eugenics movements ascribed intellectual disability as a single heritable condition and not one that can be due to a variety of genetics and other causes.

Eugenics societies sprang up across much of the Western world, with pressure being placed on the families of the intellectually disabled to encourage them to neither marry nor procreate. Arbitrary rules were established to discourage the reproduction of deficient offspring. It is only in recent years that sterilization laws have been removed from the statutes of countries such as the United States, Canada, Sweden, and France. Genetic research from British scientist Lionel Penrose, who demonstrated that eugenic strategies could only have marginal effects in reducing the number of intellectually disabled people being born at any one time, played a role in the reversal of these policies, as did the work of Lancelot Hogben and J. B. S. Haldane.

A principal figure in the eugenics movement was H. H. Goddard, director of research at the Vineland Training School for Feeble-Minded Girls and Boys in New Jersey. Goddard popularized the use of the Binet scale in America, agreeing with Binet that the tests were most effective in identifying people just below the normal range. These were then referred to as "higher grade defectives," whom Goddard christened "morons." The classification of intellectual disability, or mental deficiency, as it was popularly known, became a popular debate in the early twentieth century. Three categories emerged: "idiots," who did not develop speech and had mental ages below 3; "imbeciles," who did not become literate and had mental ages between 3 and 7; and "high-grade defectives" or "morons," as Goddard named them, who could be trained to function in society. While "idiots" and "imbeciles" could be categorized to the satisfaction of professionals, including medical practitioners and the newly developing discipline of psychologists, as having a true pathology, the third group constituted a gray area. They formed a bridge, suggested Gould (1981), between pathology and normality "and therefore threatened the taxonomic edifice" (p. 158).

While Binet had steadfastly refused to refer to his scores as "intelligence," Goddard perceived them as measures of a single innate entity, which he called "intelligence." Furthermore, he saw intelligence being completely dependent on heredity, and, more insidiously, he saw a direct link between intelligence and immorality. This was a popular eugenical theme that led to criminals, most alcoholics, prostitutes, and others living on the fringes of society to be lumped together as "morons" who were innately defectives. In linking immorality and stupidity, Goddard advocated either "colonization" or "sterilization," with a preference for the former. In institutions, such as his own at Vineland, procreation could be controlled. He even advocated that such institutions could replace the present almshouses, prisons, and even the numbers in mental hospitals. "Such colonies," he suggested, "would save an annual loss in property and life, due to the actions of these irresponsible people, sufficient to nearly, or quite, offset the expense of the new plant" (Goddard 1912:105-6).

The Reification of Intelligence

The ultimate reification of intelligence can be attributed to Lewis M. Terman (1877-1956), a professor at Stanford University, who revised Binet's 1911 scale and renamed it the "Stanford-Binet," which became the gold standard for nearly all IQ tests that followed. Terman followed Goddard in emphasizing the danger that "high-grade defectives" posed for society. His deep commitment to the value to society of mass intelligence testing is reflected in his comment that

> it is safe to predict that in the near future intelligence tests will bring tens of thousands of these high grade defectives under the surveillance and protection of society. This will ultimately result in curtailing the reproduction of feeble-mindedness, and in the elimination of an enormous amount of crime, pauperism, and industrial inefficiency. (Terman 1916:6-7)

In addition to reinforcing the low expectations for cognitive development among those with low IQ scores, the work of Terman and his colleague Yerkes (1876-1956), together with that of Sir Cyril Burt (1883-1971) in the United Kingdom, supported the concept of a racial superiority.[7] This was to have disastrous implications for African Americans and other indigenous populations who were also subjected to segregation and substandard educational and social opportunities in many parts of the world.

Results of Longitudinal Studies

Several longitudinal studies have soundly demolished the dire predictions made in the early half of the twentieth century. Notable are the works of Edgerton (1967), Edgerton and Bercovici (1976), and Edgerton, Bollinger, and Herr (1984). In his original study of 53 former patients of Pacific State Hospital in California, Edgerton's main thesis was that these persons' major motivation was to pass as ordinary people and to deny their institutional experience. However, to cope, most of them became dependent on "benefactors" who helped them to survive. Edgerton suggested that it was the *stigma* of intellectual handicap that was their biggest burden, which led them to don "a cloak of competence" to try to cover their incompetence. The management of this problem, maintained Edgerton, was the major issue for the deinstitutionalization movement that was to emerge in the 1960s.

As Clarke and Clarke (1985) observed, the prevalence of administratively defined intellectual disability peaks at the latter years of schooling, declining thereafter, almost entirely due to the eventual community adjustment for most of those with mild disabilities. However, those with more severe levels of intellectual impairment have tended to remain dependent on welfare agencies, this being the case at least until the mid-1980s. Work since then, however, has demonstrated, especially in vocational and supported living programs, that people with more severe levels of intellectual impairment do reach levels of semi-independence, which was formerly thought impossible (Parmenter 1993; Snell 1987; Wehman et al. 1988).

The effects of the assessment and classification on the field of intellectual disabilities can be viewed positively or negatively. Binet's original goal was to segregate and provide special education services for those who were identified as requiring assistance within the school environment. This initiative was to provide a basis for developing a parallel system of special education programs within the general provisions of education. However, the psychologists who followed Binet were to provide the foundations for the belief that people who fell below a certain level of IQ were ineducable. In many Western countries, it was not until well into the second half of the twentieth century that all children, regardless of disability, were deemed eligible for public education services. The pattern in developing countries has followed the same trajectory, especially as universal education for nondisabled and disabled children alike remains problematical in many of those countries.

As social welfare programs have developed, assessment and classification have been seen as an essential element for eligibility for services. On the other hand, they have been seen as encouraging the labeling processes, which have traditionally been associated with negative attitudes toward all disabled people and people with intellectual disabilities in particular. Just as the early medical scientists concentrated on the etiology of intellectual disabilities, early psychologists also became, as Clark (1974) observed, "more concerned to classify than to remedy or treat, [so] relatively little work has been done to establish how much behavioural or cognitive change can be effected in difficult groups of subnormal subjects" (p. 435).

Population Explosion in the Institutions

The promises heralded by the innovative thinking of luminaries, such as Guggenbühl and Seguin in the nineteenth century, were not to be realized in the early twentieth century for a variety of reasons. The eugenics movement, of course, led to greater numbers of marginal members of society being incarcerated for the "protection" of society generally. The severe effects of the great economic depression in the 1920s and 1930s resulted in increasing numbers of families seeking institutional care for their intellectually handicapped children because they were unable to feed and clothe them. It was common practice for families to be advised on the birth of a disabled child to immediately seek institutional care as the best solution to the "problem."

Thus, during this time, there was a burgeoning of institutional populations across the world. For instance, in the United States, institutional care increased continuously from the middle of the nineteenth century until 1967, when it peaked at 194,650 persons, or 95 per 100,000 of the general population (Lakin, Bruininsks, and Sigford 1981). Rather than places of asylum and succor, institutions became veritable "hellholes." Several commentators have described the appalling conditions evident in these institutions around the world at this time (Blatt 1981; Judge 1987). In parts of Eastern Europe, similar conditions are still to be found (Mutters 1999).

Advances in medical science, including the discovery of sulphonamides in 1935 and penicillin in 1944, had substantial effects on the morbidity and mortality of those with severe and profound levels of intellectual disability. Inmates of institutions were now kept alive in ways not previously possible. The irony is that this led to further pressures from overcrowding and extra demands on limited and, at times, ill-prepared staff. In 1965, in the United States, the average number of residents per institution peaked at 1,500 (Lakin et al. 1982). In 1962, the President's Panel on Mental Retardation assessed the status of residential programming in the United States as follows:

> The quality of care furnished by State institutions varies widely, but from the standpoint of well-qualified and adequate personnel and the availability and use of professional services and modern, progressive programs, the general level must be regarded as low. In large state institutions, the normal patterns of administration and care are compounded by overcrowding, staff shortages, and frequently by inadequate budgets. (President's Panel on Mental Retardation 1962:137-38)

The history of the place in society of persons with an intellectual disability traced thus far portrays them as essentially being on the outside or, at the very maximum, on the fringes of society. Their humanity has often been denied, they have been seen as a threat and a danger to society, they have been oppressed and segregated, and despite some enlightened attempts to provide them adequate care and succor, the perception of their "otherness" continued well into the twentieth century. However, forces for change emerging in the latter half of the twentieth century would see a shift in society's appreciation of the basic human needs of these fellow citizens.

FORCES FOR CHANGE

The Normalization Principle

Despite the enormous advances in scientific enquiry into intellectual disability in the latter half of the twentieth century, history may judge that the most significant event of the century, in the context of life changes for persons with such a disability, was the social impact of the normalization principle. In its original formulation by Swedish scholar Bengt Nirje, the principle addresses the most fundamental issue of concern—the basic humanity of people with an intellectual disability that had been historically denied them.

In this introduction to his collected papers, Nirje (1992) pointed out,

> Two concerns have interacted in my papers . . . the problems inherent in the social situation of persons with intellectual impairments or disabilities, and the problems of establishing a coherent point of view of statements with regard to action, planning and legislation affecting their conditions of life. (P. 3)

Nirje's important contribution to the field was influenced by a number of converging factors. First, he was involved in a number of service organizations, including the Association for Persons with Intellectual Impairment (1962-1970). Nirje was the social welfare officer in the Swedish Red Cross Team, which provided support for Hungarian refugees in a former military camp in Austria (1956), and he was with the Folke Bernadotte Drive for cerebral palsy, which aimed to create better child-oriented environments instead of the former hospital institutions. Nirje (1992) commented on these experiences as follows:

> Thus I had been close to the experiences of the alien, non-normal, demands-humiliations-uncertainties-fears for the future connected with life in a large collective, "mass managed," institutions—and to the efforts, strivings and deep human motivations for creating valid developmental opportunities in the society. (P. 4)

He was also closely involved at the national and international levels of policy and legal developments. In Sweden, in the early 1960s, Nirje collaborated with Karl Grunewold, inspector general of mental retardation services in Sweden, in helping to formulate the introduction in 1967 of the Act on Services and Provisions for Mentally Retarded Persons, which incorporated the ideology of normalization. Nirje admitted that one of the major inspirations for his later formulation of the principle was the pioneering work of Niels Erik Bank-Mikkelsen, the dynamic leader of the Danish state mental retardation services. Nirje recounted how he was deeply influenced by Bank-Mikkelsen's strong commitment to the legal rights of persons with intellectual disabilities and by his humanistic approach. Bank-Mikkelsen had been the driving force for the Danish law for mentally retarded citizens in 1959, the preamble to which included the words "to let the mentally retarded obtain an existence as close to normal as possible" (cited in Nirje 1992:6).

A further influence, alluded to by Nirje (1985), was his early training in the Uppsala School of Philosophy and by questions raised by Hägerström and Hedenius. Here he raised the issue that concepts of "rights" serve as a background to legislation. He asserted that human rights involve more than that which is actually covered by legislation. A final influence, suggested Nirje (1985), was Ruth Benedict's (1934) classic study *Patterns of Culture*. It was Benedict's treatise on how cultural patterns affect the development of the individual that stimulated Nirje to formulate the principle in terms of patterns of life for people with an intellectual disability. In his most recent formulation, Nirje (1992) has stated,

The normalization principle means that you act right when making available to all persons with intellectual or other impairments or disabilities pattern of life and conditions of every day living which are as close as possible to or **indeed the same as** the regular circumstances and ways of life of their communities. (P. 16)

Wolfensberger's Formulation

While Bank-Mikkelsen (1976) described normalization as the acceptance of persons with an intellectual disability of their handicap, offering them the same conditions as are offered to other citizens, a somewhat different formulation was proposed by Wolfensberger (1969, 1972) in the North American context. Basing his approach on the functionalist sociologist approach of Parsons (1951) and the interactionalist approach of Goffman (1961, 1963), Wolfensberger emphasized using normative means to establish normative behaviors. Drawing heavily on the sociology of deviance, Wolfensberger (1972) suggested that "a (potentially) deviant person should be enabled to emit behaviours and an appearance appropriate (normative) within the culture for persons of similar characteristics" (p. 28).

Wolfensberger's focus on the use of normative means to establish normative behavior was built on a different value base and conception of people from the Scandinavian approach, with quite different implications for the provision of services to support people with an intellectual disability (Perrin and Nirje 1985). Wolfensberger's reductionist approach emphasized the need for people with intellectual disability to adapt to the cultural norms of their community, in much the same way as advocated by Goffman (1963). Goffman defined the concept of "passing" as the ability of members of deviant groups to minimize their differences or signs of deviancy so they are able to "pass" undetected into society. Whereas Nirje's formulation emphasized freedom of choice and recognition of a person's integrity, in the context of the realities of life, Wolfensberger stressed the appearance of conformity and passing and the need for people to hide their deviancy. Ontologically and epistemologically, they are quite divergent conceptualizations, albeit sharing a common nomenclature.

However, it was Wolfensberger's formulation that was to have a major impact outside the Nordic region. It was his approach that was embraced by policy planners and service providers in much of the English-speaking world. The influence of his writings and public lectures was a seductive force in the deinstitutionalization movements, as governments legislated to provide support for community-based options. Of particular relevance was his development of instruments to quantitatively evaluate human services. These were appealing to government bureaucracies, which saw the need to set standards and benchmarks against which funded services for people with intellectual disabilities needed to comply (Wolfensberger and Glenn 1975; Wolfensberger and Thomas 1980).

Subsequently, Wolfensberger (1983, 2000) reformulated his approach to normalization by developing what he termed the *theory of social role valorization* (SRV), which was meant to subsume and replace the principle of normalization that he had earlier enunciated. The new formulation placed extreme importance on the concept of "deviant" groups obtaining valued roles in society.

There are a number of contradictions and paradoxes implicit in Wolfensberger's formulation. On one hand, he asserted that its "concepts and constructs [are] rooted primarily in sociology" (Wolfensberger 1969:296), yet the strong call for the person with the disability to become more competent and to acquire "valued roles" is more related to Wolfensberger's psychological training and the emerging influence of behaviorism in the 1960s and 1970s.

Clegg (1998) has argued that while normalization is often described as a philosophy, it "is no more than a set of principles which lack heuristic power . . . the power to develop and to connect with other ideas" (p. 89). It is the doctrinal nature of social role valorization that causes controversy. Wolfensberger appears, like other functionalist theorists, to conceptualize a largely homogeneous society with a set of values that are "given." It is difficult to see in a pluralistic and diverse society how SRV can be generalizable to all nations of the world. It is a moot point as to whose values one accepts.

Wolfensberger's position on choice and self-determination is interesting. While he is not opposed to the concept of self-determination,[8] he indicated that the right to choose may be in conflict with what is defined as appropriate, normalized behavior. One can appreciate that the rights of the individuals to choose certain actions must be balanced with principles such as responsible and informed behavior and duty of care, but there is still the question of who determines what is "appropriate, normalized behavior."

Clegg (1998) has suggested that ontologically, normalization has been overly narrow in perspective. She proposed that normalization has been derived from a value Taylor (1989) has termed "the affirmation of ordinary life." This idea can be traced to the Enlightenment but is nearly impossible to define. Drawing on Taylor's triaxial approach to moral ontology, respect, and dignity, as well as what gives meaning to life, Clegg pointed out that most normalization values cluster around the respect axis. This allows us, she suggested, to see both its strengths and limitations.

It may be useful to move beyond this unitary approach, to one that encompasses Taylor's (1989) other two areas of moral ontology—for instance, issues of rights and citizenship and aspects that give meaning to people's lives. Within the context of normalization, especially as promulgated by Wolfensberger, very little discussion is concerned with these areas. However, more recently, the issues surrounding rights and citizenship and a closer attention to examining the deeper personal aspects of the lives of people with an intellectual disability have become important areas of focus.

Undoubtedly, the normalization principle, in its variety of forms, has contributed much to the field in the context of the reform of the institutional era. It added a further dimension to other developments that were affecting the disability scene, such as the civil rights and independent living movements in North America. It also provided a strong belief system for the professional staff who was given the responsibility of effecting the radical change from institutional to community living. On the down side, however, it led in part to a rigid doctrinal dogmatism that eschewed critical thinking and analysis. It did not allow, in Taylor's (1989) terms, for different positions to be balanced against each other. Nor did it encourage, as Clegg (1998) suggested, the development of a "reflective researcher-practitioner" model among the various support personnel engaged in disability services. Paradoxically, the movement toward community-based services has increased, rather than diminished, the tendency to classify and administratively segregate (Simpson 1998). This is especially true in those countries where economic rationalist policies aim to reduce welfare budgets (Parmenter 1999a).

The Deinstitutionalization and Community Living Movement

The combination of philosophical and social forces, including the normalization principle, precipitated a paradigm shift, at least in the Western world, in the way services were provided to people with disabilities, including those with intellectual disabilities. Legislation was enacted that led to the gradual decline of a variety of segregationist policies in education, employment, and accommodation.

The average annual change in pace of deinstitutionalization in Scandinavian countries, the United Kingdom, and the United States in the last quarter of the twentieth century has averaged 3.8 percent compared to virtually no change (0.06 percent) among other European countries (Hatton, Emerson, and Kiernan 1995). In the Netherlands, there was an average annual increase of 0.41 percent. There is evidence, too, that while there has been a dramatic drop in the number of people who were institutionalized, there remain considerable numbers in government and private institutions in many parts of the world (Walsh 1997).

Mansell and Ericsson (1996) argued that the pace of deinstitutionalization was sustained in the 1980s because community services were no more expensive than institutional care. In a number of countries, including the United Kingdom, the United States, and Australia, access to new central government funds certainly stimulated the trend toward community-based programs. However, it was noted that in Britain and the United States, owing to central government concerns about the growth in welfare expenditure, there are growing restrictions on access to central government funds. In Scandinavia, the trend toward decentralization is placing increasing demands on local community instrumentalities. There is, therefore, an inherent danger that an institutional legacy may live on, especially as the effective community integration of people with intellectual disability has yet to be fully realized in those countries that enthusiastically embraced deinstitutionalization. In this regard, Mansell and Ericsson (1996) have asserted,

> Deinstitutionalization, then, is not just something that happened to people with intellectual disabilities and their families. It also happened to decision-makers and staff in services and to researchers. They have to shift their attention to new problems and issues in the community. . . . But they had also to recognize that institutions were the expression of beliefs in society and that their demise may leave those beliefs and the practices the underpin still to be tackled in the community. This is surely the greatest challenge for all societies: how to build and sustain social solidarity and mutual commitment among people with different needs, talents and aspirations, so that everyone may flourish and prosper. (Mansell and Ericsson 1996:252-53)

There are several challenges ahead in effecting real changes in the quality of the lives of people with intellectual disabilities and their families. Simply closing institutions does not address the factors that led to their development. We need to explore the contemporary social, economic, and political forces that are shaping social welfare policies. In particular, we need to examine the processes that lead to the effective inclusion of people with intellectual disabilities into a community that welcomes and sustains them.

The Contribution of Science

To do adequate justice to this topic, we require a much more detailed analysis than is possible in this chapter. The burgeoning of research efforts across all fields of scientific endeavor relevant to the field of intellectual disabilities, especially in the latter half of the twentieth century, is outstanding. Developments in the basic biomedical sciences and those in the social-behavioral field have made enormous contributions to our understanding of a broad range of issues, including prevention, etiology, health services, education, and community living and working.

It would not be too optimistic to suggest that current and anticipated developments in genetics and neuroscience research provide exciting windows of opportunity for doing good. However, they also provide enormous ethical challenges. Scientists, as Rioux (1997) has pointed out, come with prejudicial attitudes as to what constitutes science and the scientific method. Scientists, too, come with preconceived notions concerning the intrinsic value of persons with "inborn errors of metabolism." The very language of "normality" sends covert messages that something must be "wrong" with these people.

In his preface to Penrose's *The Biology of Mental Defect*, John Burdon Sanderson Haldane (1948), one of his most eminent colleagues in the field of biochemistry, observed that an intellectual approach to the study of biology and its importance to the etiology of intellectual disability was not enough. Apart from its practical aspects, Haldane suggested that the study of intellectual disability was of considerable philosophical importance. For instance, the question of why people are different and what determines their individuality is of the greatest interest. In this respect, Haldane's observation that Penrose's contribution to the study of human biology was as much a contribution to general culture, as it was to the study of incomplete human development, is apposite in the context of this discussion. It would appear that one of the most important challenges for science in this field in the next century is for it to be more integrated and inclusionary within the broader scientific endeavors and with humanities, economics, and the social sciences.[9] A greater synergy between these various sections of research and enquiry, together with a deeper involvement of the public sector in the development of research policies, may help reduce the ever-widening gap between research and practice that was a feature of this field in the last half of the twentieth century.

The enormous pace of discovery of new knowledge has been a factor in the slowness of its application, but political, social, and economic commitment to this marginal population has not always been sufficient to maximize the benefits scientific advances have made. For instance, we have known since the early nineteenth century the causes of goiter and cretinism.[10] Given the intense interest in the new science of human genetics and the demonstration that some cases of intellectual disability were largely genetically determined led, as indicated above, to exaggerated hopes of eugenical improvement. Penrose (1938), in his classical study, the Colchester Survey, demonstrated the multiple etiologies of the impairment. Not surprisingly, in the first half of the twentieth century, scientific efforts were directed mainly toward diagnosis of causes, assessment, and prevention, but very little effort was directed toward treatment. By 1963, Penrose reported that specific health interventions involving hormonal, dietary, and exercise treatments ameliorated the effects of specific impairments. Brain surgery for people with cerebral palsy and epilepsy was also reported in the early 1950s. Before this time, there was little emphasis on psychological and educational training, possibly with the exception for those described as "mild or borderline mental defectives."

While biological and medical efforts were predominant, there was, at this time, a growing perception that people with an intellectual disability could profit from educational programs, albeit described as "training programs." The language of the time was, in contemporary terms, patronizing and stereotypic. For instance, Penrose (1963) commented that "defectives are not naturally antisocial. They are naturally very friendly and are particularly susceptible to influence during the formative years" (p. 283). However, a closer examination of the work of trailblazers, such as Penrose, reveals a deep commitment to the essential humanity of this population and to their basic rights to exist as part of the human civilization. Penrose's (1963) exhortation that as "subcultural mentality must inevitably result from normal genetical variation . . . the genes carried by the fertile scholastically retarded may be as valuable to the human race, in the long run, as those carried by people of high intellectual capacity" (p. 295). This is germane to the current debates concerning the ethics of the implications of the human genome project (Newell 1999; Roeher Institute 1999).

A contributing factor to the fragmentation of the research effort in this field was the relative isolation of scientists and their lack of awareness of each other's work, especially across the major English-speaking countries of North America and the United Kingdom and Ireland. Although scientists in the Nordic and the Netherlands regions accessed English publications, there was little intellectual intercourse in this field across the Atlantic before the early 1960s. Language barriers also continue to be a problem for much of the Latin- and Germanic-based languages and large parts of Eastern Europe, Asia, the Middle East, and Africa, especially as English has become the major language of science.

Formation of the International Association
for the Scientific Study of Mental Deficiency

In an effort to improve the exchange of scientific knowledge, a meeting of scientists from Europe and the United States was held in London in 1960. The *Proceedings* (Richards, Clarke, and Shapiro 1962) of this conference portray the wide range of research interests across 11 aspects of intellectual disability. Of special significance was that 35 of the 97 presentations were from nonmedical disciplines, principally psychology and education. The steady growth of research on intellectual disability from these disciplines in the 1960s became even stronger in subsequent international conferences organized by the International Association for the Scientific Study of Mental Deficiency,[11] an association that formally came into being in 1964 as a sequel of the

London meeting. At the most recent Congress of the Association, held in Helsinki in 1996, the proportion of biomedical contributors was in the order of 30 percent, but the remaining 70 percent encompassed a much wider range of disciplines from the sociobehavioral sciences and a wider representation of countries (27 in 1960; 63 in 1996).

Shift in Definition of Mental Retardation

The decline of the dominance of the biomedical field was in large measure a result of the redefinition of mental retardation that included "impairment in adaptive behaviours" in addition to subaverage general intellectual functioning (Heber 1958:3). This new definition, linked with the optimism of new pedagogical techniques, supported the proposition that the effects of an intellectual disability could be reversed.[12] Interestingly, the educational initiatives of the psychologists of the 1960s and 1970s bore a remarkable similarity to those of the medico-psychologists of the nineteenth century. Simpson (1998) observed that the basic difference between the two periods was that, whereas the nineteenth-century reformers were establishing pedagogical institutions for "idiotic" children, their twentieth-century counterparts were using similar arguments to close them.

The predominant theoretical approach that the psychoeducational paradigm embraced toward the conceptualization of disability and to research and practice was one in which the disability was intrinsic to the person. This approach emphasized the utilitarian nature of programs and treatments that would make disabled people more functional for society. It was the person who must change to accommodate the needs of society; it was the person who must "pass" the test of society before his or her basic humanity was recognized and valued. A basic flaw in the psychomedical model of disability, on which many of the programs the normalization principle influenced, was its implicit assumption that there was a single set of norms appropriate for all groups (Jensen 1980). This problem was also inherent in contemporary attempts to measure quality of life (Parmenter 1996). It is suggested, therefore, that it is time to move beyond the normalization movement, as advocated by Wolfensberger, for it continues to support the objectifying and commoditization of persons with an intellectual disability. It has failed to recognize the intrinsic humanness of these people, despite their difficulties in conforming to a normative set of values that often fail to recognize the immense diversity of the human condition.[13] Yet is it too idealistic to foresee a society that will accept Nirje's (1985:67) view that integration is based on the recognition of a person's integrity, which means "to be yourself among others—to be able and be allowed to be yourself among others"? Has society reached the stage where it has, as questioned by Goodey (1996), "the ability to include people with the severest learning disabilities, to the point of not noticing, or not being anxious about, the difference between Wittgenstein and them" (p. 96)?

Integration of Biological and Behavioral Sciences

This is not to deny the positive elements of contemporary scientific advances—for instance, the integration of psychobiological processes, especially in the neurosciences. Neuroscience, suggested Schroeder (1991), represents a fusion of several scientific disciplines—biophysics, biochemistry, physiology, anatomy, pharmacology, genetics, and psychology. It also focuses on understanding the relationships between brain and behavior. An excellent example of interdisciplinary research integration is the use of the results of morphometric studies of human cerebral cortex development to influence the direction of early language development programs for children at risk for language development delay. Huttenlocher's (1990) studies of the immature cerebral cortex in humans have indicated that the growth of dendrites and synaptic connections occur during infancy and early childhood. Excess synaptic connections, however, are eliminated during later childhood years, but the abundant connections that occur during infancy may form the anatomical substrate for neural plasticity and for certain types of early learning.

This finding, Warren (1999) suggested, has profound implications for the timing of early language and cognitive development programs.

However, brain-imaging techniques, such as magnetic resonance imaging (MRI) and positron emission tomography (PET), together with chemical probes developed from the field of molecular biology, are providing powerful means for studying the complexities of the human nervous systems. The modern phrenologists are realizing the dreams of the phrenologists of an earlier era (Raichle 1999). While great advances have been made in the study of individual neurons and sensory organs, the full complexities of the human brain have remained out of reach. Other areas where the integration of the biomedical and behavioral sciences occur are in the study of behavioral phenotypes and the interaction of pharmacotherapy and behavioral therapy for people with learning and behavior handicaps.

Prevention

Modern science in this field has essentially addressed the question of how intellectual disability may be prevented. While this is a laudable objective in the eyes of many, it is not without its critics, especially as prevention raises a range of ethical and social issues. Examples of primary prevention[14] include prenatal care, including adequate nutrition, vaccination for conditions such as rubella, newborn intensive care, and public education concerning the dangers of alcohol during pregnancy, together with education for responsible parenthood. Prevention of accidents leading to head injury and general trauma in childhood would also reduce the incidence of intellectual disability, especially in developing countries where the prevalence of intellectual and other developmental disabilities is the greatest. Teratogens, especially arising as a result of environmental degradation, also are an increasing cause of congenital defects (Guthrie 1986).

Advances in the study of genetics have resulted in both primary and secondary forms of prevention. The discovery of the Fragile X (fra (x)) syndrome represents one of the major advances in the understanding of inherited causes of intellectual disability. Work in the 1970s established that this X-linked syndrome is the most common form of hereditary intellectual disability. With the advent of methods for detecting fra (x) in blood and amniotic fluid cells, population screening and prenatal diagnosis of the syndrome have become common practice. With techniques to detect carriers of X-linked intellectual disability, genetic counseling of potential parents is now an accepted practice. Detection of fetuses with chromosomal aberrations presents parents with the decision of whether to terminate or continue the pregnancy.

For some time, there has been vigorous debate surrounding the bioethical issues that relate to the prevention of intellectual disability (Campbell 1999; Harper and Clarke 1997; International League of Societies for Persons with Mental Handicap 1994; Kuhse and Singer 1985; Meininger 1999; Roeher Institute 1999). For instance, the controversial Australian ethicists Kuhse and Singer (1985) have proposed the following in *Should the Baby Live*:

> Decisions about severely handicapped infants should not be based on the idea that all human life is of equal value, nor on any other version of the principle of the sanctity of human life. . . . There is, therefore, no obligation to do everything possible to keep [them] alive in all circumstances. Instead, decisions to keep them alive—or not to do so—should take account of interests of the infant, the family, the "next child" and the community as a whole. (P. 172)

In discussing who has the authority to make this decision, Kuhse and Singer (1985) emphasized the role of the state, especially the economic costs to the state providing lifelong support for disabled infants, much in the same way health economists use the cost utility analysis concept of quality of adjusted life years (QUALYs) as a metric to decide cost-effective ways of using the health dollar (Parmenter 1996). They also argued that if parents decide that they do not wish to rear a disabled child, "there is no point in keeping handicapped children alive if, despite their potential for a worthwhile life, they end up languishing miserably in totally inadequate institutions" (Kuhse and Singer 1985:190).

This position surely begs the question of the inevitability of institutional living being the only option, and, if it is, could not something be done about the conditions that exist in them? Kuhse and Singer (1985) would argue that they are taking a rationalist, realistic approach because in many countries, the state is either unwilling or unable to provide adequate options to institutional living for this population. The alternatives of foster care and adoption are also proving to be difficult options in contemporary society. Another disincentive for parents having to make choices is the inadequacy of support that the state may be willing or able to provide. Reinders (2000) has pointed out that the ethical debate on genetics has evolved almost totally within the medical paradigm, where the lives of people affected by genetic disorders always appear in a negative light. Within this paradigm, impairments or defects inevitably lead to a life of "suffering."

The profound effects that the Human Genome Project will generally have on the future of medicine and its relevance to a range of causes of intellectual disability, in particular, place bioethical issues as one of the most important challenges this field will face in the twenty-first century. A full analysis of these issues is beyond the scope of the present discussion. Nevertheless, two points are worthy of note. First, in 1994, the International League of Societies for Persons with a Mental Handicap (now Inclusion International) published *Just Technology? From Principles to Practice in Bioethical Issues,* in which it was proposed that genetic research and its applications should be evaluated in terms of the following four principles:

The principle of justice

The principle of nondiscrimination

The principle of diversity

The principle of autonomy and informed decision making

These principles have informed Inclusion International's contribution to the United Nations Educational, Scientific, and Cultural Organization's (UNESCO's) *Declaration on the Human Genome and Human Rights,* which was finalized in 1997. The essential element of the *Declaration* resides in the balance it strikes between safeguarding respect for human rights and fundamental freedoms and the need to ensure freedom of research.

Second, the scientists involved in the Human Genome Project are aware of a number of potential dangers inherent in their new discoveries, one example being that a functional variation in a human gene is patentable. Francis Collins, director of the USA National Human Genome Research Institute, has warned that it is imperative that the public project be completed quickly, before the private sector assembles and patents databases for the common functional variants of the human genome (Collins 1999). Raichle (1999) sounded a similar warning about the maps of human cortical function.

Advances in Technology

For those with severe intellectual impairments and high-support needs, advances in technology have made significant contributions to their mobility and their ability to communicate. Technology has facilitated communicative interactions at both school and community levels and has been instrumental in their successful inclusion into regular classes, further education, and employment (Glennen and DeCoste 1997; Hunt-Berg, Rankin, and Benkelman 1994). Instructional technology, based on the principles of applied behavior analysis, transformed the quality of special education and vocational training programs that supported the full-inclusion philosophies that emerged in the latter half of the twentieth century (Bellamy et al. 1988; Snell 1987). Advances in the application of nonaversive alternatives to dealing with problem behaviors have led to more humane and enlightened approaches to helping the small yet significant numbers of people with severe challenging behaviors (Meyer and Evans 1989).

Early Intervention

One of the most significant educational and technological advances that united families and professionals in the quest for a better lifestyle for people with intellectual disabilities was the development of early intervention programs. These programs, many of which commenced soon after the birth of the disabled child, offered an alternative to institutional care. They provided support and encouragement to parents whose preference was to keep their child within the family home. This support not only facilitated the child achieving much higher levels of functioning and participation, but it also provided a strong psychological foundation for the family to integrate the child into the normal activities of family and community life (Guralnick 1997; Turnbull and Turnbull 1986). While the positive results of early intervention programs have received strong support in the research literature, Clarke and Clarke (2000) have recently warned that "theories ascribing overwhelming, disproportionate and predeterminate importances to the early years are clearly erroneous" (p. 105). They have argued that there is little support for the view that early childhood experiences are the most critical for the later development of children with an intellectual disability. For the effects of early intervention programs to be maintained, it is essential that effective educational strategies are also continued.

Changes in Nomenclature

There have been several changes in the way people with an intellectual disability have been named and categorized. Terms formerly used, such as *idiot, imbecile, feebleminded, mentally subnormal, moron,* and *retard,* are now seen as highly pejorative and stigmatizing. Likewise, organizations have responded to community pressure to use more acceptable language. Examples are the American Association on Mental Retardation (formerly "Mental Deficiency") and the International Association for the Scientific Study of Intellectual Disabilities (also formerly "Mental Deficiency"). Presently, there are committees in the United States examining replacements for the term *mental retardation.* A theory of names suggests that while names are only conventions, they are also important instruments in the construction of social reality (Stockholder 1994).

Summary of Scientific Endeavors

As indicated above, this commentary has not attempted to analyze the vast array of modern scientific endeavors across the various disciplines that contribute to the study of intellectual disabilities. What is of major significance is that as paradigms of disability have changed, so have new scientific paradigms emerged. An examination of the contents of the growing number of scholarly journals and handbooks on intellectual disability research published in the past quarter century reveals a growth in multiparadigmatic thinking and a less rigid way of conceptualizing the nature of reality.

There are promising signs of an integration of basic biological and behavioral research and evidence of a greater respect for, and understanding of, the role alternative paradigms play on the part of those engaged in basic research. However, the challenge for the scientific research community as we move further into the millennium is for a greater collaboration between researchers, policy planners, and the people most deeply affected—the persons with intellectual disability, their families, and caregivers. Successive international congresses of the International Association for the Scientific Study of Intellectual Disabilities (IASSID) have repeatedly drawn attention to the slowness with which the service field applies the research findings into practice (Parmenter 1999b). In the field of intellectual disability, many interventions currently in use are of uncertain value and have never been adequately tested. One example of this is the use of facilitated communication (Calculator 1992). With the processes of deinstitutionalization, there has been a concomitant deprofessionalization of the field. Undoubtedly, the challenges of helping a person with intellectual disability live satisfactorily in the community are greater than those required for those who were placed in an institutional environment. However, many contemporary service systems with limited budgets are forced to employ relatively untrained personnel. This is not to suggest that we return to an era of professional dominance, isolation, and a disparity in power relationships between the professionals, people with disabilities, their families, and their caregivers. One of the basic skills the service sector lacks, in many cases, is an ability to work collaboratively across disciplines and with the consumers of the service.

Self-Advocacy by People with Disabilities

The worldwide growth of self-advocacy groups, albeit currently restricted to a number of Western industrialized countries, is a further and potentially vital force in intellectually disabled people achieving equal citizenship with their nondisabled peers (Dybwad 1996). The birth of the self-advocacy movement can be traced to a convention of people with disabilities held in Vancouver, Canada, in the early 1970s. A group known as People First was formally inaugurated in Oregon in the United States in 1973 by former residents of a state institution called Fairview Training Center.

Annual meetings of this group were held throughout the 1970s and 1980s, and the movement rapidly spread across the United States and provinces in Canada. As the movement extended to other countries, such as the United Kingdom, Scandinavia, and Australia, an international conference was held in the United States in Tacoma, Washington, followed by conferences in London, Toronto, and Anchorage, Alaska. In 1998, a self-advocacy conference was held in Lebanon, sponsored by the Committee for Arab Affairs of Inclusion International. The right of people with an intellectual disability to have a voice in how they would like to live their lives is becoming increasingly recognized. They are asserting their need to be consulted on a variety of policy and service issues, including involvement in the research agenda.

Activities in Developing Countries

While this chapter has essentially addressed issues within the context of Western industrialized countries, there are striking parallels in the emergence of attitudes, services, and policies in countries that are embracing the market economy. A major focus in assisting these countries to provide a more contemporary approach, based on a human rights perspective, is the work of Inclusion International. This organization is actively involved in supporting its member associations in Africa, South America, Eastern Europe, the Middle East, the India subcontinent, and parts of Asia. In many countries, poverty, poor public health provisions, population explosion, wars, and meager educational services exacerbate the conditions of life for persons with a disability. In most cases, raising the living standards of the total population is a prerequisite for improving the position of people with a disability. There is an urgent need for epidemiological data on the prevalence of intellectual disability in these countries to enable effective planning on a global scale to be accomplished. There are indications that the World Health Organization may sponsor this much-needed research.

Limitations of the Rights Discourse

Paralleling the development of the normalization principle in its variety of forms was the emergence, especially in the Western world, of policies based on the rights of individuals. This may be traced to the French initiative in 1789 in its proclamation of the *Declaration of the Rights of Man and the Citizen*. In 1964, Harvey Stevens, in his presidential address to the First Congress of International Association for the Scientific Study of Mental Deficiency (held in Montpellier, France), placed prime importance on the inalienable rights of the individual who is mentally deficient to the same dignity as fellow human beings. In 1971, the General Assembly of the United Nations (1971) issued the *Declaration of General and Specific Rights of the Men-*

tally Retarded. This provided a moral justification for legislation that was enacted by governments of several Western countries promising opportunities for people with intellectual disabilities to be a part of normal society. In 1975, the *Declaration on the Rights of Disabled People* (United Nations 1975) was proclaimed, followed by the proclamation of the decade 1983-1992 as the "Decade of Disabled Persons." The most recent United Nations initiative in supporting the rights of disabled people was the adoption in 1993 of the *Standard Rules on the Equalization of Opportunities for Persons with Disabilities* (United Nations 1993). In the preamble to the rules, a number of United Nations resolutions are cited as constituting their political and moral foundations.

In the eyes of the major international nongovernment advocacy organizations, the realization of rights of people with disabilities is the cardinal objective to be achieved. One cannot deny the rights of disabled people to have equal opportunities to access education, employment, the physical environment, and information and communication. There is also no denying the fact that special legislation enacted in most Western countries has underpinned the provision of a wide range of supports that has enabled the fuller participation of disabled people into regular community life. However, it is suggested that rights legislation is a necessary but not sufficient condition for people with intellectual disabilities enjoying the acceptance of the community.

Reinders (1999) has argued that the moral language of rights is neither sufficient nor necessary to ground moral responsibility for disabled people. He suggested that "to claim equal rights for the disabled makes sense only on the basis of commitments that draw on other moral sources than the sources that are intrinsic to the morality of rights" (p. 2). In the case of people with intellectual disability, Reinder's essential argument is that the contemporary rights discourse is deficient in accounting for the moral features of caring practices—practices that are committed to the well-being of people who are dependent on the support of others. His concluding comments are quite apposite:

> Without people who have sufficient moral character to care, rights can do little to sustain the mentally disabled and their families. People can be forced to comply, but they cannot be forced to care. (Reinders 1999:23)

Nirje (1985) also noted,

> Laws and legislative work cannot provide total answers to problem solving and proper actions with regards to realization of human rights. These can only come into existence in the full cultural and human context. Such problems are not only practical, but also ethical. (P. 65)

As a universal approach, the rights movement runs into difficulties in cultures that do not have a social system that has a strong commitment to individualism, a phenomenon that is largely Western in origin. There are cultures that would emphasize the notion of a person's obligations to the community or tribe more strongly than the reverse. It may be more profitable to envisage a society where the principle of mutual obligation transcends the principle of individual rights.

In the latter half of the twentieth century, there were remarkable forces for change in the way society viewed and supported people with intellectual disability. The normalization principle was a major catalyst for the deinstitutionalization movement that saw thousands of people in a number of Western countries move into community living and working programs. It is important to recognize the force of the word *program,* for in many cases professionals still exerted control over the lives of these people. Spectacular developments in science have also played an important role in the emancipation of this population, but along with these developments, there are critical moral and ethical issues to be resolved. People with intellectual disabilities also commenced to speak for themselves, discovering a sense of empowerment that challenged conventional attitudes and practices, including the attribution of impairment and disability that had historically set them apart from the rest of society. The plight of people with intellectual disabilities in developing countries is becoming recognized. Much is yet to be achieved in relieving the life circumstances of people for whom the disability is an additional challenge. It is a moot point, however, whether reliance on a human rights approach will effect the greatest change in the lives of these people. The final section of this chapter will explore an approach that may see their transformation from the role of "otherness" to the achievement of the role of "citizenship" within the human family.

THE FUTURE

Throughout history, there has been a pervasive rejection of the full citizenship of people with intellectual disability, resulting in a variety of physical and psychological segregationist practices that culminated in their widespread institutionalization in the twentieth century. Movements such as normalization and human rights emerged as emancipatory forces in the last third of the twentieth century, but, as argued above, these catalysts for change are basically deficient in achieving the moral goal of full citizenship for this population. The future holds both threats and opportunities for the realization of full acceptance of persons with intellectual disability into a society that respects their "humanness" rather than their "otherness." We must be cautious, too, in not allowing the "reformer's zeal" to blind us from realities and to limit our thinking in the time warp of the deinstitutionalization era.

One of the threats at the research level is that many of the reform-oriented studies, especially in the area of community integration, are designed to answer questions posed by administrators and politicians—questions usually directed to whether reform programs are working. Insufficient interest is devoted to asking why situations are the way they are or how they can be understood from different perspectives; nor are current ideologies exposed to sufficient critical analysis.

In a sense, we are caught up in trying to solve yesterday's problems while asking questions within the narrow confines of disability research. For instance, in studying the processes and outcomes of community integration, we have not addressed the situation of people with an intellectual disability in relation to the wider society in which they live. Also, many of the issues addressed that relate to prejudice and discrimination are indeed a part of ordinary psychosocial reality and of everyday life for all people.

The Dominance of Market Ideology and Globalization of the World Economies

Undoubtedly, the economic policies of the major industrialized nations in recent years have had an impact on the provision of services for disadvantaged groups. The redistribution of income and wealth both within and between countries has resulted in a growing gap between the rich and the poor. The neoclassical economic rationalist policies, driven in part by the globalized economy, is predicated on the principle of "utility maximization," with individuals using their resources to achieve the highest level of satisfaction possible. The essential element is that people must be free to choose how they use their resources—in essence, economic reform means reducing interference by governments. In this process, strong countries can exploit the weak, while wealthy companies increase their wealth by shopping around the world for the cheapest labor. The materialization mantra is sapping the lifeblood of those elements that build social cohesion and a sense of mutual obligation toward one's fellow citizens, especially those who are marginalized and relatively powerless.

Schalock (1999) has argued that human services organizations are being increasingly challenged to provide quality services within the context of two powerful, potentially conflicting forces: person-centered values and economic-based restructured services. To justify expenditures that are measured objectively, one must demonstrate consumer outcomes. Rather than being collaboratively developed, value systems are imposed by authoritarian administrations. In much of the administratively dominated delivery systems, we are still witnessing the phenomenon Burton Blatt (1981) so eloquently exposed in his essay on the "bureaucratization of values," in which terms become mere shibboleths, devoid of their original meanings. Human services are now being operated as business replete with a panoply of "business-speak" managerialistic jargon that tends to create a veneer of efficiency but is often devoid of the warmth of sound human relationships. This is not to deny that scarce resources must be applied efficiently to achieve quality outcomes. However, who is to determine the nature of the appropriate outcomes and the method of measurement? We have reached, in many ways, the "tyranny of quality" predicted by Goode (1991).

In his book, *Voltaire's Bastards,* John Ralston Saul (1992) has argued that Western civilization is without belief for the first time since the decline of the Roman Empire.[15] Have we lost spirit and faith? Have we become more self-centered and self-indulgent? Have the richer and deeper meanings of life been leached out by the materialistic imperatives of the free market? While it may be inappropriate to look back romantically to the optimism and sense of excitement so evident in the 1960s and 1970s with the rapid growth of social policy initiatives in that period, one cannot help comparing that period with the barren social policy desert of the 1990s. There are encouraging signs, however, that a postmaterialist movement is emerging, as a reaction to the economic rationalist-driven policies of the 1980s and 1990s. People from both the industrialized and developing countries are challenging the current economic policies of governments, witnessed by the protests mounted against the World Trade Organization meeting in Seattle in 1999. Significant proportions of society are feeling alienated and isolated from the decision-making processes of governments. There is also a widespread belief that government policies are increasingly being driven by mega-transnational companies with little or no allegiance to national identities.

Environmental Degradation

In recent decades, the assault on the world's ecosystems has had and continues to have profound negative effects on the health of the world's population. The rapid growth in the production of new chemicals has increased the risk for birth defects. It is estimated that there are approximately 5 million chemicals to which our population has significant exposure. Of these, approximately 1,600 have been tested in animals for teratogenicity. About one-half of these agents have been shown to produce some form of teratogenicity (Shephard 1986). Occupational and environmental exposures to toxic solutions continue to contribute to birth defects worldwide. Lack of availability and, in some cases, lack of commitment to immunization programs such as those for rubella continue to be a major problem in the area of primary prevention. Rowitz's (1992) prediction that the human immunodeficiency virus (HIV) will become the most common infectious cause of developmental disability in the 1990s can be extended into the current century, given that the spread of this virus continues apace in large parts of Africa and Asia. Lead exposure and iron deficiency also continue to be significant causes of birth defects in both developed and developing countries. Effective nuclear waste disposal and the minimization of the risks of nuclear accidents will continue to be challenges.

Individualism

The rhetorical forces driving the free-market economy present a tantalizing and seductive similarity in their goals and processes to many of the contemporary goals for people with a disability, their caregivers, and their families. The concepts of freedom of choice, more control over one's life, release from government regulation, self-determination, and empowerment all appear to sit comfortably in both areas. The emphasis on individualism, however, presents quite a threat to a vulnerable population, such as those with intellectual disabilities. In our goal to encourage their independence, we have overlooked the essential fact that the vast majority of this population will, in many aspects of their daily lives, remain dependent on supports. Edwards (1997) has argued that the normative component of individualism compromises the integrity of intellectually disabled individuals and contributes further to their being ascribed a lower moral status than other humans. The individualistic view of the self militates against people with disabilities as dependence is viewed negatively. For example, Reinders (1999) pointed out that dependency for people with intellectual disability is the *conditio sine quo non* for their physical, mental, and spiritual well-being. The challenge, then, is for us to create environments where the interdependence of individuals is a central feature and where individuals perceive their identity and conceptualization of self in the context of a mutually dependent society.

Development of an Ethical Community

Where do the people with an intellectual disability stand in society as we move further into the new millennium? Is their position much changed from that of the previous two centuries? Have they been emancipated from the phenomenon of "otherness"? As they were before the institutional period, they are now more likely to physically be a part of society, no longer banished and segregated for their own protection and that of society. We have recognized for some time that the greatest post-deinstitutional period challenge was to help people with intellectual disability become part of a community rather than being merely physically located in it. We must also recognize that significant proportions of people with intellectual disability resided with their parents and were not placed in institutions. Many families kept their intellectually disabled sons and daughters in relative isolation from the community, fearful of negative attitudes and discrimination by neighbors and from a sense of shame because their children were perceived as less than perfectly normal human beings. On the other hand, there are families for whom the presence of a member with a disability has been an enriching experience.

How can we articulate a meaningful vision of community and social reality for this group? Paul Dokecki (1992) has argued that despite the significant movement away from dehumanizing paternalistic approaches to a greater emphasis on individual civil rights and personal autonomy, there remains a challenge for us to develop an ethical framework that will be sufficient to confront the ethical issues that will arise in the future for this population. The pervasive cult of perfectionism is still evident in present-day society nurtured by competitive individualism. We have, in many respects, maintained the power relationships so evident in the medical model of support by a power sharing with other professional groups. In this context, ethical decisions are made in a context in which professionals, deemed to be experts, make decisions. Radford (1994) has indicted the university through its authority of "science" for the rise of professionalism.

How can we foster an ethical community, as suggested by Dokecki (1992), in which the primary support roles are taken by family, friends, and extended support networks rather than by professionals? H. Rutherford Turnbull (1998) asserted that each member of a community must recognize that all are vulnerable in some aspects of our lives. As a first step, therefore, the ethical community must recognize a mutuality of need and a reciprocity of vulnerability. The ethical community would also recognize that all persons are fundamentally equal as human beings, and all persons are dependent on others in a metaphysically deep way (Edwards 1997). Dokecki's argument for the need of a concept such as "the ethical community" is strengthened by his reference to the work of Spiegelberg (1944, 1975) and Zaner (1988). Dokecki noted Spiegelberg's argument as follows:

A basic feature of being human, a feature that constitutes the basis of ethics, is that we are all subject to undeserved discriminations that produce inequalities at birth. An unde-served discrimination is an unequal lot in life, either privilege or handicap, which we in-herit through no fault or dessert of our own, in effect, through moral chance. (P. 44)

Zaner (1988) made a similar observation and has asserted that "fellowship then, not auton-omy, is basic in human life" (pp. 300-1). The movement toward supporting families and focus-ing policy research on the family's role in supporting their child with an intellectual disability is a promising sign that the development of the conception of an ethical community is not too ide-alistic to be seen as ever achievable (Dunst, Trivette, and Deal 1988; Knox et al 2000).

As we move from the era classified as modernism, epitomized by the penetration of market forces into every aspect of life and into a society characterized as "postmodern,"[16] we need to recognize, as Toulmin (1990) has suggested, that the way ahead relies less on power and force and more on moral influence. Moral influence, it is suggested, rests in part on the strengthening of human relationships that produce a social rather than a physical capital. James Coleman (1988) has suggested that "social capital . . . comes about through changes in the relations among people that facilitate action" (p. 100). The development of social capital may prove to be an antidote to the social policy agenda of most nations that are contributing in large measure to social fragmentation and the growing sense of alienation on the part of marginalized groups. The social and economic changes in the 1970s and 1980s have effectively challenged the legiti-macy of the welfare state model in which the top-down approach by governments ensured safety net provisions, especially in industrialized countries.

Mark Latham (1998), in *Civilising Global Capital,* has drawn on Amartya Sen's (1992) con-cept of "social capability" that recognizes that personal well-being relies on more than the avail-ability of material and social goods, for citizens must have the capacity to use these resources effectively. Social capability relies, suggested Latham, "on sound social relations: the recogni-tion, mutual trust and respect between people that fosters a stronger sense of social participa-tion and connectedness" (p. xxxix). In the context of support for persons with an intellectual disability and for other marginalized groups, the message for the millennium is clear. Although the latter half of the twentieth century saw tremendous advances in the physical emancipation of the intellectually disabled, we have some way to go before we see a more caring, mutually supportive, and ethical community where the aim is to promote the interrelatedness of commu-nity and human development values.

CONCLUSION

This chapter has addressed, from a historical perspective, the place in society of people with in-tellectual disability, from the prescientific era to present day. The key feature of the past 2,000 years has been society's general banishment of the intellectually disabled to a status less than full humanness. The presence of an intact intellect has traditionally been seen as the sine qua non for the recognition of full citizenship.

In tracing the range of factors that have influenced the way we view people with intellectual disability and the way support services are provided, it is interesting to note the paradox that has recently arisen between the movements of physical integration and administrative segrega-tion. As Simpson (1998) noted, "The possibility of conceptualizing the 'intellectually disabled' as comprising a discrete group, does not arise from the essence of such 'disability' nor the scien-tific study therefore, but from the precise discursive and technological conditions which sustain it" (p. 5).

Therefore, in addressing the future directions that ought to be taken in this field, it was ar-gued that the concept of the development of an ethical community could provide a framework in which to meet the broader societal challenges that face the community generally. Latham (1998), in addressing issues completely outside the realm of disability, nevertheless has an important message in the context of these broader societal challenges for people with an intellectual disability as we move into the new millennium:

> The greatest challenge . . . lies outside the realm of the State—that is, in rebuilding the foundations of mutual trust, recognition and support across the work of the non-state public sector. . . . In addressing the foundations of public mutuality, social democracy needs to give closer consideration to relationships between citizens. . . . During an era of social diversity and uncertainty, the need for new forms of commonality, in the interests shared across society, has become particularly acute. (Pp. xl-xli)

Can we meet this challenge and, in so doing, cultivate our humanity so that it includes all people?

NOTES

1. Throughout this chapter, the contemporary term *intellectual disability* will be used in preference to earlier terminology, such as *mental deficiency, mental retardation,* and *mental subnormality.* It also embraces the term *learning disability,* commonly used in the United Kingdom and Ireland.

2. Nussbaum (1997:187) noted that Nobel Prize winner economist/philosopher Amartya Sen estimated that the numbers of females in the world who are likely to have died because of their gender—whether through sex selection infanticide or through receiving nutrition and health care unequal to that given to males—to be in the order of 100 million.

3. This term was also used by Rynders (1987:2-3), who cited the allegations of "otherness" of persons with Down syndrome, such as Crookshank, who asserted in 1924 that Down syndrome represented a "regression to a non-human species (i.e., to an orangutan)," and Boyd and Fletcher in 1968, who asserted that someone with a disability such as Down syndrome is not even a person.

4. *Idiot* is a word derived from Greek, meaning a "private person." It was historically used to denote an ignorant, uneducated person. Clarke and Clarke (1974) noted that it was a term used for a considerable period of time to refer to anyone who was mentally subnormal.

5. Renowned Swedish biologist Linnaeus, in his *Systema Naturae* (1735), classified the "wild man" or "the wild child" as *Homo Ferus.*

6. Tredgold (1937), however, recognized the need to study the psychopathology of those with "amentia."

7. Mongolism, first described by Langdon Down in 1866, was a label based on the physical appearance of a particular clinical type, which together with the notion of "atavistic regression" implied that the Mongolian race was inferior (Clarke and Clarke 1974:13).

8. Self-determination is one of the ratings of the Program Analysis of Service Systems (Wolfensberger and Glenn 1975).

9. In a closing message to the 1989 Convocation of World Academics, which resulted in the publication of *Scientific Issues of the Next Century,* Claudio Martelli, deputy prime minister of the Italian government, observed that Professor Haldane, in his forecast of developments in his field of biochemistry from 1925 up until the 1990s, developed "a literary essay midway between epistemology, futurology, and experimental science" (Maltoni and Selikoff 1990:244). Haldane's evocative title, *Daedalus, or Science in the Future,* might presage the need for a similar opus that encompasses the field of intellectual disability.

10. Swiss physician Coindet (1774-1848), in a lecture to the Swiss Society of Natural Sciences, recommended iodine preparations for the treatment of goiter in 1820. In 1846, Italians Prêvost and Maffoni were the first to put forward the theory that goiter was due to iodine deficiency (Hetzel 1989).

11. Now known as the International Association for the Scientific Study of Intellectual Disabilities (IASSID).

12. This is reminiscent of the Paris Academy of Science proclamation that Seguin had solved the problem of "idiot education." Harvey Stevens, the first president of IASSMD, commented that the new definition of mental retardation suggests that it is a reversible condition (Stevens 1964:1).

13. For a detailed critique of Wolfensberger's approach to normalization, see Reinders (1997) and Simpson (1998).

14. For a comprehensive discussion of primary prevention, see the World Health Organization (1998).

15. Taylor (1989) argued that nineteenth- and twentieth-century cultures became confused about the meaning of life once religious certainties were displaced. The utilitarianism of Enlightenment thinking and the individual perspective of Romanticism could be seen as the harbingers for this shift in values.

16. Radford (1994) pointed out that some would regard postmodernity as a chimera, for we may only have moved into a more intensified version of modernity or "hypermodernity."

REFERENCES

Bank-Mikkelsen, N. E. 1976. "The Principle of Normalization." Pp. 45-50 in *Flash 2 on the Danish National Service for the Mentally Retarded,* edited by B. Nielsen. Copenhagen: Personal Training School.

Baumeister, A. A. 1970. "The American Residential Institution: Its History and Character." Pp. 1-28 in *Residential Facilities for the Mentally Retarded,* edited by A. A. Baumeister and E. Butterfield. Chicago: Aldine.

Bellamy, G. T., L. E. Rhodes, D. M. Mank, and J. M. Albin. 1988. *Supported Employment: A Community Implementation Guide.* Baltimore: Brookes.

Benedict, R. 1934. *Patterns of Culture.* Boston: Houghton Mifflin.

Blatt, B. 1981. *In and out of Mental Retardation: Essays on Educability, Disability, and Human Policy.* Baltimore: University Park Press.

Calculator, S. N. 1992. "Perhaps the Emperor Has Clothes after All: A Response to Biklen." *American Journal of Speech Language Pathology* 1:18-20.

Campbell, A. V. 1999. "Human Dignity, Human Virtue: The Lost Dimensions of Human Bioethics." Pp. 1-6 in *What Is This Thing Called Bioethics? Proceedings of the 6th National Conference of the Australian Bioethics Association,* edited by C. J. Newell. Hobart: Australian Bioethics Association.

Clark, D. F. 1974. "Psychological Assessment in Mental Subnormality. Part I, General Considerations, Intelligence and Perceptive—Motor Tests." Pp. 387-438 in *Mental Deficiency: The Changing Outlook,* 3d ed., edited by A. M. Clarke and A. D. B. Clarke. London: Methuen.

Clarke, A. M. and A. D. B. Clarke. 1974. "Criterion and Classification of Subnormality." Pp. 2-30 in *Mental Deficiency: The Changing Outlook,* 3d ed., edited by A. M. Clarke and A. D. B. Clarke. London: Methuen.

———. 1985. "Criteria and Classification." Pp. 27-52 in *Mental Deficiency: The Changing Outlook,* 4th ed., edited by A. M. Clarke, A. D. B. Clarke, and J. M. Berg. London: Methuen.

———. 2000. *Early Experience and Life Path.* London: Jessica Kingsley.

Clegg, J. 1998. *Critical Issues in Clinical Practice.* London: Sage.

Coleman, J. S. 1988. "Social Capital in the Creation of Human Capital." *American Journal of Sociology* 94:100-6.

Collins, F. S. 1999. "The Human Genome Project and the Future of Medicine." Pp. 42-55 in *Great Issues for Medicine in the Twenty-First Century: Ethical and Social Issues Arising Out of Advances in the Biomedical Sciences,* edited by D. C. Grossman and H. Voltin. New York: New York Academy of Sciences.

Crocker, A. C. 1999. "The Medical Model: A Mostly Historical Discussion." Pp. 3-9 in *Responding to the Challenge: Current Trends and International Issues in Developmental Disabilities,* edited by H. Bersani. Cambridge, MA: Brookline.

Dokecki, P. R. 1992. "Ethics and Mental Retardation: Steps toward the Ethics of Community." Pp. 39-51 in *Mental Retardation in the Year 2000,* edited by L. Rowitz. New York: Springer-Verlag.

Dunst, C., C. Trivette, and A. Deal. 1988. *Enabling and Empowering Families: Principles and Guidelines for Practice.* Cambridge, MA: Brookline.

Dybwad, G. 1996. "Setting the Stage Historically." Pp. 1-17 in *New Voices: Self-Advocacy by People with Disabilities,* edited by G. D. Dybwad and H. Bersani. Cambridge, MA: Brookline.

Edgerton, R. B. 1967. *The Cloak of Competence: Stigma in the Lives of the Mentally Retarded.* Berkeley: University of California Press.

Edgerton, R. B. and S. M. Bercovici. 1976. "The Cloak of Competence: Years Later." *American Journal of Mental Deficiency* 80:485-97.

Edgerton, R. B., M. Bollinger, and B. Herr. 1984. "The Cloak of Competence: After Two Decades." *American Journal of Mental Deficiency* 88:345-51.

Edwards, S. D. 1997. "The Moral Status of Intellectually Disabled Individuals." *Journal of Medicine and Philosophy* 22:29-42.

———. 1998. "The Body as Object versus the Body as Subject: The Case of Disability." *Medicine, Health Care and Philosophy* 1:47-56.

Gibson, J. 1968. *Locke's Theory of Knowledge and Its Historical Relations.* Cambridge, UK: Cambridge University Press.

Glennen, S. L. and D. DeCoste. 1997. *The Handbook of Augmentative and Alternative Communication.* San Diego, CA: Singular.

Goddard, H. H. 1912. *The Kallikak Family: A Study of Hereditary of Feeble-Mindedness.* New York: Macmillan.

Goffman, E. 1961. *Asylums.* Garden City, NY: Anchor.

———. 1963. *Stigma: Notes on the Management of Spoiled Identity.* Englewood Cliffs, NJ: Prentice Hall.

Goode, D. A. 1991. "Quality of Life Research: A Change Agent for Persons with Disabilities." Paper presented to the American Association on Mental Retardation National Meeting Round Table Program, June, Washington, DC.

Goodey, C. F. 1992. "Mental Disabilities and Human Values in Plato's Late Dialogues." *Archiv Für Geschichte der Philosophie* 74:26-42.

———. 1996. "The Psychopolitics of Learning Disability in the Seventeenth-Century Thought." Pp. 93-117 in *From Idiocy to Mental Deficiency,* edited by D. Wright and A. Digby. London: Routledge Kegan Paul.

Gould, S. J. 1981. *The Mismeasure of Man.* New York: Norton.

Guralnick, M. 1997. "Second Generation Research in the Field of Early Intervention." Pp. 3-20 in *The Effectiveness of Early Intervention,* edited by M. J. Guralnick. Baltimore: Brookes.

Guthrie, R. 1986. "Lead Exposure in Children: The Need for Professional and Public Education." Pp. 322-28 in *Mental Retardation: Research, Education and Technology Transfer,* edited by H. M. Wisniewski and D. A. Snider. New York: New York Academy of Sciences.

Haldane, J. B. S. 1948. "Preface." Pp. iii-iv in *The Biology of Mental Defect.* New York: Grune & Stratton.

Harper, P. S. and A. J. Clarke. 1997. *Genetics Society and Clinical Practice.* Oxford, UK: BIOS Scientific.

Hatton, C., E. Emerson, and C. Kiernan. 1995. "People in Institutions in Europe." *Mental Retardation* 33:132.

Heber, R., ed. 1958. "A Manual on Terminology and Classification in Mental Retardation." *Monograph Supplement: American Journal of Mental Deficiency* 64 (2).

Hetzel, B. S. 1989. *The Story of Iodine Deficiency: An International Challenge in Nutrition.* Delhi: Oxford University Press.

Hunt-Berg, M., J. Rankin, and D. Beukelman. 1994. "Ponder the Possibilities: Computer Supported Writing for Struggling Writers." *Learning Disability Research and Practice* 9 (3): 169-78.

Huttenlocher, P. R. 1990. "Morphometric Study of Human Cortex Development." *Neuropsychologia* 28:517-27.

International League of Societies for Persons with Mental Handicap. 1994. *Just Technology? From Principles to Practice in Bio-Ethical Issues.* Toronto: Roeher Institute.

Jensen, A. R. 1980. *Bias in Mental Testing.* New York: Free Press.

Judge, C. 1987. *Civilization and Mental Retardation: A History of the Care and Treatment of Intellectually Disabled People.* Mulgrave, Victoria, Canada: Magenta.

Knox, M., T. R. Parmenter, N. Atkinson, and M. Yazbeck. 2000. "Family Control: The Views of Families Who Have a Child with an Intellectual Disability." *Journal of Applied Research in Intellectual Disabilities* 13:17-28.

Kuhse, H. and P. Singer. 1985. *Should the Baby Live? The Problem of Handicapped Infants.* Oxford, UK: Oxford University Press.

Lakin, K., G. C. Krantz, R. H. Bruininsks, J. L. Clumpner, and B. K. Hill. 1982. "One Hundred Years of Data on Populations of Public Residential Facilities for Mentally Retarded People." *American Journal of Mental Deficiency* 87:1-8.

Lakin, K. C., R. H. Bruininsks, and B. B. Sigford. 1981. "Introduction." Pp. 28-50 in *Deinstitutionalization and Community Adjustment of Mentally Retarded People,* AAMD Monograph No. 4, edited by R. H. Bruininsks, C. E. Meyers, B. B. Sigford, and K. C. Lakin. Washington, DC: American Association on Mental Deficiency.

Latham, M. 1998. *Civilising Global Capital.* Sydney, Australia: Allen & Unwin.

Locke, J. [1690] 1959. *An Essay Concerning Human Understanding.* Reprint, New York: Dover.

Lowe, E. J. 1995. *Locke on Human Understanding.* London: Routledge Kegan Paul.

Malson, L. 1972. *The Wolf Children.* Middlesex, UK: Penguin.

Maltoni, C. and I. J. Selikoff, eds. 1990. *Scientific Issues of the Next Century: Convocation of World Academies.* New York: New York Academy of Sciences.

Mansell, J. and K. Ericsson. 1996. "Conclusion: Integrating Diverse Experience." Pp. 241-53 in *Deinstitutionalization and Community Living: Intellectual Disability Services in Britain, Scandinavia and the USA,* edited by J. Mansell and K. Ericsson. London: Chapman & Hall.

Meininger, H. P. 1999. "Dealing with the Dilemmas of Genetic Information." Pp. 53-57 in *Genome(s) and Justice,* edited by Roeher Institute. Toronto: Roeher Institute.

Meyer, L. and I. Evans. 1989. *Nonaversive Intervention for Behaviour Problems: A Manual for Home and Community.* Baltimore: Brookes.

Mutters, T. 1999. "The Situation of Mentally Handicapped Persons and Their Families in Eastern Europe." Pp. 133-42 in *Responding to the Challenge: Current Trends and International Issues in Developmental Disabilities,* edited by H. Bersani. Cambridge, MA: Brookline.

Newell, C. 1999. "Critical Reflections on Disability, Difference, and the New Genetics." Pp. 58-73 in *Goodbye Normal Gene, Confronting the Genetic Revolution,* edited by G. O'Sullican, E. Sharman, and S. Short. Sydney, Australia: Pluto.

Nirje, B. 1985. "The Basis and Logic of the Normalization Principle." *Australia and New Zealand Journal of Developmental Disabilities* 11:65-68.

———. 1992. *The Normalization Principle Papers.* Uppsala, Sweden: Centre for Handicapped Research, Uppsala University.

Nussbaum, M. C. 1997. *Cultivating Humanity: A Classical Defense of Reform in Liberal Education.* Cambridge, MA: Harvard University Press.

Parmenter, T. R. 1993. "International Perspective of Vocational Options for People with Mental Retardation: The Promise and the Reality." *Mental Retardation* 31:359-67.

———. 1996. "The Use of Quality of Life as a Construct for Social and Health Policy Development." Pp. 89-103 in *Quality of Life in Health Promotion and Rehabilitation: Conceptual Approaches, Issues and Applications,* edited by R. Renwick, I. Brown, and M. Nagler. Thousands Oaks, CA: Sage.

———. 1999a. "Implications of Social Policy for Service Delivery: The Promise and the Reality." *Journal of Intellectual and Developmental Disability* 24:321-31.

———. 1999b. "The Role of Science in Advancing the Lives of People with Intellectual Disabilities." Pp. 10-22 in *Responding to the Challenge: Current Trends and International Issues in Developmental Disabilities,* edited by H. Bersani. Cambridge, MA: Brookline.

Parsons, T. 1951. *The Social System.* Glencoe, IL: Free Press.

Penrose, L. S. 1938. *A Clinical and Genetic Study of 1,280 Cases of Mental Defect (Colchester Survey).* Special Report No. 229. London: Medical Research Council.

———. 1963. *The Biology of Mental Defect.* 2d rev. ed. New York: Grune & Stratton.

Perrin, B. and B. Nirje. 1985. "Setting the Record Straight: A Critique of Some Frequent Misconceptions of the Normalization Principle." *Australia and New Zealand Journal of Developmental Disabilities* 11:69-74.

President's Panel on Mental Retardation. 1962. *A Proposed Program for National Action to Combat Mental Retardation.* Washington, DC: Superintendent of Documents.

Radford, J. P. 1994. "Intellectual Disability and the Heritage of Modernity." Pp. 9-27 in *Disability Is Not Measles,* edited by M. Rioux and M. Bach. Toronto: Roeher Institute.

Raichle, M. E. 1999. "Modern Phrenology: Maps of Human Cortical Function." Pp. 107-18 in *Great Issues for Medicine in the Twenty-First Century: Ethical and Social Issues Arising Out of Advances in the Biomedical Sciences,* edited by D. C. Grassman and H. Voltin. New York: New York Academy of Sciences.

Reinders, H. S. 1997. "The Ethics of Normalization." *Cambridge Quarterly of Health Care Ethics* 6:481-89.

———. 1999. "The Limits of Rights Discourse." Paper presented to the Roundtable of the Special Interest Research Group (SIRG) on Ethics, International Association for the Scientific Study of Intellectual Disabilities, April, Doorn, the Netherlands.

———. 2000. *The Future of the Disabled in Liberal Society: An Ethical Analysis.* Notre Dame, IN: University of Notre Dame Press.

Richards, B. W., A. D. B. Clarke, and A. Shapiro. 1962. *Proceedings of the London Conference on the Scientific Study of Mental Deficiency.* Dagenham, UK: May & Baker.

Rioux, M. H. 1997. "Disability: The Place of Judgement in a World of Fact." *Journal of Intellectual Disability Research* 41:102-11.

Roeher Institute. 1999. *Genome(s) and Justice.* Toronto: Author.

Rowitz, L. 1992. "Predictions for the 1990s and Beyond." Pp. 353-66 in *Mental Retardation in the Year 2000,* edited by L. Rowitz. New York: Springer-Verlag.

Ryle, G. 1949. *The Concept of Mind.* London.

Rynders, J. E. 1987. "History of Down Syndrome: The Need for a New Perspective." Pp. 1-17 in *New Perspectives on Down Syndrome,* edited by S. M. Pueschel, C. Tingey, J. E. Rynders, A. C. Crocker, and D. M. Crutcher. Baltimore: Brookes.

Saul, J. R. 1992. *Voltaire's Bastards: The Dictatorship of Reason in the West.* London: Penguin.

Schalock, R. L. 1999. "A Quest for Quality." Pp. 55-80 in *Quality Performance and Human Services,* edited by J. F. Gardiner and S. Nudler. Baltimore: Brookes.

Schroeder, S. 1991. "Biological and Behavioural Interaction in Mental Retardation Research." *Psychology in Mental Retardation and Developmental Disabilities* 17:1-6.

Sen, A. 1992. *Inequity Re-Examined.* Oxford, UK: Clarendon.

Shephard, Y. H. 1986. "Human Teratogens: How Can We Sort Them Out?" Pp. 105-15 in *Mental Retardation: Research, Education, and Technology Transfer,* edited by H. M. Wisniewski and D. A. Snider. New York: New York Academy of Sciences.

Simpson, M. K. 1998. "The Roots of Normalization: A Reappraisal." *Journal of Intellectual Disability Research* 42:1-7.

Snell, M. E. 1987. *Systematic Instruction of Persons with Severe Handicaps.* Columbus, OH: Merrill.

Spellman, W. M. 1988. *John Locke and the Problem of Depravity.* Oxford, UK: Clarendon.

Spiegelberg, H. 1944. "A Defense of Human Equality." *Philosophical Review* 53:101-24.

———. 1975. "Good Fortune Obligates: Albert Schweitzer's Second Ethical Principle." *Ethics* 85:227-34.

Stainton, T. 1994. *Autonomy and Social Policy: Rights, Mental Handicap and Community Care.* Aldershot, UK: Avebury.

———. 1998. "Intellectual Disability, Oppression and Difference." Pp. 111-31 in *Countering Discrimination in Social Work,* edited by B. Lesnik. Aldershot, UK: Ashgate.

Stevens, H. A. 1964. "Overview." Pp. 1-15 in *Mental Retardation: A Review of Research,* edited by H. A. Stevens and R. Heber. Chicago: University of Chicago Press.

Stockholder, F. E. 1994. "Naming and Renaming Persons with Intellectual Disabilities." Pp. 153-79 in *Disability Is Not Measles,* edited by M. Rioux and M. Bach. Toronto: Roeher Institute.

Talbot, M. E. 1964. *Édouard Seguin: A Study of an Educational Approach to the Treatment of Mentally Defective Children.* New York: Teachers College Press.

Taylor, C. 1989. *Sources of the Self: The Making of Modern Identity.* Cambridge, UK: Cambridge University Press.

Terman, M. 1916. *The Measurement of Intelligence.* Boston: Houghton Mifflin.

Toulmin, S. 1990. *Cosmopolis: The Hidden Agenda of Modernity.* New York: Free Press.

Tredgold, A. F. 1937. *A Textbook of Mental Deficiency (Amentia).* 6th ed. London: Bailliêne, Tindall & Cox.

Turnbull, A. P. and H. R. Turnbull. 1986. *Families, Professionals and Exceptionalities: A Special Partnership.* Columbus, OH: Merrill.

Turnbull, H. R. 1998. "Are We Gaining Ground in the Pursuit of Life, Liberty and Happiness?" Keynote address to 122nd Annual Conference of the American Association on Mental Retardation, June, San Diego, CA.

United Nations. 1971. *Declaration of General and Specific Rights of the Mentally Retarded.* New York: Author.

———. 1975. *Declaration of the Rights of Disabled People.* New York: Author.

———. 1993. *Standard Rules on the Equalization of Opportunities for Persons with Disabilities.* New York: Author.

United Nations Educational, Scientific, and Cultural Organization (UNESCO). 1997. *Declaration on the Human Genome and Human Rights.* Paris: Author.

Walsh, P. N. 1997. "Old World—New Territory: European Perspectives on Intellectual Disability." *Journal of Intellectual Disability Research* 41:112-19.

Warren, S. F. 1999. "Early Communication Intervention as a Vehicle to Optimal Brain Development: Promises and Pitfalls." Keynote paper presented to the 1999 Gatlinburg Conference, June, Charleston, SC.

Wehman, P., M. S. Moon, J. M. Everson, W. Wood, and J. M. Barcus. 1988. *Transition from School to Work: New Challenges for Youth with Severe Disabilities.* Baltimore: Brookes.

Wolfensberger, W. 1969. "The Principle of Normalization and Its Implications to Psychiatric Services." *American Journal of Psychiatry* 27:291-97.

———. 1972. *The Principle of Normalization in Human Services.* Toronto: National Institute on Mental Retardation.

————. 1983. "Social Role Valorization: A Proposed New Term for the Principle of Normalization." *Mental Retardation* 21:234-39.

————. 2000. "A Brief Overview of Social Role Valorization." *Mental Retardation* 38:105-23.

Wolfensberger, W. and L. Glenn. 1975. *Program Analysis of Service Systems (PASS): A Method for the Quantitative Evaluation of Human Services.* 2 vols. Toronto: National Institute on Mental Retardation.

Wolfensberger, W. and S. Thomas. 1980. *PASSING (Program Analysis of Service Systems' Implementation of Normalization Goals).* Syracuse, NY: Training Institute for Human Service Planning, Leadership and Change Agentry, Syracuse University.

World Health Organization. 1998. *Primary Prevention of Mental Neurological and Psycho-Social Disorders.* Geneva: Author.

Zaner, R. M. 1988. *Ethics and the Clinical Encounter.* Englewood Cliffs, NJ: Prentice Hall.

Disability, Bioethics, and Human Rights

11

ADRIENNE ASCH

n 1989, Canadian philosopher Susan Wendell characterized the way bioethics literature discusses disability as follows: "Under what conditions is it morally permissible/right to kill/let die a disabled person and how potentially disabled does a fetus have to be before it is permissible/right to prevent its being born?" (p. 104). This statement aptly captures much of what bioethics has said about disability and fits the dominant view of bioethics held by those in disability studies and disability rights. Yet, despite serious problems in much of the bioethics literature for anyone with a minority group or social model of disability, the field of bioethics struggles with topics of profound importance to disability studies and to disability rights. Furthermore, some questions of bioethics pose an important challenge to both the social model and the minority group model of disability and compel people to reconsider the social, moral, and policy implications of forms of human variation.

In what follows, I review the major intersections of disability studies with bioethics, describing the principal issues that have sparked controversy between disability rights activists and scholars and those in traditional bioethics. My discussion lays out key arenas of struggle between those with a disability rights perspective and those within bioethics; it also comments on issues that have received less direct attention from within disability rights but that could benefit from a dialogue. Highlighting the critical intersections of bioethics and disability studies oversimplifies matters of considerable concern to traditional bioethics. Moreover, the two fields have not necessarily confronted issues at the same moment; rather, disability rights has reacted to bioethics literature and to dramatic, highly publicized instances of bioethics debates. Thus, I focus on issues rather than the chronology of bioethics discussion or disability response. I conclude by asking disability studies to grapple with the social justice and definitional questions posed by bioethics because they are crucial to advancing our work in disability studies and disability rights.

AUTHOR'S NOTE: I would like to express my sincere appreciation to Gary Albrecht, whose patience and persistence are much appreciated, as well as Jerome Bickenbach and David Wasserman for extremely helpful reviews of this chapter and for comments and discussions that aided me immeasurably. James Lindemann Nelson provided a careful reading with valuable suggestions under great time pressure. The research, proofreading, and support of Taran Jefferies made this chapter a reality.

DESCRIBING BIOETHICS: CONVERGENCE
AND CONTRAST WITH DISABILITY RIGHTS

What unites the field of bioethics is its concern with fundamental questions of health and illness, life and death, the relationship of medicine to nature, what constitutes a life of quality, and whether there are ever life situations that appear worse than not being alive. Bioethics shares some interesting and significant similarities with the international disability rights movement and the social/minority group models of disability—models that I will generally discuss together because they overlap on many bioethical issues (see Shakespeare and Watson, this volume).[1] Both worldwide bioethics and the worldwide disability rights movement have become known only in the past half century, and each has emerged in reaction to a dominant paradigm in the medical and helping professions. Recognition of bioethical issues first arose when people learned that in World War II Germany and in the postwar United States, physicians and scientists had abused many classes of vulnerable citizens by failing to obtain their informed consent to serve as subjects in medical research. Prisoners, concentration camp inmates, African American sharecroppers, and residents of institutions for the psychiatrically and cognitively disabled all became victims of government and professional research interests. Discovery of these abuses spurred demands for regulation, reform, and new oversight of governmental and professional behavior (Annas and Grodin 1992; U.S. National Commission for the Protection of Human Subjects of Biomedical and Behavioral Research 1978).

The early U.S. independent living and disability rights movement exemplified much the same challenge to professional domination and demands for self-determination and autonomy (Gaylin et al. 1978). Adults with disabilities and parent advocates for disabled children protested abuses by powerful government and philanthropic institutions that historically had usurped their decision-making authority, using the same language as physicians, lawyers, philosophers, and theologians who questioned the power and paternalism of medicine in conducting medical research and using new life-sustaining technologies. During the 1960s and 1970s, as the National Federation of the Blind demanded representation on boards of service agencies (Matson 1990) and as Ed Roberts and other students with disabilities challenged the paternalism of the University of California at Berkeley and created the first center for independent living, bioethics was questioning whether people who seemed near death should be sustained by technologies such as mechanical respiration or tube feeding. Even though medicine could save lives after traumatic injury or could maintain lives of people affected by cancer, stroke, and heart or kidney disease, should patients have the authority to refuse these treatments? If so, on what basis and for what reasons might it be morally acceptable and legally permissible to decline life-saving technology for oneself? If individuals could challenge professional authority for themselves, could they do so on behalf of their minor children or demented parents? Was it ever appropriate for government or professionals to limit patient or family in the realm of medical decision making?[2]

Like the new paradigms in disability scholarship and activism that have moved from demands for individual control and self-determination to calls for sweeping societal change, bioethics has recognized that the complex life-and-death decisions made by individuals and families cannot remain its only concern. Recent debate also focuses on questions about the implications of research on life-creating or life-changing technologies themselves, on questions of what constitutes a just distribution of social resources for medical care, and on which life situations should properly come under the purview of medicine. These and other bioethical issues appear regularly in the newspaper and on television, radio, in film, theater, and fiction. Should an experimental therapy for cancer be paid for by a health insurance plan? Should a health maintenance organization (HMO) refuse to cover any treatments for particular conditions, such as alcoholism, substance abuse, "gender identity disorder," depression, or infertility? When, if ever, is growth hormone therapy an appropriate treatment? Should society support research on human cloning, male pregnancy, gene modification, or extending the human life span than 100 years? Although some of these questions may ring of science fiction, others have already faced us. They all demonstrate that biology is not destiny and that we must grapple with what control we believe is appropriate to exert over our biological lives.

If Western bioethics resembles the disability rights movement in its commitments to patient autonomy, skepticism about professional power, and paternalism and championing of consumer protection, it has never accepted the claims of the movement and of recent disability scholarship in its assessment of the impact of impairment. Whether writing out of a religious or secular orientation, bioethics has tended to cast discussions about life-and-death questions in terms of contrasts between what might be called the "sanctity-of-life" and the "quality-of-life" approaches. Until the advent of means to save premature babies, young people injured in wartime or car accidents, and elderly people who had heart attacks or strokes, societies had not needed to consider whether life in such impaired conditions should be maintained. The dominant bioethics voices have argued that human life had to be respected and valued but not necessarily at any cost or in any state of impairment. Now that human mastery over nature permitted lives to be saved and sustained despite significant illnesses and disabilities, it was incumbent on individuals and societies to determine the limits to which medicine and technology should be used for these purposes. Instead of the medical question, "Can this life be saved?" bioethics invites the question, "Should this life be saved?" Medicine could now decrease mortality but only by increasing the numbers of people of all ages who would live with chronic illnesses or disabling conditions. Bioethicists have taken on the mission of supporting those who believed that the quality of the life after treatment should be a factor in medical decision making and in decision making about allocations of resources (Morreim 1995; Walter 1995). Bioethics asks the disability community the following: Is it appropriate to use technology and skill to sustain the life of someone who would have a disability?

There is not one disability response any more than there is only one bioethics response; nonetheless, the dominant message of disability studies and disability activism disputes the statements permeating most of bioethics. Bioethics writing, like the medical model of disability now being replaced by a social model, has failed to question traditional understandings of impairment, illness, or disability. In arguing that individuals should not be required to submit to unpleasant medical interventions simply because such technologies had been developed, bioethics was trying to wrest control from what it perceived to be a technology-happy medical establishment and return decisional authority to individuals. As represented in major works (Beauchamp and Childress 1994; President's Commission for the Study of Ethical Problems in Medicine and Biomedical and Behavioral Research 1982, 1983; Reich 1995), bioethics insists that individuals should be able to determine the situations under which they find life intolerable but has never challenged them to ask themselves what they found intolerable. Nor has bioethics suggested that what was unacceptable might not be inherent in quadriplegia, stroke, or a degenerative neurological disorder but instead could result from the social arrangements facing people living with such conditions. Although bioethics has been the means of challenging unbridled uses of technology and of calling for protections for participants in medical research, most bioethics literature has never contested prevailing notions of what it means to have an illness or impairment or to be a person with a disability. Rather, bioethics has presumed impaired mobility, physical deformity, sensory deficit, atypical learning style or speed, or departures from what was customary in energy, stamina, or flexibility to be the reason why people with disabilities would be less educated, less likely to be working, often in poverty, and more socially isolated than people who did not have impairments. When it concerns life with disability, most people who call themselves bioethicists have viewed having a disability from within what Gliedman and Roth (1980) and Bickenbach (1993) term the *medical* or *biomedical model,* as contrasted with a minority group (Gliedman and Roth 1980; Hahn 1983) or social model (see Shakespeare and Watson, this volume) of disability. Disability community critics of standard bioethics reject the medical model of disability, with its belief that functional impairment leads to an unacceptable, unsatisfying life. The critics do not demand to use theological or "sanctity-of-life" values; they claim that even on "quality-of-life" measures, a life with disability can be rewarding.

HEALTH, NORMALITY, DISABILITY, AND QUALITY OF LIFE

Defining terms such as *health, normality, impairment,* and *disability* continues to pose problems and cause controversy for bioethics and for disability studies. Their meanings are not clear, objective, and universal across time and place and are contentious even for contemporaries in the same culture, profession, and field. A look at the controversy within bioethics and the policy about which variations from the typical or average are impairments, which behaviors should be considered health problems, and which should be viewed as social or moral problems will reveal how difficult it is to come up with a clear and widely shared understanding. The bioethics literature contains extensive discussions about how to define health. For people such as Christopher Boorse (1987), a person is said to be healthy if the person's organism performs species-typical functions with statistically typical efficiency. Matters for debate within bioethics include whether health should be defined as the absence of disease (Boorse 1987) or as a state of well-being, as the World Health Organization proposed (Purdy 1996); whether the well-being in question includes mental and social well-being in addition to physical well-being; and whether disease can be defined neutrally or only with reference to a culture and a historical period. (Compare Boorse 1987 with Caplan, Engelhardt, and McCartney 1981; Engelhardt and Wildes 1995; Purdy 1996 for arguments about the importance of cultural and historical location in ascribing impairment; see Wasserman, this volume, for detailed discussion of this entire topic.) Virtually everyone engaged in the debate over a definition of health or impairment is convinced that individual physical, cognitive, and emotional characteristics are evaluated with reference to what is expected or desired by way of functioning and role performance for a girl or boy, woman or man. Operating within the medical framework and the worldview of bioethics, health is prized because "impairments of normal species functioning reduce the range of opportunity open to the individual . . . [to] construct [a] 'plan of life' or 'conception of the good' " (Daniels 1985:27). Congenital disability, chronic illness, traumatic injury, malnutrition, and the aging process occasion departures from "species-typical functioning" and constitute differences from both a statistical average and a desired norm of well-being, although such departures are reported to affect one-sixth to one-fourth of the world's population.

Those who embrace either the social or the minority group model of disability contend that medically oriented understandings of impairment contain two erroneous assumptions. First, the life of someone with a chronic illness or disability (used interchangeably throughout this article) is forever disrupted, as one's life can be temporarily disrupted by the flu or a back spasm. Second, if a disabled person experiences isolation, powerlessness, poverty, unemployment, or low social status, these are inevitable consequences of biological limitation. Bioethics generalizes from the problems and disorientation that some people may experience at the onset of a disability and assumes that such disruption is unchanged by rehabilitation, adaptation, mastery of new means to accomplish desired ends, or changes in the life plans one pursues. Bioethics also fails to recognize the extent to which disadvantages experienced by people with disabilities arise through society's lack of accommodation to the different methods of performing valued activities such as learning, communicating, moving, or taking in the world. On the contrary, say disability studies scholars and disability politics. First, life with disability is not the unremitting tragedy portrayed in medical and bioethics literature. Second, the culprit is not biological, psychic, or cognitive equipment but the social, institutional, and physical world in which people with impairments must function—a world designed with the characteristics and needs of the nondisabled majority in mind. An impaired arm becomes a manual disability or social handicap only because of the interaction of a particular physiology with a specific social, legal, and attitudinal environment.

In the minority group or social models of disability, rules, laws, means of communication, characteristics of buildings and transit systems, the typical eight-hour workday, and aesthetic preferences all exclude some people from participating in school, work, civic, or social life. When medicine and bioethics discuss the importance of health care, urge accident prevention, and promote healthy lifestyles, these professions perceive that a certain level of health and functioning serves as a prerequisite for the "normal opportunity range" or for an acceptable life (Daniels 1985). According to the more recent thinking, by contrast, disability is a fact of human life, and thus everyone gains if societies refashion the social and physical world to ensure the comfortable participation of all people with their diverse range of capacities. While desirable, health and medical care do not hold the keys to "the normal opportunity range" or to a satisfying life.

For the past three decades, scholars and activists in disability have argued that the problem of disability was, indeed, one of denial of civil, social, and economic rights and not one of biology and health. Yet, the attitudes toward disability and the assumptions about the impact disabled people have on families and society that abound in medicine and bioethics all compel those scholars and activists to assert that the first right of people with disabilities is a claim to life itself, along with the social recognition of the value and validity of the life of someone with a disability (D. Wasserman, personal communication, 2000).

A substantial body of literature reveals that even before legal and political advances in the United States and other nations, but certainly since then, many people with disabilities have found satisfaction in their lives that was far greater than anything expected of them by members of the health and rehabilitation professions (Albrecht and Devlieger 1999; Cameron et al. 1973; Cushman and Dijkers 1990; Eisenberg and Saltz 1991; Goode 1994; McNair 1996; National Organization on Disability 1998; Ray and West 1984; Saigal et al. 1996; Stensman 1985; Woodrich and Patterson 1983). These data reveal that people who experience disability—whether it be congenital or acquired, whether sensory, cognitive, motor, or other—can find considerable reward and satisfaction in their lives. When people with disabilities report unhappiness or dissatisfaction (a minority in every study), the sources resemble sources of unhappiness in the lives of nondisabled people—inadequacies in financial security, work, or social and personal relationships. As Albrecht and Devlieger (1999) point out, sometimes impairment-related factors, such as pain and fatigue, contribute to unsatisfying relationships or to the difficulty of holding a job, but the frustrations come from difficulty in incorporating the impairment into existing interpersonal and institutional life. Studies of "quality of life" consistently reveal that for people with disabilities, satisfaction results from achieving a harmony in their lives that can include a sense of meaning, performing expected social roles, enjoying give-and-take in their relationships, and having a sense that they live in "a reciprocal social world" (Albrecht and Devlieger 1999:984).

Unfortunately, not only do emergency room physicians, who deal with traumatically injured people, fail to appreciate that people with disabilities are able to lead satisfying lives postinjury (Gerhart et al. 1994), rehabilitation specialists also dramatically underestimate life satisfaction of people with disabilities. This is found to be true regardless of the length of time the professionals had been in the field or the number of people they had worked with (Bach and Tilton 1994). Over the years, many reasons have been offered for the gap in understanding that persists between people with and without disabilities regarding the potential for life with disability to be acceptable, rewarding, or as rewarding as the lives of people who do not report impairments. Gill (forthcoming) suggests that these persistent gaps in understanding stem from the lack of equal-status contact between clinician and patient, the crisis nature of much medical contact that rarely extends beyond the immediate medical setting, the lack of education about the social realities of life with disability in the curricula of medical professionals, and the particular psychological makeup and socialization of many who enter such professions, convinced that rationality, control of life events, and optimal workings of the human organism are the goals toward which to strive. Like many in the medical professions, bioethicists are typically highly educated individuals who prize intellect, rationality, and the goal of human health. Few bioethicists identify as people who have impairments or as members of the disability rights movement. The values and perspectives of bioethicists profoundly influence their assessments of the quality of life of persons with disabilities and in turn influence central debates about how or whether to use such assessments to settle questions of clinical decision making or resource allocation. From within the disability rights community (Carlson 1997) and from within the bioethics world (Edwards 1997; Veatch 1986), researchers have stressed that the esteem given to intellect, rationality, and self-awareness leads some to question the moral status or life quality of persons with cognitive impairments (Singer 1993, 1996; Steinbock and McClamrock 1994; Tooley 1986). It is not only cognitive impairment that calls the value of life into question. The emphasis on self-sufficiency leads others to doubt that anyone who cannot execute "normal" life tasks of eating, walking, or managing personal hygiene could enjoy life as much as someone who performs these tasks without human assistance (Shelp 1986). For other commentators, even if people themselves could find their lives acceptable, the impact of their reduced-life opportunities on family and society is thought negative and burdensome (Beauchamp and Childress 1994; Callahan 1988; Morreim 1995).

In virtually every instance of a disability rights critique of bioethics literature or of decision making in bioethics cases, the issue has revolved around the assessment of an author or a court that impairment provides a reason to deny medical intervention or to provide less treatment than would have been the case had there been no impairment. In discussions about withholding treatment from newborn infants with impairment, ending life-sustaining treatments for adults with disabilities, refusing to treat a new condition because of an individual's uncorrectable disability, or tolerating physician-assisted suicide, the disability critique is similar. Most bioethics literature and most legal decisions in bioethics cases conclude that the impairment reduces the quality and value to others and to self of the life lived and therefore justifies less effort at preservation or recovery. If people with disabilities like their lives more than others believe, it does not support ignoring the justice claims of the minority group or social models, a point taken up later in this chapter. It is a claim that substitutes myth with data that medicine and bioethics must grasp if they are to change in their handling of the many dilemmas faced by people with disabilities, their families, and the societies in which they live.

DISABILITY AND THE RIGHT TO LIVE IN THE WORLD

The disability community has expressed its outrage at mainstream bioethics when bioethics has supported claims that life with disability should not be maintained. The most prominent examples of this debate have flared in the contexts of family decision making, when people with disabilities have sought to stop treatments or to request physician assistance in dying. Family decision making about the lives of people with disabilities usually occurs in three situations:

1. decisions of parents regarding treatment for infants or minor children who will have impairments after intervention but who might die without treatment,
2. decisions by prospective parents about whether to bear children who would have disabilities, and
3. decisions about relatives who may not be able to decide for themselves about treatments.

People with disabilities may themselves choose to forego treatments that keep them alive, or they may request physician assistance to end their lives. Although all these contexts share many common themes, each situation has had its own history and deserves some separate comment.

Family Decision Making

The Case of Newborns with Impairments

In the early and mid-1980s, U.S. disability rights adherents first challenged bioethics over decisions about standards of treatment for infants born with significant disabling conditions requiring immediate medical treatment. Should physicians counsel parents of children with conditions such as Down syndrome who also have heart problems or intestinal blockages to let the infant die rather than treating the heart condition or the intestinal blockage that would leave the infant with Down syndrome? Should parents of a child with spina bifida be permitted to refuse surgery that would close the child's open spine and reduce the potential for infection? Should parents of a child with bowel obstruction consent to surgery to remove a necrotic bowel to save the child's life, even though long-term survival of a child with such an obstruction is estimated at less than 1 in 10,000? In yet another instance, should a severely premature baby be placed on a respirator against the wishes of the baby's parents if chances of survival are nearly negligible? (See Weir 1984.)

For bioethics, there were many questions embedded in these novel situations. Were infants with no chance of survival experimental subjects for physicians determining the efficacy of new treatment modalities? In situations of uncertain prognosis for low-birth-weight or premature babies, should physicians initiate treatments that might be ended if the child would never be able to go home with his or her family? Suppose parents wanted an infant to be treated aggressively but physicians declined based on assumptions of intractable pain or disability for the infant or heartache for a family raising a seriously disabled child. Should parental decision making, based on what the parents believe to be their family interest or in the interest of their minor child, take precedence over medical expertise?

Physicians, lawyers, and philosophers had discussed these issues among themselves for at least a decade (Duff and Campbell 1973; Fost 1982; Kohl 1978), and many believed it acceptable or morally desirable for parents and doctors to end the lives of infants who would remain disabled after all medical interventions. The major national ethics body believed that parents could be decision makers for their infants under most circumstances but argued that they could not refuse medical treatments that would clearly benefit babies if the reasons for their refusal stemmed from concerns about familial, as opposed to patient, well-being. Its recommendations included the following guidelines:

> Parents should be the surrogates for a seriously ill newborn unless they are disqualified by decision-making incapacity, an unresolvable disagreement between them, or their choice of a course of action that is clearly against the infant's best interests.
>
> Therapies expected to be futile for a seriously ill newborn need not be provided. . . .
>
> Within constraints of equity and availability, infants should receive all therapies that are clearly beneficial to them. For example, an otherwise healthy Down Syndrome child whose life is threatened by a surgically correctable complication should receive the surgery because he or she would clearly benefit from it. . . .
>
> The best interests of an infant should be pursued when those interests are clear.
>
> The policies should allow for the exercise of parental discretion when a child's interests are ambiguous. (President's Commission 1983:6, 7)

Interestingly, these recommendations were being crafted before members of the disability rights movement, along with the U.S. government and the general public, became acquainted with these dilemmas by Bloomington, Indiana Baby Doe and Long Island, New York Baby Jane Doe. The first, a boy with Down syndrome and an esophageal blockage, was born in 1982 and died of starvation at six days old, after his parents decided not to treat the blockage because of the advice given to them by their physician about life with Down syndrome. This event may have occasioned the specificity of the published recommendations by the President's Commission. In late 1983, parents of the girl who became known as Baby Jane Doe declined surgery for their daughter born with spina bifida and hydrocephalus because physicians advised them that without treatment, she would die more quickly.

Despite the President's Commission guidelines of 1983, professionals and the public remained deeply divided about the morality of insisting that medicine save babies who would live with disabilities. Rationales for withholding treatment focused on the physical suffering and pain of the potential treatments as well as the impairments themselves; the conviction that technology was being used to sustain children who would have short, painful, and miserable lives regardless of what was done for them; the anguish for parents who had to watch a child die slowly after enduring fruitless medical procedures; disappointment for parents who would not have the healthy child they expected and desired and might instead have to raise one who would always have disabling conditions; and belief that the millions of dollars spent for such treatments were better spent in other ways (Kuhse and Singer 1985; Shelp 1986; Tooley 1986).

Legal cases were brought on behalf of infants whose parents and physicians were refusing to provide what others perceived as beneficial treatments (*Bowen v. American Hospital Association* 1986; *Weber v. Stony Brook Hospital* 1983). Bioethicists continued to debate the merits of the President's Commission guidelines and the U.S. government's 1984 legislation deeming refusals of beneficial treatments child abuse, which was punishable by withdrawals of federal funds from hospitals that participated in such treatment denials (Child Abuse Amendments of 1984, PL 98-457). Many opponents viewed the legislation as infringing on family privacy by compelling parents to raise children who would otherwise have died without technology and who often would remain alive with significant medical problems and physical, sensory, or cognitive impairments. Many suspected that some instances of undertreatment of ill and disabled infants would be replaced with overtreatment of those who would never survive to live with their families or go to school. They suspected that the government's purpose lay not in protecting the civil rights or rights to life of the disabled infants but in using the question of disabled newborns as another weapon against those who supported abortion as a woman's right (Caplan and Cohen 1987; Murray and Caplan 1985; Rothman 1986).

Notably, people with commitments to disability rights perceived "Baby Doe" cases differently. Perhaps for the wrong reasons, the U.S. government was committed to the rights to life of infants with disabling conditions, and it thus backed the legislation that became the Child Abuse Amendments of 1984, calling for treatment of newborns unless the infant was likely to die regardless of the intervention. The intense academic, legal, and public discussion included almost no published voices from within the U.S. disability rights movement until after the passage of the 1984 legislation (Asch and Fine 1984; Asch 1986, 1987; Biklen 1987; Hahn 1987; Hentoff 1987). Perhaps because most statements appeared in disability-focused rather than bioethics publications, these views never appeared to modify the mainstream bioethics discussion of the topic. Disability critics explicitly rejected the government's pro-life agenda, pointing to the difference between a newborn infant, which no longer needed one particular woman to sustain its life, and a fetus residing in a woman's body (Asch and Fine 1984).

Concentrating on infants with treatable medical conditions who would resemble others with Down syndrome or spina bifida, the disability rights critics went beyond the patient-focused language of the President's Commission guidelines. They argued that denials of beneficial treatment represented a kind of discrimination against people with disabilities by the medical profession and frightened parents who were unable to imagine having a child with a disability as anything but a tragedy and disaster for themselves and for their nondisabled family members. After all, critics argued, when treatment for intestinal or heart problems is given to a baby without Down syndrome but denied to one who has Down syndrome, the physicians and parents based the decision on the infant's uncorrectable impairment and on their beliefs about the kind of life that the child and family would have. If denying beneficial medical treatment to a nondisabled infant constituted child neglect or abuse, denial of that same treatment to one with a disability was equally an abuse. Disability rights critics of standard bioethics discussion pointed to the social nature of the problems of disability, arguing that the baby with Down syndrome or spina bifida belonged to a despised minority that parents feared for their child and for themselves. They emphasized the stigma of disability (Goffman 1963), the "disabling images" permeating society (Gartner and Joe 1987), the erroneous belief that a disabled child or adult contributed nothing positive to family or society (Darling 1979; Fine and Asch 1988), and the notion that people with disabilities (and sometimes their families) became part of a social movement to combat their disadvantaged minority status and could draw from that movement an alternate sense of community to counteract isolation from and rejection by the majority (Asch and Fine 1984; Biklen 1987; Hahn 1987; Hentoff 1987).

Picking up this thread of the disability rights argument, the U.S. Commission on Civil Rights (1989) discussed the stigma and the minority group nature of disability in its report, titled provocatively *Medical Discrimination against Children with Disabilities:*

> The birth of an infant with a disability typically comes to them as a great shock, with feelings of depression, anger, and guilt. Because most parents have had little or no interaction with people who have disabilities, their assessments of their infants' conditions and prognoses may have little basis, and they thus turn to the attending physicians for information and recommendations. . . . Physicians with a bent toward denial of treatment for persons with disabilities can be quite insistent in conveying negative information. There appears to be near unanimity from health care personnel who support treatment in a Baby Doe situation as well as those who oppose treatment that, in all but a handful of cases, the manner and content of the medical provider's presentation of the issue will be decisive in the parental decision whether to authorize treatment.
>
> Unfortunately, there also exists misinformation among many health care personnel and bioethicists advising parents on the advances and alternatives available to children with disabilities. (P. 2)

The U.S. Supreme Court and many within bioethics reject the idea that denying treatment to newborns with disabilities constitutes any kind of legally recognizable discrimination covered by Section 504 of the Rehabilitation Act of 1973 or, by extension, the Americans with Disabilities Act (*Bowen v. American Hospital Association* 1986). They reject the discrimination argument for several reasons. First, physicians and hospitals (covered entities under antidiscrimination legislation) do not make the treatment decisions but implement those of parents. In addition, many of the infants who need some type of medical procedure require interventions unique to their impairment that no unimpaired infant would need; therefore, the situations of most critically ill, low birth weight, or premature babies differ from the paradigmatic Down syndrome complicated by treatable medical conditions that fueled the governmental and disability rights positions.

In the year 2000, most infants with Down syndrome and spina bifida born in the United States received medically indicated treatments, as did premature and low-birth-weight infants who—if they survived the treatments—became part of the disabled population. Neonatologists and bioethicists seem to believe that the contemporary question for treatment of newborn infants is one of overtreatment rather than undertreatment. Thus, the President's Commission writings, the Child Abuse Amendments of 1984, and whatever recognition the disability rights movement has achieved all have combined to ensure that most babies who can benefit from medical interventions do receive them.

Most of U.S. bioethics literature now concentrates on other topics, although there are no public retractions of views that enraged the disability rights movement. The furor over the appointment of philosopher Peter Singer to a chair in ethics at Princeton University arises from his published views about life with conditions such as Down syndrome, spina bifida, hemophilia, and other sensory, cognitive, and physical impairments. The frequently cited Singer's position is the following: "The killing of a defective infant is not morally equivalent to the killing of a person; very often it is not morally wrong at all" (Singer 1993:184). Singer acknowledges that children and adults living with these conditions may have satisfactory lives, but he continues to claim that their impairments necessarily render their lives less satisfactory than the lives of people without such impairments. Consequently, he maintains that parents would be justified in killing newborns with these conditions to replace the impaired child with a healthy one, who would bring more happiness to the family and would experience more happiness. However, he insists that once people with disabilities pass perhaps one year of age, they have the rights to life of anyone without a disability so long as they have rationality, self-consciousness, and self-awareness and can differentiate past from present or future (Singer 1999). Not surprisingly, Singer's beliefs about disabled newborns offend people with disabilities who claim a kind of social kinship with infants who might have conditions similar to theirs. Thus, Singer's insistence that his views do not apply to adults and older children who make up the membership of Not Dead Yet, ADAPT, and other similar protest groups has not mollified their opposition to his views or to the visibility and prestige accorded his work.

Prenatal Testing and Selective Abortion

As the 1980s saw bioethics and disability advocates contending over the topic of providing treatment for disabled infants, the 1990s carried out a very similar debate about the implications of the growing tendency to use many prenatal tests to get information about the status of fetuses in utero. Worldwide, disability organizations, disability rights activists, and theorists have taken up the question of how the increasing use of prenatal testing and selective abortion affects the place of people with disabilities in the world. Prenatal testing has involved no court cases or expensive and complex technologies, but the themes in the prenatal testing debate echo those on all sides of the questions about disabled newborns. By the 1990s, bioethicists, civil libertarians, health professionals, and the public generally accepted the idea that a live-born infant should get medical treatment to provide a chance at life. However, the vast majority of theorists and health professionals still argue that prenatal testing, followed by pregnancy termination if an impairment is detected, promotes family well-being and the public health. To them, it is simply one more legitimate method of averting disability in the world.

Although sometimes prenatal testing occurs outside of a plan to abort based on results of the test, most people who seek testing plan to abort the fetus if they learn of a disability (Beaudet 1990; Rinck and Calkins 1996; Wertz 1995). According to Wertz and Fletcher, who surveyed geneticists in 18 countries, in addition to the goal of helping people decide about their own family planning, most geneticists subscribe to what some view as "eugenic" goals—namely, the following:

> A majority (74%) believes that improvement of the general health and vigor of the population is important. A smaller majority (54%) subscribes to a eugenic goal, a reduction in the number of carriers of genetic disorders in the population. (Wertz 1995:1654)

Standard justifications include the following:

> Attitudes toward congenital disability per se have not changed markedly. Both pre-modern as well as contemporary societies have regarded disability as undesirable and to be avoided. Not only have parents recognized the birth of a disabled child as a potentially divisive, destructive force in the family unit, but the larger society has seen disability as unfortunate. . . . Our society still does not countenance the elimination of diseased/disabled people; but it does urge the termination of diseased/disabled fetuses. (Retsinas 1991:89, 90)

> In the absence of adequate justifying reasons, a child is morally wronged when he/she is knowingly, deliberately, or negligently brought into being with a health status likely to result in significantly greater disability or suffering, or significantly reduced life options relative to the other children with whom he/she will grow up. (Green 1997:10)

> The parent's harms . . . include emotional pain and suffering . . . loss of opportunities, loss of freedom, isolation, loneliness, fear, guilt, stigmatization, and financial expenses. . . . It might also be added that parents are harmed by their unfulfilled expectations with the birth of an impaired child. . . .
>
> Parents of a child with unwanted disability have their interests impinged upon by the efforts, time, emotional burdens, and expenses *added* by the disability that they would not have otherwise experienced with the birth of a healthy child. (Botkin 1995:36-37, emphasis added)

Parens and Asch (1999) describe the disability rights critique of prenatal testing as follows:

Rather than improving the medical or social situation of today's or tomorrow's disabled citizens, prenatal diagnosis reinforces the medical model that disability itself, not societal discrimination against people with disabilities, is the problem to be solved.... In rejecting an otherwise desired child because they believe that the child's disability will diminish their parental experience, parents suggest that they are unwilling to accept any significant departure from the parental dreams that a child's characteristics might occasion.... When prospective parents select against a fetus because of predicted disability, they are making an unfortunate, often misinformed decision that a disabled child will not fulfill what most people seek in child rearing. (P. S2)

The disability critique argues that the practice and the rationales for it are misinformed about the nature of disability and morally problematic in the attitudes they connote about both disability and parenthood. The above rationales for the practice are of three types. First, people with disabilities are more costly to society than others, and society should use its resources for children and adults who will not have impairments. Second, either the lives of disabled children are so miserable that they are not worth living at all, or they are more miserable than the lives of nondisabled children are expected to be. Third, the lives of parents and family members will be harmed by the psychological, social, and economic burdens of caring for the child, and these burdens will not be offset by the expected psychic and social rewards of raising a child without a disability.

Disability rights criticism of prenatal testing stems neither from general opposition to abortion nor from misgivings about technology. It is aimed at professional support for testing and abortion for some particular group of characteristics but not other characteristics, suggesting that health professionals, bioethicists, insurers, and policymakers believe that the births of people with some set of characteristics should be prevented. Pro-choice opposition to prenatal testing for disability shares much with those in bioethics who oppose using the technology to avert the births of children of a particular sex. Suggesting that prospective parents select against an otherwise-wanted child because of its gender or disability implies that people who exist with these characteristics might be less desirable to others and less happy themselves than people with different characteristics. The critique is aimed at changing the way that the technology is described to prospective parents, as well as at persuading professionals and parents that they have inaccurate ideas about disability and are using testing out of myth and stereotype rather than current information about how disability affects a child's or family's life.

Critics contend that this practice differs from other actions that prevent disability and should not be compared with prenatal care for women, vaccinations for children, or health promotion for everyone. Selective abortion prevents disability not in an existing human being or in a fetus likely to come to term but rather prevents disability by preventing the fetus from becoming a person with a disability. It connotes that if people do not meet a certain health standard, they should not be welcomed into the family or the world (Asch 1989; Borthwick 1994; Newell 1999). Susan Wendell (1996) expresses these views well when she writes,

I would be terribly sorry to learn that a friend's fetus was very likely to be born with ME [myalgic encephalomyelitis or chronic fatigue immune dysfunction syndrome], but I would not urge her to abort it. In other words, many people with disabilities, while we understand quite well the personal burdens of disability, are not willing to make the judgment that lives like ours are not worth living. Every life has burdens, some of them far worse than disability. (P. 154)

Most of the disability rights opposition to selective abortion comes from those who are committed pro-choice advocates who seek to persuade families and society that they do not need to abort based on disability. Critics do not seek to ban the practice, but they believe that aborting a particular fetus differs from aborting any fetus because a woman does not want a child (Fine and Asch 1982; Finger 1990; Kaplan 1994; Morris 1991; Saxton 1984; Shakespeare 1995, 1998). They respond to each of the claims offered for prenatal testing by arguing the following:

❖   Even if every disability diagnosed prenatally were followed by abortion, it would not materially reduce the prevalence of disability in the world or the need for society to change to better include those with impairments (Asch 1999).

❖   As contrasted with the claims of Green (1997) or Purdy (1995), who perceive a disability as an unacceptable infringement on a child's "right to an open future" (Feinberg 1980), people with disabilities frequently enjoy their lives and do not generally perceive them as blighted by tragedy even if their impairments impose some constraints on them. Furthermore, such constraints, as are purportedly imposed by physical, sensory, and cognitive endowments, may be diminished or eliminated by societal changes to better include all citizens (Asch 1999).

❖   Most families raising children with disabilities are not ruined by the experience, and, on average, families including disabled children fare as well as other families on measures of well-being and family functioning (Ferguson, Gartner, and Lipsky forthcoming).

Marsha Saxton (1998) expresses well the sense of offense experienced by many disability rights critics when she says,

> The message at the heart of widespread selective abortion on the basis of prenatal diagnosis is the greatest insult: some of us are "too flawed" in our very DNA to exist; we are unworthy of being born . . . fighting for this issue, our right and worthiness to be born, is the fundamental challenge to disability oppression; it underpins our most basic claim to justice and equality—we are indeed worthy of being born, worth the help and expense, and we know it! (P. 391)

Most disability rights opponents of prenatal testing and selective abortion would not claim that the practice is "eugenic" because few governments compel it (Shakespeare 1998). However, the very offer of testing for some characteristics, but not all potentially diagnosable ones, connotes that only some characteristics are worth the expense and trouble to avoid (Press 2000). Thus, prenatal testing is a social decision, expressing societal views, and a direct challenge to the societal claims to include people with disabilities as full citizens and participants in the moral and human community.

The disability critique includes the idea that the sentiments behind offering and using prenatal testing and abortion to avoid bringing children with impairments into the family and the world will ultimately undermine parental appreciation of any children they raise. Pro-choice disability critics agree that if a prospective parent makes a considered decision that the family or the child will have an unacceptable life based on parental hopes and values, abortion should be available. They caution that such assessments may be misguided about both the nature of disability and the nature of parent-child relationships. Every life, every family, and every parent-child relationship contain disappointment as well as delight, and prospective parents may be misguided and misinformed about parenthood and shortchange themselves and any children they raise by adopting a selective approach to parenthood (Asch 2000).

The disability rights challenge was little noticed by bioethics during the 1980s, but in the 1990s, bioethics has examined it, even if most mainstream bioethics and medicine remain unconvinced or hostile (Buchanan 1996; Green 1997; Purdy 1995). The most detailed and systematic dialogue between bioethics and disability studies on prenatal testing has taken place through a project sponsored by the well-known bioethics organization, The Hastings Center, and this project has resulted in a deepened understanding of the issues (Parens and Asch 1999, 2000). Without accepting all of the disability-based arguments, however, some disability organizations and bioethics panels have urged health professionals to revise the methods of providing information to people contemplating prenatal testing that would present disability in a less negative light and would discuss it from within a social as well as medical framework (Dunne and Warren 1998; International League of Societies for Persons with Mental Handicap 1994; Little People of America 1999; National Down Syndrome Congress 1994; Parens and Asch 1999, 2000; Shakespeare 2000).

Making Life-or-Death Decisions for Others

One of the first famous bioethics cases is that of Karen Ann Quinlan, a young woman who sustained brain injuries in 1975 that left her in a persistent vegetative state, unable at first to breathe without mechanical respiration and, then after breathing on her own, unable to eat except by tube feeding. For patients with impairments as multifaceted and significant as Quinlan's, the disability rights movement has not organized to oppose court decisions to terminate treatment. However, for the same reasons that people with a disability rights perspective have protested the bioethics analysis of treating newborns with impairments, they are likely to oppose views that would deny treatments to people no longer capable of making decisions because of Alzheimer's disease or stroke. They would probably oppose the reasoning of courts and philosophers who would deny treatment for cancer to people with significant cognitive impairments.

Just such cases occurred in the late 1970s and early 1980s, and state courts in Massachusetts and New York reasoned and ruled in very different ways, reflecting different assessments of how a cognitive impairment should influence treatment decisions. The highest court in the state of Massachusetts declined to authorize a man with the reported mental age of a preschool child to receive chemotherapy for his leukemia, concluding that he would not understand the purpose of the painful procedures and that they would therefore drastically reduce an already minimal set of life activities and perceived quality of life (*Superintendent of Belchertown State School v. Saikewicz* 1977). Four years later, the New York Supreme Court decided, more in keeping with a disability rights view of quality of life, that a middle-aged man with what was described as profound developmental disability with the capacities of a very young child should receive treatment for cancer. The reasoning was that without the treatment, he would die, but with it, he could maintain most of the activities he enjoyed at the state facility in which he lived (*In re Storar* 1981). In this situation, interestingly, the court ignored the expressed wishes of the man's mother, even though she reportedly visited him daily but urged that the treatments be withheld and that he be allowed to die.

In the views of many disability community commentators and some from within mainstream bioethics, even a demonstrably loving and involved family may be unable to put aside its own view of how limited life with disability is to imagine such a life from the vantage point of someone with the impairment. Cancer may seem like a way out after years of being involved with a relative who has had a lifelong cognitive impairment. The family may experience so much distress when a spouse's, parent's, or child's recent disability deprives him or her of much-valued mental capacity that they cannot appreciate life as it is left to their loved one or get beyond their own sense of grief, weariness, or burden occasioned by spending time with the person in his or her new state. For all these reasons, people with a disability rights perspective are wary of "family" as decision makers for conscious, minimally aware, or otherwise cognitively disabled people who appear to enjoy some parts of their lives. If family members must decide questions of life and death for relatives whose condition deprives them of legal authority to assert themselves, a disability rights view might insist that quality of life should be judged from the patient's current vantage point. Such a method would take account of current activities and satisfactions, rather than judging life from the perspective of the nonimpaired family members or the formerly unimpaired individual.

Current thinking in the worlds of disability and bioethics reinforces the principle of self-determination for people making major life decisions. Most cognitive impairment does not leave individuals without some means of understanding their own situation or expressing preferences about how, where, and with whom they wish to be involved (Wehmeyer 1998). Given this outcome, it should be possible for people with nearly any disabling conditions to communicate about whether they find life and medical treatments worthwhile and acceptable to them. Bioethicists Buchanan and Brock (1989) support framing questions of "competence" as ones of decisional capacity. They recognize that persons unable to examine all long-range implications of a situation might nonetheless be able to provide valuable information to ultimate decision makers about their preferences and thus meaningfully participate in decisions about their lives and well-being. Several recent discussions by professionals familiar with people who have cognitive disabilities endorse a set of methods that would enable people who may not achieve the status of legal "competence" to express their wishes and reveal their decisional capacities and views (Midwest Bioethics Center 1996; Rinck and Calkins 1996). Making complex decisions obviously requires that medical professionals, family, and others working with a developmentally disabled or communicatively impaired person take the time not only to explain diagnoses, prognoses, and possible treatments but also to ascertain the patient's questions, fears, concerns, and desires. Giving truly informed consent necessitates a high level of patient-professional conversation that all too rarely takes place even when the patient has no additional cognitive or communication disability. As Katz (1984) explains, the standard of information and conversation should not merely assume a generic "reasonable person" but should recognize the unique concerns and needs of each individual facing a treatment decision. Rinck and Calkins (1996) remind us that people with disabilities may be especially subject to conforming to the desires of others:

> Social pressures which inhibit voluntary decisions are magnified for people with disabilities who have been allowed few choices. . . . Pressure from providers or health care professionals may cause individuals to feel that, if they disagree to certain therapies, privileges will be reduced. Even when individuals with a disability do not feel coerced, there is a tendency to acquiesce. . . . It is difficult to ascertain when a decision is truly the individual's choice and not influenced by outside forces. (P. 42)

Most bioethicists contend that people could eliminate or reduce the problems of family decision making if everyone would create an "advance directive" for themselves expressing their preferences if they one day cannot make their own wishes known. Alternatively, they could name a health care proxy, who would act on their behalf. Such legal documents might assist families and health professionals to deal with treatment decisions for the millions of people who lose some of their cognitive and communicative abilities through stroke, Alzheimer's disease, or the like. However, it would not be of help to the lifelong disabled of the world. Moreover, "living wills" or advance directives pose questions about whether individuals want particular medical procedures, rather than asking people to imagine how they would feel about life after a medical intervention. They do not aid people in considering which capacities and activities represent the essential components of an acceptable life. Even the most carefully written and thorough statement is subject to misinterpretation by professionals who may be convinced that they are better at knowing the views of the impaired individual than any form could convey. From the standpoint of disability rights, the most serious flaw of advance directives is that asserted by bioethicists Dresser and Robertson (1989), who criticize the "orthodox" reliance on any advance statement of preferences. People who are not living as individuals with disabilities and cannot imagine that their lives as disabled would be satisfying make such advance statements to them. Like the President's Commission discussion of treatment decision making for infants that urges assessment of benefit from the viewpoint of the patient and not the family or the society, Dresser and Robertson urge that nondisabled people acknowledge the value of disabled life and evaluate treatment decision making from the perspective of the now-disabled individual. Dresser and Robertson's point is a valid corrective to quick assessments that "Mom would hate living like this" or "my brother's advance directive was explicit about not wanting to stay alive if he could not hear or speak" when the child or sibling observes that mother and brother appear to take great pleasure in the activities and experiences that remain possible for them. However, as Buchanan and Brock (1989), Dworkin (1994), and Nelson (1995) discuss, people care about more than their current experiences. Even a seemingly content person with significant dementia might prefer that his or her wishes not to live in a disoriented, demented state be carried out by following a validly executed advance directive.

For situations in which families typically are expected to act on behalf of those who cannot make their wishes known, disability rights adherents remain skeptical about the good faith of much purported family decision making. Fearful of covert or overt bias against a now-disabled or lifelong-disabled family member who never provided an advance directive, and convinced that people without disabilities doubt the value of life with an impairment, those holding a disability rights perspective would look to governments and courts to protect the interests of vulnerable individuals and would seek all methods to improve the chances that disabled people themselves will participate in these decisions. It is crucial for anyone seeking to advance the dignity and worth of people with all disabilities to promote their participation in life-and-death decisions and to circumscribe family decision making on behalf of those who have less than full legal authority to make their own decisions.

DECIDING ABOUT LIFE AND DEATH: DISABLED PEOPLE AS DECISION MAKERS

In 1983, just as the U.S. media brought the question of treatment for babies to the attention of the public and raised the consciousness of people with disabilities about medical treatment as a civil rights issue, a young woman with cerebral palsy and arthritis named Elizabeth Bouvia asked a hospital in California to keep her comfortable, sedated, and let her starve herself to death. Then in her 20s, Bouvia had lived with significant disability throughout her life. During the previous few years, she had been married and divorced, miscarried a wanted pregnancy, experienced her mother's illness and her brother's death, had been forced to move several times because of family problems and inadequate personal assistance services provided by the state, and was compelled to withdraw from graduate school because the dean believed her disability precluded her from becoming a master's-level social worker. Yet, when she sought help from the American Civil Liberties Union (ACLU) to support her right to die, she and the ACLU based her claim on the pain, humiliation, and difficulty of her disability. Customarily associated with championing the civil rights of minorities, the ACLU argued that Bouvia had this right to die because her disability caused her a "pitiful existence," referred to her "affliction" as "incurable" and "intolerable," and portrayed the "indignity and humiliation of requiring someone to attend to her every bodily need" (ACLU Foundation of Southern California 1983:14, 17, 35). In 1986, the California Superior Court accepted this understanding of disability and agreed that she had a right (as did any other competent adult) to end medical treatments that helped her live. The court reasoned in part,

> She, as the patient, lying helplessly in bed, unable to care for herself, may consider her existence meaningless. She cannot be faulted for so concluding. . . . Her mind and spirit may be free to take great flights, but she herself is imprisoned, and must lie physically helpless, subject to the ignominy, embarrassment, humiliation, and dehumanizing aspects created by her helplessness. (*Bouvia v. Superior Court of State of California* 1986:19, 21)

Desires of people to end their lives if they faced illness and disability were familiar to bioethics, and although mainstream bioethics considered family decision making for incompetent patients complex and controversial, North American bioethics was almost unanimous in the belief that competent individuals should be able to decide when they found treatments and life so burdensome that they wanted treatments to end, even if the end of those treatments meant the end of their lives. By the time the Bouvia case reached the courts, most bioethics professionals and most case law opposed actions of medical staff who treated patients against their expressed wishes. By contrast, bioethicists endorsed the rights of competent adults to remove themselves from medical treatments and facilities, even if by doing so they ended their lives (President's Commission 1983).

Most of the cases that bioethics had discussed, however, concerned individuals who were very likely to die from the conditions for which they needed treatment. The Bouvia situation, as well as others that engaged people from within the disability community, differed in that they concerned people who could live for decades if they continued using assistive technology. With conditions of spinal cord injury, multiple sclerosis, and amyotropic lateral sclerosis (ALS), their functional limitations resembled those of many leaders of the disability rights movement and disability studies. Bioethicists who observed the court proceedings equated Bouvia's request with those of imminently dying people who wanted to avoid prolonging their lives by a matter of days, weeks, or months. Using reasoning similar to that offered by the California courts in the Bouvia situation, the New Jersey Supreme Court in 1987 supported the decision of a woman with ALS to end her life (*In re Farrell* 1987).

Most disability movement theorists and activists then and now construe these decisions to stop treatment entirely differently. They agree that people with disabilities deserve to have their views respected. However, they argue that such end-of-life decisions arise because people with disabilities have experienced constant discrimination, denials of information about life possibilities, inability to obtain legally available services and supports, and often abandonment by family and friends. They assert that despair and depression about life prospects cause people to give up on life, just as depression and despair cause people without disabilities to end life for all sorts of reasons.

In a statement offered during 1983 regarding Elizabeth Bouvia's circumstances, the Disability Rights Coordinating Council emphasized that Bouvia's depression easily could have been the response to extreme life stresses (miscarriage, divorce, illness and death of family members). A nondisabled person would have been treated for depression under any one of these circumstances, but psychiatrists and attorneys attributed all her despair to the pain and humiliation they perceived as inevitable in someone with a significant disability. The disability rights group also pointed out that many of the constraints that Bouvia and the experts working with her attributed to her cerebral palsy actually could be traced to California's denial of the maximum amount of personal assistance services legally due her or to the discriminatory attitudes of the university that had refused to have her continue in the master's program. As in family decision making about the lives of disabled people, the disability rights view located problems not in the biology of cerebral palsy but in the society in which the person with cerebral palsy found herself. Many people with similar disabling conditions were living on their own, working, and involved in significant relationships and activities. Her problems deserved solutions to improve her life. If Bouvia were to be educated in a more welcoming institution, obtain more personal assistance to increase her access to community life, rebuild or create loving personal relationships, and accept disability as a part of her identity rather than reject it and the community of disabled people available to support her and fight with her for dignity, perhaps she might regain a sense of hope and a desire to live.

These themes play out in all the subsequent right-to-treatment and even physician-assisted suicide discussions of the past two decades. In 1984, voices of the disability community were virtually ignored by physicians, bioethics, the courts, and the media in discussing Bouvia's rights, despite eloquent statements in a major U.S. disability movement publication, *Disability Rag* (Johnson 1984). The one bioethics panel called together to examine specific questions of disability and rehabilitation published views with resonances of a disability critique of medicine's attitude toward disability and the consequent willingness to help people with disabilities end their lives. In a report on ethical issues in disability and rehabilitation, Caplan, Callahan, and Haas (1987) called for an educational model on the part of professionals working with disabled people, especially if they are treating people shortly after the onset of disability. Patient and family autonomy may be overridden in the early stages, they suggest, to aid people in having more genuine autonomy later on.

If autonomy consists in the ability to make informed, voluntary choices about the course and direction of one's own life then it is necessary for persons to understand fully the options and opportunities that are available to them. When the onset of impairment is sudden and unexpected, it may take time for persons and their families to comprehend and adapt to the reality of their condition. While such persons may be competent to make decisions, they may not fully understand or be prepared to listen to the information that health care providers or those with impairments wish to convey. In this sense it may be necessary to allow for an infringement of autonomy in the shortrun in order to ensure that subsequent choices are truly reflective of informed, voluntary deliberation. (Caplan et al. 1987:11)

Not many years after acquiring disabilities through accident or illness, several other people with disabilities have sought removal from life support systems such as ventilators and generally have been supported by bioethics and the courts. To the indignation of many in the world of disability, a well-known rehabilitation hospital permitted a man with a newly acquired spinal cord injury to be removed from his life-sustaining ventilatory support without exposing him to similarly disabled people successfully living and working in the community (Asch 1990).

Key to the different appraisal of these stories by members of the disability community is the understanding of concepts of dependence, independence, and interdependence. Asch (1990), *Disability Rag* (Johnson 1984), and the Disability Rights Coordinating Council (1983) have argued that bioethics and the courts misunderstand the meaning of independence. Like the newly disabled people themselves, professionals construe the physical inability to execute life tasks such as dressing, toileting, or moving from place to place as synonymous with dependence and leading to inevitable feelings of embarrassment and humiliation. Disability rights adherents contend that independence need not be viewed in physical terms; rather, self-direction, self-determination, and participation in decision making about one's life are more genuine and authentic measures of desirable independence or, better, interdependence. It is no more demeaning to obtain help in dressing or washing from a personal assistant than it is to get services from an auto mechanic, a plumber, or a computer technician. With personal assistance provided to people as a respected form of employment, disabled people can proudly take their places as workers, parents, community volunteers, and citizens. Dependence occurs only when disabled people are deprived of such assistance and forced to live in institutions or in homes of relatives who resent the tasks they are expected to perform. With adequate personal assistance services, methods of communication, guaranteed health care, and confidence that a disabled person can still be valued by family and community, there might be fewer requests to stop treatment (Asch 1995; DeJong and Banja 1995; Johnson 1984; Litvak, Zukas, and Heumann 1987).

Unfortunately, calls for greater involvement of people with disabilities on hospital ethics committees, use of experts with a disability rights perspective to analyze the requests of disabled people about end-of-life care, and greater use of independent living centers as training opportunities for newly disabled people and health practitioners have not yet brought greater disability sensitivity within bioethics or hospital practice (Asch 1990, 1998; Gill forthcoming). As Herr, Bostrom, and Barton (1992) discussed in their review of several treatment refusals by people with disabilities who were not terminally ill and who could conceivably have lived for decades had they been given the financial, social, and psychological tools to do so, these people believed that they had "no place to go" and that death was their only tolerable option to being imprisoned by life.

In the time that the bioethics debate shifted from ending life-prolonging treatment to physician-assisted suicide, the voice of disability rights has emerged in the discussion and has occasionally influenced the mainstream bioethics literature and legal decisions. Two strands of the ideology of the disability rights movement offer different but valuable additions to standard bioethics discussions of the proper role of the medical profession, the difficulty in establishing a prognosis of terminal illness, and appropriate safeguards to ensure the voluntariness of any request for physician assistance in dying (Annas, Glantz, and Mariner 1996). The ideological strand of disability rights that stresses self-determination and that asserts their similarity in temperament, talent, and beliefs to the nondisabled vigorously argues that disabled people are no more vulnerable to coercion, pressure from family, or victimization by society than anyone else and that they may actually benefit from legalized assistance in dying. The Coalition of Provincial Organizations of the Handicapped (COPOH) of Canada joined Sue Rodriguez in her bid to get court approval for physician assistance in her death. Bickenbach (1998) explains their reasoning this way:

> Persons with disabilities who are or will become unable to end their lives without assistance are discriminated against by the prohibition of assisted suicide since, unlike persons capable of causing their own deaths, they are deprived of the option of choosing suicide. . . . Being legally prevented from pursuing a legal option, on the basis of physical disability, is discriminatory. . . . Disabled persons have been historically victimized by stereotypical attitudes about their abilities and worth, coupled with a paternalism that has undercut their right to self-determination. Denying people with disabilities the option of suicide is an example of this unequal treatment, and must be resisted as demeaning and discriminatory. (P. 124)

Those disability theorists in the United States who stress the need for decisional autonomy are offended by what they see as the paternalism and assumption of victimization that lead some prominent members of the disability rights community to oppose legalizing physician-assisted suicide. Batavia (1997) and Silvers (1998) advocate legalization because they endorse autonomy as a supreme value and see no evidence that people with disabilities are any more likely than others in the population to succumb to external pressures to end their lives. Disability rights opponents of legalizing physician assistance in dying argue from the ideological strand that stresses inequality of the social arrangements that now prevail for people with disabilities. They contend that contemplating the legalization of the practice in a world of prejudice, unequal treatment, inadequate health care, unreliable social services, and frequent familial rejection is increasing the disadvantages of today's disabled people.

Bickenbach (1998) points out that COPOH (in supporting physician-assisted suicide) and Not Dead Yet (in opposing it) held many similar views about the devaluing of people with disabilities in the wider society and differed principally in how they perceived such a practice would influence their shared goals of improving life for disabled people. He reflects that "when an individual chooses death as the only way of escaping from an intolerable situation, it is perverse and unfair to say that this is an expression of self-determination or autonomy" (p. 128). Opponents of physician-assisted suicide point out that the way in which its supporters justify such suicide speaks to the very prejudices, stereotypes, and devaluations that have created a movement for disability rights. Quoting Bickenbach again,

> It is telling that . . . there is never any suggestion that the right to physician-assisted suicide should extend to people who do not have a severe disability. Implicit in the judgments themselves . . . is precisely the prevailing prejudicial social attitude that having a disability is a sensible reason for committing suicide.
>
> Perhaps proponents of physician-assisted suicide would be steadfast in their view even if it meant that qualified doctors could patrol school grounds waiting for despondent but mentally competent seventeen-year-olds who, having failed geography or been unable to find a date for the prom, might want to use their assisted-suicide services. (P. 130)

Opposition to the trends to approve of physician-assisted suicide sparked the formation of the direct-action protest group Not Dead Yet, which has dedicated itself to bringing the voice of the disability rights movement into the public debate about bioethical issues. Not Dead Yet joined with another U.S. protest group, ADAPT, to oppose the activities of Jack Kevorkian, the pathologist who has assisted in more than 130 deaths of people with disabilities in the past decade. They also joined to submit an amicus brief to the U.S. Supreme Court in its two cases dealing with physician-assisted suicide and to protest the hiring of Peter Singer by Princeton University.

In its amicus brief to the U.S. Supreme Court, Not Dead Yet (1995) contended that physician-assisted suicide would substantially harm existing people with disabilities as follows:

> Many doctors conclude that lives of people with severe disabilities are not worth saving, solely because of their disabilities. . . . These people represent the extent of discrimination that exists in our society; with appropriate treatment and services, many of them would be alive today. It is against the backdrop of these and other cases, reflecting society's growing support of a "right to die" for people with severe disabilities, that your amici request protection from the very real threat to the lives of people with disabilities that will result from a right to assisted suicide through active measures.

Not Dead Yet (1995) explicitly argued that if physicians were ever permitted to aid people in ending their lives, such assistance could be considered discriminatory if it were available only to terminally ill or disabled people. Singling out people with disabilities and terminal illnesses as people who might want to end their lives is itself a way to express the view that perhaps they should want to do so because their lives are understandably of less value to them and to others than would be the lives of despondent but nondisabled persons.

Not Dead Yet can take heart in knowing that some of its concerns have reached the policy and legal worlds. While not adopting all of Not Dead Yet's analysis, the U.S. Supreme Court does recognize the particular prejudices that people with disabilities already endure. In refusing to support the constitutionality of a right to assistance in dying, the court noted the "negative and inaccurate stereotypes," "societal indifference," and the "cost-saving mentality" that form the current context in which ill and disabled people decide about ending or continuing their lives (U.S. Supreme Court 1998:387). Because most of the people who have sought to end life-prolonging treatments or to obtain physician assistance in dying are people who have been disabled for only a few years, there is reason to suspect that they are indeed more vulnerable to demoralization than Silvers, Batavia, and COPOH might wish. Bioethics and disability rights need the kind of dialogue about how to respect autonomy while providing useful information and how to implement the model proposed by Caplan et al. (1987) that took place on the issue of prenatal testing through the Hastings Center and that has begun through the auspices of the University of Newcastle (Policy, Ethics and Life Sciences Research Institute 2000). What are the appropriate safeguards to forestall claims that there was no informed consent before people made life-ending decisions? In a world that asserted the value of life for everyone, regardless of health status, people with disabilities might be no more likely than any other segment of the population to consider ending their lives. In a world that still systematically reduces the life chances for people with disabilities, the disability rights movement should fear a right to physician assistance in dying when there is so little medical or social assistance in living.

EMERGING ISSUES AND NECESSARY DIALOGUES

The most bitter clash of views between disability rights and bioethics has occurred in life-and-death situations, but the clash between medical and social models of disability pervades several other areas of bioethical discussion that warrant notice here because they need attention from disability studies. Some disability theorists and activists have invoked the history of Nazi exterminations and forced sterilizations of people with disabilities to claim that contemporary debates over physician-assisted suicide or uses of prenatal testing are precursors to future wholesale state-sanctioned persecution of disabled people (Gallagher 1990). In fact, fears of a Nazi label are probably enough to keep governments and medical professionals from blatant persecutions. The devaluation and deprivation take more subtle forms that can only be acknowledged but not explored because of space limitations. The stigma and devaluation of life with disability are demonstrated in the acquittals or light sentences when professionals or family members take it on themselves to end the lives of disabled children, parents, or spouses

(Shipp 1985). In the Netherlands, a country with both universal health care and legalized physician-assisted suicide, many disabled people have died by lethal injections they themselves did not request. However, the physicians performing these acts have not been prosecuted for murder (U.S. Supreme Court 1998). Yet another example of devaluing people with disabilities arises in the continuing abuses of people with cognitive impairments who become research subjects without their informed consent (Brody 1998; Dresser 1996). Bioethicists who consider reproductive liberty and the rights to procreate as fundamental human rights have neglected the problems of people with disabilities in pursuing parenthood.

Forced sterilization still occurs to people with many disabling conditions, especially those with cognitive or emotional disability, in nations such as Australia, Spain, and Japan (Bosch 1998; Cordner and Ettershank 1997; "Japan Says Forced Sterilizations" 1997). People who need personal assistance with household and daily life activities face obstacles to parenthood if they cannot acquire any additional services to help with child care. Neither bioethics nor the disability rights movement has undertaken an in-depth discussion of what social accommodations may be justly due to those people who can experience the rewards of parenthood only with some amount of physical assistance or decisional supervision.

Stigma, Quality of Life, and Access to Health Care

Sometimes people from cultural minorities in the United States, those committed to feminist politics, and people from other parts of the world criticize standard Western bioethics for focusing on flashy, high-tech questions of acute care medicine and ignoring the day-to-day realities of creating an accessible, compassionate, and just health care system that meets ordinary needs (Flack and Pellegrino 1992; Warren 1992). A chief concern for the disability community arises in the context of access to health care itself and whether—if at all—an individual's existing impairments should influence the types of services he or she receives. Of course, physicians must be aware of someone's blood pressure or cardiac condition before prescribing certain medications or treatment regimens for other conditions; some drugs may counteract medications being taken for a different medical problem. However, disability has sometimes been used invidiously to deny people available treatments from which they could benefit. In discriminating by patient, for example, someone with Down syndrome may be denied a kidney transplant, based on a conviction that he or she could not comply with treatment requirements or an evaluation that rated life with Down syndrome as less worthy of the scarce resource than the life of someone without that impairment. In recent years, just such factors delayed or denied organ transplants, kidney dialysis, and other interventions to people with Down syndrome and dementia, based on the presence of the impairment (Goldberg 1996; Patterson 1999). Rationing by service is also a way to harm people with particular conditions if providers, insurers, or national health plans specifically exclude payment for some procedures or limit coverage so that only mild forms of a condition will be treated. Physical impairments may be treated without an annual or lifetime insurance cap, but psychological problems are subject to very low annual or lifetime caps for payment in the United States. A national health service may elect to cover treatment for some psychological disorders but not others, provide payments for treating male-factor but not female-factor infertility, or provide expensive therapies for cancer but not for AIDS.

Some commentators have examined the implications of antidiscrimination legislation for changing the heretofore unquestioned decisions of medical professionals, finding that laws such as the Americans with Disabilities Act should aid people with disabilities in asserting their claims to beneficial health care without reference to the service needed or to others' perceptions of the quality of their lives with or without treatment (Brock 1995; Mehlman, Durchslag, and Neuhauser 1997; Orentlicher 1996). Orentlicher (1996) argues that the provisions of the Americans with Disabilities Act and similar rights legislation in other countries could be used to end the disparate treatment of people with disabilities in access to services:

The equal worth of each individual suggests that we may want to give two persons equal opportunity for a particular treatment even if one would gain a smaller benefit from the treatment because of a coexisting disability. Indeed, we may want to give priority when allocating resources among different services and different patients to the persons whose health is worse to begin with even if those persons would benefit less from treatment. (P. 86)

The U.S. discussions are taking place in the context of proliferating HMOs and other managed care arrangements seeking to establish cost-saving policies. Allocation decisions that differentially (and often negatively) affect the world's people with disabilities are explicit in the guidelines of some national health service plans and are implicit in physician decisions to withhold medication or services from those considered to have significant impairments. Believing that health care expenditures must be controlled to save money for other social goals, professionals, governments, and nonprofit agencies are eager to find rational methods of allocating health care dollars and staff. Several different methods have been proposed that would allocate health care based on its presumed effect on the recipient's "quality of life" (Brock 1993). Bioethics and health policy, with input from disability studies, must grapple with the philosophical and empirical questions arising in any discussions of resource allocation schemes: Should priority be given to those considered "worst off," as Orentlicher (1996) suggests, or should priority be given to those whose presumed quality of life after care would be high? As Wasserman (this volume) explains, different allocation schemes would have vastly different results for the world's disabled population. If societies choose to provide care to improve the conditions of "the worst off," as Orentlicher proposes, people with disabilities could receive care based on being considered worst off. However, if they choose to provide care to those expected to derive the most benefit in terms of maximal quality of life, stereotypes about how disability lowers life quality could limit the care they receive.

Even if experts or nations achieved consensus on the version of social justice that should guide allocation decisions, there would be conceptual and empirical difficulties in ascertaining "quality of life," as Brock (1993) discusses in depth. However, it is worth noting the following urgent questions: From whose perspective should life quality be judged? If people with disabilities consistently indicate that their lives—even with problems—are more satisfactory to them than nondisabled people or health professionals believe, should their judgments be used in measuring life quality? If so, they might not be disadvantaged in allocation schemes because health professionals would cease being "distracted by disability" (Asch 1998). However, if nondisabled people, without experience of a particular impairment, become the judges of future life quality with impairments or if health professionals become the judges of life after impairment, this chapter and its references provide abundant evidence that people with disabilities in rich and poor nations will fare badly in allocation decisions based on expected quality of life (Brock 1993, 1995; Singer 1996; Tyson and Broyles 1996). If people in one country experience the same impairment differently based on a host of background factors such as culture, socioeconomic status, length of time with the condition, cultural beliefs, and race/ethnicity, should those background factors influence care offered to two people with the same impairment? If so, two people who could each benefit from similar treatment for hypertension, diabetes, or spinal cord injury might receive vastly different levels and types of services. The same background factors could mean that international agencies and governments might withhold available treatments from people with impairments in a poor nation that would be provided in one with greater economic resources.

David Wasserman (this volume) discusses the social justice questions that require a disability studies analysis. Yet I must reiterate how urgent it is for disability studies to oppose plans to ration care using a metric of presumed quality of life after treatment that would automatically give lower ratings to people with disabilities than to those without them. Virtually all such rationing plans could erode the gains made by the disabled population to obtain health care and other resources to ameliorate the negative impact of impairment on life and to increase opportunities for participation and equality.

CHALLENGES FROM BIOETHICS: JUSTICE, VARIATION, AND SOCIAL POLICY

Disability and Social Justice

The social and minority group models of disability claim that existing difficulties for people with impairments stem from the struggle to live in a world in which people's bodies and needs have been overlooked. Whether calling for a rights approach to social change or grounding the call in the idea that such change removes barriers for everyone regardless of current physical, sensory, or cognitive equipment, both agree that people with impairments will lag behind others unless these calls are heeded. Disability rights scholarship has not included substantial attention to articulating theories of equality and social justice that would support their demands for change. Bickenbach (1993), Bickenbach et al. (1999), Shakespeare and Watson (this volume), Scotch and Schriner (1997), and Zola (1989) have acknowledged limits of a strictly rights-based, minority group approach.

On what moral grounds should society change to better incorporate the one-sixth to one-fourth of its members who have disabilities? How much change should be expected? If access to the built environment is measured by the ease with which a person who uses a wheelchair or one who is deaf or blind can come and go freely, is that standard arbitrarily narrow in ignoring design features for those who use gurneys for mobility or in overlooking the needs of those with environmental illness to attend public events? What constitutes appropriate auxiliary services or reasonable accommodation to ensure the participation of people with significant communicative, cognitive, or emotional disabilities in education and employment? If, after all existing barriers were removed, people with some impairment appeared unable to participate in ways they would choose, what other changes should occur to foster such participation? Universal design features will benefit everyone, and thus there is value in espousing the universalizing ideas of the social or human rights models of disability. However, certain services and accommodations (Braille books, one-to-one aides in classrooms, job coaches) may not directly benefit everyone, even though they provide indirect benefits through the increased participation of all citizens. What theory of social justice supports meeting those needs of small numbers of people?

In its efforts to discuss societal obligations to provide health care to citizens, bioethics has begun tackling the real-world applications of theories of justice and equality. Although most of the bioethics discussions do not go beyond health care to address the full range of societal changes necessary to improve the lives of people with disabilities, the writings of Brock (1995); Caplan et al. (1987); Silvers, Wasserman, and Mahowald (1998); and Veatch (1986) are valuable sources with which to explore such questions. Silvers et al. represent the necessary bioethics and disability studies dialogue that points the way toward systematic explorations of considering disability in constructing theories of social justice and of elaborating the grounds for claims to societal resources for people with disabilities. Their work and that of Bickenbach (1993) should be the first in an extended series of disability, bioethics, and social justice conversations.

Human Variation

According to the scholarship of the past 30 years, disability is best understood as a civil rights and social problem and not a health problem. Yet, as just mentioned, disability studies endorses the claim that at least certain definable functional characteristics, including some differences from species-typical functioning, warrant notice and social resources to permit full inclusion. What defines an impairment, as opposed to a characteristic (e.g., eye color or race) that no one would suggest working to change? Not all departures from what is "typical" are considered impairments since being taller, stronger, quicker, and more musical than average are perceived as gifts. We call for societal change to reduce both disability discrimination and racial discrimination, but we do not imagine making physical changes in people of one heritage to provide them with another genotype or phenotypic appearance.

It seems indisputable that the inability to read print, because of a visual or perceptual processing problem, differs from the inability to read arising from poor education. Information can be conveyed by nonvisual means for people with each type of reading difficulty, but the educationally deprived person may someday read with his eyes, whereas the blind person will not. A person who is deaf will always need some method other than spoken language to communicate with someone who does not know sign language; a Turk in Germany may eventually learn German and dispense with interpreters.

Disability studies should continue to affirm that disability is not the tragedy imagined by most health professionals and bioethicists; simultaneously, it should examine the philosophical, moral, and policy implications of the difference between physiologic and nonphysiologic explanations of the inability to perform certain activities. No social changes will permit a blind person to take in a sunset using sight, although society can eliminate its fixation that without such experiences, life is pitiful.

In effect, the minority group and social models both argue that society has obligations to incorporate all its members, with their varying range of physiological, cognitive, and sensory capacities just because environments and expectations may be easier to change than the physiological equipment with which one interacts in the world. Bioethics and medicine have perceived the inability to hear a symphony because one cannot hear as psychologically and morally different from the disinterest in hearing symphonies for those who can hear. One arises from choice; the other is not anything the individual can change. Progressive disability policy recognizes obligations to remove environmental barriers to participation if not in hearing of symphonies then in communicating with others in certain situations. Society may have more obligations to help someone travel who cannot use public transit because it is inaccessible than it does to help someone travel who could use the public system but dislikes doing so. Bioethics and medicine have overstated the negative impact of any constraint on life opportunity that might arise from physiology. In its effort to point out the constraints imposed by society, disability studies may need to give more attention to examining the impact of physiological constraints and the consequences of medicine's and bioethics' belief that any constraint is necessarily bad. Even if a disabling trait puts some limits on the hypothetical open future or opportunity range of the nondisabled, why is that a problem?

Trying to pin down what counts as an impairment that matters to life activity and trying to ascertain the moral or policy implications of the impairment category remain elusive and controversial. This is especially so when linked with discussions about whether it is appropriate or unethical for individuals or families to seek correction of impairments for themselves or for minor children. People with disabilities use the health care system for conditions related and unrelated to the characteristic that renders them part of the disabled minority. People with spinal cord injury get treated for high blood pressure or cancer and try to avoid secondary conditions; someone who is blind develops Parkinson's disease and seeks treatment. As with nondisabled people, many who have disabilities take steps to stay healthy, and they support societal activities that improve the environments of homes, cities, and workplaces. They do oppose campaigns that spread false ideas about the tragedy of disability, but they do not object to efforts to improve public health (Wang 1992).

Yet what about possible efforts to "cure" or reverse disability by futuristic gene therapy, spinal cord regeneration, fetal tissue transplants, or the current cochlear implants? Such actual or potential medical interventions that would reduce functional impairment or restore species-typical function renew the exploration of what makes something an "impairment" that one might want to correct, as contrasted with a characteristic that no one would consider changing. Is being "short" a biological impairment or exclusively a socially constructed disability in a society that prizes height? There must be a place in the new paradigm of disability to discuss the question of when growth hormone might be a legitimate medical therapy and when it would be purely an enhancement (Parens 1998). If children or adults can gain some hearing from cochlear implants, are they morally obliged to have them, and should they lose access to interpreter services if they decline, as Tucker (1998) asserts? Are people morally obliged to obtain any therapies that would reduce impairment and would restore species-typical functioning? If the disability rights movement would endorse surgery for an infant with spina bifida to reduce mobility or cognitive limitations, is it equally acceptable to support parental interests in providing some hearing by virtue of a cochlear implant? Is deafness properly considered a culture and not an impairment (Crouch 1997; Lane and Grodin 1997)? When Davis (1997a, 1997b) objects to the cultural view and argues that lack of hearing places some limits on the hypothetical open future that parents should want for their children, is she making a claim that differs from a claim that parents of a child with spina bifida or a heart condition should seek treatment for such conditions to reduce the constraints that those conditions might impose? If so, why? If somatic cell gene therapy or germ-line gene therapy could safely correct detectable impairments in eggs, sperm, or embryos, should they become standard parts of medical care? Should people with disabilities support or oppose them as more versions of preventing people with disabilities from coming into the world? If some oppose such developments, do they object based on a view that disability represents a desirable form of human variation that should not be reduced by means that would reduce the births of people who might be members of the disabled population? Is having an impairment or being a person with a disability simply one form of inconsequential human variation, or even after society changes to better incorporate its disabled citizens, will impairment and disability always be seen as somehow negative or unfortunate rather than as one form of human variation? Bioethics and disability studies must work together to understand why health is valuable along with continuing to explore the meaning of impairment and disability.

Current disability studies or disability rights stresses disability as an acceptable form of human variation and urges that bioethics and the wider society learn from the disability experience about the appreciation of human diversity. It seems fitting to close this discussion of the intersections of disability studies with bioethics by affirming what bioethics can learn from disability studies. Longmore's (1995) description of the values needed for people to accept the disabled are values that, he says, would change orientations toward another regardless of disability. They would change bioethics and society in ways that could surely promote human rights for everyone: "not self-sufficiency but self-determination, not independence but interdependence, not functional separateness but personal connection, not physical autonomy but human community" (p. 9).

These values imbue the recently developed statement on bioethics by Disabled Peoples' International (2000), and it seems an appropriate conclusion to this examination of the intersection of disability and bioethics:

THE RIGHT TO LIVE AND TO BE DIFFERENT

Nothing about us without us

Up until now most of us have been excluded from debates on bioethical issues. These debates have had prejudiced and negative views of our quality of life. They have denied our right to equality and have therefore denied our human rights.

We demand that we are included in all debates and policy-making regarding bioethical issues.

We must be the people who decide on our quality of life, based on our experiences. . . .

We are full human beings. We believe that a society without disabled people would be a lesser society. Our unique individual and collective experiences are an important contribution to a rich, human society. . . .

All Human Beings are born free and equal in Dignity and Rights

Human rights are the responsibility of the state as well as the individual. Disabled people, our organizations, families and allies must work to ensure that international, regional and national legal instruments include the implementation of rights throughout all scientific advances and medical practices concerning the human genome, reproduction, assessments of quality of life, therapeutic measures and alleviation of "pain and suffering."

Biotechnology presents particular risks for disabled people. The fundamental rights of disabled people, particularly the right to life, must be protected. . . .

That no demarcation lines are drawn regarding severity or types of impairment. This creates hierarchies and leads to increased discrimination of disabled people generally.

Disabled people must join together in solidarity to ensure our voices in these life-threatening issues.

NOTES

1. As Bickenbach et al. (1999) discuss, the social and minority group models are not identical, and some differences matter for formulations of disability policy, of notions of equality, and for legal solutions to existing problems. For most of the bioethics issues discussed in this chapter, however, the differences are not as important as the similarity of approach.

2. These concerns for patient autonomy and for individual treatment and research decision making are evident in the first editions of major works in bioethics of the 1970s, the first textbook and the first comprehensive encyclopedia, respectively (Beauchamp and Childress 1979; Reich 1978).

REFERENCES

Albrecht, G. L. and P. J. Devlieger. 1999. "The Disability Paradox: High Quality of Life against All Odds." *Social Science and Medicine* 48:977-88.

American Civil Liberties Union Foundation of Southern California. 1983. *Elizabeth Bouvia v. County of Riverside* (Memorandum of points and authorities in support of application for temporary restraining order and permanent injunction). Los Angeles: Author.

Annas, G. J., L. H. Glantz, and W. K. Mariner. 1996. "Brief for Bioethics Professors Amicus Curiae Supporting Petitioners, No. 95-1858 and No. 96-110." In *Supreme Court of the United States, October Term, 1996, Dennis C. Vacco, et al., Petitioners, v. Timothy E. Quill, et al., Respondents. And State of Washington, Petitioners v. Harold Glucksberg, et al., Respondents* [Online]. Available: www.bumc.bu.edu/www/sph/lw/Brief.htm. Accessed January 19, 2000.

Annas, G. J. and M. A. Grodin. 1992. *The Nazi Doctors and the Nuremberg Code: Human Rights in Human Experimentation.* New York: Oxford University Press.

Asch, A. 1986. "On the Question of Baby Doe." *Health PAC Bulletin* 16 (6): 6, 8-10.

———. 1987. "The Treatment of 'Handicapped Newborns': A Question with No Simple Answers." *Disability Studies Quarterly* 7:1-4.

———. 1989. "Reproductive Technology and Disability." Pp. 69-124 in *Reproductive Laws for the 1990s*, edited by S. Cohen and N. Taub. Clifton, NJ: Humana.

———. 1990. "The Meeting of Disability and Bioethics: A Beginning Rapprochement." Pp. 85-89 in *Ethical Issues in Disability and Rehabilitation: An International Perspective*, edited by B. S. Duncan and D. Woods. New York: World Rehabilitation Fund, World Institute on Disability and Rehabilitation International.

———. 1995. "Disability: Attitudes and Sociological Perspectives." Pp. 602-8 in *Encyclopedia of Bioethics*, edited by W. T. Reich. New York: Simon & Schuster.

———. 1998. "Distracted by Disability." *Cambridge Quarterly of Healthcare Ethics* 7:77-87.

————. 1999. "Prenatal Diagnosis and Selective Abortion: A Challenge to Practice and Policy." *American Journal of Public Health* 89:1649-57.

————. 2000. "Why I Haven't Changed My Mind about Prenatal Diagnosis and Selective Abortion: Reflections and Refinements." Pp. 234-58 in *Prenatal Testing and Disability Rights*, edited by E. Parens and A. Asch. Washington, DC: Georgetown University Press.

Asch, A. and M. Fine. 1984. "Shared Dreams: A Left Perspective on Disability Rights and Reproductive Rights." *Radical America* 18 (4): 51-58.

Bach, J. R. and M. C. Tilton. 1994. "Life Satisfaction and Well-Being Measures in Ventilator Assisted Individuals with Traumatic Tetraplegia." *Archives of Physical Medicine and Rehabilitation* 75:626-32.

Batavia, A. I. 1997. "Disability and Physician-Assisted Suicide." *New England Journal of Medicine* 336:1671-73.

Beauchamp, T. L. and J. F. Childress. 1979. *Principles of Biomedical Ethics*. New York: Oxford University Press.

————. 1994. *Principles of Biomedical Ethics*. 4th ed. New York: Oxford University Press.

Beaudet, A. L. 1990. "Carrier Screening for Cystic Fibrosis." *American Journal of Human Genetics* 47:603-5.

Bickenbach, J. E. 1993. *Physical Disability and Social Policy*. Toronto: University of Toronto Press.

————. 1998. "Disability and Life-Ending Decisions." Pp. 123-32 in *Physician Assisted Suicide: Expanding the Debate*, edited by M. P. Battin, R. Rhodes, and A. Silvers. New York: Routledge.

Bickenbach, J. E., S. Chatterji, E. M. Badley, and T. B. Ustun. 1999. "Models of Disablement, Universalism and the International Classification of Impairments, Disabilities and Handicaps." *Social Science and Medicine* 48:1173-87.

Biklen, D. 1987. "Framed: Print Journalism's Treatment of Disability Issues." Pp. 79-96 in *Images of the Disabled, Disabling Images*, edited by A. Gartner and T. Joe. New York: Praeger.

Boorse, C. 1987. "Concepts of Health." Pp. 359-93 in *Health Care Ethics: An Introduction*, edited by D. VanDeVeer and T. Regan. Philadelphia: Temple University Press.

Borthwick, C. 1994. *Prevention of Disablement*. North Blackburn, Australia: Collins Dove.

Bosch, X. 1998. "'Voluntary' Sterilisations in Spain Clarified in New Legislation." *Lancet* 352:124.

Botkin, J. 1995. "Fetal Privacy and Confidentiality." *Hastings Center Report* 25 (5): 32-39.

Bouvia v. Superior Court of State of California, Court of Appeal of the State of California, Second Appelate District, Division Two, 2d Cir. No. B019134 (1986, April 16).

Bowen v. American Hospital Association, 54 LW 4579 (U.S. Sup. Ct., June 9, 1986), affirming American Hospital Association v. Heckler, 585 F. Supp. 541 (S.D.N.Y.).

Brock, D. 1993. "Quality of Life Measures in Health Care and Medical Ethics." Pp. 95-132 in *Quality of Life*, edited by A. Sen and M. C. Nussbaum. New York: Oxford University Press.

————. 1995. "Justice and the ADA: Does Prioritizing and Rationing Health Care Discriminate against the Disabled?" *Social Philosophy and Policy* 12:159-85.

Brody, B. A. 1998. *The Ethics of Biomedical Research: An International Perspective*. New York: Oxford University Press.

Buchanan, A. E. 1996. "Choosing Who Will Be Disabled: Genetic Intervention and the Morality of Inclusion." *Social Philosophy and Policy* 13:18-46.

Buchanan, A. E. and D. W. Brock. 1989. *Deciding for Others: The Ethics of Surrogate Decisionmaking*. New York: Cambridge University Press.

Callahan, D. 1988. "Families as Caregivers: The Limits of Morality." *Archives of Physical Medicine and Rehabilitation* 69:323-28.

Cameron, P., D. G. Titus, J. Kostin, and M. Kostin. 1973. "The Life Satisfaction of Nonnormal Persons." *Journal of Consulting and Clinical Psychology* 41:207-14.

Caplan, A. L., D. Callahan, and J. Haas. 1987. "Special Supplement: Ethical and Policy Issues in Rehabilitation Medicine." *Hastings Center Report* 17 (4): S1-S20.

Caplan, A. L. and C. Cohen, eds. 1987. "Special Issue: Imperiled Newborns." *Hastings Center Report* 17 (6): 5-32.

Caplan, A. L., H. T. Engelhardt, and J. J. McCartney, eds. 1981. *Concepts of Health and Disease: Interdisciplinary Perspectives*. Reading, MA: Addison-Wesley.

Carlson, L. 1997. "Beyond Bioethics: Philosophy and Disability Studies." *Disability Studies Quarterly* 17:277-83.

Child Abuse Amendments, PL 98-457 (1984).

Cordner, S. and K. Ettershank. 1997. "Australia's Illegal Sterilisations Revealed." *Lancet* 349:1231.

Crouch, R. A. 1997. "Letting the Deaf Be Deaf: Reconsidering the Use of Cochlear Implants in Prelingually Deaf Children." *Hastings Center Report* 27 (4): 15-21.

Cushman, L. A. and M. P. Dijkers. 1990. "Depressed Mood in Spinal Cord Injured Patients: Staff Perceptions and Patient Realities." *Archives of Physical Medicine and Rehabilitation* 71:191-96.

Daniels, N. L. 1985. *Just Health Care: Studies in Philosophy and Health Policy.* Cambridge, UK: Cambridge University Press.

Darling, R. B. 1979. *Families against Society: A Study of Reactions to Children with Birth Defects.* Beverly Hills, CA: Sage.

Davis, D. S. 1997a. "Cochlear Implants and the Claims of Culture? A Response to Lane and Grodin." *Kennedy Institute of Ethics Journal* 7 (3): 253-58.

———. 1997b. "Genetic Dilemmas and the Child's Right to an Open Future." *Hastings Center Report* 27 (2): 7-15.

DeJong, G. and J. Banja. 1995. "Disability: Health Care and Physical Disability." Pp. 615-22 in *Encyclopedia of Bioethics,* edited by W. T. Reich. New York: Simon & Schuster.

Disability Rights Coordinating Council. 1983. *Elizabeth Bouvia v. County of Riverside (Declaration of Carol Gill).* Los Angeles: Author.

Disabled Peoples' International. 2000. "The Right to Live and to Be Different." Paper presented the DPI Conference on Disabled People, Bioethics and Human Rights, February, Solihull, UK.

Dresser, R. S. 1996. "Mentally Disabled Research Subjects: The Enduring Policy Issues." *Journal of the American Medical Association* 267:67-72.

Dresser, R. S. and J. A. Robertson. 1989. "Quality of Life and Non-Treatment Decisions for Incompetent Patients." *Law, Medicine and Health Care* 17:234-44.

Duff, R. S. and A. G. M. Campbell. 1973. "Moral and Ethical Dilemmas in the Special-Care Nursery." *New England Journal of Medicine* 289:890-94.

Dunne, C. and C. Warren. 1998. "Lethal Autonomy: The Malfunction of the Informed Consent Mechanism within the Context of Prenatal Diagnosis of Genetic Variants." *Issues in Law and Medicine* 14:165-202.

Dworkin, R. 1994. *Life's Dominion: An Argument about Abortion, Euthanasia, and Individual Freedom.* New York: Random House.

Edwards, S. D. 1997. "The Moral Status of Intellectually Disabled Individuals." *Journal of Medicine and Philosophy* 22:29-42.

Eisenberg, M. G. and C. C. Saltz. 1991. "Quality of Life among Aging Spinal Cord Injured Persons: Long Term Rehabilitation Outcomes." *Paraplegia* 29:514-20.

Engelhardt, H. T., Jr. and K. W. Wildes. 1995. "Health and Disease: Philosophical Perspectives." Pp. 1101-6 in *The Encyclopedia of Bioethics,* edited by W. T. Reich. New York: Simon & Schuster.

Feinberg, J. 1980. "The Child's Right to an Open Future." Pp. 124-53 in *Whose Child? Children's Rights, Parental Authority, and State Power,* edited by W. Aiken and H. Lafollette. Totowa, NJ: Littlefield, Adams.

Ferguson, P., A. Gartner, and D. Lipsky. Forthcoming. "The Experience of Disability in Families: A Synthesis of Research and Parent Narratives." In *Prenatal Testing and Disability Rights,* edited by E. Parens and A. Asch. Washington, DC: Georgetown University Press.

Fine, M. and A. Asch. 1982. "The Question of Disability: No Easy Answers for the Women's Movement." *Reproductive Rights National Network Newsletter* 4 (3): 19-20.

———. 1988. "Disability beyond Stigma: Social Interaction, Discrimination, and Activism." *Journal of Social Issues* 44 (1): 3-21.

Finger, A. 1990. *Past Due: A Story of Disability, Pregnancy and Birth.* Seattle, WA: Seal.

Flack, H. E. and E. D. Pellegrino, eds. 1992. *African-American Perspectives on Biomedical Ethics.* Washington, DC: Georgetown University Press.

Fost, N. 1982. "Passive Euthanasia of Patients with Down's Syndrome." *Archives of Internal Medicine* 142:2295.

Gallagher, H. G. 1990. *By Trust Betrayed: Patients, Physicians, and the License to Kill in the Third Reich.* Arlington, VA: Vandamere.

Gartner, A. and T. Joe, eds. 1987. *Images of the Disabled: Disabling Images.* New York: Praeger.

Gaylin, W., I. Glasser, S. Marcus, and D. Rothman. 1978. *Doing Good: The Limits of Benevolence.* New York: Pantheon.

Gerhart, K. A., J. Koziol-McLain, S. R. Lowenstein, and G. G. Whiteneck. 1994. "Quality of Life following Spinal Cord Injury: Knowledge and Attitudes of Emergency Care Providers." *Annals of Emergency Medicine* 23:807-12.

Gill, C. J. Forthcoming. "Health Professionals, Disability, and Assisted Suicide: An Examination of Empirical Evidence." *Psychology, Public Policy, and Law.*

Gliedman, J. and W. Roth. 1980. *The Unexpected Minority: Handicapped Children in America*. New York: Harcourt Brace.

Goffman, E. 1963. *Stigma: Notes on the Management of Spoiled Identity*. New York: Oxford University Press.

Goldberg, C. 1996. "Her Survival Proves Doubters Wrong: Retarded Woman Recovers from Transplant She Had Been Denied." *New York Times*, March 3, p. 12.

Goode, D., ed. 1994. *Quality of Life for Persons with Disabilities: International Perspectives and Issues*. Cambridge, MA: Brookline.

Green, R. 1997. "Prenatal Autonomy and the Obligation Not to Harm One's Child Genetically." *Journal of Law Medicine and Ethics* 25 (1): 5-15.

Hahn, H. 1983. "Paternalism and Public Policy." *Society* (March-April): 36-46.

———. 1987. "Public Policy and Disabled Infants: A Sociological Perspective." *Issues in Law and Medicine* 3:3-27.

Hentoff, N. 1987. "The Awful Privacy of Baby Doe." Pp. 161-80 in *Images of the Disabled, Disabling Images*, edited by A. Gartner and T. Joe. New York: Praeger.

Herr, S. S., B. A. Bostrom, and R. Barton. 1992. "No Place to Go: Refusal of Life-Sustaining Treatment by Competent Persons with Physical Disabilities." *Issues in Law and Medicine* 8:3-36.

In re Farrell, 108 N.J. 335, 529 A.2d 404 (1987).

In re Storar, 52 N.Y.2d 363, 420 N.E.2d 64, 438 N.Y.S.2d 266 (1981).

International League of Societies for Persons with Mental Handicap. 1994. *Just Technology? From Principles to Practice in Bio-Ethical Issues*. North York, Ontario: Roeher Institute.

"Japan Says Forced Sterilizations Merit No Payment, No Apology." 1997. *New York Times*, September 18, p. A12.

Johnson, M., ed. 1984. *Disability Rag* (February-March).

Kaplan, D. 1994. "Prenatal Screening and Diagnosis: The Impact on Persons with Disabilities." Pp. 49-61 in *Women and Prenatal Testing: Facing the Challenges of Genetic Testing*, edited by K. H. Rothenberg and E. J. Thomson. Columbus: The Ohio State University Press.

Katz, J. 1984. *The Silent World of Doctor and Patient*. New York: Free Press.

Kohl, M., ed. 1978. *Infanticide and the Value of Life*. New York: Prometheus.

Kuhse, H. and P. Singer. 1985. *Should the Baby Live? The Problem of Handicapped Infants*. New York: Oxford University Press.

Lane, H. and M. Grodin. 1997. "Ethical Issues in Cochlear Implant Surgery: An Exploration into Disease, Disability, and the Best Interests of the Child." *Kennedy Institute of Ethics Journal* 7:231-52.

Little People of America. 1999. *Position Statement on Genetic Discoveries in Dwarfism* [Online]. Available: www2.shore.net/~dkennedy/dwarfism_genetics.html.

Litvak, S., H. Zukas, and J. E. Heumann. 1987. *Attending to America: Personal Assistance for Independent Living*. Berkeley, CA: World Institute on Disability.

Longmore, P. K. 1995. "The Second Phase: From Disability Rights to Disability Culture." *Disability Rag* 16 (September/October): 4-11.

Matson, F. 1990. *Walking Alone and Marching Together: A History of the Organized Blind Movement in the United States, 1940-1990*. Baltimore: National Federation of the Blind.

McNair, D. 1996. "My Quality Is Not Low." *Bioethics Forum* 12 (3): 11-16.

Mehlman, M. J., M. R. Durchslag, and D. Neuhauser. 1997. "When Do Health Care Decisions Discriminate against Persons with Disabilities?" *Journal of Health Politics, Policy and Law* 22:1385-1411.

Midwest Bioethics Center and University of Missouri–Kansas City Institute for Human Development Task Force on Health Care for Adults with Developmental Disabilities. 1996. "Health Care Treatment Decision-Making Guidelines for Adults with Developmental Disabilities." *Bioethics Forum* 12 (3): S1-S8.

Morreim, E. H. 1995. "Life, Quality of: Quality of Life in Health-Care Allocation." Pp. 1358-61 in *Encyclopedia of Bioethics*, edited by W. T. Reich. New York: Simon & Schuster.

Morris, J. 1991. *Pride against Prejudice*. London: The Women's Press.

Murray, T. H. and A. L. Caplan, eds. 1985. *Which Babies Shall Live? Humanistic Dimensions of the Care of Imperiled Newborns*. Clifton, NJ: Humana.

National Down Syndrome Congress. 1994. *Position Statement on Prenatal Testing and Eugenics: Families' Rights and Needs*. Prepared for and approved by the Professional Advisory Committee [Online]. Available: members.carol.net/~ndsc/eugenics.html.

National Organization on Disability. 1998. *Harris Survey of Americans with Disabilities* [Online]. Available: www.nod.org/press.html#poll. Accessed August 29, 1999.

Nelson, J. L. 1995. "Critical Interests and Sources of Familial Decision-Making Authority for Incapacitated Patients." *Journal of Law, Medicine and Ethics* 23 (2): 143-48.

Newell, C. 1999. "The Social Nature of Disability, Disease, and Genetics: A Response to Gillam, Persson, Holtug, Draper and Chadwick." *Journal of Medical Ethics* 25:172-75.

Not Dead Yet. 1995. "Amicus Curiae Brief of Not Dead Yet and American Disabled for Attendant Programs Today in Support of Petitioners, No. 95-1858." In *Supreme Court of the United States, October Term, 1995, Dennis C. Vacco, et al., Petitioners, v. Timothy E. Quill, et al., Respondents* [Online]. Available: www.acils.com/NotDeadYet/amicus1.html. Accessed January 19, 2000.

Orentlicher, D. 1996. "Destructuring Disability: Rationing of Health Care and Unfair Discrimination against the Sick." *Harvard Civil Rights—Civil Liberties Law Review* 31:48-88.

Parens, E. 1998. *Enhancing Human Traits: Ethical and Social Implications.* Washington, DC: Georgetown University Press.

Parens, E. and A. Asch. 1999. "The Disability Rights Critique of Prenatal Genetic Testing: Reflections and Recommendations." *Hastings Center Report* 29 (5): S1-S22.

———, eds. 2000. *Prenatal Testing and Disability Rights.* Washington, DC: Georgetown University Press.

Patterson, R. 1999. "Rationing Access to Dialysis in New Zealand." *Ethics and Intellectual Disability Newsletter* 4 (1): 3-4.

Policy, Ethics and Life Sciences Research Institute, University of Newcastle. 2000. *Reproductive Choices, Disability Rights.* Newcastle upon Tyne, UK: Author.

President's Commission for the Study of Ethical Problems in Medicine and Biomedical and Behavioral Research. 1982. *Making Health Care Decisions.* Washington, DC: Government Printing Office.

———. 1983. *Deciding to Forego Life-Sustaining Treatment: A Report on the Ethical, Medical, and Legal Issues in Treatment Decisions.* Washington, DC: Government Printing Office.

Press, N. 2000. "Assessing the Expressive Character of Prenatal Testing: The Choices Made or the Choices Made Available?" Pp. 214-33 in *Prenatal Testing and Disability Rights*, edited by E. Parens and A. Asch. Washington, DC: Georgetown University Press.

Purdy, L. M. 1995. "Loving Future People." Pp. 300-27 in *Reproduction, Ethics, and the Law: Feminist Perspectives*, edited by J. C. Callahan. Indianapolis: Indiana University Press.

———. 1996. "A Feminist View of Health." Pp. 163-82 in *Feminism and Bioethics: Beyond Reproduction*, edited by S. M. Wolf. New York: Oxford University Press.

Ray, C. and J. West. 1984. "Social, Sexual and Personal Implications of Paraplegia." *Paraplegia* 22:75-86.

Reich, W. T., ed. 1978. *Encyclopedia of Bioethics.* New York: Simon & Schuster.

———, ed. 1995. *Encyclopedia of Bioethics.* 2d ed. New York: Simon & Schuster.

Retsinas, J. 1991. "Impact of Prenatal Technology on Attitudes towards Disabled Infants." Pp. 75-102 in *Research in the Sociology of Healthcare*, edited by D. Wertz. Westport, CT: JAI.

Rinck, C. and F. Calkins. 1996. "Challenges across the Lifespan for Persons with Disabilities." *Bioethics Forum* 12 (3): 37-46.

Rothman, B. K. 1986. "On the Question of Baby Doe." *Health PAC Bulletin* 16 (6): 7, 11-13.

Saigal, S., D. Feeny, P. Rosenbaum, W. Furlong, E. Burrows, and B. Stoskopf. 1996. "Self-Perceived Health Status and Health-Related Quality of Life of Extremely Low-Birth-Weight Infants at Adolescence." *Journal of the American Medical Association* 276:453-59.

Saxton, M. 1984. "Born and Unborn: The Implications of Reproductive Technologies for People with Disabilities." Pp. 298-312 in *Test-Tube Women: What Future for Motherhood?* edited by R. Arditti, R. D. Klein, and S. Minden. Boston: Pandora.

———. 1998. "Disability Rights and Selective Abortion." Pp. 374-95 in *Abortion Wars: A Half Century of Struggle, 1950-2000*, edited by R. Solinger. Berkeley: University of California Press.

Scotch, R. K. and K. Schriner. 1997. "Disability as Human Variation: Implications for Policy." *Annals of the American Academy of Political and Social Science* 549:148-59.

Shakespeare, T. 1995. "Back to the Future? New Genetics and Disabled People." *Critical Social Policy* 15:22-35.

———. 1998. "Choices and Rights: Eugenics, Genetics and Disability." *Disability and Society* 13:665-81.

———. 2000. "Arguing about Disability and Genetics." *Interaction* 13 (3): 11-14.

Shaw, M. W. 1984. "Presidential Address: To Be or Not to Be, That Is the Question." *American Journal of Human Genetics* 36:1-9.

Shelp, E. E. 1986. *Born To Die? Deciding the Fate of Critically Ill Newborns.* New York: Free Press.

Shipp, E. R. 1985. "Mistrial in Killing of Malformed Baby Leaves Town Uncertain about Law." *New York Times*, February 18, p. A14.

Silvers, A. 1998. "Protecting the Innocents from Physician-Assisted Suicide: Disability Discrimination and the Duty to Protect Otherwise Vulnerable Groups." Pp. 133-48 in *Physician Assisted Suicide: Expanding the Debate,* edited by M. P. Battin, R. Rhodes, and A. Silvers. New York: Routledge.

Silvers, A., D. Wasserman, and M. Mahowald. 1998. *Disability, Difference, Discrimination.* Lanham, MD: Rowman & Littlefield.

Singer, P. 1993. *Practical Ethics.* New York: Cambridge University Press.

———. 1996. *Rethinking Life and Death: The Collapse of Our Traditional Ethics.* New York: St. Martin's Griffin.

———. 1999. "Ethics, Health Care and Disability: A Discussion with Peter Singer and Adrienne Asch." Personal communication on October 12, Princeton University, New Jersey [Online]. Available: www.princeton.edu/WebMedia/special.

Steinbock, B. and R. McClamrock 1994. "When Is Birth Unfair to the Child?" *Hastings Center Report* 24 (6): 15-21.

Stensman, R. 1985. "Severely Mobility-Disabled People Assess the Quality of Their Lives." *Scandinavian Journal of Rehabilitation Medicine* 17:87-99.

Superintendent of Belchertown State School v. Saikewicz, 370 N.E.2d 417 (Mass. 1977).

Tooley, M. 1986. *Abortion and Infanticide.* New York: Oxford University Press.

Tucker, B. P. 1998. "Deaf Culture, Cochlear Implants and Elective Disability." *Hastings Center Report* 28 (4): 6-14.

Tyson, J. E. and R. S. Broyles. 1996. "Progress in Assessing the Long-Term Outcome of Extremely Low-Birth-Weight Infants." *Journal of the American Medical Association* 276:492-93.

U.S. Commission on Civil Rights. 1989. *Medical Discrimination against Children with Disabilities.* Washington, DC: Author.

U.S. National Commission for the Protection of Human Subjects of Biomedical and Behavioral Research. 1978. *Belmont Report: Ethical Principles and Guidelines for the Protection of Human Subjects of Research.* Washington, DC: Government Printing Office.

U.S. Supreme Court. 1998. "*Washington et al. v. Glucksberg et al.*: Text of the Supreme Court decision, June 26, 1997." Pp. 377-422 in *Physician Assisted Suicide: Expanding the Debate,* edited by M. P. Battin, R. Rhodes, and A. Silvers. New York: Routledge.

Veatch, R. M. 1986. *The Foundations of Justice: Why the Retarded and the Rest of Us Have Claims to Equality.* New York: Oxford University Press.

Walter, J. J. 1995. "Life, Quality of: Quality of Life in Clinical Decisions." Pp. 1352-58 in *The Encyclopedia of Bioethics,* edited by W. T. Reich. New York: Simon & Schuster.

Wang, C. 1992. "Culture, Meaning, and Disability: Injury Prevention Campaigns and the Production of Stigma." *Social Science and Medicine* 35:1093-1102.

Warren, V. L. 1992. "Feminist Directions in Medical Ethics." Pp. 32-45 in *Feminist Perspectives in Medical Ethics,* edited by H. B. Holmes and L. M. Purdy. Indianapolis: Indiana University Press.

Weber v. Stony Brook Hospital, 60 N.Y.2d 208, 211 (1983); 456 N.E.2d 1186, 1187 (1983); 469 N.Y.S.2d 63, 64 (1983); 464 U.S. 1026 (1983); 95 A.D.2d 587, 589 (1983); 467 N.Y.S.2d 685, 686-87 (1983), 329-31.

Wehmeyer, M. L. 1998. "Self-Determination and Individuals with Significant Disabilities: Examining Meanings and Misinterpretations." *Journal of the Association of Persons with Severe Handicaps* 23:5-16.

Weir, R. F. 1984. *Selective Nontreatment of Handicapped Newborns: Moral Dilemmas in Neonatal Medicine.* New York: Oxford University Press.

Wendell, S. 1989. "Toward a Feminist Theory of Disability." *Hypatia* 4 (2): 104-24.

———. 1996. *The Rejected Body: Feminist Philosophical Reflections on Disability.* New York: Routledge.

Wertz, D. C. 1995. "Medical Genetics: Ethical and Social Issues." Pp. 1652-56 in *Enclyclopedia of Bioethics,* edited by W. T. Reich. New York: Simon & Schuster.

Woodrich, F. and J. B. Patterson. 1983. "Variables Related to Acceptance of Disability in Persons with Spinal Cord Injuries." *Journal of Rehabilitation* 49:26-30.

Zola, I. K. 1989. "Toward the Necessary of Universalizing of a Disability Policy." *The Milbank Quarterly* 67 (Suppl. 2, Pt. 2): 401-28.

Disability Studies and Electronic Networking

12

ELLEN LIBERTI BLASIOTTI

JOHN D. WESTBROOK

IWAO KOBAYASHI

Electronic networking has been extremely useful to the field of disability studies. This field has been aided by the exchange of views among scholars internationally. Also, many databases and Web sites provide a wealth of resources for scholars to use in conducting research activities and for people with disabilities to use in daily living. This chapter argues that electronic networking will continue to serve a vital role for disability studies in the future, refining and enhancing communication, discussion, and debate, as well as forming virtual communities of disability researchers who share knowledge, techniques, and even research subjects through the Internet and World Wide Web. The Internet and World Wide Web have been instrumental in forming new global communities, unfettered by political and social boundaries. The Internet has empowered people with disabilities, who look and act no differently than any other "surfers." These computer-based modalities serve to inform research and to consume research results as never before. The effects of their political empowerment have already been felt, as has their usefulness as an electronic market for services, products, and information. However, while electronic information networking is rapidly changing and offers new opportunities, the extent to which people with disabilities will "automatically" benefit is unclear. Sensitivity to the impact of new technologies is important in understanding the growing digital divide. The opportunities afforded are countered by potential problems and must be carefully studied.

BURGEONING ELECTRONIC INFORMATION

Like the public airwaves, cyberspace is a public medium that offers new communication and information opportunities. For those with access to a computer and online services, electronic communications, such as electronic mail (e-mail), listservs, chat rooms, discussion forums, and World Wide Web sites, are laterally connecting growing numbers of us to one another without involving intermediary institutions or individuals. The outlook for the future is even more intriguing. Devices will be wireless and handheld. The Internet will be ubiquitous.

Electronic communication offers the chance for rapid, free personal expression. Many complain that the "Information Superhighway" is too crowded and that the wealth of available information is often overwhelming. Today, most electronic communication technologies require almost all users to "filter" or sort through information received to determine what to process, consider, and possibly use. To an increasing degree, listservs and other group communication functions are being used to limit messages or facilitate this filtering process. Portals to targeted information "type https" have significantly increased in numbers and use. Portals to disability-related information and organizations are growing in number and are easily located through common public search engines.

INFORMATION FOR PEOPLE WITH DISABILITIES

Researchers and government agencies that sponsor programs for people with disabilities have taken great pride in making available online a wealth of information for people with disabilities. The National Rehabilitation Information Center (NARIC), sponsored by the National Institute on Disability and Rehabilitation Research (NIDRR) of the U.S. Department of Education's Office of Special Education and Rehabilitative Services, has provided a disability research collection since 1978. Over the years, consumers overtook researchers as primary users of the research information. In addition, in response to an increasingly powerful disability community, NIDRR decided that NARIC should make its abstracts of collected research be available online for searching (www.naric.com).

Even more directly, members of the disability consumer movement in the United States demanded the opportunity to search for information on assistive technology provided by ABLEDATA (also sponsored by NIDRR). They wanted to see the range of devices available and to determine for themselves what would be best for them, rather than to be "fed" by information brokers. Like the NARIC experience, collections of consumer-directed information are fully searchable on the World Wide Web (www.abledata.com/index.htm). The site is constantly being redesigned to be "consumer friendly." There has been a shift in information handling from the approach of a traditional librarian to that of a customer-directed approach. In addition to information about equipment and manufacturers in the United States, ABLEDATA has provided a wealth of links to Web sites in Europe, Africa, Australia, North America, and Asia.

Principally, because of electronic networking, ABLEDATA has served to foster a similar Web site in Japan—SenSui. Contacts in the 1980s with ABLEDATA by a student with a disability in Japan inspired him to build a similar site for consumers in his own country. Access to the "Web" in Japan had been limited to researchers who belonged to research institutes or universities. Information for consumers was almost nonexistent. All of the disability resources for consumers were available through listservs, netnews, and FTP resources from the United States and European countries. To construct a system of this type with information about Japanese equipment and manufacturers, Dr. Iwao Kobayashi constructed SenSui: Information Resources for People with Disabilities in Japan and has been managing it since January 1995 (www.sd.soft. iwate-pu.ac.jp/sensui).

Similar to most consumer-directed Web sites, SenSui provides information, free software to improve accessibility, and links to other disability-related sites throughout the world on important disability-related topics. It provides online consultation services and documentation from important meetings. The pairing of SenSui with ABLEDATA has provided many opportunities for cross-cultural communication. Kobayashi has continued to write and present papers with his counterparts from ABLEDATA, and this electronic linkage has served to form the basis for joint presentations at international meetings in Hawaii, Greece, and Germany.

Sean Lindsay (2000), in a recent editorial in the *Disability Times,* characterized this type of activity as follows:

> Until recently, the disability community online was primarily served by dozens of small, noble, but hopelessly under-funded services, most of which spun out of existing service providers or efforts of passionate individuals. . . . Some of these services were moderately

successful in their areas of expertise, but they lacked the cash necessary to explore some of the greater possibilities of the Internet.

This has now changed. Recently, a new phenomenon—well-capitalized megasites (or portals) for the disability community—have been launched with much fanfare. Some examples are the following:

WeMedia (www.wemedia.com)

Half the Planet (www.halftheplanet.com)

CanDo (www.cando.com)

CanOnline (www.CanOnline.com)

These sites come with the financing to mount complex, inclusive information sites, with services such as listings of accessible real estate, travel opportunities, disability news, research briefs, and other offerings in one "comprehensive" package. The hope is that by focusing on a disability consumer niche market, they can be successful commercially. This seems to be quite appealing at the present time, and many "names" in the disability movement are directors or affiliates of these sites. The subtle appeal of this is that it appears to offer a legitimization of the disability community as a commercial and political powerhouse. This is in contrast with past years when, for example, the apparent lack of a commercial base for devices designed by rehabilitation engineering centers consigned them to the category of "orphan technologies."

WeMedia describes itself as a "unique online community of e-commerce offering the disabled community more than $1 trillion in purchasing power—greater choice and freedom when purchasing goods and services." It has drawn together many services, which are, in fact, available to anyone on the Web. It gathers special-interest information and offers not-for-profit organization members assistance in developing and serving free Web sites, e-mail, chat rooms, and other online services. Half the Planet offers articles about new technology, political activity, housing and jobs for disabled people, and other services and information. For these and similar sites, "free" services and information are mixed with commercial messages and links to particular vendors.

According to Lindsay (2000), in 1998, all of electronic journalism was seized with the "portal wars" of such companies as Yahoo!, Excite, and others. In 1999, many health portals, such as OnHealth and WebMD, were similarly battling for users. They competed with the Mayo Clinic and C. Everett Koop's Web sites. More business-based sites were PlanetRx and Drugstore.com, which sold products. Some of the underfunded ones, such as Koop's, appear at present to be going under. Lindsay cites some patterns of use:

Once people invest time in learning to use one Web site, they are less likely to try another.

People only access health information when they need it.

People are not confident about divulging medical information or about paying for health and medical services online.

The more important the purchase, the less likely it will be made over the Internet.

It is not easy to "monetize" an audience that is drawn by free information.

Lindsay (2000) believes that the two principles most important to being economically successful are content and community. The idea is to keep them "coming back for news, articles, and community discussions," and later they will come back to buy something because they feel they can trust the site. It will be interesting to watch these sites in the future.

INFORMATION FOR RESEARCHERS, STUDENTS, AND PROFESSIONALS

Researchers and disability professionals do not seem to be caught up in these commercial ventures. Although they look at the commercial sites, there is a plethora of other places for them to enter the electronic networks to find sought-after information. More focused sites attempt to address the information needs of particular communities of interests. Some are organized and sponsored by specific disability organizations, such as The Arc (www.thearc.org), or professional groups, such as the American Occupational Therapy Association (AOTA) (www.aota.org). Other sites address individual issues such as "community-based rehabilitation" or "disability statistics." Counties and cities, such as London, have Web pages that provide information on disability for those living or visiting within a specific geographical boundary.

There is a worldwide community of those interested in disability studies. Many are connected only by this medium, rather than by face-to-face contact. Disability researchers in the United States and those in Great Britain, for example, participate regularly in electronic discourses about their research. Preeminent as one of the world's leading disability studies centers, the University of Leeds (United Kingdom) provides "mailbase." This electronic information program of the Disability Research Unit in the School of Sociology and Social Policy at the University of Leeds (www.mailbase.ac.uk) is one of the most active discussion channels for disability research.

Because disability studies is interdisciplinary by nature, the dialogue has been enriched by collaborators from many countries and fields such as the humanities, medicine, law, architecture, rehabilitation, political science, sociology, and anthropology. While in earlier days, these discussions might have been among participants gathered at a pub after an international conference, today, this challenging and testing of ideas often take place over the "Information Superhighway." Various "factions" of disability studies researchers have chosen to make resources available to particular interest groups. For example, professors in the humanities offer curricula and discussions online (www.georgetown.edu/crossroads/interests/ds-hum/index.html).

In addition to the academics who participate in these online discussions, people with disabilities often provide their experiential testimony, facilitating the formulation of research questions. The Canadian Centre on Disability Studies provides the "Disability Studies Web Ring," which helps to engage researchers and students in intellectual discourse. The Society for Disability Studies (SDS) is committed to developing theoretical and practical knowledge about disability and promoting the full and equal participation of persons with disabilities in society. The Global Applied Disability Research and Information Network (GLADNET) brings together research centers, universities, enterprises, government departments, trade unions, and organizations representing disabled people—all committed to the common goal of advancing competitive employment and training opportunities for persons with disabilities.

All of these sites attempt to filter information to save time and effort. There are also more traditional printed informational compendia and guides available. One such example by Julia Stock and Robert Drake (2000) is *Data Sources for Social Researchers,* which includes printed sources, CD-ROM databases, and key social science Web sites worldwide. More than 200 references to key sources of primary and secondary data are listed. Special sections on the European Union, United States, United Kingdom, and other major European countries, as well as subject sections on anthropology, sociology, social work, and social policy, are included. Intended for researchers and academics, the sources in the guide, prepared by social policy specialists, provide students and researchers with useful starting points in their search for secondary sources and data. The Internet sources chosen are considered by the authors to be stable and valid.

LOOKING BACK, LOOKING FORWARD

If the fruit of disability studies and other disability research is to be ensured a fully credible and lasting place in academia, it is important for disability studies researchers to become good disseminators. While many think that just making information "available" is enough, there is a great difference between distribution and dissemination or utilization of information. Changes in information dissemination in the past decade have accelerated the process at a rate that dwarfs 5,000 years of human history.

Modern information dissemination began when the oral storytelling tradition converted to the written word, which was, in fact, the "original independent data-transfer medium" (Rojas 2000). This allowed knowledge to progress beyond what could be remembered by the human mind at any one time. Most accounts credit the invention of written language to Sumeria around 3200 B.C. The separation of language from speech by writing allowed knowledge to be documented and transmitted, even if its originator had died or was remote.

The first writers toted clay tablets with their writings on them, and then wax tablets became prominent and remained popular until the eleventh century (even after the invention of papyrus paper 2400 B.C.). However, papyrus in the form of scrolls enhanced the collection and transfer of information. The Egyptians spread knowledge and their rule through this medium. Literacy, however, was still restricted because of the fragility of the scrolls. Also, this medium was restrictive of lengthy discourse and voluminous data. The development of codes helped condense information to a more manageable form.

By the fourth century, it was recognized that the "epics, religious teachings, histories, philosophical musings and legal codes," which had been in the form of scrolls, could not be "easily accessed or transported efficiently in codex forms" (Rojas 2000:274). Paper, which had been invented in China in the first century B.C., made its appearance in Europe in the Middle Ages. It replaced the more delicate and expensive parchment and vellum. Coupled with this was, of course, the invention of movable type by Johannes Gutenberg in the fifteenth century, which made the book available to more than the elite classes. According to Professor Gary Holland of the University of California at Berkeley,

> Within the first 50 years after the development of printing, approximately 25,000 titles were published. Even if the print runs were just 200 or 500 books, the number of books that existed in Europe was mind-boggling compared with just a few years before. (Rojas 2000:274)

The Enlightenment period proceeded full bore in Europe. The next five and a half centuries further increased the acceleration of information, and, with the invention of the telegraph by Samuel Morse in 1844, "information could move as quickly as the fastest human could travel" (Rojas 2000:277).

Of course, even with telephones, television, and radio, books remained the key to knowledge dissemination. They helped to "archive and transport knowledge" (Rojas 2000:277). The computer was the next vehicle. However, it took 10 or more years for computers to be both powerful and portable enough. The Internet and "networked intelligence" have now allowed the storage and instant communication of more knowledge than can be held in any single computer, not to mention any single library. This type of knowledge is soon to be available in one's hand.

Paul Edwards, an associate professor at the University of Michigan's School of Information, speculates that "once handheld devices with high-speed Internet connections become commonplace, the amount of information that can be held in one's hand will soon be nearly infinite, and we will likely see a sharp decrease in the value placed on memory and history." He states, "Children in five years will ask why they should bother to learn facts and dates, when those can be accessed from an Internet-connected, handheld computer, anywhere instantaneously" (Edwards 2000:224).

Bandwidth is the next crucial medium for knowledge exchange. "Broadband wireless communication is expected to eclipse demand for cable modems and DSL, with 26 per cent growth this year, according to internal numbers for Sprint's Broadband Wireless Group" (Edwards 2000:226). Europe has led the United States in the development and use of portable information devices.

The development of "standards," such as Bluetooth (named after a Danish king in the tenth century who had poor orthodontia), will allow wireless devices to provide seamless communications, whether one is in an office or a residence. Connectivity will be constant (Edwards 2000:226).

Electronic books should replace print revisions, according to Martin Eberhard, the erudite founder of NuvoMedia. His opinion is "that by 2005 people will be much more comfortable carrying an electronic book than a dog-eared paperback." Companies will also change the business from such media enterprises as broadcasting to the "copyright, content and delivery business" (Eberhard 2000:234).

With all of the "noise" generated by the myriad of information sources and techniques available electronically, disability studies research disseminators must ensure that their information "survives the cut" of filtering processes. This will require effective information disseminators, among other things, to "tailor" the content of messages to the needs of specific, identifiable users. Despite the powerful flexibility of modern-day electronic communication technologies, too many Web sites encourage only passive information gathering, without constructing information for learning or developing messages for particular user audiences and known informational needs. While plural uses of the Internet are good, developing an "online virtual community" requires a focused message with a known audience of intended users.

DISTRIBUTION OR DISSEMINATION?

The principles of effective and efficient dissemination practice must be more widely understood and applied in the disability community. Ironically, the advent of the electronic Information Superhighway presents both opportunities and barriers to effective information dissemination and utilization by people with disabilities and many others. New electronic information technologies promote a clearer common understanding of the differences between dissemination and simple distribution. Distribution refers to the act of moving information from one point to another, while dissemination implies a process that has utilization as its intended outcome. While the differences may seem subtle on the surface, their accomplishment is remarkably difficult.

There have been significant differences in the dissemination of research findings and outcomes generated by electronic networking. Increasingly, the outcomes of research are being widely shared electronically, often at a much faster pace than ever before in history. Traditionally, the dissemination process for findings required years of documentation, the presentation of conference papers, and the preparation and publication of peer-reviewed journal articles. This information trajectory is now often short-circuited with the direct, electronic publication on the World Wide Web of tentative, preliminary, or final research results.

The task of dissemination is to bridge the gap between research and practice. Part of the challenge is that dissemination has fallen prey to the very dilemma it seeks to address. That is, research on dissemination, or knowledge utilization, as it is frequently called, has yielded a wealth of information about what does and does not work. However, most of those understandings have not moved from the academic research community to the "practice" community. As a result, most dissemination practices are still based on a mechanistic belief that the only task is to "get the word out" or simply distribute the information.

Klein and Gwaltney (1991) cite the notion common in the dissemination literature of the 1960s and 1970s that was touted by the federally constituted Dissemination Analysis Group in 1977. This work identified four functions or types of dissemination:

> spread, which is defined as the one-way diffusion or distribution of information;
>
> choice, a process that actively helps users seek and acquire alternative sources of information and learn about their options;

- exchange, which involves interactions between people and the multidirectional flow of information; and
- implementation, which includes technical assistance, training, or interpersonal activities designed to increase the use of knowledge or R&D or to change attitudes or behavior or organizations or individuals.

Clearly, knowledge is not an inert object to be "moved" and "received" but rather a fluid set of understandings shaped both by those who originate it and by those who use it (Louis 1992). Using knowledge is an active learning process. Dissemination research shows that knowledge users shape and filter information according to their prior experience and understandings. Effective electronic information dissemination must recognize this "constructivist" approach in tailoring basic elements in the process of dissemination. The use of knowledge acts on information relating it to existing knowledge, imposing meaning and organization on experience and, frequently, monitoring understanding throughout the process (Hutchinson and Huberman 1993).

FIVE BASIC ELEMENTS OF EFFECTIVE DISSEMINATION

In considering the complexities of dissemination through electronic and other channels, it is useful to recognize the following five basic elements that enhance or preclude knowledge utilization. These elements include the following:

- the content or message that is selected for dissemination (this includes the knowledge or product and any needed supporting information or materials);
- the dissemination source, that is, the agency, organization, or individual responsible for creating the content or conducting the related dissemination activities;
- the medium, that is, the ways in which the content is described, "packaged," and transmitted;
- the user, or intended user, of the information to be disseminated; and
- the context, or circumstances and conditions, that must be met to access or acquire the information (e.g., cost, materials, or computers to access electronic Web-based information).

Also, to achieve the goal of knowledge use—rather than simple distribution—those involved in the dissemination activity must know about and be responsive to the target audiences for whom their information content is intended. Saying this, it is also important to recognize that "change" or action on information that is disseminated can be a complex consideration. Values are involved in all decisions of this sort.

INVOLVING USERS OF ELECTRONIC COMMUNICATIONS

In a study of 34 projects that developed software tools to advance internal productivity in four large U.S.-based electronics firms, Leonard-Barton and Sinha (1990) found that, in addition to the quality and cost of the technology and its initial compatibility with the user environment, two managerial processes were important in explaining different levels and types of successful implementation. The first of these was the degree and type of user involvement in the design and delivery of the system. The second was the degree to which the project participants deliberately altered the technology and also adjusted the user environment in a process of mutual adaptation (Leonard-Barton 1995).

Similar to the current view that a participatory action model leads to better research, effective disability studies disseminators must know and involve their intended user group in a variety of ways as they are shaping communications strategies. Moreover, the ways in which intended users are involved in shaping electronic communication systems (e.g., Web sites), informational systems, retrieval archives, and databases, among others, appear to be related to the overall communication "power" of the integrated set of basic elements of dissemination: user, content, medium, context, and source.

Because *user involvement* is not a precise term, care must be taken by disseminators in shaping the involvement process. Characteristics of sampling intended users correlate to the resulting quality of a dissemination effort. Some factors are the following:

- selection of users based on their knowledge, experience, or representativeness of the larger intended user group;
- inclusion of differing forms and levels of expertise that may be related to the use of the informational content;
- distribution of users according to geographical, cultural, language, ethnic, economic, and social lifestyle affiliations; and
- desire or willingness of potential users to use new information or to change old patterns of behavior or thinking as a result of new information dissemination.

Too frequently, electronic information disseminators do not consider the "attendant" level of information that may be needed by most intended users, if they are to actually apply or implement the information shared with them. This type of "cold" dissemination, without previous user involvement, is successful only if the new information is completely self-explanatory, requiring only intuitive notions and flexibility in how it may be applied, or if the intended users receiving the new information are already knowledgeable in all areas needed to assess and implement the new information or innovation successfully. This rarely happens.

Effective information disseminators must also be cognizant of the irony of mass communications such as those afforded through electronic technologies such as the Internet. Specifically, some experts recommend that disseminators carefully consider the size of the user audience that they will be able to address effectively (Dentler 1984). Clearly, the greater degree to which electronic dissemination practices conform to a careful matching of the intended user with the desired content, medium, and context through a respected source, the greater the likelihood that the intended user will be able to assess and use the disseminated information. A thoughtful and responsive codevelopment process strengthens the integration of elements critical to successful dissemination practices.

Many are familiar with the adage "information is power." New electronic communication technologies offer great opportunities for creating equitable access to electronic information. In addition, social attention appears to recognize a need and a benefit to this equity in access in ways that are new and powerful.

To a growing degree, the outcomes realized through research are becoming available through the World Wide Web. For example, in 1995, about 25 percent of the research projects funded by the U.S. Department of Education's National Institute on Disability and Rehabilitation Research had information available through the Web. At the end of 1999, however, a little more than 80 percent maintained Web sites to share information about their activities and outcomes.

THE "DIGITAL DIVIDE"

The increasing prominence of the Internet-based technologies makes it imperative for disability studies researchers and disseminators to address this dynamic new medium. There is growing evidence that Internet usage is affecting all people, including those with disabilities (Zajac 1998). However, it must be noted that while more people are using computers, many persons with disabilities may still lack access to a computer (NCDDR 1997). Also, given the high correlation between disability and poverty (Seelman and Sweeney 1995), many people with disabilities may not be able to afford a home computer and online services.

The National Telecommunications and Information Administration (NTIA) in the U.S. Department of Commerce has compiled data regarding the use of the Internet among the U.S. population and has found significant trends that should be known by those intending to use electronic media for dissemination purposes. Highlights of the NTIA (1999) findings indicate the following:

- The "digital divide" for Internet use between those at the highest and lowest educational levels widened by 25 percent from 1997 to 1998.
- Of those with college degrees, 61.6 percent now use the Internet, while only 6.6 percent of those with an elementary school education or less use the Internet.
- Those with college degrees or higher are 10 times more likely to have Internet access at work as persons with only some high school education.
- Almost 60 percent of home Internet users report using it to search for information.
- Approximately one-third of Americans reported using the Internet in 1999.
- Approximately 8 percent of Americans reported using the Internet primarily through public libraries as their access point.
- U.S. households earning incomes more than $75,000 a year are 20 times more likely to have home Internet access than those at the lowest income levels.
- Hispanic households in the United States are roughly half as likely to own a computer as white households and nearly 2.5 times less likely to use the Internet.
- Hispanic and African Americans in the United States are less likely to have access to the Internet from any location (home, school, work, or library) than whites are from home.
- Native Americans access the Internet at a rate of 18.9 percent, which is less than the national average in the United States.
- At every income level, households in rural areas in the United States are significantly less likely—sometimes half as likely—to have home Internet access than those in urban or central city areas.

However, there is growing access to computers and to the Internet. Plans have been formulated to allow for computers in every classroom in the United States or for every schoolchild in Japan. Free access to the Internet through public libraries, the presence of WebTV, decreasing costs for portable devices, and wider bandwidth will likely help ameliorate this situation. In the United States, President Clinton announced on April 4, 2000, an initiative to provide for 1,000 computer centers and a large volunteer effort to help eliminate the digital divide in the United States. He stated,

> I want you to understand that while most people talk about the digital divide—and it is real and it could get worse—I believe that the computer and the Internet give us a chance to move more people out of poverty more quickly than at any time in all of human history.

The U.S. president described a scene from a trip to India where, even in a remote village, the mother of a newborn can go to a public building and print out instructions on caring for her newborn. She could take with her the government-sponsored information with significant visual content, which, in his estimation, would be equal to what she might be given at a hospital of great renown.

It is expected that people in developing countries or rural areas of the United States, where Internet access is not currently widely available, will be helped by the business community. Business is financing the availability of direct service lines (DSL), wider bandwidth, and satellite systems that will carry larger amounts of information at greater speed. Satellite systems operating high above developed areas can also be extended to cover undeveloped areas (Gates 1999).

The "digital divide," however, is not just between technological "haves" and "have-nots." Additional concerns must be raised about technical literacy and the ability to use electronic communication and information dissemination capabilities. Modern dissemination strategies must recognize that new digital communication technologies offer powerful opportunities and tools that can radically change the nature of "informed decisions" made by those with access to the World Wide Web.

Use of the Internet as a dissemination medium has moved from 13.5 million adults in the United States in 1995 to more than 58 million or 30 percent of the U.S. adult population in 1998 (Birdsell et al. 1998). An estimated 700 million pages of content are available on the Internet, addressing a great range of topics, including aspects of disability, chronic health conditions, and independent living (Blasiotti 1999; NCDDR 1999; Novak and Hoffman 1998).

GLOBAL READINESS

Access and utilization of the Internet's resources are uneven from the global perspective. The extent to which the Internet offers useful and available information globally depends on an infrastructure and awareness level that, in certain countries, is still developing. For example, the Center for Democracy and Technology (2000) reports its conclusions regarding Internet access in Central and Eastern Europe.

❖ Internet usage was growing throughout the region but remained very low compared to Western Europe. Estimates of users ranged from a high of 500 per 10,000 in Slovenia to less than 1 per 10,000 in Belarus and Moldova. While Russia had at least 185,000 hosts (essentially, domain names ending in .ru) as of December 1999, Finland, a country with 1/30th the population, had more than twice that many.

❖ A major barrier to Internet usage in many countries is the poor state of the underlying telecommunications infrastructure. Most people, particularly residential users and nongovernmental organizations (NGOs), currently are dependent on telephone dial-up connections to the Internet. Throughout the Central and Eastern Europe region, teledensity rates are low, service quality is often poor, and there are long waiting lists for installation of new telephone lines.

❖ A second major barrier to Internet usage is the practice of per-minute charges for local calls, which makes connection time prohibitively expensive for many.

❖ In much of Central and Eastern Europe, due to the influence of the European Union (EU), telecommunications policy is focused on privatization and competition. These are necessary but are not sufficient conditions for the expansion of access to both basic telecommunications and Internet services. Much more needs to be done to open up the telecomm and Internet markets to true competition.

❖ Countries seeking to join the EU must commit to universal service. This is an important lever over national governments but so far has not been reflected in concrete definitions of universal service or "affordability." Under EU directives, the concept of universal service has been extended to Internet access.

❖ Given the rapid technological changes that are afoot and the global boom in Internet development, there is an urgent need for the EU and other international and regional bodies to adopt more effective policies to promote affordable access to noncommercial users.

❖ A range of alternative access technologies, including wireless, fixed wireless, satellite, and cable modem, hold the promise of overcoming landline telephone infrastructure deficiencies.

While the Center for Democracy and Technology (2000) report focuses on the Central and Eastern European region, its findings and conclusions have broader relevance to the growing debate over the digital divide from a global perspective.

BELLS, WHISTLES, AND ACCESSIBILITY

For disseminators of disability studies information, another major "divide" is caused by problems with the physical accessibility of information channels. It is imperative that accessibility be planned and included in the formulation of all products. Alschuler (1998) pointed out that accessibility could mean more than accommodation to a physical disability.

Good accessibility means making full use of content when one or more senses is turned off or turned down. This applies to the tens of millions of people with physical disabilities, but it also applies to others. What renders a person with "normal" vision, hearing, and motor and cognitive abilities "disabled"?

- the use of a Lynx browser on a character-based terminal;
- the use of a browser in a hands-free, eyes-busy environment, such as a moving vehicle;
- aging—after age 65, approximately 70 percent of the population acquires some form of access-related disability.

If you define *disability* as a permanent or temporary restriction on the use of sight, sound, color, and motor skills, we are all disabled to some degree. Our degree of "disability" will increase as we age and as Web browsing goes onboard in cars and in the operating rooms and permeates more corners of our daily life.

Most societies appear to be sensitive to the accessibility needs of people with disabilities. While some countries have enacted legislation officially safeguarding rights and privileges for people with disabilities, most societies appear to recognize that frequently, accommodations made for people with disabilities benefit many others in the society as well. These legislative responses to disability will be addressed in this volume.

The power of the World Wide Web to accommodate text, graphics, animation, video, audio, video and audio, and other simultaneous strands has the potential either to facilitate or to complicate Web site accessibility. The use of nontext forms of communication must also be accompanied by alternate formats for communicating the same information, generally to maximally meet the accessibility needs of computer users accessing Web pages with screenreaders or other forms of assistive or adaptive technologies. Web site designers need to be informed about accessibility issues to provide these alternate forms or strands of information.

Advances in software development offer hope that Web site construction may someday be more "automatically" accessible. Today, however, the accessibility of most Web sites rests in the knowledge and sensitivity of Web site designers. Enhancing Web site designers' awareness and sensitivity in this area can be challenging due to the fact that many have not had formal training to perform such work but have, instead, learned through their own experience. Thus, Web sites of disability-related entities have an additional responsibility to demonstrate in functional ways how Web sites can be maximally accessible to all users, including those with disabilities.

WORLD WIDE WEB CONSORTIUM

Accessibility of the World Wide Web for people with disabilities has been of concern to many in the private and corporate worlds. The World Wide Web Consortium (W3C) was founded to develop common protocols that could be used by Web designers, computer programmers, and Web-based information specialists to promote access to information for all users through the WWW. Some technologists and information specialists recognized that the rapid growth and development of the Information Superhighway afforded the opportunity to open many new possibilities for people with disabilities. Or, through inattention to the needs of people with disabilities and others, the Superhighway can create a rich information treasure that is inaccessible to some.

The W3C was founded in October 1994 at the Massachusetts Institute of Technology's Laboratory for Computer Sciences. The W3C added a European presence in cooperation with France's National Institute for Research in Computer Science and Control in April 1995, and in August 1996, Keio University in Japan became the third cohosting institution for the W3C. In 1999, the W3C had approximately 270 commercial and academic members that included computer hardware and software manufacturers and vendors, telecommunications and Internet service provider companies, and a variety of information, corporate, government, and academic entities.

The W3C has led the way to accessibility of the WWW by establishing common specifications that promote concerns and features for accessibility. Sensitive information disseminators using the World Wide Web or related HTML technologies will, at the least, be aware of the recommendations of the W3C. Each entity within the disability community that establishes and maintains a WWW presence, knowingly or unknowingly, serves as a model for Web site accessibility.

Web site accessibility is a construct that changes as new software, hardware, and related technologies become available. In addition, complete accessibility for all potential users of the Internet is at the end of the accessibility continuum. Ultimate, complete, and everlasting Web site accessibility, in other words, does not exist. Web site designers must continue to sensitively consider new technologies and their implications in terms of accessibility.

CYBERTALK AND SOCIAL CHANGE

E-mail and other Internet information technologies can serve as a unique tool for people with disabilities and others to engage directly in advocacy and social change activities. In the area of disability studies, Disabled Peoples' International, for example, has helped inform the research by bringing the disability experiences of people from many countries into the research equation. What is important is not only its breadth of scope but also its influence. Organizations—large and small—are more "equalized" through these technologies, especially in terms of the promotion of disability policy and related social change issues.

This also holds true for the "recruitment" of people with disabilities in the disability studies research area. Researchers are collaborating across international boundaries to study the sociopolitical status of such persons in various countries. The data and testimony brought to disability studies through electronic participation can add immensely to the richness of the literature. Although only a handful of researchers may be able to spend time abroad in legal research or studying legislation similar to the Americans with Disabilities Act (two NIDRR-sponsored Switzer Fellows have done this), electronic discourse and the use of databases, newspaper articles, and formal archives of various countries can all be accessed with immediacy.

As a "living classroom," the political activity of disability advocates can not only be gathered on the Internet but can also be observed and documented in this medium. Concerning the vital contribution the Internet has made in promoting civic participation, Steve Case, founder of America Online, commented in October 1998 as follows:

> We must use this medium to increase civic participation. . . . One of the first goals of this effort should be the development of an index of benchmarks—"leading indicators"—if you will that can measure the Internet's contributions to our social, political, and economic lives.

As a regular information medium, the Internet can shape public attitudes and could be strengthened to more greatly affect policy. It is a method through which new concepts, such as the "new paradigm of disability," can gain wider acceptance. Although the regular media are constrained by editorial policies and responses to economic influences, such as advertisers or their market niche, the Internet provides for freedom of expression.

Because much of the political work is being done by what we in the United States call "nonprofits" (in other places, they may be NGOs), it may be instructive to pay attention to the December 1998 report, *Democracy at Work: Nonprofit Use of Internet Technology for Public Policy Purposes*. The OMB Watch contends that

> the Internet (and its resulting technologies) has become a tool that considerably equalizes the potential of both large and smaller nonprofits to increase their visibility and engage potential volunteers and supporters. The amount of resources—including funding, staff availability, and time—make a big difference, however, in the tools available for organizations to utilize in their public policy activities. (OMB Watch 1998:37)

As a means for greater political organization and activity, the Internet does not currently seem to be living up to its promise, at least as reported by not-for-profit agencies, which are the organizations likely to be active on behalf of people with disabilities. The C. S. Mott and Surdna Foundations funded a study to analyze how nonprofit organizations use newer information technologies to engage in public policy activities. The findings of the study clearly reflect the state-of-the-art of Internet use among disability-related nonprofits as well as others. The results were issued in 1998 and generally reflected the following Internet use characteristics.

❖ The Internet is not currently widely used as a major policy-shaping tool. Although Web sites of nonprofit organizations have demonstrated enormous growth, the technology, including associated electronic mail capabilities, has not grown into a consistent policy tool. Most nonprofits use the Internet to make documents available that have already been distributed in another—usually print—format.

❖ Far greater numbers of nonprofits have the capability to use the Internet than are currently using it for public policy activities. While thousands of nonprofits engage in public policy activities, few are using the Internet in these activities.

❖ Web site information of nonprofits is not consistently maintained or kept up-to-date.

❖ The Internet is a more inactive, passive form of public policy networking than listservs. Some argue that the Internet and use of Web pages are far too passive to be an effective and powerful advocacy tool.

❖ Nonprofits are currently using only a narrow range of the full panoply of options available as Internet technologies. Listservs, frequently only used as automated distribution systems, were the most common tool used in public policy activities.

❖ Interactivity is not a common characteristic of Internet use by nonprofits engaged in public policy activity. Although robust Internet technologies supporting chat rooms, discussion forums, bulletin boards, and virtual reality exchanges exist today, limited use is made of them.

❖ Establishing a consistent and easily recognizable identity on the Internet is important to support a higher frequency of use and access through search engines.

❖ A significant number of nonprofits do not use the Internet due to knowledge, tool, and skill barriers related to Internet Web site design, development, and maintenance.

❖ Internet Web sites of nonprofits suggest organizational contexts and characteristics to viewers and users of the site. For example, nonprofits reflect conservatism by using high-end Internet tools to coordinate contacts to members of Congress for various public policy issues. Nonprofits appear progressive by emphasizing the use of currently available Internet tools to help grassroots efforts initiate and conduct public policy activities.

❖ Funding assistance to develop and maintain public policy Web sites is difficult to obtain. Most foundations—frequent funders of public policy activities—do not frequently use Internet Web sites and do not frequently fund Internet advocacy activities.

Clearly, the Internet affords many new opportunities to those engaged in public policy debate and activities and could be more aggressively used by the disability studies community to effect change. Schwartz (1996) outlines three major advantages that promote advocacy activity through the medium of the Internet. These include the following:

▪ the ability to very rapidly send complex materials and related information to general and specific audiences,
▪ the opportunity to communicate with large numbers of people simultaneously with limited per-person costs and time allocation, and
▪ the ability to have ongoing and long-term discussions with selected individuals or groups of individuals in specific "threads" or areas.

CHANGING TERRAIN OF INFORMATION ACCESS AND RESOURCES

The "almost instant" online publishing of research results can be beneficial in making the information demanded by people with disabilities available sooner in the research continuum. However, the immediacy and lack of standards for judging information internationally lead to the potential for serious problems through the promotion of faulty and even potentially destructive concepts. The Internet and related electronic forms of information exchange are creating new demands and expectations on the part of those seeking information.

This demand is creating some unexpected changes in information resources. For example, in August 1999, the secretary of the U.S. Department of Commerce announced plans to eliminate the National Technical Information Service (NTIS), which had been a major repository for government-sponsored research information. The secretary worked with Congress to close the NTIS as a major source of information while still hoping to preserve public access to scientific and technical reports. After extensive review and analysis, it was determined that the core function of NTIS, providing government information for a fee, was no longer needed in this day of advanced electronic technology. While the agency previously sold government documents in microfiche and paper formats, this became an unprofitable pursuit, as agencies and groups posted their reports on the Internet for free. These changes in the information marketplace have made obsolete the need for some "libraries" or information clearinghouses to continue operation.

Clearly, new technology will result in changes in the information resource terrain. The transition from print to electronic formats will cause some previously "successful" resources to be less than profitable or, perhaps, unnecessary in the age of free information exchange. This may affect government support for disability studies research.

POTENTIAL CONCERNS ABOUT THE QUALITY OF INFORMATION

While electronic information systems, such as the Internet, bring substantial opportunities for rapid information exchange, traditional communication channels also appear "challenged" to keep pace and maintain their standards of quality. For example, early in 1999, Dr. Harold Varmus, director of the National Institutes of Health (NIH), announced a proposed plan to publish new biomedical research results electronically through the Internet, using a new Web site called E-biomed. Varmus argued that the plan would propel research results into the arena for use much more quickly than traditional academic journal pathways. He also proposed that a portion of the information on the Web site would be peer reviewed, while some of it would not be.

Dr. Arnold Relman, editor-in-chief of the *New England Journal of Medicine*, was vocally opposed to the plan, considering it a risky endeavor. He contended "that immediately publishing official research without accompanying expert commentary and interpretation could lead to mistakes, inaccuracies and misinterpretation." This is not a new debate for persons in the medical and rehabilitation fields. As pressure has increased for the public release of research information, traditional research information sources have grappled with the choice of speed over traditional peer review procedures. Relman noted that it was more important for new research findings to be "thoroughly reviewed, not hastily published" (*San Jose Mercury News*, 1999).

EVALUATING WEB-BASED INFORMATION

This "instant credibility debate" is new for many fields and could affect disability studies because of the nature of findings and their direct relationship to disability consumers. Disability information disseminators have kept an eye on the medical community in this regard. There have been a number of attempts over the past several years to devise guidelines that help users of Web-based information evaluate medically oriented research available through the Internet. Similar evaluative assistance has been suggested for information related to medical rehabilitation results (Blasiotti 1992).

For example, NIDRR sponsored establishment of the National Center for the Dissemination of Disability Research (NCDDR) (www.ncddr.org) in 1995 as a pilot project. In establishing its Web site, the NCDDR jointly constructed a component of the Web site to highlight information produced by the NIDRR-funded Model Spinal Cord Injury Systems (MSCIS) (www.ncddr.org/rpp/hf/hfdw/mscis) projects. Working with a representative peer group of the MSCIS dissemination committee, the NCDDR identified information for posting that was deemed "worthy" and ready for wider distribution.

In 1998, the *Journal of the American Medical Association* included an article titled "Rating Health Information on the Internet: Navigating to Knowledge or Babel?" The authors focused on sites that had been distinguished by awards, citations, or other quality ratings or approvals. The criteria suggested for evaluation of the Web-based health information included the following:

mentioning information about the academic and professional background of the authors;

attributions for references and other related sources for information-gathering instrumentation used;

disclosure, if appropriate, of Web site ownership, sponsorship, advertising, underwriting, commercial funding arrangements, other support, or potential conflicts of interest.

The authors located 47 instruments developed to rate health information Web sites. Only 13 of the instruments included descriptions of the rating criteria. During the six-month period following the initiation of the survey, 9 of the instruments with previously available criteria ceased to make them available. In addition, 3 of the rating instrument developer organizations decided to stop rating health information Web sites. The authors concluded,

Even if desirable, however, the next question is if it is possible to evaluate the information on the Internet. The successful development of instruments to evaluate health information on the Internet is not an easy task. Evaluation of just the content, for instance, presents the same challenges by those evaluating the quality of randomized controlled trials published in paper-based journals, including the lack of a "gold standard" for quality and the controversy around its definition. ("Rating Health Information" 1998:614)

In August 1999, *The Washington Post* reported that a team of Michigan researchers had reviewed some 400 Web sites for information on a rare form of cancer, Eking sarcoma. The researchers found that 6 percent of the sites contained erroneous information, and many of them contained misleading information. Of the remainder, survival rates cited ranged from 5 to 85 percent, creating concern that individuals using these sources of information might refuse treatment. The leader of the research team, Dr. Sybil Biermann, an orthopedic surgeon, stated,

I think the Internet is a really positive development, but there are perils in the lack of peer review and promulgation of bad information. When patients come in to discuss information with their doctor, I recommended that doctors ask patients if they got their information via the Internet. Thus, the doctors can assess their patients level of misinformation and provide needed guidance and support. (Boodman, 1999:207)

In November 1999, *Red Herring* reported on the privacy challenge as well as the "judging" question. In an article aptly titled, "Faustian Bargain or Valuable Exchange?" (Oh 1999), this confluence of technical information and consumer interest was discussed. One popular site allows those with cancer to input specific details of their condition and, in return, obtain information specifically related to their case. The Cancer Profiler provides information from peer-reviewed articles from the *Journal of the American Medical Association,* and it "weighs treatment options." The site developers consider this a filter for the information, and they also consider that they have a second review by a medical editorial board.

Some of the information concerns the preference for drug over surgery and others. However, as in most commercially backed sites, this one's primary source of revenue is "fees paid by an undisclosed number of drug developers." In return for their capitalization of the site, companies can access the aggregated database. Although this site will not have commercial banner ads on its site, it provides its sponsors with market information. Although the site provides what appears to be targeted information, it might also be providing very private information to other sources. One of the reported activities of the site is informing a user in one city that he or she may be a good candidate for a research study in another.

This site has tried to find some ways to ensure the privacy of its users, including applying for a "TrustE Web Seal." This seal is supposed to signify that the site has met at least minimum standards for the insurance of privacy. However, it is noted that these measures are not "true guarantees." It remains to be seen if this site, like the commercial sites mentioned earlier, can prove economically successful to retain its partners in the pharmaceutical industry.

INTERNET 2

Increasing traffic on the Internet has caused growing pains and roadblocks for some attempting to use the Internet for information collection and research. Internet service providers (ISPs) are struggling to offer adequate communications bandwidth while maintaining profitable applications. Problems are occurring, however, due to the continuing exponential growth of the medium over a relatively short period of time.

In response to this and the growing commercialization of the Internet, a plan to develop another version of the Internet was conceived. In early October 1996, 34 research universities convened and agreed to establish the Internet 2 Project. The goal of the Internet 2 Project is to coordinate the activity of the universities and several government and industry partners to develop the next stage of the electronic Internet medium. The Internet 2 Project goals are the following: (1) to establish a leading-edge networking infrastructure for the national research and higher education community, (2) to encourage and support the development of a new generation of applications to fully use the capabilities of the Internet technology, and (3) to improve the reliability and ease of use of the Internet technology for all members of the academic community. The Internet 2 mission is to

facilitate and coordinate the development, deployment, operation, and technology transfer, of advanced, network-based applications and network services to further the United States' leadership in research and higher education and accelerate the availability of new services and applications on the Internet. (www.Internet2.edu)

The Internet 2 Project is expected to evolve over the next three to five years. Beta applications and other trials will surely be a part of the Internet 2 development process. Innovative applications are planned that will enhance collaboration in research linking instruments, data, students, and teachers; development of virtual laboratories that enhance real-time access to remote instruments and supercomputing centers; digital libraries that will contain extensive video and audio collections; and large-scale computation capabilities. Internet 2 advancements promise to revolutionize uses of the Internet technology.

DISABILITY, ELECTRONIC INFORMATION, AND THE FUTURE

Without doubt, the way in which disability is perceived and defined in the future will be changing. Today, some authors (see Fujiura 1999; Seelman and Sweeney 1995) are discussing factors in our global society that are contributing to new or emerging disabilities. Factors such as violence, poverty, environmental toxicities, and accidental injuries—to name a few—are contributing to disabilities in increasing numbers. The nature of services and related information that individuals with these types of emerging disabilities may require will be evolving in the twenty-first century and challenging the service delivery and informational systems.

In addition, increased attention is being paid to the environmental factors that contribute to the mobility and integration of people with disabilities into their communities. The way in which physical environments are built and the degree to which these factors constitute "barriers" for some people with disabilities will continue to gather increased scrutiny by consumer groups, policymakers, and service providers.

It also appears clear that the expectations for electronic information systems to inform, provide services, and foster personal and targeted social interactions will continue to increase. Publicly funded informational resources will continue to feel pressure to offer current, timely, and pertinent assistance and access to desired information. Electronic formats for sharing and archiving this information will continue to increase and allow a growing expectation for on-demand comprehensive electronic forms of information and related assistance. This expectation will certainly continue to forge change.

ELECTRONIC LEARNING

The use of electronic media and information resources affords new possibilities in the learning process. Those engaged in disability studies should become familiar with and make use of this tool, which is increasing the "audience" of learners. For people with transportation difficulties engendered by their disability or perhaps their remote setting, distance learning is opening up the world of disability studies to them. This has the potential for great impact on disability studies curriculum development (international scope, accessibility, people with undetermined skill levels, and others). Clearly, as some researchers are finding out, the Internet and attendant information allow learning to occur through a variety of new communication and information-gathering procedures.

Some writers have mused on the changes of the "new learning" over traditional formats such as lecture and memory recitation. In fact, there has been much discussion—much of it on the Internet on the future shape of the "university." One futurist, Don Tapscott (1998), has described a learning model that is based on discovery rather than instruction:

The new model shifts from teacher-centered to learner-centered education. In the past, education has tended to focus on the teacher, not the student. This is especially true in post-secondary education where the specific interests and background of the teacher strongly influence the content. Much of the activity in the classroom involves the teacher speaking and the student listening. Learner-centered education begins with an evaluation of the abilities, learning style, social context and other important factors about the student that affect learning. It would extensively use software programs which can structure and tailor the learning experience. It would be more active, with students discussing, debating, researching and collaborating on projects. The new university emphasizes learning how to navigate and how to learn and think, rather than absorbing materials, preparing youngsters for lifelong learning. This includes learning how to synthesize, not just analyze. (P. 6)

Certainly, an extensive range of resources are at the disposal of modern-day students. These can be accessed in a timely fashion for a variety of purposes. Combining Internet searches with database resources and materials, along with electronic mail to and from content experts, creates rich information capacities.

ELECTRONIC INFORMATION DISSEMINATION IN THE TWENTY-FIRST CENTURY

The use of the Internet can be expected to grow exponentially for the foreseeable future. In addition, the availability of information and the number of Web pages available through the Internet will markedly increase.

Futurists have forecast a variety of possibilities for cyber-communication into the twenty-first century. Some of these include the following:

❖ The self-contained personal computer, as we knew it at the end of the twentieth century, will be replaced by "networked intelligence," and e-commerce will abound. The Internet will be where computing is done, and people will be able to widely share it through WebTV, cheap terminals, and other means of access. Bandwidth will continue to increase and will speed up communications and be readily available in homes through cable services (Harris 1999).

❖ Research will change as a result of the changes in electronic access to information. In the past, scientists—even more than other knowledge workers—have spent the vast majority of their time collecting data and only a small part of their time applying it. Better tools will enable researchers to apply most of their brainpower to the tough problems rather than to data collection and verification.

❖ The Internet will become a hotbed of political activism and a revolutionary organizing tool. It will enable users to discuss coordinated actions and facilitate mobilization while also allowing more people to express their personal views. Technoliteracy connotes the inherent political power of networks (Harris 1998).

❖ The increased use of electronic networks for telemedicine, telerehabilitation, telehealth, and telehome health care will become common tools used to address professional personnel shortages and expand service capacity.

Clearly, electronic information dissemination will significantly contribute to the growth and change of our global society in the twenty-first century. Although the technology and associated information promise to remove some barriers for people with disabilities, it also may create new, unforeseen obstacles.

CONCLUSION

Exponential growth is occurring in the use of electronic networking to access Internet-based information and communications resources. The field of disability studies must focus on the effects of this growth in the lives of people with disabilities. Clearly, new networking technologies offer great potential that could facilitate or limit the integration of people with disabilities into broader circles of social, business, cultural, and educational activity. Radical changes appear possible—and perhaps probable—in how disability studies research will be conducted in the future and how people with disabilities will participate in shaping both disability studies research and curricula.

REFERENCES

Alschuler, L. 1998. "Making Your Website Accessible." *ZDNet* [Online]. Available: www.zdnet.com/devhead/stories/articles/0,4413,1600180,00.html.

Birdsell, D., D. Muzzio, D. Krane, and A. Cottreau. 1998. "Web Users Are Looking More Like America." *The Public Perspective* 9 (3): 33-35.

Blasiotti, E. 1992. "Disseminating Research Information to Multiple Stakeholders: Lessons from the National Institute on Disability and Rehabilitation Research." *Knowledge* (March): 305-19.

———. 1999. 147Dr Vincent Cerf visits NIDRR." *The Research Exchange* 4 (2). Austin, TX: Southwest Educational Development Laboratory [Online]. Available: www.ncddr.org/du/researchexchange/v04n02/.

Boodman, S. 1999. "Medical Web-Sites Can Steer You Wrong: Study Finds Erroneous and Misleading Information on Many Pages Dedicated to a Rare Cancer." *The Washington Post*, August 10, p. Z07.

Case, S. 1998. Luncheon address by Steve Case, Chairman and CEO of America Online. National Press Club, October 26, Washington, DC.

Center for Democracy and Technology. 2000. *Bridging the Digital Divide: Internet Access in Central and Eastern Europe* [Online]. Available: www.cdt.org/international/ceeaccess/report.shtml.

Clinton, W. J. 2000. Remarks by the President at the Digital Divide Kick Off. The White House, Office of the Press Secretary, April 4, Washington, DC.

Dentler, R. 1984. "Putting Knowledge to Work: Issues in Providing Affective Educational Dissemination." Paper presented at the annual meeting of the Council for Educational Development and Research, November, Phoenix, AZ.

Eberhard, M. 2000. "Pocket Projector: The E-Book Might Be the Next Portable Device You Can"t Live Without." *Red Herring* 78:234.

Edwards, P. 2000. "Briefing: Handheld Devices." *Red Herring* 78:224-26.

Fujiura, G. 1999. *Quality of Life for Persons with Disabilities in the United States.* Chicago: McCormick Tribune Foundation.

Gates, B. 1999. *Business and the Speed of Thought: Using a Digital Nervous System.* New York: Warner.

Harris, B. 1999. "Don Tapscott: Main Street Tomorrow." *Government Technology* [Online]. Available: www.interlog.com/~blake/tapscott.htm.

Harris, E. 1998. "Quote of Evan Hershaw-Plath, Founder of Protest.Net." *Wall Street Journal* [Online]. Available: interactive.wsj.com.

Hutchinson, J. and M. Huberman. 1993. *Knowledge Dissemination and Utilization in Science and Mathematics Education: A Literature Review.* Washington, DC: National Science Foundation.

Klein, S. and M. Gwaltney. 1991. "Charting the Education Dissemination System." *Knowledge* (March): 241-65.

Leonard-Barton, D. 1995. *Wellsprings of Knowledge: Building and Sustaining the Sources of Innovation.* Boston: Harvard Business School Press.

Leonard-Barton, D. and D. Sinha. 1990. "Dependency, Involvement, and User Satisfaction: The Case of Internal Software Development." Working Paper No. 91-008, Harvard Business School, Boston.

Lindsay, S. 2000. "The Disability Portal Wars: Competing to Define and Conquer the Disability Community." *Disability Times.com* [Online]. Available: www.disabilitytimes.com/2000/04/18/editorial.

Louis, K. 1992. "Comparative Perspectives on Dissemination and Knowledge Use Policies." *Knowledge* (March): 287-304.

National Center for the Dissemination of Disability Research (NCDDR). 1997. *Report of NCDDR Consumer Survey.* Austin, TX: Southwest Educational Development Laboratory.

———. 1999. *Disability, Diversity, and Dissemination: A Review of the Literature on Topics Related to Increasing the Utilization of Rehabilitation Research Outcomes among Diverse Consumer Groups.* Austin, TX: Southwest Educational Development Laboratory.

National Telecommunications and Information Administration (NTIA). 1999. *Falling through the Net: Defining the Digital Divide.* Washington, DC: U.S. Department of Commerce.

Novak, T. and D. Hoffman. 1998. *Bridging the Digital Divide: The Impact of Race on Computer Access and Internet Use* [Online]. Available: www2000.ogsm.vanderbilt.edu/papers/race/science.html.

Oh, J. 1999. "Faustian Bargain or Valuable Exchange?" *Red Herring* 72:49-50.

OMB Watch. 1998. *Democracy at Work: Nonprofit Use of Internet Technology for Public Policy Purposes.* Washington, DC: Author.

"Rating Health Information on the Internet: Navigating to Knowledge or Babel?" 1998. *Journal of the American Medical Association*, February 28, p. 614.

Rojas, P. 2000. "A Brief History of the Development of Portable Information." *Red Herring* 73:272-77.

San Jose Mercury News. 1999. Reuters [Online]. Available: www.mercurycenter.com/svtech/news/breaking/internet/docs/5288651.htm

Schwartz, E. 1996. *NetActivism: How Citizens Use the Internet.* Los Angeles: Songine Studios.

Seelman, K. and S. Sweeney. 1995. "The Changing Universe of Disability." *American Rehabilitation* 21 (3): 2-13.

Stock, J. and R. Drake. 2000. *Data Sources for Social Researchers.* London: Hazeldene.

Tapscott, D. 1998. "Reinventing the University: Thirty Years from Now Big University Campuses Will Be Relics." *NewsScan Exec* [Online]. Available: www.newsscan.com/exec/spring1998/reinventing.html.

U.S. Department of Commerce. 1999. "Commerce Secretary William M. Daley Announces Intention to Close National Technical Information Service" [Press release]. Washington, DC.

Zajac, A. 1998. "In Online Access, a Great Divide." *Chicago Tribune,* June 22 [Online]. Available: http://archive.chicago.tribune.com/cgi-bin/slwebchi.pl?DBQUERY=zajac&DBLIST=ct98&NITEMS=25%3A25&SORT=r%3Ah.

II

EXPERIENCING DISABILITY

Divided Understandings

13

The Social Experience of Disability

CAROL J. GILL

THE BRIDGE

I feel calm,
  then I stagger
    and stumble.
I want to be graceful.
  When I meet
someone new, I feel shy,
  my muscles start
jerking and I stutter.
  I need harmony
  between inner me
  and outer me.
People see the outer me,
  off balance,
  out of kilter,
  and drooling. Ah,
but I am learning to confront
  my rage and despair
  and I have friends
  who support me as
  I solve the daily
  challenges of creating
  an independent life.
  I imagine a bridge
  between outer and inner,
between stranger and friend,
  between you and me.

          —Mariana Ruybalid

T he bridge symbolizes a poignant theme in disabled persons' autobiographical accounts: their desired connection with others. Ironically, the image of the bridge in the introductory poem highlights a troubling disjuncture between the worlds of disability and nondisability that many disabled individuals find central to their social experience. This chapter examines the area of disconnect beneath the bridge—specifically, the tense gap between disabled people's "insider" experience of disability and "outsiders'" convictions about what that experience must be.

THE DILEMMA: "MY DISABILITY IS HOW PEOPLE RESPOND TO MY DISABILITY"

The ideas presented in this chapter evolved from a wide-ranging exploratory review of theoretical and empirical work on "the experience of disability." Although an examination of "experience" reasonably involves inquiry at the individual level, it also invites analysis at the social level. This review was, in fact, guided by the conviction that rigorous investigation of the personal and interpersonal experiences of members of a minority group yields crucial information about social forces and cultural values affecting the group. In light of current criticism within disability studies of an exclusive sociopolitical rendering of disability (Hughes and Paterson 1997), sources were also reviewed that extend the inquiry to personal experiences of impairment and embodiment.

The resulting analysis draws primarily from three information sources:

1. conceptual papers addressing the experience of disability, many of them authored by individuals with disabilities;
2. formal social science and rehabilitation research addressing the disability experience and related themes;
3. personal accounts of persons with disabilities.

The interrelatedness of these three knowledge sources, particularly the consistency of themes across them, is arresting. One does not venture far into an exploration of the disability experience before noticing that isolation, invisibility, tension, and struggle are recurring topics whenever and however disabled persons are asked about their lives (French 1993; Zola 1982). Despite conventional public perceptions, these negative universals of the disability experience rarely issue directly and exclusively from impairments or related functional limitations (Olkin 1999). In fact, the entity that disabled persons feel most isolated *from*, invisible *to*, and in tense struggle *with* is generally a person with whom they try to interact (employer, neighbor, salesperson, physician, case manager) but who draws unfounded assumptions about their experience and therefore cannot understand who they really are. In a damaging self-fulfilling cycle of judgment, many nondisabled observers naively contribute to a real tragedy of disability—the interpersonal impasse—by clinging steadfastly to the presumption that to live with an impairment is to linger in a tragic state. Stated more directly by Craig Vick, an informant in Gelya Frank's (1988) anthropological study of disability, "My disability is how people respond to my disability" (p. 111).

Several well-known conceptual frameworks have been advanced to describe and explain the disability experience, including disabled people's experience of estrangement and tension in the world of social relations, what that experience means to them, and how they respond to it. Some of the most frequently cited theories and related constructs, such as stigma, adaptation to functional loss, and liminality, will be presented and evaluated with respect to both their contributions and their shortcomings in accounting for the data. This discussion culminates in a proposal to reframe the dilemma of disabled people's experienced social disconnection as a conflict of values, perspective, and identity rather than in the more passive terms of adjustment or stigma management.

In particular, it will be argued that a central feature of the disability "insider" experience is a persistent and disquieting sense of mistaken identity. Across a range of situations and interpersonal relationships, disabled persons find that the identities they forge and present to the world are commonly dismissed by others in favor of stereotypical identity ascriptions. Consequently, a significant part of the disability experience centers on disabled persons' tireless efforts to set the record straight and to reestablish their real identities. These efforts and the stakes attached to them are examined in the context of theory. The ways in which this dynamic differs from the experience of other marginalized and misperceived groups is also considered. Overall, this chapter is dedicated to disabled people's indefatigable strivings for integrity in both *self* and *social* relations. It acknowledges not their need for functional integrity, or normality, but their critique and expansion of that concept and their impressive industry in bridging the divide between their self-views and public perceptions of them, between their inner and outer worlds.

In writing this chapter, I have worried that it may convey the impression that the disability experience is essentially negative and immutable or that interaction between disabled and nondisabled people is hopeless—neither of which I believe. This topic encompasses some of the hardest realities confronted by disabled persons regarding their place in the world of social relations and their ambiguous status as minority group members scattered throughout the matrix of the dominant nondisabled majority culture. After delving into the pertinent conceptual, empirical, and narrative literatures, however, it became clear that searching for a positive spin on this subject might not only imperil the scholarship but would also render a disservice to people with disabilities who have no choice but to confront these hard realities daily. Furthermore, the disability experience is, more accurately, various group, subgroup, and individual experiences. Many are frankly positive. We need to know more about these and the conditions under which they occur. However, the positive stories will be all the more compelling if set into an honest analysis. That analysis begins with a review of the most frequently cited theories bearing on the experience of disability.

A CHRONOLOGY OF "CLASSIC" THEORY
ON THE DISABILITY EXPERIENCE

Beatrice Wright and Value Transformation

Formal study of the disability experience seemed well launched in the period following World War II. The widely cited work of Beatrice Wright (1960) and her colleagues from Kurt Lewin's school of field psychology, such as Roger Barker, Tamara Dembo, and Gloria (Ladieu) Leviton, had underscored the importance of social context in understanding the experience of disabled persons (Fine and Asch 1988). Interwoven throughout Wright's description of the *individual's* efforts to integrate disability into a positive sense of self was an explicit acknowledgment of disability as a devalued status imposed on persons *collectively*. According to Wright, disabled people react to functional impairment not in simple ways, determined directly by individual physiology, but in complex, socially reasonable ways that are powerfully influenced by cultural values and others' behavior.

Wright's classic text, *Physical Disability: A Psychological Approach* (1960), and her revised text, *Physical Disability—A Psychosocial Approach* (1983)—retitled to strengthen its emphasis on the interaction between individual and society—richly showcased the words and perspectives of individuals experiencing physical and sensory impairment. Her appreciation for the disability voice complemented her criticism of observer negative bias in interpreting the disability experience. In this regard, she wrote, "We must again remind ourselves how seriously mistaken outsiders can be when led astray and deluded by the compelling nature of their own values and perspective" (Wright 1983:159).

One of Wright's most enduring contributions to our grasp of the disability experience was her attention to values and their transformation during the disability adjustment process. Her theory of value change, extending seminal groundwork by Dembo, Leviton, and Wright (1956), posited a set of mechanisms to address the following paraphrased question: In a society that values unblemished appearance and function, how can an individual come to accept functional limitation or loss without absorbing a sense of shame and inferiority?

One mechanism employed by self-accepting disabled persons, according to Wright (1983), is the enlargement of their scope of values, accomplished by developing interest in still attainable goals and by reaching beyond what has been lost. Another mechanism is the subordination of the values of body appearance and performance, which she referred to as "physique," to qualities of human worth that are still within grasp, such as personality attributes and the willingness to expend effort. Another is the "containment" of disability effects to prevent the perceived "spread" of limitation to the entire self. Here Wright advocated what these days might be called the deconstruction of disability stereotypes through efforts to separate the functional consequences of impairment from overgeneralized or incorrectly ascribed limitations. In explaining this process, she presented some ideas about the complexity and context dependence of the disability experience that seem surprisingly consistent with contemporary disability rights and disability culture ideology, including the notion that "not all effects [of impairment] are negative," and two statements significantly italicized by the author that conclude her discussion of containment: "*A disability involves certain limitations in certain situations. The source of limitation is due to barriers imposed by society and not only to personal incapacity*" (Wright 1983:178). The remaining mechanism of value change addressed by Wright is the transformation of comparative-status values, the assessment of one's qualities in comparison to the qualities of others or in comparison to cultural norms, into asset values, the assessment of qualities in terms of their contribution to one's life. An example would be skill in using adaptive equipment. Although outside observers immersed in comparative-status values may judge the use of such devices as inferior compared to "normal" functioning, persons with disabilities regard them as assets because they have learned to appreciate the benefit derived from their use.

In this conceptualization of the experience of disability, the contribution of impairment, or "physique," and the contribution of the social environment were equally weighted. Disability encompassed both a personal and a social struggle. The personal challenge was to confront functional losses, possibly even to mourn them, and then to develop goals and values compatible with remaining abilities. The social challenge was to navigate, forebear, or oppose the negative attitudes and obstacles constructed by those who overvalue physique, fear impairment, and focus inordinately on functional and aesthetic loss.

The idea that the disability experience involves a significant transformation of values and an affirmative surrender of dominant cultural standards is noteworthy in at least two respects. First, it is supported by empirical evidence and by the subjective reports of persons with disabilities. In fact, as suggested by research and narrative discussed later in this chapter, value transformation is one of the outstanding common denominators of the disability experience. Second, it marks a critical locus of divergence between insiders and outsiders of the disability experience. The overhaul of priorities and worldview prompted by the functional and social exigencies of disability is the point at which many disabled individuals veer sharply from nondisabled associates in their understanding of disability and its consequences for daily life.

Wright and her colleagues established an impressive body of disability research and conceptual analysis that, given its historical context, was far-reaching and progressive. Before their work, after all, psychoanalytic formulations of the experience of disability had focused primarily on somatic dysfunction and its presumed direct threat to healthy self-development.[1] Although predating the emergence of disability studies as an academic field, the work of Wright and her associates presaged a social model research paradigm in two key respects: It was grounded in the perspectives of persons with disabilities, and its context was disabled people's social devaluation.

The stage had thus been set, it seemed, for investigating the individual's experience of disability as knowable only in the context of the sociopolitical status of disabled people as a group. This potential for a fuller exploration of the disability experience in social context was, however, only partially realized in the immediately succeeding years. Investigations of the disability experience were primarily taken up by either sociologists or rehabilitation clinicians whose studies correspondingly clustered around two constructs: stigma and adjustment.

Stigma, Deviance, and Social Role Learning

Erving Goffman's (1963) sociological analysis of stigma and its consequences in socially marginalized groups is frequently cited as foundational in disability literature reviews. His interpretation of the social experience of disability has been influential for so long, in fact, that disability studies scholars from several disciplines collaborated in the late 1980s to produce a special issue of the *Journal of Social Issues* (Fine and Asch 1988) dedicated to the theme of moving disability research "beyond 'stigma.' "

Goffman (1963) drew a stark picture of strained relations between disabled and nondisabled people. According to his observations, a major aspect of the experience of disability is the ongoing struggle to ward off potential interpersonal devaluation caused by one's social classification as less than normal, at best, and less than human, at worst. If stigma, an attribute that triggers social discreditation, can be minimized or submerged during social interaction through strategies such as using humor, proving competence, or hiding difference, the individual may "pass" as socially acceptable. If stigma cannot be successfully managed, the individual is consigned to the margins of humanity and often internalizes the stigmatized, spoiled identity as somehow deserved. Goffman described in detail the social implications of publicly noted deviance. For example, persons with detectable impairments may be subject to rude questions or comments and denied the privacy that "normal" adults are generally accorded in public. In some cases, they may be granted superficial acceptance as long as they remain mindful of their tenuous status and take care not to exceed the tacit limits of social tolerance. More extremely, disabled persons may be treated as nonpersons, dismissed as incapable of the same feelings, goals, and role responsibilities as nondisabled people. Goffman wrote extensively of the particular dilemma of the "discreditable," persons with a nonvisible stigma that could be potentially discovered, contrasting them with the "discredited," persons with obvious stigma. Whereas the central social demand of visible stigma is managing the tension of encounters, Goffman theorized, the central social demand of hidden stigma is managing information about oneself to avoid discreditation.

One of Goffman's contemporaries, Fred Davis (1961), gathered data that substantiate both the strained nature of encounters between disabled and nondisabled persons and the effort expended by disabled persons to minimize that strain. His study described strategic behaviors adopted by disabled persons to "disavow deviance" and to establish their common humanity in interactions with others. Davis theorized that social interaction is threatened by the public's routine perceptions of disabled persons as " 'different,' 'odd,' 'estranged from the common run of humanity,' etc.; in short, other than normal" (p. 122). Such perceptions, he believed, are expressed in a "pronounced stickiness of interactional flow and in the embarrassment of the normal by which he conveys the all too obvious message that he is having difficulty relating to the handicapped person as he would to 'just an ordinary man or woman' " (p. 122).

Davis (1961) interviewed adults whose impairments included orthopedic conditions, blindness, and cosmetic facial conditions, asking how they handled social relationships affected by societal attitudes toward disability. On the basis of the informants' responses, the investigator concluded that new relationships between disabled and nondisabled persons move through sequential stages of deviance disavowal involving both parties. In the first stage, called *fictional acceptance,* nondisabled persons superficially treat disabled persons as equals. This surface acceptance may become an end in itself, thus fossilizing the relationship at a barren and limited level. Davis observes, "As with the poor relation at the wedding party, so the reception given the handicapped person in many social situations: sufficient that he is here, he should not expect to dance with the bride" (p. 127).

If the first stage proceeds smoothly, however, the disabled person may begin to disclose sufficient personal information to challenge stereotypes and to encourage the nondisabled person to identify in terms of shared interests and perspectives. Davis (1961) referred to this stage as *breaking through*. Particularly interesting in light of this chapter's opening poem, he describes several strategies employed by his informants for "bridging fictional acceptance." They include deliberate reference to their involvement in "normal" activities, the interjection of in-group disability terminology in conversation as an ice-breaking tactic, displays of wit and charm, particular attention to or agreement with topics introduced by the nondisabled person, and the leveraging of the "normalization potential" of being seen with an attractive nondisabled companion.

If breaking through succeeds, Davis (1961) explained, the nondisabled person relates to the disabled person as though he or she were nondisabled—a goal Davis presumed is desirable to most disabled persons. The final stage of deviance disavowal is *institutionalization of the normalized relationship*. The relationship has been redefined as normal; the work of this stage is to sustain this redefinition as the nondisabled associate is incrementally exposed to some of the less than "normal" realities of life with disability. Specifically, the disabled person must assist the nondisabled associate in acquiring a repertoire of responses to bumps in the road such as inaccessible buildings and unsolicited help from strangers to facilitate a gradual qualification of the normalized relationship without upsetting it.

Although both Goffman and Davis considered, albeit parenthetically, the case of "deviant" people who deliberately opt to forego the struggle for acceptance by "normals," neither presented this possibility in a positive light. In *Stigma*, Goffman (1963) initially discussed positive minority group pride as démodé and later argued that individuals who politically reject "normal" culture in favor of alliance formation with similarly stigmatized persons not only risk calling attention to their differences, thereby reinforcing their social disconnection, but also operate according to the very propensity to categorize that they find objectionable. Davis dedicated merely a footnote to the discussion of disabled persons who refuse to court nondisabled persons for acceptance, reporting that his informants spoke of such individuals with mixed feelings: admiration for their moral courage but disapproval of their willingness to risk exacerbating negative attitudes toward disabled people, thus reducing chances of future public acceptance.

In his analysis of disability as a social role, presented in the book *The Making of Blind Men*, Robert Scott (1969) theorized that blind people's needs for assistance hold them captive to the transmutational philosophies and practices of the powerful blind services system. In the process of qualifying for and receiving services, he maintained, blind persons are rewarded for adopting the attitudes and behaviors expected of them by service professionals, and they are punished for viewing themselves in ways that contradict the professionals' own views of blind people. Ultimately, they are conditioned to be dependent and compliant, a social role that is systematically learned but which the public views as the natural outcome of impaired sight. The blind role, then, is a particular instance of the master tragic identity imputed to all disabled people. Scott noted the economic and political underpinnings of this phenomenon. For example, in communities where the number of available clients is low and interagency competition is high, he pointed out, professionals are likely to endorse intervention strategies that tether profitable clients to the facility rather than encouraging independence. Furthermore, agencies that sequester blind clients are likely to be well supported by communities that wish to avoid integrating blind citizens into mainstream life.

In contrast to Goffman and Davis, Scott (1969) devoted considerably more than a footnote to the discussion of blind people who disagree with the social role assigned to them by service professionals and the public. He described several forms of resistance. According to Scott, resisters may selectively adopt a facade of compliance in interactions with others for the sake of expediency or to avoid being labeled as ungrateful or bitter, dropping the role when circumstances permit. Alternatively, they may knowingly exploit the blind role to their advantage, as in the case of beggars. Scott describes yet another possibility:

> Another way that blind men cope with discrepancies between putative and personal identity is to resist and negate the imputations of others at every turn. By doing so, personal integrity is preserved, but the cost is very high. It requires an enormous commitment and expenditure of energy to resist these forces, and the blind man who does so inevitably alienates himself from other people. (Pp. 23-24)

The theoretical frameworks advanced by Goffman, Davis, and Scott all focus on handicapping responses of the social environment to human difference. All suggest that the public's unwillingness to regard disabled persons as equals serves the interests of the nondisabled community in some consequential way (e.g., as reassurance of normality or superiority), as insulation from the anxiety-provoking fact of human vulnerability, or even as a means of maintaining a rewarding professional career. These are blunt, plain-speaking theories. Their description of nondisabled people's role in disabled people's marginalization is unflinching, exemplified by this declaration in the concluding chapter of Scott's (1969) book: "Blind men are not born, they are made" (p. 121). Acknowledgment of the devalued status of disabled people in these theories is equally forthright, exemplified by Davis's (1961) bluntness in asking his disabled informants how they handled the imputation that they were not "normal, like everyone else" (p. 121).

These three frameworks also concur in assigning a hapless status to disabled individuals who would oppose society's negative view of them. The implication is that such individuals act as solitary dissidents who provoke social disapproval or even retaliation with little hope of gain. The conformist majority, in the meantime, is sentenced to the quieter but ceaseless tension between two options: abiding stereotypic ascriptions or asserting personal integrity at the risk of personal harm.

Although the 1970s was a period of increasingly visible disability rights activism, most published disciplinary scholarship on disability began to edge away from forthright social analysis. According to prominent disability studies scholars within social psychology (Fine and Asch 1988; Meyerson 1988), disability research shifted in the decade following the initial publication of Beatrice Wright's (1960) book toward a more impairment-centered, individual coping framework. Increasingly, researchers focused on the impact of impairment on the individual's emotional status and the well-being of his or her significant associates, her or his efforts to compensate for functional loss, and the performance of roles, such as worker, student, or family member, rather than on the contribution of society to the creation of disability problems (Eisenberg, Griggins, and Duval 1982; Fine and Asch 1988). Increasingly, explicit discussion of the social dynamics of disability in academic journals and books yielded, for the most part, to a growing interest in the process of intrapersonal psychological adjustment to disability.

Disability Adjustment as Adaptation to Loss

The disability adjustment literature is voluminous and has been dominated by various stage models describing the individual's progressive adaptation to impairment-related loss, the stated or implicit goal of which is a return to a best approximation of "premorbid" levels of personality adjustment. The typical stages and their corresponding emotional states, such as denial, anger, depression, and acceptance, are still commonly referenced in disability curriculum and rehabilitation practice (see Livneh 1986 for an overview of major stage models). According to this framework, the individual's inner experience of disability can be wretched or tranquil, depending on his or her current level of adaptation and its associated emotional state. The individual's relationship to others is similarly mediated by his or her progress through the stages toward adjustment to disability. An individual who reaches emotional resolution and accepts the losses of disability is well positioned for interpersonal success. The person who denies or rails against the losses of disability is less likely to relate well to others.

After two decades of research designed to validate stage models of disability adaptation, however, there is little clinical or empirical evidence of an orderly or characteristic sequence of reactions to disability. In fact, a summary of empirical and clinical findings on adaptation to illness and disability recently compiled by two leading rehabilitation researchers (Livneh and Antonak 1997) reveals few conclusive results beyond the consistent discovery that emotional distress is a common (but not universal) initial response to disability and that it tends to diminish over time. The researchers report that rehabilitation clinicians and investigators are increasingly turning their interests toward a complex process of adaptation to illness and functional loss, involving changes in the body, body image, self-concept, and interactions between the person and the environment. It is interesting to note, however, that despite this encouraging indication that rehabilitation researchers are focusing more attention on social determinants of disability, Livneh and Antonak (1997) frame the following question as particularly deserving of more investigation: "How are persons with various chronic illnesses and disabilities affected by their conditions?" (p. xv).

Paradoxically, as the focus of research on the disability experience shifted from the external world to the internal emotional life of the individual, research methodology shifted from the subjective toward the objective—away from available experiential accounts toward the operationalization and standardized measurement of constructs such as adjustment. Studies that collected objective data from large numbers of subjects seemed to hold the promise of cross-sample comparison and generalizable conclusions that could not be drawn from small sets of anecdotal records. Standardized procedures beckoned the elimination of subjective bias, including the personal opinions of disabled subjects about their self-esteem and quality of life. Although there were exceptions, the major role of the disabled individual in research changed from key informant to object of study.

Robert Murphy and the Theory of Liminality

In counterpoint to the attenuation of subjectivity in disability research, however, persons with disabilities, empowered by the disability rights and independent living movements, began to accelerate their production and publication of experiential accounts in autobiographies, anthologies, and participatory research reports (Browne, Connors, and Stern 1985; Campling 1981; Carillo, Corbett, and Lewis 1982; Duffy 1981; Zola 1982). In this context, disabled anthropologist Robert Murphy (1990) published *The Body Silent,* his eloquent self-study of the disability experience. Among his many contributions and insights, some of which will be discussed in the next section, he linked the social experience of disability to the anthropological concept, liminality. For Murphy, liminality referred to the marginal status of individuals who have not yet passed a test of full membership in cultures that adhere to a strict progression through rites of passage. Such individuals, Murphy observes, are shut out of the formal social system until they prove worthy of membership. Caught in a transitional state between isolation and social emergence, they do not count as proven citizens of the culture. In a sense, they are sociologically dead and, therefore, considered socially dangerous (Murphy et al. 1988). The apparent solution is for society to sequester them and interact with them in ritualized ways, thus confining such individuals, no matter how successfully autonomous and productive they may become, to the "twilight zones of social indefinition" (Murphy et al. 1988:237).

Murphy argued that "liminality" was a construct superior to "deviance" or "stigma" in describing the disability experience. Whereas the phenomenon of stigmatization is predicated on a static behavioral or physical marker and differentiates little between the experiences of a multiplicity of stigmatized groups, liminality is grounded in cultural symbolism and allows for the processual, shifting nature of socially constructed meanings affecting particular social groups

(Murphy et al. 1988). Furthermore, liminality implies not simply the failure to comply with a cultural standard, such as normality, but a pervasive, indeterminate limbo-like state of being in the world that is "the antiphony of everyday life" (Murphy 1990:135). This pervasive exclusion from ordinary life and denial of full humanity, Murphy believed, aptly characterizes the social experience of disabled people.

EVIDENCE ON THE SOCIAL EXPERIENCE OF DISABILITY

The preceding overview of "classic" theory has surveyed much of what has been *thought* by social scientists in the past half century about the experience of disability. This section examines what has been *discovered* about that experience, particularly with respect to social relations. Evidence from various disciplinary literatures and first-person accounts will be presented and discussed in relation to key components of theory.

Evidence of the Divide

Goffman's (1963) and Davis's (1961) thesis that relations between disabled persons and nondisabled persons are marked by strain, misunderstanding, and disconnection is supported by a wide range of data sources. Authors with disabilities, in particular, commonly treat this idea as a "given" that has been so firmly established by group consensus that it needs no further documentation or support. Robert Murphy (1990) described disability as a "disease of social relations" (p. 4), adding, "Social relations between the disabled and the able bodied are tense, awkward, and problematic. This is something that every handicapped person knows" (p. 86). Throughout his book, he elaborated on this theme. For example, he wrote of feeling a "profound sense of removal" from society, family, and friends; of a mental and physical "quarantine" imposed by society on disabled persons; and of disability leading to "social death."

Summarizing the results of their interviews with disabled persons, Murphy and colleagues reported that "handicapped people of every condition complain that they act as if we were contagious" (Murphy et al. 1988:238), and wheelchair users know that in public places, they are commonly "noticed by everyone and acknowledged by nobody" (p. 239). Studies investigating communications between nondisabled and disabled interactants confirm patterns of avoidance, strain, and depersonalization (Asch 1984). Compared to communication patterns between nondisabled interactants, communication behaviors of nondisabled persons vis-à-vis disabled persons include abbreviated interactions, less eye contact but more staring, less smiling, more indicators of anxiety, more distancing speech patterns, and less information seeking about the other person (Fox and Giles 1996). Listing a variety of avoidant reactions that disabled persons commonly encounter from others, including turning away and ignoring, Adrienne Asch (1988) concluded that "studies of the behavior of the nondisabled toward the disabled demonstrate a variety of responses that, at the very least, hinder ordinary social interaction" (p. 159).

The empirical literature on perceptions of disability also generally supports Wright's (1960) concept of "negative bias" in public and professional attitudes toward disabled people. Nondisabled persons' responses to research measures indicate that they expect disabled people to be socially introverted, unstable, depressed, and hypersensitive (Emry and Wiseman 1987). Australian disability advocate Elizabeth Hastings (1981) lists prejudice as a major feature of the disability experience, evidenced by public expectations that disabled people are dependent and frightened. Such assumptions are resistant to disconfirmation because the public tends to discount as nonrepresentative of their group those disabled persons who behave counter to stereotype (Fox and Giles 1996; Hastings 1981). Studies indicate that nondisabled persons express less willingness to interact with disabled people and impute a lower quality of life to disabled people than do others with disabilities (Albrecht and Devlieger 1999).

Social distancing between disabled and nondisabled persons may be intensified when the disability involves communication (Albrecht, Walker, and Levy 1982) or emotional status (Esses and Beaufoy 1994) or if disabled individuals are perceived as contributing to their own misfortune. In this vein, a study of the multiple components of disability attitudes indicated that attitudes toward persons with depression and persons with AIDS are more negative than attitudes toward amputees (Esses and Beaufoy 1994). The investigators suggest that some of the difference might be caused by attributions of control over the emergence of the disability.

Interpersonal intimacy may be a critical variable in the quality of relationships between disabled and nondisabled persons. Murphy (1990) observed that colleagues who did not know him well before his disability seemed more uncomfortable in his postdisability presence than did his closer friends. However, he acknowledged that many disabled persons experience disturbed interactions with their most intimate associates, even family, and that this can be particularly damaging because family symbolizes refuge and support. Murphy et al. (1988) discussed the gulf between disabled persons and family members who lack knowledge of the social problems of disability, mentioning one informant in their study who preferred being returned to the hospital rather than staying at home because he found his parents' lack of understanding of his disability experience extremely distressful. Other researchers confirm disabled people's frequent experience of estrangement within their families. In writing about the embodied experience of disability, Toombs (1994) observed that strangers may be repelled by persons who use equipment or move awkwardly, but intimate associates who share the disabled person's past "find it hard to adjust to the new self. The relationship has to be redefined, reconstituted" (p. 347). A sense of alienation within the family may be a particularly detrimental aspect of the disability experience for some individuals. According to DeLoach and Greer (1981), the reaction of friends and family to one's disability is significantly related to self-acceptance. Li and Moore (1998) hypothesize that friends' and family members' difficulty in accepting a loved one's disability may help explain why late-onset disability was associated with lower disability acceptance in their study than was congenital disability.

Although some studies suggest that negative disability attitudes may be amenable to the corrective influence of increased contact and familiarity with disabled persons, proximity and length of association may not necessarily engender congruence between insiders' and outsiders' perceptions of disability. Disparate viewpoints often persist despite opportunities for significant contact, not only in families but also among those who choose to affiliate with disabled persons. For example, some rehabilitation experts who have dedicated their lives to working closely with disabled people express the view, frequently disputed by informants with long-term disabilities, that functional limitations necessarily limit enjoyment of life.[2]

Responding to the Divide

In addition to evidence confirming a common social disconnect between disabled and nondisabled persons, there is compelling evidence of disabled people's motivation to bridge the divide. Cahill and Eggleston (1994) studied the experience of wheelchair users in public interactions using participant observation, interviews, and analysis of published autobiographical accounts. The investigators found that such encounters demand a good deal of emotional control from wheelchair users who must not only suppress their own frustration in response to public treatment but also help nondisabled persons manage their discomfort. Belying stereotypical images of disabled persons as weak and dependent, the investigators concluded that wheelchair users shoulder the primary responsibility for positive relations with others. They use humor to put others at ease, tactfully ignore others' lack of tact, respond graciously to others' intrusive curiosity, and routinely sacrifice their interpersonal equality to accept unsolicited help from others who need to feel superior through helping. In short, they expend considerable energy to help nondisabled persons feel positive about interacting with disabled people.

These findings suggest that disabled people work hard to smooth public interactions. The results are less clear in explaining why disabled interactants work so hard. Are they attempting to pass as acceptable to the nondisabled culture they covet, as Goffman (1963) theorizes? Do they wish to convince potential friends that they are, indeed, normal, as Davis (1961) proposes? Cahill and Eggleston (1994) uncovered information that may, at least, help explain why many disabled individuals are reluctant to forego their socially prescribed role and to assert their authentic selves: They have good reason to fear mistreatment. Wheelchair users who refuse help or express indignation over prejudicial treatment risk being identified as "ungrateful, testy, and uncivil" (p. 309). Some encounter threatening public retaliation. Although disabled people who work to keep their relations with the public peaceful often report that they feel torn between their inauthentic public persona and their genuine private feelings, most choose to bear internal stress rather than external confrontation.

To read others' attitudes toward them, disabled persons often develop proficiency in observing and analyzing nonverbal reactions (Hahn 1997). Braithwaite (1990) interviewed 24 visibly disabled adults about their communication encounters with nondisabled people. The participants reported that many nondisabled persons were uncomfortable around them and expressed their distress through such behaviors as fidgeting, lack of eye contact, physical distancing, staring, expressions of sympathy, avoidance, or acting as though the disability does not exist. In response, participants deliberately employed strategies to promote their acceptance, such as talking about "normal things," managing curious questions, and taking control of helping behaviors in ways that signaled their full personhood.

Nonvisible or partially apparent impairments are often associated with additional layers of social tension. British author and activist Sally French's (1993) thoughtful narrative on growing up with "partial sight" discusses disability denial as a systematically learned mechanism of social survival: "By denying the reality of my disability I protected myself from the anxiety, disapproval, frustration and disappointment of the adults in my life" (p. 70). She describes the amount of hard work, discomfort, and self-denial that disabled persons tolerate to assure others that they are just fine. It is particularly difficult for others to grasp ambiguous disabilities, such as partial sight, where help may be needed in unexpected ways despite "normal" appearances. In such cases, disabled individuals may alter their behavior significantly to avoid disappointing or confusing observers, such as French's reluctance to openly read a book in front of strangers who had just watched her use a white cane to cross the road.

Other nonvisible conditions, such as multiple chemical sensitivity/environmental illness (MCS/EI), are associated with a complex of public misunderstandings and attributions that contribute to social estrangement while adding to the inherent difficulties of the impairment. In addition to the stress of managing fluctuating, unpredictable, but debilitating episodes of lost function as well as the vigilance and hard work required to avoid situations that may aggravate functional difficulties, persons with such conditions must address public doubts about the legitimacy of their impairment (Gibson 1993). This may engender feelings of hopelessness, isolation, and self-doubt that widen the gulf between the individual and the social environment. Despite their commitment to narrowing that gulf, disabled people's efforts to ease interactions with others do not always lead to hoped-for connections. Hastings (1981) describes the difficulty of reaching beyond surface relations:

Luckily, disabled people have usually learnt how to set other people at ease and steer them through the rough spots. However, we know that what else is going on in the stranger's mind is harder to deal with, for what is going on is the underlying assumption that we are not as human as they are. (P. 110)

Nonperson Status and Other Ascribed Identities

Hasting's (1981) frank and unsettling remarks prompt a critical question relating to the theories of Goffman, Davis, and Scott: Are disabled persons fated to receive and internalize denigrating identity ascriptions? On the basis of his own disability experience and his observations of others, Murphy (1990) concluded that acquiring a disability typically precipitates the loss of familiar social roles and the assignment of a negative identity, such as social burden, object of charity, perpetual dependent, or quasi-human. Marilyn Phillips's (1990) analysis of personal experience narratives from 33 individuals with physical and sensory impairments led her to conclude that much of her informants' experiences of disability were predicated on the cultural view of disabled persons as "damaged goods," a socially assigned identity that they believed was perpetuated by the media and medical and rehabilitation systems. Some disabled writers suggest that no matter how capable and giving disabled individuals may be, they are likely to be viewed as weak, childlike, suffering, and needy (Karp 1999). Those traits, in turn, are directly linked to the individual's impairment (Olkin 1999). Typecasting based on impairment places disabled persons in a defeating bind. As long as their impairment remains incurable, they become the incurably tragic—the dominant spoiled identity of disability.

The dilemma of identity for disabled people is arguably central to their well-being. Theories of personality development suggest that the harmonious integration of major aspects of an individual's being into a signature identity allows that person to feel whole and valid (Gill 1997; Landau 1998). However, when individuals receive persistent messages that part of them is unacceptable, when others treat them in a manner that dismisses or contradicts who they are, or when they feel compelled to submerge their authentic selves to project a more acceptable image, they experience a sense of disintegration that can thwart self-determination and self-esteem (Gill 1994, 1997). French (1993) describes the impact on her self-image of being expected to appear and function as something she was not—namely, nondisabled:

> The adults would also get very perturbed if ever I looked "abnormal." Being told to open my eyes and straighten my face, when all I was doing was trying to see, made me feel ugly and separate. (P. 69)

Contradictions between personal and public identities are particularly burdensome and damaging to the self-concept. Studies of intellectually gifted young people, for example, indicate that they often feel pressured to conceal their intelligence to avoid being typecast as freaks by other young people. The price of belonging is high. Leading a dual life—smart on the inside, average on the outside—serves to alienate such individuals from everyone, including themselves (Gross 1998).

In certain ways, many disabled persons are forced to lead dual lives. First, they are repeatedly mistaken for something they are not: tragic, heroic, pathetic, not full humans. Persons with a wide range of impairments report extensive experience with such identity misattributions. Second, disabled people must submerge their spontaneous reactions and authentic feelings to smooth over relations with others, from strangers to family members to the personal assistants they rely on to maneuver through each day.

Although the public's presumption of tragic victimhood tends to trump the authentic identities of most disabled people, this dynamic may be even more overwhelming for persons with impairments that affect communication or expression. Lacking a bridge "between inner and outer" (Ruybalid 1999), such individuals may have fewer options to bring their inner experience to the surface, signal their identity to observers, and forestall the tide of stereotype. Persons with nonvisible impairments, on the other hand, are faced with the omnipresent dilemma of deciding when and how much to reveal about their socially "discreditable" status.

There are strong indications, however, that many disabled people are no longer, if they ever were, captive receptors of stigmatized identity. Gelya Frank's (1988) intensive anthropological study of individuals with "congenital limb deficiencies" documented their capacity to critique and oppose the negative attributions that bombarded them on a steady basis during the course of development. Instead of pining for normality or covering their stigma to gain acceptance from others repelled by their differences, her informants openly presented themselves in public activities and forged empowered identities that integrated disability into their sense of autonomy and wholeness. Frank interpreted her findings as a critical challenge to stigma theory.

Studies on the relationship between social categorization and self-concept of persons with developmental disabilities suggest that they, like Frank's informants, can be aware of stigma without inevitably internalizing or even reacting to it (Finlay and Lyons 1998). Interviews with developmentally disabled persons indicate that although they demonstrate awareness of their labels when asked about them, they generally are not likely to describe themselves spontaneously in terms of disability. Although this tendency has been explained by some researchers as an example of psychological defensiveness against stigma or, alternatively, as the result of caregivers' tendencies to shelter disabled individuals from knowledge of their impairment, others suggest that externally imposed labels may simply lack salience and utility for those living inside the experience. Furthermore, social identities based on disability can be viewed as fluid; whether they are accepted or rejected may depend on the social demands of any particular interaction (Rapley, Kiernan, and Antaki 1998). Intellectually disabled persons, like everyone else, encounter a variety of positive experiences that may serve both to nudge disability from a central position in the self-concept and to fortify them against the impact of stereotyping and social devaluation (Mest 1988). Consequently, they may be more likely than outside observers to take for granted that they can have impairments *and* view themselves as whole or ordinary.

Transformation of Values

A pervasive theme in disability research and narrative is the transformative power of the disability experience. Disability generally disrupts the expected life course (Bury 1982) and, as Wright (1960) postulated, prompts a reassessment of norms and values. Reflecting on her own embodied experience of multiple sclerosis, Kay Toombs (1994) theorizes that disability represents "not simply an episode in the life narrative, but rather a major transformation of the narrative" (p. 345) and "a profound transformation of the self" (p. 338).

Preferences and values are not fixed but may differ dramatically between persons in different circumstances or cultures and may shift dramatically for a particular individual depending on alterations in life circumstances. Significant relationships, satisfying roles, and existential or spiritual meaningfulness of experience all serve to help individuals reorganize priorities, relinquish past reference points for normality, and find value in life with disability (Leplege and Hunt 1997; Olkin 1999). Research on life satisfaction of people who encounter functional loss indicates that they find positive meaning in the disability experience and adjust their perceptions and values over time in a manner that accords with their capacities and preserves satisfaction with life as it is (Bach and McDaniel 1993; Bury 1991; McMillen 1999).

This process was supported by a study that compared 325 chronically ill or disabled persons with 504 nondisabled individuals on the task of rating 82 "life values" on the dimensions of "importance" and "attainment" (Montgomery, Persson, and Ryden 1996). Although both groups agreed on the importance of most life values, the disabled participants assigned lower importance to relatively less attainable values involving health and mobility, such as the ability to walk. Stensman (1985) found that persons with mobility disabilities ranked functions such as "to walk" and "get dressed on one's own" as less important than functions related to communicating, thinking, and relating socially. Moreover, their rankings of physical functions were lower than nondisabled persons' rankings of the same functions. Kennisto and Sintonen (1997) found a similar pattern when they compared persons with spinal cord injuries and the general population in the assignment of values to life dimensions. A qualitative investigation of health beliefs of people with physical disabilities suggested that they had come to understand constructs such as health differently from nondisabled persons, de-emphasizing the biological and emphasizing subjective feelings (Watson et al. 1996).

These studies generally support Wright's (1960) conceptualization of value change. In response to permanent disability, individuals stretch the boundaries of what is important to them. They place greater value on areas of life that are open to exploration and that they may have underappreciated before acquiring an impairment. They relinquish or redefine unattainable comparative-status standards, such as normality, that no longer have meaning, and they adopt new goals that fit their lives.

In addition to a transformation of *values*, there is growing evidence that many disabled people undergo a crucial cognitive or *conceptual* transformation. They change the way they understand and think about disability. According to Hahn (1997), a relatively uniform phenomenon across different people is their tendency to view the world differently after disability, leading to insights and understandings about major life experiences that differ from the views of nondisabled peers. Arthur Frank (1991, 1995) has written eloquently about the growing number of individuals who experience chronic conditions in a way that has transformed their worldview, in that they develop a keener perception of life's details and a fuller understanding of the common human experience. This transformation becomes an essential part of their identity and connects them to others with similar experiences.

Increasingly, persons with disabilities from various backgrounds are learning to think about disability as a social justice issue rather than as a category of individual deficiency. Surveys indicate that disabled Americans who are young enough to have been influenced by the disability rights movement are more likely than their older counterparts to identify as members of a minority group—namely, the disability community (Longmore 1995a, 1995b). Many disabled individuals discover and adopt a social model framework both to conceptualize their own problems and to relate them to the problems of all disabled people as a socially oppressed group. This conceptual shift leads, in turn, to a critical shift in how they view themselves (Gill 1994, 1997). The informants in Phillips's (1990) study, for example, reported experiencing an emancipatory impact on self-image of adopting social philosophies of disability. Their belief in social minority status was associated with their rejection of stigmatized status. The investigator observed that they had begun to disavow the desirability of normalization while affirmatively embracing "difference" in place of "deviance" (Phillips 1985).

Deindividualizing the problems of disability and learning to understand the social determinants of their devalued status reinforce disabled people's tendency to feel valid and whole as they are. Applying Wright's (1960) terminology to disability identity, these developments support disabled people's efforts to "contain" impairment-related social devaluation and to prevent its "spread" to the entirety of their identities. These paradigmatic shifts in understanding disability also pave the way to identifying with other disabled people and entering into collective action against unjust attitudes and practices. In addition to mobilizing for political change, people with disabilities are organizing to set the record straight about who they are collectively. They are broadcasting their identities by developing and implementing far-reaching disability awareness education, excavating and celebrating disability history, engaging in media activism, and writing articles, books, plays, and television scripts about the disability experience. Most affirmatively, they are declaring positive identity through disability pride and disability cultural activities, including projects focusing on the peer mentoring of young disabled people.

DISCUSSION OF THE EVIDENCE

Multiple sources of evidence about the disability experience confirm the prevalence of a disturbing division of understanding between disabled people and nondisabled people in the world of social relations. In effect, many disabled persons spend much of their lives grappling with a sense of mistaken identity that dominates and diminishes their experience. Disabled people are aware of this; they write about it, talk about it, and regret it deeply. Simply stated, they want acknowledgment of who they are, and they seek this from family, acquaintances, and strangers on the street. When, instead, they repeatedly intercept entrenched misconstruals of who they are and what it means to be disabled, they swing into action to correct the wrong impressions and to reestablish their identities. They wage an exhausting struggle to be known. The stakes are high, for how can they be accepted for who they are unless they are knowable as they are?

Caught in the "Twilight Zone"

Although they know themselves to be full participants in the human community, with strengths, desires, foibles, and triumphs common to all people, disabled persons are typically viewed as existing outside the boundaries of common human experience. Like the protagonist in a science fiction story who is erroneously pronounced missing or dead because others cannot detect vital signs of his or her existence, many disabled persons contest vigorously the dismissal of their personhood. Sources reviewed in this chapter indicate that disabled people use much of their finite supply of energy and skills to signal their presence, their viability, and their humanity to those around them, yet in the social limbo that Murphy calls the "twilight zone" (Murphy et al. 1988:237), they may remain eerily unrecognized. In sum, a core element of the experience of disability is being seen as something you are not, joined with the realization that what you are remains invisible.

Arguably, in addition to psychological and social stress, the public's misreading of the disability experience contributes to disabled people's well-documented struggles with employment discrimination, educational segregation, and environmental barriers. A tragic victim, after all, is not likely to be considered a strong job candidate, a capable learner, a wise consumer, or an equal citizen of the community. Furthermore, the attribution of victimhood to disabled persons separates them from the greater social fabric that they want and expect to remain part of, notwithstanding their differences from social norms. Sufferers, however noble, are not likely to be welcomed as helpful neighbors, reliable friends, desired lovers, or competent parents or spouses.

Differences from Other Minority Groups

The dilemma of disabled people's mistaken identity may seem at first no different from the social stereotyping of other marginalized groups. Although all forms of intergroup misperception may share common elements, four distinguishing features of the disability experience are noteworthy.

Public misperceptions of disabled people are embedded in a confusing mix of conflicting positive and negative emotions. Because open devaluation of disabled people would collide with prevailing values of protection and charity toward the afflicted (Murphy et al. 1988; Roth 1983), the public's negative disability attitudes may be projected through a confusing blend of emotions, including admiration and nurturance. Consequently, disability prejudice is seldom expressed overtly in the way racial bigotry or antigay views are communicated (Hahn 1997). Nonetheless, paternalism taints relations between nondisabled and disabled people and reinforces the inferior position of the latter (Roth 1983).

In contrast to race and gender, negative ascriptions based on disability can be superficially linked to "real" human differences. Impairment-related problems, such as pain and troubling limitation, are part of the disability experience for many individuals and cannot be reduced to social construction. When such difficulties are overgeneralized or interpreted in isolation from other aspects of the individual's life, however, they evoke a distorted wholesale disparagement of the disability experience (Asch 1998).

Disabled people's problem of mistaken identity pervades sancta where most marginalized groups can expect to be understood. In contrast to racial/ethnic minority group members who generally share their marginalized status and experience with relatives, many disabled people feel isolated and typecast within their own families. Similarly, minority communities and progressive political groups are not necessarily shelters from oppression for disabled people. Disabled persons of color and disabled gay people, in fact, have reported marginalization within all of their minority communities: ethnic/racial, gay/lesbian/bisexual/transgender, and disability (Tsao 1998; Vernon 1998). Women with disabilities have reported that many progressive women's groups who organize aggressively against racism, sexism, homophobia, and seemingly all dimensions of oppression nonetheless openly convey defamatory views of life with disability (Klein 1997; Morris 1991).

Unless they have developed a political or cultural consciousness that centralizes difference, most disabled people identify as typical. Disabled people generally lack preparation to be continually conscious of minority status and its life consequences in the way that growing up in a marginalized racial/ethnic community informs community members about racism. Moreover, most disabled people think of themselves as ordinary because impairments recede in importance as they are integrated into daily routines. Disabled psychologist Rhoda Olkin (1999) expresses this orientation when she says, "In our world abnormal *is* normal" (p. vii). It can be repeatedly jolting for individuals who identify as ordinary to be persistently categorized as extraordinary or pathetic by those whom they regard as peers, even intimates.

These four points underscore the ambiguity and isolation that pervade the social experience of disabled people. Like other marginalized people, they are targets of negative and inaccurate ascriptions. In contrast to other minority groups, however, they have few guideposts to define their social treatment and few supports to oppose it. They rarely encounter the clarity of contempt associated with racism and homophobia because others consciously suppress that sentiment, harbor mixed feelings, or both. Furthermore, disability ascriptions are not as clearly lacking foundation as they are for other marginalized groups because although it is true that disabled persons are not defined by their impairments, their impairments can be quite salient. It is more difficult to refute a distortion of fact than an outright fiction. Finally, in contrast to members of other minority communities, it is hard for disabled persons to grasp their dilemma because it is often perpetrated even by the persons with whom they identify and from whom they expect affirmation, not dismissal: family members, contemporaries, and fellow seekers of justice.

To be irrationally disdained by others, to feel it every day of your life, and to share that experience with both intimates and a substantial community are clearly horrible. That is the reported social experience of many minority people in encounters with the dominant culture. On the other hand, to be silently, smilingly dismissed as someone pathetic and strange and encounter dismissal even in cultural milieux you call your own is confusing and dispiriting. That is the standard social experience of disabled people in the nondisabled world they inhabit.

Suggested Directions for Inquiry

From all accounts, the problem of relations between the disabled and nondisabled worlds is not a small rift of communications but a deep divide. It encompasses both intellectual and affective components, in that it is based on *misconceptions* about the experience of disability and conflicting *values* between disabled and nondisabled peoples about what constitutes a worthy life. If the experience of disability transforms people, its social and functional presses make them different from most people who do not experience disability differently in their fundamental understandings about human difference and associated values. It will take more than an adjustment of expectations, sensitivity pointers, or a more tolerant attitude from either side to bridge this gap. It will take an honest appraisal of the problem, including its gravity, scope, and complexity, and it must start with a more coherent grasp of what is known and what needs investigation.

Subjectivity

For future research to be useful, investigators will need to invite, not dismiss, the perspective of those who experience disability. Although it may seem absurd that anyone would need to argue on behalf of subjectivity in research on the disability experience, there are indicators that this recommendation needs articulation. In discussing the lack of progress in empirical work on disability adaptation, for example, rehabilitation researchers Livneh and Antonak (1997) call for more psychometrically sound operationalized measures that correspond to the researcher's conceptualization of key constructs while minimizing "respondent reactivity." They list strategies for bypassing the "biasing" effects of subject response style and sensitization, including the use of concealed observation, the use of deception about the purpose of the measures, and the adoption of physiologic measures in which the subject is an "inactive participant" (p. 451).

British disability studies scholar and activist Michael Oliver has criticized past sociological work on stigma for remaining too far removed from the lived experience of people with disabilities (cited in Rapley et al. 1998). Braithwaite (1990) reports that most previous research on communication between disabled and nondisabled persons has been limited because it was conducted exclusively from the perspective of nondisabled persons. Murphy et al. (1988) call for the analysis of disability as a symbolic system that, they assert, has been neglected partly because the perspectives of disabled people have been omitted. A number of researchers, many of them disabled persons, link the exclusion of the disability perspective to the dominance of the medical model in guiding research design (Asch 1998; Murphy et al. 1988; Reindal 1995, 2000; Toombs 1994). Murphy et al. conclude that the meanings of disability must be seen as culturally and historically changing rather than fixed in biology:

> Such a new freedom of attitude is a precondition for the manumission of the disabled from the misunderstandings of their situation held by the public, by health professionals, and even by themselves. (P. 242)

The value of subjective measures lies in tapping new information about the experience of disability and in respecting the power of the disability voice, but such measures are often criticized when they conflict with conventional judgment (Brown and Vandergoot 1998). Asch (1998), for example, discussed a research report in which the investigators virtually discredited positive assessments of health-related quality of life reported by disabled persons (Tyson and Broyles 1996, cited in Asch 1998). Their responses were interpreted as "inflated" or influenced by denial, a skepticism that was not extended to the positive assessments of nondisabled subjects. Brown and Vandergoot (1998) found that subjective quality-of-life judgments might diverge considerably from external measures. For examples, persons with "severe" brain injuries tend to rate quality of life more favorably than do those with less extensive impairments. This relationship contradicts conventional wisdom predicting a positive association between functional status and life quality. An explanation offered to explain the findings is that persons with greater cognitive impairment may be less aware of changes in pre- versus postdisability functioning. This naïveté argument, however, fails to account for similar findings for other disability groups (Gill forthcoming).

It should be noted that the tide seems to be turning and that calls for participatory research are emerging in many fields. Rapley et al. (1998) report that anthropology and sociology have turned to qualitative methods and have accepted the primacy of lay knowledge, beliefs, and experience for informing researchers about embodiment. In an article recently appearing in the *Journal of the American Medical Association,* Leplege and Hunt (1997) point out that standard research and survey questionnaires, such as quality-of-life measures, may not capture critical elements of disabled persons' experience and the meanings they attach to their experience. Regardless of their impeccable psychometric properties, the authors warn, measures that force the respondent to choose between alternatives that reflect not her or his actual experience but rather the professional's framework for organizing that experience may inhibit the full discovery of critical information.

In privileging the disability voice, however, researchers must realize that the disability experience warrants multiple and complex representation. The experiences of disabled persons with intersecting minority identities predicated on race, gender, sexuality, and age must be included in efforts to expand theory and empirical knowledge in this area.

Investigating the Resisters

An aspect of the disability experience that has received little attention is the decision of many disabled persons to renounce the struggle for acknowledgment and acceptance from others who consistently fail to understand them. The recognition of others' mistaken perceptions of them and their resistance to the negative views surrounding them is a common theme in disabled people's accounts. For example, in a recent report of qualitative research on disabled persons' perceived quality of life (Albrecht and Devlieger 1999), the following compelling statements from three informants appeared in just the brief transcript selections presented in the Results section:

I don't care what others think when they see me. I live my own life and can do about anything. If I can do it, then what's the difference? (P. 982)

People look at me with my chronic obstructive pulmonary disease and think what a poor bastard. I'm glad I'm not in his shoes. They don't understand. Visually, you see an oxygen bottle, impairments and limits, but the spirit is boundless. (P. 983)

Other people can't understand why I am so happy. They don't have the same appreciation of life. (P. 983)

These sentiments ring with a timber reminiscent of statements found throughout disability narratives, such as the spontaneous statement of a participant in Phillips's (1985) study, "There is nothing *wrong* with me!" (pp. 48-49), and radio/television journalist John Hockenberry's (1995) declaration, "You must accept me as I see myself." Concepts such as disability pride and culture, once controversial, are becoming mundane elements of the disability lexicon.

Although Goffman and Davis barely noted them in the 1960s, stigma resisters are a rapidly expanding breed that commands interest. How do they think about concepts such as disability and normality as they construct identity? What facilitates their disengagement from reigning cultural values and their adoption of alternative values, particularly regarding productivity, independence, and beauty? How do they avoid succumbing to isolation? What factors encourage or impede their affiliation with other disabled persons? What are the benefits of such affiliation? Are there core disability values or worldviews? Is there a disability culture? Hahn (1997) points out that disabled people have demonstrated remarkable strength and achievement in the face of environmental obstacles and social exclusion. He suggests that rather than conceptualizing disability as a case of loss, those who seek to understand disability should view it as an identity and as an experience that can engender creativity and an enhanced appreciation of commonly neglected aspects of everyday life. There is undoubtedly a wealth of information about values change, identity construction, resilience, and empowerment to be learned from those who decide they are valid and whole citizens of the human community despite failing society's yardstick for functional and aesthetic acceptability.

Positive Relationships

Little is known about disabled people's positive relationship experiences (Asch 1984). Despite the negative trends in the literature, many disabled persons have enjoyed salutary connections with nondisabled family members, friends, intimate partners, health professionals, and employers. In their narratives, disabled individuals describe key allies in their lives who seem devoid of disability prejudice but who know and despise it when they see it. They make the effort to learn who their disabled associates are in their full glory and their full ordinariness. In disability cultural parlance, these nondisabled friends and relatives are the ones who "get it."

These relationships raise intriguing questions about disability and intergroup relations. What qualities of the individuals, social networks, and the interaction itself are important for sustaining such connections, bridging differences, and moving relationships beyond superficial acceptance? What are the defining features of genuine allies to the disability community? How are they found or developed?

The Place of Impairment in the Social Experience of Disability

By honoring subjectivity and remaining closer to the experience of disabled persons in their research, disability studies scholars cannot escape the realization that bodies matter. Whether grappling with pain and the unwanted limitations of impairment or reveling in the carnal expression of cultural aesthetic subversion, the disability experience is undeniably embodied (Hughes and Paterson 1997). A series of provocative articles and Internet discussions among disability studies scholars continue to criticize not only the traditional medical and rehabilitation models of disability but also the newer hegemony of the impairment (biological) versus disability (social oppression) binary.

Future research on the social experience of disability should examine impairment-related factors such as visibility, type of impairment (including those affecting communication, expression, control of movement), preventability, and age of acquisition in influencing public perceptions, attributions, and social interaction. The manner in which individuals process and incorporate their experience of impairment into public and personal identities and expressions of pride is also a promising area for exploration.

CONCLUDING THOUGHTS

As disabled people warm to concepts such as disability identity, pride, and culture, they are reconstructing values about deviance and actively exploring rather than subordinating their interest in "physique." They are exiting liminal twilight zones by conjuring new rituals of validation, and they are taking their bodies with them. They are building connections to each other purposefully—not merely clustering with costigmatized peers by default—exchanging fresh ideas and patinated stories as well as continuing political goals. Graciously, they are sending word of this out to the larger world as they go. Still working hard to be known, they continue to forge bridges in all directions: to the nondisabled world, to each other, and to the self.

NOTES

1. Although some psychoanalytic theorists acknowledged the importance of social environment in mediating the psychological hazards of physical difference, they emphasized a direct link between functional impairment and impairment of the self. For example, in his discussion of "organ inferiority," Alfred Adler (1917) explained, "The possession of definitely inferior organs is reflected upon the psyche—and in such a way as to lower the self-esteem" (p. 3).

2. Henry Betts (2000), acknowledged by many as the preeminent pioneer in rehabilitation medicine, recently defined disability as "a term used to describe people who have a physical or mental impairment that interferes with their ability to lead a happy, productive life" (p. 218). Frederic Kottke, a prominent rehabilitation clinician and textbook author, stated, "The disabled patient has a greater problem in achieving a satisfactory quality of life. He has lost, or possibly never had, the physical capacity for the necessary responses to establish and maintain the relationships, interactions, and participation that healthy persons have" (Kottke 1982:60).

REFERENCES

Adler, A. 1917. *The Neurotic Constitution.* New York: Moffat, Yard.

Albrecht, G. L. and P. J. Devlieger. 1999. "The Disability Paradox: High Quality of Life against All Odds." *Social Science & Medicine* 48:977-88.

Albrecht, G. L., V. Walker, and J. Levy. 1982. "Social Distance from the Stigmatized: A Test of Two Theories." *Social Science and Medicine* 16:1319-27.

Asch, A. 1984. "The Experience of Disability: A Challenge for Psychology." *American Psychologist* 39:529-36.

———. 1988. "Disability: Its Place in the Psychology Curriculum." Pp. 156-67 in *Teaching a Psychology of People,* edited by P. A. Bronstein and K. Quina. Washington, DC: American Psychological Association.

———. 1998. "Distracted by Disability." *Cambridge Quarterly of Healthcare Ethics* 7:77-87.

Bach, C. A. and R. W. McDaniel. 1993. "Quality of Life in Quadriplegic Adults: A Focus Group Study." *Rehabilitation Nursing* 18:364-67.

Betts, H. B. 2000. "Disabled." *World Book Encyclopedia*. Vol. 5. Chicago: World Book.

Braithwaite, D. O. 1990. "From Majority to Minority: An Analysis of Cultural Change from Ablebodied to Disabled." *International Journal of Intercultural Relations* 14:465-83.

Brown, M. and D. Vandergoot. 1998. "Quality of Life for Individuals with Traumatic Brain Injury: Comparison with Others Living in the Community." *Journal of Head Trauma Rehabilitation* 13:1-23.

Browne, S. E., D. Connors, and N. Stern, eds. 1985. *With the Power of Each Breath: A Disabled Women's Anthology*. Pittsburgh, PA: Cleis.

Bury, M. R. 1982. "Chronic Illness as Biographical Disruption." *Sociology of Health and Illness* 4:167-82.

———. 1991. "The Sociology of Chronic Illness." *Sociology of Health and Illness* 13:451-68.

Cahill, S. A. and R. Eggleston. 1994. "Managing Emotions in Public: The Case of Wheelchair Users." *Social Psychology Quarterly* 57:300-12.

Campling, J. 1981. *Images of Ourselves: Women with Disabilities Talking*. London: Routledge Kegan Paul.

Carillo, A. C., K. Corbett, and V. Lewis, eds. 1982. *No More Stares*. Berkeley, CA: Disability Rights Education and Defense Fund.

Davis, F. 1961. "Deviance Disavowal: The Management of Strained Interaction by the Visibly Handicapped." *Social Problems* 9:120-32.

DeLoach, C. and B. G. Greer. 1981. *Adjustment to Severe Physical Disability: A Metamorphosis*. New York: McGraw-Hill.

Dembo, T., G. L. Leviton, and B. A. Wright. 1956. "Adjustment to Misfortune: A Problem of Social-Psychological Rehabilitation." *Artificial Limbs* 3:4-62. (Reprinted in 1975 in *Rehabilitation Psychology* 22:1-100.)

Duffy, Y. 1981. *All Things Are Possible*. Ann Arbor, MI: A. J. Gavin.

Eisenberg, M., C. Griggins, and R. Duval, eds. 1982. *Disabled People as Second Class Citizens*. New York: Springer.

Emry, R. and R. L. Wiseman. 1987. "An Intercultural Understanding of Ablebodied and Disabled Person's Communication." *International Journal of Intercultural Relations* 11:7-27.

Esses, V. M. and S. L. Beaufoy. 1994. "Determinants of Attitudes toward People with Disabilities." *Journal of Social Behavior and Personality* 9:43-64.

Fine, M. and A. Asch. 1988. "Disability beyond Stigma: Social Interaction, Discrimination, and Activism." *Journal of Social Issues* 44:3-21.

Finlay, M. and E. Lyons. 1998. "Social Identity and People with Learning Difficulties: Implications for Self-Advocacy Groups." *Disability & Society* 13:37-51.

Fox, S. A. and H. Giles. 1996. "Interability Communication: Evaluating Patronizing Encounters." *Journal of Language and Social Psychology* 18:265-90.

Frank, A. W. 1991. *At the Will of the Body: Reflections on Illness*. Boston: Houghton Mifflin.

———. 1995. *The Wounded Storyteller: Body, Illness, and Ethics*. Chicago: University of Illinois Press.

Frank, G. 1988. "Beyond Stigma: Visibility and Self-Empowerment of Persons with Congenital Limb Deficiencies." *Journal of Social Issues* 44:95-115.

French, S. 1993. " 'Can You See the Rainbow?': The Roots of Denial." Pp. 89-77 in *Disabling Barriers—Enabling Environments,* edited by J. Swain, V. Finkelstein, S. French, and M. Oliver. Newbury Park, CA: Sage.

Gibson, P. R. 1993. "Environmental Illness/Multiple Chemical Sensitivities: Invisible Disabilities." *Women & Therapy* 14:171-85.

Gill, C. J. 1994. "A Bicultural Framework for Understanding Disability and Family." *Family Psychologist* 10 (4): 13-16.

———. 1997. "Four Types of Integration in Disability Identity Development." *Journal of Vocational Rehabilitation* 9:39-46.

———. Forthcoming. "Health Professionals, Disability, and Assisted Suicide: An Examination of Empirical Evidence." *Psychology, Public Policy and the Law.*

Goffman, E. 1963. *Stigma: Notes on the Management of Spoiled Identity.* Englewood Cliffs, NJ: Prentice Hall.

Gross, M. U. 1998. "The 'Me' behind the Mask: Intellectually Gifted Students and the Search for Identity." *Roeper Review* 20:167-74.

Hahn, H. 1997. "An Agenda for Citizens with Disabilities: Pursuing Identity and Empowerment." *Journal of Vocational Rehabilitation* 9:31-37.

Hastings, E. 1981. "The Experience of Disability." *Australian Journal of Developmental Disabilities* 7:107-12.

Hockenberry, J. 1995. *Moving Violations: War Zones, Wheelchairs, and Declarations of Independence.* New York: Hyperion.

Hughes, B. and K. Paterson. 1997. "The Social Model of Disability and the Disappearing Body: Towards a Sociology of Impairment." *Disability & Society* 12:325-40.

Karp, G. 1999. *Life on Wheels: For the Active Wheelchair User.* Sebastopol, CA: O'Reilly.

Kennisto, M. and H. Sintonen. 1997. "Later Health-Related Quality of Life in Adults Who Have Sustained Spinal Cord Injury in Childhood." *Spinal Cord* 35 (11): 747-51.

Klein, B. S. (with P. Blackbridge) 1997. *Slow Dance: A Story of Stroke, Love, and Disability.* Berkeley, CA: Page Mill.

Kottke, F. J. 1982. "Philosophic Considerations of Quality of Life for the Disabled." *Archives of Physical Medicine and Rehabilitation* 63:60-62.

Landau, E. 1998. "The Self—The Global Factor of Emotional Maturity." *Roeper Review* 20:174-78.

Leplege, A. and S. Hunt. 1997. "The Problem of Quality of Life in Medicine." *Journal of the American Medical Association* 278:47-50.

Li, L. and D. Moore. 1998. "Acceptance of Disability and Its Correlates." *Journal of School Psychology* 138:13-25.

Livneh, H. 1986. "A Unified Approach to Existing Models of Adaptation to Disability. Part I—A Model Adaptation." *Journal of Applied Rehabilitation Counseling* 17:5-16.

Livneh, H. and R. F. Antonak, eds. 1997. *Psychososcial Adaptation to Chronic Illness.* Gaithersburg, MD: Aspen.

Longmore, P. K. 1995a. "Medical Decision Making and People with Disabilities: A Clash of Cultures." *Journal of Law, Medicine & Ethics* 23:82-87.

———. 1995b. "The Second Phase: From Disability Rights to Disability Culture." *Disability Rag* (September/October): 4-11.

McMillen, J. C. 1999. "Better for It: How People Benefit from Adversity." *Social Work* 44:455-68.

Mest, G. M. 1988. "With a Little Help from My Friends: Use of Social Support Systems by Persons Retardation." *Journal of Social Issues* 44:117-25.

Meyerson, L. 1988. "The Social Psychology of Physical Disability: 1948 and 1988." *Journal of Social Issues* 44:173-88.

Montgomery, H., L. O. Persson, and A. Ryden. 1996. "Importance and Attainment of Life Values among Disabled and Non-Disabled People." *Scandinavian Journal of Rehabilitation Medicine* 30 (4): 233-40.

Morris, J. 1991. *Pride against Prejudice.* Philadelphia: New Society.

Murphy, R. F. 1990. *The Body Silent.* New York: Norton.

Murphy, R. F., J. Scheer, Y. Murphy, and R. Mack. 1988. "Physical Disability and Social Liminality: A Study in the Rituals of Adversity." *Social Science & Medicine* 26:235-42.

Olkin, R. 1999. *What Psychotherapists Should Know about Disability.* New York: Guilford.

Phillips, M. J. 1985. " 'Try Harder': The Experience of Disability and the Dilemma of Normalization." *The Social Science Journal* 22:45-57.

———. 1990. "Damaged Goods: Oral Narratives of the Experience of Disability in American Culture." *Social Science and Medicine* 30:849-57.

Rapley, M., P. Kiernan, and C. Antaki. 1998. "Invisible to Themselves or Negotiating Identity? The Interactional Management of 'Being Intellectually Disabled.' " *Disability & Society* 13:807-27.

Reindal, S. M. 1995. "Discussing Disability: An Investigation into Theories of Disability." *European Journal of Special Needs Education* 10:58-69.

———. 2000. "Disability, Gene Therapy and Eugenics: A Challenge to John Harris." *Journal of Medical Ethics* 26:89-94.

Roth, W. 1983. "Handicap as a Social Construct." *Society* 20:59-60.

Ruybalid, M. 1999. *Daring to Write.* Huntington, WV: University Editions.

Scott, R. A. 1969. *The Making of Blind Men.* New York: Russell Sage.

Stensman, R. 1985. "Severely Mobility-Disabled People Assess the Quality of Their Lives." *Scandinavian Journal of Rehabilitation Medicine* 17:87-99.

Toombs, S. K. 1994. "Disability and the Self." Pp. 337-57 in *Changing the Self: Philosophies, Techniques, and Experiences,* edited by T. M. Brinthaupt and Richard P. Lipka. Albany: State University of New York Press.

Tsao, G. 1998. *Growing Up Asian American with a Disability* [Online]. Available: www.rehab.uiuc.edu/archive/ss/9899/growing.html.

Tyson, J. E. and R. S. Broyles. 1996. "Progress in Assessing the Long-Term Outcome of Extremely Low Birthweight Infants." *Journal of the American Medical Association* 276:492-93.

Vernon, A. 1998. "Multiple Oppression and the Disabled People's Movement." Pp. 201-10 in *The Disability Reader,* edited by T. Shakespeare. London: Cassell.

Watson, J., S. Cunningham-Burley, N. Watson, and K. Milburn. 1996. "Lay Theorizing about 'the Body' and Implications for Health Promotion." *Health Education Research* 11:161-72.

Wright, B. A. 1960. *Physical Disability: A Psychological Approach.* New York: Harper & Row.

———. 1983. *Physical Disability: A Psychosocial Approach.* New York: Harper & Row.

Zola, I. K. 1982. *Missing Pieces: A Chronicle of Living with a Disability.* Philadelphia: Temple University Press.

Mapping the Family

14

Disability Studies and the Exploration of Parental Response to Disability

PHILIP M. FERGUSON

Imagine Eric and his family for a moment. Eric is eight years old, has a bright smile and an active curiosity, and finds it hard to sit still for very long. He sometimes has trouble following directions and is beginning to throw temper tantrums, according to his parents. Oh yes, Eric has Down syndrome. Now, imagine Eric and his family in three different years: 1950, 1980, and 2010. How might the scenarios differ even if Eric stays the same?

In 1950, one can imagine Eric's parents facing the daunting task of finding an educational program of any kind for Eric and other "Mongoloid" children. Like many families in this era, Eric's parents are often encouraged, even pressured, to institutionalize Eric. They are warned of the dangers that Eric poses to the healthy development of his nondisabled brothers and sisters and are offered psychological counseling to cope with their tragedy. Even other parents themselves are publishing such advice:

> The inability of many parents to commit hopelessly retarded children to institutional care has created untold social problems, particularly in families where there are other, normal children. The family that is fortunate is the one in which the parents eventually recognize the hardships to which they are subjecting themselves and their child, and have the courage and the opportunity to commit the child to an institution. ("When a Child Is Different" [1951] 1969:89)

To start the town's first early intervention program in the basement of the local church, Eric's parents had to go door-to-door to find other families with similarly disabled children. Now that Eric is school age, the family is again facing some stark choices. Some schools have "ungraded classes," but the children in those classrooms are labeled "educable mentally retarded." Eric's level of intellectual disability is thought to be more severe. He falls into the range of so-called trainable mental retardation, and the local school system chooses not to serve these children. For Eric's family, the choices seem to be the state institution with its dubious commitment to education or a gradually expanded preschool program that seems be evolving into a self-contained school.

Move to 1980. Things look different for Eric and his family. Eric still has the bright smile and other traits, but his parents hear the term *mongolism* less and less often. A federal law enacted five years earlier mandated a free, appropriate public education for Eric and all other disabled children in something referred to as "the least restrictive environment." Eric's parents are told that means a self-contained class in an elementary school. Rather than run their own program in a church basement, Eric's parents are part of a planning team that includes a variety of special educators and therapists as well as a director of special education. They are asked to participate in a "parent training" program to teach them the basics of "behavior modification" and help them cope with the practical demands of their tragedy.

Various model intervention programs have been established with accompanying parent involvement training components. The need is especially obvious in infant and preschool programs, where it has been shown that parent application of instructional technologies can aid in the improvement of certain developmental deficits. . . . Moreover, improvement has been not only in relation to student-centered variables, but family adjustment problems have been ameliorated as well, with corresponding facilitation toward normalization. (Sternberg and Caldwell 1982:27)

Each of Eric's therapists at his school provide a detailed home program for the parents, along with data sheets for the parents to complete and turn in weekly to track Eric's performance. Eric's school is located in a nearby city, not his hometown, and he rides the "short bus" to school with the other "handicapped" children.

Now jump to the year 2010. Let's be realistically optimistic and imagine that this first decade of the new millennium has brought a host of changes for Eric and his family. Eric's smile seems brighter than ever. He attends school a few blocks from home with other children from his neighborhood. Eric's family has worked closely with the school principal and classroom teachers to arrange a system of supports and educational strategies. Eric spends most of his day in the general classroom along with his friends (disabled and nondisabled) from the neighborhood. The teachers all have high expectations for the diverse group of students in Eric's class. Eric now has an official label of "intellectual disability," but most often the teachers just speak of him as one of their third-grade students. Eric's parents both work, but the school finds ways to connect with them and other families in the community. Eric's parents have joined an advocacy group of parents and adults with disabilities and take pride in their membership within the disability community. They find themselves echoing the sentiments expressed by another parent of a child with Down syndrome almost 15 years earlier:

My job, for now, is to represent my son, to set his place at our collective table. But I know I am merely trying my best to prepare for the day he sets his own place. For I have no sweeter dream than to imagine—aesthetically and ethically and parentally—that Jamie will someday be his own advocate, his own author, his own best representative. (Bérubé 1996:264)

Why create these three vignettes? Certainly, I hope the stories suggest how much things have changed over the past half century or so in the way we think and talk about children with disabilities and their families. Society in general, especially the community of educators and parents, thinks very differently about disabilities than was true even 10 years ago, much less 50 years or more. The vignettes could have shown equal variation by moving across cultures rather than decades. Whether looking at the same society at different times or at different cultures at the same time, the variation in social response to disability and family can be dramatic. However, as important as the extent and substance of the differences themselves, what I also want to emphasize is the constancy of the change itself. The futility of searching for some singular profile of *the* family of a child with a disability emerges forcefully in even the most cursory review of how drastically policies and practices have evolved over a few generations or a few cultures.

As the vignettes about Eric illustrate, then, interactions between families and professionals always occur within a social and historical context. The linkages that doctors, therapists, and educators try to establish with families inevitably reflect assumptions about the nature of family life itself. These assumptions, in turn, are at least partially shaped by what the research says about how families respond to disability. One indicator of the rapid growth of disability studies is how unsurprising this contextual claim now seems. It is commonplace now to argue that a family's reactions to having a child with a disability are inescapably embedded within a sociohistorical context. As with all human endeavor, how a family interprets the meaning of disability cannot help but reflect to some degree the larger context of social attitudes and historical realities within which that interpretations emerges.

Research on families of children with disabilities does not escape this context of assumptions and perspectives specific to a given time and place. It should come as no surprise, then, that the implicit and explicit assumptions that have guided family research in the past primarily reflect the social and historical context within which that research was conducted. This is not surprising unless one assumes that the influence of cultural values and social policy somehow stops at the door of the diagnostic lab. Family research has found its place within the emerging perspective of disability studies by increasingly accepting the assumption that it is not a specific set of parental reactions to disability that is inevitable but the influence of social contexts in shaping those reactions.

In what Anthony Giddens (1984) has called the "double hermeneutic" that is intrinsic to the social sciences, family researchers try to interpret the interpretations of families. They are, in a sense, domestic geographers, mapping the territory in which parents and children locate themselves.

It is precisely this shared activity of "map making" that ties both family and researcher to a specific time and place. They share a cultural terrain whose boundaries of meaning and myth change just as disability itself is always being redefined. With that in mind, what follows is not really a summary of a steadily expanding knowledge base about parents, children, and disability. I would rather characterize it as a conceptual atlas of disputed territory, showing how the landscape of family research has changed over time and with some interpretation of where the roads to the future seem to be heading.

This chapter has four major sections. First, I will provide an all-too-sketchy account of how professionals and researchers have portrayed families of children with disabilities over the past 200 years or so in Europe and North America. Next, I present a conceptual matrix that helps organize and locate some of these major interpretive approaches. Third, I discuss the relatively recent attempts to both widen and deepen the exploration of family responses to disabilities. Finally, I will provide a somewhat speculative synthesis of how family research will find its place within this emerging field of disability studies. Specifically, I will argue that the intersection of social history and social psychology is leading us down some promising lines of theory development and research agendas.

MAPPING THE PAST: A HISTORY OF PROFESSIONAL PROFILES OF FAMILIES AND DISABILITY

The vignettes imagining the social context of policies and practices surrounding Eric and his family over the past 50 years or so emphasized how substantially things have changed in that relatively short span of time. These changes become even more impressive when one looks at them within a much wider historical focus. When one takes a longer historical view, the changes in North American society since the 1970s seem strikingly sudden and dramatic. What this longer view also uncovers, however, is a professional approach to parents that seems remarkable for its persistent pessimism rather than the incremental optimism of the past few decades.

Approximately 10 years ago, my colleague Adrienne Asch and I began a review of the published narratives written by parents and persons with disabilities with what struck us as some simple truths. "The most important thing that happens when a child with disabilities is born is that a child is born. The most important thing that happens when a couple becomes parents of a child with disabilities is that a couple becomes parents" (Ferguson and Asch 1989:108). However, a review of the history of professional responses to the birth of such a child shows patterns of research and practice that have, until recently, assumed that the disability itself inevitably overwhelmed all other considerations. The literature is replete with parental "horror stories" of how they were informed of their child's disability. Parents remember a clinical portrayal of their child, dominated by the medical perspectives and prognoses (Engel 1993), with little or no information about the positive contributions that many parents and other family members talk about receiving from a child with disability (Behr, Murphy, and Summer 1992; Turnbull, Guess, and Turnbull 1988). The direction of the logic shifted over the years, but the supposedly tragic connotations of such births were consistently presented as inherent and immutable.

The durability of this predominantly negative approach to families and disability is most impressive when comparing the similarity in accounts of parents from vastly different eras of medical and educational knowledge. One of the earliest of these accounts can be found in the journals of Hester Thrale in 1775. Thrale (a friend of Samuel Johnson whose diaries of life in eighteenth-century London are well known to literary critics and historians interested in that period) tells how the doctor had provided her a blunt diagnosis that her two-year-old son was a "fatuous idiot," with dismal prospects for a life worth living. Moreover, she reports, the doctor told her he had just not had the heart to tell her sooner.

> [Dr.] Bromfield told me today he was *always* apprehensive about his Intellects, & that he said so to Old Nurse while I was in Wales last summer. I proposed the Cold Bath [one of the many versions of "hydrotherapy" in vogue at the time]; "any thing dear Madam" replied he, "that may contribute to quiet your Mind, but while you are trying every Means to preserve the Life of little master I fear your truest Friends will scarce be able to wish You Success." Melancholy Conversation. (Hyde 1977:116)

Some 200 years later, another English parent reports a strikingly similar conversation with her physician:

> The doctor cleared his throat and spoke very quietly. "I am so sorry to have to tell you this, but I'm afraid that our tests show that it is extremely unlikely that your daughter will ever be educated, or for that matter, that she will ever be able to recognize you as her parents. (Copeland 1973:11)

However, beneath this pattern of unrelenting pessimism and tragedy, there were some important shifts that occurred as specialized professionals began to emerge in the nineteenth and twentieth centuries. The tragedy remained, but the location of its source and nature started to move.

The Nineteenth Century

The end of the eighteenth century in London, as portrayed in Hester Thrale's family journal, actually represented something of a transition period in the emergence of professional explanations of parental responses to disability. As the Enlightenment took hold, the presence of disability in God's universe acquired newly scientific explanations. Yet burgeoning confidence in scientific and medical knowledge coexisted with a persistent moralistic gloss on the occurrence of such blatant evidence of original sin as the birth of disabled children. Even for someone of Thrale's elevated and educated social status, the sense of shame at having a disabled child was vivid and (as seen in the doctor's reaction) reinforced by the designated experts of the era. Thrale reflected the common belief that she must be responsible for her child's condition, which, from other passages from the diary, sounds like what might now be diagnosed as hydrocephalus:

In the midst of this Distress [i.e., the deaths of her mother and one of her other children] I have brought a Baby, which seems to be in measure affected by my Vexations; he is heavy stupid & drowsy, though very large.... I see no Wit sparkle in his Eyes. (Hyde 1977:85)

For the poor, the assignment of blame for such births was even more blatant. The presence of disabled children was not so much God's plan as parents' sinful, or at least ignorant, behavior, increasingly couched in the terms of biological discovery that was coming to dominate Enlightenment discourse.

Throughout the nineteenth century in Europe and in North America, this curious mixture of moralistic blame and scientific explanation for disability continued to become more and more refined and specialized. Even as the specializations in education, psychology, and neurology emerged throughout the century, parents were consistently presented as ethically and biologically responsible (especially those both poor and female). What has been called an "entrepreneurial model" of family life increasingly emphasized "self-discipline and firm, internalized moral codes" (Farber 1986:7). Home life was to be a "haven in a heartless world" (Lasch 1977) of capitalist competition. As such, any distractions from the moral and social code were seen as inevitable burdens on the economic success of the family. Poverty became the outcome of indolence and deviation from the moral code. As such, poverty itself was a symptom that could be passed on to children in an endless cycle of family degeneracy (Demos 1970; Katz 1983).

Of course, the blame had always been there for parents. What was new in the optimism of the nineteenth-century scientists and social engineers was the belief that the knowledge was now available to intervene and prevent such generations of depravity and social expense. Educators, psychologists—or alienists, as they were known then (e.g., Cooter 1981)—criminologists, and social reformers all claimed more and more public responsibility for raising children, especially if they were disabled. With "proper" methods of modern science and religious background, the cycle of poverty and disability could be broken. In a sense, parenting children became much too important to be left to parents. Parents, after all, were the amateurs. At the same time, parents quickly heard the new social message demanding "perfect" children. No longer, said the experts, could failure be condoned in raising productive offspring.

This common link in professional responses to families can be seen in superficially disparate developments in the United States, such as the emergence of the kindergarten and the congregate asylum for increasingly specialized categories of disability and social deviance. The professional argument behind both policy reforms was that such initiatives were needed to remove vulnerable children from the evil influence of "lowbred idleness" present in their homes. Henry Barnard, one of America's most respected advocates of public education, argued for kindergartens (and universal public schooling generally) as the only way to overcome the unfortunate influence of the retrograde family. The most dangerous families for Barnard were the poor and immigrant households increasingly concentrated in the nation's major cities. In 1851, Barnard listed his reasons for wanting early schooling for children of these classes.

No one at all familiar with the deficient household arrangements and deranged machinery of domestic life, of the extreme poor and ignorant, to say nothing of the intemperate—of the examples of rude manners, impure and profane language, and all the vicious habits of low-bred idleness, which abound in certain sections of all populous districts, can doubt that it is better for children to be removed as early and as long as possible from such examples and placed in an infant or primary school, under the care and instruction of a kind, affectionate, and skillful female teacher. (Barnard 1865:294)

A parent both poor and with a disabled child was even more at a risk of professional accusation. Society demanded "perfect" children, yet that, by definition, was what a child with an intellectual or physical disability could supposedly never be. If parents of nondisabled children were, in general, not to be trusted to raise their children, even less adequate were parents of disabled youngsters. The comparison becomes clear in the words of a contemporary of Barnard, Samuel G. Howe. An equally activist reformer, Howe specialized in issues affecting people with visual and intellectual disabilities. In a report for the Massachusetts state legislature, he gave his opinion on the causes of "idiocy" (as intellectual disability was called then).

> The moral to be drawn from the prevalent existence of idiocy in society is that a very large class of persons ignore the conditions upon which alone health and reason are given to men, and consequently they sin in various ways; they disregard the conditions which should be observed in intermarriage; they overlook the hereditary transmission of certain morbid tendencies; they pervert the natural appetites of the body into lusts of divers kinds,—the natural emotions of the mind into fearful passions,—and thus bring down the awful consequences of their own ignorance and sin upon the heads of their unoffending children. (Howe [1846] 1976:34)

Whether in the specific guise of reform schools, asylums, and residential schools for increasingly specific disabilities (blindness, deafness, epilepsy, idiocy, insanity, infantile paralysis), there was a common push throughout the nineteenth and early twentieth centuries, then, to institutionalize social programs that would remove children with disabilities from their parents. The only way to break the connection between poor parents and disabled children was to allow professionals to assume the parental role within the walls of their facilities (Ferguson 1994; Katz 1983; Rothman 1971). This carried over into the rapid spread of special education classes in public school systems after the turn of the century (Tropea 1993).

This does not mean that parents were totally passive in this social process. Recent correlations of institutional admission patterns with neighborhood census data show that "the explosion in accommodation for idiots, lunatics, and persons of unsound mind in nineteenth-century Europe and America was driven by families of all social and geographical backgrounds" (Wright 1998:203). However, as even these studies suggest, it was the professional promises of an increasingly dramatic cure or amelioration of troubles previously thought beyond remediation that found an eager audience in families struggling to support their loved ones with little prospect of permanent relief or even temporary respite. In the face of professional claims of specialized knowledge (not to mention the economic relief for many families provided by the state's assumption of the costs of daily care), it is probably more surprising that the clamor from families for institutional remedies was not more unanimous. Instead, we have the historical reality that even at the height of institutionalization in the United States, institutional and educational professionals complained of parental resistance to calls to place their children in institutional settings (Ferguson 1994). In 1915, Elizabeth Irwin of the Public Education Association in New York City testified before a state commission examining the status of services in the state for people with mental retardation. She reported visiting all of the "ungraded" classes (as the special education classrooms were often called at the time) in New York City in 1912 and 1913 in a effort to convince parents of children with intellectual disabilities to institutionalize them. Her testimony laments the resistance to her proposals that she received from the parents. Only 20 of 100 cases actually agreed to send their children to asylums. Out of those 20, Irwin regretfully reported, only two children stayed in the asylum for more than a year (New York State Commission 1915:115). What Irwin saw as the irrational resistance of parents to offers of institutional support might also be interpreted as parental resistance to unwanted professional control and disruption of their lives. I would argue that the explanation of historian Ellen Dwyer comes closest to the response of most families: "Asylums were places of last, not first, resort" (Dwyer 1987:3). To professionals of the era who made families the object of their studies, this response was a source of concern rather than one of admiration.

A Shift in Blame: 1920 to 1980

The circular logic that associated poverty with pathology rather than social inequity reached its depths in the pseudo-science of the eugenics movement in the early twentieth century (Reilly

1991; Selden 1999; Smith 1985; Zenderland 1998). However, overlapping with this "surgical solution" (Reilly 1991) to the perceived threat of imbecility, there began a shift in focus among family specialists in medicine, education, and the new field of social work. Among this group, the emphasis was no longer on how poor and probably disabled parents breed poor and inevitably disabled children. These professionals shifted their attention to how disabled children inevitably damaged the families into which they were born. What remained constant was the proclaimed need for trained professionals to displace parents as proper nurturers of children with disabilities.

Increasingly in the years up to World War II, educators, psychiatrists, and social workers all invoked a "medical model" (in which disability—or dependency of any kind—is wholly perceived as an individual defect or disease) by which to justify their takeover of parental functions. These experts were the "doctors" to a "sick society." One historian of the family has described the process as one whereby the "helping professions" invaded the family, convinced parents to rely on new scientific techniques and outside advice, and thereby dissipated the family's ability to overcome any special circumstances (Lasch 1977). Lasch (1977) summarized the vicious circle in which families found themselves spinning:

> Having first declared parents incompetent to raise their offspring without professional help, social pathologists "gave back" the knowledge they had appropriated—gave it back in a mystifying fashion that rendered parents more helpless than ever, more abject in their dependence on expert opinion. (P. 18)

While this approach to families as *damaged by* children with a disability never totally displaced the earlier view (in which it was the families doing the damage to the children), it did come to dominate the field of family research in the second half of the century. In part, this simply reflected the explosion of family research itself. For those interested in therapeutic intervention with the family rather than the child, the object of research understandably shifted to diagnosis over blame. One rather crude measure of this new specialization is the rapidly rising number of research articles on families published in professional journals. The increase in articles on families with "special needs" (most of which dealt with families of children with disabilities living at home), immediately following World War II, is striking. In the 8-year period from 1945 to 1953, almost as many research studies were cited (232) as in the preceding 45 years combined (280) (Dempsey 1981:7). Clearly, a growing cadre of professionals, as well as the professors who trained them, felt as though they had more to say about families of children with disabilities.

As the published research continued to grow, at least until the 1980s, one feature persisted as a foundational belief for professional portrayals of parents. Whether they preferred to emphasize attitudinal categories (e.g., guilt, denial, displaced anger, grief) or behavioral ones (e.g., role disruption, marital cohesiveness, social withdrawal), most family researchers assumed that disability distorted the connection between child and parent in ways that were both intrinsic and harmful (Darling and Darling 1982; Ferguson and Ferguson 1987; Lipsky 1985; Turnbull and Summers 1987). The challenge for researchers was to catalogue and sequence the evidence of parental damage and to argue for the efficacy of this or that therapeutic intervention. In other words, the medical model that increasingly dominated approaches to disability was extended to families as well.

MAPPING THE MAPS: A CONCEPTUAL MATRIX OF PROFESSIONAL INTERPRETATIONS OF FAMILIES

Since the 1960s, there has been a veritable floodtide of literature pertaining to parental adjustment to a child with a disability. To make sense of it all, it may be helpful to create a conceptual matrix to help group the major approaches to interpreting families. To create the matrix, one can view research on family reactions as efforts to answer one (or both) of two basic questions:

1. What is the *nature* of parental reaction to having a child with a disability?
2. What is the *source* of this reaction?

Until recently, most researchers reflected their academic training and disciplinary orientation (e.g., psychology, sociology, social work) by tending to answer the first question in either *attitudinal* or *behavioral* categories. Certainly with the advent of social psychology and ecological approaches, a firm separation of emphasis on emotional or behavioral terminology has become much less common, and one finds research that cuts across the realms of both internalized feelings and externally observable actions. However, it is still useful as an idealized typology to distinguish these orientations toward parents.

For the second question, another binary distinction (crude but fundamental) can be found. Regardless of whether family researchers have interpreted the underlying nature or essence of parental reactions in attitudinal or behavioral categories, they have tended to describe the source of those reactions as either inherent (*normative*) to the impact of disability on the family or as *contextually* determined by a variety of influences internal and external to the family.

A comment about paradigms in the social sciences is appropriate here before discussing this particular conceptual matrix. Paradigms in the natural sciences tend to disappear as they are replaced by a new consensus (e.g., it is rare to run across published research on why the flat earth paradigm really works). Social science paradigms are different. While certainly new policies and programs come to reflect the dominant social worldviews of any given era, the remnants and representatives of the previously dominant perspectives do not disappear. So, theological, moral, and medical explanations of disability continue to have their adherents even as the social/environmental model of disability studies continues to gain acceptance.

This is certainly the pattern that family research has followed. Some of the categories of answers to the basic questions that I have just described are less common now than they used to be. Others have never been dominant but may become so in the future. They all continue to exist, however, waxing and waning from era to era. It is hoped, however, that locating these answers within a conceptual schema can help reveal some of the underlying themes in professional characterizations of families. Combining these characterizations yields a two-by-two matrix (see Figure 14.1) that conceptually locates much of the research on families and disability in the past decade or so. Moreover, the durability of these answers suggests that they each must continue to resonate with some parents and support providers.

The Psychodynamic Approach: The Neurotic Parent

Although much less dominant today than in previous decades, the single largest body of professional literature on parents views them from a psychodynamic frame of reference that traces its roots back to Freudianism. It is in the language of this psychological culture that the most common descriptions of the "typical" parent of a child with a disability are stated. Hostility, denial, grief, guilt, defense mechanisms of all types, and a positive goal of acceptance are all prominent terms in the traditional profile of parental reactions. These researchers primarily used attitudinal categories to characterize the neurotic paths families followed. If families expressed displeasure with doctors or other professionals over the supposed lack of support, this was presented as merely the displaced anger that was originally directed at the disabled child (Pinkerton 1972; Zuk 1962). Of course, one could suggest that by interpreting displays of parental hostility as based on the intrinsically neurotic reaction to the birth or diagnosis of a child with a disability, professionals may avoid examining the inadequacies of their own performance. Justifiable anger toward an inadequate system of formal services is implicitly removed as an available parental response.

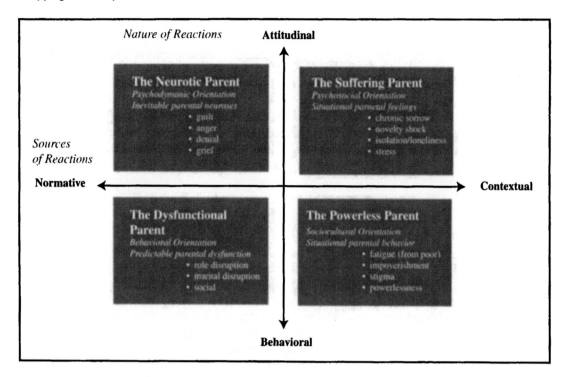

Figure 14.1. Professional Portrayals of Parental Reactions

On the other hand, if instead of anger the parent seemed too passive in the face of inadequate services, then this was seen as an outgrowth of underlying guilt or denial (McKeith 1973). As a category, denial arises most often in research on cognitive or emotional categories of disability (e.g., mental retardation, autism, learning disability). The argument is that the often vague nature of diagnosing and labeling such disabilities is lost on parents who simply refuse to acknowledge the reality that something is wrong with their child (Stanhope and Bell 1981; Wetter 1972). More recently, both research and parent narratives suggest that what was formerly interpreted as denial is more often a rejection of certain terminology or labels (Heifetz 1980).

Guilt is probably the most commonly invoked category of neurotic response within the psychodynamic interpretive box. Indeed, guilt is seemingly unavoidable within this perspective because it can occur supposedly as either the cause or effect of other emotions. Even parent involvement itself has been interpreted as based in an underlying guilt reaction by parents that they are somehow responsible for their child's disability. Researchers attributed active parent involvement and dedication to the welfare of their child as prima facie evidence of a deep-seated need to compensate for the same underlying guilt complex (Solnit and Stark 1961).

Apathetic or involved, angry or accepting—there was a professional explanation of the pathology behind any conceivable parental response (Lipsky 1985). In many ways, this pathologizing process is at the heart of the so-called medical model that many in the disability community now disavow as dehumanizing and reductionist. All parent reactions are reduced to neurotic symptoms of the disability. Life is medicalized, and pathology becomes the focus of professional interest whether the person involved is the child with the disability or the family of that child. The dominance of the process can be seen in educational as well as medical settings. Bruce Engel (1993) found the process repeatedly described by parents he interviewed about their interactions with professionals:

Whereas parents tend to perceive the whole child and to emphasize capabilities, the professionals tend to perceive the child in terms of those "defects," those aspects of the child that deviate from the norm and justify the child's classification as "handicapped" or "disabled." (Pp. 811-12)

The pathologizing is extended to parents by dismissing their emphasis on a child's capabilities as merely the symptoms of denial rather than adaptation (Drotar et al. 1975). It is a therapeutic "Catch-22" in which whatever response parents provide, the assumption of damage can be seen as verified. As Lipsky (1985) wrote,

> Not only do the perspectives discussed [of researchers and professionals] have serious limitations, not only are they severely overgeneralized and overapplied, but they increase the likelihood that no matter which role a family plays, it will be deemed unsatisfactory by one or more professional. In other words, both sides of the coin show pathological behavior. (P. 615)

The Behavioral Approach: The Dysfunctional Parent

In the 1960s and 1970s, research on families reflected the larger shift in the social sciences to a preference for behavioral approaches and categories over the previously fashionable psychoanalytic tradition. However, despite the conceptual reorientation, the assumptions of inevitability about family responses to a child with disability remained largely unchallenged. In one of the largest and best-known studies from this era, Farber (1962) found that the families who institutionalized their children identified as mentally retarded were much more relaxed, harmonious, and integrated. They participated more in activities outside the house. However, subsequent studies showed the danger of professional assumptions about what was normative and what was not. The question unasked by Farber was whether the erratic or nonexistent community support services for families in the 1950s and 1960s might explain the observed social withdrawal and marital breakdown better than (or at least as well as) any inherently disruptive influence of the disabled child living at home. Indeed, a less well known but revealing study from the same era discovered that when disabled children living at home were in day programs or schools, marital integration was much higher than in families without such services (Fowle 1968). What Farber interpreted as normative and unavoidable was, in fact, found to be situational and contingent.

The behavioral emphasis in family research had its applied side in the elaboration of what Turnbull and Summers (1987) have labeled the "parent as intervenor." The solution to the inevitable dysfunctional tendencies in parents was to systematically instruct parents in the instructional technologies and therapeutic exercises that would allow parents to emulate the skills of the professionals. Instead of putting the parent on the couch to "work through" various defense mechanisms, the behavioral approach put parents to work as paraprofessionals whose jobs were to carry over the intervention strategies devised by the experts.

At its best, this approach can help parents develop practical coping strategies that will allow them to interact effectively with their children. Moving away from the attitudinal obsessions of the psychoanalysts, the behaviorists offered parents more practical advice about how to help the child learn to hold a spoon or how to reinforce positive social skills that the child needed to participate in family activities. At its worst, however, the behavioral approach assumed that parents wanted to turn their homes into classrooms. Again, Turnbull and Summers (1987) make the connection that too many behaviorists had to earlier views of parents. "Is not the assumption that parents should be intervenors a direct outgrowth of the older assumptions that parents have deficits to be corrected, and that parents should be service providers?" (Turnbull and Summers 1987:294).

In both attitudinal and behavioral research, the causal connections between disabled child and damaged family continued to dominate throughout the 1970s and into the 1980s. The extremes to which this passion for pathology was taken can be seen in the title of one research piece that appeared in 1981 just before the tide of family research began to shift once again. In an article titled "Parentalplegia" (Murray and Cornell 1981), the authors provide perhaps the most transparent version of the dominant logic:

Children having conditions of mental retardation or other handicaps involving physical deficiencies are likely to be *causes* of a secondary handicapping condition involving the parents. . . . The authors have chosen the term parentalplegia to describe a secondary psycho-physiological (stress induced) condition that evolves among parents of handicapped children. Parentalplegia seems to be caused by an inability on the part of parents to adjust to the handicap of their children. (Murray and Cornell 1981:201)

The Psychosocial Approach: The Suffering Parent

As a steady counterpoint to the psychodynamic drumbeat of Bettelheim (1967) and others, the psychosocial approach emphasized the interplay of parental emotions with the environmental circumstances in which the family found itself. The attitudinal labels change. Guilt, anger, and denial are replaced by terms such as *stress, loneliness,* and *chronic sorrow.* The focus here expands from the almost exclusive attention to the mother-child dyad within the psychodynamic orientation to a much more contextual approach that presages the more complex analyses of family systems theory and constructivism.

One of the first examples of this approach is Olshansky's (1962) classic description of "chronic sorrow" (Wikler, Wasow, and Hatfield 1981). Instead of neurotic grief and guilt, chronic sorrow was offered as a normal, understandable reaction to an unexpected and, in many ways unwanted, situation. Indeed, it would be the absence of such regret and sorrow that should provoke professional concern, not its presence. The abnormal aspect of such grief is, argued Olshansky the social worker, more often in the psychologist's assumptions than in the parent's emotions. What is important is how responsive the parent's environment is to this initial reaction.

Perhaps an even better example of this psychosocial orientation to parental reactions is a pattern described by Wolfensberger (1983) as "novelty shock." Novelty shock differs from the psychodynamic accounts of grief at the "loss of the expected perfect child." The emphasis of the novelty shock interpretation is that an unanticipated event occurs, producing initial reactions of bewilderment, confusion, and dismay. Instead of the disability itself, the crucial factor is now seen as the social communication of information and interpretive stances taken by professionals and other family members.

Compared to the psychodynamic approach, the contextual emphasis of the psychosocial approach provided a healthy corrective to the excessively medicalized categories of inevitable neuroses. Emotions arise in various shapes and forms; what parents feel is the product of myriad influences, not any single factor. Parental reaction to a child with a disability is more or less adaptive depending on the social context. The psychosocial perspective, then, holds that there is no one natural way or sequence of ways for parents to respond.

The Sociopolitical Approach: The Powerless Parent

Perhaps the least common approach of the four options discussed here is the sociopolitical approach. Indeed, this contextual orientation arose mainly out of parent narratives themselves rather than professional inquiry (Featherstone 1980; Ferguson and Heifetz 1983; Massie and Massie 1975). The behavioral emphasis on marital role disruption, social withdrawal, and other terms transforms into a focus on more socially imposed outcomes of disempowerment, stigma, and fatigue. Socially inflicted problems have also been identified in economic terms of impoverishment. Poor families of children with disabilities get less attention and lower quality services than do well-to-do families. Middle-class families are sometimes impoverished due to financial needs associated with certain disabilities.

Over the past 10 years, then, family researchers have increasingly come to assume that it is not a specific set of parental reactions to disability but the influence of social contexts in shaping those reactions that are inevitable (Bérubé 1996; Gartner, Lipsky, and Turnbull 1991; Harry

1992; Hayden and Heller 1997; Patterson 1993; Turnbull and Turnbull 1990). Underlying the approach is the emphasis on the interconnection between external resources (or lack of them) and family adaptation to a disability. This approach emerged in the 1970s as part of the general disability advocacy movement. While translating into political activism for its practical applications, the approach found its niche within family research as part of the stress and coping literature in social psychology. It is this evolution that has come to dominate family research over the past decade. It has changed the direction of family research in ways that have finally abandoned the "blaming" efforts of the past. It has helped shift the emphasis from how families respond to disability to one that also emphasizes how society responds to families.

THE EMERGENCE OF THE ADAPTATIONAL CONTEXT

What has prompted family research to take such a dramatically new direction over the past 10 to 20 years? Of course, social and historical forces continue to influence the questions that family researchers are asking today. As the stories of Eric illustrate, we have seen over the past four decades a dramatic evolution in both policy and practice of our attitudes and support for individuals with disabilities and their families. The emergence of the disability rights movement finds its legal reflection in legislation from Section 504 of the Vocational Rehabilitation Act to the Americans with Disabilities Act. The growth of inclusive education for children with disabilities in our nation's schools is traceable through the elaboration of legal concepts such as "least restrictive environment" and "zero rejection" found in the Education of All Handicapped Children Act and its extension to early childhood in PL 99-457 (both now encompassed in the Individuals with Disabilities Education Act). Early intervention programs, based in the public school system in many states, now extend down to the youngest infants. Most students with disabilities now spend most of their day in general education classrooms (U.S. Department of Education 1999). Finally, it has been demonstrated by both educational and human service policy initiatives that people with even the most significant and multiple disabilities can be supported as active members of school and community, productively participating in the daily life of their society. Medicaid waivers have been extended in most states, allowing more and more children with multiple disabilities and chronic health conditions to stay at home with their families rather than be institutionalized.

I mention these developments for a reason, as they are part of the context that both generates and reflects the questions that today's researchers try to answer about families and disability. One of the most prominent of these researchers, Marty Krauss of Brandeis University, has summarized the implications well:

> For decades, researchers examining families of children with disabilities explicitly assumed a high degree of pathology in family functioning. . . . These studies may have served a useful purpose in focusing attention on the enormous difficulties experienced by families who received little or no public services to support their caregiving efforts. . . . However, substantial strides have been made in publicly supported early intervention systems, educational inclusion policies, and family support programs over the past decade. . . . Thus, studies conducted prior to the early 1980s are based on a different cohort of families than those who have participated in research conducted within the context of current service initiatives. (Krauss 1993:393)

Over the past 20 years, the most influential developments in research on the effects of a child with a disability on parents and other family members have arisen in three key areas:

The adaptive family: models of stress and coping (or adaptation)
The evolving family: models of family life course development

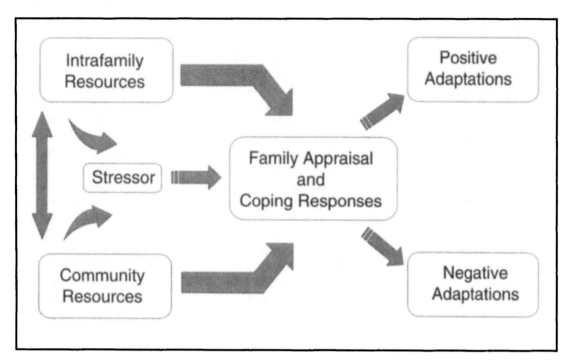

Figure 14.2. Model of Family Stress and Adaptation
SOURCE: Singer and Irvin (1989:6).

■ The active family: the importance of routine activities for understanding family perspectives

Only a summary sketch of these three research themes is possible here. However, even a cursory outline reveals the important changes that recent research and social context have made to interpret the meaning of disability in people's lives.

The Adaptive Family

Within the broad field of social psychology, research has centered on developing a theoretical representation of how families adapt to the potentially stressful situation of having a child with a disability. With this focus, researchers have steadily refined and elaborated the classic ABCX model originally developed by Reuben Hill (1949, 1958). Essentially, this model describes "family crisis" (X) as an interactive outcome of three factors: A, an initial "stressor event"; B, a family's resources for dealing with crises; and C, how the family defines the stressor (Behr et al. 1992; Patterson 1993; Singer and Irvin 1989).

Later modifications of the original ABCX model of family adaptation to stress have emphasized the distinction between internal and external resources available to families. For example, availability of effective family support programs makes a significant difference in how well a family copes with the financial stress sometimes associated with having a child with a disability (Singer and Irvin 1989). However, even the distinction of external and internal resources is embedded within a sociohistorical context of social policy and cultural assumptions (see Figure 14.2). Two additional areas of refinement in understanding the adaptive family can be identified.

Recognizing Resilience

First, over the past few years, the use of the revised ABCX model and other models of family adaptation and resilience has allowed researchers to recognize and interpret many successful coping strategies and positive adaptations that families report (Antonovsky 1993; Behr and Murphy 1993; Kazak and Marvin 1984; Summers, Behr, and Turnbull 1989; Turnbull and Turnbull 1990). The shift in emphasis away from solely negative family outcomes is important. Most researchers have abandoned the tally sheet mentality that adds up responses to record how bad (or good) it is for families to have a child with a disability. The research question is no longer one of listing the "unfortunate consequences" of an "unquestioned tragedy."

The old question has not been replaced by one seeking to discover purely positive family responses. Instead, most of the more sophisticated research on family stress today tries to understand the factors that contribute to some families adapting more successfully than other families. Family researchers overwhelmingly agree that the adaptational profile of families who have children with disabilities basically resembles that of families with children without disabilities (Baxter, Cummins, and Polak 1995; Knoll 1992; Krauss 1993; Krauss and Seltzer 1993; Lie et al. 1994; Taanila, Kokkonen, and Jarvelin 1996). That is, families of children with disabilities, on average, fare no better or worse than families in general. Some families flourish; some flounder. Most go up and down, depending on a complex array of personal and social factors, many of which have nothing to do with the presence of a disability. Again, Krauss (1993) provides a summative judgment on the effect within the field of this growing research base:

> There is increasing recognition that many families cope effectively and positively with the additional demands experienced in parenting a child with a disability. . . . The most recent literature suggests that families of children with handicaps exhibit variability comparable to the general population with respect to important outcomes such as parent stress . . . family functioning . . . and marital satisfaction. . . . Thus, although no one disputes the highly stressful effects on both mothers and fathers of learning that their child has a disability, research is now focused on understanding the factors associated with the amelioration of the "crisis" and on the similarities and differences between mothers and fathers in their perceptions of and responses to the experience of parenting a child with special needs. (Pp. 393-94)

Finding a Pattern

Second, researchers have made the adaptive model dynamic by recognizing that the ABCX cycle of responding to crisis is often cyclical and cumulative within a family. How a family responds to one stressor will influence how the family responds to subsequent stressors (McCubbin and Patterson 1983). Moreover, researchers have tried to capture not only the importance of a family's initial or "elementary" appraisal of the various elements of the crisis but also a "secondary" appraisal of their own capacity and resources. That is, the model now usually incorporates not only the resources for dealing with the crisis but also how the family appraises its resources for dealing with a crisis (Patterson 1993). What this elaborated model allows is a dual focus. Researchers look at how families respond differently in terms of their behavior, as well as how the cognitive interpretations that families place on those behaviors shape their response.

For example, several interesting studies have compared families of children with Down syndrome to families of children with other disabilities or with no disabilities. In one study, Cahill and Glidden (1996; see also Van Riper, Ryff, and Pridham 1992) matched samples of families of children with Down syndrome with families of children with other disabilities and found no significant differences in family and parental functioning. The authors suggest that this counters a persistent stereotype that children with Down syndrome are easier to raise than children

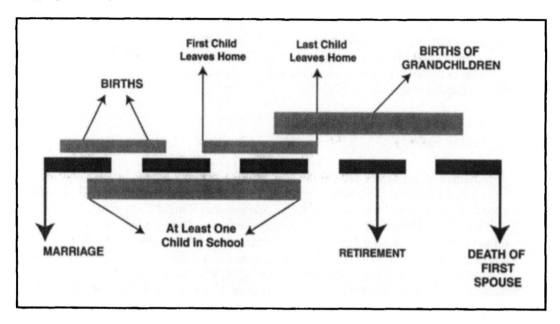

Figure 14.3. Example of Typical Nuclear Family Life Cycle Timeline

with other disabilities. Not only was there no "adjustment advantage" to rearing a child with Down syndrome but

> the average level of functioning for all families was quite good. On most variables, scores were at or near norms based on families in general, not [just] those engaged in rearing children with developmental disabilities.... Most families who are rearing children with disabilities are demonstrating effective coping with this task. (Cahill and Glidden 1996:158)

The Evolving Family

The adaptive shift from a normative to a situational understanding of response to disability has also allowed recognition of where a family is in its own life course. As with much of social science research, once a finding is pronounced, it seems strikingly obvious: Families have a life course of their own, in addition to the life course of each family member. Researchers have begun to recognize the importance of identifying where a family is in its life course. Particularly important in our own era is the question of how a particular family may have departed from a specific life course pattern (e.g., grandparents becoming primary caregivers for a grandchild). Other questions are equally critical. How many children are in the family? How many are at home? Are both parents alive and available to the children? These and other elements of family development inevitably shape how family members perceive a specific source of potential stress (see Figure 14.3) (Fewell and Vadasy 1986; Turnbull, Summers, and Brotherson 1986).

This emergence of the life course perspective has supported the "discovery" of older parents by researchers and is especially relevant for secondary and transition support programs for students with disabilities and their families. Until recently, almost all research on family response to a child with a disability focused on families with young children. Studies that followed families across a life span or that specifically sought older parents of adults with disabilities have opened up fascinating information about why some families are more resilient than others and how extended coping with chronic illness or disability affects families over time. New questions emerge because the frame has expanded. Do families tend to adapt over time to having a child with a disability so that stress goes down as the child gets older? Or do years of parenting simply wear parents down, eroding their resiliency into lives in which nerves are exposed and tensions bared? One recent study of parents older and younger than age 55 actually found higher levels of adjustment in the older group, supporting the "adaptational" over the "wear-and-tear" hypothesis (Hayden and Heller 1997).

The Active Family

A third area of important development in family research has been in the elaboration of activity-based approaches to family adaptation. Some of the most exciting work here has been the study of "ecocultural niches" by Thomas Weisner and Ronald Gallimore and colleagues (Gallimore et al. 1996; Gallimore et al. 1989; Gallimore, Goldenberg, and Weisner 1993; Gallimore, Weisner, et al. 1993; Nihira, Weisner, and Bernheimer 1994; Weisner 1997; Weisner, Beizer, and Stolze 1991). This research combines a social ecology approach to families that is most familiar, perhaps, in Bronfenbrenner's (1979) concentric circles. The circles illustrate the simultaneous influences and interrelatedness of multiple levels of analysis (from "micro" characteristics of individual families to "macro" features of cultural mores and social variables).

The problem with this model has been how to use it in practice. If everything is potentially relevant to understanding how a family functions, then where does one begin to focus attention for research or intervention? The ecocultural niche approach responds to this problem by focusing on family routines and daily activities as the crucible within which a multiplicity of influences is forged into a family's adaptation to the "hassles" of daily life. These family routines, or "activity settings," serve as the unit of analysis for understanding the social construction process that families use to shape the meaning of disability in their lives. For families of children with disabilities, the critical contexts become those routines that involve parents and children together.

> Children's activity settings are the architecture of everyday life, not a deliberate curriculum; they are homely and familiar parts of a family's day: preparing meals, eating dinner, cleaning up, and dozens of mundane routines in which adult-child interaction is embedded. (Gallimore et al. 1989:217)

It is critical to note that what is important is not so much the activity settings themselves but how a family constructs those activities or portrays them to others. What type of narrative account does a mother offer about a day in the life of her family? Within that account—if properly "read"—one can find many levels of culture, background, and personal values embedded in a mealtime, an outing, or a weekend morning. For example, deaf parents of a deaf child might interpret their child's first signs not merely as the beginnings of communication but as the continuation of a linguistic and cultural heritage that makes them proud that their child is deaf. In such a family, disability (if that even continues to be an appropriate term) is celebrated rather than lamented (Corker 1996). In another family, perhaps the activity level of a child at mealtime might seem to outsiders as symptomatic of an official diagnosis of attention deficit/hyperactivity disorder. However, the family's expectations and norms might find such energy acceptable and appropriate, placing more value on assertive enthusiasm than quiet compliance. The behavior that is seen as disruptive in the classroom is deemed acceptable at the dinner table.

A Summary of Findings

The emergence of these three new interpretations of families as adaptive, evolving, and active has helped expand and deepen our current approach to families of children with disabilities. What do we know now about the range of family reactions to having a child with a disability? Several key points emerge from a thorough reading of recent research on family adaptation to raising a child with a disability.

❖ What is perhaps most universally agreed on is that family responses to disability are immensely variable. As one recent synthesis of the research concluded,

> What we are beginning to realize is that maternal and family reaction to disability, and to mental retardation in particular, is highly variable, so that it is difficult and inaccurate to talk about "families of children with retardation" in a general sense. Within the universe of families of children with retardation, there is a greater range in the nature and extent to which individual mothers report maladaptation. (Shapiro, Blacher, and Lopez 1998:625)

❖ A dominant body of research finds aggregate patterns of overall adjustment and well-being to be similar across groups of families with children with or without disabilities. This pattern, however, does show some adaptational differences over the family life course from the birth of the first child to the death of the last parent.

❖ Research recognizes a significant number of parents who report numerous benefits and positive outcomes associated with raising a child with disabilities. These include coping skills (adaptability), family harmony (cohesiveness), spiritual growth or shared values, shared parenting roles, and communication. Of course, parents in general have long cited such benefits to raising children. What is new is that researchers have finally overcome their disbelief that some parents attribute these benefits to the presence of the disability itself.

❖ Study of the research does not deny that having a child with a disability can be a stressful event. The research continues to examine why some families are more resilient than others in adapting to this stress and identifies the patterns of adjustment that families adopt.

❖ Some research suggests that factors, such as level of disability (e.g., cognitive disability with pervasive support needs) or family structure (e.g., single parents, family size), may not be as critical as other factors (e.g., presence or absence of self-injurious or challenging behavior, social support, family income). Differential patterns may exist along ethnic, religious, and cultural lines.

❖ Family perspectives on having a child with a disability are clearly revealed in family accounts of daily routines and activities.

MAPPING THE FUTURE: ISSUES AND CHALLENGES FOR FAMILY RESEARCH

I began this chapter with a series of vignettes about Eric to capture the significant progress made over the past few decades in support for and collaboration with families who have children with disabilities. Of course, significant challenges remain. I want to conclude this chapter by mapping out some future directions that need continued attention by both family researchers and educators.

A Need for Family Narratives

The turn toward contextual adaptation in family research and the model of ecocultural niches brings to light the need for family researchers to pay attention to the first-person narrative accounts that families offer. There is a greater need than ever to understand how the accounts that families provide match the conceptual developments in research. That is, most research in this area understandably uses research constructs and measures specifically designed to fit the structure and categories of the model being tested. However, a parallel need exists to collect less-structured versions of family life to explore how well the model of ecocultural niches fits when families generate the terms and categories of their own narratives. Despite the growth over the past decade of qualitative techniques, such as semistructured interviewing in family research, a need persists for more extended narrative accounts from parents and other family members that capture the full range of details of daily life and family history.

Researchers who rely on more interpretive methods have been content to collect and analyze the stories that pack all of that history and culture into a shared family narrative (Engel 1993). The elaboration of the stress and adaptation models and the family life span orientation have allowed researchers to rediscover the rich body of information available in the stories that families have always been willing to tell about their experience. These stories are useful as more than simple accounts of the recent (or not-so-recent) past. As anthropologists have always known, the stories and myths that we adopt to explain our origins as part of a family or a culture always tell as much about our current situation as our past. What we choose to remember and the stories with which we frame those memories always help to "clarify the circumstances at the time the story is retold" (Engel 1993:797). In telling us about their lives "then," families are telling us equally as much about their lives "now."

Cross-Cultural Competence and Family Diversity

Until recently, most research on families of children with disabilities tended to gloss over the situational complexities and cultural variables that surround and ground all families. Much research and practice made rather global claims about the inevitable—and always negative—responses of families to having a child with a disability. One result of this emphasis has been to neglect (until recently) families of non-European racial and cultural backgrounds.

Freed from the nuisance of contextual variation, research for decades got by with little more than rhetorical acknowledgments that maybe somewhere down the research road, conclusions about disability and families should be based on subjects in addition to white middle-class mothers. Obviously, we need to move faster and farther down that road. Regardless of where one comes down on the continuum of cultural relativism, the immense variety of beliefs and practices reflects the equally broad variety of ways that specific families interpret specific disabilities.

Surely the differences in cultural attitudes, social supports, and personal beliefs across countries should be associated with different patterns of family response to disability. What is most surprising is how little of this comparative research has actually been conducted. However, we do have a growing body of self-contained studies within individual countries that can be examined. The research of this type that does exist suggests that the anticipated differences do appear when one looks at separate studies done in different countries. For example, one study of Scandinavian mothers of children with Down syndrome (Ryde-Brandt 1988) found "little evidence of depression or anxiety, revealed normal social and emotional contacts, and observed the negative feelings experienced at birth of the child almost invariably changing in a positive direction" (Shapiro et al. 1998:622-23). On the other hand, a study of mothers in India found evidence of much greater perceived burden and social isolation (Singhi et al. 1990).

Rather than treat such findings as contradictory, the future of family research promises to use such differences as keys to the cultural construction of the meaning of disability within families. The differences may not be solely related to levels of formal social support. There is some evidence that extended kinship networks are also effective in reducing perceived stress, and such networks are often stronger in non-European cultures (Shapiro at al. 1998).

Both family and disability are cultural constructs, which does not mean they are simple social conventions such as being polite or the Big Ten athletic conference. This does imply that neither family nor disability can be considered in the abstract for long. Rather, what the anthropologist Clifford Geertz (1973) refers to as "thick description" is needed that will put substance to the terms. The problems we have in agreeing on universal definitions of either family or disability stem from this cultural specificity and descriptive detail. The field of disability studies is increasingly trying to assume the challenge of providing this narrative richness and exploring the cultures of disability and family (Goode 1994; Ingstad and Whyte 1995; Mallory et al. 1993). Important studies of the double-minority status of being nonwhite and disabled in America are now appearing (Baxter et al. 1990; Blacher 1996; Kalyanpur and Rao 1991; Madiros 1989; O'Connor, 1993). A great need remains, however, for multicultural studies that explore the diversity of experiences of disability.

Parenthood and the Familial Location of Disability

This chapter has addressed family research but has actually focused on nondisabled parents of disabled children. However, even as I have tried to map the professional portrayal of family reactions to disability, there is also a need to map the location of disability within the family. Throughout this chapter, I have noted how a disability studies perspective has perhaps gained enough influence that it is no longer surprising to find arguments that understand the interaction of disability and family life within a sociohistorical context. It is less common to ask how that interaction is influenced, depending on which member of the family has the disability. If disability can be located along a historical timeline, it can also be located on a map of family relationships. Yet comparisons of how this movement of the disability from the mother to the father to the son or daughter within family units are, to our knowledge, almost nonexistent in the social science literature. Social psychological research on how families cope with the stress of disability usually means families of children with disabilities. Recently, similar research has begun to appear that focuses on the coping skills of disabled parents (Barker and Maralani 1997; Berkeley Planning Associates 1997). Little, if any, of this research has asked the next comparative question of how those experiences differ as the location of the disability moves from one family member to another.

Of course, the variations in this direction quickly multiply. The experiences of an adult with a disability who then becomes a parent might significantly differ from those of a parent who subsequently becomes disabled. The comparable situation with children might be couples who adopt children whom they know to be disabled compared with the experiences of parents who did not know in advance that their children would have a disability. One could also include additional family relationships (siblings are perhaps the most obvious) where the disability could move around. Finally, all of these variations must be coupled with more traditional demographic variables (race, gender, and class) as well, in the search for explanatory factors.

A map of the future is always full of speculation and uncharted territory. What disability studies has allowed for family research is an opportunity to redefine its boundaries and to set off and explore exciting new vistas previously thought unreachable or unimportant. If the vignette of Eric in 2010 is to come true, however, we must, as a field, link our research to our reforms. We must apply what we are learning about disability as a concept to what we want to know of families. We must learn to use the history of our mistakes as a beacon to illuminate our future research. Most important, we must hasten the journey. There are families waiting for our discoveries.

REFERENCES

Antonovsky, A. 1993. "The Implications of Salutigenesis: An Outsider's View." Pp. 111-22 in *Cognitive Coping, Families, and Disability*, edited by A. P. Turnbull, J. M. Patterson, S. K. Behr, D. L. Murphy, J. G. Marquis, and M. J. Blue-Banning. Baltimore: Brookes.

Barker, L. T. and V. Maralani. 1997. *Challenges and Strategies of Disabled Parents: Findings from a National Survey of Parents with Disabilities.* Oakland, CA: Berkeley Planning Associates.

Barnard, H. 1865. "Extracts from the Sixth Annual Report of the Superintendent of Common Schools to the General Assembly for 1851." *Journal of American Education* 15:293-313.

Baxter, C., R. A. Cummins, and S. Polak. 1995. "A Longitudinal Study of Parental Stress and Support: From Diagnosis of Disability to Leaving School." *International Journal of Disability, Development and Education* 42:125-36.

Baxter, C., K. Poonia, L. Ward, and Z. Nadirshaw. 1990. *Double Discrimination: Issues and Services People with Learning Difficulties from Black and Ethnic Minority Communities.* London: Kings Fund Centre.

Behr, S. K. and D. L. Murphy. 1993. "Research Progress and Promise: The Role of Perceptions in Cognitive Adaptation to Disability." Pp. 151-63 in *Cognitive Coping, Families, and Disability,* edited by A. P. Turnbull, J. M. Patterson, S. K. Behr, D. L. Murphy, J. G. Marquis, and M. J. Blue-Banning. Baltimore: Brookes.

Behr, S. K., D. L. Murphy, and J. A. Summer. 1992. *User's Manual: Kansas Inventory of Parental Perceptions.* Lawrence: University of Kansas, Beach Center on Families and Disability.

Berkeley Planning Associates. 1997. "Parent with Disabilities." *Disability Studies Quarterly* 17:172-79.

Bérubé, M. 1996. *Life as We Know It: A Father, a Family, and an Exceptional Child.* New York: Pantheon.

Bettelheim, B. 1967. *The Empty Fortress.* New York: Free Press.

Blacher, J. 1996. "Fathers, Families, Retardation and Cultural Context." Paper presented at the NICHD Conference on Developmental, Ethnographic, and Demographic Perspectives on Fatherhood, June, Bethesda, MD.

Bronfenbrenner, U. 1979. *The Ecology of Human Development: Experiments by Nature and Human Design.* Cambridge, MA: Harvard University Press.

Cahill, B. M. and L. M. Glidden. 1996. "Influence of Child Diagnosis on Family and Parental Functioning: Down Syndrome versus Other Disabilities." *American Journal of Mental Retardation* 101:149-60.

Cooter, R. 1981. "Phrenology and British Alienists, ca. 1825-1845." Pp. 58-104 in *Madhouses, Mad Doctors, and Madmen: The Social History of Psychiatry in the Victorian Era,* edited by A. Scull. Philadelphia: University of Pennsylvania Press.

Copeland, J. 1973. *For the Love of Ann.* London: Arrow.

Corker, M. 1996. *Deaf Transitions: Images and Origins of Deaf Families, Deaf Communities and Deaf Identities.* London: Jessica Kingsley.

Darling, R. B. and J. Darling. 1982. *Children Who Are Different: Meeting the Challenges of Birth Defects in Society.* St. Louis, MO: C. V. Mosby.

Demos, J. 1970. *A Little Commonwealth: Family Life in Plymouth Colony.* New York: Oxford University Press.

Dempsey, J. J. 1981. *The Family and Public Policy: The Issue of the 1980s.* Baltimore: Brookes.

Drotar, D., A. Baskiewicz, N. Irvin, J. Kennell, and M. Klaus. 1975. "The Adaptation of Parents to the Birth of an Infant with a Congenital Malformation: A Hypothetical Model." *Pediatrics* 56:710-17.

Dwyer, E. 1987. *Homes for the Mad: Life inside Two Nineteenth-Century Asylums.* New Brunswick, NJ: Rutgers University Press.

Engel, D. M. 1993. "Origin Myths: Narratives of Authority, Resistance, Disability, and Law." *Law & Society Review* 27:785-826.

Farber, B. 1962. "Effects of a Severely Mentally Retarded Child on the Family." Pp. 227-46 in *Readings on the Exceptional Child: Research and Theory,* edited by E. P. Trapp and P. Himelstein. New York: Appleton-Century-Crofts.

———. 1986. "Historical Context of Research on Families with Mentally Retarded Members." Pp. 3-23 in *Families of Handicapped Persons: Research, Programs and Policy Issues,* edited by J. J. Gallagher and P. M. Vietze. Baltimore: Brookes.

Featherstone, H. 1980. *A Difference in the Family.* New York: Penguin.

Ferguson, P. M. 1994. *Abandoned to Their Fate: Social Policy and Practice toward Severely Retarded People in America, 1820-1920.* Philadelphia: Temple University Press.

Ferguson, P. M. and A. Asch. 1989. "Lessons from Life: Personal and Parental Perspectives on School, Childhood, and Disability." Pp. 108-40 in *Schooling and Disability: Eighty-Eighth Yearbook of the National Society for the Study of Education,* Vol. II, edited by D. P. Biklen, D. L. Ferguson, and A. Ford. Chicago: National Society for the Study of Education.

Ferguson, P. M. and D. L. Ferguson. 1987. "Parents and Professionals." Pp. 346-91 in *Introduction to Special Education,* edited by P. Knoblock. Boston: Little, Brown.

Ferguson, P. M. and L. J. Heifetz. 1983. "An Absence of Offering: Parents of Retarded Children and Their Experiences with the Clergy." *Pastoral Psychology* 32:49-57.

Fewell, R. R. and P. F. Vadasy, eds. 1986. *Families of Handicapped Children: Needs and Supports across the Life Span.* Austin, TX: ProEd.

Fowle, M. 1968. "The Effect of the Severely Retarded Child on His Family." *American Journal of Mental Deficiency* 13:468-73.

Gallimore, R., J. Coots, T. Weisner, H. Garnier, and D. Guthrie. 1996. "Family Responses to Children with Early Developmental Delays: Part III—Accommodation, Intensity, and Activity in Early and Middle Childhood." *American Journal of Mental Retardation* 101:215-32.

Gallimore, R., C. N. Goldenberg, and T. Weisner. 1993. "The Social Construction and Subjective Reality of Activity Settings: Implications for Community Psychology." *American Journal of Community Psychology* 21:537-61.

Gallimore, R., T. S. Weisner, L. P. Bernheimer, D. Guthrie, and K. Nihira. 1993. "Family Responses to Young Children with Developmental Delays: Accommodation Activity in Ecological and Cultural Context." *American Journal of Mental Retardation* 98:185-206.

Gallimore, R., T. S. Weisner, S. Z. Kaufman, and L. P. Bernheimer. 1989. "The Social Construction of Ecocultural Niches: Family Accommodation of Developmentally Delayed Children." *American Journal of Mental Retardation* 94:216-30.

Gartner, A., D. K. Lipsky, and A. P. Turnbull. 1991. *Supporting Families with a Child with a Disability: An International Outlook.* Baltimore: Brookes.

Geertz, C. 1973. *The Interpretation of Cultures.* New York: Basic Books.

Giddens, A. 1984. *The Constitution of Society: Outline of a Theory of Structuration.* Berkeley: University of California Press.

Goode, D., ed. 1994. *Quality of Life for Persons with Disabilities: International Perspectives and Issues.* Cambridge, MA: Brookline.

Harry, B. 1992. *Cultural Diversity, Families and the Special Education System: Communication and Empowerment.* New York: Teachers College Press.

Hayden, M. F. and T. Heller. 1997. "Support, Problem-Solving/Coping Ability and Personal Burden of Younger and Older Caregivers of Adults with Mental Retardation." *Mental Retardation* 35:364-72.

Heifetz, L. J. 1980. "From Consumer to Middleman: Emerging Roles for Parents in the Network of Services for Retarded Children." Pp. 349-84 in *Parent Education and Intervention Handbook,* edited by R. R. Abidin. Springfield, IL: Charles C Thomas.

Hill, R. 1949. *Families under Stress.* New York: Harper & Row.

———. 1958. "Generic Features of Families under Stress." *Social Casework* 49:139-50.

Howe, S. G. [1846] 1976. "Remarks on the Causes of Idiocy." Pp. 31-60 in *The History of Mental Retardation: Collected Papers,* vol. 1, edited by M. Rosen, G. Clark, and M. Kivitz. Reprint, Baltimore: University Park Press.

Hyde, M. 1977. *The Thrales of Streatham Park.* Cambridge, MA: Harvard University Press.

Ingstad, B. and S. R. Whyte, eds. 1995. *Disability and Culture.* Berkeley: University of California Press.

Kalyanpur, M. and S. S. Rao. 1991. "Empowering Low-Income Black Families of Handicapped Children." *American Journal of Orthopsychiatry* 61:523-32.

Katz, M. 1983. *Poverty and Policy in American History.* New York: Academic Press.

Kazak, A. E. and R. S. Marvin. 1984. "Differences, Difficulties and Adaptations: Stress and Social Networks in Families with a Handicapped Child." *Family Relations* 33:67-77.

Knoll, J. 1992. "Being a Family: The Experience of Raising a Child with a Disability or Chronic Illness." Pp. 9-56 in *Emerging Issues in Family Support,* edited by V. J. Bradley, J. Knoll, and J. M. Agosta. Washington, DC: American Association on Mental Retardation.

Krauss, M. W. 1993. "Child-Related and Parenting Stress: Similarities and Differences between Mothers and Fathers of Children with Disabilities." *American Journal of Mental Retardation* 97:393-404.

Krauss, M. W. and M. M. Seltzer. 1993. "Current Well-Being and Future Plans of Older Caregiving Mothers." *The Irish Journal of Psychology* 14 (1): 48-63.

Lasch, C. 1977. *Haven in a Heartless World: The Family Beseiged.* New York: Basic Books.

Lie, H. R., M.-C. Borjneson, B. Lagerkvist, R. Rasmussen, J. H. Hagelsteen, and J. Lagergren. 1994. "Children with Myelomeningocele: The Impact of Disability on Family Dynamics and Social conditions: A Nordic Study." *Developmental Medicine and Child Neurology* 36:1000-9.

Lipsky, D. G. 1985. "A Parental Perspective on Stress and Coping." *American Journal of Orthopsychiatry* 55:614-17.

Madiros, M. 1989. "Conception of Childhood Disability among Mexican-American Parents." *Medical Anthropology* 12:55-68.

Mallory, B. L., R. W. Nichols, J. I. Charlton, and K. Marfo. 1993. *Traditional and Changing Views of Disability in Developing Societies: Causes, Consequences, Cautions.* Durham: University of New Hampshire, Institute on Disability.

Massie, R. and S. Massie. 1975. *Journey.* New York: Knopf.

McCubbin, H. I. and J. M. Patterson. 1983. "The Family Stress Process: The Double ABCX Model of Adjustment and Adaptation." *Marriage and Family Review* 6:7-37.

McKeith, R. 1973. "Parental Reactions and Responses to a Handicapped Child." Pp. 131-41 in *Brain and Intelligence,* edited by F. Richardson. Hyattsville, MD: National Education Consultants.

Murray, J. N. and C. J. Cornell. 1981. "Parentalplegia." *Psychology in the Schools* 18:201-7.

New York State Commission. 1915. *Report of the State Commission to Investigate Provision for the Mentally Deficient.* Albany, NY: J. B. Lyon.

Nihira, K., T. S. Weisner, and L. P. Bernheimer. 1994. "Ecocultural Assessment in Families of Children with Developmental Delays: Construct and Concurrent Validities." *American Journal of Mental Retardation* 98:551-56.

O'Connor, S. 1993. *Multiculturalism and Disability: A Collection of Resources.* Syracuse, NY: Syracuse University, Center on Human Policy.

Olshansky, S. 1962. "Chronic Sorrow: A Response to Having a Mentally Defective Child." *Social Casework* 43:190-93.

Patterson, J. M. 1993. "The Role of Family Meanings in Adaptation to Chronic Illness and Disability." Pp. 221-38 in *Cognitive Coping, Families, and Disability,* edited by A. P. Turnbull, J. M. Patterson, S. K. Behr, D. L. Murphy, J. G. Marquis, and M. J. Blue-Banning. Baltimore: Brookes.

Pinkerton, P. 1972. "Parental Acceptance of a Handicapped Child." *Developmental Medicine and Child Neurology* 12:207-12.

Reilly, P. R. 1991. *The Surgical Solution: A History of Involuntary Sterilization in the United States.* Baltimore: Johns Hopkins University Press.

Rothman, D. J. 1971. *The Discovery of the Asylum: Social Order and Disorder in the New Republic.* Boston: Little, Brown.

Ryde-Brandt, B. 1988. "Mothers of Primary School Children with Down's Syndrome." *Acta Psychiatrica Scandinavia* 78:102-8.

Selden, S. 1999. *Inheriting Shame: The Story of Eugenics and Racism in America.* New York: Teachers College Press.

Shapiro, J., J. Blacher, and S. R. Lopez. 1998. "Maternal Reactions to Children with Mental Retardation." Pp. 606-36 in *Handbook of Mental Retardation and Development,* edited by J. A. Burack, R. M. Hodapp, and E. Zigler. New York: Cambridge University Press.

Singer, G. H. S. and L. Irvin. 1989. "Family Caregiving, Stress, and Support." Pp. 3-25 in *Support for Caregiving Families: Enabling Positive Adaptation to Disability,* edited by G. H. S. Singer and L. K. Irvin. Baltimore: Brookes.

Singhi, P. D., L. Goyal, D. Pershad, S. Singhi, and B. N. S. Walia. 1990. "Psychological Problems in Families of Disabled Children." *British Journal of Medical Psychology* 63:173-82.

Smith, J. D. 1985. *Minds Made Feeble: The Myth and Legacy of the Kallikaks.* Rockville, MD: Aspen.

Solnit, A. J. and M. H. Stark. 1961. "Mourning and the Birth of a Defective Child." *Psycho-Analytic Study of the Child* 16:523-37.

Stanhope, L. and R. Q. Bell. 1981. "Parents and Families." Pp. 688-713 in *Handbook of Special Education,* edited by J. M. Kauffman and D. R. Hallahan. Englewood Cliffs, NJ: Prentice Hall.

Sternberg, L. and M. L. Caldwell. 1982. "Parent Involvement and Training." Pp. 27-43 in *Educating Severely and Profoundly Handicapped Students,* edited by L. Sternberg and G. L. Adams. Rockville, MD: Aspen.

Summers, J. A., S. K. Behr, and A. P. Turnbull. 1989. "Positive Adaptation and Coping Strength of Families Who Have Children with Disabilities." Pp. 27-40 in *Support for Caregiving Families: Enabling Positive Adaptation to Disability,* edited by G. H. S. Singer and L. K. Irvin. Baltimore: Brookes.

Taanila, A., J. Kokkonen, and M.-R. Jarvelin. 1996. "The Long Term Effects of Children's Early-Onset Disability on Marital Relationships." *Developmental Medicine and Child Neurology* 38:567-77.

Tropea, J. L. 1993. "Structuring Risks: The Making of Urban School Order." Pp. 58-90 in *Children at Risk in America: History, Concepts, and Public Policy,* edited by R. Wollons. Albany: State University of New York Press.

Turnbull, A. P. and J. A. Summers. 1987. "From Parent Involvement to Family Support: Evolution to Revolution." Pp. 289-306 in *New Perspectives on Down Syndrome,* edited by S. M. Pueschel, A. C. Crocker, and D. M. Crutcher. Baltimore: Brookes.

Turnbull, A. P., J. A. Summers, and M. Brotherson. 1986. "Family Life Cycle: Theoretical and Empirical Implications and Future Directions for Families with Mentally Retarded Members." Pp. 58-90 in *Families of Handicapped Persons: Research, Programs, and Policy Issues*, edited by J. J. Gallagher and P. M. Vietze. Baltimore: Brookes.

Turnbull, A. P. and H. R. Turnbull III. 1990. *Families, Professionals, and Exceptionalities: A Special Partnership*. Columbus, OH: Merrill.

Turnbull, H. R., III, D. Guess, and A. P. Turnbull. 1988. "Vox Populi and Baby Doe." *Mental Retardation* 26:127-32.

U.S. Department of Education. 1999. *Twentieth Annual Report to Congress on the Implementation of the Individuals with Disabilities Education Act*. Washington, DC: Author.

Van Riper, M., C. Ryff, and K. Pridham. 1992. "Parental and Family Wellbeing in Families of Children with Down Syndrome: A Comparative Study." *Research in Nursing and Health* 15:227-35.

Weisner, T. S. 1997. "The Ecocultural Project of Human Development: Why Ethnography and Its Findings Matter." *Ethos* 25:177-91.

Weisner, T. S., L. Beizer, and L. Stolze. 1991. "Religion and Families of Children with Developmental Delays." *American Journal of Mental Retardation* 95:647-62.

Wetter, J. 1972. "Parent Attitudes toward Learning Disabilities." *Exceptional Children* 39:490-91.

"When a Child Is Different." [1951] 1969. Pp. 85-91 in *If Your Child Is Handicapped*, edited by W. C. Kvaraceus and E. N. Hayes. Reprint, Boston: Porter Sargent.

Wikler, L., M. Wasow, and E. Hatfield. 1981. "Chronic Sorrow Revisited: Parent vs. Professional Depiction of the Adjustment of Parents of Mentally Retarded Children." *American Journal of Orthopsychiatry* 51:63-70.

Wolfensberger, W. 1983. *Normalization Based Guidance, Education and Supports Families of Handicapped People*. Downsview, Ontario: National Institute on Mental Retardation.

Wright, D. 1998. "Family Strategies and the Institutional Confinement of 'Idiot' Children in Victorian England." *Journal of Family History* 23:190-208.

Zenderland, L. 1998. *Measuring Minds: Henry Herbert Goddard and the Origins of American Intelligence Testing*. New York: Cambridge University Press.

Zuk, G. H. 1962. "The Cultural Dilemma and Spiritual Crisis of the Family with a Handicapped Child." *Exceptional Children* 28:405-8.

Disability and Community 15

A Sociological Approach

MICHAEL P. KELLY

This chapter considers the individual with impairment and his or her experience of that impairment in the community. This chapter also links the personal experience of impairment with the social factors that create disability. It is argued that the community is the place where disability is constructed and experienced. The implications of the changing nature of social structures for those personal experiences are highlighted. The argument is based on a number of theoretical sociological approaches: a materialist conception of the human condition, a phenomenological account of the experience of the human condition, an interactionist exposition of the concepts of self and identity, and a focus on the disjunction between the social and technical divisions of labor in the contemporary world. The literature on which the argument is based includes some of the classical sociological writings of Weber, Marx, and Durkheim. The argument also rests on some of the more significant sociological writings of the twentieth century. Authors such as Mead, Parsons, Braverman, Goffman, Berger, and Schutz are explored for their contemporary relevance to understanding disability in the community. The concept of community that is used is neither bounded by geography nor neighborhood but is instead defined with reference to the life-world (Schutz 1970). The life-world of impairment and disability is therefore the initial focus.

The argument of this chapter begins by developing a conceptual means to understand personal experience and community. The concept that is used is called the *life-world*. The idea of the life-world helps to illuminate different aspects of personal experience. Personal experience becomes social experience in relationships with other people. A model is presented to help us understand these relationships. This model demonstrates the way people behave toward one another and what happens when one person dominates a relationship with another. Dominance of one person over another, it is argued, is what turns impairment into disability. The concept of *self* is then introduced as a way of understanding the manner in which people can feel both linked to and separated from the communities they inhabit. How communities respond to persons, who are in some sense seen as different, is considered, using the idea of *identity*, especially negative public identity. The manner in which identities are linked to social structures is described using the term *division of labor*. Two kinds of division of labor are contrasted. These are the technical division of labor, which is associated with productive work, and the social division of labor, which refers to broader patterns of social organization. The social significance of barriers to participation in the technical division of labor is noted. The connection between such barriers and negative public identities is explored. The fact that the idea of the technical division of labor has exerted a profound influence on many sociologists is outlined. Specifically, the assumptions that undertaking paid work is normal and that a life without work is deviant are seen to have been a highly influential assumption in writings about illness. This assumption, it is suggested, is unhelpful. In contemporary societies, the significance as well as the complexity and structure of the division of labor is changing. The way that these changes may affect identities is described, and the likely impact on personal experience is drawn out.

LIFE-WORLDS, COMMUNITY, AND THE DIVISION OF LABOR

The life-world is defined as follows. Most people inhabit a social world in which they interact with other people. Some of these others they meet with on a regular and repetitive basis. This includes those with whom they share their domestic and work arrangements. Others still may be more casual acquaintances. The level of intimacy is not the crucial issue. It is the repetitive and routine nature of some of the contacts with others that is important. The repetition of contact with people and the meanings given to those contacts constitute the life-world. These contacts may be geographically proximate. Throughout most of human history, the life-world was bounded by immediate territory. However, imaginary, deceased, and anticipated future people as well as totems, gods, and spirits may also be significant in some people's life-worlds. In an era of rapid, cheap, and efficient communication, the life-world expands dramatically, as it did with the inventions of printing, postage, railways, motor cars, telephones, television, airplanes, and, more recently, information technology.

The community is the everyday life-world of contacts—direct and indirect, real, imaginary, or virtual—that an individual has. Domestic life, work, and leisure may be the most important components of many people's life-worlds, but community cannot be defined solely with reference to these types of attachments. The potential variability is enormous. It is the repetitive and routine contacts in the life-world that is the defining characteristic of the experience of community. This chapter examines the nature of that experience for persons with impairments.

Schutz (1967, 1970) conceptualized the life-world as a series of concentric circles. The innermost circle is the one in which the everyday contacts and routines are highly predictable and are therefore taken for granted. It is important to note that this innermost circle of the life-world may not be, and Schutz never suggested it would be, a place that is benign and cozy. It may be violent and bullying. It may be cold and unforgiving. It may be unpleasant and chronically difficult. It will be the place where discrimination and disadvantage are experienced. However, it constitutes the center of the existence of the person. The types of life-worlds that are grimly malign have been described in those diagnosed with paranoia (Cameron 1943; Lemert 1962) and in prisons and psychiatric hospitals (Cohen and Taylor 1972; Goffman 1968). Other writers have described a more mundane private sphere (notably Berger and Berger 1976), and there is a rich anthropological and sociological tradition exploring ordinary everyday examples (Bott 1971; Dennis, Henriques, and Slaughter 1956; Goldthorpe et al. 1969; Salaman 1974). The key Schutzian point relates to the central realities and experiences of everyday life as the principal focus for sociological analysis of community. To understand how this conception clarifies the position of people with impairment and how impairment leads to discrimination and disadvantage, one should highlight the points of disjunction of the innermost circles of the life-world and those circles proximate to it. This is where the community transforms impairment into disability.

Schutz (1970) described the concentric circles of the life-world as zones of relevance. The closer to the center, the greater the relevance is of what goes on there to the "I." The values and prescriptions of immediately proximal circles to the center are important. The stocks of knowledge or assumptions that an individual has of those parts of the life-world are crucial resources for making sense of things (Schutz 1967). However, these assumptions do not apply in more distant outer circles of the life-world. The stocks of knowledge held by others, which exist in the outer zones of relevance of the life-world, might be understandable, but they do not have immediacy. The important qualifier to this argument applies where the "I" has proximal zones of relevance where the assumptions, values, and prescriptions are well understood and indeed relevant—but are fundamentally opposed or different—to the worldview held personally by the "I." This, it is suggested, is potentially the condition of someone with impairment.

The differences in proximal zones of relevance in the life-world might therefore be very significant indeed. Impairment may be conceptualized as a differential opportunity (life chance) to control one's life-world, which is materially determined by the physical body. Differences in zones of relevance in the life-worlds are the social manifestation of differences in physical life chances. The meaning of this in the life-world is differential experiences of power, exploitation, and access to resources. At the abutment of zones of relevance of the life-world, the significance of experience of discrimination and disadvantage, as well as the physical experience of pain and suffering, is located. It is not that communities are historically motivated agents that discriminate against people with disabilities. Communities do not exist as historically motivated actors. What happens is that the central life-world of the compromised life chance of someone with impairment is in opposition to those of others in the proximate zones of relevance of the life-world.

The way this works may be schematically described by using the concept of interaction. Sociologists use the term *interaction* to refer to the behavior or actions that people engage in with each other, rather than when they are on their own. Interaction is behavior between people. The term is used to mean that the actions of people in the company of others are more than the sum of two individuals' separate actions. What happens between people is a product of a process of communication. The communication involves physical things such as gesture or voice or some other medium of communication. The parties involved are not only communicating; they are also able to think about what they are involved in. They can also think about what the other people involved are doing and thinking. This allows them to appraise what is happening. Because they can think about what is going on, they can modify their own conduct, if they want to, in response to their evaluation of the situation (Mead 1934; Schutz 1967).

The easiest way to imagine this is to think about two people, A and B, meeting for the first time. Where they meet, what led up to that meeting, and their expectations (if any) of what will happen provide the starting point. Whether they meet in a railway carriage as fellow travelers, in a dark alley, or at a cocktail party will provide very different beginnings for what might then ensue. Their gender, age, ethnicity, and whether they have some obvious impairment will provide signals to either party as to what might happen next. Yet none of the potential possibilities of what might occur can be worked out from first principles alone. It is only as some type of communication takes place that A and B will begin to make sense of how they may or may not connect with each other. When A does or says something, B's response is conditioned by what was initially observed in A, as well as by what was seen and heard. This does not happen in some automatic cause-and-effect way but rather is a process of unfolding understanding. That understanding may become shared, or it may not. So, if the first gesture by A is to pull a knife, offer a drink, shake hands, utter some general greeting, or remark about the weather, it will set things off in a particular direction. The participants will then negotiate from different positions of power and influence with each other. Both A and B will be thinking about the other, observing what he or she is doing and saying, and observing the responses to his or her own actions. Movement, words, deportment, voice tone and pitch, dress, touch, smell, and physical proximity all contribute to the process. This occurs at particular times and in physical places. Time and place, together with the other aspects of communication, allow those involved (as well as other people who might observe what is going on or might hear about it later) to make some sense of it. Obviously, interaction often involves more than two people, and therefore the levels of complexity are potentially very great. Also, interaction is not limited to face-to-face contact. It can take place through any medium, which allows for mutual generation of meaning and understanding.

In summary, interaction with intimates in the immediate life-world and with others who enter it from time to time is both symbolic and communicative. When humans interact, they have the capacity to think about what they are doing, think about what they are going to do, and tell other people what they have done, what they are going to do, and why they have done it (Mills 1940). They possess the ability to anticipate and observe the impact on others and what they are doing and saying. Also, they mostly assume that the others with whom they are interacting engage in the same processes of thinking and anticipation (Schutz 1970). Humans have the ability to place themselves in the mind's eye of their fellows and to imagine how they appear to others (Blumer 1962; Mead 1934).

In the simplest interaction, the dyad, the individual will more or less consciously offer a version of the self to the other. This will be done in a variety of ways: in what is said; in movement, dress, and the use of props; and in the words themselves (Mead 1934). In all of these activities, the self attempts to provide a version of reality that the other person will agree with or at least recognize. This is to achieve some goal or purpose that he or she has in mind. He or she also anticipates the responses of the other to his or her performance (Goffman 1969). In repetitive interaction with familiar others, behavior becomes so routine that little preparatory thought needs to go into the presentation of self. It is habitual and unself-conscious. On other occasions, when the responses of others are difficult to anticipate, the person will be self-conscious. He or she may have to give a great deal of thought to what to wear and say and how he or she will behave. In between the extremes of taken-for-grantedness and self-consciousness, a range of presentations of self are possible.

In whatever way the self is presented to others, the person making the presentation stakes some claim to be taken seriously in what she or he is doing. Presentation of self is about appearance, authenticity, and assurance in the performance (Goffman 1969). At their most mundane, these claims to be taken seriously may be nothing more than to be recognized as a man or a woman. It might be much more complex, though, and such presentations are linked to the division of labor and roles played in the division of labor such as parent, neighbor, brain surgeon, or computer programmer. If others acknowledge the legitimacy of the claims being made, then interaction will proceed routinely and unproblematically. *Unproblematically* does not mean without conflict or pain but rather that the rules of the interaction are mutually understood. Each party can assume that the other has roughly the same idea about what is going on as the other. They both respond to and legitimize the version of self being offered.

If, however, the other denies the claims for legitimacy being made by the person presenting the self, then interaction will need to be renegotiated. This is because the parties involved do not share assumptions about the legitimacy of the situation. When the other legitimates claims made in interaction, then the interaction is grounded in authority and social order. Authority, according to Weber (1947), is where the rights of one party in the interaction to behave in particular ways toward the other are accepted as legitimate. *Legitimacy* means that in a dyadic relationship, certain claims to status, knowledge, or resources have to be acknowledged as rightful for interaction to proceed routinely and for the taken-for-granted aspects of what is going on to remain taken for granted (May and Kelly 1982).

The opposite of authority in social relationships is power (Weber 1947, 1948). In some relationships, the person in a subordinate position neither acknowledges nor legitimates nor willingly follows the demands made by superordinate others. Nevertheless, if one party is in a position to force the other to do what he or she wants, despite resistance, then the relationship is one of power. When power affects a simple dyadic relationship, the subordinate does not regard the position, the actions, or the claims of the other as legitimate. Through various mechanisms, from threat and coercion to actual violence, the superordinate gets his or her way. In these situations, the superordinate party denies the legitimacy, in full or in part, of the subordinate. Social order exists by control rather than consent.

Power and authority link to material resources. These, in turn, link to the social division of labor. The social division of labor is the manifestation of the differences in the distribution of resources in the social world (Braverman 1974). The experience of power or authority in relationships (i.e., of the social division of labor) is the outcome of maneuvers between self and others and is experienced and witnessed subjectively in the life-world. At its most abstract and schematic, this is the position in which people with an impairment find themselves. They are in a relationship of power in which they are subordinate. Their claims to be taken seriously as people with legitimate claims to citizenship, involvement in the world of work, involvement in sexual activities, and involvement in the division of labor and the social world are denied. Their experience in the center of their own life-world is not legitimated. Simultaneously, the aspect of the person, which attracts the attention of the other, is the impairment. When the other responds to the impairment (rather than the person) or when, outside of the dyad, in the broader world of everyday contacts, the response is to the impairment, this is the exercise of power. At that point, the impairment becomes a disability. Disability is the experience of power that subordinates, marginalizes, and excludes. Subordination, marginalization, and exclusion are felt and experienced in the life-world as the inner world collides with the proximal zones of relevance where assumptions about self of the inner life-world are not shared.

This is a simple version of a complex reality, and a very broad range of other social possibilities exists. Empirically, there will be widespread differences in social life, in response to impairment and of the experience of disability, as indeed there are many billions of possibilities in human contact. However, the dyad and the articulation of the presentation of self, as well as the power-authority responses described, allow the core of the experience of marginalization and exclusion and its experience in the life-world to be explained. Within the life-world, the locus of that experience of marginalization and disadvantage is the self.

THE SELF AND THE BODY

At its simplest, self is nothing more or less than the view that each of us has in our mind's eye of who and what we are (Ball 1972). Assuming a conscious adult, each of us has an account in our head about our self. This may be little more than a loosely linked set of attributes such as warm-hearted, kind, or talkative. These labels are self-attributed and constitute a borrowing from the various possibilities that human life generates. The self-attributions need not have anything to do with labels applied externally by others. They may bear only the most passing resemblance to what the world at large thinks.

In sociological terms, self is not a psychological thing having biological or physical substance. Instead, self may be conceptualized as a set of verbal routines bounded in the grammars of language, which are given substance in talk about self and in turn are the basis of our thoughts about who and what we are (Kelly 1992). We become conscious of the self because of our ability to talk about it as if it were a thing separate from the subjectivity that is the experience of the self (Kelly and Dickinson 1997). The various narratives that people use to articulate their own sense of who and what they are in the world, as well as to make sense of actual and vicarious experiences, give shape to self. Certain narrative styles give rise to different views of the self and of different attempts to present the self to the external world. The narrating "I" is at the center of such stories. Not infrequently, this produces a sense of the grammatical "I" being coterminous with the self. As narrative structures and styles are cultural resources, it follows that the sense of self will be sociohistorically and culturally diverse. Self has both a changing and a continuous structure (Ball 1972).

Self is historically and culturally variable. So, what it is to have a sense of self as a seventeenth-century Polynesian fisherman, a nineteenth-century naval cadet, or a contemporary airline pilot, for example, will be different. To be a man or woman, young or old, black or white, or disabled or able-bodied will mean different things at different historical times and cultural places. As well as being historically and culturally variable, the self is malleable in the same person through one's life span. As people move from situation to situation, from social context to social context, as they interact with different people, they act out different social roles. Indeed, as they witness their own subjectivity, their sense of self changes (Kelly 1992). As people age and when they get ill, their sense of self changes.

Self may be said to change in two important ways: in space and in time. Ball (1972) refers to the situated self and the substantial self. The situated self is the changing self. It is that sense that people have of who and what they are at a particular moment and in a specific context. Certain situational factors assume salience and significance, which define how the self is experienced at any moment. In a single day, we may move in and out of many different physical spaces in the company of many different others. In a lifetime, our position in the life cycle and the capacities of our physical bodies change. These local saliences and changes in the life cycle will dominate the situated self, the discourse we use to describe to ourselves, and what we think and feel about ourselves. So, when someone walks into a shop to buy a newspaper, this transient experience of being a shopper, although central to the short period of the exchange of money and goods, will have a high but short-term salience. As they move on to their next appointment (e.g., a secret assignation with a lover), then their sense of self changes again. We might assume, for example, that the salience of the chemistry between a person and his or her lover would be of greater significance than that between customer and shopkeeper. It may have an even greater salience if one's sense of who and what one is also is tied up with the guilt that one feels about deceiving one's spouse.

Time also exerts a malleable effect on self but usually in a more gradual way. When we are 9 years old, in contemporary society at least, we generally have a clear sense of being a child. At age 29, we tend to have a clear sense of being a grown-up. At age 49, most people begin to recognize that they are changing. They may need spectacles to read. They cannot run as fast as they could at age 19. They perhaps feel less sexually vigorous. By age 69, the process of change tends to lead to people having a view of themselves as getting old or older. Leaving aside the fact that young children can sometimes behave in very mature ways and that adults can on occasion be childish, the aging process has an impact on self, regardless of our attempts to resist it. Aging can be linked to loss of function up to a point of significant impairment. Impairments themselves affect our sense of who and what we are, although the physical environment, the space rather than the time aspect of self, is the situation that transforms loss of function into a disability. The potential impact of this on the self is therefore considerable. Significant impairments may be rendered more functionally important in the aging process. When the physical space adds to the impairment, as an experience of being separate from the world, it is felt more acutely.

Ball (1972) also described the substantial self. This means that despite changes in immediate situations and changes that take place in the self because of the aging process, we mostly recognize that we are the same person who was a nine-year-old child, an adolescent, someone in the prime of life, and now someone whose functions are diminishing. We also know that if we are a clandestine lover, the guilt is more insistent when we return home. This is precisely because we are the same person who now sits quietly watching television with his or her spouse and plays with the children but who not long before was declaring love for someone else. We are also the same person who did 101 humdrum tasks since we bought our newspaper earlier that day.

In summary, the sense of who and what we are is experienced by most sober and conscious humans as having continuity through time and space. The sense of continuity around a particular body and autobiography are defining characteristics of subjectivity, at least in the Western world. They also create the sense of self and body as the same thing and also provide an empirical experience in which mind and body are both separate yet part of the same thing. The "I" at the center of the mind-body experience can easily create a taken-for-granted life-world in which the self is experienced as having a concrete reality sui generis.

SELF IN THE WORLD: SELF AGAINST THE WORLD

In lay terms, the concept of the self is easy to understand, by virtue of its apparent coterminosity with the body and autobiography through time and space. The experience of self in most mundane circumstances appears to be the experience of body and indeed to be one and the same thing. The body, moreover, gives a sense of physical unity and continuity in the world. The self is, in that everyday mundane sense, embodied. The body provides an important locus of experience and is a mechanism for mediating the world. However, it is not helpful to go too far down this "lay" line of reasoning. Sociologically, the self is not the same thing as body. For example, the self not infrequently experiences itself as in some way separate from the body it inhabits. For example, this may happen when bodily movements are uncontrolled (as in the muscle spasms that occur prior to falling asleep); when we dream; in moments of semiconsciousness induced by drugs, alcohol, or hemiplegia; and in illness when the control of bodily functions may be lost. The sense of separation from the body is highly noticeable in response to certain types of very invasive surgery, such as coronary artery bypass and organ transplantation (Radley and Green 1985). The subjective "I" can also easily get outside of its own body. It can inspect its own subjectivity and treat its sense of self as an object, for all intents and purposes, like any other object in the environment. It can also view its own body in the same way. In other words, to see our selves as we imagine others see us is a process relating to the self and a process relating to the body.

The self, as just indicated, also experiences a sense of separation from others as the impact of space and time is felt on the self. In its most extreme, the sense of self as separate from or against the world may be found in people who entertain paranoid delusions (May and Kelly 1992). Yet the sense of being separate from the world is a process that is essential to the experience of self for all individuals. What happens is that through narrative talk and self-indications, the self accounts for and makes sense of the world of everyday experience. We construct the world in our mind around our self (around our inner circle of the life-world). The sad fact, however, is that the world has a material reality that does not conform to the social constructions the self may make of it. Like the developing child, we constantly, if figuratively, bump into the material world, and it hurts. This is when others deny the presentation of self. Our everyday experience is of hurt and discomfort. The paranoid person accounts for these experiences in terms of conspiracies, and sane people call them delusions. Yet all humans develop accounts in which they mend the gaps between their sense of self and social, physical, and material reality (Mills 1940; Scott and Lyman 1968; Sykes and Matza 1957). The sense of being apart from and set against the world is a common human experience. Conceptualizing the idea of identity is helpful.

The term *identity* is sometimes assumed to be interchangeable with the term *self*, and the terms are sometimes juxtaposed as self-identity. It is more convenient, however, to separate the ideas of self and identity in the way Ball (1972) has done. In a very simple distinction, Ball defines identity as the public label that is applied to the person, whereas the self consists of the ideas each of us has about who and what we are. Those public labels (identities) may relate to social roles and statuses in the division of labor or may simply be attributions made in interaction or more generally to groups in the population. In any event, these labels are the ways the person is defined by others at particular points in time and place. Identity is ego as known to others, whereas self is ego as known to ego (Ball 1972). Of course, self and identity may overlap in significant ways, in respect of key social variables. So ego's sense of being a man is usually congruent with others' views of him as a man. Similarly, ego's sense of being a middle-aged, white, middle-class male may be entirely congruent with the public identities that are imposed by the world at large on that person (Kelly 1992).

None of this is immutable, and most individuals seem to spend some time attempting to manipulate the identities that others may attribute to them. This includes the relatively trivial attempts to conceal true chronological age, which are engaged in by teenagers wishing to appear older than they really are and the middle-aged trying to look younger or slimmer. It also includes the kinds of confidence trickery that Goffman (1969) described and the more thorough-going attempts that individuals sometimes make to present their gender or their racial grouping as different from the way they think others will perceive it to be.

The more interesting phenomenon from a sociological viewpoint is when self and identity are discordant (i.e., the sense of self, which the individual has and presents to others, is denied in social interaction by others). This is the heart of the issue in relation to disability. When the community in the near zones of relevance of the life-world respond to the impairment, they are constructing a social identity (disability) that draws on a set of cultural and social understandings about illness and disability. The sense of self of the person with the impairment is precisely that—*with* the disability, not *the* disability. The disability is not denied as a significant difficulty or as a significant diminution of resources, but the self, which is presented, is *more* than the disability. However, if the community members construct the disability as the all-powerful social identity, the attempts by self to construct it any other way will be thwarted in the normal run of interaction. This again is about power. However, that power is not just at a macro level in which the issue is scarce resources; it is about power in the micro life-world where self and identity collide or, put another way, where the individual human agent hits the social structure.

The place where individuals with impairment deal with others is in their life-world, and the consequences of those interactions are disability. The sense of otherness and strangeness created within the life-world by the disjunction between self and identity constitutes the fundamental life problem for all humans. It is rendered the more acute for some people because of impairment. The central life problem for all people, disabled or otherwise, is how to cope with a material and social world that is hostile, frequently disordered, and disorderly and how to cope with the anxieties that this creates. The problems are greatly exacerbated when the identities constructed in the community are highly discordant with the self.

Humans have to connect with the world as a part of the lived everyday experience of being in the world. Schutz (1967) called this "intersubjectivity." By this, he refers to the sense of shared subjectivity, which in reality can never be fully shared. We can never know what even the most intimate of our acquaintances really thinks about something or the way they see and experience the world. However, we normally assume that, more or less, what they see and experience and how they make sense of the world are much the same as the way that we do. The times in life when we experience that sense of being in the world and, at the same time, of not being in the world are at the point when intersubjectivity breaks down. Schutz argued that the task that had to be accomplished in everyday interaction was to engage with others as if they shared the same assumptions and understandings of the world as self. The person with an impairment has to do this, even when the community manifestly operates with very different assumptions about the nature of the world and the person with an impairment's place within it.

When intersubjectivity breaks down, the experience is of being in the world, but separate from it, or of being in the community but not part of it. However, the self has to engage with this highly problematic and ambiguous world as if it were not like this and as if they were not separate from it. The person with impairment therefore has to operate with a double level of meaning. It is important to note that this is not an issue limited to disability, but the problem is critical in the case of disability.

This is very familiar sociological territory. Because Marx wrote about alienation, many sociological and other theorists have made separation of self from the world an integral part of their social theories (Marx 1961). It provides us with the means to open up a set of other issues: Life is inherently problematic for all human actors (Lazarus 1969). The illusion that it might be otherwise is promoted in advertising, ideology, and religion, and true believers, political or religious, will create for themselves a transcendent reality in which the illusion is taken to be true. However, the emollients of advertising, ideology, and religion can only ever provide comfort. They cannot transform the world, although they make dealing with it a little easier. Access to resources, especially and particularly differential access to resources in the world at large, means that not everyone experiences it in the same way. Differential material resources, including the functioning of the human body, are the central fact of human existence in one form or another for us all. The analysis here is dependent on the idea of the body as a differentially available resource, like a Weberian life chance or a Marxian inequality.

Because sociologists sometimes talk about social structure as if it were a motivated human agent, it is easy to miss the fundamental issue that experiences of discrimination and prejudice are not found in the reifications of abstract entities, such as social structure, but rather are experienced in the epicenter of the life-world—the "I." This is where the pain and suffering caused by the exercise of power is really felt. This is at the interface with the community as it reaches into the life-worlds of people with disabilities and, for that matter, everybody else. The interface with the community is the point when life-worlds meet, and it is the point when the social definitions of disability are contested. This collision with the world is the case for all human beings, but the difference is that the division of labor has evolved in such a way that the battle is not joined with the parties as equal. The resources are one-sided because of the form that the division of labor takes.

HOMO FABER AND THE DIVISION OF LABOR

One of the defining characteristics of the human species is its creativity and ingenuity. Humans possess the knowledge, the tools, and the imagination to confront the material world in which they live and to change it in ways that their imaginations dream of. *Homo faber* is the term to describe the capacity to think of things differently from the way they are in the present and to bring various forces to bear on the material world to alter it in line with imagination (Berger 1964). The division of labor is important because it arises in the attempt to control the material world and is one of the tools for attempts at control.

Human beings exist in many material worlds. They inhabit a physical universe, which is geological, meteorological, cosmic, and botanical, for example, and one that is the product of human endeavor or work itself. To survive, people have to engage with and protect themselves from that physical environment. This physical world is usually experienced as external to the individual and frequently as a determining force on his or her life. Until relatively recent times, even the most advanced human societies were at the mercy of powerful physical forces that were paramount in the life and death of individuals. Climate, geology, and microbiology constrained human life. It is only in the most recent past that the species has, through ingenuity and fashioning of tools, managed to keep these powerful forces at bay. However, such control is contingent. The appearance of human control over the physical world through technical means may appear to be a reality, but it is always a precarious control of the physical universe. The physical world is full of reminders that the efficacy of human dominance is tenuous. The irritating malfunctions of contemporary technologies, such as cars, washing machines, and computers, as well as the full force of nature in hurricanes, earthquakes, or floods, show that the assumption of human omnipotence is dangerously naive. Nevertheless, one of the most successful ways the species has brought this dangerous material world at least partly under control is through cooperation. This cooperation is the basis of the division of labor.

The idea of productive and cooperative activity is central to the concept of the division of labor (Glover and Kelly 1987). An important characteristic of human beings is the capacity to produce goods and services beyond basic subsistence needs in relationships with other humans and the physical environment. The social division of labor is the particular ways the producers and consumers of different goods and services within a society are differentiated from and interrelated with each other (Braverman 1974). The various forms, which the social division of labor takes, generate the different types of social and political organization found in societies. The degree to which different forms of communities relate to each other and to the social system as a whole is a manifestation of the social division of labor. The ways in which different groups and individuals, such as minorities, the young, the old, men and women, and the people with impairments, link together is a form of the division of labor. The social division of labor is a neutral concept, but its impact and its effects are far from neutral. The dynamics of exclusion, the basis of power, and the positioning of classes and other social divisions in society all stem from the form that the social division of labor takes. In general terms, people with disabilities have found themselves relatively disadvantaged and marginalized in the social division of labor historically and contemporarily. As argued above, this is experienced in the face-to-face interactions in the life-worlds within specific communities.

The *technical division of labor* (as against the social division of labor) refers to the specific productive configurations or arrangements in work organizations (Braverman 1974). In preindustrial society, these may well be difficult to distinguish from the social organization of community life, in agriculture or craft working. In industrial society, the distinction is clearer. Scots political economist Adam Smith most famously described the technical division of labor. He considered the division of labor in manufacturing and enunciated the principles of the division and subdivision of tasks and functions and the link of this division to efficiency. He concluded that it was more efficient for a task to be divided and subdivided and for there to be further subdivision than for someone to complete the whole task on his or her own (Smith 1976).

Marx (1971) developed this theme further. He was fascinated by the productive energy of capitalism and with the forces released by machinery combined with a specialized division of labor. For Marx, the great irony and trick of capitalism was its ability to produce plenty but to deny the wealth created by the many being shared among them. These principles are at the heart of Marx's theory of surplus value and at the center of his analysis of capitalism. The important critical leap in Marx's thinking was to extend the analysis beyond the economic into the social and political. Critically, Marx argued for the principle that the very structure of society in the form of its class system emerged directly from relations arising in the technical division of labor. The relationship of participants in productive activity in the technical means of production and the form of the exploitative relationships that emerge establish the social division of labor (Marx 1971).

Marx (1971), on the division of labor, provides an insight into the dynamics of exploitation. At its heart is a materialist conception of the basis of human life. The technical division of labor allows cooperative and productive engagement with the material world. The shape of society is the *social division of labor* (Braverman 1974). When a disjunction exists between the social and technical divisions of labor, conflict emerges in a sharp and acute form. This is vitally important to understanding contemporary developments for all marginalized, disenfranchised, exploited, and discriminated groups. In this conception, the person with the impairment, by virtue of limited life chances, may not play a full role in the technical division of labor. This, in turn, leads to marginalization in the social division of labor. However, the issue is more complex in contemporary societies.

The Division of Labor and Work in the Contemporary World

What all the classical writers on the division of labor shared was an agreement about the importance of work (Durkheim 1933; Marx 1971; Smith 1976). Contemporary technologies offer some interesting possibilities about the development of the division of labor and, in turn, impairment, disability, and community. Work roles, given their position in the technical division of labor and their consequences for the social division of labor, are assumed in most classical and much contemporary sociology to be the cornerstones of the social structure (Parkin 1972). The dominance of such thinking is demonstrated by the fact that most accounts about the dispossessed start from an analysis of their exclusion from the technical division of labor and their consequent disempowerment in the social division of labor. The paradigmatic case is people with disabilities. De facto, such people were wholly or mostly excluded from the productive process or at least grudgingly allowed a minor role in disadvantaged labor markets.

However, the underlying assumption of such theorizing is that full employment is the norm, that work roles are central in terms of personal and system integration, and that such work roles are enduring and lifelong. This assumption is based on the highly specific sociohistorical example of industrial societies, especially the Western European and North American economies of the first half of the twentieth century. It is based on an economic world in which there is an industrial base, when the primary and secondary sectors of the economy are relatively labor intensive, when the nature of the social systems in such societies was relatively stable, and when it seemed that this state of affairs was a crowning achievement of progress (or the heart of capitalist exploitation, depending on your point of view).

Several points need to be made. First, outside the industrialized West, this model did not apply. Second, even in the industrialized West, the model only had limited application. As far as paid employment was concerned, it applied principally to adult men. Female participation rates in the economy, defined in terms of paid employment, were less than men in general, and so are we to assume either the model did not really apply to them or that some other kind of model or set of assumptions should have been brought to bear? Women are discounted as real participants in the social world by virtue of being outside of the technical division of labor. What about children, the dispossessed, the unemployed, the aged, and those in large parts of continental Europe who were located in a rural agrarian tradition? In other words, the underlying assumption of the theory was based on a minority of the population, even in those societies that are or were the most technically advanced at a particular point in time.

Such was the deeply engrained nature of the assumption about the centrality of paid work that writers in many branches of sociology used the occupational structure and the division of labor as a metaphor to describe other aspects of social life. The doyen of medical sociology, Parsons (1951), builds the idea of the centrality of work, derived from an understanding of the division of labor into the epicenter of his theory of the sick role. One of the core ideas of the sick role is that of exemption from normal social role responsibilities, the principal responsibility being engagement with paid work. To be sick, according to Parsons, is to disengage from the productive part of the technical division of labor and to settle, albeit temporarily, in a specialized part of the social division of labor—the sick role.

This has had very important consequence for the theories of medical sociology and disability. If the assumption is challenged that work is or should be the central life activity of humans, a very different account of illness and disability emerges. Much of the early work on chronic illness, for example, focused on the impact of the loss of opportunity to work consequent on the illness. The illness was thus conceptualized as a double deficit. There was the illness itself and the pain and suffering that accompanied it, as well as the losses associated with the inability to fulfill normal social role responsibilities. One of the core ideas of the sick role is exemption from normal social role responsibilities. The principal responsibility from which people who are sick are exempted is engagement with paid work. Subsequently, theorists of chronic illness borrowed heavily from the discourse about the centrality of work and even used the idea of the illness *career* as a guiding principle in the construction of ideas about illness. In this regard, illness and disability are theorized as deficits when measured against a standard of normality in which work and adulthood (for men) are synonymous, and loss of work is about the detachment from society and the principal anchor points in the social structure.

This kind of thinking led Parsons (1951) to describe illness as deviance at an individual and social level and as a disturbance to the normal functioning of the individual and society. It is helpful to note that this way of theorizing does not conceptualize illness or disability as aspects of life chances (and hence as dimensions of stratification) or as aspects of the distribution of power and legitimacy in the social structure. Neither does this kind of reasoning allow for an embedding of the person who is ill in the social structure (which a life chance approach would). Instead, it effectively places the ill or disabled person outside of the social structure proper, by virtue of his or her unproductiveness, deviance, and special character, which follow from the illness itself. The community may reject the person, and the person may feel alienated and separate from the community, but that is not the same as being deviant and outside society in any sense other than not being able to work.

Recent debates about postmodernity and about postmodernism serve to highlight the particular view of industrial society and the roles of work within it, central to this kind of thinking (Kelly and Field 1998). At the heart of an understanding of disability using traditional sociological reasoning is that having a disability is a state of physical being that results in a state of economic, social, and psychological being that is not wholly integrated into the dominant civil society. The argument might be made that this is the inevitable consequence of material physical difference. It might also be argued that the material conditions of existence might or must be changed. However, at the center of the argument is a model of society in which equilibrium is possible, either as Parsons (1951) argued, by managing the deviance of difference in various ways, or, as other writers have argued, by overturning politically the oppressive structures (Oliver 1990).

In contemporary society, the fixed nature of work roles cannot be assumed, however. The transition from a manufacturing-based economy to a predominantly service-based economy, as well as developments in information technology, automation, and the introduction of more flexible work patterns, has led to the widespread disappearance in the West of industrial work dependent on a predominantly male, low-skilled manual workforce. Jobs linked to primary production and manufacturing have declined in large numbers. New types of segmented labor markets have emerged in which part-time, short-term work in retail leisure and services is increasingly common (Edwards 1979). There is greater participation by women in the total labor market. The growth of global markets has been accompanied by diminished state intervention in many aspects of economic and social life.

Against this background, key aspects of the social division of labor have altered in their significance. Class, age, and gender, which were arguably once the fundamental and accepted axes of social structure and identities created around the life-world, have become more fluid and less deterministic. Gender identities have become less rigid and coercive, and cultural identities based on ethnicity are more prominent, highlighting a range of legitimate diversity not previously acknowledged. As these aspects of the social division of labor evolve in ways that articulate increasing diversity, fashion and image have become increasingly important in a world of global mass communications.

The experience of having impairment may also change as the life-worlds change and fragment within the social division of labor. Television, video, mobile phones, and the Internet provide a means of changing and expanding life-worlds. The new private mass media and do-it-yourself communications have shifted and expanded the life-world by creating a new type of experience. They expand the potentially knowable and give a new basis for intersubjectivity. The face-to-faceness of community relationships has been changed and also expanded as a consequence of modes of communications, which allow communication globally. This has and will continue to play a role in the fragmentation and unification of social life. The privatization of entertainment and the global possibilities of cyber-friendships produce a life-world that is not geographically defined and potentially at least is not class, gender, or ethnicity bound. In one very interesting development, communication between people with shared experiences of illness is very easy now without the constraints of official definitions (by the medical profession or other dominant groups). This may facilitate, in a much more direct way, the development of alternative views of the illness potentially contrary to mainstream thinking, in a way that erstwhile patient support or self-help groups were not able to do very easily.

Another aspect of this fragmentation process relates to identities. In the era when the social division of labor was relatively fixed and stable, the numbers of identities—the public knowable aspect of the person that an individual could adopt—were circumscribed often quite rigidly within communities. The anchor points of social roles in communities were limited to occupation, gender, age, and perhaps religion. These identities had an enduring quality through time. Geographical and social mobility were limited, and such identities were lifelong. Having a disability or a chronic illness mirrored the core identities in the social structure. Having a disability became the dominant identity, at least as far as officialdom, medicine, and perhaps the rest of the community were concerned. The medical and social services were the arbiters of the identity and how it should be constructed. Arguably, the fragmentation of identities in contemporary Western and North American societies means that the constraints of an earlier era are no longer so absolute.

One particularly important aspect of this is what might be termed the *celebration of difference*. Drawing inspiration from antiracist, feminist, and postmodern discourses more generally, the disability movement has celebrated difference in an attack on what is defined as the ideological assumption that difference is bad (Oliver 1996; Shakespeare 1996). This leads not only to a kind of relativism in the aesthetics of appearance (long inspired by the avant-garde) but also to the political demand for a tolerance and acceptance of difference. In turn, this generates, through the appearance of new discourses of self, alternative ways of constructing meaning about the world to provide for different ways of having a disability or a chronic illness. Once upon a time, the hegemony of the medical and social services to define what the role should be led to some extraordinary coercive regimes (Scott 1969). The new discourse of difference is not just about changes in identity and changes in community relations; it is also about the creation of life-worlds in which difference is both a reality and a choice.

However, there is still the question of the technical division of labor and, more specifically, the technology on which many of the changes described depend. Information technologies have changed the nature of the technical division of labor at the workplace and opened the possibility of distance working, home working, and remote access. They also open up possibilities for entry into the labor market for many people who could not separate home and work for mobility or health reasons. Yet the new technologies have a range of other liberating potentials in terms of being the tools themselves of functional replacement in which the material life chances of the body are limited. The technology is the potential to replace the lost or absent resource. There are quantum issues too. A wheelchair or a prosthetic limb has to be negotiated as part of identity, but that negotiation becomes much easier when the technology offers direct, easy, and effortless control by the person using it, rather than when it requires constant assistance to be of any use.

What of resources? The technology is not inexpensive, and persons living in the contemporary West are more likely to see its use sooner than are persons in developing countries. Obviously, someone has to pay for it. Here, prediction is probably unwise, but the previous two decades have seen the costs of the technology fall steeply while its power has increased. There is evidence that the Internet, for example, is growing at a rate that will make global possibilities of reality sooner than could have been imagined even a few years ago. The class and cultural biases that affect access to the mass media of communications are likely to have an impact, but it is far from clear where the line of access, which is economically determined, will actually fall. The model of innovation here is more likely to be that of the video player and the computer game, which, in a society such as Britain, have spread rapidly through all sectors of the class system, rather than something such as air travel, which has more restricted use. Also, it is not just the technologies of mass communication; it is the technology of mobility and prosthetics for which we are probably at the very earliest stages of development.

CONCLUSION

The community then ceases to be something in which the dominant motif is neighborliness and proximity. If we use the definition of community described at the beginning of this chapter as the life-world, we have a much better way of conceptualizing actual and potential changes in community relationships. If we acknowledge the significance of the social division of labor, take note of its traditional link to work, and then see the possibilities that changes to the technical division of labor facilitate, both to the nature of work itself and to the social division of labor, then we begin to see interesting practical possibilities. Go further and question the centrality of work as a full-time activity within the social division of labor and think in terms of the extra productivity that new technologies potentiate, and then a range of possibilities, theoretical and practical, may be discerned.

The new social arrangements offer freedom and liberation in ways that theorists of alienation could scarcely have thought possible two or three decades ago. The nature of politics also changes in such an environment. It has been argued that in contemporary Western society, issue-based politics has replaced class-based politics (Crook, Pakulski, and Waters 1992). So, green issues, environmental issues, and food scares become the bread and butter of political life, while issues of class exploitation remain submerged. Likewise, worker resistance moves from outright industrial confrontation through strikes to a more simple disengagement with the work and, within the workplace, a greater emphasis on legislation and legal contracts.

However, contemporary society is more than just the occupational structure destabilized. The nature of sociability has altered in subtle ways too. With the demise of the engagement with work, people seem much freer to create lifestyles of their own choosing, and there is evidence that this is exactly what many have decided to do. Changing patterns of sexual partnering, cohabitation, child rearing, and gender identities have all been explored and tried out not just by persons in the margins of society or those who are excluded in various ways but also by those at the center of our political establishment. This is not to say that marriage is no longer popular, nor to deny that many people live in conventional arrangements. It is to say that some of the easy certainties of life in the middle of the twentieth century seem to have given way to growing uncertainties. Impairment means diminished life chance. Diminished life chance is experienced in the technical division of labor as exclusion and in the social division of labor as marginalization. This is felt as a disjunction between self and identity in the life-world and is transformed into disability. If the technical division of labor changes, if life-worlds expand, and if public identities fragment, then the impact on life chances may be different. They may not necessarily be better, but sociological theory allows a means to plot their progress.

This chapter has shown, by using a number of traditional sociological concepts, that it is possible to theorize disability in the community. A number of core ideas were presented. First, the life-world was defined with reference to the subjectivity of the self. It was identified as the locus of pain, suffering, and alienation from others. Second, community was described as the intersection of self's subjectivity in the life-world and public identities imposed by others. The interactive processes, which lead to the application of negative labels, were outlined. Third, power and authority in interaction were shown to be embedded in understandings of legitimacy in interaction and especially the nature of presentation of self. Fourth, the social division of labor was defined as the outcome of social relationships as well as an important constraint on them. The social division of labor is linked to the consequences of power and authority relationships in social interaction. Fifth, the technical division of labor was described with reference to technical and technological artifacts and the location of productive paid work. It was argued that impairment became disability at the point when others denied the claims made by the self in the community. It was noted that this traditionally has had implications for exclusion from the technical division of labor and hence from paid work, and it also has had considerable effects in the social division of labor. It was suggested that with the transformation of the technical division of labor and the concomitant changes in the social division of labor, the continuity of these arrangements and indeed the theoretical arguments that underpin them should be questioned.

REFERENCES

Ball, D. W. 1972. "Self and Identity in the Context of Deviance: The Case of Criminal Abortion." Pp. 158-83 in *Theoretical Perspectives on Deviance,* edited by R. A. Scott and J. D. Douglas. New York: Basic Books.

Berger, P. 1964. "Some General Observations on the Problem of Work." Pp. 211-41 in *The Human Shape of Work: Studies in the Sociology of Occupations,* edited by P. Berger. New York: Macmillan.

Berger, P. and B. Berger. 1976. *Sociology: A Biographical Approach.* Rev. ed. London: Penguin.

Blumer, H. 1962. "Society as Symbolic Interaction." Pp. 179-92 in *Human Behavior and Social Processes,* edited by A. Rose. London: Routledge Kegan Paul.

Bott, E. 1971. *Family and Social Network*. 2d ed. London: Tavistock.

Braverman, H. 1974. *Labor and Monopoly Capital: The Degradation of Work in the Twentieth Century*. New York: Monthly Review Press.

Cameron, N. 1943. "The Paranoid Pseudo-Community." *American Journal of Sociology* 49:32-38.

Cohen, S. and L. Taylor. 1972. *Psychological Survival: The Experience of Long-Term Imprisonment*. London: Penguin.

Crook, S., J. Pakulski, and M. Waters. 1992. *Post-Modernisation: Change in Advanced Society*. London: Sage.

Dennis, N., F. Henriques, and C. Slaughter. 1956. *Coal Is Our Life: An Analysis of a Yorkshire Mining Community*. London: Eyre and Spottiswoode.

Durkheim, E. 1933. *The Division of Labour in Society*. New York: Free Press.

Edwards, R. C. 1979. *Contested Terrain: The Transformation of the Workplace in the Twentieth Century*. New York: Basic Books.

Glover, I. A. and M. P. Kelly. 1987. *Engineers in Britain: A Sociological Study of the Engineering Dimension*. London: Allen & Unwin.

Goffman, E. 1968. *Asylums: Essays on the Social Situation of Mental Patients and Other Inmates*. London: Penguin.

———. 1969. *The Presentation of Self in Everyday Life*. London: Penguin.

Goldthorpe, J., D. Lockwood, F. Bechoffer, and J. Platt. 1969. *The Affluent Worker in the Class Structure*. Cambridge, UK: Cambridge University Press.

Kelly, M. P. 1992. "Self, Identity and Radical Surgery." *Sociology of Health and Illness* 14:390-415.

Kelly, M. P. and H. Dickinson. 1997. "The Narrative Self in Autobiographical Accounts of Illness." *Sociological Review* 45:254-78.

Kelly, M. P. and D. Field. 1998. "Conceptualising Chronic Illness." Pp. 3-20 in *Sociological Perspectives on Health, Illness and Healthcare*, edited by D. Field and S. Taylor. Oxford, UK: Blackwell.

Lazarus, R. 1969. *Patterns of Adjustment and Human Effectiveness*. New York: McGraw-Hill.

Lemert, E. 1962. "Paranoia and the Dynamics of Exclusion." *Sociometry* 25:2-20.

Marx, K. 1961. *The Economic and Philosophic Manuscripts of 1844*. Moscow: Foreign Languages Publishing House.

———. 1971. *The Grundrisse*. Edited by D. McLellan. London: Macmillan.

May, D. and M. P. Kelly. 1982. "Chancers, Pests and Poor Wee Souls." *Sociology of Health and Illness* 4:279-301.

———. 1992. "Understanding Paranoia: Toward a Social Explanation." *Clinical Sociology Review* 10:50-70.

Mead, G. H. 1934. *Mind, Self and Society: From the Standpoint of the Social Behaviorist*. Edited by C. W. Morris. Chicago: University of Chicago Press.

Mills, C. W. 1940. "Situated Actions and Vocabularies of Motive." *American Sociological Review* 5:904-13.

Oliver, M. 1990. *The Politics of Disablement*. Basingstoke, UK: Macmillan.

———. 1996. "Rehabilitating Society." Pp. 95-109 in *Understanding Disability: From Theory to Practice*, edited by M. Oliver. Basingstoke, UK: Macmillan.

Parkin, F. 1972. *Class, Inequality and the Political Order: Social Stratification in Capitalist and Communist Societies*. St. Albans, UK: Paladin.

Parsons, T. 1951. *The Social System*. London: Routledge Kegan Paul.

Radley, A. and R. Green. 1985. "Styles of Adjustment to Coronary Graft Surgery." *Social Science and Medicine* 20:461-72.

Salaman, G. 1974. *Community and Occupation: An Exploration of Work-Leisure Relationships*. Cambridge, UK: Cambridge University Press.

Schutz, A. 1967. *The Phenomenology of the Social World*. Translated by G. Walsh and F. Lehert. Evanston, IL: Northwestern University Press.

———. 1970. *On Phenomenology and Social Relations: Selected Writings*. Edited by H. Wagner. Chicago: University of Chicago Press.

Scott, M. B. and S. Lyman. 1968. "Accounts." *American Sociological Review* 33:46-62.

Scott, R. A. 1969. *The Making of Blind Men: A Study of Adult Socialization*. New York: Russell Sage.

Shakespeare, T. 1996. "Disability, Identity, Difference." Pp. 94-113 in *Exploring the Divide: Illness and Disability*, edited by C. Barnes and G. Mercer. Leeds, UK: The Disability Press.

Smith, A. 1976. *An Inquiry into the Nature and Causes of the Wealth of Nations*. Edited by R. H. Cambell and A. S. Skinner. Oxford, UK: Clarendon.

Sykes, G. M. and D. Matza. 1957. "Techniques of Neutralisation: A Theory of Delinquency." *American Sociological Review* 22:664-70.

Weber, M. 1947. *The Theory of Social and Economic Organisation.* Translated by A. M. Henderson and T. Parsons. London: Collier Macmillan.

———. 1948. "Class, Status, Party." Pp. 180-95 in *From Max Weber: Essays in Sociology,* edited by H. Gerth and C. W. Mills. London: Routledge Kegan Paul.

Welfare States and Disabled People

16

ROBERT F. DRAKE

This chapter is concerned with the impact of welfare states on disabled people in Western, industrialized countries. I deal first with competing definitions of the concept of the "welfare state" and then explore the development of welfare. I argue that two key aspects are of particular importance in fashioning the experiences of disabled people. These are the structure of income distribution through welfare and the supremacy of a medical understanding of disablement.

In formulating their social security systems, many Western states have distinguished between contributory (earnings-related) benefits and noncontributory (often, means-tested) benefits. When employees have been able to subscribe to schemes that provide earnings-related benefits, their subsequent nonwork income is generally above subsistence level and, in some countries, such as Sweden and Germany, could be very close to their erstwhile level of earnings (Ginsburg 1993; Wilson 1993). However, many disabled people may not have done paid work at all and may not have contributed either to earnings-related schemes or to private insurance. Many thus rely on "safety net" systems of social assistance or "flat-rate" allowances (Oliver and Barnes 1998). The main point here is that states may keep noncontributory levels of benefit deliberately low to discourage benefit dependency on social security and encourage unemployed people back into work (Andrews and Jacobs 1990). The option of resuming work may be closed to some disabled people, who may consequently command only low levels of income for much of their lives (Berthoud, Lakey, and McKay 1993).

The second key aspect of the relationship between welfare states and disabled people has been the prevalence of medical understandings of disability. In subscribing to a medical model of disability, both society at large and the institutions of health and social services have regarded disabled people as "defective" in some way. The project of medicine has been to treat, ameliorate, or "normalize" disabled people according to prevailing understandings of physiological and cognitive norms (Barnes, Mercer, and Shakespeare 1999; Oliver 1990; Symonds and Kelly 1998).

In this chapter, I argue that a key historical effect of these two systems (social security benefits and medicine) has been either the conceptual or, indeed, the actual segregation of disabled people from society at large. Public responses ranged from fear to pity and from punishment to "care" (Hevey 1992; Oliver 1990). Disabled people have been stigmatized through the powerful mechanisms of conformity that operate as part of everyday life to secure the cohesion of society (Becker 1963; Giddens 1993; Goffman 1969, 1970; Lemert 1962). Only in more recent times have we witnessed a reappraisal of welfare policy. A new civil rights paradigm is emerging in which the problems faced by disabled people are recognized as sociopolitical in origin. Increasingly, the environment, as opposed to the individual, is becoming the focus for change (Oliver 1996).

The final section of this chapter assesses some of the tangible impacts of welfare on disabled people. I begin by discussing the economic consequences that flow from dependency on benefits or low-paid work. I then turn to social and environmental outcomes, including aspects of education and growth, domicile, location, transportation, and mobility. Finally, I consider political implications for disabled people.

WELFARE STATES

In writing about welfare states, scholars often begin by warning how difficult the concept is to define. Lowe (1993), for example, tells us that there is "no agreement amongst historians or social scientists over when the first welfare states were established or what the term actually means" (p. 9). In a similar vein, Hill (1993) contends that attempts at welfare state macrotheory have yielded only low levels of specificity and are of limited utility in applied studies. One of the key problems, perhaps, is the diversity in the extent of welfare provision. Some states, particularly the Scandinavian countries, have built extensive and universally available systems of welfare (Ginsburg 1983, 1993; Gould 1988, 1993). Other states engage in what Mabbott and Bolderson (1999) called "residualism." In places such as the United States and Hong Kong, citizens are expected to make their own provision through private insurance or reliance on the family. Administrations thus adopt a far more residual role, providing only means-tested and basic (safety net) services to the most vulnerable in the population (Mabbott and Bolderson 1991; McLaughlin 1993).

Welfare states have emerged principally in societies with high levels of democratic participation and industrialization (Ashford 1986; Esping-Andersen 1990; Hill 1993). Within a functional analysis, Mishra (1977) saw welfare states as instruments of social reform, social administration, and social engineering. However, others, in stressing the differences between national welfare states, have explained considerable degrees of divergence by referring to unique historical circumstances in their evolution (Cochrane and Clarke 1993; Fraser 1984; Jones 1991). Finally, some scholars have analyzed welfare states according to their main (and common) purposes. From this perspective, Blakemore (1998) and Baldock et al. (1999) define welfare systems in terms of the range of institutions that together determine the welfare of citizens. These institutions usually include health, education, housing, and social security or income maintenance.

I do not wish to deny the utility of any of these approaches. Each reveals its own insights about state welfare in the contemporary world. However, as the task in this chapter is to mainly assess the relationship between welfare states and disabled people, I will concentrate on the evolution and the impact of welfare states in just two key respects: income and health. Clearly, disabled people's experience of social institutions will vary over time and among states. The precise outcomes of policies will differ from country to country, as will the consequences that flow from them. It is possible, nevertheless, to discern some common impacts.

THE EMERGENCE OF STATE WELFARE

Public services come into being for a number of reasons, although specific circumstances may have varied among nations. Several common economic, social, and political influences led to the development of welfare states in the twentieth century. With the growth of capitalist economies and international competition between states, each saw the need for fit and healthy workers and strong military forces (Searle 1971; Semmel 1960). In every population, however, there were those who could not meet these requirements, and, at least in part, state welfare emerged as a response to this problem (Alcock 1993; Novak 1988; Spicker 1993).

In Britain, for example, early social research by Hyndman (1911), Booth (1903), and Rowntree (1901) revealed that as Queen Victoria's reign came to a close, some 30 percent of her subjects dwelt in perpetual poverty. There were other concomitant social problems such as high perinatal mortality rates, poor nutrition in the workforce, poor housing, overcrowding, disease, and dependency in old age (Burnett 1986; Finer 1999; Gauldie 1974; Lewis 1980; Stedman Jones 1971).

Governments came under pressure to intervene from the findings of social research, the records of medical officers of health, and the documentation supplied by philanthropists and charities. These were supplemented by protests from militant trade unions representing the unskilled laboring classes; from the birth of radical political groups, such as the Social Democratic Federation and the Labour Party; and from new political voices emerging from the extension of the franchise through the reform acts of 1832, 1867, and 1884 (Harris 1972; Jenkins 1994; Rose 1972).

Governments had been content to leave the "problem" of the poor, the marginalized, and disabled people to philanthropists and were reluctant to intervene in what were seen as individual tragedies. Unsurprisingly, therefore, the first official responses were both ad hoc and fragmented. Nevertheless, between 1906 and 1914, the Liberal administrations of Campbell Bannerman and (from 1908) Asquith introduced unemployment and sickness benefits, subsidized school meals, provided regulations for the training of midwives and services for the medical inspection of schoolchildren, and extended educational opportunities and Britain's first old-age pension (Hay 1978; 1975; Rowland 1971). Through the interwar years, a more incisive understanding of the causes of poverty was developed by William Beveridge (1942), leading ultimately to the formulation of his plans for social security based on mutual insurance (Timmins 1995).

In addition, the two world wars gave impetus to the development of health services and enhanced the status of the medical professions. In 1918 and 1919, hundreds of thousands of men returned from the Great War permanently impaired. Many of them had been gassed or blinded in the trenches of Paschendale, Ypres, the Somme, and all along the Western front. The combatant nations felt they had moral obligations toward their war wounded (Bourke 1996). Initial policy responses were, however, rather uncoordinated, haphazard, and not particularly generous (Sainsbury 1993). There are two key points here. First, as with industry and commerce, the strength of the armed forces depended on the successful reproduction of a healthy, well-nourished, and "able-bodied" population. Health services had thus to deal with both the requirements and the consequences of war. Second, the creation of so many disabled people in wartime was met with a rapid expansion of health services. Society's response to disability was naturalized within the context of medicine.

In sum, welfare states were intended to provide health services and education to underpin a nation's military, industrial, and economic requirements. Welfare states were also a product of social concerns, about overcrowding, poor housing, and poverty. Finally, they were responses to political pressure from radical groups and threats to the social fabric in the form of protest and riot.

DISABLED PEOPLE IN THE EARLY WELFARE STATE

How was it, then, that in large numbers, disabled people came to rely on welfare for their livelihoods? There can be no natural or preordained reason for the fact that so many found themselves dependent on the benefaction of the state.

To deal first with economic factors, Finkelstein (1981) argues that much of the responsibility for disabled people's plight rested with the gradual change in the nature of work that resulted from the industrialization of the Western world. Prior to the advent of heavy industry, disabled people enjoyed legitimate, valued, and productive roles within their local communities. However, as production became increasingly mechanized and required greater speed, they were gradually excluded from work because new tools and instruments were built to designs that could, by and large, be used only by people who had no significant physiological impairment. Those who could not work were quickly differentiated from those who would not work, but both groups were segregated from mainstream society (Ryan and Thomas 1980; Topliss 1979).

While the "idle" and "undeserving" were met with deterrent (and sometimes brutal) measures, the "deserving" poor might hope for philanthropy from the well-to-do (Ditch 1991; Owen 1965). Punitive regimes took different forms in different countries. In Britain, prior to and during the nineteenth century, a pauper family no longer able to provide for itself might be committed to the dreaded institution of the workhouse, an establishment in which families would be segregated in large dormitories, given meager rations, and put to sweated labor or loaned out to local farmers as additional labor (Crowther 1983; Novak 1988). There is also evidence that between the 1780s and 1860s, at least some disabled people were convicted as criminals and transported to Australia (Hughes 1987).

While some disabled people might be incarcerated as paupers or criminals, others would have been counted among the deserving poor and have received alms or asylum (Kirkman Gray [1905] 1967). In Britain, philanthropy became a major part of Victorian society, and as far as disability was concerned, charitable and voluntary activity became increasingly organized within the worldview of medicine (Jones 1991; Nightingale 1973). This legacy has meant that even today, a significant proportion of voluntary organizations still include some specific medically defined condition in their names (the Spina Bifida Association, the National Schizophrenia Fellowship, the Parkinson's Disease Society, the Muscular Dystrophy Society, the Alzheimer's Disease Society). These organizations continue to define their membership in similarly diagnostic and delimited terms (Brilliant 1990; Drake 1992a, 1994, 1996b; Stanton 1970).

MODERN STATE WELFARE

Clearly, the growth of state involvement and the particular shape that it took differed from country to country. However, I have argued elsewhere (Drake 1999) that we may commonly detect four overlapping strands in the evolution of disability policies and the development of welfare services more generally. These are containment, compensation, care, and citizenship. Reference has already been made to early policies in the British context where containment stood as a preeminent aim. It entailed the removal of disabled people from the community into prisons, workhouses, almshouses, or hospitals. I have also discussed the idea of "compensation" as it applied to people injured at work or wounded in World War I and World War II and who, according to the origin of their impairments, might expect differential forms of help from the state. These benefits might include war pensions, disability allowances, tax or other relief, and health and rehabilitation services (see Drake 1999:49-57).

In more recent times, the third strand of policy response, "care," came to the fore. Here I refer to the development, particularly in the latter part of the twentieth century, of more tangible, widespread, and direct state programs. Such programs include daycare services, "special" education, sheltered employment, occupational skills training, health care, prosthetic services, community-based personal social services, and broader social assistance or social security programs, providing more specific forms of financial support according to an individual's condition (Hill 1993; Lowe 1993). The extent to which such services have been developed and the degree to which they cohere vary between states. Common wisdom has it that in the half century following World War II, Sweden and the Scandinavian countries created perhaps the most extensive welfare programs (Ginsburg 1983, 1993; Gould 1988; Ronnby 1985). A second group, of which Britain was typical, produced piecemeal and rather uncoordinated services inaugurated at different levels of government and managed by differing departments of state (Barnes 1991; Lowe 1993; Oliver 1990, 1991; Timmins 1995). Yet other countries, such as the United States, Canada, and Australia, looked as much to civil rights mechanisms as to social services (Drake 1999; Tucker 1994) (see below).

These different approaches have resulted in wide variation in expenditure. Certainly, there are clear differences in the proportions of gross domestic product (GDP) devoted to social security (Organization for Economic Cooperation and Development [OECD] 1999). Even so, in the past three or four decades, care services have expanded rapidly in many countries. For example, the number of welfare staff in Sweden increased from 35,000 in 1960 to 160,000 by 1975 (Ronnby 1985). In Britain, there were 7,828 welfare workers in 1959. By 1995, the whole-time equivalent staffing of English social services departments had reached 233,862 (Department of Health 1996).

The prime focus of health and social services continues to be on disability as a personal condition. Welfare is still significantly about changing the individual to fit into the social and physical environment rather than altering the social, political, and physical contours of society. Following the International Year of Disabled People in 1981, however, some administrations began to respond to the challenge of national disability movements that governments must recognize disability as a civil rights issue (Barnes 1991; Crow 1990; Hasler 1993; Pagel 1988). New kinds of laws emerged, particularly in the United States, which were aimed less at extending welfare provision than at securing a framework of legal rights through which disabled people might achieve greater and ultimately equal access to the key institutions of civic and public life (Scott 1994). It is to this concentration on legal and environmental change that I refer when I speak of a fourth orientation of policy: the development of citizenship.

Citizenship is not an easy concept to define, but many writers see "participation" as being the crux of the matter. For Barbalet (1988), citizenship defines who is and who is not a member of a society. Similarly, Turner (1993) contends that membership is realized in a set of practices concerned with law, justice, economics, and culture. Voet (1998) argues that of all these, a share in governance is perhaps the most critical. While some scholars, such as Marshall (1992), stress the *rights* conferred by citizenship, others, such as Scruton (1982) and Joseph and Sumption (1979), underline the *responsibilities* that citizens owe to the state. We may say, then, that when a person has no access to governance, society, or an economy, when he or she neither fulfills duties toward a state nor enjoys rights guaranteed by it, then such a person has no citizenship. I should add, however, that there are questions of degree here. Without being destroyed completely, a person's citizenship could be damaged or infringed on. For example, inequality of opportunity can enhance the life chances of some and increase their privilege in exercising economic and political power. However, at the same time, others may be excluded from political, economic, and social structures, thereby diminishing the scope of their potential and actual participation in society (Baker 1987; Tawney 1964). Unsurprisingly, many marginalized groups, including disabled people, frequently describe themselves as being oppressed and treated like "second-class citizens," meaning that they regard their citizenship as being of a quality inferior to that enjoyed by the majority (Brisenden 1986; Campbell and Oliver 1996).

Few, if any, nations can claim to have achieved comprehensive and well-integrated ("joined-up") sets of policies, which together secure the full inclusion of disabled people in contemporary society. It remains more typical to encounter welfare policies and systems that are residual, piecemeal, and far from exhaustive (Howard 1999). Why, then, has it proved so difficult to create legislation that guarantees the citizenship of disabled people? In the next section of this chapter, I argue that both historical and current conceptualizations of "welfare" play a large part in this failure. Indeed, the term itself may be formulated in accordance with doctrines that are to some extent antithetical to citizenship.

WELFARE AND CITIZENSHIP:
A CLASH OF PRINCIPLES?

In seeking to define (or to redefine) *welfare,* contemporary governments have sought to reconcile principles that are abrasive with respect to each other. On one hand, there has been a desire (or at least a perceived duty) to support "those in genuine need." (Of course, what is critical here is the definition applied by governments to the term *genuine need* and the subsequent nomination of groups deemed to fall within the chosen definition.) On the other hand, governments have been determined to protect capitalism and support the work ethic by blocking or excluding from welfare programs all those thought to be abusing or defrauding the welfare system. These restrictive aims are explicit, for example, in the guidance issued in the United States by the Social Security Administration:

> Disability under Social Security is based on your inability to work. You will be considered disabled if you are unable to do any kind of work for which you are suited and your disability has lasted or is expected to last for at least a year or to result in death. Some consider this a strict definition of disability and it is. (Social Security Administration 1997:4)

The program assumes that working families have access to other resources to provide support during periods of short-term disabilities, including workers' compensation, insurance, savings, and investments.

Two key mechanisms are commonly used in judging whether claimants are entitled to benefits: means testing and medical evaluation. When an allowance, benefit, or other form of help is means-tested, the applicant must disclose to the authorities private information about income, savings, and property. If the applicant's wealth exceeds some given figure, the claim for the particular benefit is rejected. Some states extend the calculation beyond the individual to take into account resources available within the immediate family, and some states look to the extended family as well before making a benefit available (Jones 1993; McKay and Rowlingson 1999).

The second testing mechanism of particular relevance to disabled people is medical evaluation. In addition to diagnosis by doctors nominated by the state, there may also be extensive inquiry (often involving intimate questions or examination) into the capacities and incapacities of a claimant. "How many steps can you take without a stick or chair?" "Can you wash yourself without help?" "Are you able to use the lavatory unaided?" The answers to such questions, plus reports from doctors, are critical in determining whether particular resources or allowances are made available to a claimant (Kirk 1999).

The desire to minimize welfare expenditure is epitomized in policies such as the "workfare" program pursued in Wisconsin (Kaus 1995; Mead 1997; Rector 1997; Scully 1998). It is also evident in recent alterations to British social security law restricting access to incapacity benefits and other disablement allowances (Berthoud 1995; Berthoud et al. 1993; Digby 1989; House of Commons 1998; Walker 1991). Here, the emphasis is clearly on the more selective targeting of allowances and other benefits. In asking how disabled people experience welfare in any particular state, much of the answer will thus depend on the criteria on which welfare stands and the structures through which a system is delivered. In sum, welfare systems have, as a prime concern, the need to restrict access to protect economic (wealth-producing) structures. These same structures militate against disabled people's access to work and thus to resources.

Clearly, then, we may detect a certain measure of incongruity between the principles governing welfare as an aid to citizenship, on one hand, and as protection for the economy, on the other. I explore the potential contradiction brought about by these desiderata more fully in the next section.

SEMANTIC AND STRUCTURAL CONTEXTS OF WELFARE

Welfare systems built on (medically inspired) definitions of disability will comprehend disability as stemming from individual, as opposed to social and environmental, causes (Barnes et al. 1999; Barnes and Mercer 1996; Priestley 1999). As a result of that understanding, attempts at change will be focused primarily on disabled individuals as opposed to disabling environments. Typically, then, welfare systems may make little impact on the political, social, economic, and physical environments in which they have evolved. These same environments can be alien to disabled people and may serve to impede their citizenship and participation in society. Indeed, the general purpose of welfare is to accommodate and sustain disabled people within these prevailing environments. Welfare services may therefore aim to restructure a person's physiology, for example, through invasive surgery or the provision of prosthetic aids or adaptations (see, e.g., Blumberg 1991). Or again, welfare may involve interventions aimed at producing changes in personality or cognition, for example, through the use of behavior modification techniques or "normalization" programs (see the critique by Chappell 1992). Finally, welfare may simply be used to palliate an individual by using services such as occupational or "diversion" therapy, leaving many disabled people unqualified and underemployed (Hyde 1996; Walker 1982).

Nevertheless, opportunities for disabled people to create their own self-governed structures have grown in recent years. Examples include the work of the Derbyshire Coalition of Disabled People (Priestley 1999), user governance in social work projects (d'Aboville 1991), user-directed residential services (Brown and Ringma 1989), and user-managed mental health projects (Barker and Peck 1987; Levy 1986). As opposed to actual self-governing projects, the notion of "participation" in the management of the welfare state has been more problematic. In joining preexisting welfare setups, particularly those in the statutory sector, disabled people have often found that they lack authority over and within them and have little control of the predominantly nondisabled personnel who manage and operate welfare programs (Beresford and Croft 1993; Drake 1997; Pithouse and Williamson 1997; Welsh Office 1989).

Finkelstein (1980:17) explained this powerlessness of disabled people by arguing that in any helper-helped relationship, the "helpers," by dint of their superordinate position, are able to exercise greater influence over defining the problem to be solved. When there is dissonance between society and a minority of citizens, the strong tendency is to locate pathology in the person or group rather than in the surrounding status quo. The basis on which "welfare" is offered, therefore, is one that demands of disabled people not only acquiesce in helper-based definitions of the welfare relationship.

Several researchers have noted how in practice disabled individuals often adjust to these circumstances by adopting roles and expectations appropriate to the dependency thus created (Albrecht 1976; Albrecht and Levy 1981; Rose and Black 1985; Safilios-Rothschild 1970; Scott 1970). Moreover, Bloor (1986) highlights the fact that the construction of dependency may occur not as a result of any overt use of power by welfare staff but by means of "social orchestration":

Because of their practised grasp of community life, their skills as group therapists, but pre-eminently because of their pre-existing and continuous superordinate position staff were able to relinquish directive control of events but nevertheless predict, shape and act upon subsequent developments. A position of power converts mere anticipation of events into a capacity to orchestrate. (P. 319)

Clearly, then, when disabled people lack authority within welfare structures, a key consequence is their concomitant lack of control over the purposes of such structures and the distribution of resources within them. Inasmuch as welfare systems are subservient to economic systems, it is not surprising to find that disabled people receive low levels of financial support compared with their nondisabled counterparts who derive their incomes from employment. Even disabled people who have work tend to receive lower pay than nondisabled counterparts.

SUMMARY

Welfare states have developed as a response to poverty and "need," but they also constitute mechanisms designed to protect vital state interests and national economic goals. Frequently, states intervened in "private" need principally because the sheer scale of want threatened to undermine the health of modern industry and trade. Medicine received the imprimatur of the state to diagnose and then deal with the "needs" of disabled people. These "needs" were (and, in large measure, continue to be) defined in terms of individual as opposed to environmental disorders, deficits, and disadvantages.

Given such origins, we may see how contemporary welfare systems struggle to respond to disabled people's calls for citizenship and equality of opportunity. Against this background, it becomes easier to comprehend welfare not only in its ostensible roles of rehabilitation and support but also as a force for conformity and control. In the next section, I argue that the understanding on which welfare systems are based and the structures and forms they take may offer some material help, but along with tangible and useful aid, there are other, less desirable outcomes for disabled people.

OUTCOMES

The experiences of disabled people will depend on how welfare states are configured. Do they integrate or segregate? Are there equitable levels of income as between disabled and nondisabled people? How is citizenship conceived, and how far is it guaranteed? What power relationship is there between service users and providers? Clearly, welfare services may be liberating or constraining. The outcomes will depend on (1) the influence of disabled people over policy and purposes, (2) their position (if any) within management hierarchy, and (3) their involvement and experiences at the point of service delivery. I have said that the experience of welfare is contoured by the meanings and principles that shape any particular regime and by the mode of its delivery. I have also argued that at least two divergent aims vie for preeminence—the ostensible goal of providing support and the contiguous desire to control and, possibly, to exclude. In this part of the chapter, my aim is to consider three key areas in which there are outcomes for disabled people. These are economic consequences, social outcomes, and political implications.

Economic Consequences

Old soldier Jack Brayley, age 76, was just about surviving on £51 ($83) per week. The money had to stretch to cover rent, gas, electricity, water, and rates bills. He spent about £15 ($24) per week on food. He had no television because he could not afford the license. "I'm an invalid and I've been on a low income for some years," said Mr. Brayley. "When I didn't have money, I used to stay in, because I don't believe in cadging [borrowing]." ("Old Soldier's Pride" 1996:4)

Typically, noncontributory systems of financial benefits (social security or social assistance) provide resources very near to or actually below the lowest levels of wages earned by people in work (Alcock 1993). Generally, the work available to disabled people tends to be lower paid and of lower status than that available to their nondisabled counterparts. So, for example, McNeil (1999) reports an average difference between the earnings of severely disabled people and nondisabled people in America of more than $10,000 per annum. (The difference between salaries of people whose impairment was not severe and nondisabled people's earnings was more than $5,000 per annum.) The same is true in Britain, where the weekly wage of disabled male workers represents only 81 percent of the average enjoyed by nondisabled males (Berthoud et al. 1993; *Hansard* 1989). More recent data from Blackaby et al. (1998) reveal that most disabled people earn less than their nondisabled counterparts, primarily because they occupy jobs demanding fewer skills and qualifications, and confirm Barnes's (1991) contention that they have less access to the more professional and well-paid posts. Indeed, disabled people tend to earn less than nondisabled people, even when they are doing similar (or even identical) jobs (Martin and White 1988). Finally, when they have work, many disabled people are "underemployed" (Royal Association for Disability and Rehabilitation [RADAR] 1993; Walker 1982).

In 1996, about 77 percent of nondisabled people were in paid work. This compares with just 32 percent of disabled people (Sly 1996). By gender, only about one-third of disabled men and about 29 percent of disabled women have jobs (Lonsdale 1990; Martin, White, and Meltzer 1989). There is substantial evidence, then, that both the level and the duration of unemployment among disabled people in Britain have been consistently higher than those experienced by nondisabled people (Clark and Hirst 1989; Glendinning 1991; Hirst 1987; Hyde 1996; Lonsdale 1986; Townsend 1979).

Some welfare systems, particularly in Scandinavia, seek to provide "sheltered" work or to help disabled people find work on the open market. This is also true in Britain, where the Department of Social Security employs disablement resettlement officers (DROs) and personal advisers. As Barnes (1991) points out, however, intercession with employers by DROs has the drawback of emphasizing difference by suggesting that disabled workers need special pleading, that they are in some sense inferior to nondisabled workers. The evidence is, however, to the contrary that, ceteris paribus, disabled people perform at least as well as and are often more reliable than their nondisabled counterparts (see Barnes 1991, chap. 4).

The key remaining question concerns those disabled people whose impairments may be so severe as to prevent them from taking up work even in the most conducive and best-adapted environment. As early as the 1970s, groups such as the Disablement Income Group and the Union of Physically Impaired against Segregation (UPIAS 1976) called for disablement incomes at a level that would allow these disabled people to maximize their citizenship to the fullest potential (Oliver and Barnes 1998). Other writers, such as Abberley (1996), have questioned the centrality of work as the (almost) sole arbiter of social status and access to economic resource and call for new ways of valuing people's lives and contributions to society. Income is an important element in determining disabled people's access to the social world. But just as critical is the configuration of the environment itself.

Social and Environmental Outcomes

What annoys me is, we can't even get in . . . corners, access, getting there by bus . . . there's always small corridors to go round. ("Peter," in Drake 1992b:225)

We are disabled by buildings that are not designed to admit us . . . the disablement lies in the construction of society, not in the physical condition of the individual. (Brisenden 1986:176)

I have said that welfare tends, in so many of its guises, to be focused on individual lives rather than the contours of the social and physical environment. In these circumstances, changes are wrought at the individual level rather than social and environmental levels. Perhaps a key outcome in terms of individuals' experiences of welfare is that present policies and configurations may do little if anything to diminish the environmental obstacles that constitute disabling barriers.

Given its focus on individual causation, welfare commonly offers "solutions" in the form of personal aids, adaptations, and allowances so that individuals can negotiate their "given" surroundings, thus leaving those conditions unaltered. Social work in Britain, for example, is described as a "personal social service." Its aim is to provide "professional" help in solving "personal" problems. There is, however, no welfare agency whose task it is to alter the environment in which obstacles arise. The key areas, vital to participation in society, include growth (particularly educational growth), movement (including transport), and location (including domicile and access to buildings that serve the public).

Education

The historical expectation that disabled people might lead lives segregated from society at large meant that such education as they might receive fitted them poorly for subsequent life beyond the institution (Barton 1986, 1988). In many countries, more recent educational policies have favored the integration of disabled children into mainstream schooling. However, some commentators have asked whether such moves have aimed for genuine integration or simply aided the preservation of two sorts of education (for disabled and nondisabled persons), albeit under one roof (Barton 1986, 1988, 1989; Barton and Tomlinson 1981; Fulcher 1989).

I have already outlined some of the economic consequences that may flow when there is inferior education and lack of equality of opportunity. Potentially, there are also, however, consequences in other areas of life. When a disabled child is educated separately and less extensively than his or her nondisabled counterparts, he or she may enjoy fewer choices later on. Many careers, particularly those in the professions, demand specific qualifications, skills, and training. Those who do not possess the necessary attainments find the doors of such professions (e.g., accountancy, teaching, engineering, and the law) closed to them (Langdon-Down 1996).

Location and Domicile

When welfare services are targeted on individual as opposed to environmental change, they may fail to combat restrictions imposed on disabled people by the broader society. An important example of this effect occurs in housing with respect to both location and type. Choice between public housing and the private market, or between rented accommodation and home ownership, is only possible when disabled people command sufficient resources to be able, if they wish, to opt for house purchase and private ownership. However, Barnes et al. (1999) and Harris, Sapey, and Stewart (1997) show that most dwellings are not only beyond the pockets of disabled people but are also physically inaccessible. Goldsmith (1976) has argued that buildings are constructed by and for people who move around on two legs, not those who use sticks or wheels. In Britain, for example, between 1984 and 1989, local authorities and housing associations built some 168,665 "mainstream" homes but only 1,840 houses accessible to wheelchair users. The private house-building sector built no wheelchair-accessible homes at all (Barnes 1991).

Nor are aids and adaptations always readily obtainable. In a survey of some 700 complaints toward local authority services, RADAR (1994) quoted as reasonably common the experience of a disabled man who claimed he had been subjected to emotional blackmail over his request for a stair-lift. If his local authority supplied him with a stair-lift costing several thousand pounds, he was told, this would deny other disabled people things they need. Since the interview, he has fallen down the stairs on three occasions.

The resulting domestic and urban environment is the product of what Imrie and Wells (1993) have called "design apartheid." Because specially adapted housing tends to be built in clusters and because state or local authority housing for rent tends also to be marshaled in estates in particular quarters of towns and (inner) cities, the upshot is a segregation of various groups or classes within a population. This is an effect that Forrest and Murie (1991) have termed *social polarization.*

Transport

While access to social settings may have improved generally, it remains true that in many Western societies, public transport is only partially accessible to disabled people. The United States and Sweden are leading the way here, but in Britain, only now are bus companies being forced to make new vehicles accessible. In Britain, it may take 15 years or more (as old buses are replaced) before disabled people are able to travel as freely as their nondisabled counterparts (Greater London Association of Disabled People [GLAD] 1994). In 1994, only 70 of 5,000 London buses were accessible to wheelchair users (*Hansard* 1994). The use of trains and other vehicles remains problematic. Only about 25 percent of the London taxi fleet is accessible, a much lower proportion of taxis than in other cities (Barnes 1991).

Welfare systems may provide some vehicles. Frequently, however, these are minibuses available only at prescribed times and on predetermined routes, and they are often restricted to supplementing other services such as day centers or lunch clubs. Even voluntary "dial-a-ride" schemes have limited coverage, and, as I point out elsewhere,

> Charities . . . provide specially adapted minibuses whose use is confined principally to designated groups of disabled people characterised as being in need and deserving of help. These agencies are content to see their benefaction prominently advertised on the exteriors of the vehicles they supply. Through this act of identification, charities draw a distinction between those who use . . . philanthropic transport and those who do not. (Drake 1996a:151)

The point here is that there is a value difference not only in the *form* of the transport but also in the *social status* ascribed to clients by dint of their use of that transport.

When traditional welfare focuses on the person and when disability is defined in individual ("medical model") terms, it deals only indirectly (if at all) with environmental restrictions in movement and location. When antidiscrimination legislation is absent, these restrictions remain undealt with.

It follows that when disabled people also have less influence in government and wield little political authority, it becomes harder for them to change either the orientation of welfare or the disabling environment itself. Questions of political participation are thus of critical importance, and it is to these that I now turn.

Political Implications

Citizenship depends in large measure on political participation and on the ability to exercise at least some power with respect to deciding the prevailing norms and values of a society. In theory, welfare policies and practices, as well as those involved in the welfare professions, either could tend toward the exercise of control (by seeking to impose conformity to prevailing social and behavioral norms) or could attack the environmental structures that constrain disabled people. The latter course of action raises a dilemma for those who earn their living as welfare staff, for such a change of focus carries with it the implication that they must cede some or all of their own authority to their clients. There is often resistance to the idea of transferring—or even sharing—power.

> The sort of, old contract, if you like, was, "we're the helpful, competent, able people, you give up everything to us, you're the needy ones and we'll do it for you." So it involves quite a shift in that contract and that *status quo* it's quite a subversive movement in a

way—it hinges on power, and the [name of authority] are a very powerful body who actually don't like a lot of the stuff that's going on. ("Elaine," in Drake 1992b:235)

Here, then, I consider some possible impacts of welfare systems on the political participation of disabled people. There are, perhaps, three main points at issue: the expression of political preferences (voting), standing for office, and serving in office (exercising political authority).

Perhaps the most immediate obstacles to exercising political influence are absence from the electoral register and a lack of access to polling stations. Fry (1987) has shown that low numbers of disabled people actually cast their votes, and both Enticott, Graham, and Lamb (1992) and Barnes (1991) have demonstrated that low turnout is exacerbated in Britain by inaccessible polling booths and because many disabled people (those in residential accommodation or hospitals) may fail to appear on the electoral register because their names have been omitted from the lists.

Voting is, in any case, a very blunt method of political participation. People who are elected to serve have a far stronger and more intimate access to power. However, a number of constitutions have historically excluded at least some portion of the disabled population from standing for office. In Britain, people are debarred if they have an incapacity due to physical or mental disability—specifically, "idiots, lunatics, and persons under the age of 21, in all of whom the law supposes a want of mental capacity or discretion" (Wollaston 1970:38-39). Schofield (1955) recorded that "deaf and dumb persons are ineligible for Parliament" (p. 83), but it is unclear whether such an opinion would be confirmed today. There are, nevertheless, impediments to the candidature of many disabled people, and even once elected, neither Parliament nor the great majority of town halls across Britain have been designed to accommodate disabled representatives. The Americans with Disabilities Act may have made matters easier for their counterparts in the United States.

Given the difficulties I have just outlined, it is not surprising that the number of disabled people elected as councilors or members of Parliament is very low. For example, only one of some 650 current members of British Parliament is a wheelchair user. Only one, a government minister, is blind, and one other, the chair of the all-party disablement group in the House of Lords, is hearing impaired. It is a sign of their absence from the political scene as a group that the few prominent disabled people who succeed become widely known and recognized. Even then, there is no guarantee that the successful few will share the aspirations of their peers. Nor would they claim to represent them.

Without political power, it has been difficult for disabled people to achieve movement in policy away from the guiding principle of "welfare" toward the principles of "citizenship" and "rights." One response to exclusion has been "direct action." Some disabled people have rejected welfare and have demanded equality, access, and participation, thus bringing home forcibly their arguments by civil disobedience. For example, they have carried out actions such as stopping buses in busy city centers, occupying radio or television studios, and conducting marches and demonstrations at parliaments and political headquarters (Crow 1990; Morris 1991).

CONCLUSION

In the nineteenth and early twentieth centuries, disabled people were judged against "able-bodied" social norms and requirements. Many were segregated or actually expelled from mundane society. I have shown how in Western industrialized states, this early policy of "containment" gave way in the post–World War II period to a search for other responses to disability. The construction of social services and community care policies took *integration* for their watchword. There came into being services based on the domestic, rather than institutional, settings. Several approaches were adopted in the search for solutions. In Sweden, an extensive welfare state came into being that provided income, social and health services, adapted accommodation, and employment training organizations such as the AMS (Arbetsmark-nadsstyrelsen). The United States, in a civil rights approach, led the way with antidiscrimination laws, such as the Americans with Disabilities Act in 1990. In Britain, welfare has been developed in a somewhat more piecemeal and fragmented way. The Disability Discrimination Act of 1995 is far weaker than its American counterpart, but new forms of resources, such as the Independent Living Fund and Disability Working Tax Credit, are aimed at enhancing the scope of disabled people's lives. In many countries, access to public transport is gradually improving and is facilitating greater independence for disabled people through access to society and to work. However, considerable social and environmental change is still required before it can be said that disabled people enjoy equal access and opportunity in modern Western societies.

Welfare states have come a long way since the days of the almshouse and the workhouse, but it remains true that disabled people still encounter restricted access to several key civil and social structures in many countries. As of this writing, for example, it is still legal in Britain to discriminate against disabled people in areas such as the military and higher education (Rights Now 1994). Equally, a common factor in advanced industrial and technological states has been the subservience of welfare to the requirements of capital. Governments have been keen to avoid undermining incentives to work, and this has meant that they have sought to ensure that incomes and other resources derived from programs of social assistance remain lower than commensurate rewards to be gained from employment. Such an approach has direct consequences for those disabled people excluded from work due either to the severity of a physiological or cognitive impairment or as a result of the contours of work itself. Other obstacles have included the absence of equal opportunity or other appropriate legislation, the lack of access to training, or the prejudicial attitudes of some employers. For whatever reasons, disabled people in general command fewer resources than their nondisabled counterparts. The upshot has been that they have been reliant on welfare structures.

I have argued that, hitherto, the prime focus of health and social service organizations has been the individual rather than the environment. Change (therapy, treatment, rehabilitation) has been located within the body or mind of the disabled person. From this perspective, we may interpret "welfare" as a mechanism formulated by and protective of prevailing (nondisabled) norms and values. Insofar as the flow of power is asymmetrical, both the concept and conduct of welfare preserve existing social and political norms from radical challenge by defining the values and condition of disabled people as being aberrant and by affirming the status quo.

Across Europe, Australasia, and North America, the response has been the growth of pressure groups run by disabled people themselves. In many countries, "disability movements" have gained considerable influence and have argued for inclusive social and physical environments and for equality of opportunity (Albrecht 1992; Campbell and Oliver 1996; Zola 1994). These calls have been accompanied by campaigns for antidiscrimination legislation.

The policy research and action that are now required must build on those innovations that have sought to liberate disabled people. For example, in Britain, innovations such as the Independent Living Fund passed some control of resources to disabled people themselves rather than to intermediaries acting on their behalf. In the United States, the Americans with Disabilities Act strengthened considerably the civil rights and legal redress available to disabled people in cases of discrimination. Clearly, then, the key research questions for the future must focus on citizenship and civil rights. How can we devise policies to remove environmental barriers and attitudinal discrimination? How best can welfare services be designed so that control rests as much (if not more) with recipients than with providers? Finally, how can we ensure that disabled people have access to the resources that are necessary for citizenship?

In the nineteenth century, states declared certain elements in their populations to be deviant and dealt with them (often very harshly) as "problem people." In the twentieth century, the paradigm shifted. People faced problems, and states inaugurated services aimed at helping these individuals to remedy or ameliorate their problems. In the twenty-first century, many nations are recognizing that (at least in part) the way we choose to build our societies (both physically and with respect to attitudes) can cause problems for some citizens. Now the focus for change is shifting away from the individual toward the contours of what Swain et al. (1993) have called "the disabling environment."

REFERENCES

Abberley, P. 1996. "Work, Utopia and Impairment." Pp. 61-82 in *Disability and Society: Emerging Issues and Insights,* edited by Len Barton. Harlow, UK: Longman.

Albrecht, G. 1976. *The Sociology of Physical Disability and Rehabilitation.* Pittsburgh, PA: University of Pittsburgh Press.

———. 1992. *The Disability Business: Rehabilitation in America.* Newbury Park, CA: Sage.

Albrecht, G. and J. Levy. 1981. "Constructing Disabilities as Social Problems." Pp. 11-32 in *Cross National Rehabilitation Policies: A Sociological Perspective,* edited by G. L. Albrecht. Beverly Hills, CA: Sage.

Alcock, P. 1993. *Understanding Poverty.* London: Macmillan.

Andrews, K. and J. Jacobs. 1990. *Punishing the Poor: Poverty under Thatcher.* London: Macmillan.

Ashford, D. E. 1986. *The Emergence of the Welfare States.* Oxford, UK: Blackwell.

Baker, J. 1987. *Arguing for Equality.* London: Verso.

Baldock, J., N. Manning, S. Miller, and S. Vickerstaff. 1999. *Social Policy.* Oxford, UK: Oxford University Press.

Barbalet, J. M. 1988. "Citizenship, Class Inequality and Resentment." Pp. 36-56 in *Citizenship and Social Theory,* edited by B. S. Turner. Newbury Park, CA: Sage.

Barker, I. and E. Peck, eds. 1987. *Mental Health Services.* London: Good Practices in Mental Health.

Barnes, C. 1991. *Disabled People in Britain and Discrimination.* London: Hurst.

Barnes, C. and G. Mercer. 1996. *Exploring the Divide, Illness and Disability.* Leeds, UK: The Disability Press.

Barnes, C., G. Mercer, and T. Shakespeare. 1999. *Exploring Disability: A Sociological Introduction.* Cambridge, UK: Polity.

Barton, L. 1986. "The Politics of Special Educational Needs." *Disability, Handicap & Society* 1 (3): 273-90.

———. 1988. *The Politics of Special Educational Needs.* London: Falmer.

———. 1989. *Integration: Myth or Reality?* London: Falmer.

Barton L. and S. Tomlinson. 1981. *Special Educational Needs, Policy, Practices and Social Issues.* London: Harper & Row.

Becker, H. 1963. *Outsiders.* New York: Free Press.

Beresford, P. and S. Croft. 1993. *Citizen Involvement: A Practical Guide for Change.* London: Macmillan.

Berthoud, R. 1995. "Social Security, Poverty and Disabled People." Pp. 77-88 in *Removing Disabling Barriers,* edited by G. Zarb. London: Policy Studies Institute.

Berthoud, R., J. Lakey, and S. McKay. 1993. *The Economic Problems of Disabled People.* London: Policy Studies Institute.

Beveridge, W. 1942. *Social Insurance and Allied Services.* London: Her Majesty's Stationery Office.

Blackaby, D., K. Clark, S. Drinkwater, D. Leslie, P. Murphy, and N. O'Leary. 1998. *Earnings and Employment Opportunities for People with Disabilities: Secondary Analysis Using the Census, General Household Survey and the Labour Force Survey.* Swansea, UK: University of Wales, Swansea.

Blakemore, K. 1998. *Social Policy: An Introduction.* Buckingham, UK: Open University Press.

Bloor, M. 1986. "Social Control in the Therapeutic Community: Re-Examination of a Critical Case." *Sociology of Health and Illness* 8:305-24.

Blumberg, L. 1991. "For Who among Us Has Not Spilled Ketchup?" Pp. 34-42 in *Women and Disability,* edited by E. Boylan. London: Zed.

Booth, C. 1903. *Life and Labour of the People of London.* 17 vols. London: Macmillan.

Bourke, J. 1996. *Dismembering the Male: Men's Bodies, Britain and the Great War.* London: Reaktion.

Brilliant, E. 1990. *The United Way: Dilemmas of Organized Charity.* New York: Columbia University Press.

Brisenden, S. 1986. "Independent Living and the Medical Model of Disability." *Disability Handicap & Society* 1 (2): 173-78.

Brown, C. and C. Ringma. 1989. "New Disability Services: The Critical Role of Staff in a Consumer-Directed Empowerment Model of Service for Physically Disabled People." *Disability, Handicap & Society* 4 (3): 241-57.

Burnett, J. 1986. *A Social History of Housing*. London: Routledge Kegan Paul.

Campbell, J. and M. Oliver. 1996. *Disability Politics: Understanding Our Past, Changing Our Future*. London: Routledge Kegan Paul.

Chappell, A. 1992. "Towards a Sociological Critique of the Normalisation Principle." *Disability, Handicap & Society* 7 (1): 35-51.

Clark, A. and M. Hirst. 1989. "Disability in Adulthood: Ten Year Follow Up of Young People with Disabilities." *Disability, Handicap & Society* 4: 271-83.

Cochrane, A. and J. Clarke, eds. 1993. *Comparing Welfare States*. London: Sage.

Crow, L. 1990. *Direct Action and Disabled People: Future Directions*. Manchester, UK: Greater Manchester Coalition of Disabled People.

Crowther, M. A. 1983. *The Workhouse System, 1834-1929: The History of an English Social Institution*. London: Methuen.

d'Aboville, E. 1991. "Social Work in an Organisation of Disabled People." Pp. 64-85 in *Social Work, Disabled People and Disabling Environments*, edited by M. Oliver. London: Jessica Kingsley.

Department of Health. 1996. *Health and Personal Social Services Statistics for England*. London: Her Majesty's Stationery Office.

Digby, A. 1989. *British Welfare Policy: Workhouse to Workfare*. London: Faber & Faber.

Ditch, J. 1991. "The Undeserving Poor: Unemployed People, Then and Now." Pp. 24-40 in *The State or the Market, Politics and Welfare in Contemporary Britain*, edited by M. Loney, R. Bocock, J. Clarke, A. Cochrane, P. Graham, and M. Wilson. London: Sage.

Drake, R. F. 1992a. "Consumer Participation, the Voluntary Sector and the Concept of Power." *Disability & Society* 7 (3): 267-78.

———. 1992b. "A Little Brief Authority? A Sociological Analysis of Consumer Participation in Voluntary Agencies in Wales." Ph.D. dissertation, University of Cardiff, Wales.

———. 1994. "The Exclusion of Disabled People from Positions of Power in British Voluntary Organisations." *Disability & Society* 9 (4): 461-80.

———. 1996a. "A Critique of the Role of the Traditional Charities." Pp. 147-66 in *Disability & Society: Emerging Issues and Insights*, edited by L. Barton. London: Longman.

———. 1996b. "Charities, Authority and Disabled People: A Qualitative Study." *Disability & Society* 11 (1): 5-24.

———. 1997. "Disability, User Participation and the Governance of Voluntary Agencies: Behind the Facade." Pp. 85-102 in *Engaging the User in Welfare Services*, edited by A. Pithouse and H. Williamson. Birmingham, UK: Venture.

———. 1999. *Understanding Disability Policies*. London: Macmillan.

Enticott, J., P. Graham, and B. Lamb. 1992. *Polls Apart: Disabled People and the 1992 General Election*. London: Spastics Society.

Esping-Andersen, G. 1990. *The Three Worlds of Welfare Capitalism*. Cambridge, UK: Polity.

Finer, C. J. 1999. "Trends and Developments in Welfare States." Pp. 15-33 in *Comparative Social Policy, Concepts Theories and Methods*, edited by Jochen Clasen. Oxford, UK: Blackwell.

Finkelstein, V. 1980. *Attitudes and Disabled People: Issues for Discussion*. London: Royal Association for Disability and Rehabilitation.

———. 1981. "Disability and the Helper/Helped Relationship: An Historical View." Pp. 58-64 in *Handicap in a Social World*, edited by A. Brechin, P. Liddiard, and J. Swain. London: Hodder & Stoughton.

Forrest, R. and A. Murie. 1991. *Selling the Welfare State*. London: Routledge Kegan Paul.

Fraser, D. 1984. *The Evolution of the British Welfare State*. London: Macmillan.

Fry, E. 1987. *Disabled People and the 1987 General Election*. London: Spastics Society.

Fulcher, G. 1989. "Integrate and Mainstream? Comparative Issues in the Politics of These Policies." Pp. 6-29 in *Integration: Myth or Reality?* edited by L. Barton. London: Falmer.

Gauldie, E. 1974. *Cruel Habitations*. London: Allen & Unwin.

Giddens, A. 1993. *Sociology*. Cambridge, UK: Polity.

Ginsburg, H. 1983. *Full Employment and Public Policy: The United States and Sweden*. Lexington, MA: Lexington Books.

———. 1993. "Sweden: The Social Democratic Case." Pp. 173-204 in *Comparing Welfare States*, edited by Allan Cochrane and John Clarke. London: Sage.

Glendinning, C. 1991. "Losing Ground: Social Policy and Disabled People in Great Britain 1980-1990." *Disability, Handicap & Society* 6:3-19.

Goffman, E. 1969. *The Presentation of Self in Everyday Life*. Harmondsworth, UK: Penguin.

———. 1970. *Stigma: Notes on the Management of Spoiled Identity*. Harmondsworth, UK: Penguin.

Goldsmith, S. 1976. *Designing for the Disabled*. London: Royal Institute of British Architects.

Gould, A. 1988. *Conflict and Control in Welfare Policy: The Swedish Experience*. London: Longman.

———. 1993. *Capitalist Welfare Systems: A Comparison of Japan, Britain and Sweden*. London: Longman.

Greater London Association of Disabled People (GLAD). 1994. *London Disability Guide*. London: Author.

Hansard. 1989. 6th June, col. 69.

Hansard. 1994. 11th March, col. 566.

Harris, J. 1972. *Unemployment and Politics, 1886-1914*. Oxford, UK: Oxford University Press.

Harris, J., B. Sapey, and J. Stewart. 1997. *Wheelchair Housing and the Estimation of Need*. Preston, UK: University of Central Lancashire.

Hasler, F. 1993. "Developments in the Disabled People's Movement." Pp. 278-84 in *Disabling Barriers, Enabling Environments*, edited by J. Swain, V. Finkelstein, S. French, and M. Oliver. London: Sage.

Hay, J. R. 1975. *The Origins of the Liberal Welfare Reforms, 1906-1914*. London: Macmillan.

———. 1978. *The Development of the British Welfare State, 1880-1975*. London: Edward Arnold.

Hevey, D. 1992. *The Creatures Time Forgot*. London: Routledge Kegan Paul.

Hill, M. 1993. *The Welfare State in Britain: A Political History since 1945*. Aldershot, UK: Edward Elgar.

Hirst, M. 1987. "Careers of Young People with Disabilities between the Ages of 16 and 21." *Disability, Handicap & Society* 2:61-75.

House of Commons. 1998. *Social Security Committee, Second Report*. London: Her Majesty's Stationery Office.

Howard, M. 1999. *Enabling Government: Joined Up Policies for a National Disability Strategy*. London: Fabian Society.

Hughes, R. 1987. *The Fatal Shore*. London: Collins Harvill.

Hyde, M. 1996. "Fifty Years of Failure: Employment Services for Disabled People in the United Kingdom." *Work, Employment and Society* 12 (4): 683-700.

Hyndman, H. M. 1911. *Record of an Adventurous Life*. London: Macmillan.

Imrie, R. and P. Wells. 1993. "Disablism, Planning and the Built Environment." *Environment and Planning C: Government and Policy* 11 (2): 213-31.

Jenkins, T. A. 1994. *The Liberal Ascendancy*. London: Macmillan.

Jones, C., ed. 1993. *New Perspectives on the Welfare State in Europe*. London: Routledge Kegan Paul.

Jones, K. 1991. *The Making of Social Policy in Britain 1830-1990*. London: Athlone.

Joseph, K. and J. Sumption. 1979. *Equality*. London: John Murray.

Kaus, M. 1995. "The Latest Thing in Welfare: Tommy's New Tune." *New Republic*, September 18 and 25, pp. 25-27.

Kirk, N. 1999. *The Benefits Guide, 1999/2000*. London: National Homeless Alliance.

Kirkman Gray, B. [1905] 1967. *A History of English Philanthropy*. Reprint, London: P. S. King & Son.

Langdon-Down, G. 1996. "Why Justice Is Blind but There Are No Blind Justices." *The Independent*, February 21, p. 21.

Lemert, E. 1962. *Human Deviance, Social Problems and Social Control*. Englewood Cliffs, NJ: Prentice Hall.

Levy, L. 1986. *Finding Our Own Solutions: Women's Experience of Mental Health Care*. London: Women in MIND.

Lewis, J. 1980. *The Politics of Motherhood*. London: Croom Helm.

Lonsdale, S. 1986. *Work and Inequality*. Harlow, UK: Longman.

———. 1990. *Women and Disability: The Experience of Physical Disability among Women*. London: Macmillan.

Lowe, R. 1993. *The Welfare State in Britain since 1945*. London: Macmillan.

Mabbott, D. and H. Bolderson. 1991. *Social Policy and Social Security in Australia, Britain and the USA*. Aldershot, UK: Avebury.

———. 1999. "Theories and Methods in Comparative Social Policy." Pp. 34-56 in *Comparative Social Policy*, edited by J. Clasen. Oxford, UK: Blackwell.

Marshall, T. H. 1992. *Citizenship and Social Class*. London: Pluto.

Martin, J. and A. White. 1988. *Surveys of Disabled People in Great Britain: Report No. 2. The Financial Circumstances of Disabled Adults Living in Private Households*. London: Office for Population Censuses and Surveys.

Martin, J., A. White, and H. Meltzer. 1989. *Disabled Adults, Services, Transport and Employment.* London: Office for Population Censuses and Surveys.

McKay, S. and K. Rowlingson. 1999. *Social Security in Britain.* London: Macmillan.

McLaughlin, E. 1993. "Hong Kong: A Residual Welfare Regime." Pp. 105-40 in *Comparing Welfare States,* edited by A. Cochrane and J. Clarke. London: Sage.

McNeil, J. 1999. *Americans with Disabilities, 1991-92: Data from the Survey of Income and Programme Participation.* Washington, DC: U.S. Department of Commerce Economics and Statistics Administration, Bureau of the Census.

Mead, L. M. 1997. *From Welfare to Work.* London: Institute for Economic Affairs.

Mishra, R. 1977. *Society and Social Policy: Theories and Practice of Welfare.* London: Macmillan.

Morris, J. 1991. *Pride against Prejudice.* London: The Women's Press.

Nightingale, B. 1973. *Charities.* Harmondsworth, UK: Penguin.

Novak, T. 1988. *Poverty and the State.* Philadelphia: Open University Press.

"Old Soldier's Pride." 1996. *South Wales Evening Post,* April 24, p. 4.

Oliver, M. 1990. *The Politics of Disablement.* London: Macmillan.

———, ed. 1991. *Social Work, Disabled People and Disabling Environments.* London: Jessica Kingsley.

———. 1996. *Understanding Disability: From Theory to Practice.* London: Macmillan.

Oliver, M. and C. Barnes. 1998. *Disabled People and Social Policy.* London: Longman.

Organization for Economic Cooperation and Development (OECD). 1999. *Public Sector Consumption 1996.* Paris: Author.

Owen, D. 1965. *English Philanthropy, 1660-1960.* Oxford, UK: Oxford University Press.

Pagel, M. 1988. *On Our Own Behalf.* Manchester, UK: Greater Manchester Coalition of Disabled People.

Pithouse, A. and H. Williamson, eds. 1997. *Engaging the User in Welfare Services.* Birmingham, UK: Venture.

Priestley, M. 1999. *Disability Politics and Community Care.* London: Jessica Kingsley.

Royal Association for Disability and Rehabilitation (RADAR). 1993. *Disability and Discrimination in Employment.* London: Author.

———. 1994. *Disabled People Have Rights.* London: Author.

Rector, R. 1997. "Wisconsin's Welfare Miracle." *Policy Review* 82 (March-April) [Online]. Available: www.policyreview.com/mar97/rector.html.

Rights Now. 1994. *What Price Civil Rights?* London: Rights Now Campaign.

Ronnby, A. 1985. *Socialstaten.* Lund, Sweden: Studentlitteratur.

Rose, M. E. 1972. *The Relief of Poverty.* London: Macmillan.

Rose, S. and B. Black. 1985. *Advocacy and Empowerment: Mental Health Care in the Community.* London: Routledge Kegan Paul.

Rowland, P. 1971. *The Last Liberal Governments.* 2 vols. London: Barrie & Jenkins.

Rowntree, S. 1901. *Poverty: A Study of Town Life.* London: Macmillan.

Ryan, M. and F. Thomas. 1980. *The Politics of Mental Handicap.* Harmondsworth, UK: Penguin.

Safilios-Rothschild, C. 1970. *The Sociology and Social Psychology of Disability and Rehabilitation.* New York: Random House.

Sainsbury, S. 1993. *Normal Life: A Study of War and Industrially Injured Pensioners.* Aldershot, UK: Avebury.

Schofield, A. 1955. *Parliamentary Elections.* London: Shaw.

Scott, R. 1970. "The Constructions of Conceptions of Stigma by Professional Experts." Pp. 255-90 in *Deviance and Respectability,* edited by J. D. Douglas. New York: Basic Books.

Scott, V. 1994. *Lessons from America: A Study of the Americans with Disabilities Act.* London: Royal Association for Disability and Rehabilitation.

Scruton, R. 1982. *A Dictionary of Political Thought.* London: Pan.

Scully, S. 1998. "Wisconsin Works on Welfare." *Washington Times,* August 18 [Online]. Available: www.ncpa.org/pi/welfare/wel43a.html.

Searle, G. R. 1971. *The Quest for National Efficiency.* Oxford, UK: Blackwell.

Semmel, B. 1960. *Imperialism and Social Reform.* London: Allen & Unwin.

Sly, F. 1996. "Disability and the Labour Market." *Labour Market Trends,* September, 413-24.

Social Security Administration. 1997. *Social Security Disability Benefits.* Washington, DC: Author.

Spicker, P. 1993. *Poverty and Social Security: Concepts and Principles.* London: Routledge Kegan Paul.

Stanton, E. 1970. *Clients Come Last.* Beverly Hills, CA: Sage.

Stedman Jones, G. 1971. *Outcast London.* Oxford, UK: Oxford University Press.

Swain, J., V. Finkelstein, S. French, and M. Oliver, eds. 1993. *Disabling Barriers, Enabling Environments.* London: Sage.

Symonds, A. and A. Kelly, eds. 1998. *The Social Construction of Community Care*. London: Macmillan.

Tawney, R. H. 1964. *Equality*. London: Allen & Unwin.

Timmins, N. 1995. *The Five Giants: A Biography of the Welfare State*. London: Fontana.

Topliss, E. 1979. *Provision for the Disabled*. Oxford, UK: Blackwell & Martin Robertson.

Townsend, P. 1979. *Poverty in the United Kingdom*. Harmondsworth, UK: Penguin.

Tucker, B. 1994. "Overview of the DDA and Comparison with the ADA." *Australian Disability Review* 3 (94): 23-27.

Turner, B. S., ed. 1993. *Citizenship and Social Theory*. Newbury Park, CA: Sage.

Union of Physically Impaired against Segregation (UPIAS). 1976. *Fundamental Principles of Disability*. London: UPIAS & the Disability Alliance.

Voet, R. 1998. *Feminism and Citizenship*. Thousand Oaks, CA: Sage.

Walker, A. 1982. *Unqualified and Underemployed*. London: Macmillan.

Walker, R. L. 1991. *Thinking about Workfare: Evidence from the USA*. London: Her Majesty's Stationery Office.

Welsh Office. 1989. *Still a Small Voice: Consumer Involvement in the All Wales Strategy*. Cardiff, UK: Author.

Wilson, M. 1993. "The German Welfare State: A Conservative Regime in Crisis." Pp. 141-72 in *Comparing Welfare States,* edited by Allan Cochrane and John Clarke. London: Sage.

Wollaston, H., ed. 1970. *Parker's Conduct of Parliamentary Elections*. London: Charles Knight.

Zola, I. K. 1994. "Towards Inclusion: The Role of People with Disabilities in Policy and Research Issues in the United States—A Historical and Political Analysis." In *Disability Is Not Measles*, edited by M. Roux and M. Bach. North York, Ontario: Roeher Institute.

Advocacy and Political Action

17

SHARON BARNARTT
KAY SCHRINER
RICHARD SCOTCH

DISABILITY AND POLITICAL ACTION

As is addressed throughout this volume, people with disabilities frequently occupy marginalized social and economic positions in contemporary societies. In recent decades, people with disabilities have increasingly sought to participate collectively in broader decisions about public policy. These political initiatives have taken a variety of forms, depending on the nature of existing political institutions in various national settings and on the nature of the issues in question. In this chapter, we will attempt to describe the diverse nature of disability politics and political advocacy, drawing particularly on areas that have been the subject of established scholarship in disability studies.

In the medical model traditionally used to characterize disability in Western culture, disability is an individualized condition dispersed across the general population rather than a collective one and thus would not naturally serve as the basis for collective political activity (Scotch 1988). In this model, disability is a chronic pathology or impairment associated with an incapacity to perform bodily functions or activities of daily living. This incapacity is considered to be an organic fact that must be overcome through medical intervention, compensated for by rehabilitation, or responded to with social welfare benefits and services. Gatekeeping, which by definition determines who is and is not entitled to claim the label of disabled, is managed by medical and rehabilitative professionals and is nominally apolitical and not considered an appropriate realm for public debate.

In the medical model of disability, the primary role for politics is reallocative, to secure resources for medical and rehabilitative research and services and for benefits and services. Such politics are typically practiced by nondisabled advocates for people who have disabilities rather than by people with disabilities themselves.[1] Such political initiatives frequently emphasize the

AUTHORS' NOTE: Communication concerning this chapter should be directed to Richard Scotch, Associate Professor of Sociology and Political Economy, School of Social Sciences, University of Texas at Dallas, Box 830688, Richardson, TX 75083-0688; e-mail: scotch@utdallas.edu. We would like to acknowledge the assistance of Gary Albrecht, Michael Bury, and the anonymous reviewers for their many helpful suggestions and insights as this chapter was being prepared.

incapacity associated with disability and the moral blamelessness for their conditions of those who are unable to help themselves. These kind of political appeals often feature tales of woe about poster children (of all ages) whose lives will be ruined by their impairments unless help is found, particularly help in the form of a cure.

Such political appeals have often been quite successful, and efforts have been made to medicalize a number of conditions to entitle those who have them to a flow of benefits and services for the "deserving" poor (Fox 1977). In the United States, for example, Congress has often appropriated more funds to research on targeted diseases and conditions than had been requested for biomedical research at the National Institutes of Health in response to advocacy by those affected by various illnesses. Many public officials are reluctant to appear insensitive to appeals by those perceived as helpless and blameless.

At issue in such political discourse is often the moral entitlement of those who are "afflicted," being based on random victimization rather than their own choices and behavior. Questions of personal responsibility are opposed to medical definitions in debates over public funding benefiting people with conditions widely considered to be morally ambiguous, such as HIV/AIDS, psychiatric disorders, obesity, teen pregnancy, or learning disabilities.

Nonmedical models of disabilities are associated with different political forms, issues, and dynamics. A social model of disability conceptualizes disability as a social construction that is the result of interaction between physical or mental impairment and the social environment. Technology, architecture, and spatial organization all reflect concepts of what is "normal" and how "normal" people function, as do cultural attitudes and institutional processes (Higgins 1992). These social characteristics help to define who is "disabled" and who is "normal" and what constitutes an appropriate social response to those who have a disability (see, e.g., Goffman 1963).

In such a social model, people with disabilities may be grouped together into common medical, educational rehabilitative, human service, and custodial systems, but the establishment of such systems and the definition of who is to be considered disabled vary across cultures and historical periods. Gatekeeping under a social model of disability is not solely the province of professionals but can be contested by many within society, including people with disabilities themselves.

The politics of disability takes far different forms within the social model than would be expected in the medical model. Political issues are not simply allocative, although disputes over resources are found here too but may also include conflict over what social roles can appropriately be played by individuals who have disabilities and how the state should support or restrict those roles through its policies. A social model of disability would lead one to expect political conflict over such issues—over what is the appropriate role for people with disabilities in education, employment, public services such as transportation, economic development, and participation in civic life.

By characterizing the social isolation and enforced dependency of people with disabilities as the result of social choices rather than as inevitable results of impairment, the social model suggests analogies between the social status of people with disabilities and other marginalized groups, such as racial and ethnic minorities, women, or gays and lesbians. Within this political framework, disability politics can encompass disputes over civil rights (Scotch 1984). Similarly, politics encompasses conflicts over the role of disabled people collectively in the governance of service systems and other institutions addressing the disability community and the role of individuals with disabilities in shaping and controlling the services they receive.

There is a long history of state policies affecting people with disabilities,[2] but the creation and operation of these policies have typically been on behalf of people with disabilities rather than with their direct participation. In recent decades, this exclusion has ended with active involvement sought and frequently achieved by advocates who have disabilities themselves and who are considered to be legitimate representatives of the broader disability community.[3]

Some efforts to redefine the social position of people have occurred through legal advocacy in the courts, particularly in the United States. Enabled by the distinctive American constitutional and legal framework and building on the civil rights advocacy that fought racial segregation through federal lawsuits in the post–World War II era, a number of class action suits were successfully pursued in the late 1960s and 1970s on behalf of children denied public school education because of their disabilities,[4] people with disabilities receiving inappropriate treatment in residential institutions,[5] and others denied fair treatment because of their disabilities. These lawsuits were often the product of public interest law centers such as the Mental Health Law Project, the Center for Law and the Handicapped, and the Public Interest Law Center of Philadelphia.

Key judicial rulings helped to establish legal protections for disabled people and helped to foster the growing disability rights movement in the United States. Gerry and Benton (1980) have written that prior to the mid-1970s in the United States,

> only in the courts had active conflicts arisen between those who insisted that disabled children and adults had a right to be free of discrimination and those who argued that the very notion of rights was likely to destroy the good will and charity which had allowed disabled people to advance as far as they had. (P. 3)

Yet in the absence of more broadly based political advocacy, litigation-based political strategies tend to be episodic and non-self-enforcing (Carty 1978) and to have limited capacity to effect institutional change (Horowitz 1977). Legal advocacy is a crucial component in ensuring that broader public policies are applied appropriately to individual cases, and legal organizations such as the Disability Rights Education and Defense Fund (DREDF) have been valuable resources in the protection of individuals with disabilities. In the United States, parent groups have been very effective in securing court decisions that have established the rights of children with disabilities to public education and to decent treatment in institutional settings. Nevertheless, we would contend that such advocacy is most effective when it is part of a wider political mobilization of people with disabilities on their own behalf, a process that requires both social solidarity and collective action.

Beyond the United States, there have been a number of other important efforts to secure legal rights for people with disabilities (Jones and Marks 1999a). Legal protections have been enacted in Australia (Jones and Marks 1999b), Canada (Rioux and Frazee 1999), and the United Kingdom (Doyle 1999). In 1994, Sweden established an Office of the Disability Ombudsman to promote full participation and equality for people with disabilities (Wastberg 1999). There have also been efforts through the United Nations (UN) to develop an international legal framework to serve as a model of legal protections for disabled people, beginning with the *Standard Rules on the Equalization of Opportunities for Persons with Disabilities,* adopted by the UN General Assembly in 1993 (Michailakis 1999). It is unclear, however, what the short-term impact of these laws has been in actually improving the actual conditions facing people with disabilities.

THE SOCIAL BASIS FOR COLLECTIVE POLITICAL ACTION

Having a disability does not in itself lead to participation in collective political action with others who have disabilities (Scotch 1988). Many political constituencies form out of geographic communities or out of already socially cohesive groups. Disabilities are spread spatially and demographically across the general population, although many disabilities are concentrated among those with the least economic, social, and political resources in their societies. Disability per se is not generally tied to a distinct social structure within society (Barnartt 1996), and in most societies, it is only in recent history that disability activists have acted on their own behalf as a political interest group. For example, as recently as 1985, Harlan Hahn wrote of the United States, "There is no organized constituency of disabled voters comparable to groups that have been formed by blacks, Hispanics, women, and aging citizens" (Hahn 1985a:309-10). In the past few decades, however, political organization and activity among people with disabilities have increased in many nations through both social movement organizations and, increasingly, efforts focused on electoral politics.

While some disability advocates commonly refer to "the disability community," those who actively identify with this community include only a minute portion of the substantial number of people with disabilities in any society. One barrier to collective action is the stigma associated with disabilities. Hahn (1985a) writes, "Persons with disabilities often are understandably reluctant to focus on that aspect of their identity that is most negatively stigmatized by the rest of society and to mobilize politically around it" (p. 310).

However, when disability is created as a social category, particularly through public policy and the provision of health and social services, those as having a disability can become a distinct interest group that may become capable of mobilization. Policy interventions may literally bring people with disabilities together to receive services, facilitating interaction and laying the groundwork for the formation of a collective identity. Rehabilitation facilities, independent living centers, disabled student service networks, and recreational programs have all helped to build solidarity among disabled people.

There are numerous examples of people with disabilities engaged in protests or forming organizations on their own behalf. For example, in Spain in 1894, graduates of the Madrid School for the Blind formed an organization, Centro Protectivo e Instructor de Ciegos, to protest the segregation of the blind and their reliance on begging (Vaughn 1998). In 1935, several hundred unemployed disabled people in New York City formed the League of the Physically Handicapped to protest their exclusion from public jobs through the Works Progress Administration (Longmore 1997). In Great Britain, Finkelstein (1981) reports that following World War II, there was a "rapid growth" in the numbers and size of organizations of people with disabilities.

In the past four decades, political activity by individuals with disabilities and organizations of disabled people has particularly increased. To some extent, political activity has been directed toward increasing the level or scope of government benefits. However, significant activity also has been directed toward the goals of equal access, community integration, and independent living.

Among the explanations that have been offered for this increase are emerging medical and assistive technologies that have supported independence for many people with disabilities, changing ideologies of treatment that have encouraged noninstitutional service strategies, and the models of other minority movements in the 1960s and 1970s that advocated inclusion and social change (Scotch 1989).

Underlying the increasing political mobilization of people with disabilities has been an evolving but distinctive ideology that explains their marginal societal status in sociopolitical terms (Barton 1992; Hahn 1985b). Under a sociopolitical perspective, disadvantage and marginality are characterized as the products of a hostile and disabling environment that must be challenged by political, legal, and social efforts. These efforts are often framed by the political culture of the nation in which they occur. In the United States, for example, political goals have been articulated in terms of individual rights, and those goals have served as a model for movements in a number of other countries. Yet in some other societies, protests may be framed differently, for example, on models of social solidarity or group rights. One particularly thoughtful review of different conceptual bases for disability policy that focus on rights is Jerome E. Bickenbach's (1993) *Physical Disability and Social Policy*.

ELECTORAL POLITICS: PEOPLE WITH DISABILITIES AS VOTERS

Among the countries that have democratic systems of government characterized by periodic and free elections for positions in representative institutions, "universal" suffrage, competing political parties, and accountability of elected officials, participation in elected politics is an avenue for people with disabilities to secure their political voice.[6] These countries include the many nations that represent the "third wave" of democratization.

Not much is known about the electoral process in any democratic nation. Only a handful of studies have addressed this topic, and these were conducted in the United States. These studies indicate that U.S. citizens who have disabilities are much less likely to register and vote than are nondisabled individuals (Schur and Kruse 2000; Shields, Schriner, and Schriner 1998).[7] In addition, this research challenges how well political science findings about "who votes" apply to the disability community. People with disabilities are much *less* likely to vote as they age as compared to nondisabled individuals, who are much *more* likely to vote as they grow older. Furthermore, when other socioeconomic variables such as age, education, and income are controlled for, having a disability is a significant negative factor in determining whether an individual votes (Shields et al. 1998). This new knowledge strongly suggests that the research on political behavior is incomplete without considering whether individuals have a disability—at least in the United States.

Notwithstanding the relative lack of information regarding participation rates and patterns, it seems likely that a study of electoral participation in any nation will begin with a similar set of questions. A primary concern will be accessibility of the polling place. Individuals with disabilities may encounter a variety of architectural barriers. In the United States, election officials admit that some 14 percent of states' election sites are inaccessible to individuals with mobility impairments (a figure that might be higher if it were based on evaluations conducted by a knowledgeable and disinterested party and if the accessibility criteria included those relevant to people with communication, cognitive, and emotional impairments).[8]

Another issue is the receptivity and responsiveness of election officials. At times, election officials may become sufficiently frustrated with meeting accessibility needs that they urge the disabled voter to vote absentee. Some individuals with disabilities view absentee voting as an inferior form of participation. People with cognitive impairments, blindness, or deafness are sometimes subjected to challenges or encounter election officials who are uninformed about their accommodation needs or who resist taking the necessary steps to make the voting process or polling place accessible. Blind voters have complained that election officials have limited understanding of methods necessary to accommodate them, and deaf individuals have made similar claims. A related issue is the role of family members in the voting process. A recent story published in an English magazine recounts conversations with parents, some of whom believe their disabled children can and should vote and others who confess to marking their children's ballots for them ("Invisible Voters" 1992).

In addition to these physical and attitudinal barriers, policy barriers may affect participation. In the United States, for example, 44 states disenfranchise some individuals with cognitive and emotional impairments (Schriner, Ochs, and Shields 1997). Other countries have similar prohibitions. England's Representation of the People Act 1983 disenfranchises people who have been involuntary admitted to mental hospitals ("Invisible Voters" 1992). Similarly, the constitution of Albania prohibits voting by individuals who have been adjudicated as incompetent.

The dearth of information regarding the voting behavior of people with disabilities and the policies that may affect their turnout suggests a pressing research agenda for the next decade. What are the experiences of people with disabilities when they go to the polls? Do these vary by country and, if so, how? Are the opportunities for participation better in some countries than others? What accommodations and modifications are necessary to ensure that they have the same opportunities and protections as other citizens? What policies are required to encourage them to vote and protect that right to self-governance? These inquires must be made to develop the knowledge base necessary to promote the participation of people with disabilities in democratic governance.

One particularly thorny set of questions surrounds the issue of competent voting. Democratic theorists typically assume that excluding individuals based on "mental incompetence" or some similar term of definition accomplishes the necessary task of ensuring that electors are competent. Robert Dahl (1989), for example, a prominent American theorist, argues that such individuals are like children and, like children, should be excluded from the electorate.

These theoretical treatments of the competence standard raise several significant questions. The first and most central is the following: What *is* competence with respect to voting? The answer to this question has evaded theorists and policymakers because of the difficulty of saying with certainty what is the minimum set of skills and knowledge one must possess to be entrusted with self-rule. This question will be answered differently depending on the political institutions involved. Taking part in direct democracy presumably places more demands on the individual than does participating in a representative democracy (though, it could be argued, direct democracy also encourages the development of such skills and knowledge to a greater degree than does representative democracy). Irrespective of these differences, however, the question of *defining* the competencies necessary for participation and developing a *valid and reliable scheme* for separating the incompetent from the competent remains a daunting challenge.

Second, is it *necessary* to adopt legal prohibitions against voting by incompetent people, or do laws against influencing others' votes through bribery or other criminal acts provide equivalent protections against the incompetent voter? Finally, if we must have laws that disenfranchise individuals based on mental competency, what is the most objective way to identify these persons? The U.S. experience, we would suggest, is not the approach that should be taken. In most U.S. states, some individuals with cognitive and emotional impairments are disenfranchised—but, undoubtedly, some individuals who are truly unable to competently case a ballot are not identified through this statutory scheme, and others who truly are competent to vote are disenfranchised. The potential constitutional deficiencies of the laws in many U.S. states, when coupled with the difficulties in determining the abilities necessary to define voting competence, call for a closer look at the issue of competence and its place in democratic theory and practice. The competence standard is perhaps the purest example of the political nature of the disability category.

PARTICIPATION OF PEOPLE WITH DISABILITIES AS CANDIDATES AND ELECTED OFFICIALS

Another item for the research agenda arises when considering the issue of disability in the broader context of campaigns and elections. Knowledgeable observers report that persons with disabilities hold or have held elected offices in several countries,[9] but there is little if any scholarly inquiry regarding the way disability is portrayed in campaigns. This may be a crucial factor in shaping the electorate's response to people with disabilities and the "problem" of disability. Information observations of U.S. politics indicate that disability is often an issue in campaigns, particularly contests for the presidency. In the 1996 campaign, for example, the Republican Party candidate, Senator Robert Dole, a World War II veteran, lost the use of his arm from an injury sustained in combat. His disability was labeled a "badge of honor." The Democratic Party candidate, Bill Clinton, was not disabled, but the Democratic national convention featured an address by Christopher Reeve, an actor who became quadriplegic after a riding accident. Reeve, a controversial figure in the U.S. disability community (Stanglin 1996), issued a plea for funding for research to cure paralysis. In neither of these instances was civil rights for people with disabilities a major focus of the campaign message, although in both parties' campaigns, disability rights was a minor emphasis.

To the extent that people with disabilities can exercise some influence of their portrayal in campaigns, they will be able to influence the outcomes of elections and the public policies that elected officials propose and adopt. Achieving this level of influence will require complete access to campaign activities, which will only be possible if the electoral system is more accessible to people with disabilities. Television and radio ads, printed material, and live events should be conducted in such a way that individuals with all kinds of impairments can obtain information necessary to be well informed but are often not. Moreover, because they tend to be less affluent than nondisabled individuals, people with disabilities around the world are less likely to have the wherewithal to contribute money, time, or other resources to political candidates. Because disabled people have fewer resources and opportunities to be heard in the electoral process, they may continue to have a lower visibility in elections, particularly in those democracies where having such resources greatly influences the degree of access to the political process.

REPRESENTATION

The issue of representation is also important. The mere presence of disabled individuals in elected bodies by no means ensures that "disability issues" will be represented in those institutions' decisions. In Uganda, for example, the constitution (newly written in 1995) guarantees representation by reserving five seats in parliament for persons with disabilities. *Disability International* reported that a deaf man, Alex Ndeezi, was recently elected to the national parliament and became the first deaf parliamentarian in Africa. Ndeezi has become a "leading defender of gender balance and marginalized groups" (Mutabazi 1997) and joins four other individuals with disabilities in the national parliament.[10]

This strong national presence of persons with disabilities is quite remarkable and has occurred in many nations around the world with growing democratic participation in government. In the Soviet Union, along with a number of other political organizations founded in the wake of the Helsinki Accords in the late 1970s, the Action Group to Defend the Rights of the Disabled in the USSR was founded in 1978 to advocate for legal rights for Soviets with disabilities (Raymond 1989). In the Philippines, a national political party was recently established to represent the interests of disabled persons (Venus Ilagan, personal communication, March 1, 1999).

Nevertheless, issues often occur concerning who can legitimately represent the interests of people with disabilities. Many individuals with disabilities have questioned whose interests are actually advanced by politically engaged nondisabled professionals who serve disabled people and have contended that only people with disabilities should speak exclusively on their own behalf. Others have questioned whether parents or other family members of disabled individuals should be seen as a part of the "disability community" and allowed to represent that community in political forums. These questions become even more complex when applied to individuals with severe cognitive or psychiatric impairments who may have difficulty articulating their own interests in political discourse.

LOBBYING AND PRESSURE GROUPS

In addition to participation as elected officials or through political parties, disabled people in many nations have formed organizations whose purpose is to represent the disability community and influence governmental bodies responsible for the enactment and implementation of public policy. In recent decades, a number of umbrella organizations have been formed to coordinate political activity and speak with one voice on behalf of the disability community. In Great Britain, for example, the British Council of Organisations of Disabled Peoples (BCODP) formed in 1981 (Campbell and Oliver 1996) to represent 80 organizations and approximately 200,000 Britons with disabilities (Gooding 1994:160). In the United States, the American Coalition of Citizens with Disabilities was organized in 1975, with 19 constituent groups, and it has since been replaced by several longstanding and ad hoc coalitions of disability organizations engaged in political advocacy. In Canada, the Coalition of Provincial Organizations of the Handicapped (COPOH) was founded in 1976 with affiliates from most Canadian provinces.[11] In Denmark, De samvirkende Invalideorganisationer (DSI) has been active in promoting the integration into Danish society of Danes with disabilities for decades (Jorgenson 1982).

Parallel to the formation of these national coalitions has been the creation of cross-national coalitions. Some international groups have organized around specific disabilities, such as the African Union of the Blind, founded in 1987, whose activities have been supported by the Norwegian Association of the Blind and Partially Sighted (Vaughn 1998:131). In 1981, Disabled People's International (DPI) was formed, an international cross-disability coalition of more than 110 organizations, including many from developing nations in Latin America, Africa, and Asia (Driedger 1989). DPI, which is led by people with disabilities, has been especially active in advocating for disability rights in international governmental, particularly nongovernmental activities, and in supporting the development of organizations of people with disabilities around the world. Pelka (1997) quotes Joshua Malinga, a former DPI chairperson from Zimbabwe, who remembered the 1980 organizational meeting of DPI in Singapore:

> It was at this meeting that most of us from Africa first understood what was meant by a 'disability rights movement.' We had never thought about disabled rights as a cause, to the disabled community as a community. . . . It was a shift from looking at disability as a health issue, to looking at it as a human rights issue. (P. 103)

Perhaps the most established political role for disability advocates has been in the United States, where a number of organizations maintain active lobbying roles in Washington and many state capitals. Scotch (1984, 1989) and Percy (1989) have described the extensive and significant role of representatives of disability organizations in the United States in disability policy development in the 1970s and 1980s. Bowe (1992) writes that "in Sweden and Denmark . . . the State has given over most of the control of many disability policies to organized representatives of people with disabilities" (p. 45). Organizations of people with disabilities in many other countries, including Canada, Singapore, England, Ireland, and the Netherlands, have participated in the reformulation of outdated disability policies (Miller, Chadderdon, and Duncan 1981).

Most American disability policies since the mid-1970s, including the landmark Americans with Disabilities Act, were drafted with the active participation of representatives of organizations of disabled people (Pfeiffer 1993). In addition, in the 1990s, many appointed government officials responsible for making and enforcing government disability policies were recruited to their posts from organizations of people with disabilities. In a number of instances, the prior connections among government appointees from the disability movement have meant that the longstanding absence of communication and cooperation among competing public bureaucracies has been overcome.

While access to positions of power and influence has had many important benefits for the disability community, it has often created dilemmas for those holding them, who must balance their loyalties to their constituencies with the practical considerations of public policymaking. Nevertheless, because so many aspects of life for people with disabilities are shaped by public policy, institutionalized participation in policy debates within government appears to have incorporated the experience of disability into many policy decisions. When regular participation does not occur, however, disability advocates may need to turn to more contentious nonelectoral political action to represent their own interests.

SOCIAL MOVEMENTS OF PEOPLE WITH DISABILITIES

There has been little scholarly attention paid to social movement activities occurring in the disability community. There are books written by advocates (e.g., Hartman and Johnson 1993), books presenting an advocate's point of view (e.g., Woodward 1982), journalistic accounts of the awakening of the disability community (e.g., Kleinfield 1977; Shapiro 1993), and accounts of specific protests (e.g., Christiansen and Barnartt 1995). Within general scholarly anthologies about social movements (e.g., Goldberg 1991), the disability movement does not show up, with one exception (Johnson 1983). Only a few scholarly articles have analyzed the general issue of social movements in the disability community from a social movement perspective.

In this section, we examine movement politics in the disability community, with a particular focus on the United States. Movement politics, referred to within some of the literature as contentious politics (Tarrow 1996), occurs outside of normal political institutions, mobilizes participants on the basis of beliefs, involves long-term political actions that seek social change, and uses tactics and strategies that are other than "politics as usual" (Meyer 1993). This form of politics is resorted to by those with little influence within mainstream political institutions (Piven and Cloward 1979), although social movement organizations may combine it with less disruptive tactics such as lawsuits, letter-writing campaigns, or voter registration drives. Most organizations of people with disabilities, however, choose a less disruptive political style. Oliver (1990) writes of this choice for the disability movement:

> Should it settle for incorporation into state activities with the prospect of piecemeal gains in social policy and legislation with the risks that representations to political institutions will be ignored or manipulated? Or should it remain separate from the state and concentrate on consciousness-raising activities leading to long-term change in policy and the empowerment of disabled people, with the attendant risks that the movement may be marginalized or isolated? (P. 128)

Actors who participate in contentious politics tend to be angry, emotional, and demanding. They are protesting issues about which they feel so strongly that they are willing to engage in risky behavior and angry rhetoric, even if they sometimes alienate potential supporters. Disability protestors have been willing to confront public officials, block traffic, occupy public places and government offices, or be arrested for their causes. In 1972, for example, members of the cross-disability group, Disabled in Action, blocked traffic in the New York financial district. In 1977, disabled protesters occupied federal government offices in 10 cities around the United States to demand that the delayed regulations for Section 504 of the Rehabilitation Act be issued (Scotch 1984). In 1981, in Canada, coordinated national protests were organized by the Council of Canadians with Disabilities to advocate for a human rights amendment to protect the civil rights of Canadians with disabilities (Pelka 1997). Through much of the 1980s, members of American Disabled for Accessible Public Transit (ADAPT) chained themselves to buses and disrupted meetings of the American Public Transit Association to protest inaccessible public transportation. In 1988, deaf students at Gallaudet University in Washington, D.C., forced the closure of their campus for a week, demanding that a deaf person be hired as university president (Christiansen and Barnartt 1995). British organizations of people with disabilities have engaged in similar disruptive tactics; Gooding cites a 1993 *New Statesman* report of a national register maintained by the Direct Action Network of more than a thousand disability activists willing to take part in civil disobedience (Gooding 1994).

Typically, protests involve not just short-term objectives but also a sense of shared purpose based on a vision of an alternative to existing social arrangements. The goal of an inclusive, barrier-free society may motivate disability activists beyond the specifics of an exclusionary policy or demeaning practice. Len Barton (1992) writes,

> A politics of disability can draw some lessons from feminist thought and practice. For example, connecting the personal with the political so that what has been depicted in mainly individual terms can be viewed as a social predicament. Making their standpoints known to themselves and to others is a central part of the agenda. . . . This can be a means of developing a stronger individual and collective sense of worth and effort. (P. 9)

While mainstream research in politics has traditionally tended to view protests and other nonelectoral political activities as ineffective, social movement research suggests that protest activity, particularly when it is disruptive, may be successful in influencing public policy

(Gamson 1990; Piven and Cloward 1979). Disability movements appear to be influential in securing short-term policy goals and in changing the terms of the larger debate over how government and society at large ought to address the role of people with disabilities.

CONTENTIOUS ACTIONS IN THE AMERICAN DISABILITY COMMUNITY: A CASE STUDY

While disability movements have formed in many nations around the world, the movement in the United States is probably the most extensive and the one with the longest and broadest history of contentious disability politics. This section presents empirical results from a study by Barnartt and Scotch (forthcoming) of protests in the disability community from 1970 to 1999. That study used media and other reports of 646 specific instances of protest activity by disability activists in the United States.[12] The reports were compiled from 4 newspapers of national scope, which covered the entire period; more than 100 newspapers with more limited geographical or temporal scope; and some non-newspaper sources, including books, disability periodicals, and disability-related e-mail discussion lists. The published media reports were identified by the use of Internet search engines as well as other methods (see Barnartt and Scotch [forthcoming] for further methodological details). Using event history analysis, this research focuses on the actual protest event, not on protesters or social movement organizations. Variables that represented characteristics of the protests, such as location, date, target, and issue, were created, and the data were coded and entered into computer files for quantitative analysis.

Here we examine patterns of movement that political action has taken over time, changes in types of issues over time, changes in organizational involvement over time, and changes in types of organizations over time. Table 17.1 shows the numbers of protests in each year.

No reports of protests could be located for 1971 or 1972. From 1972 through 1987, the number of reported protests fluctuated between 4 (1978) and 18 (1977). After 1987, contentious political activity began to explode, with at least 18 protests every year. In 1987, there were 10 reported protests, but the next year, there were 41. The highest levels of protest were in 1991, 1992, and 1997, with 55, 57, and 80 protests, respectively.

These figures are contrary to the perception of many journalists (Lembke 1975; Schultz 1977) and academics (Anspach 1979; Treanor 1993), who perceived an increasingly active disability movement to exist by the mid-1970s. The numbers in Table 17.1 suggest that significant political power was unlikely to have derived from the small numbers of protests. By 1975, there had been only 20 marches or other forms of disruptive protest. The new phenomenon of visibly disabled people engaging in disruptive protests resonated within the national media, however, and led to the perception, by journalists and scholars, that there was an active and politically powerful social movement of people with disabilities.

What made protest activity begin in 1972, and how do we explain the fluctuations in the numbers of protests in subsequent years? Even when the social stage is set for collective action, as seemed to be the case by the end of the 1960s, collective action is unlikely to occur without some proximate cause. There must be the emergence of some specific grievance that sparks collective action. According to our database, the central political issue that provoked protests by disability activists from 1972 to 1977 was the struggle to pass and implement the Rehabilitation Act of 1973, particularly the provision in that law that prohibited discrimination on the basis of disability in federally supported programs, Section 504 (Scotch 1984). These highly visible protests were conducted by a broad cross-disability coalition, a somewhat new development in the disability movement. In 1972, protests in New York and Washington focused on President Nixon's two vetoes of earlier versions of this law. Many protests in 1976 and particularly 1977 urged the release of federal regulations implementing Section 504, which had been held up for

Table 17.1   Disability Protests by Year

Year	Number
1972	9
1973	6
1974	5
1976	7
1977	18
1978	4
1979	10
1980	8
1981	14
1982	5
1983	13
1984	9
1985	17
1986	13
1987	10
1988	41
1989	39
1990	35
1991	55
1992	57
1993	49
1994	18
1995	29
1996	40
1997	80
1998	26
1999[a]	30

a. Through July 26 only.

several years by cautious federal officials (Scotch 1984). Although the officials involved denied any connection, after a delay of more than three years, the Section 504 regulations were issued following these widely publicized disability protests. The apparent success of the protestors fueled the growth of the movement.

The Rehabilitation Act success contributed to a growing willingness in the disability community to plan and participate in disruptive collective action. In 1981, protests occurred in response to cuts in social programs by the Reagan administration.

However, at least two other issues showed up in the early 1980s that might have been expected to attract disability protests but did not. One was the controversy over the so-called

Baby Doe regulations. These regulations related to the extent to which hospitals must keep babies with several physical impairments alive or, alternatively, when a hospital could let such an infant die.[13] The other was a controversy over the right of a woman named Elizabeth Bouvia, who had severe physical impairments, to take her own life. This controversy also involved the extent to which hospitals should or could keep someone alive—by force, if necessary—who did not want to stay alive. There were no protests identified by the searching mechanisms used here that focused on either of these cases.[14] However, the organization Not Dead Yet refers to this situation as the basis for its establishment.

The surge in protest activity that began in 1988 does not have a single cause. Rather, there seems to be several factors at work. One cause may have been the success of the Deaf President Now (DPN) protests at Gallaudet University. Gallaudet, a university in Washington, D.C., serving deaf students, had never been led by a deaf president, and students demanded that the university trustees select one in a series of large-scale demonstrations (Christiansen and Barnartt 1995). Partly as a result of that protest, there appears to have been a change in political culture regarding disability around that time, which resulted in more sympathy and empathy for disability issues in Congress than had heretofore been seen (Altman and Barnartt 1993). This change in political culture may have brought with it an opening up of the political opportunity structure (Tarrow 1994), which was supportive of the introduction of the Americans with Disabilities Act (ADA) into Congress. The responsiveness of the American government to disability protests also may have increased with the transition from the Reagan to the Bush administration, which included more officials with some connection to disability (Altman and Barnartt 1993). This opening of the political opportunity structure may have been perceived by activists as something to be exploited with increased protest activity.

In addition, the introduction of the first version of the ADA in Congress in 1988 probably spurred some protest activity; it clearly provided a target for some protests. Although there is little evidence of a huge increase in protests specifically aimed at the ADA, some of the protests between 1988 and 1990 were aimed at its issues. A few protests had demanded one or more of the provisions that were eventually included in the law, especially the transportation provisions, but the numbers of these protests are smaller than one might have expected. Between the introduction of the ADA into Congress and the fact that there was now also a track record of widely publicized and successful protests, we have the beginnings of an explanation for the rise in the numbers of protests.

The large numbers of protests in 1992 and 1993 may be explained in part by protests against telethons that many disability advocates consider demeaning and exploitative of disability as tragic and catastrophic. In 1992, there were 18 such protests, and in 1993, there were 10. The large numbers of protests in 1997 are partially explained by the events of August 9, 1997. On this day, ADAPT sponsored protests against Greyhound in 40 cities across the country ("Protesters Serve Notice" 1997). Although the number of protests in 1998 decreased somewhat, the number of protests for the first half of 1999 suggested that protest activity has not begun to die down.

Analysis of the specific protest issues does not tell us enough about why the levels of protest waxed and waned or why they increased overall during this period. To do that, we examine changes over time in several other factors. Some disability movement researchers (e.g., Longmore 1997; Young 1998) claim that the current disability movement is more cross-disability than it had been in the past because of the presence of cross-disability organizations such as the American Coalition of Citizens with Disabilities (ACCD), which was founded in 1974. They further imply that this is one reason for the increasing number of protests during this time. Longmore (1997) states that current disability protests exemplify "an ecumenical ideology of disability issues and an inclusive definition of disability identity" (p. 97).

Table 17.2 shows the percentages of protest demands that were cross-disability by decade. It shows that there was considerable variation by decade, with the largest percentage of cross-disability demands showing up in the earliest decade (56 percent). The number of protest demands that were cross-disability was substantially lower in the 1980s (22.5 percent), although the numbers increased again in the 1990s (50 percent).

Table 17.2   Percentage of Demands That Were Cross-Disability, by Decade

Decade	Percentage	Number
1970s	55.7	34
1980s	22.5	38
1990s	50.4	210

Table 17.3   Percentage of Protests That Had Organizational Involvement, by Decade

Decade	Percentage	Number
1970s	55.7	34
1980s	68.9	104
1990s	64.1	241

ORGANIZATIONAL INVOLVEMENT

Table 17.3 shows the percentages of protests that were conducted by organizations by decade. It shows that while about 55 percent of the protests were conducted by organizations in the 1970s, this increased to almost 69 percent in the 1980s. However, in the 1990s, organizational involvement decreased slightly to about 64 percent of protests. Thus, while more protests were conducted by organizations than were not, organizational involvement in protests was somewhat variable. It did increase from the earliest decade, but, overall, it seems to be lower than in other social movements. (However, that is somewhat difficult to evaluate because many studies of social movements analyze only organizational records.)

In addition, patterns of organizational involvement changed. By the 1990s, there were more state-level branches of national organizations and more organizations that participated in so few protests that they were not coded separately, as well as at least eight new organizations participating in protests than had occurred in the 1970s and 1980s (data not shown).

One of the largest changes has to do with ADAPT's role in protests. ADAPT is one of the most well-known organizational players in the American disability community. Organized in 1984, this organization's initial goal was to promote accessible public transit systems; it has more recently become focused on guarantees of personal assistance services to support disabled people living in the community. (Its acronym originally stood for Americans Disabled for Public Transit; with its change of focus, the acronym now stands for Americans Disabled for Attendant Programs Today.) ADAPT was a major organizational player in protests that occurred in the 1980s; it organized about two-thirds of those protests, which had organizational involvement. However, the proportion of organizational-led protests attributed to ADAPT decreased after 1990, when ADAPT-led protests constituted only a little more than 40 percent of such protests.

Increases in organizational involvement, after the early years of a movement, can occur for several reasons. Existing organizations can become radicalized and begin to view their organizational goals as being most readily attained through protest. Alternatively, new organizations can emerge whose stated purpose is to produce social change and engage in collective action in order to produce that change. In a climate of successful collective action, it is less likely that an organization already involved in collective action will cease to do so, although it is imaginable if an organization decides to devote its resources to other aspects of social change.

CHANGES IN ORGANIZATIONAL TYPE

Rather than there being one social movement organization or even a few organizations that represent the diverse community of potential beneficiaries of these protests, a large number of organizations have been involved in disability-related protests. Organizations can vary on many dimensions. One of these is whether the focus is on a single issue or multiple issues. Organizations can also vary on a dimension that might not have an analog in other social movements—that of how many types of impairments they appeal to or recruit from. If we add this to the dimension of numbers of issues their scope encompasses, we can create a two-dimensional characterization of organizations: single-disability, single-issue organizations; multiple-disability, single-issue organizations; single-disability, multiple-issue organizations; and multiple-disability, multiple-issue, or cross-disability organizations. (Because there were no single-disability, single-issue organizations, this category is not included in this discussion.)

Multiple-disability, single-issue organizations focus on one specific issue but appeal to people who have a variety of types of impairments. ADAPT is one such organization. Its issue initially was the fairly narrow issue of accessibility of public transportation systems. Although a single, narrow issue, it was one that appealed to people who may have had a variety of types of mobility impairments as well as to some people with other types of impairments, such as blind people. However, there are also a number of other multiple-disability, single-issue organizations. One such organization is Not Dead Yet, whose opposition to assisted suicide is based on the notion that it is easier for society to assist the disabled in killing themselves than it is to assist them to live independent and productive lives with disabilities; they object to any legalization of assisted suicide for this reason. Another organization is Jerry's Orphans. This organization protests the portrayal of people with disabilities in telethons, Jerry Lewis's involvement in the telethons, and some of his statements about disability, such as his statement that he would rather be dead than be disabled. Other such organizations include The FDR in a Chair Campaign, which focused on how President Franklin Delano Roosevelt was to be portrayed in a new memorial, which opened in 1997. Concrete Change focuses on the accessibility of housing, and Concerned Rail Corridor Riders focuses on the accessibility of trains in the Chicago suburbs. All of these organizations are multidisability, in the sense that their issue relates to more than one type of impairment, but their rallying cry involves a single issue.

Single-disability, multiple-issue organizations focus on multiple issues, but these issues are of interest primarily to people with one type of impairment. Such organizations do not recruit from all sectors of the disability community, and the issue or issues that form their central concern are not applicable to people with all types of impairments. Such organizations include the National Association of the Deaf (NAD), the National Federation of the Blind (NFB), the American Council of the Blind (ACB), and Support Coalition International (SCI), an organization that focuses on issues related to psychiatric disabilities.

Multiple-issue, multiple-disability groups are not homogeneous. Rather, the category includes several subcategories. Some, such as the American Coalition of Citizens with Disabilities (ACCD) and Disabled in Action (DIA), have attempted to represent people with all types of impairments on issues, such as laws or discrimination patterns, which have the potential for affecting all disabled people. They truly attempt to be cross-disability organizations.

Other organizations such as The Association for the Severely Handicapped (TASH) and The ARC (The Association of Retarded Citizens) do not represent all people with impairments. Rather, they represent people with a number of types of impairments on a number of types of issues. TASH focuses on people, primarily children, with multiple impairments or extremely se-

Table 17.4   Type of Organization, by Decade

| | % (N) | | | | | | | |
| | Multiple Disability, Single Issue | | Single Disability, Multiple Issue | | Cross-Disability | | Totals[a] | |
Decade	Percentage	Number	Percentage	Number	Percentage	Number	Percentage	Number
1970s	0.0	(0)	11.4	(4)	88.6	(31)	100	(35)
1980s	62.5	(70)	2.7	(3)	34.8	(39)	100	(112)
1990s	52.7	(133)	8.3	(21)	38.9	(98)	99.9	(252)

a. Two organizations were coded when possible; therefore, the totals for this table do not equal the totals shown in Table 17.3.

vere impairments, while The ARC focuses on issues relevant to people with mental retardation, no matter what its source. Thus, these groups are multiple impairment, multiple issue, but they are not comprehensively cross-disability in their coverage.[15]

Table 17.4 shows that multiple-disability, single-issue groups were nonexistent in the 1970s. However, such groups comprised a majority (62.5 percent) of groups leading protests in the 1980s. Their "market share" dropped in the 1990s, to a little more than half of the protests. Organizations that we have been characterized as being single disability, multiple issue only conducted a minority of protests in any decade. However, they conducted comparatively more in the 1970s (11 percent) than in the other two decades. Clearly, this type of organization has never been a major player in the protest arena. Cross-disability organizations, contrary to the prognostications mentioned above, conducted most of the protests only in the 1970s, when they conducted almost 90 percent of all protests with an identified organization. Since then, this type of organization has conducted less than 40 percent of all reported protests.

Thus, we see that not only were more organizations becoming active in the protest arena as the cycle of protest heated up, but they also represented a different type of organization. These new organizations solved, to some extent, the problem posed by the political separation that was engendered by the medical community's division of impairment types (Zola 1983). Focusing on all types of impairments was clearly an impossible task, unless there were to be hundreds of disconnected groups. If so, that was not a strategy that would create the types of communication and interaction networks that would most facilitate collective action. So these groups coalesced around crosscutting issues, which affected many impairment groups. They organized around the issue instead of the type of impairment. Three of these issues were public portrayals of individuals with disabilities, fundraising telethons, and assisted suicide; the groups that formed around these issues were The FDR in a Chair Campaign, Jerry's Orphans, and Not Dead Yet, respectively.

This appears to have been an important solution to the problem posed by some types of separation engendered by the physical fact of impairment. These new groups were not as all-encompassing as were groups active in the 1970s, such as Disabled in Action or ACCD, either in the scope of their issues or in their desired membership. They were, however, much more inclusive than were the single-disability groups. For example, none of these new groups and none of their issues appealed to deaf people or appear to have attempted to recruit them. Or, if they did, it was most likely to have been without success since their issues are not the issues to which most deaf people are attracted. These issues were also unlikely to resonate with people with psychiatric impairments or who saw themselves as psychiatric survivors.

Clearly, then, the pattern of organizational structure of the protests that have been held in the disability community has undergone changes in recent years. These changes made the successful mobilization of larger numbers of aggrieved activists possible since they expanded the scope of issues while not limiting themselves to impairment groups that might have small populations—or would have small populations of potential activists.

CONCLUSION: A RESEARCH AGENDA
ON DISABILITY POLITICS

In this chapter, we have sought to provide a broad overview of the breadth and variety of organized political action by people with disabilities, focusing in particular on participation in electoral politics and on the activities of disability social movements. As discussed above, while there is a long history of political activity by and on the behalf of people with disabilities, disability politics has become far more widespread in the post–World War II era, particularly in the past three decades of the twentieth century. This has been building on the example of similar movements for self-determination and inclusion by other politically marginalized social groups around the world.

The growing ubiquity of disability politics, however, has not led to a corresponding body of scholarship. While there have been a number of important theoretical works on how disability can be viewed as a political phenomenon, there is only a modest body of empirical research beyond a number of anecdotal case studies. The problem is twofold. Within mainstream social science disciplines, such as political science, sociology, and history, disability in general and the politics of disability in particular are rarely considered. In these fields, disability is largely neglected in research compendia, professional journals, and curricula both in liberal arts and specialized graduate courses. Even when disability politics is addressed in the social sciences, it is often from a perspective largely uninformed by the experience of disability or the insights of disability studies scholarship. To address this vacuum, professional societies, graduate training programs, academic journals, and authors of textbooks that deal with politics and government should be pressed to incorporate disability issues and the political concerns and strategies of people with disabilities into their institutional activities. One model for activity is the American Sociological Association, which has recently published a collection of syllabi and instructional materials for teaching the sociology of disabilities (Schlesinger and Taub 1998). Many of the materials included in this compilation address disability politics. Another model is the 1993-1994 special issues of the *Policy Studies Journal* on disability policy edited by Sara D. Watson and David Pfeiffer, particularly the 1994 issue that dealt with disability politics and practice (21:4 Winter 1993 and 22:1 Spring 1994). These issues included articles by a number of prominent political scientists and other researchers on a variety of disability-related topics in politics and policy.

Within the growing field of disability studies, consideration of political factors, broadly defined, has been central and has shaped much of the discourse since the early 1980s, particularly in Great Britain and in the United States (Hahn 1993). However, much of this body of work involves theoretical analysis informed by personal accounts. As has been noted at several points in this chapter, there is very little systematically gathered empirical data on political action by people with disabilities, whether through voting, seeking political office, or social movement activity. Much of the data that do exist deal only with the United States. While there is tremendous value in individual case studies, the development and pursuit of a collective research agenda on political action within disability studies would help build a more coherent and comprehensive body of knowledge on disability politics. And while some disability studies scholars would object to the assumptions and methodologies of mainstream political and social science, there would be value in applying these established analytical techniques to achieve a better understanding of the political status and behavior of people with disabilities.

What should this research agenda include? Topics for which far more research is needed include the following:

■ voting studies and examination of barriers to political participation;

■ examinations of how lobbying and pressure group activity shape disability policy;

■ research on recruitment, mobilization, and leadership within and across social movement organizations;

■ analyses of the effectiveness of alternative political strategies and tactics; and

■ historical studies of important organizations and political leaders within disability
movements.

While there is not enough known about those countries where the most research has been focused, the United States and Great Britain, there is also a tremendous need for studies of disability politics in other nations, particularly in Africa, Asia, and Latin America, and a general need
for comparative political research. Political theory and public law would also be productive
fields for analytical work on disability politics on topics such as distributive justice, democratic
theory, and equal protection. In short, there is an important need for studies relating to disability in every subfield within the overall study of government and politics. The bibliography that
follows provides some valuable models for this needed work.

NOTES

1. The literature commonly makes the distinction between organizations *for* people with disabilities, which are
often led by nondisabled individuals and typically include charitable organizations or professional associations, and
organizations *of* people with disabilities, whose membership and leadership are predominantly composed of individuals who themselves have disabilities (see, e.g., Oliver 1983:134-36).

2. In *The Disabled State,* Deborah Stone (1984) has examined how disability is defined as the basis for eligibility
for public welfare in the United States, Germany, and Great Britain. A very broad cross-cultural and broadly historical
overview that addresses some apparent social constants in law and disability is provided in Scheer and Groce (1988).

3. One broad analysis of recent disability policies in the United States and Great Britain and the politics that have
shaped them is provided by Caroline Gooding in her 1994 book *Disabling Laws, Enabling Acts: Disability Rights in
Britain and America.*

4. For example, *Pennsylvania Association for Retarded Children v. Commonwealth of Pennsylvania* (1971) established a right to appropriate education for children with mental retardation, and *Mills v. Board of Education*
(1972) extended this right to all children with disabilities. These rulings served as the basis for the 1975 Education for
All Handicapped Children Act, now known as the Individuals with Disabilities Education Act.

5. For example, *Wyatt v. Hardin* (1971) established a right to treatment for individuals involuntarily committed
to public mental institutions, and *New York State Association for Retarded Children v. Carey* (1975) established a constitutional right to protection from harm for children in institutions for mental retardation.

6. We will not discuss more participatory forms of democracy such as direct democracy. Nor will we discuss the
arguments that democracy, when limited to the political sphere, is insufficient. These arguments portray purely political forms of democracy as inconsistent with broader values of economic and social equality. Some proposed that the
democratic process be extended to social and economic relations. It is also argued that democracies, which are
thought to be purely political, do in fact govern economic and social relations without this fact being widely understood or admitted.

7. In the 1994 midterm election, 56 percent of people with disabilities were registered to vote, as compared with
71 percent of nondisabled individuals; only 33 percent of people with disabilities reported voting, as compared to 54
percent of nondisabled individuals (Shields et al. 1998).

8. Only some countries have legal guarantees that polling places will be accessible. The Canadian province of
Ontario, for example, does not require that election places be architecturally accessible, nor does it require that interpreters be present during election periods (Fraser Valentine, personal communication, April 7, 1999). The U.S. Americans with Disabilities Act requires that all activities of state and local governments, including the conduct of elections,
be accessible, but the program accessibility standard is, in practice, quite weak (Schriner, Batavia, and Shields forthcoming).

9. These include Joshua Malinga of Zimbabwe, who was mayor of Bulawayo (Barbara Duncan, personal communication, February 26, 1999); Joseph Sinyo of Kenya, a member of the national parliament (Barbara Duncan, personal communication, February 25, 1999); Kalle Konkkola, who has served on the city council of Helsinki, Finland (Barbara Duncan, personal communication, March 3, 1999); Midori Hirano, who was elected to 1998 to the Kumamoto prefecture in Japan (Barbara Duncan, personal communication, March 10, 1999); a Philippine congressman, Ernesto Herrera (Venus Ilagan, personal communication, March 1999); and several individuals with disabilities who have served or are serving in the national parliament of South Africa (Lucy Wong-Hernandez, personal communication, February 26, 1999).

10. Approximately 47,000 Ugandans with disabilities serve in the country's governing bodies. This total includes about 40,000 who have been elected at the village level (Jenny Kern, personal communication, March 1, 1999).

11. In 1985, COPOH renamed itself the Coalition of Citizens with Disabilities (CCD).

12. Data were also collected on foreign protests. However, only 57 protests in other countries were located; the countries most likely to be represented were the United Kingdom (23 protests), Canada (6), Germany and Italy (4 each), and France (3). Other countries had fewer than 3 protests.

13. Although the disability community did not use this situation as an occasion for disruptive collective action, many disability groups were involved in the court cases that confronted this issue (Pelka 1997:37-38).

14. The one exception was a protest about the Elizabeth Bouvia situation—but this was clearly aligned with the "right-to-life" movement rather than with any disability movement ("Picketers at Hospital" 1987).

15. There are other organizations in all of these categories, but they are not, or have not so far been, involved in contentious politics. One relatively new organization, which attempts to be multiple disability, multiple issue, is the American Association of People with Disabilities.

REFERENCES

Altman, Barbara and Sharon N. Barnartt. 1993. "Moral Entrepreneurship and the Passage of the ADA." *Journal of Disability Policy Studies* 4 (1): 21-40.

Anspach, Renee. 1979. "From Stigma to Identity Politics: Political Activism among the Physically Disabled and Former Mental Patients." *Social Science and Medicine* 13A:765-73.

Barnartt, Sharon. 1996. "Disability Culture or Disability Consciousness?" *Journal of Disability Policy Studies* 7 (2): 1-20.

Barnartt, Sharon and Richard Scotch. Forthcoming. *Social Movements in the Disability Community*. Washington, DC: Gallaudet University Press.

Barton, Len. 1992. "Disability and the Necessity for a Socio-Political Perspective." Pp. 1-14 in *Monograph 51: Disability and the Necessity for a Socio-Political Perspective*. Durham, NH: World Rehabilitation Fund.

Bickenbach, Jerome E. 1993. *Physical Disability and Social Policy*. Toronto: University of Toronto Press.

Bowe, Frank. 1992. "Commentary." Pp. 45-46 in *Monograph 51: Disability and the Necessity for a Socio-Political Perspective*. Durham, NH: World Rehabilitation Fund.

Campbell, Jane and Michael Oliver. 1996. *Disability Politics: Understanding Our Past, Changing Our Future*. London: Routledge Kegan Paul.

Carty, Lee A. 1978. "Advocacy." Pp. 144-64 in *Disability and Rehabilitation Handbook*, edited by Robert M. Goldenson. New York: McGraw-Hill.

Christiansen, John and Sharon Barnartt. 1995. *Deaf President Now: The 1988 Revolution at Gallaudet University*. Washington, DC: Gallaudet University Press.

Dahl, Robert A. 1989. *Democracy and Its Critics*. New Haven, CT: Yale University Press.

Doyle, Brian. 1999. "From Welfare to Rights? Disability and Legal Change in the United Kingdom in the Late 1990s." Pp. 209-26 in *Disability, Divers-ability, and Legal Change*, edited by Melinda Jones and Lee Ann Basser Marks. The Hague, the Netherlands: Kluwer Law International.

Driedger, Diane. 1989. *The Last Civil Rights Movement: Disabled People's International*. New York: St. Martin's.

Finkelstein, Victor. 1981. *Attitudes toward Disabled People*. New York: World Rehabilitation Fund.

Fox, Renee. 1977. "The Medicalization and Demedicalization of American Society." Pp. 9-22 in *Doing Better and Feeling Worse: Health in the United States*, edited by John H. Knowles. New York: Norton.

Gamson, William. 1990. *The Strategy of Social Protest*. 2d ed. Belmont, CA: Wadsworth.

Gerry, Martin and J. Martin Benton. 1980. "Section 504: Expanding Educational Opportunities." Unpublished paper.

Goffman, Erving. 1963. *Stigma*. Englewood Cliffs, NJ: Prentice Hall.

Goldberg, R. A. 1991. *Grassroots Resistance: Social Movements in Twentieth Century America*. Prospect Heights, IL: Waveland.

Gooding, Caroline. 1994. *Disabling Laws, Enabling Acts: Disability Rights in Britain and America*. London: Pluto.

Hahn, Harlan. 1985a. "Introduction: Disability Policy and the Problem of Discrimination." *American Behavioral Scientist* 28 (3): 293-318.

———. 1985b. "Towards a Politics of Disability Definitions, Disciplines, and Policies." *Social Science Journal* 22 (4): 87-105.

———. 1993. "The Potential Impact of Disability Studies on Political Science (as Well as Vice Versa)." *Policy Studies Journal* 21 (4): 740-51.

Hartman, T. S. and M. Johnson. 1993. *Making News: How to Get News Coverage for Disability Rights Issues*. Louisville, KY: Advocado.

Higgins, Paul C. 1992. *Making Disability: Exploring the Social Transformation of Human Variation*. Springfield, IL: Charles C Thomas.

Horowitz, Donald L. 1977. *The Courts and Social Policy*. Washington, DC: Brookings Institution.

"Invisible Voters." 1992. *New Statesman & Society* 5 (197): 19-20.

Johnson, R. A. 1983. "Mobilizing the Disabled." Pp. 82-97 in *Social Movements of the 60's and 70's*, edited by Jo Freeman. New York: Longman.

Jones, Melinda and Lee Ann Basser Marks. 1999a. "Law and the Social Construction of Disability." Pp. 3-24 in *Disability, Divers-ability, and Legal Change*, edited by Melinda Jones and Lee Ann Basser Marks. The Hague, the Netherlands: Kluwer Law International.

———. 1999b. "Disability, Rights and Law in Australia." Pp. 189-208 in *Disability, Divers-ability, and Legal Change*, edited by Melinda Jones and Lee Ann Basser Marks. The Hague, the Netherlands: Kluwer Law International.

Jorgenson, I. Skov. 1982. "Independent Living for Handicapped Persons in Denmark." Pp. 7-29 in *Independent Living: An Overview of Efforts in Five Countries: Denmark, Federal Republic of Germany, Yugoslavia, Costa Rica, and Japan*, edited by Denise Galluf Tate and Linda M. Chadderdon. East Lansing: University Center for International Rehabilitation, Michigan State University.

Kleinfield, Sonny. 1977. *The Hidden Minority: A Profile of Handicapped Americans*. Boston: Little, Brown.

Lembke, D. 1975. "Handicapped: A Pushy New Political Force." *Los Angeles Times*, July 16, pp. 1+.

Longmore, Paul. 1997. "Political Movements of People with Disabilities: The League of the Physically Handicapped, 1935-1938." *Disability Studies Quarterly* 17 (2): 94-98.

Meyer, D. S. 1993. "Protest Cycles and Political Process: American Peace Movements in the Nuclear Age." *Political Research Quarterly* 46:451-79.

Michailakis, Dimitris. 1999. "The Standard Rules: A Weak Instrument and a Strong Commitment." Pp. 117-30 in *Disability, Divers-ability, and Legal Change*, edited by Melinda Jones and Lee Ann Basser Marks. The Hague, the Netherlands: Kluwer Law International.

Miller, Kathleen S., Linda M. Chadderdon, and Barbara Duncan, eds. 1981. *Participation of People with Disabilities: An International Perspective: Selected Papers from the 1980 World Congress of Rehabilitation International*. East Lansing: University Center for International Rehabilitation, Michigan State University.

Mills v. Board of Education, 348 F. Supp. 866 (D.D.C. 1972).

Mutabazi, Pascal. 1997. "Deaf Politician Elected in Uganda." *Disability International* 9:10.

New York State Association for Retarded Children v. Carey, 393 F. Supp. 715 (E.D.N.Y. 1975).

Oliver, Michael. 1983. *Social Work with Disabled People*. London: Macmillan.

———. 1990. *The Politics of Disablement*. London: Macmillan.

Pelka, Fred. 1997. *The ABC-CLIO Companion to the Disability Rights Movement*. Santa Barbara, CA: ABC-CLIO.

Pennsylvania Association for Retarded Children v. Commonwealth of Pennsylvania, 324 F. Supp. 1257 (E. D. Pa. 1971).

Percy, S. L. 1989. *Disability, Civil Rights, and Public Policy: The Politics of Implementation*. Tuscaloosa: University of Alabama Press.

Pfeiffer, David. 1993. "Overview of the Disability Movement: History, Legislative Record, and Political Implications." *Policy Studies Journal* 21 (4): 724-34.

"Picketers at Hospital Protest Judge's Decision." 1987. *The Denver Post*, January 24, p. B3.

Piven, F. F. and R. Cloward. 1979. *Poor People's Movements: Why They Succeed, How They Fail.* New York: Random House.

"Protesters Serve Notice on Greyhound." 1997. *Ragged Edge* (September/October):6.

Raymond, Paul D. 1989. "Disability as Dissidence: The Action Group to Defend the Disabled in the USSR." Pp. 235-52 in *The Disabled in the Soviet Union: Past and Present, Theory and Practice,* edited by William O. McCagg and Lewis Siegelbaum. Pittsburgh, PA: University of Pittsburgh Press.

Rioux, Marcia H. and Catherine L. Frazee. 1999. "The Canadian Framework for Disability Equality Rights." Pp. 171-88 in *Disability, Divers-ability, and Legal Change,* edited by Melinda Jones and Lee Ann Basser Marks. The Hague, the Netherlands: Kluwer Law International.

Scheer, Jessica and Nora Groce. 1988. "Impairment as a Human Constant: Cross-Cultural and Historical Perspectives on Variation." *Journal of Social Issues* 44 (1): 23-38.

Schlesinger, Lynn and Diane E. Taub, eds. 1998. *Syllabi and Instructional Materials for Teaching Sociology of Disabilities.* Washington, DC: American Sociological Association.

Schriner, K., A. I. Batavia, and T. Shields. Forthcoming. "The Americans with Disabilities Act: Does it Secure the Fundamental Right to Vote?" *Policy Studies Journal.*

Schriner, K., L. Ochs, and T. Shields. 1997. "The Last Suffrage Movement: Voting Rights for People with Cognitive and Emotional Disabilities." *Publius* 27 (3): 75-96.

Schultz, T. 1977. "Handicapped: A Minority Demanding Its Rights." *New York Times,* February 13, pp. 8+.

Schur, L. A. and D. L. Kruse. 2000. "What Determines Voter Turnout? Lessons from Citizens with Disabilities." *Social Science Quarterly* 81 (2): 571-87.

Scotch, Richard K. 1984. *From Good Will to Civil Rights: Transforming Federal Disability Policy.* Philadelphia: Temple University Press.

———. 1988. "Disability as the Basis for a Social Movement: Advocacy and the Politics of Definition." *Journal of Social Issues* 44 (1): 159-72.

———. 1989. "Politics and Policy in the History of the Disability Rights Movement." *The Milbank Quarterly* 67 (Suppl. 2, Pt. 2): 380-400.

Shapiro, J. 1993. *No Pity: People with Disabilities Forging a New Civil Rights Movement.* New York: Times Books.

Shields, T., K. F. Schriner, and K. Schriner. 1998. "The Disability Voice in American Politics: Political Participation of People with Disabilities in the 1994 Election." *Journal of Disability Policy Studies* 9 (2): 53-76.

Stanglin, Douglas. 1996. "Disability Protest." *U.S. News and World Report* 121 (9): 20.

Stone, Deborah A. 1984. *The Disabled State.* Philadelphia: Temple University Press.

Tarrow, S. 1994. *Power in Movement: Social Movements, Collective Action and Politics.* New York: Cambridge University Press.

———. 1996. "Social Movements in Contentious Politics: A Review Article." *American Political Science Review* 90 (4): 874-83.

Treanor, R. B. 1993. *We Overcame: The Story of Civil Rights for Disabled People.* Falls Church, VA: Regal Direct.

Vaughn, C. Edwin. 1998. *Social and Cultural Perspectives on Blindness: Barriers to Community Integration.* Springfield, IL: Charles C Thomas.

Wastberg, Inger Claesson. 1999. "The Office of the Disability Ombudsman in Sweden." Pp. 131-38 in *Disability, Divers-ability, and Legal Change,* edited by Melinda Jones and Lee Ann Basser Marks. The Hague, the Netherlands: Kluwer Law International.

Woodward, J. 1982. *How You Gonna Get to Heaven if You Can't Talk with Jesus: Depathologizing Deafness.* Silver Spring, MD: T. J. Publishers.

Wyatt v. Hardin, 325 F.Supp. (M.D. Ala. 1971).

Young, Jonathan. 1998. "The President's Committee on the Handicapped and the Origins of Cross-Disability Organizing." Paper presented at the annual meeting of the Society for Disability Studies, June, Oakland, CA.

Zola, Irving K. 1983. "The Evolution of the Boston Self Help Center." Pp. 143-53 in *A Way of Life for the Handicapped,* edited by G. Jones and N. Tutt. London: Residential Care Association.

Health Care Professionals and Their Attitudes toward and Decisions Affecting Disabled People

18

IAN BASNETT

MY STARTING POINT

My pager went off. It was a nurse from the ward. "Hi, Dr. Basnett. Patient from ITU for you to admit." "OK. What's the problem?" I asked. "Chest infection. Oh, and he's paralyzed, been in before." I walked confidently to the patient's bed, and said, "Hi, I'm Dr. Basnett. I have to take some details and examine you." "Yeah," he replied with disinterest in an east London accent. I used a piece of cotton wool to examine his nervous system and felt a sense of horror come over me. "You can't feel anything below here on your shoulder? You can't move your legs at all—how much can you move your arms? I see not much. How long have you been like this?" As I continued, I became more horrified. This man was in his late 20s and was quadriplegic. Sensation, with all its pleasure and pain, was completely absent. Below the shoulders may just as well not exist for this man. How could he do anything that was fun or valuable? Life, as I understood it then, couldn't exist. I didn't bother to ask him. I was stumbling and awkward with no understanding of disability. I didn't know, nor could I have imagined, how he got out of bed at all, let alone how he did it daily and drove to work.

That was in the early 1980s. I next met this man in a spinal unit in 1985, as I was pushed to the computer next to him in occupational therapy. A few months earlier, I had severed my cervical spinal cord playing rugby, and I was quadriplegic—slightly more impaired than was my former patient. He sized me up, as patients in spinal units do, coming to a quick assessment of my "level." He didn't recognize me, without my stethoscope, white coat, and veneer of assurance. I couldn't bring myself to remind him. He told me he was in for a short stay with a skin problem but was looking forward to getting home. He was moving soon, and he had just started driving again.

AUTHOR'S NOTE: Some of the thinking and experiences that helped develop this chapter are thanks to a Commonwealth Fund Harkness Fellowship to the United States, spent at University of California, San Francisco (UCSF). I am grateful to the editors, together with Professor Ed Yelin, UCSF and Jane Campbell, who read earlier drafts of this chapter and provided helpful comments. I am also grateful for Professor Donald Patrick's thoughts on quality-of-life measurement.

This chapter is, in part, a personal account of my journey from medical student and physician to disabled physician and member of the disability movement. However, I will use this as a vehicle to reflect on my own medical training, practice, and attitudes in relation to disability. Later, I will contrast this with my experiences as a disabled person. I will draw on some of the evidence of the impact of training on health care professionals and their attitudes toward disability and discuss why this matters and how it can change how disabled people are viewed. I argue that the predominant influences on health professionals are the norms of society, often reinforced by training and practice and biased predominantly by seeing disabled people when they are sick. As in my case, health professionals can develop a view of disability that is at substantial variance from its reality for many disabled people. This can affect vital decisions involving health professionals that affect disabled people. These range from decisions at an individual clinical level, a policy level (including rationing), and at a health system level. I describe my own experiences as a medically qualified disabled person and contrast this with my earlier attitudes and beliefs. I conclude by making some proposals for improving medical training and health care for disabled people. Although I discuss health care in general terms, I will concentrate on medical health professionals. The chapter reveals my own conflicts resulting from a background that is medical and sometimes curative.

TRAINING HEALTH PROFESSIONALS

My medical training was traditional and typical—biomedical and hospital dominated. The disabled people I came into contact with were usually ill or institutionalized. I was taught about body systems and their failures but rarely about the interaction between our bodies, the environment, and society. A few social science and public health classes aside, treatment of the individual was essentially dominant. I had one memorable afternoon with an occupational therapist. We ran around with empty wheelchairs, "learning about obstacles." Many of us used it as an opportunity to play "bumper chairs."

In my clinical training, I remember one patient very well, a young disabled man who was regularly admitted to the acute ward for respite care. I understood nothing of the environment from which he came, rarely saw him dressed, and learned only how his nervous system was failing him. The attitude of the ward staff and physicians was universally benign, regarding him with great fondness, but rather like one might be fond of a respected and much-loved pet. The consultant, who had known him longest, was perhaps a little more enlightened. I presented his case to the consultant, explaining the onset of his disease and concluded by saying, "He gradually went downhill from there." The consultant forced me to ask a little about this young man's aspirations and discovered that he was able and had a great deal more insight than me (which wasn't difficult). However, the consultant's view of this young man was that he was an intelligent man whose life was a tragedy as a result of his disease and subsequent disability, and he deserved the best care. I remember the difficulty I had persuading the young man's primary care physician to assist with his anticoagulation. The physician viewed it as "overactive" intervention given his disability. For me, this was part of the tide of disempowered disabled people in hospital or residential settings that we witnessed as students.

Some studies, although now rather dated, have shown medical students to be more uncomfortable, more uncertain, and spending less time with disabled people than they spend with patients who don't have disabilities (Kleck et al. 1968, 1969, quoted in Hordon 1994). Some research from Australia and Leeds has shown increasingly positive attitudes to disability during medical training, although lacking long-term follow-up (Hordon 1993; Mitchell et al. 1984). However, a cross-sectional study found that the attitudes of senior students and junior doctors were no better than those of junior medical students (Duckworth 1988). Other research has found increases in cynicism (Rezler 1974; Wolf et al. 1989), loss of humanity (Diseker and Michielutte 1981), and loss of empathy (Perricone 1974). In a review, French (1994) concludes that the attitudes of health professionals are similar to the attitudes of the general public and may become more negative as professional education proceeds. Some studies (but not all) and commentators have concluded that the nature of the contact between health professionals and disabled people is what matters. They suggest that contact as caregivers leads to more negative attitudes toward disabled people, in contrast to contact with disabled people as equals (Donaldson 1980; Eberhardt and Mayberry 1994; French 1994), and point out the power imbalance in this relationship (Eberhardt and Mayberry 1994; Roush 1986). It is likely that attitudes formed in these sorts of situations highlight functional limitations and the differences of disabled people, rather than contact, which emphasizes the strengths and similarities of disabled people. It is noticeable how little research there is in relation to training physicians; this may be partly explained by some professional groups specializing more in disability (e.g., occupational therapists). However, I suspect it also reflects the low priority accorded to disability and that it is usually considered in terms of medically defined impairments.

My experience and the evidence suggest that for many physicians, the medical, individual, and tragic view of disability (Oliver 1990) is reinforced at the end of their training. It could be argued that, given that this dominates most Western societies, it would be unreasonable to expect the medical profession to be any different. Frequent contact with disabled people has not changed that. And why should it? Contact is often when people are sick, and physicians have been subjected to an intensely individualistic and biomedical model. There are others who would be less generous, particularly as medical training has increasingly become enlightened, taken a more holistic approach, and included more social science and disability studies. They might also say that given their role, health professionals have no right to be simply a mirror of society and should be more enlightened. We will see whether the dominance of the individualistic, medical model in the health professions proves to be a cohort effect that changes as society and medical training changes and there is a new generation of doctors.

The evidence suggests that it will be more complicated than that. Others have argued that the dominance of the individualistic interpretation of disability is partly a result of those with an interest in doing things to and writing about disabled people (with the medical profession center stage), promulgating that view (Oliver 1990:62). After all, in answer to the question "Who benefits?" an individualistic model clearly suits the health profession, particularly the medical profession. It emphasizes the importance of their skill and assists in their professional dominance. The need to provide interventions that cure the individual or provide psychological and physical adjustment to disability is reinforced. Thus, it could be argued that health professionals are not just passive mirrors of society, taking an individualistic interpretation and accentuating it, but are also active promoters of a paradigm that strengthens their own role. That will make understanding disability in terms of social control and oppression much more difficult for individuals trained in that environment. Although medical training is becoming more community based and holistic, few courses are taking disability awareness seriously. To most physicians, the possibility that they are acting as agents of social control and oppression, however passively, is abhorrent and likely to produce an abreaction!

WHY DOES THIS MATTER?

For disabled people, the training, attitudes, and behavior of health professionals toward them are all vital because of the important role health professions play in many disabled people's lives (often with physicians dominant). These roles include providing health or social care, acting as a gatekeeper to treatment, influencing health policy and society, and training future professionals (see examples below, and see Altman 1981 and French 1994 for a description of the relationship between attitudes and behavior). Negative attitudes can lead to avoidance, anxiety, overprotectiveness, pity, segregation, and alienation (Goddard and Jordan 1998). Discrimination toward disabled people has been documented in some of the professional literature (Biley 1994; Scullion 1999), although more formally recognized in nursing. This perhaps demonstrates a greater awareness and openness to the concept, rather than an absence of discrimination by the medical and other professions. Discrimination, negative attitudes, segregation, stigmatization, and poor service provision have been documented in many users' accounts and reports (see Beardshaw 1988; Biley 1994; "Cabbage Syndrome" 1990; French 1994; Hadley and Gough 1997; Lindow and Morris 1995; National Health Service [NHS] Executive 1997; Sutherland 1981). Persistently emphasizing the dependency of disabled people in attitudes and interactions may encourage disabled people to accept dependency and adopt that role, making it more difficult to achieve independence (Altman 1981; French 1994). Discriminatory attitudes, or a simple lack of awareness of the lives disabled people lead and their quality, mean that the behavior of some professionals and the decisions they make may be questionable. Extreme examples of this are decisions made regarding the beginning and end of life.

To return to my personal journey, I was a junior physician with, as far as I knew, no significant impairment. My transformation into someone with a very significant impairment was sudden but also had a number of ironies beyond "my patient," whom I introduced at the beginning of this chapter.

Nearly two years before my accident, a friend had a sporting accident that resulted in quadriplegia. I remember visiting him in the spinal unit, where I was later to become a patient. At the time, I was shocked to see someone in such a state. He was unable to move independently, and I had last seen him standing in a pub. I met him a few times later as his physical condition improved, and I remained utterly convinced this was a tragedy of the most profound kind. For some time, I found it difficult to move beyond that and to consider my friend as the same person, let alone understand anything more complex.

I describe this coincidence not to dwell on the irony itself, which is relatively common to people who acquire impairments during adult life as a product of chance and recall bias. I want to use it to illustrate my personal starting point, emotionally as well as conceptually. My reaction was the common one, so common others might describe it as "natural." Although I was a physician, I was not informed by the perspective of disabled people. This persisted whether I was dealing with an anonymous patient as I described above or someone I knew much more personally, prior to impairment.

I have discussed how many physicians are not trained to understand the perspective of disabled people and make any good judgments about quality of life. This is compounded by the biased view most physicians have of disabled people because most contact is limited to when we are sick or suffering from the most severe health problems. I showed earlier how I was horrified by what I imagined to be the experience of disabled people, which I encountered in my practice. Now, 15 years after becoming disabled, I find myself completely at home with the concept, of effectively being me! At the time of the injury that caused my impairment, I remembered my girlfriend reminding me how important physical activity and sport were in my life and that "I'd rather be dead if I could not play sport." She couldn't understand why I was "taking it so well." Of course, at the time of an acute injury, one has no choice, and you develop coping mechanisms. Now I know that my assessment of the potential quality of life of severely disabled people was clearly flawed.

Was I alone in being so profoundly and inappropriately pessimistic about life as a disabled person? The evidence would suggest not. In the United Kingdom, variance between disabled people and physicians was confirmed in a study of people with multiple sclerosis (Rothwell et al. 1997). The study revealed that physicians specializing in neurology were significantly more likely to believe that physical impairment was an important determinant of quality of life than were disabled people. Disabled people placed more weight on vitality, wellness, and mental health. Physicians also underestimated the quality of life of disabled people (suggested in an earlier study by Gardner et al. 1985). Similarly, in an earlier study in the United States, given a hypothetical situation, providers of emergency care imagined a strikingly more negative quality of life and outcome with quadriplegia than those actually reported by quadriplegics (Gerhart et al. 1994). For example, 92 percent of people with quadriplegia reported being glad to be alive, whereas only 18 percent of emergency care providers imagined they would be glad to be alive if they were quadriplegic. Eighty-six percent of people with quadriplegia reported their quality of life was average or above average, but only 17 percent of the providers imagined their quality of life would be average or above average. Similarly, the providers underestimated the actual self-esteem of people with quadriplegia and the extent to which they socialize and have sexual relations. When asked what interventions they would want if they were quadriplegic, 22 percent of providers would want nothing done to ensure their survival, and 23 percent would only want pain relief. The authors describe the sentiment they unearthed as a "better-off-dead" mentality. Importantly, those who imagined a poorer quality of life as a quadriplegic were significantly less likely to intervene actively. In a study of neonatal outcomes, a sample of adolescents and parents rated the health-related quality of life of disabled children higher than physicians and nurses working in neonatal tertiary centers (Saigal et al. 1999). The study used hypothetical cases, and some of the adolescents had been extremely low birth weight infants.

Discrimination and the relative ignorance of the quality of life raise fundamental questions when physicians are involved in decisions about access to health care. These could include appropriate aids or adaptations, whether to keep a disabled infant alive, "do not resuscitate" measures on disabled children, whether to operate on a child with Down syndrome, health policy and allocating resources, and the debate over assisted suicide.

Decisions about health services affecting disabled people are made at a number of levels. At the highest level, the values, structure, and functions of the health care system may enable or disable disabled people. This may be a function of the fundamental values being applied in the system. For example, in social care in the United Kingdom, a belief that empowering individuals is important has led to the institution of user-led direct payments for independent living—a substantial step forward for disabled people. In contrast, a dominance of a medical model and clinical effectiveness, defined only in medical terms, may have an adverse impact on disabled people. Other aspects of health care systems, such as capitation in a highly marketized system, can adversely affect disabled people (see DeJong and Basnett, this volume). Also, at a policy and health program level, decisions about resource allocation can adversely affect disabled people.

DECISIONS MADE AT A "PATIENT LEVEL"

As I have discussed, the attitudes, actions, and decisions of the clinicians working within a health care system have an important impact on disabled people. My professional outlook, my personal interactions with other disabled people, and medical decisions were recently brought into conflict in a "beginning-of-life" decision, in which a friend was involved. My friend, who is 41 years old and has a severe impairment, was asked to support the parents of a baby with similar impairment. In a complex legal case, a fight ensued with a hospital whose blanket policy was that it is inappropriate to ventilate severely impaired children. In the court case, a clinical expert stated that the baby's disability was "too terrible to lead a quality life," and she would need "total bodily care for the rest of her life." My friend leads a very full life, has been married, and is one of the leading advocates within the disability movement, frequently working with government ministers on legislation. She has had health problems; especially when as a baby, she needed ventilation on several occasions. Clearly, there was no guarantee this baby's life would replicate that of my friend. However, this seemed to be a case of perspective. Clinicians see more disabled people when they are ill. There is a selection bias toward those needing most medical support and a lack of insight into the quality of lives of disabled people. The evidence given reflects a view that requiring personal support is a failure rather than an appropriate accommodation to facilitate independent living (Asch 1998). The hospital has since changed its policy and treats each case on its merits and in discussion with the parents. Similar cases have gone to the courts in the United States, including the Baby Doe case. In 1982, an infant with a tracheoesophageal fistula and esophageal atresia (a surgically remediable link between the esophagus and trachea and blockage of the esophagus) was allowed to die (Fost 1999; Pless 1983).

Decisions at the beginning of life about the degree of medical intervention appropriate for a neonate often have to be made quickly and still are frequently dominated by neonatologists

(Raeside 1997), although they are becoming increasingly collaborative (Fost 1999)—sometimes with the support of ethics committees. With the increasing survival of sickly and low-weight babies, these decisions are becoming more commonplace. However, what is not clear is the ethical framework and assumptions about the quality of life of disabled people that inform those decisions. While neonatologists have the expertise to make accurate neurological and physiological assessments, their views regarding the future quality of life and prognosis of infants may be biased by their own prejudice and experience and may differ considerably from parents and adolescents (Saigal et al. 1999). Of course, the vast majority of these decisions are made without great controversy, often with the advice of a neonatologist being accepted by other staff and parents (Raeside 1997), and increasingly neonatologists are receiving training in ethical issues. However, if the neonatologist's view on life with a disability and the likely prognosis are biased by training and caseload (concentrating largely on sicker children and seeing them when they are sick), the validity of that judgment requires testing. The viewpoint described by Shearer (1992) that "a child with a disability is a tragedy not only to the child, but for [his or her] family" (p. 277) may indeed be prevalent. These issues are necessarily complicated by the fact that decisions made at the beginning of life cannot involve the neonate and therefore the potential disabled child and adult. When there is conflict, these cases are increasingly coming to the courts. In the United States, the regulations resulting from the Baby Doe case indicate that the prospect of "future disability" should play no role in treatment decisions. However, there is still room for considerable discretion in deciding when treatment is futile or inhumane, and in practice the debate has shifted away from conditions such as Down syndrome onto much sicker, much more severely impaired infants.

Similarly, decisions made when adult disabled people are ill or near to the end of life place valuation of the quality of disabled people's lives in sharp relief. These may range from decisions about which interventions are made or maintained in an illness or increasing or maintaining interventions to maintain life, which is most commonly discussed with respect to ventilation. As with the majority of other clinical decisions, most are made by a clinician or clinicians, sometimes in reference to a wider team, varying in the extent to which the disabled person is involved.

The treatment that a disabled colleague endured in a U.K. hospital provides a striking example of how the medical profession is still getting these things wrong (this case was featured in a TV program, *From the Edge* [Bowler 1999]). My colleague, who is reasonably healthy and a wheelchair user, was admitted to hospital, unwell with a chest infection. With no more than a few words with her, no consultation with her partner, and no prior knowledge of her life, a junior doctor recorded in her notes that "in view of her poor quality of life and the underlying medical condition [spinal muscular atrophy, not the most severe type] she should not be considered for resuscitation." Fortunately, my colleague, who is a lawyer and was vice chair of the local community trust (NHS provider of community health care), recovered, and she continues to lead a very full life. What appears to have happened here is what Asch (1998) describes as the substitution of an ill-informed social judgment about disability for a medical one. Whatever the medical arguments about performing cardiopulmonary resuscitation in this case, the premise on which it was taken, a poor quality of life because of disability was wrong.

The current debate on assisted suicide and disabled people in the United States is, in some ways, related to this, although theoretically driven by individuals' choices. The proponents of assisted suicide believe that for many people, particularly those with terminal illness, offering the option of death is moral and humane. For some disabled people, the debate has largely been framed in terms that give cause for great concern (Asch 1998). For example, in the case of Elizabeth Bouvia, a young woman with cerebral palsy, the judge described her existence as "pitiable." She had suffered a series of bereavements, including dismissal from college by a dean who thought she could not be a social worker because of her disability—together with the loss of educational opportunities and attendant care services. However, submissions supporting her assisted suicide focused on her physical circumstances and largely ignored whether other interventions, such as improved analgesia, attendant support, and reinstatement in a college, might improve her life. Similarly, David Rivlin, a man with quadriplegia, decided to end his life when he learned that a lack of funding for attendants meant that he would be unable to leave the nursing home. Recently and most notorious is the Thomas Youk case. Youk was a man with amyotrophic lateral sclerosis, killed by Dr. Jack Kevorkian, a crime for which Kevorkian was convicted of murder.

The underlying assumption for many of the proponents of assisted suicide for disabled people is that life as a disabled person is of a very poor quality, and therefore it is rational and logical for some disabled people to wish to terminate their lives. This has been challenged on a number of fronts. Gill (1992) points out that for nondisabled people, the desire to commit suicide is often considered irrational and a sign of mental illness. She contrasts this with several cases of assisted suicide in disabled people, in which the interventions offered are limited and the debate is framed in a totally different way.

In contrast, others have maintained that allowing disabled people the right to take their lives is a natural extension of their fight for rights. This idea has support among disabled people (Batavia 1997). For me, this ignores the social and financial context in which disabled people often find themselves and thus the extent to which this is a rational decision or one borne of desperation in a discriminatory society. In other words, health services assisting with killing the disabled person are the wrong intervention. In terms of formulating a policy, whether assisted suicide should be legal for disabled people should rest on the balance of benefit and harm. Notwithstanding the possibility of careful regulation, while one can envisage situations in which there might be benefit, in my view the potential harm to individuals and social attitudes outweighs that.

In the case of my colleague whose quality of life was described as poor, the judgment was simply wrong. In some cases of assisted suicide, disabled people are experiencing a very poor quality of life, but that is because of the absence of personal care and other support.

ALLOCATION DECISIONS MADE AT A "POPULATION LEVEL"

Decisions made at a population or health care intervention are becoming increasingly important as health care systems grapple with the problem of perceived infinite demand and limited resources, and physicians are frequently involved in the process. Clearly, by its nature, much of this debate is not taking place at an individual level and does not directly relate to my personal "journey." However, because of its importance and my relationship with a changing attitude toward disability, I will spend some time reflecting on it.

Tools are being developed, including the quality-adjusted life year (QALY) and the disability-adjusted life year (DALY), to compare the impact of diseases with the utility of different health care interventions. The QALY is a composite figure, combining the extra years of life and the extra quality of life obtained from health care interventions. Interventions can then be ranked in terms of cost per QALY. The DALY is also an amalgam of mortality and disability in assessing the overall "burden" of disease. Perfect health has a weight of 0, death has a weight of 1, and impairments have varying weights allocated. For example, angina has a weight of 0.223; quadriplegia, 0.895. The utility assessments of health states in QALYs are usually determined using standard gamble or time trade-off techniques among largely healthy people (described in Nord et al. 1999). For DALYs, the weights were determined with professional health care providers using the person trade-off method (Üstün et al. 1999).

A number of criticisms have been made of QALYs, DALYs, and similar tools, not least their impact on disabled people. For example, Silvers (1995) points out that QALYs systematically value one year of a disabled person's life less than somebody without a disability, conflicting with the beliefs underlying civil rights and civil rights legislation. Harris (1987, 1995) objects on grounds of "double jeopardy." It is unfair that an individual who is already unfortunate is then less likely to receive treatment that may be life saving or may relieve his or her misfortune. Furthermore, even if accurate judgments about quality or length of life are made, does that equate with value? Singer et al. (1995) reject this argument on an number of fronts. QALY maximization is about the maximization of QALY gain and not, per se, based on an individual's starting point; the absence of a rational base to make decisions if one rejects utilitarian comparisons; and the view that in ranking things such as suffering, an approach should be taken, influenced by the absence of future suffering rather than the present or past suffering. He also argues that decisions about resource allocation should be taken from behind a "Rawlsian veil of ignorance." In other words, they should not be influenced by potential personal gain.

DALYs have been severely criticized too. Sayers and Fliedner (1997) argue that this single measure obscures more than it tells us. For example, it cannot account for economic, family, and social differences between communities, which equity requires us to consider. DALYs clearly suffer from being weights assigned by health professionals with all the shortfalls I described above. In a small study, Üstün et al. (1999) found some similarity in the way health professionals and disabled people from a range of countries ranked the disabling effect of a variety of health conditions. However, there were also systematic differences large enough to shed doubt on the universality of the rankings. Furthermore, ranking alone tells us nothing about absolute assessment effects, which may vary widely.

For my part, I can see at least three objections to QALYs, DALYs, and similar measures as they apply to disabled people. First, I address the principle that extra years of life or the quality of life of disabled people are worth less than the able-bodied. Like most current methods for assigning values to health states for preference weighting, including the Oregon experiment or other cost-effective measures, QALYs systematically equate reduced levels of functioning with a lower quality of life. This is wrong. There is no evidence of a broad consensus supporting a purely utilitarian approach. Indeed, even Singer et al. (1995) point out that evidence from Australia suggests that many believe other elements of justice, above and beyond the purely utilitarian, should be brought into play when deciding about the allocation of resources. Nord et al. (1999) quote more evidence of public preferences, suggesting that ability to benefit should be balanced by concerns about equity and severity of impairment. Given that we are operating in a society where there is already considerable discrimination and lack of understanding of the quality of life of disabled people, it is difficult to believe that a just solution will be produced. Second, as Harris (1995) points out, is there any reason why or consensus for equating a lower quality of life with a lower value? A third objection is that even if one accepted that some sort of utilitarian system of redistribution should contribute to decisions developed based on the ability to benefit, the basis for the formal tools and the views of many involved in making these decisions are substantially flawed with respect to disability. While the view that potential personal benefit should not influence decisions has some merit, these decisions also need to be informed by a proper understanding of the life disabled people lead and the potential for a high-quality life, given appropriate support.

The Oregon Health Plan, which was proposed in 1992, brought many of these arguments to the fore. The plan was regarded by many as a rational and inventive way of rationing health care. However, it was opposed by disabled people in the United States on the basis that it violated their civil rights. They sought support from the Americans with Disabilities Act (ADA) for this because it denied people with existing or potential disabilities equal health care (on the basis that they were less likely to benefit). Although debated (Hadorn 1992; Orentlicher 1994), initially these objections were accepted at the federal level. However, the Oregon plan was later approved after many of the structural features were removed (Silvers 1995).

The Oregon Health Plan is not unique internationally; health care systems in other countries, such as New Zealand and Australia, have developed mechanisms to make similar utilitarian judgments (Feek et al. 1999). For example, the New Zealand guidelines for chronic renal dialysis normally exclude anyone older than age 75 or with a serious disease or disability that is likely to affect their quality of life. Perhaps most important, health care systems throughout the world make judgments based on similar considerations but do so without making those judgments and choices explicit. With a few exceptions, this is the case in the NHS in the United Kingdom. From time to time, individual cases are highlighted or tested in the court where doctors are making decisions based on assumptions about the current or future quality of life of disabled people involved. The apparent restriction of heart surgery and transplants for children with Down syndrome is a case in point (Down Syndrome Association 1999; Phillips 1999; Rogers 1999).

An important tool for making judgments about health care interventions, at a program and an individual level, is clinical effectiveness or evidence-based medicine.[1] This has assumed much greater importance over the past 10 years and affects clinical care, health policy, and research priorities. In principle, the concept is sound; numerous studies have documented the prevalence of treatment—at best ineffective, at worst harmful (Chalmers 1991; Sackett and Rosenberg 1995). Physicians had often provided treatments, believing they were effective, not realizing the influence of bias and random variation in their observations. This led to the expression, "Lies, dam lies and clinical impressions." After all, why should health care systems pay for, or people be subjected to, ineffective treatments? This approach has gained great acceptance with an international collaboration established to produce systematic reviews of the evidence (Chalmers 1993). It has also become an increasingly important element of health policy, particularly in the United Kingdom (Department of Health [DOH] 1998; Sheldon and Chalmers 1994), with purchasers becoming increasingly fastidious in the approval of any intervention in which the evidence of clinical effectiveness is lacking.

As I say, in principle, I have no problem with this approach. If there is a choice, I would rather have treatments that have been shown to "work well." However, there are difficulties. In this context, I am most concerned about the evidence on which judgments are based and who is making the judgments. The evidence is largely based on clinical trials in which the outcomes measured are often decided by physicians or other health care professionals, although some quality-of-life measures are being included. With breast cancer, for example, there is often evidence of the effect of treatment on relapse-free survival and survival. Less often is there evidence on quality of life, and rarely is there evidence of things that women have said are important, such as self-esteem, appearance, and sex life. Some of the supporters of clinical effectiveness recognize this deficit whereby the perspective of the user is not included in the sort of research question addressed or the outcome measures used (Chalmers 1998). To quote Chalmers, who discussed perinatal research, "Whose priorities are being addressed in the perinatal research agenda?" Not that of women, he argues, and he calls for more trials with women as collaborators, not as subjects (Chalmers 1991). Thus, particularly for disabled people, where the intervention is often not related to an acute life-threatening event but is longer term, the outcomes need to be subtler and include what users want from treatments. Hickey et al. (1996) developed this principle in the trial of treatment for HIV/AIDS. Until that happens, much of the evidence is incomplete and is dominated by physicians' perspectives.

MY TRANSFORMATION, OR CROSSING THE DIVIDE

The accident that resulted in my disability led me to an intensive care unit, then to two spinal units where I experienced the spectrum of health care in all respects. Initially, I needed high-tech, intensive medical intervention, followed by care in a friendly but ramshackle old fever hospital and then a newer spinal unit that had benefited considerably from charitable donations. My interactions with staff also ranged from the enabling to profoundly disabling.

Of course, my personal experiences may be informative but not necessarily generalizable. First, it is possible that my worst experiences were bad luck, although I observed those around me and some of the most oppressive elements were the result of a universal policy. Second, my recall is undoubtedly affected by the fact that I was going through my own "personal tragedy." Third, as a physician, I was bound to be different, whether I wanted it or not. I talked the language and knew more about the implications of what was going on, and some of the staff, particularly physicians, felt more empathy with me than they might otherwise have done. Finally, other health care providers may have been doing much better, and indeed things may have improved over time.

Notwithstanding all this, my first exposure "on the receiving end" was an education. Initially, I spent six months in hospital, and the staff became used to me as another patient and stopped telling the new nurses that I was a physician. Petty, depersonalizing policies were often the most wearing. I remember rebelling against wearing my wristband with its name and number. After a few months, I knew everyone, and they knew me! However, although one could get away with removing the wristband, nurses could not issue medication without one reciting one's hospital number! Some of the nurses were as frustrated as I was, but with hindsight, the policy is even more extraordinary than it seemed at the time.

Not surprisingly, given my background and the general mores of society, my view of disability was medical at the time, centered on my own recovery, or the lack of it. Like many physicians, I knew very little of what is experienced as a patient—the day-to-day interactions with porters, nurses, and physiotherapists. The interactions I did know about—those with physicians—were much rarer and were usually ritualized as part of ward rounds. This felt very different from the receiving end! Staff varied, of course. As my "patient career" progressed, I came into contact with more physicians whom I had known before my disability. Their reactions varied. Some were embarrassed; many did absolutely everything they could to help me through the system. Many of those I had known before my impairment shared and substantially reinforced my then view of what had happened as a personal tragedy. With others treating me, I observed paternalism and disempowerment of disabled people. My first serious experiences as a recipient of health care began to refashion my thinking about the health care professions and their approach. Despite now being relatively senior within my profession, I continue to experience health professionals who are much more comfortable if they are in control of me and my health care.

My experiences of physicians as people exercising substantial control over my options were entirely new and disturbing, often provoking in me personal anger. It made me understand the power physicians possess when patients seek our help and in other situations (see the previous discussion on end-of-life decisions).

INDEPENDENT LIVING

While I was in the spinal unit, I met the social worker whose job was to facilitate my discharge. I was in my mid-20s and had lived away from parents for some years. It was obvious to me that I should continue to do the same. Unfortunately, it was more complicated than that. There were no immediate options for achieving the independence I sought. We looked at the costs of private staff for the hours of care I needed. The costs came to more than I could afford. The social worker proposed that I live with my parents who would "care" for me. When I rejected that, she presented me with a series of glossy brochures for residential homes, all set in the countryside and pictured bathed in sunshine—not for me. So, I returned home to my parents, who were supportive and loving as ever, although living with them was a different matter. My drive for living independently did not come from any exposure to disability groups or from the independent living movement. It came from having lived like that before and naively assuming that it should be straightforward to do it again. My shock, and then depression, at discovering the real world was an important step in my understanding disability. Until then, most of my other problems had been medical or eating and drinking when there was no staff to help. I had seen those problems as inevitable, given the combination of my impairment and the staffing of NHS hospitals. However, this was fundamental. I could not live where and with whom I chose and make decisions about when to get up and go to bed.

After my "release" from the cosseted world of the spinal unit, I slowly began to rediscover the world. As others have remarked about Vietnam veterans returning from the war, my expectations had been framed by my previous life without a disability. I was fortunate that I had qualified and worked prior to my disability. Together with farsighted and accommodating mentors, this eased my reentry into the workforce.

With the promise of work came the necessity to develop some sort of "independent living package." Indeed, I did my utmost to link the two, because despite loving my parents, I did not want to live with them permanently. So, having secured a promise of employment away from home, I began to negotiate through a social worker to set up some kind of independent living package. After some false starts and a few leaps in the dark, I began to live independently and started to work. At the time, I was incredibly grateful for the social care package that was developed and run by a care manager. Although I met the staff before they started and theoretically had a power of veto, in practice, I had limited control over shift lengths, their roles, and who was employed. As a result, at times I was institutionalized in the community, organizing my life around the shifts of personal assistants (PAs).

After some years of struggling with an expensive package, which was largely controlled by social services, with encouragement and support from other disabled people, I transferred to a user-controlled scheme. Higher levels of satisfaction and quality and increased cost-effectiveness in user-controlled schemes have been found in a number of studies (Beatty et al. 1998; Doty, Kasper, and Litvak 1996; Oliver and Zarb 1993; Zarb and Nadesh 1994). For me, this was a revolutionary change. This scheme allowed me to employ and manage PAs myself. Initially, I had substantial concerns about managing the budget and hiring and managing staff. The flexibility and increased freedom changed my life. Once again, I had some choice over when I went to bed and when I went out in my van, and I had support during the day. I went from relying on nearly 30 percent agency staff to rarely requiring agency staff. Independent living gave me confidence, enabled me to participate more fully in society, and gave me a chance to influence local health and social care provision.

My achievement of independent living reflects my catching up late on a movement that had begun some years before, partly through centers for independent or integrated living (CILs) and led by disabled people (see Davis 1993; Hasler 1993; Oliver 1990). The disability movement had a profound effect on society and access. It is a way of living, but it also proved to be the genesis and hub around which disabled people have organized and expressed themselves as part of the disability rights movement. In the more rights-based culture of the United States, this was partly reflected in the adoption of antidiscrimination legislation much earlier than in many other developed countries.

Independent living has been linked to "other contemporary movements, such as civil rights, consumerism, self-help, de-medicalization, and de-institutionalization" (DeJong 1983:5, quoted in Oliver 1990; Rodwin 1994). To what extent has this movement influenced the mainstream provision of health care and social support? As an individual, I became more involved, less excluded, more confident, and unwilling to accept the status quo. I had the practical support enabling me to participate. This reflects the disability movement more broadly, in which disabled people were less likely to be institutionalized, more confident, and better able to organize, and power is transferred from professionals. Thus, independent living became and remains a major potential change agent for health and social services for disabled people—partly through its direct effect on community care services, enabling disabled people to have more control over their lives (e.g., via direct payments), and partly as the movement itself emancipated disabled people, leading them to challenge health policy. This also forced health professionals to consider disabled people differently. At a minimum, some accepted disabled people were no longer dependent and simply in need of help. Others were even willing to accept disabled people as "experts" who could assess their own needs, help assessing the needs of others, and had control over decisions about their health care. Once disabled people were freed from residential care and with adequate personal assistance support, they had the means to organize and assert themselves as a group and to challenge discrimination.

However, although the disability movement and independent living movement have begun to exert its influence, there is still some way to go. Discussing disability policy in the United Kingdom, Priestly (1999) characterizes two approaches: The disability movement views disability as a form of discrimination or social oppression, whereas the bulk of disability policy emphasizes individualism, dependency, and otherness. Much health and community care policy and practice continue to reflect the individualistic, tragedy approach. Why? Well, I suspect for a number of reasons. First, attitudes of society as a whole are slow to change, and some health professionals reflect that, reinforced by medical approaches to their training. Second, there continues to be small numbers of disabled people in the health professions; disabled people continue to be disempowered. (ADAPT estimates 2 million disabled Americans are institutionalized against their will.) Third, because disabled people are disempowered by attitudes in society and financial, physical, employment, and other barriers, disability will feel like a "tragedy" for many disabled people at some stage. This may be especially true of older disabled people. Fourth, disabled people, or at least activists in the "disability movement," have not seen health care issues as a priority until recently. Finally, some disabled people have reinforced the medical, individualistic approach, for example, via some impairment-specific organizations.

SELF-IDENTIFICATION AS DISABLED

When I moved into the community, I began a journey that many disabled people would recognize. For a long time, I felt very uncomfortable in the presence of disabled people, particularly anyone with a learning disability or speech impairment. It was impossible not to "pathologize" disabled people, my medical training making guessing the impairment an irresistible mental game. I saw myself as essentially normal, although having a "problem" with my arms and legs.

Over time, a number of things happened. I began to mix more with disabled people as friends and colleagues. I became increasingly aware that the barriers I encountered in my life need not be there—they were the products of poor design, unwillingness to accommodate me, and so on, but they were what disabled me. I became unhappy with being described, either as an individual or in more general references to disabled people, as a tragedy or "the result of an awful accident," being "in the state you're in" or, alternatively, as extremely brave. I began to feel insulted. It no longer fit my self-image. Many disabled people will recognize this as a gradual growing in confidence as a disabled person and self-identification as disabled (Oliver and Barnes 1998:71-76).

This journey toward a clearer understanding of disability took some years. I also had the advantage of being someone who was living life as a disabled person. It may be that my prejudices and ignorance about disability were more profound than the average physician, but I doubt it. This underscores the difficulty that individual physicians face in understanding disabled people, given the values of the society we live in and the training most medical students undergo. However, the medical profession has profound responsibilities, not only as providers of health care but also as powerful decision makers in disabled people's lives (e.g., the provision or withdrawal of treatment from disabled neonates and infants, the provision of equipment or services, and end-of-life decisions, including euthanasia).

As I became more involved in the "disability community" of local and national organizations of disabled people, I became involved with challenging, lobbying, and helping to form legislation on direct payments.

Perhaps the most important piece of legislation affecting disability in the United States is the Americans with Disabilities Act. It has had its most profound effects on physical access, transport, and, to a lesser extent, employment. Health care and personal care featured less prominently in the initial framing of the act, and it has not profoundly altered the nature of U.S. health care. However, it has had an impact. It was successfully cited in challenging the initial Oregon Health Plan and in the Baby Doe case. More recently, it has had an impact on long-term care. In the United States, judges have confirmed that states have a responsibility to provide long-term care in the most integrated setting, although this continues to be challenged.

In the United Kingdom, unsatisfactory antidiscrimination legislation came into force in 1996 and is being implemented in stages. This places certain duties on the health service with respect to access and the employment of disabled people but is unlikely to otherwise profoundly affect the delivery of health care. Currently, the government and disability advocates are debating the extent to which the latest antidiscrimination legislation will affect health and social care. The civil service is resisting allowing antidiscrimination to affect health and social care, fearing the implications (personal communication from a disabled member of the task force, who was set up to establish antidiscrimination legislation in disability together with the supporting structures, May 1999, although ultimately the task force made recommendations that include health and social care, and the Disability Rights Commission has included this in its three-year strategy). Whether you view this as a justified wariness of subjecting health and social care to further possible legal intervention or inappropriately defending discriminatory practice depends on your viewpoint.

In both the United States and the United Kingdom, it appears that antidiscrimination legislation is not going to produce whole-scale changes in health services. However, in some specific areas, there may be substantial change, for example, with respect to states providing long-term care in the "most integrated setting" in the United States. In the United States, there is an acceptance that it will require physicians and others making decisions about health care provision and rationing to ensure that the disabled are not unfairly discriminated (Hadorn 1992; Orentlicher 1994). In the United Kingdom, the impact remains to be seen.

In summary, it is possible to discern two intertwined influences on health and social care. The independent living movement has enabled more disabled people to live independently, influencing social attitudes. The same movement has encouraged campaigning for antidiscrimination legislation.

CONCLUSION

I have used my own experience of transforming from a junior physician with no significant impairment to someone with a very significant one as a tool to illustrate the limitations of health professionals in their dealings with disabled people. That transformation is by no means unique. Wainapel (1999) thoughtfully describes his move between the two cultures and illustrates how physicians are often negative about disability, seeing inability before ability and frustrated by the lack of a prospect of cure and ill-informed about simple accommodations. However, it is not common to become disabled and then become part of the disability movement, embracing the concept of disability as a product of the interface between people and the environment. The corollary of that is that it displaces the primacy of my years of training in medicine.

Using the example of my own experience, I have demonstrated how little I understood of disability as a junior doctor and how inappropriately negative my attitudes were. By supplementing this with vignettes and the published evidence, I have demonstrated that this was not limited to me. Some of the influences on health care professionals, including society as a whole, medical training that concentrates on disease and individuals, and the bias toward seeing disabled people only when they are sick, do not equip physicians well enough to contribute to the health care of individual disabled people. Nor does it help them to make decisions at other levels affecting disabled people. During my relatively short clinical career, I was undoubtedly ambivalent toward disabled people, with very little insight into the potential for a good quality of life. My training and subsequent experience tended to reinforce this. Given that disability in its broadest terms forms a large part of the day-to-day work of many health care physicians, this is a disturbing conclusion. There is evidence that the results of this are often inappropriate attitudes and care for disabled people. Of course, this should be moderated by the fact that despite training and negative influences in society, many physicians manage to provide an excellent service and have enlightened attitudes. There are also other examples of health care programs that offer some hope (Master et al. 1996; Silburn 1993).

However, at the level of the individual physician providing care, to ensure that the sort of substantial changes are made that I believe are necessary, a number of things need to happen. Much more emphasis should be placed in training in the broader influences of health and disability outside the health care systems. More emphasis should be placed on understanding the impact of attitudes and the environment on people with impairments and how that can be disabling. Finally, focus should turn toward empowering disabled people as patients in the relationship with physicians. There is some progress being made in some of these areas. For example, patient power is becoming an increasingly potent force within health care. However, the balance of power still remains firmly with health care professionals at all the levels in which they are involved with decision making. In the United Kingdom, the British Medical Association (BMA) is proposing that more responsibility lie with individual physicians in "end-of-life" decisions (BMA 1999) to the concern of some disabled people (Davis 1999). Providing some balance to the individualistic, medically dominated approach to training will be a major undertaking, although in the United Kingdom, the placing of more medical student training in primary care may help this.

Another way of making health and social care services more accessible and appropriate for disabled people is employing more disabled health care professionals. That alone is not a panacea, and to consider it so can be more damaging. Disabled health care professionals can of course perform their jobs poorly and behave inappropriately toward patients. However, given appropriate support and training, which need to be ongoing, disabled health care professionals have much to offer, but there is evidence that this is not being taken up, nor are the opportunities for training as broadly available to disabled people as they should be (French 1993).

In an effort to allocate resources most effectively and efficiently, health systems around the world are grappling with different tools, and physicians are influential in the debate. Ensuring that health services provide effective care is laudable, and evidence-based medicine has much to commend it. However, as I have demonstrated, the evidence base itself is currently flawed, lacking assessment of many outcomes that matter to disabled people. Some countries have adopted policies that seem, frankly, discriminatory (e.g., in New Zealand). Others have tried hard to develop policies for rationing that include a range of perspectives (e.g., the Oregon experiment), although still proving discriminatory in the first instance. The problem seems to be that most current methods for assigning values to health states for cost-effectiveness work systematically and equate lower functioning with a lower quality of life. This is wrong conceptually and ignores the interaction between a disabling society and environment, as well as the person with impairments. In addition, persons with less room to improve on most preference-based outcome measures are at a disadvantage compared with others who have a greater chance of improvement. This introduces a bias and puts people whose health can only improve a limited amount at a disadvantage in terms of QALYs gained.

Patrick describes four ways of dealing with that (D. Patrick, personal communication, 2000): First, do not undertake cost-effectiveness work. There is an argument for that with respect to disability, given the attitudes in society. Second, leave disabled people out of the system (unlikely to happen). Third, adopt Nord's approach (Nord et al. 1999), positively weighting functioning in disabled people. Fourth, create a weighting system that permits disabled people to add their own evaluation. However, there are clearly difficulties in producing a tool that accurately reflects disabled people's quality of life and their likely outcomes.

The independent living movement and antidiscrimination legislation in some countries have considerably advanced many disabled people. The effects of the independent living movement on health services have been twofold. Of itself, it has empowered disabled people to be more active consumers and commentators on health care policy. It has also meant that many more disabled people are living independently, rather than in institutions.

One of the central tenets of the independent living movement is that the disability people face is largely attributable to the effect of attitudes and the environment on people with impairments. This begs the following question: Do health services have any role in supporting disabled people? Clearly, disabled people disproportionately use health services. Open to question is whether enough attention is given to the broader determinants of disability. While health policy in the United Kingdom has yet to catch up with this, there is an increasing recognition that many of the broader determinants of public health lie outside health services.

Therefore, what is the role of medicine and rehabilitation? To take McKeown's (1979) and Illich's (1979) general reflections on the role of medicine, it is a chimera—at best achieving marginal improvements—and there is more to be gained by addressing broader problems within society.[2] In my view, the "medical model" of disability is displaced from being the sole explanation of disability; that does not mean medicine and other health care and rehabilitation should not have a role in empowering disabled people.

To realize its potential though, people need to rethink the approach adopted by health services. This includes the balance between trying to change disabled people's impairments and providing them with the tools to manage in a disabling society.

Some projects have integrated a "social model" approach, addressing the environment and aids as part of an integrated approach to independent living. Their work focuses on society as the problem, not the disabled person. However, they report having encountered opposition from members of the rehabilitation teams (Silburn 1993). Physician training also needs substantial rethinking, not simply the addition of a few disability awareness courses. Furthermore, clearly the experience of disabled people with health care cannot be disassociated from society as a whole.

Different cultures and systems of medical care have a different impact on disabled people's experiences. For example, the greater rights-based U.S. culture provides everyone with access to the health care system, where ability to pay is an important determinant; as long as one has adequate insurance or cash, there is substantial individual autonomy (albeit moderated by the growth in managed care). In contrast, in much of Europe, there is a more collectivist approach, largely funded via central insurance or taxation, which aims for universal access but is more paternalistic in its approach.

In more general terms, disabled people's experiences with health care are part of discrimination and the disabling effects of society. Oliver (1990) introduces the idea that adjustment, with respect to disability, should not be the individual coming to terms with her or his impairment but society adjusting to the changed requirements of an individual. There is an important corollary for the medical profession. Perhaps society and health professionals need "rehabilitation" more than disabled people do.

NOTES

1. *Evidence-based medicine,* a clinical learning strategy developed at McMaster Medical School in Canada in the 1970s, aims to ensure that clinical decisions are based on critically appraised research findings (Rosenberg and Donald 1995).

2. Later analyses (e.g., Bunker 1995) point toward a more significant contribution for medicine.

REFERENCES

Altman, B. M. 1981. "Studies of Attitudes towards the Handicapped: The Need for a New Direction." *Social Problems* 28:321-37.

Asch, A. 1998. "Distracted by Disability." *Cambridge Quarterly of Healthcare Ethics* 7:77-87.

Batavia, A. J. 1997. "Disability and Physician Assisted Suicide." *New England Journal of Medicine* 336:1671-73.

Beardshaw, V. 1988. *Last on the List: Community Services for People with Physical Disabilities.* London: King's Fund.

Beatty, P. W., G. W. Richmond, S. Tepper, and G. DeJong. 1998. "Personal Assistance for People with Physical Disabilities: Consumer-Direction and Satisfaction with Services." *Archives Physical Medicine and Rehabilitation* 70:674-77.

Biley, A. M. 1994. "A Handicap of Negative Attitudes and Lack of Choice: Caring for Inpatients with Disabilities." *Professional Nurse* 9 (12): 786-87.

British Medical Association. 1999. *Withholding and Withdrawing Life-Prolonging Medical Treatment: Guidance for Decision Making.* London: British Medical Journal Books.

Bunker, J. 1995. "Medicine Matters after All." *Journal of the Royal College of Physicians of London* 29 (2): 105-12.

"Cabbage Syndrome." 1990. *Lancet* 336:91-92.

Chalmers, I. 1991. "The Perinatal Research Agenda: Whose Priorities?" *Birth* 18:137-41.

———. 1993. "The Cochrane Collaboration: Preparing, Maintaining, and Disseminating Systematic Reviews of the Effects of Health Care." *Annals of the New York Academy of Sciences* 703:156-63.

———. 1998. "Unbiased, Relevant, and Reliable Assessments in Health Care." *British Medical Journal* 317:1167-68.

Davis, A. 1999. "Guidelines Dismay Disabled People Unable to Speak for Themselves." *British Medical Journal* 319:705.

Davis, K. 1993. "On the Movement." In *Disabling Barriers—Enabling Environments,* edited by J. Swain, V. Finklestein, S. French, and M. Oliver. London: Sage.

DeJong, G. 1983. "Defining and Implementing the Independent Living Concept." Pp. 4-27 in *A First Class Service: Quality in the New NHS,* edited by N. Crewe and I. Zola. London: Department of Health.

Department of Health (DOH). 1998. *A First Class Service: Quality in the New NHS.* London: Author.

Diseker, R. A. and R. Michielutte. 1981. "An Analysis of Empathy in Medical Students before and following Clinical Experience." *Journal of Medical Education* 56 (12): 1004-10.

Donaldson, J. 1980. "Changing Attitudes towards Handicapped Persons: A Review and Analysis of the Evidence." *Exceptional Children* 46:504-14.

Doty, P., J. Kasper, and S. Litvak. 1996. "Consumer-Directed Models of Personal Care: Lessons from Medicaid." *The Milbank Quarterly* 74:377-499.

Down's Syndrome Association. 1999. *Access All Areas: Down's Syndrome, a Health Guide.* London: Author.

Duckworth, S. C. 1988. "The Effect of Medical Education on the Attitudes of Medical Students towards Disabled People." *Medical Education* 22:501-5.

Eberhardt, K. and W. Mayberry. 1994. "Factors Influencing Entry-Level Occupational Therapists' Attitudes toward Persons with Disabilities." *American Journal of Occupational Therapy* 49:629-35.

Feek, C. M., W. McKean, L. Henneveld, G. Barrow, W. Edgar, and R. J. Paterson. 1999. "Experience with Health Care Rationing in New Zealand." *British Medical Journal* 318:1346-48.

Fost, N. 1999. "Decisions Regarding Treatment of Seriously Ill Newborns." *Journal of the American Medical Association* 281:2041-42.

French, S. 1993. "Disabled Health and Caring Professionals." Pp. 201-9 in *Disabling Barriers—Enabling Environments,* edited by J. Swain, V. Finklestein, S. French, and M. Oliver. London: Sage.

———. 1994. "Attitudes of Health Professionals towards Disabled People: A Discussion and Review of the Literature." *Physiotherapy* 80:687-93.

Bowler, E., assistant producer. 1999. *From the Edge.* 1999. London: BBC 2, September 7.

Gardner, G. P., R. Theocleous, J. W. Watt, and K. R. Krishnan. 1985. "Ventilation or Dignified Death for Patients with High Level Tetraplegia." *British Medical Journal* 291:160-222.

Gerhart, K. A., J. Koziol-McLain, S. R. Lowenstein, and G. G. Whiteneck. 1994. "Quality of Life following Spinal Cord Injury: Knowledge and Attitudes of Emergency Care Providers." *Annals of Emergency Medicine* 23:807-12.

Gill, C. 1992. "Suicide Intervention for People with Disabilities: A Lesson in Inequality." *Issues in Law & Medicine* 8:37-53.

Goddard, L. and L. Jordan. 1998. "Changing Attitudes about Persons with Disabilities: Effects of a Simulation." *Journal of Neuroscience Nursing* 30:307-13.

Hadley, R. and R. Gough. 1997. *Care in Chaos: Frustration and Challenge in Community Care.* London: Cassel.

Hadorn, D. C. 1992. "The Problem of Discrimination in Health Care Priority Setting." *Journal of the American Medical Association* 268 (11): 1454-59.

Harris, J. 1987. "QALYfying the Value of Human Life." *Journal of Medical Ethics* 3:118.

———. 1995. "Double Jeopardy and the Veil of Ignorance—A Reply." *Journal of Medical Ethics* 21:151-57.

Hasler, F. 1993. "Developments in the Disabled People's Movement." In *Disabling Barriers—Enabling Environments,* edited by J. Swain, V. Finklestein, S. French, and M. Oliver. London: Sage.

Hickey, A. M., G. Bury, C. A. O'Boyle, F. Bradley, F. D. O'Kelly, and W. Shannon. 1996. "A New Short Form Individual Quality of Life Measure (SE1QoL-DW): Application in a Cohort of Individuals with HIV/AIDS." *British Medical Journal* 313:29-33.

Hordon, L. D. 1993. "The Effect of Medical Training on Attitudes to Disabled People." *British Journal of Rheumatology* 32:151.

———. 1994. "Attitudes of Medical Students to Disabled People." *British Journal of Rheumatology* 33:203-4.

Illich, I. 1979. *Limits to Medicine: Medical Nemesis: The Expropriation of Health.* Harmondsworth, UK: Penguin.

Lindow, V. and J. Morris. 1995. *Service User Involvement: Synthesis of Findings and Experience in the Field of Community Care.* Layerthorpe, UK: York.

Master, R., A. Dreyfus, S. Connors, C. Tobias, Z. Zhou, and R. Kronick. 1996. "The Community Medical Alliance: An Integrated System of Care in Greater Boston for People with Severe Disabilities and AIDS." *Managed Care Quarterly* 4 (2): 26-37.

McKeown, T. 1979. *The Role of Medicine: Drama, Mirage or Nemesis.* Oxford, UK: Blackwell.

Mitchell, K. R., M. Hayes, J. Gordon, and B. Wallis. 1984. "An Investigation of the Attitudes of Medical Students to Physically Disabled People." *Medical Education* 18:21-23.

National Health Service (NHS) Executive. 1997. *Patients Disabled? The Care of Disabled People in Hospital: Conference Report.* London: Department of Health.

Nord, E., J. L. Pinto, J. Richardson, P. Menzel, and P. Ubel. 1999. "Incorporating Society Concerns for Fairness in Numerical Valuations of Health Programmes." *Health Economics* 8:25-39.

Oliver, M. 1990. *The Politics of Disablement.* London: Macmillan.

Oliver, M. and C. Barnes. 1998. *Disabled People and Social Policy: From Exclusion to Inclusion.* London: Longman.

Oliver, M. and G. Zarb. 1993. "Personal Services." *Community Care*, July 22.

Orentlicher, D. 1994. "Rationing and the Americans with Disabilities Act." *Journal of the American Medical Association* 271:308-14.

Perricone, P. J. 1974. "Social Concern in Medical Students: A Reconsideration of the Eron Assumption." *Journal of Medical Education* 49 (6): 541-46.

Phillips, M. 1999. "The Hospital Gods Who Decide Whether We Die." *Sunday Times*, July 25, p. 17.

Pless, J. E. 1983. "The Story of Baby Doe." *New England Journal of Medicine* 309:664.

Priestly, M. 1999. *Disability Politics and Community Care.* London: Jessica Kingsley.

Raeside, L. 1997. "Ethical Decision-Making in Neonatal Intensive Care." *Neonatal Care* 13:157-59.

Rezler, A. 1974. "Attitude Changes during Medical School: A Review of the Literature." *Journal of Medical Education* 49:1023-30.

Rodwin, M. A. 1994. "Patient Accountability and Quality of Care: Lessons from Medical Consumerism and the Patients' Rights, Women's Health and Disability Rights Movements." *Americal Journal of Law & Medicine* 20:147-67.

Rogers, L. 1999. "Hospital Refuses New Heart to Down's Child." *Sunday Times*, July 25, p. 7.

Rosenberg, W. and A. Donald. 1995. "Evidence Based Medicine: An Approach to Clinical Problem-Solving." *British Medical Journal* 310:1122-26.

Rothwell, P. M., Z. McDowell, C. K. Wong, and P. J. Dorman. 1997. "Doctors and Patients Don't Agree: Cross Sectional Study of Patients' and Doctors' Assessments of Disability in Multiple Sclerosis." *British Medical Journal* 314:1580-83.

Roush, S. E. 1986. "Health Professionals as Contributors towards Attitudes to Persons with Disability: A Special Communication." *Physical Therapy* 66:151-54.

Sackett, D. L. and W. M. C. Rosenberg. 1995. "The Need for Evidence Based Medicine." *Journal of the Royal Society of Medicine* 88:620-24.

Saigal, S., B. L. Stoskopf, D. Feeny, W. Furlong, E. Burrows, P. L. Rosenbaum, and L. Hoult. 1999. "Differences in Preferences for Neonatal Outcomes among Health Care Professionals, Parents, and Adolescents." *Journal of the American Medical Association* 281:1991-97.

Sayers, B. M. and T. M. Fliedner. 1997. "The Critique of DALYs: A Counter-Reply." *Bulletin of the World Health Organisation* 75:383-84.

Scullion, P. 1999. "Challenging Discrimination against Disabled Patients." *Nursing Standard* 13 (18): 37-40.

Shearer, A. 1992. "Disability: Whose Handicap?" P. 277 in *Milton Keanes: Health and Disease: A Reader,* edited by N. Black, D. Boswell, A. Grey, S. Murphy, and J. Popay. London: Sage.

Sheldon, T. and I. Chalmers. 1994. "The UK Cochrane Centre and the NHS Centre for Reviews and Dissemination: Respective Roles within the Information Strategy of the NHS R+D Programme, Co-ordination and Principles Underlying Collaboration." *Health Economics* 97:11-25.

Silburn, L. 1993. "A Social Model in a Medical World: The Development of the Integrated Living Team as Part of the Strategy for Younger Physically Disabled People in North Derbyshire." Pp. 218-26 in *Dis-*

abling Barriers—Enabling Environments, edited by J. Swain, V. Finklestein, S. French, and M. Oliver. London: Sage.

Silvers, A. 1995. "Damaged Goods: Does Disability DisQALYfy People from Just Health Care." *Mount Sinai Journal of Medicine* 62:102-11.

Singer, P., J. McKie, H. Kuhse, and J. Richardson. 1995. "Double Jeopardy and the Use of QALYs in Health Care Allocation as the Double Jeopardy Argument." *Journal of Medical Ethics* 21:144-50.

Sutherland, A. T. 1981. *Disabled We Stand.* London: Souvenir.

Swain, J., V. Finklestein, S. French, and M. Oliver, eds. 1993. *Disabling Barriers—Enabling Environments.* London: Sage.

Üstün, T. B., J. Rehm, S. Chatterji, S. Saxena, R. Trotter, R. Room, J. Birkenbach, and the WHO/NIH Joint Project CAR Study Group. 1999. "Multiple-Informant Ranking of the Disabling Effects of Different Health Conditions in 14 Countries." *Lancet* 354:111-15.

Wainapel, S. 1999. "A Clash of Cultures: Reflections of a Physician with a Disability." *Lancet* 354:763-64.

Wolf, T. M., P. M. Balson, J. M. Faucetti, and H. M. Randall. 1989. "A Retrospective Study of Attitude Change during Medical School." *Medical Education* 23:19-23.

Zarb, G. and P. Nadesh. 1994. *Cashing In on Independence: Comparing the Costs and Benefits of Cash and Services.* Derby, UK: British Council of Disabled People (BCODP)/Policy Studies Institute (PSI).

The Role of Social Networks in the Lives of Persons with Disabilities

19

BERNICE A. PESCOSOLIDO

> You should give Lia medicine to take for a week but no longer. After she is well, she should stop taking the medicine. You should not treat her by taking her blood or fluid from her backbone. Lia should also be treated at home with our Hmong medicines and by sacrificing pigs and chickens. We hope Lia will be healthy, but we are not sure we want her to stop shaking forever because it makes her noble in our culture, and when she grows up she might be a shaman.
>
> —Fadiman (1997:260)

In all societies, people experience illness and live with their disabilities in communities; even when they access the health care system, it is a human service system. Lia, a Hmong child with a seizure disorder, and her family understand and confront her seizure disorder with a set of attitudes and beliefs that stand in opposition to the dominant medical culture in the United States where her family now resides. These social forces, from the ethnic group to the medical context to the larger society, shape the recognition and response to problems. Too often, we have neglected to consider that what makes people's experience in the community and in treatment systems "success" or "failure" are intimately tied to the kinds of relationships forged and maintained in those contexts.

A social network perspective offers a way to break down these large, critical components into a set of ongoing ties that chart people's experiences. The basic premise of social network theory, in contrast to most economic, psychological, and public health models, is that individuals shape their everyday lives through consultation, suggestion, support, and nagging from others. Furthermore, it suggests that social networks set a context in formal organizations and institutions among those who work in or are served by them that affects what people do, how they feel, and what happens to them.

Within this tradition, there are four ideas and corresponding literatures of relevance. First, sociological, psychological, anthropological, and, more recently, economic research support

AUTHOR'S NOTE: This research is supported by the National Institute of Mental Health (grants R24MH51669 and K02MH42655). I would like to thank Fred Hafferty and Barbara Wolf for introducing me to the larger world of disability studies. Furthermore, Mary Hannah, as always, provided expert clerical assistance on this chapter.

the general idea that social networks are basic building blocks of human experience. We will consider that here only to the extent that it offers an introduction to concepts, measurement, and findings. Second, within that literature, a body of work focuses on health. This is central to the introduction of ideas about how social networks affect the lives of people who confront, respond to, and live with health problems. Third, even more specifically, within the social science and medical literatures on social networks and health, there has been a tradition of research on disability, most often targeting chronic health conditions, such as HIV/AIDS and Alzheimer's disease (Cohen, Teresi, and Blum 1994; Cook 1988). Fourth, there is small and more recent literature on issues of social networks and physical impairments (Morgan, Patrick, and Charlton 1984).

In sum, this chapter presents a basic introduction to the social network perspective, its terms and its foci. It introduces one approach that frames issues of recognition, reaction, and outcome to problems in light of the existing and subsequent changes in the "community" that surround individuals (Pescosolido 1991, 1992; Pescosolido, Boyer, and Lubell 1999). Furthermore, it provides a review of social network findings relevant to issues of health, illness, and disability, often with a focus on chronic mental illness. Descriptions of existing research are organized as a socially dynamic process, focusing on how social networks influence recognition of health problems, the options to deal with them, the way treatment is provided, and their effects on outcomes.

THE BASIC PREMISE OF SOCIAL NETWORKS RESEARCH AND ITS ROLE IN HEALTH AND DISABILITY STUDIES

Today this illness, these voices are still a part of my life. But it is I who have won, not they. A wonderful new drug, caring therapists, the love and support of my family and my own fierce battle—that I know will never end—have all combined in a nearly miraculous way to enable me to master the illness that once mastered me. (Shiller and Bennett 1994:7)

Lori Schiller's story of her life with schizophrenia illustrates the idea that many "others" are important, a notion that has become central in epidemiological and health services literatures, policymaking, and public understanding. However, as Berkman (1986) points out, its incorporation into research is quite recent, beginning with Cassel's (1976) classic article laying out a wide range of factors in the social environment that could affect "host resistance." Much existing research, then, has been on the role of social support and social networks on mortality, documenting that social isolation increases the risk of death. In the Alameda County study, for example, more social network ties were associated with lower morbidity and mortality (Berkman and Syme 1979). The effects, however, were weaker for women and nonwhites than for white men (House, Robbins, and Metzner 1982; Schoenbach et al. 1986). House et al. (1982) caution that such findings may not represent the lack of importance of social ties for these latter groups. Rather, persons with these social characteristics are more likely to create, sustain, and, ironically, be less aware of the social ties that deeply embed them in their families, jobs, or communities. This point will be discussed later in the recommendations for future research.

Because there has been no shortage of the use (or misuse) of the concept of social networks in health care research in the past 20 years, understanding the basics that are common to all of the various approaches offers a foundation for thinking about their role in disability studies. Many different kinds of studies mark the impact of social relationships. For example, in the arena of mental health disabilities, studies target self-help (Segal, Silverman, and Tempkin 1995; Zinman, Harp, and Budd 1987), caretakers (Tausig, Fisher, and Tessler 1992), social support (Cresswell, Kuipers, and Power 1992; Froland et al. 1979), natural support networks (Hammer 1983), peer support (Cook, 1988), and even the treatment alliance (Solomon, Draine, and

Delaney 1995). Despite theoretical and methodological differences, all tap some type of social network tie or treatment system in the community that can affect both the response to and outcomes for persons with disabilities. To begin, then, a shared understanding of the basic concepts and tenets of the network approach is in order.

Most important, a social network approach builds on a set of concepts and ideas about the centrality of social interactions influencing the attitudes, beliefs, and behaviors of "social actors." Table 19.1 provides a brief overview of the most frequently used terms in the social network perspective. Often, social networks map the connections that individuals have to one another. They can also map relationships among organizations to examine the "cracks" in the social service system (e.g., McKinney, Morrissey, and Kaluzny 1993; Morrissey et al. 1994) or to examine the trading alliances between countries to chart the world economic system (Ragin 1987). The central focus is always on the relationships between a social actor (often referred to as "ego" or the "focal" person or organization) and the social actors with whom they having a certain type of relationship (i.e., ties "sent") or from whom they receive a mention as an interaction partner (i.e., ties "received" from an "alter"). There is no standard way to chart network relationships—they may be derived from a list on a survey, wherein an individual is asked to name those persons who they share information with, trust, admire, or dislike. They may come from observing the behavior of individuals, for example, who they talk to in their workgroup. They may come from checking which organizations have referral agreements, contracts, or shared personnel. Deciding which types of social networks are of interest and how to elicit the ties becomes a critical issue. In surveys, the selection of the "stem question" or "network generator" can determine, for example, whether research taps into a personal support network, a trail of contacts in a search for information, or a set of formal treatment arrangements. The network generator can elicit ties sent (e.g., "On whom do you depend for advice?") or ties received (e.g., "Who depends on you for advice?").

In general, three overall characteristics of social networks are central to mapping the nature of relationships. The first and most often used is network *structure*. That is, we are concerned with the overall size of the network, the different types of relationships that people can have (e.g., kin, confidant, member of the same church), and whether social ties have more than one basis of connection (i.e., multiplexity in which a tie may be a spouse and a coworker). We are also concerned with how tightly knit the social network is (i.e., density or how well all people listed know one another). The scope or range of ties refers to how broadly based ties are. Individuals who have only family members as network ties have limited scope or range, while those who report ties at work, church, and the gym have greater network range. For example, individuals with mental health problems in Puerto Rico are less likely to access the formal health care system if they report a large social network on whom they can depend for advice and care in the community (Pescosolido et al. 1998). Among Puerto Ricans on the island, problems are considered to reside squarely in the family; it is this group that holds the responsibility for care of its members. Medical or mental health care is a last resort. This contrasts sharply with the social networks in other cultural groups on the U.S. mainland, where Charles Kadushin (1966) documented the opposite. On the Upper West Side of Manhattan, informal social networks, which he called the "Friends and Supporters of Psychotherapy," were likely to encourage the regular and routine use of the mental health system for emotional problems.

The strength of the tie may tap access to different kinds of social networks. In his study of job hunting on the East Coast of the United States, Granovetter (1973) found that men who had only strong ties seemed to be disadvantaged compared to men who had both strong and weak tie relationships. Weak ties, those that are infrequent and not of central importance to an individual (an old high school or college friend), are critical because they allow individuals access to other social networks and, as a result, to new and different information. Strong ties are likely to share similar knowledge and common access to opportunities. Only by tapping into other networks, even in a transient and almost happenstance manner (e.g., running into someone in a grocery store), did job hunters gather new information.

The form, shape, or "geometry" of the network reflects only one aspect of what is important about social networks. In addition, network *content* is important because it taps into the quality

Table 19.1   Some Basic Terms in Social Network Research

	Definition	Examples
General terms		
Network tie	A social actor mentioned or observed to have a connection with another	Ego = focal person or organization; alter = person or organization mentioned as a "contact"
Stem question/ network generator	Question designed or protocol to elicit names of specific kinds of network ties	Who are the people you discuss important matters with? Who are the people who nag you about your medication?
Network structure	Characteristics that describe the form of the network or the geometry of ties	Size, frequency of contact, multiplexity, density, strength of tie, scope/range
Network content	Characteristics that describe the substance of the network, the things that flow across the ties	Valence (positive, negative); attitudes, beliefs held; cultural meetings
Network function	Characteristics that describe the things that network ties do	Emotional/social supports, instrumental aid, appraisal, regulation/monitoring
Terms specific to health and health care		
External or outside social networks	Community ties, network ties that exist outside of the health care sector	Family/kin, friends/peers, acquaintances, culture of daily life or community
Internal or inside social networks	Ties that are formed to professionals within the health care sector	Providers/alliance, case managers, support personnel, cultural climate of treatment organization
Interface of external and internal networks	The nature of the interconnections between individuals, the community, and the treatment system	Support groups, family programs, cultural "fit" between ideas/attitudes in the lay and professional networks

and substance of social networks. If we conceptualize the structure of the network as a set of connections between people, then content represents the types of things that flow from or to each person. Two analogies may be useful in making the distinction clear. From a biological perspective, aspects of size and density make up the skeleton of social relationships. The attitudes, beliefs, and practices are the muscle, blood, and skin of social networks. From an engineering perspective, the structure of the network represents the power grid or electrical lines connecting power sources. The content of networks represents the energy that passes through those conduits.

The now vast literature on "social support" essentially captures the substantive dimension of social networks—whether individuals provide care, nurturing, or assistance of one sort or another. However, what flows along these ties has a valence (or "charge") that can be positive or negative. In fact, the little research that has explored the presence of negative ties in people's lives has found them to have powerful effects on health (e.g., Berkman 1987; Pagel and Becker 1987).

One of the strongest sets of networks in the disability arena has been the development of lobby groups, consumer groups, and interest groups that form around a disease or impairment (e.g., the National Alliance for the Mentally Ill [NAMI], the AIDS Awareness Network, and the RAG Ring with its *Ragged Edge Magazine* and online counterpart, the *Electric Edge*). Belonging to NAMI, for example, with its emphasis on the biological and brain dysfunction theories of the etiology of mental illness, pushes individuals and their families toward medical solutions and pharmacological interventions and away from psychoanalytic theories and therapies that historically focus on the role of the mother's behavior in "causing" mental illness (e.g., the "refrigerator" mother).

There are also specific *functions* that networks serve—emotional support (e.g., care, concern), instrumental aid (e.g., lending money, providing transportation, baby-sitting), appraisal (e.g., evaluating a problem or solution), and monitoring (e.g., making sure a person with diabetes watches his or her diet and takes insulin shots) (Pearlin and Aneshensel 1986). As Umberson (1987) found for married men, it is not only the support that comes with marriage that is essential to men's health but also the kind of regulatory behavior that wives exert in watching their husbands' health habits. Although love and caring are important, so too are nagging and monitoring.

External and Internal Social Networks

For issues surrounding disability, it is important to draw a dichotomy: the difference between "external" and "internal" social networks (Pescosolido et al. 1998). This distinction is simplistic but necessary because too often, epidemiologists, providers, and services researchers see social networks as something "out there" in the community. A wide array of meanings exists among the diverse cultural groups in most societies, and many are not in line with the dominant culture (e.g., the Chinese in Malaysian society). Many clinical researchers and providers accept this rich diversity in the community. However, they fail to see the relevance for the work that they themselves do in clinics, rehabilitation centers, and even support groups. Social networks are interesting and important but, from the perspective of the researchers and providers, outside the purview of and removed from what actually happens in formal health care. This cultural bias, derived from the notion of the "objectivity" of science in Western societies, overlooks the powerful culture that the medical model creates. Social networks exist inside treatment programs and are built or not built as providers do clinical interventions. All health care is provided through human communication, with or without human touch, aided by human compassion or devoid of it (Hohmann 1999; Pescosolido et al. 1998). The manner in which health protocols are established brings a set of values and ways of "knowing" and "doing" that represent its own culture.

The randomized clinical trial, for example, assumes that all "manualized" treatment[1] will or should work in the same way on all of the individuals who have been carefully selected according to inclusion criteria. The scientific medical image, then, is one of a generic client treated by a generic provider; they appear to be as replaceable as parts in a well-oiled machine. However, the types of bonds formed, or the lack thereof, between clients and providers or even among providers themselves are powerful social factors and can have important effects on what happens when individuals face disabilities. Even the earliest research on hospitals (Coser 1952) suggests that the effect of the social environment on how health care services are provided can affect the quality of the delivery of services and the relationships among doctors and nurses. Wright (1997) documents that in psychiatric units in the United States, whether the staff reports a sense of social support among coworkers finds its way into whether family is treated as an important part of the treatment process. Specifically, only when nurses, doctors, and aides felt a stronger sense of collaboration were they likely to include families in decisions and even conversations about their loved ones.

The social network perspective, then, requires an understanding of not only community network ties but also of those that may be formed in health care and rehabilitation settings. Three sets of connections result:

1. external social networks that map the community social relationships that individuals have,

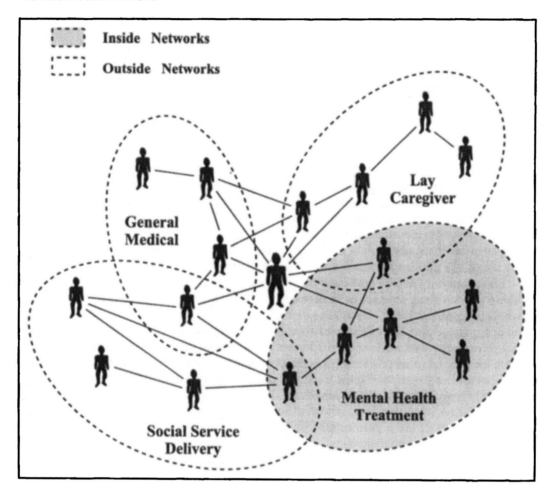

Figure 19.1. Hypothetical Social Relationships of Individuals with Serious Mental Illness in the Community

2. internal social networks that describe the social relationships among providers and their clients during clinical interventions or in the development of long-term plans for living in the community,

3. the interface of these two networks systems, which shape the implementation of interventions and clients' responses to them (e.g., adherence).

Figure 19.1 depicts the many kinds of social circles relevant to the lives of persons with disabilities.

External social networks represent the more usual notion of "community ties." Originally, these social networks were circumscribed by the places people lived, and social relationships were often constrained by social customs that prohibited relationships across gender, class, or even age lines (Simmel 1955). More recently, these networks have taken on many more forms, including relationships formed over computer networks (see Sharf 1997 on cancer). For this reason, it is better to think of external social networks as "personal communities of meaning," however formed and maintained. Instead of trying to describe some amorphous entity such as *the* community, social network theorists contend that people live their lives in smaller worlds. These worlds can be mapped as *their* community by noting the structure, function, and content of social ties people acquire, forge, or have forced on them (Fischer 1982; Pescosolido and Rubin 2000; Wellman 1982).

Internal social networks help to open up the "black box" of what goes on in formal organizations designed to assist people with disabilities by seeing them, at least in part, as the human provision of care (Pescosolido 1996a, 1996b). Social networks in medical facilities are not treatment but are any diagnostic instrument, medication, or manipulation delivered to individuals by human providers in a human service organization. Clinical interventions determine "what" is offered, while internal social networks (provider and organizational networks) shape "how" it is implemented. The social network perspective puts a human face on issues of access, system barriers, intervention, continuity, and adherence by conceptualizing the actions of real people.

Furthermore, those who work in organizations form social networks of cooperation and conflict and face administrations of support and constraint. The nature of the work network that is formed in a medical care setting can influence, for example, whether programs succeed or fail. In his study of "outcomes" for children with serious emotional problems, Glisson (1994) found that the single most important factor influencing children and their families' lives was the degree to which members of the service team were allowed to innovate, be flexible in addressing the child's needs, and have the ability to respond to larger social issues.

Inside and outside networks meet at the interface of community and treatment networks. These ties can work together or in opposition, for example, to make assisted living and the whole independent living movement a success or failure. When persons with disabilities have no or sparse social networks, the role of bonds forged between the person and health care or social service providers will be more important, in and of themselves, in assisting the person to form meaningful social relationships in the community. When persons have community social ties that are in agreement with the treatment philosophy, approach, or providers, internal and external networks form a strong web of care. When they are in conflict about the nature of the problem, its causes, or even potential solutions, internal and external networks clash (Pescosolido et al. 1998; Pescosolido, Wright, and Sullivan 1995). Gottlieb (1992) contends that many mental health treatments, including social support interventions, have failed because there is a discrepancy between the "culture" of treatment and the "culture" in which community relationships take place.

The Basic Tenets of a Social Network Perspective

Underlying most social network research is a basic set of assumptions and propositions that can be summarized as follows (see Pescosolido et al. 1998 for greater detail):

1. Social network theory and research aim to understand human behavior through the social relationships those individuals have with each other.

2. Social network theory and research stand in contrast to other approaches that focus on individuals alone, mental events, cognitive maps, or technological determinism, for example (White 1992). It does not ignore these others factors but sees them as critically tied to ongoing social relationships in the larger context of individuals' lives.

3. Social network theory and research offer a way to think about abstract influences such as "society," "the community," and "the system" by looking to the set of social interactions that occur within them.

4. Social network interactions have structure, content, and function (see Table 19.1).

5. Social interactions can be positive or negative, not simply "social support." Network ties can be helpful or harmful; they can integrate individuals into a community and, just a powerfully, place stringent regulations on behavior that isolate them from others.

6. It is not the case that "more is better" with regard to social networks. Having too much oversight, whether positive or negative, can be stifling and repressive (Durkheim 1951). Also, "strong" ties are not necessarily optimal because the "weak" ties that individuals have often act as a bridge to other social groups with different information, resources, and insights.

7. The effect of the structure, content, and functions of social networks needs to be considered separately because how they come together is important. For example, having many network ties that offer care has a very different impact on persons with disabilities than having many network ties that are indifferent or hostile.

8. Sociodemographics characteristics, such as age, sex, race/ethnicity, and social class, cannot be used as indicators of existing social networks because historically their role in placing limits around interaction partners is decreasing (Pescosolido and Rubin 2000). Among physically disabled people living in an inner London borough, for example, marital status is a poor proxy for the existence of social support (Morgan et al. 1984). However, this not to say that sociodemographic characteristics do not affect social networks (see below). Particularly in more traditional cultures, age and gender can circumscribe allowable relationships among individuals. Social class may facilitate some people's access to the Internet while putting others at a disadvantage.

INTRODUCING SOCIAL NETWORKS INTO THE STUDY OF HEALTH AND PHYSICAL IMPAIRMENTS: THE SOCIAL ORGANIZATION STRATEGY FRAMEWORK AND THE NETWORK EPISODE MODEL

Everyone has got one, or will, and they will likely have them a lot longer than anyone realizes. . . . Thus my first forewarning . . . is that they are not so clearly about "someone else's problem." (Zola 1993:802)

Irving Zola's wisdom on the nature of disabilities requires that we think about the role of social networks in disability in a very general sense, not simply as related to health and medical care. To that end, one needs to think about social networks primarily as part of a general perspective on social life and decision making and only secondarily as a way to think about treatment systems. It has become fashionable of late to explain human behavior and people's actions to solve social problems in terms of a rational choice perspective. In this approach, an individual is seen as engaging in a cost-benefit analysis. While very elegant and sophisticated, this approach tends to neglect the critical role that others play in social life. A complementary approach (and the one introduced here) is the social organization strategy (SOS) perspective. It sees social interaction, rather than individual mental calculus, as the basis of social life. It is not enough to see the influence of social networks as one more factor in the individual's weighing of the costs and benefits of action. Rather, social interaction often determines whether individuals have a choice to make, whether and how they are pushed in a particular direction, and whether they recognize problems and see certain actions as within the range of acceptable possibilities.

Some may argue that this approach flies in the face of free will or individual rights, making people powerless social puppets. But the SOS approach does not see irrationality as the opposite of rationality in the narrow sense. Rather, individuals are pragmatic, social, and knowledgeable with a cultural tool kit from which to draw. Often, they can draw from routinely available scripts, without intense engagement in a cost-benefit analysis. They can improvise, and, most important, they can sometimes be forced into one direction or another. This approach shifts the focus from the individual to the individual in patterned interaction with others. It is through this regular contact that people have with one another that they learn about, come to understand, and attempt to handle difficulties they confront (Pescosolido 1992).

Finally, it offers a real way to see how the larger social context, organizational structures, and institutional landscapes affect people's lives and their options by seeing them occur through the human contact at each level. Individuals, as they confront disabilities, are "neither puppets of some abstract structure, nor calculating individualists; people both shape and are shaped by social networks" (Pescosolido 1992:1109).

This overall perspective can be used to develop models tailored to particular issues. The network episode model (NEM) (Pescosolido 1991; Pescosolido, Boyer, and Lubell 1999) was designed to address issues of service use and outcomes for individuals with serious health problems, most specifically for mental health impairments. Its adaptation to the broader issues of disabilities requires some adjustment, but the fundamental points remain the same. That is, the NEM starts with a basic idea. Dealing with any health problem or physical disability is a social process that is managed through the contacts (or social networks) that individuals have in the community, the treatment system, and the social service agencies (including support groups, churches, community recreation centers). How people respond to disabilities is as much a process of social influence as it is a result of individual action; it is both a social and personal process.

In the NEM, individuals act using commonsense knowledge that they draw from past experience, from proactively talking to others and from reactively responding to the comments of others when impairments or other health problems associated with them occur. The NEM, in line with the SOS framework, questions whether every action in coping with a disability is a result of the complicated cost-benefit calculus typical of many other approaches (e.g., for reviews, see Gochman 1997; Pescosolido 1992). There may be times when people have to sit and weigh the costs and benefits of a whole list of factors (e.g., when faced with a serious decision about living arrangements). But, in general, people face disabilities in the course of their day-to-day lives by interacting with other people who may recognize (or deny) a problem, send them to (or provide) treatment, and support, cajole, or nag them about appointments, medications, or lifestyle.

Figure 19.2 shows a revised version of the NEM and its four basic components—the disability career, social support system, treatment system, and social context.

Unlike many other models, the NEM is focused on the "career" of a person who faces a health or physical impairment. For example, it conceptualizes the use of social or health care services *not* as a single, yes-no, one-time decision but as the patterns and pathways of practices and people consulted as a result of disabilities or in response to an episode of illness, which may or may not result from the disability. Pictured as the "middle stream" (right side of Figure 19.2), the "disability career or illness" marks all of an individual's attempts to cope with the onset of an "episode," charting what individuals do and when they do it.

What is an "episode"? Given the context of some disabilities, this raises questions. For chronic health impairments, the answer is relatively simple. The "career" marks the time from when the symptoms first occur and follows them through as one more strand in the "life course." An episode occurs when there is a "flare-up," an acute set of health problems that need to be addressed. For physical impairments, the issues are more complicated. Again, the disability career coincides with the onset of the impairment. While there may be periods of acute health problems that may accompany the impairment, a broader and more reasonable view of episodes must be developed. This is where resorting back to the SOS framework is useful. Episodes can be conceptualized as any problem, related directly to the impairment, which requires a concerted effort of problem solving. So the negotiation of accommodations to a workplace for a person in a wheelchair can be considered an episode in this model. But to return to the model's original focus, the NEM does not target the typically narrow issue of whether individuals use formal health services (e.g., "Did individuals access the system? What was their volume of use over a six-month period?"); the NEM targets three different kinds of phenomena or "dependent variables." Patterns of care describe the combination of advisers or practices used during the course of coping with a disability or illness episode. For example, some individuals may depend only on formal health care services; others may become involved in the disability movement, seeking advice and suggestions from others with experience in the social and medical

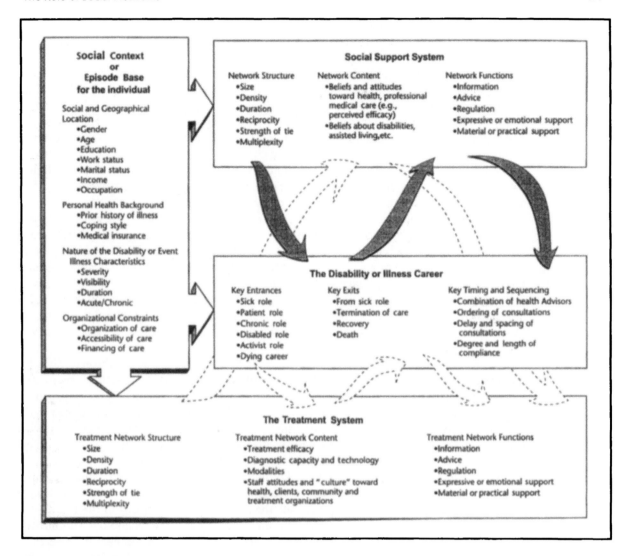

Figure 19.2. The Revised Network Episode Model
SOURCE: Pescosolido and Boyer (1999).

worlds. Pathways add the element of order, that is, the sequences of advisers or practices used to deal with a disability or confront an acute episode of health problems during the disability career. Are requests for formal medical services different if the person seeks that care first, followed by self-help groups, versus contacting these groups first and then entering the medical care system? Only by following individuals and mapping out the nature of the contacts they make, the experiences they have, and the outcomes that result (health, social, and otherwise) can we understand the lives of persons with disabilities and how they cope with problems as they arise. Because this is a relatively new conceptualization, we have little information about either patterns or pathways to care, in general, and none that could be found on physical disabilities from a search of the social science and medical literatures (see the review in a later section).

Whatever the patterns or pathways, disability careers are not assumed to occur in a vacuum in the NEM. They are embedded in personal lives and changing communities. The NEM conceptualizes the idea of "community" through the idea of a dynamic social support system (top stream, Figure 19.2). It does this through breaking down the community into the set of social networks that individuals have. The structure (e.g., size), content (e.g., beliefs about and experiences with the medical system), and functions (e.g., support or coercion) of social networks mark the wide range of people who might be consulted regarding a disability. At any time, network advisers may or may not be consulted, they may or may not be a stable set, or they may or may not be consistent in their advice.

In any case, the nature of encounters that people have in their day-to-day lives helps to provide meaning to issues surrounding the health or physical impairment. For example, if individuals see mental health impairments as crises of faith, as bad marriages, as stress in child rearing, or as any of a number of other things beside illness, they may visit faith healers, spiritualists, or clergy (Lubchansky, Egri, and Stokes 1970; Rogler and Hollingshead 1961). If they or others around them see the problem as a result of "bad character" rather than illness, they might seek out police and lawyers (Cummings and Harrington 1963; Hiday 1992; Link et al. 1999). If they conceptualize their "problem" as physical illness (e.g., fatigue associated with depression), they may visit physicians, try an exercise regime, or start taking vitamins.

The NEM, following on the general tenets of social network theory, suggests that all these characteristics of social networks have to be taken into account to give us a sense of how much influence is being exerted on the person with a disability and to determine the trajectory or direction of that "push." For example, is the influence toward or away from organized groups that emphasize the need for larger social changes to allow persons with disabilities to exercise their rights as members of the community (e.g., becoming an activist in the disability rights movement)? That is, the size of a network calibrates the potential amount of influence that can be leveraged, but the beliefs and experiences of individuals in social networks guide them in a particular direction.

Because the NEM is oriented to understanding how individuals move through different kinds of systems of care, and given the dominance of the formal health care sector in many contemporary societies, the "bottom stream" in Figure 19.2 attempts to depict the reciprocal influence of the formal treatment system on the lives of persons with disabilities and on their social support systems. While some kind of "scientific" treatment system exists in every society, what that system looks like, who has access, what is offered, and how difficult it is for people to get care can be very different, even within the same society (Andersen 1995). The NEM conceptualizes the medical system as a changing set of providers and organizations with which individuals may or may not have contact. Similar to the community and the disability career, it changes over time—perhaps on a very different scale than the other two streams in the NEM—but changing nonetheless in response to the problems people have, the technology and medical knowledge that exists, the resources that society makes available, and community preferences and demands (e.g., see Albrecht 1992 on the "disability business").

In the same way that social networks can help us break down the community into the set of contacts people have, the network perspective allows us to unpack what happens to people when they access the formal treatment sector and how their experiences affect whether they come back, follow medical advice, or give positive or negative reports to others about their experiences in the medical care system. The treatment system can be important in shaping network contacts for persons with disabilities, their families, and other people who become involved (e.g., social service workers, activists). Like the community, the treatment system can provide a rich set of helpful, supportive people for individuals, or it can allow for contacts that are only brief, impersonal, and antagonistic. The kinds of social networks that exist in treatment settings create a climate of care, affecting the work of the medical providers and shaping reactions of individuals who come for assistance (Pescosolido 1996a, 1996b; Pescosolido et al. 1995).

The left side of Figure 19.2 represents the foundation, the larger social context, and the starting point for all three changing dynamic streams of the disability career, the social support system, and the treatment system. All are anchored in the social locations, histories, and past or current problems that people have. For example, sociodemographic characteristics can affect the kinds of network ties people have. Women, for example, tend to have more social network ties and to be more involved in caretaker networks than men (Cook 1988; Thoits 1995). The history, severity, and nature of the health or physical impairment shape the disability career and the extent to which individuals in the social support system and even the treatment system experience "burnout" (Tausig et al. 1992; Wright 1994). In fact, a number of studies (e.g., Bowling and Browne 1991) find that health status itself is a more important predictor of outcomes such as emotional well-being than are social networks. However, even individuals' evaluation of their health status depends, to a great extent, on consultation with and response to the information, reactions, and beliefs of others.

In sum, the NEM offers a dynamic approach, rooted in the community and its institutions, to understand the lives of persons with disabilities. It incorporates ideas from other existing models but insists that we understand what happens to people in both the short and long run. It proposes that the social interactions that we have with one another, even within large and sometimes daunting social institutions such as the medical care system or the workplace, form the basis of our actions and outcomes. Rather than one more "contingency" or "utility," the NEM sees interaction in social networks as the underlying mechanism at work, thereby contextualizing the response to disabilities in everyday life. The types of social networks characteristic of an historical era reflect and shape the structure of social relations, the social construction of health and social problems, and the societal response to them (Pescosolido and Rubin 2000).

WHAT WE KNOW: THE ROLE OF SOCIAL NETWORKS IN RECOGNIZING AND DEALING WITH THE ONSET OF HEALTH AND PHYSICAL IMPAIRMENT

"Fred is very, very sick," Rebecca's husband explained, "He has schizophrenia." "You're full of shit," said Gary, "There's nothing wrong with my brother. You're the one who's sick." And he walked out of the house and has never talked to Rebecca or her husband since. And if he talks about them, he doesn't use their names. (Winerip 1994:100)

There are two fundamental but closely connected issues addressed in this section on the role that others, such as Fred's brother, play during early phases of the disability career. First, how do individuals or those around them come to see that there may be a problem? Deny a problem? Second, and often intertwined with it, how do they respond and what kinds of assistance do they activate in response? From drug and alcohol abuse (D'Annuo and Price 1986), to cancer (Funch and Mettler 1982; McKinney et al. 1993), to Alzheimer's disease (Pillemer and Suitor 1993), to mental health and illness (Meeks and Murrell 1994; Wellman 1982), and to HIV/AIDS (Wright and Shuff 1995), the role of community ties has been seen as central to the causes of and responses to problems. A longitudinal study in Finland, for example, found that interpersonal conflict at work, combined with marital conflicts at home, produced higher rates of work disability (Appleberg et al. 1996). A review of previous research on African Americans found that both kin and nonkin networks play a role in defining the significance of personal problems as well as providing access to professional services (Taylor and Perkins 1996)—specifically, in disseminating health information to prevent obesity in African American women (Melnyk and Weinstein 1994).

These findings are not limited to the United States or to industrial countries. In Ecuador, the existence of complex social networks has been documented, which helps to interpret disease and structure responses that combine Western, traditional, religious, and lay family healing options (Pedersen and Coloma 1983). In Africa, traditional healers are being seen as an important part of the struggle against AIDS because they have considerable authority, including the ability to reinterpret cultural categories and endow behavior with new meaning (Schoepf 1992).

Health researchers have always recognized that individuals draw advice and assistance from what Kleinman (1980) calls "lay" and "folk" systems of care as well as the formal health care system. However, a serious effort to incorporate social networks into models of health and illness behavior began in the 1970s with Freidson's (1970) theory of the "lay referral system."

Freidson conceptualized the size (extended or truncated) and network beliefs about scientific medical care (congruent or noncongruent) as affecting the probability of using lay, folk, or professional care. Following up on these insights, a number of consistent findings emerge. First, larger networks hold a greater capacity for care and often result in lower use of the formal system. For example, larger social networks are negatively related to institutionalization for the elderly (Steinbach 1992). In fact, when members of intense social networks decide to move elderly persons into residential care homes, medical researchers have evaluated the cases as more serious than other cases (Bear 1990). Second, those outside the family network are often critical in getting people into formal health care (e.g., Taylor and Perkins 1996). Police, neighbors, coworkers, friends, and even bystanders are more likely to suggest medical attention than those inside the family circle (Calnan 1983; Clausen and Yarrow 1955).

Networks have been shown to affect not only whether individuals use the formal health care system but also how they use it. While the likelihood of hospitalization for persons experiencing a psychotic episode decreased with network size, the number of services actually used for those who did enter the system actually increased with larger reported network size (Becker et al. 1997). Among the elderly in Israel, respondents with the most diversified networks (e.g., with the greatest network range) made the greatest use of health services, while those with networks limited to family members used services least (Litwin 1997). Finally, those with psychiatric disabilities who had the fewest community support networks were also likely to report the most ties to the social service system (Meeks and Murrell 1994).[2]

WHAT WE KNOW: THE ROLE OF SOCIAL NETWORKS IN "TREATMENT"—RECEIVING CARE FOR DISABILITIES WITHIN THE MEDICAL SYSTEM

I signed up for five years of psychoanalysis and that was destructive to me. The woman who became my analyst completely misunderstood the problems. She kept criticizing me. . . . She wasn't right for me anyway. She wasn't very good. And the analysis really hurt me. (Karp 1996:117)

I think he's the best doctor I've ever had. He just knows what the hell I'm talking about. He's empathetic but he's not, you know, coddling. . . . You know, we're on the same wave length. (Karp 1996:117)

While these internal networks have received far less attention, these statements by individuals suffering from depression provide a strong sense of the importance of social networks in care. Three types of relationships or social network ties are important here. They are ties between individuals and providers (client-provider), among providers within organizations (provider-provider), and among providers across organizations (agency-agency). These ties create instrumental and affective resources that can be brought to bear during the course of treatment.

The idea that the type of relationships forged in a health care setting affects what happens to individuals is hinted at in studies of how the "quality" of instruction on exercises influenced individuals with arthritis (Dexter and Brandt 1993). Such relationships were also examined in studies of the "alliance" formed in mental health treatment between clients and providers (Solomon et al. 1995) and with the success of both child and adult mental health programs that focus on creating and sustaining contacts between the "person" and the "system" through community-based care (e.g., Glisson 1994; McFarlane et al. 1996; Stein and Test 1980). Furthermore, the "compliance" literature suggests that patients' perceptions of their integration into the treatment setting are at least as powerful predictors of repeat utilization and acceptance of medical regimes as are sociodemographic characteristics (e.g., see Blackwell's 1976 review; see also Hall and Dornan 1988; Scarpaci 1988). This involves dissecting the "working alliance," broader than the doctor-patient relationship, to understand when, why, and which type of alliances result in greater quality of life, satisfaction with care, lower symptomatology, and more positive attitudes toward taking medication. For example, in a cardiac rehabilitation program, those individuals who reported positive social network interactions with staff had increased motivation to follow recommended changes in health behaviors. Those who reported value conflicts with staff reported less motivation (Fleury 1993). The staff's perception of clients' social networks affects outcomes as well. For example, in Britain, persons with psychiatric disabilities who have been hospitalized but who reported larger social networks were more likely to be selected for "community reprovision" (i.e., treatment in community-based care) (Jones 1993).

The shift from "activity-passivity" or even "guidance-cooperation" models of the physician-patient interaction to a "mutual participation" model (Szaz and Hollender 1984) has occurred, to a large extent, by the challenge of disabilities, particularly long-term health impairments such as mental illness and HIV/AIDS. They require a serious and extended look at the nature of the interactions that exist between medical providers and their patients and among the medical care providers themselves. Case management, now a mainstay in these and other areas, brings the importance of inside social networks to the fore. The ability to build a relationship of contact, trust, support, and practical assistance is fundamentally shaped by the nature of the case management approach. Different case management models mark out the regular and routine contacts that providers are supposed to establish with one another and with clients, setting varying levels of therapeutic, personal, and community involvement (Hargreaves et al. 1984; Rose 1992). When a team model is in operation, social interactions in the team strengthen the range and potential of internal social networks (see Pescosolido et al. 1995 for a review of case management models in a network perspective).

Furthermore, case management highlights the fuzzy line between inside and outside networks and emphasizes the increasingly important role of social network "bridges" as managed care shifts responsibility from treatment in hospitals and clinics to community-based care (Pescosolido and Kronenfeld 1995). In one of Detroit's community programs, for example, social networks of the village health workers were critical to program success (Schultz et al. 1997). The Save Our Sisters project, focused on breast cancer in the African American community, developed "natural helpers" (lay advisers) whose role was to assist with social supports in the community, negotiate with professionals, and mobilize community support (Eng 1993; Eng and Smith 1995). However, Gartner (1996) found that friction between self-help groups and professional help sources came from differences in the type of knowledge considered "legitimate" in each group. The focus on personal experience and peer support in the former versus objective knowledge and scientific methodology in the latter prohibited close cooperation.

Although the coordination (or lack thereof) among medical and social services agencies has always marked whether there is a seamless continuum of care or serious "cracks" in the system, the emergence of managed care has also increased the focus on the network connections across organizations (i.e., interorganizational structure) (Alba 1982; Knoke 1990). These structures determine resource and information flows across systems and organizations, and they influence the behavior of individuals who are connected to or operate within them. Not surprisingly from a network perspective, internal social network ties among providers that go across organizations (interprofessional networks) appear to be more important than either those that exist within an organization or those that are formally mandated by policy or contract (i.e., the "boundary spanners") (Aldrich and Herker 1977; DiMaggio 1991). For example, the receipt of supplemental security income (SSI) among homeless individuals with psychiatric disabilities actually increased social networks compared to those who did not receive it (Estroff et al. 1997). Furthermore, Social Security disability applicants and beneficiaries with mental illness who received case management from rehabilitation specialists were more likely to find a job than did those who received routine mental health services (Okapaku et al. 1997). As the length and number of hospital admissions increased for persons with chronic psychiatric disability, the number of networks remained the same, but the number of relatives and friends decreased, replaced by persons met through the mental health system (Holmes-Eber and Riger 1990;

Pescosolido, Wright, and Lutfey 1999). However, as Meeks and Murrell (1994) note, these relationships tended to be nonreciprocal. Participation in support groups for families of persons with psychiatric disabilities increased their knowledge of mental illness and also resulted in more active participation in the treatment process (Shapiro et al. 1983).

WHAT WE KNOW: THE ROLE OF SOCIAL NETWORKS IN MAINTENANCE AND OUTCOMES

I didn't think about the deaf any more than you'd think about anybody with a different voice. "Oh," she said emphatically, "those people weren't handicapped. They were just deaf." (Groce 1985:5)

Nora Groce's (1985) study of hereditary deafness on Martha's Vineyard provides the quintessential example of how the larger culture shapes the way that disabilities are experienced and given meaning. Because of the close-knit set of social networks on the island and the frequency of the disability, sign language became a standard skill of all island residents. Social networks in the "receiving" community, then, become a critical factor in outcomes.

One of the most fascinating and puzzling findings of the World Health Organization's (WHO's) International Study of Schizophrenia is the difference in outcomes between the "developed" and "developing countries" (Jablensky et al. 1992). Specifically, in Nigeria, Colombia, and India, individuals with schizophrenia were more likely to have a "remitting" course, be symptom free, function without social impairments, and spend less time in psychiatric hospitals in the two years following the original evaluation. The researchers investigated whether the particular type or course of the disease was influential (e.g., whether the individuals in the developing countries were more likely to have "acute transient psychoses") but found that wanting. Rather, they suspect and marshal some evidence of the role of differences in the level of social interaction between individuals in the study and key people in their social environments.

Furthermore, Rogers, Hassell, and Nicolaas (1999) point out that the capacity and willingness of other people to substitute works tasks in the community affect the degree to which individuals can use self-care as a strategy for staying at home rather than in the hospital. They call for a "shared agenda" between professionals inside the system and community members outside the system because smaller networks are associated with longer disability status (see also Anderson et al. 1984).

Finally, recent research suggests that what may distinguish successful from unsuccessful forms of community-based care may be just that—the types of social relationships formed or not formed among individuals, families, other caretakers, providers, and communities. Surprisingly, initiatives with state-of-the-art clinical programs failed, as did those that assumed that organizational change would trickle down to individuals (Pescosolido 1996a; Pescosolido et al. 1998). Many that succeeded are low-tech by comparison. Those programs that either allowed providers to be flexible in bringing tailored solutions to the individual's day-to-day problems of community living or those that attended to the relationships among providers, family members, key individuals in the community (e.g., landlords, work supervisors, neighbors), *and* clients have shown better outcomes (e.g., in the area of psychiatric disabilities, see assertive community treatment for adults and service coordination for children) (Glisson 1994; McFarlane et al. 1996; Stein and Test 1980). For example, continuous treatment teams (CTT) and assertive community treatment (ACT) link individuals with serious mental illness (primarily schizophrenia) to a team of providers (at an ideal ratio of 40:10) who range from psychiatrists, nurses, housing specialists, social workers, and peer counselors. This program requires that providers go into the community. Ideally, the team reviews the situation for each client daily, assesses the needs, and develops a contact plan, which may include shopping, laundry, and negotiating with landlords—in essence, replacing the social safety net.

More generally, Charmaz (1991) argues that both camaraderie and competition, which often characterize rehabilitation programs, offer "incentives." They promote "accountability" to fellow travelers as well as spouses, providers, and others. In sum, successful models mark profound differences in the reconstruction and management of community relations for people whose social networks have been damaged, altered, or simply inadequate to deal with the new challenges that chronic illness or disability present. They have, more or less, succeeded in reconstructing the "community" for clients by creating a synthetic, professionally based set of social network ties that are flexible and resilient and fostering the development of other community ties for individuals (Pescosolido et al. 1995). They buoy the ability of those whose interactional skills and former ties have been damaged in an era that requires individuals to maintain and create their ties to social circles (Pescosolido and Rubin 2000). The team structure also prevents burnout for providers, increasing the likelihood that individuals with health and physical impairments can have some continuity of care and that they are less dependent on their relationship with one provider as in standard case management. Reviewing articles on psychosocial support, Matarese and Salmon (1997) conclude that "adjunctive medical treatment" (e.g., support groups) with a "spirit of community" improves not only outcomes but also perceptions of and responses to associated medical problems. Among Puerto Rican women with schizophrenia, those who have a network with greater range (neighbors, friends, professionals) rather than just family reported better outcomes (Garrison 1978). Finally, Stein, Rappaport, and Seidman (1995) find that the greater the congruence between the perceptions of persons with psychiatric disabilities and their network ties about the situation, the better individuals' social and psychological functioning.

WHAT NEEDS TO BE DONE: QUESTIONS AND METHODS FOR FUTURE DISABILITY STUDIES

A lot of people realize they need help. But a lot of people be sayin', "well you know they went to the crazy house." You know, something like that, you know, but, no one's ever criticized me and I think people think more of me now, you know, cause I told my pastor that I was in a hospital, you know, and um, he said, "that's good," you know, "I'm glad to see that you're seeking help so you can get on with your life," you know . . . it takes a lot for a man to break down and say "okay, I need help." (Indianapolis Network Mental Health Study: Case 171) (Pescosolido, Brooks-Gardner, and Lubell 1998)

The first generation of network studies has been promising. They have provided evidence that others around us are important for our health and well-being, as reflected in the statement of our respondent in Indianapolis. But, not surprisingly, they raise as many questions as they have provided this important lead. We have begun the work of providing a new conceptual framework, but much remains to be done. Moving to a model that acknowledges the complexities of people's day-to-day lives requires new ways of thinking about study design, methods of data collection, and analytic methods. What is the best way to find out who important network ties are (i.e., the question of appropriate name generators)? Can we settle for just asking how many ties do people have and what they, in general, think, provide, and suggest? Or do we have to enumerate who those people are and exactly what they do? How do we observe or measure "weak" ties, which seem to have such a crucial information function?

Berkman (1986), drawing from the work on the Tecumseh Community Study (House et al. 1982), suggests that we still have not developed adequate measures of social support and social networks. Measures tend to be general and rather crude, not allowing an examination of the specific kinds of ties or qualities that are essential to health. Furthermore, we are only beginning to examine methodological issues of validity and reliability of instruments (O'Reilly 1988). And we are only starting to examine how social networks change, in general (Suitor, Wellman, and Morgan 1996; Wellman, Tindall, and Nazer 1996), or when they are under stress (Leik and Chalkley 1996).

We must also confront the issue of the causal relationship, not just the association, between social networks and health status. That is, the ability to form and maintain social ties may be the result of health, illness, and disability problems, not simply factors implicated in their cause (Berkman 1986). Mental health, for example, affects social relationships. Calling this a social selection process, Johnson (1991) argues that this has been neglected in favor of the other causal direction (i.e., social networks cause mental health). However, the NEM suggests that neither, in itself, is an adequate conceptualization because we can expect a continuous flow of change and a reciprocal influence.

We need to understand the efficacy of social networks. Some suggest that it is biological. In a study of middle-aged men in Finland, Helminen et al. (1997) found that men with lower social participation had higher mean values of plasma fibrinogen than men who had higher scores in overall support. McIntosh et al. (1996) found similar effects for platelet status, both of which are implicated in cardiovascular impairments. Others suggest that it is social and psychological. Rosenfield and Wenzel (1997) conclude that supportive and negative relationships appear to work by affecting individuals' self-esteem. Hammer (1983) suggests that the underlying mechanism is social feedback.

Finally, how can we facilitate the development of social networks in treatment settings and communities for persons with disabilities? What are the policy implications and recommendations? Little work has been done here, but what has been done is suggestive. Simkiss and Floyd (1995) found, for example, that in the United Kingdom, job placement assistance capacities are so strained for people with visual disabilities that the Royal National Institute for the Blind Employment Network is considering a computerized solution. Would such a plan improve outcomes or reduce them because they remove the human social connection? How could the computer be used to facilitate social interactions? Sharf (1997) finds that women's communication on the Breast Cancer List (an online discussion group) provided information and support, which led to greater feelings of empowerment.

These studies and the issues they raise have only begun to open the door to the potential of naturally occurring and deliberately constructed social networks to improve the lives of persons with disabilities.

NOTES

1. In manualized treatment, the exact protocol (including technologies, medications, and provider behavior) are laid out in a fashion that is standardized and to be followed exactly by providers.

2. Of course, there is research that either does not find a network effect in terms of protecting individuals for disease and disability or finds detrimental effects of networks (e.g., for a good summary, see Rogers et al. 1999: 112-13).

REFERENCES

Alba, Richard D. 1982. "Taking Stock of Network Analysis: A Decade's Results." *Sociology of Organizations* 1:39-74.

Albrecht, Gary. 1992. *The Disability Business: Rehabilitation in America*. Newbury Park, CA: Sage.

Aldrich, Howard and D. Herker 1977. "Boundary Spanning Roles and Organization Structure." *Academy of Management Review* 2:217-30.

Andersen, Ronald. 1995. "Revisiting the Behavioral Model and Access to Care: Does It Matter?" *Journal of Health and Social Behavior* 36:1-10.

Anderson, C. M., G. Hogarty, T. Bayer, and R. Needleman. 1984. "Expressed Emotion and Social Networks of Parents of Schizophrenic Patients." *British Journal of Psychiatry* 144:247-55.

Appleberg, Kirsi, Kalle Romanov, Kauko Heikkila, Marja-Liisa Honkasalo, and Markku Koskenvuo. 1996. "Interpersonal Conflict as a Predictor of Work Disability: A Follow-Up Study of 15,348 Finnish Employees." *Journal of Psychosomatic Research* 40:157-67.

Bear, M. 1990. "Social Networks and Health: Impact of Returning Home after Entry into Residential Care Homes." *The Gerontologist* 30:30-34.

Becker, Thomas, Graham Thornicroft, Morven Leese, Paul McCrone, Sonia Johnson, Maya Albert, and David Turner. 1997. "Social Networks and Service Use among Representative Cases of Psychosis in South London." *British Journal of Psychiatry* 171:15-19.

Berkman, Lisa F. 1986. "Social Networks, Support, and Health: Taking the Next Step Forward." *American Journal of Epidemiology* 123:559-62.

———. 1987. "Assessing Social Networks and Social Support in Epidemiological Studies." *Revue d'Epidemiologie et de Sante Publique* 35:46-53.

Berkman, Lisa. F. and S. L. Syme. 1979. "Social Networks, Host Resistance and Mortality: A Nine-Year Follow-Up Study of Alameda County Residents." *American Journal of Epidemiology* 109:186-204.

Blackwell, Barry. 1976. "Treatment Adherence." *British Journal of Psychiatry* 129:513-31.

Bowling, A. and P. D. Browne. 1991. "Social Networks, Health, and Emotional Well-Being among the Oldest Old in London." *Journal of Gerontology* 46:S20-S32.

Calnan, M. 1983. "Social Networks and Patterns of Help-Seeking Behaviors." *Social Science and Medicine* 17:25-28.

Cassel, J. 1976. "The Contribution of the Social Environment to Host Resistance." *American Journal of Epidemiology* 104:107-23.

Charmaz, Kathy. 1991. *Good Days, Bad Days: The Self in Chronic Illness and Time.* New Brunswick, NJ: Rutgers University Press.

Clausen, John and Marian Yarrow. 1955. "Pathways to the Mental Hospital." *Journal of Social Issues* 11:25-32.

Cohen, C., J. Teresi, and C. Blum. 1994. "The Role of Caregiver Social Networks in Alzheimer's Disease." *Social Science and Medicine* 38:1483-90.

Cook, J. A. 1988. "Who 'Mothers' the Chronically Mentally Ill?" *Family Relations* 37:42-49.

Coser, Rose Laub. 1952. "Authority and Decision-Making in a Hospital: A Comparative Analysis." *American Sociological Review* 23:56-63.

Cresswell, C. M., L. Kuipers, and M. J. Power. 1992. "Social Networks and Support in Long-Term Psychiatric Patients." *Psychological Medicine* 22:1019-26.

Cummings, E. and C. Harrington. 1963. "Clergyman as Counselor." *American Journal of Sociology* 69:234.

D'Annuo, Thomas and Richard A. Price. 1986. "Linked Systems: Drug Abuse and Mental Health Services." Pp. 233-76 in *The Organization of Mental Health Services,* edited by W. Richard Scott and Bruce L. Black. Beverly Hills, CA: Sage.

Dexter, Phyllis and Kenneth Brandt. 1993. "Relationships between Social Background and Medical Care in Osteoarthritis." *Journal of Rheumatology* 20:698-703.

DiMaggio, Paul A. 1991. "The Micro-Macro Dilemma in Organizational Studies." Pp. 34-47 in *Macro-Micro Interrelationships,* edited by Joan Huber. Newbury Park, CA: Sage.

Durkheim, Emile. 1951. *Suicide.* New York: Free Press.

Eng, E. 1993. "The Save Our Sisters Project: A Social Network Strategy for Reaching Rural Black Women." *Cancer* 72 (Suppl.): 1071-77.

Eng, E. and J. Smith. 1995. "Natural Help Functions of Lay Health Advisors in Breast Cancer Education." *Breast Cancer Research and Treatment* 35:23-29.

Estroff, Sue E., D. L. Patrick, Catherine Zimmer, and William S. Lachicotte. 1997. "Pathways to Disability Income among Persons with Severe, Persistent Psychiatric Disorders." *The Milbank Quarterly* 75:495-532.

Fadiman, Anne. 1997. *The Spirit Catches You and You Fall Down.* New York: Noonday.

Fischer, C. 1982. *To Dwell among Friends.* Berkeley: University of California Press.

Fleury, J. 1993. "An Exploration of the Role of Social Networks in Cardiovascular Risk Reduction." *Heart and Lung* 22:134-44.

Freidson, Eliot. 1970. *Profession of Medicine.* New York: Dodd Mead.

Froland, C., G. Brodsky, M. Olson, and L. Stewart. 1979. "Social Support and Social Adjustment: Implications for Mental Health Professionals." *Community Mental Health Journal* 15:82-93.

Funch, D. P. and C. Mettler. 1982. "The Role of Social Support in Relation to Recovery from Breast Surgery." *Social Science and Medicine* 16:91-97.

Garrison, V. 1978. "Support Systems of Schizophrenic and Nonschizophrenic Puerto Rican Women in New York City." *Schizophrenia Bulletin* 4:561-96.

Gartner, Audrey. 1996. "Professionals and Self-Help: The Uses of Creative Tension." *Social Policy* 27:47-52.

Glisson, C. 1994. "The Effect of Services Coordination Teams on Outcomes for Children in State Custody." *Administration in Social Work* 18:1-23.

Gochman, David S. 1997. *Handbook of Health Behavior Research*. Vol. 1, *Personal and Social Determinants*. New York: Plenum.

Gottlieb, B. 1992. "Quandries in Translating Social Support Concepts to Intervention." Pp. 293-309 in *The Meaning and Measurement of Social Support,* edited by H. Veiel and U. Baumann. New York: Hemisphere.

Granovetter, Mark. 1973. "The Strength of Weak Ties." *American Journal of Sociology* 78:1360-80.

Groce, Nora Ellen. 1985. *Everyone Here Spoke Sign Language: Hereditary Deafness on Martha's Vineyard*. Cambridge, MA: Harvard University Press.

Hall, Judith A. and Michael C. Dornan. 1988. "What Patients Like about Their Medical Care and How Often They Are Asked." *Social Science and Medicine* 27:935-39.

Hammer, M. 1983. " 'Core' and 'Extended' Social Networks in Relation to Health and Illness." *Social Science and Medicine* 17:405-11.

Hargreaves, William A., Richard E. Shaw, Richard Shadoan, E. Walker, Robert W. Surber, and Jessica Gaynor. 1984. "Measuring Case Management Activity." *Journal of Nervous and Mental Disease* 172:296-300.

Helminen, Annelie, Tuomo Rankinen, Sari Vaisanen, and Rainer Rauramaa. 1997. "Social Network in Relation to Plasma Fibrinogen." *Journal of Biosocial Science* 29:129-39.

Hiday, V. 1992. "Coercion in Civil Commitment: Process, Preferences and Outcome." *International Journal of Law and Psychiatry* 15:359-77.

Hohmann, Ann A. 1999. "A Contextual Model for Clinical Mental Health Effectiveness Research." *Mental Health Services Research* 1:83-91.

Holmes-Eber, P. and S. Riger. 1990. "Hospitalization and the Composition of Mental Patients' Social Networks." *Schizophrenia Bulletin* 16:157-64.

House, J. S., C. Robbins, and H. L. Metzner. 1982. "The Association of Social Relationships and Activities with Mortality: Prospective Evidence from the Tecumseh Community Health Study." *American Journal of Epidemiology* 116:123-40.

Jablensky, A., N. Sartorius, G. Ernberg, M. Anker, A. Korten, J. E. Cooper, R. Day, and A. Bertelsen. 1992. *Psychological Medicine*. Washington, DC: American Psychological Association.

Johnson, T. P. 1991. "Mental Health, Social Relations, and Social Selection: A Longitudinal Analysis." *Journal of Health and Social Behavior* 32:408-23.

Jones, D. 1993. "The TAPS Project 11: The Selection of Patients for Reprovision." *British Journal of Psychiatry* 19 (Suppl.): 36-39.

Kadushin, Charles. 1966. "Friends and Supporters of Psychotherapy: On Social Circles in Urban Life." *American Sociological Review* 31:786-802.

Karp, David A. 1996. *Speaking of Sadness: Depression, Disconnection and the Meanings of Mental Illness*. New York: Oxford University Books.

Kleinman, Arthur. 1980. *Patients and Healers in the Context of Culture*. Berkeley: University of California Press.

Knoke, David. 1990. *Political Networks*. New York: Cambridge University Press.

Leik, R. K. and M. A. Chalkley. 1996. "On the Stability of Network Relations under Stress." *Social Networks* 19:63-74.

Link, Bruce G., Jo C. Phelan, Michaline Bresnahanm Ann Stueve, and Bernice A. Pescosolido. 1999. "Public Conceptions of Mental Illness: Labels, Causes, Dangerousness, and Social Distance." *American Journal of Public Health* 89:1328-33.

Litwin, Howard. 1997. "Support Network Type and Health Service Utilization." *Research on Aging* 19:274-99.

Lubchansky, Isaac, Gladys Egri, and Janet Stokes. 1970. "Puerto Rican Spiritualists View Mental Illness: The Faith Healer as Paraprofessional." *American Journal of Psychiatry* 127:88-97.

Matarese, Susan M. and Paul G. Salmon. 1997. "The Spirit of Community in Adjunctive Medical Treatments: Humanizing Trends in the Care of the Ill." *Midwest Quarterly* 38:329-37.

McFarlane, W. R., E. Lukens, B. Link, R. Dushap, S. A. Deakins, M. Newmark, E. J. Dunne, B. Horen, and J. Toran. 1996. "Multiple-Family Groups and Psychoeducation in the Treatment of Schizophrenia." *Archives of General Psychiatry* 52:679-87.

McIntosh, William, Howard B. Kaplan, Karen S. Kubena, Robyn Bateman, and Wendall Landmann. 1996. "Platelet Status, Stress and Social Support in the Elderly." *Applied Behavioral Science Review* 4:39-54.

McKinney, Martha M., Joseph P. Morrissey, and Arnold D. Kaluzny. 1993. "Interorganizational Exchanges as Performance Markets in a Community Cancer Network." *Health Services Research* 28:459-78.

Meeks, S. and S. A. Murrell. 1994. "Service Providers in the Social Networks of Clients with Severe Mental Illness." *Schizophrenia Bulletin* 20:399-409.

Melnyk, M. G. and E. Weinstein. 1994. "Preventing Obesity in Black Women by Targeting Adolescents: A Literature Review." *Journal of the American Dietetic Association* 94:536-40.

Morgan, M., D. L. Patrick, and J. R. Charlton. 1984. "Social Networks and Psychosocial Support among Disabled People." *Social Science and Medicine* 19:489-97.

Morrisey, J. P., M. Calloway, W. T. Bartko, M. S. Ridgeley, H. H. Goldman, and R. J. Paulson. 1994. "Local Mental Health Authorities and Service System Change: Evidence from the Robert Wood Johnson Program on Chronic Mental Illness." *The Milbank Quarterly* 72:49-80.

Okapaku, Samuel O., Kathryn H. Anderson, Amy E. Sibulkin, J. S. Butler, and Leonard Bickman. 1997. "The Effectiveness of a Multidisciplinary Case Management Intervention on the Employment of SSDI Applicants and Beneficiaries." *Psychiatric Rehabilitation Journal* 20:34-41.

O'Reilly, P. 1988. "Methodological Issues in Social Support and Social Network Research." *Social Science and Medicine* 26:863-73.

Pagel, M. D. and J. Becker 1987. "Social Networks: We Get by with (and in spite of) 'Little Help from Our Friends.'" *Journal of Personality and Social Psychology* 53:793-804.

Pearlin, L. I. and C. S. Aneshensel. 1986. "Coping and Social Supports: Their Functions and Applications." Pp. 417-37 in *Applications of Social Science to Clinical Medicine and Health Policy*, edited by D. Mechanic and L. H. Aiken. New Brunswick, NJ: Rutgers University Press.

Pedersen, D. and C. Coloma. 1983. "Traditional Medicine in Ecuador: The Structure of the Non-Formal Health Systems." *Social Science and Medicine* 17:1249-55.

Pescosolido, B. A. 1991. "Illness Careers and Network Ties: A Conceptual Model of Utilization and Compliance." *Advances in Medical Sociology* 2:161-84.

———. 1992. "Beyond Rational Choice: The Social Dynamics of How People Seek Help." *American Journal of Sociology* 97:1096-1138.

———. 1996a. "Bringing the 'Community' into Utilization Models: How Social Networks Link Individuals to Changing Systems of Care." *Research in the Sociology of Health Care* 13A:171-97.

———. 1996b. "Bringing People Back in Why Social Networks Matter in Effectiveness Research." Paper presented at the CEI Workshop of the American Public Health Association, November, Washington, DC.

Pescosolido, B. A. and C. A. Boyer. 1999. "How Do People Come to Use Mental Health Services? Current Knowledge and Changing Perspectives." Pp. 392-411 in *A Handbook for the Study of Mental Health*, edited by A. V. Horwitz and T. L. Scheid. New York: Cambridge University Press.

Pescosolido, B. A., C. A. Boyer, and K. M. Lubell. 1999. "The Social Dynamics of Responding to Mental Health Problems: Past, Present and Future Challenges to Understanding Individuals' Use of Services." In *Handbook for the Sociology of Mental Health*, edited by C. Aneshensel and J. Phelan. New York: Plenum.

Pescosolido, B. A., C. Brooks-Gardner, and K. M. Lubell. 1998. "Choice, Coercion, and 'Muddling Through': Accounts of Help-Seeking from 'First-Timers.'" *Social Science and Medicine* 46 (2): 275-86.

Pescosolido, B. A. and J. J. Kronenfeld. 1995. "Health, Illness and Healing in an Uncertain Era: Challenges from and for Medical Sociology." *Journal of Health and Social Behavior* 36:5-33.

Pescosolido, B. A. and Beth A. Rubin. 2000. "The Web of Group Affiliations Revisited: Social Life, Postmodernism and Sociology." *American Sociological Review* 65:52-76.

Pescosolido, B. A., E. R. Wright, M. Alegría, and M. Vera. 1998. "Formal and Informal Utilization Patterns among the Poor with Mental Health Problems in Puerto Rico." *Medical Care* 36:1057-72.

Pescosolido, B. A., E. R. Wright, and K. Lutfey. 1999. "The Changing Hopes, Worries and Community Supports of Individuals Moving from a Closing Long-Term Care Facility." *Journal of Behavioral Health Services and Research* 26:276-88.

Pescosolido, B. A., E. R. Wright, and W. P. Sullivan. 1995. "Communities of Care: A Theoretical Perspective on Case Management Models in Mental Health." Pp. 37-80 in *Advances in Medical Sociology*, edited by Gary Albrecht. Greenwich, CT: JAI.

Pillemer, Karl and J. Jill Suitor. 1993. "It Takes One to Help One: Effects of Status Similarity on Well-Being." LCI Working Paper No. 93-01, Life Course Institute, Cornell University, New York.

Ragin, Charles C. 1987. *Comparative Methods: Moving beyond Qualitative and Quantitative Strategies.* Berkeley: University of California Press.

Rogers, Anne, Karen Hassell, and Gerry Nicolaas. 1999. *Demanding Patients: Analysing the Use of Primary Care.* Buckingham, UK: Open University Press.

Rogler, Lloyd and August Hollingshead. 1961. "The Puerto-Rican Spiritualist as Psychiatrist." *American Journal of Sociology* 67:17-21.

Rose, Steven. 1992. "Case Management: An Advocacy/Empowerment Design." Pp. 271-97 in *Case Management and Social Work Practice,* edited by S. Rose. New York: Longman.

Rosenfield, Sara and Suzanne Wenzel. 1997. "Social Networks and Chronic Mental Illness: A Test of Four Perspectives." *Social Problems* 44:200-16.

Scarpaci, Joseph L. 1988. "Help-Seeking Behavior, Use and Satisfaction among Frequent Primary Care Users in Santiago de Chile." *Journal of Health and Social Behavior* 29:199-213.

Schiller, Lori and Amanda Bennett. 1994. *The Quiet Room: A Journey out of the Torment of Madness.* New York: Warner.

Schoenbach, V. J., B. H. Kaplan, L. Freedman, and D. C. Kleinman. 1986. "Social Ties and Mortality in Evans County, Georgia." *American Journal of Epidemiology* 123:577-91.

Schoepf, B. G. 1992. "AIDS, Sex and Condoms: African Healers and the Reinvention of Tradition in Zaire." *Medical Anthropology* 14:225-42.

Schultz, Amy J., Barbara A. Israel, Adam B. Becker, and Rose M. Hollis. 1997. " 'It's a 24-Hour Thing . . . a Living-for-Each-Other Concept': Identity, Networks, and Community in an Urban Village Health Worker Project." *Health Education and Behavior* 24:465-80.

Segal, S. P., C. Silverman, and T. Tempkin. 1995. "Characteristics and Service Use of Long-Term Members of Self-Help Agencies for Mental Health Clients." *Psychiatric Services* 46:269-74.

Shapiro, R. M., S. M. Possidente, K. C. Plum, and A. F. Lehman. 1983. "The Evaluation of a Support Group for Families of the Chronically Mentally Ill." *Psychiatric Quarterly* 55:236-41.

Sharf, Barbara E. 1997. "Communicating Breast Cancer On-Line: Support and Empowerment on the Internet." *Women and Health* 26:65-84.

Simkiss, P. and M. Floyd. 1995. "Developing a Computerized Information System for Visually Disabled People to Assist with Job Placement." *International Journal of Rehabilitation Research* 18:133-41.

Simmel, Georg. 1955. *Conflict and the Web of Group Affiliations.* New York: Basic Books.

Solomon, P., J. Draine, and M. A. Delaney. 1995. "The Working Alliance and Consumer Case Management." *Journal of Mental Health Administration* 22 (2): 126-33.

Stein, C. H., J. Rappaport, and E. Seidman. 1995. "Assessing the Social Networks of People with Psychiatric Disability from Multiple Perspectives." *Community Mental Health Journal* 31:351-67.

Stein, L. I. and M. A. Test. 1980. "An Alternative to Mental Hospital Treatment. Part 1—Conceptual Model, Treatment Program, and Clinical Evaluation." *Archives of General Psychiatry* 37:392-97.

Steinbach, U. 1992. "Social Networks, Institutionalization and Mortality among Elderly People in the United States." *Journal of Gerontology* 47:S183-90.

Suitor, J. J., B. Wellman, and D. L. Morgan. 1996. "It's about Time: How, Why, and When Networks Change." *Social Networks* 19:1-8.

Szasz, Thomas and Marc Hollender. 1984. "Models of the Doctor-Patient Relationship." Pp. 111-15 in *The Sociology of Medicine and Illness,* edited by Richard A. Kurtz and Paul Chalfant. Boston: Allyn & Bacon.

Tausig, M., G. A. Fisher, and R. C. Tessler. 1992. "Informal Systems of Care for the Chronically Mentally Ill." *Community Mental Health Journal* 28:413-25.

Taylor, K. E. and R. E. Perkins. 1996. "Identity and Coping with Mental Illness in Long-Stay Psychiatric Rehabilitation." *British Journal of Clinical Psychology* 30:73-85.

Thoits, Peggy A. 1995. "Stress, Coping and Social Support Processes: Where Are We? What Next?" *Journal of Health and Social Behavior* 36:53-79.

Umberson, Debra A. 1987. "Family Status and Health Behavior: Social Control as a Dimension of Social Integration." *Journal of Health and Social Behavior* 28:306-15.

Wellman, B. A. 1982. "Studying Personal Communities." Pp. 61-80 in *Social Structure and Network Analysis,* edited by P. Marsden and N. Lin. Beverly Hills, CA: Sage.

Wellman, B. A., R. D. Tindall, and N. Nazer. 1996. "A Decade of Network Change: Turnover, Persistence and Stability in Personal Communities." *Social Networks* 19:27-50.

White, Harrison C. 1992. *Identity and Control.* Princeton, NJ: Princeton University Press.

Winerip, Michael. 1994. *9 Highland Road: Sane Living for the Mentally Ill.* New York: Pantheon.

Wright, Eric R. 1994. "Caring for Those Who 'Can't': Gender, Network Structure, and the Burden of Caring for People with Mental Illness." Ph.D. dissertation, Indiana University.

————. 1997. "The Impact of Organizational Factors on Mental Health Professionals' Involvement with Families." *Psychiatric Services* 48:921-27.

Wright, Eric R. and Michael I. Shuff. 1995. "Specifying the Integration of Mental Health and Primary Health Care Services for Persons with HIV/AIDS: The Indiana Integration of Care Project." Working Paper No. 2, Indiana Consortium for Mental Health Services Research, Indiana University.

Zinman, S., H. T. Harp, and S. Budd, eds. 1987. *Reaching Across: Mental Health Clients Helping Each Other.* Riverside: California Network of Mental Health Clients.

Zola, Irving K. 1993. "In the Active Voice: A Reflective Review Essay on Three Books." *Policy Studies* 21:802-5.

Inclusion/Exclusion

20

An Analysis of Historical and Cultural Meanings

JEAN-FRANÇOIS RAVAUD

HENRI-JACQUES STIKER

Questions of inclusion versus exclusion of disabled persons cannot be separated from questions relative to the global processes of social cohesion or social dissociation. The way in which a society situates and treats the disabled is not independent of the way in which it constructs social bonds or dissolves them.

However, each society (and, in a broader sense, each culture) has its own fashion of integrating or excluding certain categories or certain subjects, that is, of creating social links or denying them. We must thus expect the meanings of words and practices not to remain the same over time (in the history of societies) or across space (the synchronic diversity of cultural eras). There are numerous ways of posing and answering the question of the social bond and thus of addressing inclusion and exclusion. There is not just a single set of problems relative to the inclusion and exclusion of disabled persons.

Consequently, our objective in this chapter is to avoid being restricted to a single reductive vision of the problem, whether this perspective is French, British, or North American. We shall strive to reveal the different historical and cultural facets of inclusion and exclusion and to show their origins and effects, which are both diverse and most often ambivalent. This sociological and historical observation raises a conceptual problem. The terms *inclusion* and *exclusion* operate in tandem and can be understood only in relation to one another. For any definition of inclusion, there is a corresponding definition of exclusion. This means that it is necessary to determine who are affected by exclusion and inclusion, determine what disabled persons are excluded from or what they are included in, and how and to what degree they are in or out at different times and in different social groupings.

Now that the general framework of our approach is set out, we shall proceed as follows. With point of departure in some major theories of the social bond, we will show the difference between societies that could be called premodern and those we recognize as modern societies. The aim of this distinction is to reveal that our present societies are continuously in search of processes and procedures; that is, they are unable to maintain a stable state inherited from tradition but swing ceaselessly between different models. We will lay out the structure of these models and the mechanics of these global processes using a sociological inquiry.

From the perspective of the consequences of this state of affairs in our societies, we will illustrate current forms of exclusion and inclusion and establish a typology of praxis. This typology will, in turn, illuminate our premise that the modalities of inclusion and exclusion are variable, ambivalent, and often connected, in that some of the modalities of premodern societies still crop up in modern societies.

Returning to the way in which the question of inclusion and exclusion is generally posed today, we will show the relevance and value of this historical and sociological distancing for the future of advocacy and action in the sphere of persons with disabilities. Today's problems can be profitably illuminated by a consideration of the problems of every society, even though the contemporary situation is a specific one, and history does not offer lessons.

THE FUNDAMENTAL SOCIAL PROCESSES OF EXCLUSION AND INCLUSION

Mechanical Inclusion, Organic Inclusion

These terms obviously derive from Durkheim. The French thinker, one of the fathers of sociology, had clearly seen that in modern societies of increasing complexity, one of the central phenomena was the division of labor or, in a broader sense, social division (Durkheim 1930). Unlike Spencer, who analyzed this fact from the perspective of the utility that could be gained thereby, Durkheim called attention to the increase in the "social and moral density of societies"—in other words, "the number of persons who are in effective relations with each other, with the same population volume" (Durkheim 1930:214). With such an augmentation, the system of social roles becomes increasingly differentiated and entails constant shifts in the system of norms and values. An evolutionary process is thereby initiated, in the sense that the fundamental forms of "mechanical" or "mimetic" solidarity, which were those of traditional societies, more and more give way to forms of solidarity that are "organic" or "complementary." But the latter entail increasing individualism, which conflicts with the priority that had traditionally been given to the social whole.

Durkheim's distinction is pertinent on several counts. It permits us to emphasize the dynamic character of contemporary societies as well as the permanent challenge that confronts them. On one hand, we can stress the risks of social dissociation, which are greater than in traditional societies and, on the other hand, the possibilities they have, by virtue of their organic nature, of increased integration of the new and alien.

The second interest in recalling Durkheim is to alert us to the fact that in the present global space, social groups may still proceed from a mechanical form of solidarity or at least be caught between a modern dynamic and powerful tradition. This is not to say that all trace of the "mechanical" is absent, even at the very heart of our global Western world, where exchange is continuous and rapid and technology dominant. We do well to recall that these are processes. To the extent that the ruptures are not absolute, we could interrogate African and Asian societies. We are not sufficiently competent in these matters, but there are enough indications that in such cases, the premodern and the modern are interdependent and connected.

The third point of interest in Durkheim's distinction is that it assists us in seeing the difference between exclusion *from* a society and possible exclusion *within* society. Societies founded in mechanical solidarity are indeed strongly integrated but are not able to admit "foreign bodies." When they exclude, they do so in radical fashion and are often incapable of assimilating the new. Modern societies have a very great capacity for inclusion but, on the other hand, are in danger of pulling apart by creating enclaves within themselves.

Before turning our focus fully to contemporary societies, we shall briefly describe those societies that proceed from mechanical solidarity.

Early Societies

In societies characterized by mechanical solidarity, which can be compared to the holistic societies of Louis Dumont (1966) or what Tönnies (1979) called the *Gemeinschaft,* the individual is a constituent of an irreducible whole. The individual has his or her fixed place, determined at birth, and in this sense is completely integrated. The individual is a cog in a set of gears. There is no question of changing one's place, which would jeopardize the global mechanism, leading to severe sanctions against the cog that no longer fills its function. In such societies, persons with infirmity may be integrated and may have a definitive and entirely predetermined place, but without having any claim to free participation in society. This was the case of crippled buffoons at princely courts: The role that was devolved onto them also enclosed them. Take the example of the dwarf Joseph Boruwlaski (1788), who, at the height of the eighteenth century (the threshold of the modern era), illustrates the kind of inclusion of which we are speaking. In the society of the ancien régime, he had his place as a Polish princess's *Joujou*: pet and entertainer. He was integrated—on condition of not pretending to leave his situation, which was fixed once and for all. The day he laid claim to love, marriage, and an independent life, he was rejected and condemned to wander through Europe. Nothing had been foreseen, in social terms, that would assist emancipation. Today, persons of short stature are still subject to depreciating figurations, but the right to live and work among others is no longer denied them. On the other hand, if they want a place, they have to struggle for it, for if society is legally "open," all of its spaces are conceived on a scale dictated by the average stature of its citizenry as a statistical norm: transportation, public counters, equipment, and the layout of controls. It is here that the issue of accommodation arises. The gap between the dwarf, *Joujou,* and persons of short stature today is great because we have passed from a society with mechanical solidarity, which assigned an invariable place to its members and thus included them in a certain fashion, to a society that *works* for their integration but scarcely succeeds because it has surrendered its social mechanics in favor of organicity.

Thus, we can establish a first meaning for the concept of integration in the following terms: a place, a single place, and a fixed place in a whole that has no intention of modifying itself. The person who does not have a place of this kind is literally not part of society. He or she may be the stranger, whose assimilation is problematic and presupposes, when it possibly occurs, recognition of similarity and a partial integration by means of a subgroup (Simmel 1908). However, most often, one can scarcely say whether the individual is excluded or included because he or she cannot enter into the society, being so completely "other." This person is excluded through negative rather than through positive action. Barbarians could not become Romans, foreigners could not become citizens of Athens (except through a very special procedure), and so on.

The positive act of exclusion, on the other hand, can occur in the case when the individual raises the issue of his or her "integration." Here we could speak of disintegration in some cases, in the sense that the disruptive element will be destroyed (the death penalty in some societies for certain kinds of behavior can be explained in this way). The typical example is antiquity's treatment of infants born deformed: Their strangeness, referencing a divine warning, and a fear of deviance within the species and of more or less imminent misfortune led to the well-known "exposure" beyond the social space. We are dealing with a society, however capable it was of strongly integrating its citizens, that could not tolerate the "stranger," who is then excluded *from* society. In this kind of mechanical solidarity, a term such as *inclusion* is inadequate or, at a minimum, too weak. One has one's place or one does not, but there is no real process of "being included in." When solidarity is of the mechanical kind, belonging is a factor of the idea of community. One must be similar, a relative, or a neighbor. Nor can we speak of exclusion *within* society, for these societies, however hierarchical they may be (and thus encompass the status of the privileged as well as the status of pariah), assign each group and each individual a place. Even if the superior "castes" are not mixed with the inferior, all social strata are integrated into the whole.

Today, there remain but a few societies that exhibit pure mechanical solidarity. Colonization, economic development, the international doctrine of human rights, and democratic trends have combined to produce many mixed cultural environments, positioned between centuries-old tradition and modernization at work. The inclusion that we have called mechanical is now, in global terms, behind us. However, we do well to bear it in mind, for societies cannot be voided of their holistic character because they are always something more structured than a myriad or even a sum of individuals. Even when the whole no longer exclusively directs the collective arrangements of a society, there still exists an imperative for cohesion and minimal conformity.

Modern Societies

In societies characterized by organic solidarity, which may be compared to the individualistic societies of Louis Dumont or the *Gesellschaft* of Tönnies, there is a tendency for the individual to be isolated. What must be emphasized here is that these societies have to construct their solidarity and their modes of integration. They cannot fall back on the idea of a place for each determined by tradition and culture. They are under pressure to offer individuals a place allowing evolution. Integration is a long road, and there is a reiterated obligation to make new advances because the division of labor and social division entails the constant introduction of new *procedures* (legislative, institutional, financial), so that individuals are not left to the rigors of competition and isolation. In other words, in modern Western societies, we are moving toward the idea of a *process of integration* and are no longer focused on places and statuses that are determined once and for all. When these processes loosen, individuals are at risk of being left adrift, subject to what Durkheim (1930) called *anomie*. There are no longer sufficient common arrangements to sustain the social bond. Moreover, on the global level, there must be sufficient commonly shared mental representations that these processes can be maintained. This is what Durkheim called the collective consciousness. This notion is one of Durkheim's most contested ideas, but it indicates that societies are made up of representations as much as of concrete practices. Sociology has developed these ideas at considerable length, as has the Chicago school with Goffman (1963) and Becker (1963), particularly with reference to persons with disabilities.

It is useful to ask why modern societies are thus simultaneously engaged in the task of inclusion and at risk of disaggregation. Societies displaying mechanical solidarity, almost completely holistic, are also societies that may be qualified as religious in the sense that they conceive of themselves in relation to an exteriority or believe that their foundation and fundamental rules are derived from elsewhere, in the divine. These are heteronomous societies (from *heteros,* "other," and *nomos,* "law") in the sense that law is based in a radical alterity. In all traditional societies, the way of addressing the question of disability depends on maintaining a connection with the transcendental, with the beyond, and with the gods or the dead (Stiker 1982, 1999). Western societies, on the other hand, are characterized by having broken with the notion of heteronomy. They base themselves in their own immanence. They have become autonomous. Theories of the social contract, whatever the manner of conceiving this contract, are theories of society's autonomy. This is because the origin of civil society, in contrast to the state of nature, derives from a "contract" on which humans agreed among themselves to secure their existence and raise the possibility of living together. Admittedly, not all theories of the social contract will lead to the establishment of democracy. There is a huge gulf between Hobbes and Spinoza. Yet all of them institute society on an immanent foundation. Even the absolute monarchies of seventeenth-century Europe, although they were regimes more onerous in terms of subjection than many others, inaugurated this new way of conceiving society (Gauchet 1985). This passage from heteronomy to autonomy is not the only product of the new political thought first evidenced in the early seventeenth century. It is also to be referred to as the birth of scientific thought, in which people could think and know the world by its own means without recourse to revelation. Galileo's famous "But it does move," when he compared his discovery to dominant theological discourse, is significative of all emancipation from collective reference to an exteriority. To this must also be added the individual's conquest of autonomy and not only that of society as such. This affirmation and claim had their specific origin in the Reformation, which permitted each individual conscience to interpret scripture independently of established religious authority and dogmatic definition. The autonomy of the individual also includes the capacity to be an economic agent and to create one's own place and role, as Max Weber (1920) has emphasized.

All these factors then contributed to the emergence of societies that, relying only on themselves and on the strength of constituent individuals, are entirely responsible and accountable for people living together. This equally explains why they are vulnerable and why the risk of marginalization, even social abandonment or exclusion, is so great. This is the greatness and weakness of democracies that are all continuously working at the process of integration. Here, we would distance ourselves from the thesis that emerges from a reading of Michel Foucault. Foucault (1961, 1975) described exclusionary measures that took the form of the confinement of the insane or the incarceration of the criminal. In so doing, he gives the impression that since the seventeenth century, Western societies would be characterized only by exclusion. This fails to take into account the very powerful revolutionary movement toward political equality. This is not the place for the full discussion of Foucault's thought that would be needed to explore all its contrasted aspects. What is certain, however, is that since the end of the eighteenth century, Western societies have experienced a thrust toward inclusion because they were so obliged by virtue of their very founding principles (Gauchet 1995).

Let us explore in greater detail this idea of society as a "construction site for democracy," illuminating clearly the nature and degree of the inclusion or exclusion of the persons with disabilities in our contemporary societies.

Constructing Inclusion in Modern Societies and Its Contradiction

The Normalization Process

One of the major procedures in the attempt at integration is normalization. Let's be sure we have an exact sense of this concept. It is not a question of leading all members of a society to an ideal model of humanity, as was the case in certain earlier philosophies or religions. Stoicism and the imitation of Christ may serve as examples. It is a question of defining the mean, comparing deviations from this mean, and trying to diminish such deviations to bring individuals closer to the mean.

Our societies no longer have a single ideal of the human being or of the citizen any more than they have one conception of a fixed and definitive form for the social order. As a consequence, a system of reference that permits minimal conformity and basic social cohesion becomes the effective mean in practical terms. Society's approach is based in statistics and probability theory.

This manner of inclusion is clearly illustrated in the case of persons with disabilities. For children with mental retardation to be admitted to school, they need to be able to follow lessons and thus reach the required level of competence. If they fail to reach this level, they are placed in separate institutions, which are supposed to bring them (back) to the norm. In the event of impossibility, they risk being segregated for almost their entire lives. For disabled adults to have access to employment in the business environment, they must acquire the equivalent autonomy and vocational competence, and this too must match the mean. These efforts, unquestionably beneficial, to reeducate the body and mind are also aimed at reducing the gap between the disabled and the able-bodied individuals. To be, to do "like others," is the objective of such rehabilitation. In addition, it is on this idea of deviation from the norm that the notions of the notorious *International Classification of Impairment, Disability, and Handicap*, proposed by the World Health Organization (WHO) in 1980, is founded. *Disability* is equated to any restriction or lack of ability to perform an activity in the manner or within the range considered normal for a human being (which human being, if not the one taken as the reference?). Handicap is in turn defined as a disadvantage that limits or prevents the fulfillment of a role that is normal (depending on age, sex, and social and cultural factors) for a given individual. The normalization imperative could not be more evident.

We would do well to recall Goffman (1963). In humorously describing the average American by showing that anyone found at odds with one of his or her characteristics was considered deficient and more or less to blame, Goffman analyzed the weight of the statistical norm with acuity. He wrote,

> For example, in an important sense there is only one complete unblushing male in America: a young, married, white, urban, northern, heterosexual Protestant father of college education, fully employed, of good complexion, weight, and height, and a recent record in sports. Every American male tends to look out on the world from this perspective, this constituting one sense in which one can speak of a common value system in America. Any male who fails to qualify in any of these ways is likely to view himself—during moments at least—as unworthy, incomplete, and inferior; at times he is likely to pass and at times he is likely to find himself being apologetic or aggressive concerning known-about aspects of himself he knows are probably seen as undesirable. The general identity values of a society may be fully entrenched nowhere, and yet they can cast some kind of shadow on the encounters encountered everywhere in daily living. (Pp. 128-129)

Similarly, Norbert Elias (1965) shows that between the *established* and the *outsiders,* the distinction is based less on problems of characteristic features than on the disparity in credo, values, and established "habitus." It is racism without race. If there is still a problem of identity, there is first and foremost the difference with respect to accepted norms.

The will toward normalization must be referred to another force that permeates our contemporary societies: the appeal of the universal. Modern Western societies, driven by the necessity of establishing the conditions of inclusion on their own to further cohesion and reduce inequalities, have thought that their forms of sociability were the most advanced. In this they pursued, perhaps without being too aware of it, the Christian universalism that formerly justified the conversion of nations and the wholesale imposition of Christian civilization. However, this is clearly not our present problem. What is certain is that democratic principles (the celebrated notions of liberty-equality-fraternity) seem destined to rule the world, just like our production modes, with free trade, salaried employment, and all the other components of industrial society. Topping it all, the individualism of success, performance, and pursuit of well-being also seems universal. The assimilation model is suited to summarizing a powerful thrust in our societies and is a model that plays a determining role in the social treatment of disabled people.

The Assimilation Model

The point of departure is the undeniable universality of humanity. The human species is a unity. The other can only be another "I." In principle, there are no limits to the rights of human beings as such. This is the great triumph of democratic revolutions, both French and American. Yet we move very quickly from recognition of equality to a desire for sameness. The other is destined to become like me, for I represent the universal human. In concrete terms, this slippage from the universal to pseudo-universalism is frequent, whereas the universal ought to remain only a regulating idea. This was the temptation of many an empire: One form of life or one ideology is raised to the status of universal and seeks to impose itself against an insurmountable diversity. In a case such as the former Soviet Union, this is more than evident. The Stalinist mold sought to impose uniformity, and after its failure, nationalities and nationalism were instantly reborn. The temptation is a constant one and is also seen in the pretension of Western nations to be the guardians of an order that is above all their own, as in that of certain Middle Eastern countries, to impose their politico-theological conceptions.

In more empirical fashion, the assimilation model generates more or less this discourse: There are common values, common objectives, canons of conduct, and a mean that we must strive to approach. The task consists of doing everything to rejoin this consensual and uniformizing communality. There is a certain French-style republicanism here: The republic defines its points of reference and its criteria, often enviable or even grandiose (secularism, social rights, educational system, public morale, and equality of rights). Yet, in turn, one must accept to live according to these norms, and this kind of republican environment can become "blind to differences."

In this model, we are on the way toward forceful integration. Each element must conform enough to assume its place in the good order of the whole. In return, the powerful denial of anything "other" keeps us in check. The other can be annulled. In its fullest expression, this model leads to the rule of "in-difference."

As it concerns persons with disabilities, this model seems to take into account such an orientation as positive discrimination. This statement may appear paradoxical because such a measure isolates and stigmatizes. One has to be labeled "handicapped" to benefit from the special measures reserved for this population. The legislator has foreseen a series of aid measures (financial) and special means of training or work (sheltered institutions of all kinds) in consideration of the fact that people in difficulty, due to an impairment, represent a vulnerable population for which special dispositions are required for them to "catch up with the bunch" and not be left adrift. We can clearly see how this perspective leads social environments to become disinterested and think themselves dispensed from the day-to-day integration of disabled persons.

This compensation for disability sometimes entails social isolation, rehabilitation, training, and work, all of which is under the rubric *adapted*. However, what must be emphasized is that this segregating effect is first and foremost the consequence of a will toward assimilation. This discrimination, which we will metaphorically and euphemistically call a *detour*, has as its objective a return to ordinary life or, if this is really not possible, at least a behavior and mode of life close to the average citizen's. If it were not for the appeal of these norms and common habitus, many of these efforts would not be sustained.

Let there be no misunderstanding about our analysis. Our purpose is not to discredit this pull toward conformity or the assimilation of disabled persons into the mainstream. The assimilation model is a powerful stimulant toward equality and integration. We seek only to point out that it is one of the points of reference that has a pronounced effect on attitudes toward persons with disabilities. The critical point is this: If we go too far in the direction of assimilation and thus fall into what could be called "assimilationism," we will end up rejecting the other in his or her irreducible difference, in the right to be oneself or to be as one is. We end up rejecting the richness of these multiple ways of being human. We end up being drawn into what psychoanalysis knows so well—denial. Denial is always dangerous, for what is denied surges up again and can at times advance its claims with violence. An obvious example is found in the proscription of deaf sign language. It has returned in full force but has also obliged the Deaf community to "bang on the table."

Contradictions

The will to assimilate, which finds its major process in normalization, entails a series of contradictions and runs up against social phenomena that are moving in a quite different direction.

The normalization process collides with the increasing complexity of our societies. As concerns disabled persons, if we have succeeded in eradicating certain impairments or diseases, such as poliomyelitis (at least in the West), we have seen quadriplegia increase, seen brain injury become a major form of injury, and are now confronted with instances of multiple disability. These examples permit us to pinpoint two facts: Society, by its very development, multiplies risk, and medical technology saves and prolongs "cases" that otherwise would have disappeared. Moreover, the risks are due as much to the evolution in behavior (e.g., sexual risk) as to technical evolution (traffic accidents, among others).

We must also insist on the innumerable consequences of lengthened life. Here, too, we confront problems in the sphere of disability that were unknown a few decades ago. We have won many additional years of life for those with Down syndrome or muscular dystrophy, but we must face the problems that accompany their reaching adulthood with questions of employment and, at a more advanced age, the complex problem of their aging and of adequate services.

In short, present-day society can no longer lay claim, as it did more easily in the case of victims of accidents at work or wounded veterans, to an inclusion or even an erasure of the consequences of these deficiencies.

However, this is not the essential. We must analyze the new processes of social exclusion in wealthy societies and the rising tide of claims to identity.

When the Social Bond Is Broken

From a functionalist perspective, exclusion results in dysfunctionalities in a society whose norms bar the way to integration for populations that do not correspond to the norm or do not do so sufficiently. The new phenomenon is that for some 20 years, Western societies have found themselves in a paradoxical situation in that they continue to produce great wealth but no longer have any means of ensuring sufficient employment. The production of wealth (material and immaterial goods, financial products) does without labor resources more and more. Unemployment has become endemic, as if it were one of the preconditions for society's functioning. In addition, habits and customs have changed (divorce, single-parent families, substantial vocational mobility), and a considerable amount of people no longer find a sufficient foundation in human relationships. Economic instability and the fragility of relationships rise in tandem (Castel 1995). Clearly, the loss of revenue, to the point of having no revenue at all, and the degeneration of relationships, to the point of complete isolation, are processes; as a consequence, they can come to a halt and even recede. This is why public policy, thanks to more or less shifting measures, occasionally succeeds in maintaining these populations in social inclusiveness. Yet at other times and quite frequently, a precariousness takes over, a kind of social substatus. The affected populations are continuously in the process of losing and regaining income or relationships. Unemployment, like employment, is intermittent. If they prevent people from falling into absolute, permanent poverty, they do not permit true integration, in the sense of lasting participation in the enjoyment of material and cultural goods. When the two processes—unemployment and loss of relationships—come to a head, then the fundamental social bond is breached, even lost. Then one receives little or nothing from society and no longer contributes to its wealth and social development. Finally, one is supernumerary and superfluous. In historical terms, it is not carved in stone that this situation cannot change or even be reversed. The exclusion of today, as it is historically situated, is not a fixed destiny. The problem of exclusion today is much more a problem of the social bond than a problem of poverty. Substantial populations are at constant risk of finding themselves removed from what constitutes the very basis of social belonging, that is, exchange. Exchange is what Marcel Mauss (1923) analyzed so well in the category of the gift. The degradation of the social bond, for a considerable percentage of the population of so-called advanced societies, foils the work of inclusion, which is nonetheless inscribed in the ongoing democratization that characterizes them.

Are disabled persons affected by these processes of social dissociation, what the French sociologist Robert Castel (1995) calls "disaffiliation"?

When there are no specific measures (special programs or affirmative action), there is a great risk of seeing those struck by illness or accident being drawn into the vortex of exclusion, in the sense in which it has been analyzed above. This is less true when public authorities—in the form of allowances, institutions, and human and technical assistance—direct specific attention to them. Yet no one is free from being swept off by the processes of which we have spoken. When this happens to disabled persons, the situation is aggravated by the usual barriers that block their route and by their lack of access (physical, psychological, cultural) to social spaces. We should stress the difference between exclusion in the sociohistorical sense described above, due to conditions that the future may well change even if the end is not presently in sight, and exclusion from certain goods, places, or services. This nonaccessibility has a dimension that is more constant but also is more commonplace because it is the lot shared by a great number of citizens—in fact, by everyone at one time or another. The social barriers are certainly more numerous and more insurmountable in the case of deficiencies, but they are determined to a greater extent by the political will for accommodation, which could be brought to a successful conclusion if we persevered and brought appropriate technologies into play. In any event, this type of exclusion is not dependent on central mechanisms that are part of the world economy and established customs, as is the type we have called disaffiliation. We would prefer to call it segregation because it entails moving people to the side, and this also is an obstacle to the full participation of citizens.

Identity Traps

We called attention to another factor—that of claims to identity. Our perspective will be the problem of profound deafness. Let us summarize the argument of the Deaf community. First, we are speakers like other speakers, and we have a language. Admittedly, it is a language of gestures and signs and not of sounds and words, but it is a whole and distinct language. We also have, through this medium, a way of thinking, of situating ourselves, of being in the world. In short, we have a culture. Our "inferiority" is nothing other than oppression and can be compared to that of minority cultural communities in the simple numerical sense or because they are too alien to the dominant and dominating culture. From this position, we easily see how the notion of disability and impairment begins to withdraw, become a secondary feature, or is completely dropped.

Second, the deaf are deaf, just as some people are black or white and are male or female. To wish to transform this condition is as absurd as wanting to make a white person black or a woman a man. One part of the eugenics movement, fearful of seeing a "deaf race" evolve, proposed forbidding marriage between deaf people and called for sterilization (Bell 1883).

This condition entails a mode of communication and signifying of its own—sign language—and also a specific and original culture. Withdrawing a deaf child from his or her natural community is an inadmissible violation. In *Mask of Benevolence*, Harlan Lane (1992) writes,

> Even if we could take the children destined to be members of the African-American, or Hispanic-American, or Native American, or Deaf American communities and convert them with bio-power into white, Caucasian, hearing males—even if we could, we should not. (P. 237)

The possible is not the desirable, and the ethical debate over cochlear implants is there to prove the topicality of the question. Nor should we ask a deaf person to express himself or herself in oral speech like hearing people. Deafness is not a limitation; it is a biological characteristic that has given rise to a specific culture (Lane 1984). This position reflects a vision of identity that can be translated into the notion of minority. The sociological concept of minority, in fact, stresses the ethnic and cultural aspects of difference, well beyond the question of number. Minorities are composed of

> individuals who have a common history and culture (and often a common national origin), who transmit their membership along lineage lines, who are in a position to demand signs of loyalty from some of the members, and who are in a relatively disadvantaged position in society. (Goffman 1963:145)

From this background, we can understand how deaf people and all kinds of disabled people have formulated the slogans of "deaf pride" and "disability pride." It is a matter of pride to belong to a cultural minority, to a group that not only has nothing to be ashamed of but can also make valid claims for its own characteristics.

The characteristics of the Deaf community lend themselves well to the American "culturalist" interpretation of the situations of blacks, women, and Hispanics. The question of the deaf can stand as symbol of very broad problematics and rejoins those of cultural communities and, more generally speaking, of different identities in a society that cannot allow itself fragmentation but ought to be capable of creating social bonds, cohesion, and integration. Our societies are thus confronted with the question of managing differences.

The Differentiation Model

In contrast to the assimilation model discussed above, a model of differentiation has been formulated.

The first form of the differentiation model is the *hierarchical* one. This submodel seems more predominant in European history than in that of North America but is, on the other hand, very close to many holistic and religious societies. Specificity and difference are recognized and may even be accepted. However, according to the logic of genus and species, a common human genus is defined here, within which a series of points of view are situated that correlate with at least one distinctive feature. From the reference point of sex, the distinction would be man/woman; from that of biological conformity, the distinction would be able/disabled; and from the reference point of appearance, the distinction would be whites/people of color. Yet once these "species" are established, they are not thereby all considered equal. They are situated on a scale of positions and values. This is one means of integrating differences, for they are made to hold together in a coherence that is at the same time a system of subjection and submission. For example, man and woman represent two ways of being human. Yet man will dominate woman because the social roles attached to these roles result in one having a greater precedence, dignity, and importance than the other (political role vs. domestic role, productive role vs. nurturing role, authoritative role vs. affective role). In his *Souci de soi* (*Concern for Oneself*), Michel Foucault (1984) shows that relations between the sexes in ancient Greece, just like relations between adult men and younger men, for that matter, are dictated by social position, which determines rights and liberties. This is a kind of cohesion through hierarchy. The Roman Catholic Church has offered us the purest model of this conception. The clergy are different from laity but enjoy a dominant position. Christian people are a genus, but in this genus there are two great species, clergymen and laymen. In each of these species (which can then in turn play the role of genus), there are subspecies. The clergy is divided into bishops and priests, the laity into consecrated laymen (men in orders who are not priests), and laymen in secular life, and these latter groups are divided into men and women. A fine pyramid is created, from the summit where the clergy is to the base with its simple laypeople. This grand terrestrial hierarchy must then correspond to a no less grand celestial hierarchy. All the differences have a place on a scale of values. The common and equal nature as children of God in no way precludes different situations that are differently valorized.

Our example may appear ethnocentric since Roman Catholicism is not a universal reference point. The hierarchical model can also be illustrated by Indian caste society. The massive fact of social hierarchy by means of the caste system is too well known to need emphasis. We should, however, stress that it is only from a basis in diversity and differentiation that national integration is possible. The caste system is not, per se, antidemocratic. India is a democracy, a very specific one admittedly, but a real one. The hierarchy of status, inegalitarian in its very essence, does, however, leave room for the autonomy of the individual will. Each person is responsible for his or her acts. The principle of caste, like that of "states of life" in Catholicism, neither isolates nor encloses in a group that would dictate decisions to all its members. It opens onto a network of possible relationships in which each person must constantly take initiatives to improve or maintain his or her status, gain influence, build personal prosperity, and ensure survival. On the other hand, this maneuvering space around the hierarchized positions does introduce a real possibility for participation in a common life. The hierarchical model, because it has its point of departure in difference, is not incapable of permitting a modern form of integration and inclusion.

The example of India also permits us to comment on our opening words. Louis Dumont (1966) put the caste system beside holistic societies, which we in turn compared to those displaying mechanical solidarity. We said that this solidarity was characteristic of ancient societies. Yet it should be noted that the lines of reality are not so sharply drawn. It is not only that India's holism is in evolution, for we are witnessing a living, contemporary society, but also that holism is not entirely synonymous with mechanical solidarity. There can be mixed forms and also very original forms of conceiving inclusion and possibly producing exclusion. This can be said in support of our intention to make a number of distinctions in a question as complex as that treated here.

The hierarchical model makes it possible to suppress differences by an initial acceptance of similarity, although one that is strictly controlled. This is, of course, a means of consolidating differences that already exist. Here we link up with the analysis of Robert Castel (1995), when he shows that throughout European history, the categories of "handicapology" are constant ones. There are always groups that, unable to meet their needs through their labor, are legally exempted from such labor and are assisted. The disabled have always been so seen. Even when they are not excluded, they have a well-established inferior position. Even if it is not impossible to break out of the category of the permanently assisted, both mental and social structures are, in practical terms, opposed to it.

Still, in the universe of differentialization, we meet a second model, that of *juxtaposition*. It is, no doubt, the most frequent in countries with a British heritage. This is the model with a degree of tolerance in the sense of accommodation. They are what they are, and we are who we are; their culture is that way, and ours is this way. We have no cause to subjugate them or render them inferior, but we really have nothing to do with them. The recognition of a difference is pushed far enough for each person to exist on his or her own, a stranger in the midst of a group of strangers. There is a certain kind of nationalism reflected in this model. Foreigners have the right to exist as long as they stay out of our space. There is no integration. It is a jigsaw puzzle, a mosaic, as much from the international point of view, which leads to the rejection of any kind of transnational organization, as from a state's internal point of view, which leads to fragile unions (Yugoslavia). This model can be wedded to a form of democracy, as we see in the multiculturalist thought of the United States, but left to its own logic, it destroys all common space, and, within a nation, it would destroy its foundation. Federalism attempts to surmount the disadvantages of this model from which, in a certain sense, it issues. When groups, classes, or cultures are in simple juxtaposition, an opposition of values necessarily arises, which will hamper the social order and, above all, reinforce the preexistent social structure.

This model is more reflective of a possible tendency in the treatment of persons with disabilities than a policy that has been applied in history. Yet it would move in the direction of what we could call the "Indianization" of disabled persons, borrowing the example of reserves for Native Americans. Fortunately, the extermination of Native Americans has come to an end, a policy that placed them in a situation of radical difference, of terminal exclusion, but now they are situated apart, a sequestration in the very name of their difference. There are a number of people who would not be unhappy to exploit this form of segregation if it led to a purification, a purging of their group space.

In its most extreme form, which we will call *differentialism*, this model states that you are other and you have nothing to do with me, unless it is to submit to placement on a scale of values where I am more perfect than you. Let's make no mistake, juxtaposition, like hierarchy, is a way of putting some people at the top and letting it be thought that these people alone represent the universal. Misfortune always follows when a social group (or a state or a nation) believes itself to be the sole realization of the universal, while the universal is only a panomara, all of whose aspects are singular. There can exist only parts of the universal. Once a people or an ethnicity takes itself for the universal, perversion is at work and can lead to the worst consequences.

Returning to the question of the deaf, a possible surplus of identity could shore up an exacerbated differentialism. The reasoning of the deaf, when taken to extremes, reflects the juxtaposition model but in a radical form that mixes two approaches that are not comparable. Deaf culture exists but has been forged, like all cultures, in the historical process. It is not a "natural" fact. On the other hand, the fact of being deaf, like being black or white or being a man or a woman, is a natural fact. Yet can we draw cultural consequences from a natural feature? This is all the more chancy when we recognize that this kind of confusion has served as basis for so much exploitation and racism: "They" have natural features of such a kind that they can have no part in our evolved white culture! Locking a group into its natural features amounts to establishing it in a closed specificity and preparing the ground for all the extreme forms of cultural identity, ultraculturalism, and even group fanaticism. By virtue of wishing to affirm our own identity—however undeniable it is—we risk being enclosed in our own ghetto and finding ourselves excluded at the very interior of the society to which we, by our own logic, belong.

To conclude our discussion of the contradictions and tensions of normalization and of the models of assimilation and differentiation, we shall summarize the different senses of inclusion and exclusion that we have met.

The doubtless, most dynamic notion of inclusion leaves room for an effort toward adjustment, acceptability and acceptance, and social participation. The notion of integration presupposes conformity and alignment, which are always experienced as the domination or even oppression of the group that defines the norms or of the majority over the minority. Being included may represent a situation in which you are a part, in an organic way, without necessarily being forced to conduct yourself according to a rigid norm.

Otherwise, inclusion (or *insertion,* as it is sometimes called in French, with a rather different thrust) can prove to be weak, a synonym for simple presence, simple admittance, and simple tolerance. One can be supported without being recognized. One can be received without being incorporated. We have seen that the semantics differ according to the sociological and linguistic contexts. Being fully recognized as an equal, a partner, or a participant with the same dignity and of the same quality as any other is called *integration* rather than *inclusion.* Yet these are translations of French terms, and what is true of one language is not true of all. We must perhaps resign ourselves to the impossibility of translating from one language to another terms that are charged with such historical and cultural weight.

In inverted fashion, exclusion in contemporary societies designates several phenomena: radical exclusion from society; segregation *in* society; discrimination, also within, as concerns access to social goods and spaces; and disaffiliation and withdrawal from social exchange.

According to historical times and praxis, inclusion and exclusion may take on differing significations. They are not univocal or unambiguous terms and are not historically fixed. There is diversity in exclusion and diversity in inclusion. We will illustrate this diversity and show the indivisible relationship between the two aspects by establishing a typology. To one form of exclusion corresponds another form of inclusion or, at a minimum, a certain tendency toward inclusion. This typology is necessary to do justice to a whole series of practices that we have thus far not been able to mention.

A DRAFT TYPOLOGY OF THE DIVERSE FORMS OF EXCLUSION AND INCLUSION WITH REFERENCE TO THE SOCIAL TREATMENT OF DISABILITY

In the first part of this chapter, we saw the multiple facets of inclusion and exclusion, both processes and states. The analysis of different models has made it possible to resituate these notions with reference to other theories of the social bond and its possible dissolution (marginality, deviance). Anthropologist Robert Murphy (1987) employs the concept of liminality to express the fact that in all societies, disabled persons live in a state of social suspension. They are neither ill nor well, neither dead nor alive, neither really excluded nor really included in society (Murphy 1987).

These failures of inclusion or integration that may be experienced by disabled people are translated as the loss of or difficulty in access to a place in society, as a permanent move to the sidelines. The study of the historical treatment of disability (Stiker 1982, 1999), as well as anthropological studies of this same theme (Ingstadt and Reynolds Whyte 1995), show that the exclusion of disabled persons through time and across civilizations has assumed and still assumes extremely diverse forms within the host society. We shall then try to draw up a typology of different forms of exclusion, whether they are social, geographical, economical, cultural, or judicial while comparing the forms of inclusion that seek to offset them.

From the more radical forms of exclusion, such as extermination or abandonment, there is a continuum representing exclusion *from* society to the diverse forms of exclusion *within* society, through segregation, marginalization, or discrimination. We can observe that each of these types of exclusion, even if it has been characteristic of some ancient society, nonetheless displays survival in our contemporary Western societies. Moreover, it appears possible in such a typology to establish correspondences between each form of exclusion *within* society and a form of inclusion in it.

Exclusion through Elimination

The most extreme form of social exclusion is death. One of the first types of exclusion that can be identified is exclusion through elimination. The elimination of disabled persons can be effected in a direct way by putting them to death or indirectly through abandonment or the deprivation of care. We may also consider that elimination, not of persons but of disability, may be considered before life. This raises the timely questions posed by the termination of pregnancy when a deficiency is identified in the fetus and even before conception with the latest developments in genetic engineering. Eugenicist theories show the possible link of continuity between the practice of elimination in ancient societies and the praxis of contemporary societies linked to the most recent technological developments.

This radical form of exclusion of persons with disabilities, the ultimate one, is then situated at the level of the most fundamental principle, that of life itself. In Greco-Roman antiquity, the practice of exposing deformed infants offers an example. The fear of seeing the species deviate from its true course (eugenicism) is projected onto deformed births, even if such deformation is to modern eyes quite minimal. Such births are interpreted as a baleful sign sent by the gods that must be officially expelled from the social space and returned to its senders (Stiker 1997, 1999). Infants coming into the world with deformities are left outside inhabited space, on fallow land, in a rut, or along a stream. In short, they are not socialized. Although they are not sacrificed in a formal rite of immolation, they are ritually abandoned. This practice, which we are not encouraged to believe was ever implemented on any massive scale, given what we know of the cities of antiquity, is a form of elimination, even if we could in one sense connect it with abandonment. The myth of Oedipus, one of the founding myths of the West, certainly constitutes one of the best illustrations of the ancient practice that was exposure.

However, it is probably Nazi Germany that offers the most extreme example of the extermination of disabled persons. Thus, some 200,000 people (in particular, those with a mental illness or congenital malformation) were exterminated in the hospitals and death camps because of their disability (Burleigh 1994).

From another perspective, the ethical debate over euthanasia or assisted suicide deserves to be mentioned here as representative of the most current way of reposing the question of the elimination of disabled persons. "Quality of life" has become a key notion in public health, and some economists will go so far as to speak of the "price of human life." The value accorded to human life is conditioned by social representations of disability and, in our Western societies, is influenced by the existence of severe forms of impairment. This value may be judged negatively, with life under certain conditions being considered not worth living, which then justifies a certain number of medical practices that surround the beginning or end of life. On such a basis, it becomes possible in some countries to put a person to death in fully legal fashion. What is under discussion here is not, of course, the freedom of individual choice of life or death for a severely impaired person but the fact that social pressure, by reducing disability to a dimension of personal tragedy, makes it acceptable to accommodate disabled persons in their desire for death. Death, in this sense, is qualified as "natural," whereas for nondisabled persons, everything would be done to convince them of the transitory nature of such a wish and to prevent any attempt at suicide. In other words, the latter group is considered depressed and treated as such, while members of the former will possibly be offered themselves in suicide the help that they were unable to obtain in daily life.

Even though these are interventions before birth, it is possible to include medical measures that aim at precluding the birth of a disabled child in this discussion of exclusion through elimination. These methods share the radical nature of the foregoing and raise the question of the very humanity of disabled persons. A decision to terminate a pregnancy through medical means can be taken after prenatal diagnosis or a strong presumption resulting from an echography of a fetus anomaly or a risk of birth of a disabled child. With new genetics and preimplantation screening, it becomes possible to identify a certain number of genetic diseases even before pregnancy. The question of elimination can be raised in these terms, and we then speak of the eradication of Down syndrome or muscular dystrophy, for example. Thus, we could see societies emerge that have been "cured" of certain genetic diseases, but this prospect is accompanied by a certain concern over the limits that will have to be put in place to regulate such an evolution. Certain associations of persons with disabilities may have spoken in this context of genocide and crimes against humanity.

The eugenicist perspectives opened by the possibilities of genetic screening are certainly among the most difficult ethical problems that democratic societies will have to face in the near future.

Lastly, the sterilization of mentally disabled women, which has occasionally been practiced, although often illegally, can also be associated with these measures addressing procreation.

Exclusion through Abandonment

The practices of abandonment can be distinguished from elimination by the fact that they do not entail death or at least not in such direct fashion. Practiced in antiquity, the form of exclusion through abandonment recurs in contemporary forms of social death—social abandonment.

There is no lack of examples of the practice of abandoning people: children born deformed, victims of multiple injuries, and very dependent elderly persons. Abandonment can take different routes; it can be the transfer of parental authority to another agency, leaving in God's hands the fate of a newborn, but the more modern fashion is anonymous delivery in view of adoption.

Abandonment, then, is not something specific to ancient societies. A French study has shown that parallel to the increasingly widespread success in the prenatal diagnosis of Down syndrome, the number of such infants who are abandoned at birth has increased in France in recent years (Dumaret et al. 1998). The hypothesis can then be advanced that more widespread prevention methods are accompanied by a decrease in the social acceptability of this type of disability.

To abandon something or someone is to cease to be concerned with it, to deprive it of care. Here we return to the question of passive euthanasia, which consists of no longer providing all possible care to a newly born infant, an accident victim, or an elderly person when he or she is considered as too severely disabled or risk becoming so.

The surplus population thesis has been advanced as one of the chief explanations of exclusion by abandonment (Oliver and Barnes 1998). The evolution in European thought in the nineteenth century, with the emergence of liberal utilitarianism and social Darwinism, raises the question of the place of individuals who are too weak, too dependent, or incapable of meeting their needs without assistance.

Decisions not to attempt resuscitation and to disconnect life support systems are certainly the modern face of this form of abandonment, which quite simply consists of ceasing to look after someone. We can also see that the duties and responsibilities of family and of society may diverge here.

Exclusion through Segregation or Differentiated Inclusion

Segregation and the various practices of sequestration constitute one of the most widespread forms of exclusion. This *geographical* exclusion, in the generic sense of the word, can be found, with immediate topical relevance, across eras and cultures. This is also a form of social treatment that, by clearly setting out an inside and an outside, is very close to the basic meanings of inclusion and exclusion. The point here is that this separate treatment does not necessarily occur outside the community but frequently at its very center. Lastly, we may note that this kind of segregation may be more or less constraining and may entail a greater or lesser deprivation of personal freedom.

In his *L'histoire de la folie à l'âge classique* (*A History of Insanity in the Age of Reason*), Michel Foucault (1961) describes in convincing detail what he calls, after the creation of the Hôpitaux Généraux in France in 1662, the Great Confinement of the seventeenth century. Most European countries have known a parallel evolution, such as Britain with its workhouses.

The first institutions for disabled people were often intended for the deaf and the blind. The confinement of the mentally ill or deficient against their will (legislated in 1838 in France and 1845 in Britain) is a particularly characteristic example of the kind of social control that would henceforth be imposed on this population through the power accorded to physicians. In Western European countries, this movement toward the institutionalization of disabled persons would last until the 1970s.

In the sphere of disability, the term *institution,* which we relate to the question of segregation, refers to a kind of establishment that is most often structured on a residential basis to treat, train, and intern disabled people. Thus, it has been possible to speak of total institutions (Goffman 1961). The institutions created by the first educators in the domain of persons with infirmity are of this type. The Abbé de l'Épée (1712-89) founded a school for the deaf, with whom he learned to make himself understood by means of sign language. Valentin Haüy (1745-1822) founded the Institution for Blind Children (l'Institution des Jeunes Aveugles) in Paris and conceived of letters printed in relief that would permit the blind to read, before Louis Braille (1809-52), a blind teacher, devised the systematic code that still bears his name. In the same period, Jean Marc Gaspard Itard (1774-1838) tried to educate a feral child, Victor of Aveyron. His failure in this attempt did not prevent Édouard Séguin (1812-80), his successor, from inventing a pedagogy designed for mentally retarded children. The creation of special establishments—which Séguin promoted in America, especially since he was poorly received in France—was based on the segregation model, despite their passion for education, in the broadest sense of the word.

Similarly, Philippe Pinel (1745-1826), well known for having freed the insane from their chains, affirmed the curability of the "mad" and laid the basis for modern psychiatry. However, he did not envisage his famous "moral treatment" other than within the sequestering walls of the hospital. In our time, the greater part of treatment, placement, training, and education is still effected within the framework of institutions. Severely criticized by the antipsychiatry and deinstitutionalization movements, such as at Basaglia in Italy, institutions have been the object of heated criticism on the part of numerous organizations of disabled persons. Thus, in Great Britain, the Union of the Physically Impaired against Segregation (UPIAS) describes segregated residential institutions as the "ultimate human scrapheaps." It adds that thousands of people, whose only crime is being physically impaired, are sentenced to these prisons for life. . . . For the vast majority, there is no alternative, no appeal, no remission of sentence for good behavior, no escape, except the escape from life itself. (UPIAS 1976)

One of the constant features of the institutionalization of disabled people has been the separation of the sexes. This repression of sexuality, thus precluding all procreation, can be associated with the practices of sterilization and the eugenicist issues treated above. It must be stated that the theories of degeneracy that were developed in the nineteenth century saw a major solution to such degeneration in barring disabled persons from reproduction. If the decline of institutionalization was furthered by strong advocacy based on humanistic arguments, it is probable that economic arguments and the waning of the welfare state really precipitated this evolution. However, this segregating institutional environment was part of the matrix that generated the movements of rebellion and protest by disabled people against these structures, which they considered primarily responsible for their oppression, and their will to gain control over services that concerned them.

This form of exclusion through segregation may also affect more limited aspects of social life, such as education, employment, and transportation. Thus, there are specialized schools for disabled children, sheltered workshops for disabled workers, and specialized forms of transportation for persons with disabilities.

One of the paradoxes is that what is often seen as a segregating "detour" (e.g., in the form of temporary separate schooling) is often presented as having integration as its ultimate goal. In fact, such segregation is today most often conceived of as a provisional bypass to regain the mainstream, to participate more fully in society, even if it should happen that this detour never does come back around. Thus, the intention is not to exclude but to include at a future date. The goal of sequestration is no longer confinement, as in the seventeenth century, but a mediated inclusion.

Exclusion through Assistance or Conditional Inclusion

The reference to employment and productive capacity permits us to address another form of exclusion—exclusion through assistance, an "economic" form of exclusion, which has permeated the entire question of social policy since the end of the Middle Ages. In fact, the lot of the crippled is linked to the social treatment of poverty during the entire medieval period.

The distinction erected in the countries of Western Europe since the Middle Ages between the meritorious poor, who included persons with deficiencies as well as the able-bodied indigent, sought to distinguish those who were exempt from work and those who were obligated to it. For the former, recognition of incapacity would open the way to the possibility of being assisted. Measures to combat begging condemned the second group to repression: deportation, forced labor, and the banishment of vagabonds.

Assistance is a form of close-up protection, intended, for example, for other inhabitants of the village, and concerns those who by virtue of their inability to work cannot meet their needs. Christian values, including charity, dominate what we may call the Christian West. Disability recalls the suffering of Christ, and the charity that it stimulates enables practicing Christians to atone for their sins. The church plays a major role in the development of individually targeted assistance, initially through the intermediary of its convents, monasteries, and other religious institutions and then through specialized institutions such as hospitals, hospices, and orphanages. This protective role of the church was also an aspect of its power. Until the French Revolution, the church may be said to have been the principal organ for the provision of assistance. The counterpart to such aid is that disabled persons were obliged to show the most complete humility toward their benefactor.

Welfare activity and good works marked the history of the social treatment of disability until the twentieth century.

If the relationship to work is a determining factor in understanding the economic role of disabled people, work represents, beyond its connection with production, a justification for inscription in the social structure. Thus, failure to participate in any productive activity and isolation from other human relationships combine their negative effects to generate exclusion or rather disaffiliation (Castel 1995). Inversely, the combination of stable work and solid functioning relationships creates the conditions for integration. Between the two lies a zone of social vulnerability.

Assistance is a form of economic exclusion that defines those who are "useless to society." It also introduces a relationship of subordination and dependence between persons helped and their benefactors. The individual so aided is divested of all responsibilities, such as that of working in exchange for submission to a status of inferiority. This surrender of obligations or "irresponsibility" is the source of marginalization and calls the very idea of citizenship into question.

Some theorists of disability consider that exclusion from the world of work is the ultimate cause of other, differing forms of exclusion that disabled people experience (Oliver and Barnes 1998). Some among them argue that criteria for citizenship cannot be based in social unusefulness. The passage of assistance into the secular sphere did not resolve this inequality of position, which is now being challenged from the perspective of civil rights. On the other hand, present-day dissociation from systems of economic production often entails exclusion from systems of compensation and social protection.

Assistance or, to invert the terminology, social security and welfare are admittedly weak forms of participation in society. They confer a social substatus. Yet to assist is not to exclude because those who are helped are part of society by the very fact that society is concerned about them. At times, as during the medieval period, this substatus is even necessary for the well-to-do because it offers them the opportunity to win eternal salvation. However, those helped are part of society only on condition that they stay in their place. Georg Simmel (1908) has clearly shown that poverty does not consist of being without resources but of being assisted, with such assistance being the very means of ensuring social cohesion on this level. Assistance is basically a sociological relationship and has an indispensable function. This is why social assistance policies do not have the elimination of poverty as their objective, as one might believe, but its integration into the system, to the benefit of the latter.

Exclusion through Marginalization
or Inclusion through Normalization

In the precise sense of the word, *marginalization* is the process of moving to the side as a consequence of a refusal to accept or of an impossibility of accepting currently recognized rules of operation. The marginalized are defined by transgression of or protest against the values and habitus of the community. Whether it is a decision to put oneself outside boundaries (e.g., the criminal, the panhandler) or rejection by the dominant group (e.g., the prostitute, the teenager whose parents' oppression forces him or her into delinquency), marginality is always characterized by a lifestyle that cannot be accommodated within the behavioral norms that are in force. Its origin may lie in a conflict over rights (rights recognized and rights denied), in the absence of rules (total permissiveness on the part of parents, leading youngsters to set up their own rules), or in a conflict of values (a person no longer wants to live according to the law of consumption and goes into self-imposed exile in a autarkical way of life). Disabled persons who may find themselves rejecting norms that are applied to them or who are rejected for not "playing the game" are susceptible to being drawn into this process of marginalization. Yet this is not the general case because their desire for integration in society most often makes them accept the common rules. The fundamental problem is that of norms. To be included, you must achieve and accept a certain degree of conformity.

The key concern of rehabilitation (called *réadaptation* in French) is to reduce this deviation from the norm. Action on the individual who is to be reintroduced into the mainstream is accompanied by the desire to efface any difference. The individual must act "like others," even if this requires technical aids, various devices, or prostheses.

However, this same concern to reduce deviance laid the groundwork for the kind of normalization procedures developed by Wolfensberger (1972) for mentally retarded persons.

Exclusion through Discrimination or Progressive Inclusion

The last type of cultural or juridical exclusion that must be addressed is exclusion through discrimination.

To discriminate is to single out, put a social group to one side, and restrict its rights. These distinctions made in social life at the expense of disabled persons may be judged unacceptable because they violate social norms and the principle of equality before the law, even if in other societies and at other times they are or were current.

To define *discrimination* as the act of treating equal individuals inequitably shows to what extent this concept is tied to modern society, which puts equality at the center of its code of values. In societies based on differences in status or caste, discrimination is a neutral, descriptive notion, devoid of all pejorative connotation as we in Western societies would see it.

With the development of civil rights, most modern democracies instituted judicial protection against negative discrimination as a function of criteria relative to the impairments of an individual. If the intentional discrimination of individuals is then proscribed in the United States, Great Britain, Australia, and New Zealand, this does not preclude, in these very same countries, the existence of statistical discrimination on the level of the population of disabled persons. It has thus been possible to show that in France, despite a law promoting the employment of disabled workers by means of an obligatory quota system for both private and public sectors, disabled persons continue—all other things being equal—to experience discrimination in their search for employment (Ravaud, Madiot, and Ville 1992).

However, discrimination may also be positive and have the restoration of equality as its goal. It is interesting for French researchers to note to what extent the current English phrase *affirmative action* differs in this respect. Positive discrimination can be effected by social assistance measures in cases determined according to extrinsic characteristics (tied to income, for example). It can also be ensured by authoritarian measures (which raises the question of personal freedom) or by preferential measures (e.g., policies of employment quotas favoring disabled workers, women, or certain ethnic minorities). It may also be conceived of as a compensation measure and justified on the basis of distributive justice, which is not without its paradox because it is not the injured individual who benefits from the compensation (Auroux 1990). It has an inherent defect since it necessarily arises only after negative discrimination, in that it must temporarily violate the principle of equality on which it is based. It can thus be defended for reasons of social utility (the employment of disabled persons may at times be part of a company's communications and public relations policy).

We can see the contradictions inherent in the principle of nondiscrimination, which tends to be generalized. In the struggle against negative discrimination, it makes vulnerable the systems that are based on protective and compensatory measures.

The principal question that is posed today in Western countries is the nature of the citizenship that disabled persons may enjoy. Modern politics excludes the possibility of distinguishing among different categories of persons in the public sphere. Behind these questions of discrimination and exclusion, we discern the principle of equality of citizens before the law as the moral ideal of a democratic nation. We do well to state precisely the limits of this equality before the law: right to identical treatment, right of access, right to equal opportunities, and right to an identical quality of life. We can see to what extent, in a society that has become segmented, that the perspective that is assumed will depend on the conception that we have of justice and social inequalities.

This typology is of course quite schematic, and there are numerous intermediary forms between each of these modalities of exclusion and inclusion. Thus, the very existence of people who are judged to be socially and economically useless is deeply interwoven with eugenicist practices of elimination. Discrimination is not just cultural or judicial exclusion but also economic exclusion.

However schematic, this typology makes it possible to identify differences in the reactions of cultures to anomalies such as impairments—reduce them, control them physically, avoid them, catalog them as dangerous, or adopt them as rituals—as described by Mary Douglas (1966).

Exclusion needs to be perceived from a global perspective that encompasses the view of the excluded and that of the entity that rejects him or her. Because, contrary to contemporary representations, exclusion is not an abstract, inexorable phenomenon, without actors, nor is it ultimately an inevitability due to entry into a new global economy. As Norbert Elias (1965) illustrated in his study of the logic of exclusion, it is clear that exclusion is also inscribed in a society's power relationships.

Lastly, the tension between the two approaches to disability policy that we have characterized as differentialist and universalist is not without consequences for the social situation of disabled people. The first calls for a right to difference—for specificity, even a minority group identity—and the second invokes the universality of human rights and rejecting all particularism. The former carries the latent risk of segregation, the latter of inequalities.

A CHALLENGE TO DEMOCRATIC SOCIETIES

The models of exclusion and inclusion that we have reviewed, as well as the multiple forms of integration and segregation, raise the fundamental question of what form true democratic inclusion would take. According to us, addressing this question offers the real prospect, the real future for a just stance on the issue of disabled persons. The word *just* must be understood in its two senses of justice and justness, that is, cover what is theirs by right and was is right for their specific case.

We shall base our discussion on two thinkers who have recently sought to conceive of a way beyond the opposition between the policy of assimilation (whose proponents are called "liberals" in the United States) and the turn inward to group identity issues or communitarianism. Kymlicka (1995), whom we would qualify as a moderate liberal, attempts to find room for expressions of collective identity, taking as point of departure the irrefutable principles of individual citizenship. Charles Taylor (1992), on the other hand, who would be a similarly moderate communitarian, looks for ways to recognize publicly specific cultures without neglecting the equality of citizens. We shall not develop these lines of thought here, centered as they are on the problems of cultural communities relatively linked to the North American context. Yet it is important to see how the search is being conducted—by Michaël Walzer (1988) as another example—for a differentiated citizenship, a democracy of participation, the conjunction of individual citizenship with a policy of support for minorities and singular identities—in short, a democratic pluralism.

It seems that, to a greater or lesser degree, these forms of relating to the "other" have in turn or at the same time been able to exert influence on the way the disabled are treated. Their lot seems to have always swung between subjection, indifference, and denial. Denial is apparent in the older forms of radical exclusion or in the more modern forms of unnuanced segregation and also, very subtly, in the form of a passion for assimilation through normalization at all cost. Subjection is shown when the crippled served some "other purpose": offering salvation for the charitable, playing the fool, being exhibited as freaks, or, in more contemporary fashion, partaking of policies for population management, business, or justifications for the existence of the disabled service industry. Indifference, when placed in what Murphy (1987) calls liminality, is neither included nor excluded, neither rejected not accepted. Either the disabled are left to the care of the welfare establishment according to a roundabout principle of nondiscrimination, or they are protected and assisted according to the arrangements of a compensatory discrimination that are not brought to a full conclusion.

The positions adopted by disabled persons themselves may favor one model or another and entail the perverse side effects of each. Minority activism at times takes on the trappings of overdriven differentialism, as discussed above. Will Kymlicka's (1995) idea, according to which the recognition of separate collectivities would not be unconditional and according to which the individuals of a group ought to be free equally to enter and leave it, would be to propose a kind of communitary extremism.

Inversely, one form of discourse on the abolition of differences and the claim to be like others may derive from an assimilationist model that is not just euphoric. There is also a way of stressing the "social model," which is not without its drawbacks. The social model has become the means of referencing a train of thought that tries to think of disability from the side of the social barriers of every order that constitute it, by abstracting its corporeal and individual dimension (Barton and Oliver 1997). It is the state of society alone that creates disability, its material and mental state. Even if the diffusion of this model has had undeniable pedagogical merit by throwing into relief dominant social praxis, the risk now is of "disembodying" disability by neglecting its corporeality and the dimension of individual experience. Once the social barriers are abolished, what would be left of disability would be only banal differences (moving in a wheelchair instead of walking, not recognizing certain communication signs but having others in their place). To approach disability from the quarter of impairment is to see it upside down and to attribute difficulties to the individual, which, when we think about them, have to do only with the managing "in act" of the environment. If we followed this logic to its end, we would come to a common space that we could, metaphorically, call so desexed that all expressions of particularity, including cultural ones, would be swept away. In the name of individual citizenship, there would no longer be any collective identities. In fact, if we assert our disabled identity, with a view to abolishing social barriers, we presuppose a certain collective identity; otherwise, there is only a swarm of individuals. Under which flag would people then gather? It seems that it is impossible to disregard the fact that two poles have to be maintained: civic universalism, on one hand, and groups and differentiated individuals, on the other. What is fundamental in the struggle to abolish social barriers and in advancing the claim to be like others is to reassert the need to create truly common social space and truly common access (a universal design). What is fundamental in the affirmation of a certain specific identity is to obligate this social space, which will never be an incarnation of the universal, to compensate on an ongoing basis for the weaknesses of certain people by putting at their disposal what they need to occupy, just as they are, this common space.

To take the example of schooling, disabled children would have their specific needs met but within the framework of regular classes and classrooms, with all the necessary support. As Stainback and Stainback (1990) write,

> Full inclusion does *not* mean that special educators are no longer necessary; rather it means that special educators are needed even more to work with regular educators in teaching and facilitating challenging, supportive, and appropriate educational programs for all students. However, special educators do need to be integrated into, and in effect, become "regular or general" educators in the mainstream who have expertise in specific instructional, curricular, and assessment areas. (P. 4)

The example of schools clearly shows the concrete applications of what we have formulated in more abstract fashion. We could go on at greater length concerning the business world and daily life. Imagine if we introduced a sufficient number of professionals trained in disability *into work environments* so that accessibility became total; all the structures of sheltered employment would become useless. What is necessary in this utopian vision is the conversion of corporate officers. Yet having a utopia before one's eyes is not without its effects, as history shows us. Let us imagine that in city neighborhoods, "social workers" were present on a daily basis, discussing and working with all the vital resources (associations and various service agencies) and with all those who were active there (storekeepers, tradespeople, professionals). Many disabled persons could maintain themselves and live among others. Daily democracy has a fine, wide path ahead of it. The necessary precondition for the progressive realization of such a utopia is the existence of political will. The role of the citizen is indispensable here in influencing elected representatives and administrative officers but also in convincing groups of disabled people to move openly and boldly in this direction. We are often very short of the mark. All the more reason to get started.

In the meantime, many efforts already begun must be reaffirmed and amplified: the creation of services to accompany children and their families throughout the schooling process; the development of ergonomic services (in the widest sense of the term) to adapt urban spaces, transportation, and work stations; the training of professionals in the areas of public health and social work in the issues of disabled people; public advocacy campaigns to combat stigmatization, prejudice, and stereotypes; and the presence of well-informed persons at the moment of birth of a disabled child. We cannot give an exhaustive list.

This model is a challenge for what we as French speakers would call any truly republican, truly democratic space: to establish relationships that presuppose and respect particular terms of existence, invent various combinations of such terms, and take into account all forms of alterity. If we wanted an image for such a model, we could find it in language where all the differences (since there is only that) oppose and interconnect with one another to constitute meanings, meanings that are always open since the combinations are infinite. In turn, each language, however alien to the others, can still manage to be translated into another language, not completely transferred but translated, with some of the inevitable betrayal of original meaning. Disabled persons cannot be reduced to a social identicalness (the deviant, the marginalized) or to an identity based in able-bodiedness. Their existence in the world is singular (and singular in differing ways, depending on the persons and their impairments), but they can translate our experience into theirs and vice versa.

It should be possible to install a common, shared space where there would no longer be any hierarchy but where we would no longer be separated, without being reduced.

This is what Diderot envisaged in his famous *Lettre sur les aveugles à l'usage de ceux qui voient* ("Letter on the blind for the use of the sighted," 1749), when he shows that Saunderson, or the celebrated blind man of Puiseaux, was an "anthropological variety." This is what a literary critic, well experienced in disability, expressed at the end of a conference devoted to the topic of disability in literature:

In light of all this, it should be evident that traditional literary images of the afflicted contribute little or nothing toward creating attitudes which might make possible in actuality a society in which the disabled would be recognized as representing not some absolute, unendurable Other, but one pole on a human spectrum, in which differences of perception and agility separate not merely one individual from another, but one stage from another in each individual's life: from the total dependency of infancy to the gradual crumbling of our powers in old age. . . . In such a utopian society, worked for as well as dreamed by committed professionals and amateurs of goodwill, all means of information retrieval and transport would be redesigned to accommodate such differences. And on a psychological one, even the most debilitating handicaps would be perceived as constituting not a departure from but another assertion of the almost infinitely varied human "norm." Even pain and early death would come to be faced head-on, tragically and joyously, rather than sniggered at in embarrassment, turned away from in terror or denied in pity. (Fiedler 1982:68-69)

CONCLUSION

We have chosen to address the question of exclusion and inclusion as evidenced in the principal forms of "relationships with others" in our organic societies, which have to create their own processes for cohesion and social equalization. Limiting ourselves to what could be called the primary degree of opposition between exclusion and inclusion would have been only to skim the surface of the attendant phenomena.

Evidence supports the notion that every citizen—and certainly even more a disabled citizen—is excluded from some places, from some social goods, and even from some *rights* (to culture, leisure, education), at least in part. Intolerable as this may be, it is proof that society is not egalitarian. This is the rationale that justifies the present claims and the concrete action toward their realization. Persons with a "disability," more than any others, are the living proof of iniquity and inequality. On this level, the specifics of inequality between the able and the disabled are of degree and not of nature. We are all targets for inequitable and unjust treatment—disabled people often to a greater degree than others. Still, the struggle for disabled people is of the same nature as for all those who do not have the access to social goods that is their due. It is the social dimension of citizenship that is called into question.

The most serious question is to ask whether the "rights to" (to free expression, to freedom of movement, to the vote)—that is, the universal rights of human beings—are being denied to the disabled. In certain countries, perhaps, but doubtless also because they are being denied to all individuals. In countries where citizens have rights, these specific rights are not being denied to disabled persons, even though certain guardianship systems could be criticized from this perspective. The disabled are not excluded from "political" citizenship.

As we can see, analysis does not support a brutal assertion to the effect that "disabled people are excluded people" because exclusion itself is a process. It can take different forms, always relates to a social context, can be effected by degrees, and can be common to many other individuals and groups.

On the other hand, situating the issue of disabled people with reference to models, schematics, reference points, the principles of a given society, and so on has the advantage of greater intelligibility. This is the case not only because, as in the preceding instance, the persons with disabilities are situated in a global movement of which they are the symptom, but still more because neither their singularity nor their quality as citizens is effaced.

REFERENCES

Auroux, S. 1990. "Les notions philosophiques." P. 669 in *Encyclopédie Philosophique Universelle*. Paris: Presses Universitaires de France.

Barton, L. and M. Oliver. 1997. *Disability Studies: Past, Present and Future*. Leeds, UK: The Disability Press.

Becker, H. S. 1963. *Outsiders*. New York: Free Press.

Bell, Alexander Graham. 1883. *Memoir upon the Formation of a Deaf Variety of the Human Race*. New Haven, CT: National Academy of Sciences.

Boruwlaski, J. 1788. *Mémoires du célèbre nain Joseph Boruwslaski, gentilhomme polonais*. London.

Burleigh, M. 1994. *Death and Deliverance: Euthanasia in Germany 1900-1945*. Cambridge, UK: Cambridge University Press.

Castel, R. 1995. *Les métamorphoses de la question sociale, une chronique du salariat*. Paris: Fayard.

Douglas, Mary. 1966. *Purity and Danger*. London: Routledge Kegan Paul.

Dumaret, A.-C., C. De Vigan, C. Julian-Reynier, J. Goujard, D. Rosset, and S. Aymé. 1998. "Adopting and Fostering Babies with Down Syndrome: A Cohort of 593 Cases." *Prenatal Diagnosis* 18:437-45.

Dumont, L. 1966. *Homo hierarchicus, le système des castes et ses implications*. Paris: Gallimard.

Durkheim, Émile. 1930. *De la division du travail social*. Paris: Presses Universitaires de France.

Elias, N. 1965. *The Established and the Outsiders*. London: Sage.

Fiedler, Leslie A. 1982. "Pity and Fear: Images of the Disabled in Literature and the Popular Arts." *Salmagundi* 57:57-69.

Foucault, Michel. 1961. *L'histoire de la folie à l'âge classique*. Paris: Plon.

———. 1975. *Surveiller et punir*. Paris: Gallimard.

———. 1984. *Le souci de soi. Histoire de la sexualité 3*. Paris: Gallimard.

Gauchet, Marcel. 1985. *Le désenchantement du monde*. Paris: Gallimard.

———. 1995. *Pour une autre histoire de la folie*. Published with Gladys Swain, *Dialogue avec l'insensé: essai d'histoire de la psychiatrie*. Paris: Gallimard.

Goffman, Erving. 1961. *Asylums: Essays on the Social Situation of Mental Patients and Other Inmates*. Harmondsworth, UK: Penguin.

———. 1963. *Stigma: Notes on the Management of Spoiled Identity*. Englewood Cliffs, NJ: Prentice Hall.

Ingstadt, B. and S. Reynolds Whyte. 1995. *Disability and Culture*. Berkeley: University of California Press.

Kymlicka, Will. 1995. Multicultural Citizenship. In *A Liberal Theory of Minority Rights*. New York: Oxford University Press.

Lane, Harlan. 1984. *When the Mind Hears: A History of the Deaf*. New York: Random House.

———. 1992. *The Mask of Benevolence*. New York: Knopf.

Mauss, Marcel. 1923. *Essai sur le don. Forme et raison de l'échange dans les sociétés archaïques. Année Sociologique. Seconde série, t. I*. Re-ed. 1950 and 1983 in *Sociologie et anthropologie*. Paris: Presses Universitaires de France.

Murphy, Robert. 1987. *The Body Silent: A Journey into Paralysis*. New York: Holt.

Oliver, M. and C. Barnes. 1998. *Disabled People and Social Policy: From Exclusion to Inclusion*. London: Addison-Wesley.

Ravaud, Jean-François, B. Madiot, and I. Ville. 1992. "Discrimination towards Disabled People Seeking Employment." *Social Science and Medicine* 35 (8): 951-58.

Simmel, G. 1908. *Der Arme*. Munich: Duncker & Humblot.

Stainback, William and Susan Stainback. 1990. *Support Networks for Inclusive Schooling: Interdependent Integrated Education*. Baltimore: Brookes.

Stiker, Henri-Jacques. 1982. *Corps infirmes et sociétés*. Paris: Aubier.

———. 1997. *Corps infirmes et sociétés*. Rev. ed. Paris: Dunod.

———. 1999. *A History of Disability*. Ann Arbor: University of Michigan Press.

Taylor, C. 1992. *Multiculturalism and "the Politics of Recognition."* Princeton, NJ: Princeton University Press.

Tönnies, F. 1979. *Gemeinschaft und Gesellschaft: Grundbegriffe der reinen Soziologie*. Darmstadt, Germany: Wissenschaftliche Buchgesellschaft.

Union of the Physically Impaired against Segregation (UPIAS). 1976. *Fundamental Principles of Disability*. London: Author.

Walzer, Michaël. 1988. *Sur la tolérance*. Paris: Gallimard.

Weber, Max. 1920. *Gesammelte Aufsätze zur Religionssoziologie*. Tübingen: Mohr.

Wolfensberger, W. 1972. *The Principle of Normalization in Human Services*. Toronto: National Institute of Mental Retardation.

World Health Organization (WHO). 1980. *International Classification of Impairment, Disability, and Handicap: A Manual of Classification Relating to the Consequences of Disease*. Geneva: Author.

III

DISABILITY IN CONTEXT

Disability Culture

21

Assimilation or Inclusion?

COLIN BARNES
GEOFF MERCER

S ince the 1970s, a disabled people's movement has become established as a political force worldwide. It has confronted the orthodox view that disability should be defined in terms of individual impairment that requires medical treatment. In contrast, disability theory and practice argue that this movement arises from society's failure to remove the wide-ranging social, economic, and environmental barriers that underpin the social exclusion of disabled people and the denial of their basic citizenship rights—what has been termed a *social model of disability* (Finkelstein 1980; Oliver 1983, 1990). This has been complemented by concerted campaigns against the negative stereotypes contained in media and cultural representations. The politicization of disabled people has also highlighted the significance of an alternative disability culture, which celebrates a positive disabled identity and consciousness.

This chapter has four main objectives:

1. to review the analysis of culture and its relationship to society, the economy, and politics;
2. to outline the representation of disability in mainstream culture;
3. to explore the generation of disability cultures;
4. to examine the development of the disability arts movement and its implications for disability culture.

These issues will be illustrated with examples from both U.K. and U.S. cultures.

ANALYZING CULTURE

Sociological studies of culture have adopted a broad interpretation to include symbolic aspects of human society, such as beliefs, rituals, customs, and values, as well as work patterns, leisure activities, and material goods. "Culture consists of the values the members of a given group hold, the norms they follow, and the material goods they create" (Giddens 1989:31). While values are "abstract ideals," norms encompass the rules or guidelines for what is acceptable in social life. This highlights a diffuse view of culture as a shared "way of life." The emphasis is on culture as a "signifying system" through which practices, meanings, and values are "communicated, reproduced, experienced and explored" (Williams 1981:13).

To become a member of a society, one must learn or be socialized into its cultural assumptions and rules, including what (or who) is considered "normal" and typical and categorized as "different." H. G. Wells, in a short story published in 1904, tells of a man called Nunez who falls off a mountain into an isolated valley populated entirely by people with congenital blindness. He presumes that "in the Country of the Blind, the One-eyed Man is King" (Wells 1979:129). In practice, the efforts of Nunez to help the people are rejected by the community, which is sustained by its own distinctive cultural norms and values.

In the conditions of complex industrial societies, cultures rest on something less than complete uniformity among its members. Moreover, such cultures are not static but typically exhibit a degree of flux:

> A culture has two aspects: the known meanings and directions, which its members are trained to; the new observations and meanings, which are offered and tested. These are the ordinary processes of human societies and human minds, and we see through them the nature of a culture: that it is always both traditional and creative. (Williams 1989:4)

The exact form of the relationship between culture and society, particularly its material base, has attracted considerable theoretical debate, stretching back to the writings of classical social theorists, such as Marx, Weber, and Durkheim. In the "orthodox" Marxist variant, the ownership and control of the means of production provide the explanatory key. In some accounts, this leads to a crude determinism in which culture, ideas, and other aspects of what is called the superstructure reflect conditions in the material base. This highlights the political significance of culture as a "dominant ideology" that justifies or obscures social inequalities and perpetuates the oppression of one social group by another. More recent analyses have taken inspiration from a diverse range of social theories, particularly critical theory and neo-Marxism, feminism, poststructuralism, and postmodernism.

The Frankfurt school is generally credited with initiating studies of the media and culture in the 1930s located within critical theory. Its focus was multidisciplinary and spanned a political economy of the media (and the "culture industries"), an analysis of texts, and studies of the social and ideological effects of the media (mass culture) on audiences (Kellner 1989). While the primary focus was on the role of mass culture in promoting working-class passivity and stabilizing industrial capitalism, other studies explored the ways in which some "high" culture offered possibilities for stimulating social and political criticism. It was not until the late 1960s that such issues were picked up and reformulated with a revival of interest in the work of the Italian Marxist, Antonio Gramsci (1971, 1985). His analysis of capitalist domination stressed not only the significance of coercion but also the achievement of "hegemony"—by "willing consent"—through the dominant group's direction of the production and consumption of cultural activities.

Gramsci's influence is very evident in the British cultural studies approach associated with Stuart Hall and his colleagues in the Centre for Contemporary Cultural Studies (CCCS) at the University of Birmingham (Hall 1980; Hall and Jefferson 1976). A further important contributor has been Raymond Williams (1958, 1980, 1981), who developed the notion of cultural materialism. Their work has helped spark a vibrant cultural studies literature. It dismisses the notion of an all-enveloping culture and explores instead the "relative autonomy" between the dominant or "hegemonic" culture and the economy, society, and polity.

The CCCS analysis also stressed the importance of hierarchical and antagonistic social divisions located in gender, race, and generations. These subordinate groups generate "subcultures" or "counterhegemonies" that lead to a form of cultural conflict with the dominant social group. Early studies concentrated on the more spectacular youth subcultures of the post-1960s period (i.e., teddy boys, mods, rockers, skinheads, and punks). In "resisting" adult culture, disillusioned, working-class youth find opportunities in the increasing consumerism of the late-twentieth-century Western capitalist societies to create their own meanings through peer group relations, style, and leisure activities (Hall 1992; Hall and Jefferson 1976).

Most recently, the analysis of late-twentieth-century society, with its emphasis on cultural difference and pluralism, has been at the heart of a burgeoning influence of postmodernism within the cultural studies literature (Inglis 1993). The emphasis on class conflict and struggle has been displaced by a much broader discourse on social and cultural difference, including race, sexuality, and age as well as disability (Hall 1997; Woodward 1997). This heralds a transition in cultural politics—what Stuart Hall in analyzing black culture refers to as a shift "from a struggle over the relations of representation to a politics of representation itself" (Hall 1988:27-28). This suggests that in the continuing campaign against the marginalization and subordination of disabled people, there is an emerging conflict over identity and competing interpretations of what it means to be a "disabled person" within the imagined "disability community." The political struggle assumes new forms that are manifested in the arena of cultural representation.

In the writings of the French "poststructuralist" Michel Foucault, the history of ideas about medicine, madness, and sexuality are analyzed as sociocultural products of particular epochs. His notion of "discursive practice" focuses on the ways in which individual subjects are constituted by discourse (by the ways we talk about them), which itself is structured by a "power/knowledge" complex. That is, the authority to define or describe people or events occupies a significant role in social regulation. This suggests an examination of the "invention" of disability in nineteenth-century medical discourse and of the relationship between "able-bodied normality" and the disabled "other," as increasingly defined by professional knowledge and practice (Hughes and Paterson 1997).

As a sign of the changing times, one of the first books in Britain to challenge the "able-bodied" orthodoxy by disabled people was Paul Hunt's (1966) edited collection, *Stigma: The Experience of Disability*. In his own essay, Hunt argues that disabled people "are set apart from the ordinary" in ways that represent them as a direct "challenge" to commonly held societal values. They are "unfortunate, useless, different, oppressed and sick" (Hunt 1966:146). This characterizes disability in industrial capitalist societies as a "personal tragedy" in which

> people's shocked reaction to the "obvious deviant" stimulates their own deepest fears and difficulties, their failure to accept themselves as they really are and the other person simply as "other." (Hunt 1966:152)

This sets the scene for a struggle by disabled people to supplant oppressive representations with others that reflect their own experiences and values. It heralds the generation of a disability culture, which expresses and sustains a positive disabled identity. From this perspective, disability culture acts as a means of politicizing and cohering disabled people. In contrast, the recent influence of poststructuralist and postmodernist theory has been to highlight the importance of "difference" and multiple identities. This suggests a focus on disability subcultures and provokes debates about the possibilities for unified political action within the disabled population.

CULTURAL REPRESENTATIONS OF DISABILITY

Historically, the characterization of disabled people in mainstream culture has stressed their significant "abnormalities." These are variously used as sources of "entertainment" or to induce and confirm the fears and abhorrence in the nondisabled population. In ancient Greece and Rome, it would almost seem as if no fashionable household was complete without a generous sprinkling of dwarfs, mutes, cretins, eunuchs and hunchbacks, whose principle duty appears to have been to undergo degrading and painful humiliation in order to provide amusement at dinner parties and other festive occasions. (Garland 1995:46)

Evidence of society's fascination with perceived bodily abnormalities persisted throughout the Middle Ages. Many royal courts in Europe retained people of short stature as "court jesters" or kept a complement of "fools," including people with cognitive impairments and learning difficulties, as well as others who feigned "idiocy" to provide amusement. It was also common practice for people with perceived "deformities" and intellectual impairments to be put on display at village fairs on market days, festivals, and holidays, "and peasant parents are known to have toured the countryside displaying for money recently born infants with birth defects" (Gerber 1996:43). The public exhibition of the inmates of "madhouses," such as Bedlam, continued this practice.

By the nineteenth century, such displays had developed into "freak shows," which offered a "formally organized exhibition of people with alleged physical, mental or behavioural difference at circuses, fairs carnivals or other amusement venues" (Bogdan 1996:25). These flourished in Europe and North America in the nineteenth century and in the early part of the twentieth century. They were complemented by the so-called "Ugly Laws" in the United States, which placed social restrictions on those whose physical appearance might offend or frighten "normal" people (Bogdan 1996; Gerber 1996). The freak shows were undoubtedly the site for the exploitation and degradation of people with impairments, although some disabled performers enjoyed public celebrity status and sometimes earned corresponding financial rewards (Bogdan 1996).

While public acceptance of the freak show markedly declined in the early twentieth century, other cultural forms took over. These continued to reflect and confirm negative stereotypes and provide ample rationalization for treating disabled people as "defective" (Battye 1966; Campling 1981; Shearer 1981) or in a "liminal" state. "Neither fish nor fowl; they exist in partial isolation from society as undefined, ambiguous people" (Murphy 1987:112). Indeed, at the end of the century, as Susan Sontag graphically illustrates, the cultural meanings associated with "dread diseases," such as cancer and HIV/AIDS, are so powerful that "it is hardly possible to take up one's residence in the kingdom of the ill unprejudiced by the lurid metaphors with which it has been landscaped" (Sontag 1991:3).

Yet while illness and impairment are often the catalyst for stigma and dread, there is a converse reaction to romanticize their impact on the production of "high culture." For example, in the nineteenth century, tuberculosis or "consumption" became closely associated with individual creativity and artistic sensitivity, as with a number of well-known novelists and poets, including Robert Louis Stevenson, Katherine Mansfield, and John Keats. From this standpoint, some sickness or impairment is credited with adding to the appeal or the insight of the artist (Sontag 1991). This linkage continues through to contemporary musical performers, including Ray Charles, Stevie Wonder, and Hank Williams.

Yet overall, it is the negative cultural stereotyping of people with impairment that rules as the "norm." A series of American studies of representations of disabled people document this pattern across different forms of media culture (Biklen and Bogdan 1977; Clogson 1990; Haller 1995; Klobas 1988; Kurtz 1981; Zola 1985). One of the most cited collections, *Images of the Disabled, Disabling Images* (Gartner and Joe 1987), provides a comprehensive critique. In his contribution, Laurence Kriegel (1987) concludes, after reviewing sources as diverse as *Lady Chatterley's Lover* and *Moby Dick,* that

the world of the crippled and disabled is strange and dark, and it is held up to judgment by those who live in fear of it. The cripple is the creature who has been deprived of his ability to create a self. . . . He must accept definition from outside the boundaries of his own existence. (P. 33)

This argument is echoed in John Schuchman's (1988) survey of images of deafness or "pathological myths" in Hollywood films. Other writers document how this disabling imagery extends to popular cartoon series (Longmore 1987).

Content analyses of the British media programs provide a similar picture. For example, Guy Cumberbatch and Ralph Negrine (1992) monitored television output for six weeks during 1988. Their central findings, reinforced by more recent studies (Ross 1997), are that television programs consistently adhere to a "personal tragedy" approach. The most prevalent story lines linked disabled people with medical treatment or cure, together with programs focusing on their "special achievements." More widely, the representations of disabled people were highly stereotypical, depicting them not as ordinary members of society and part of the "drama of life" but using them to evoke emotions of pity, fear, or admiration. Newspaper reporting of disability has attracted parallel criticism (Smith and Jordan 1991). A limited number of themes dominate newspaper coverage, with health, fund-raising, charity, and personal and individual interest stories most widespread. This unites tabloids and broadsheets, even if the former are particularly prone to dramatize and sensationalize.

A summary audit of the media's preference for "crippling images" includes a fondness for "wonder cure" stories, the role of charity appeals, the invisibility of disabled people on television, the stereotyped portrayal of disabled characters, and the underemployment of disabled people in TV and radio (Karpf 1988). The most frequently documented cultural stereotypes represent the disabled person as pitiable and pathetic, as an object of violence, as sinister and evil, as atmosphere or curio, as "super-cripple," as an object of ridicule, as their own worst and only enemy, as a burden, as sexually abnormal, as incapable of participating fully in community life, and as "normal" (Barnes 1992). While the latter stands apart as the sole positive viewpoint, it remains the least widely expressed, and its representation of "normality" largely ignores the social exclusion of disabled people. The overall effect is clear:

> The general culture invalidates me both by ignoring me and by its particular representations of disability. Disabled people are missing from mainstream culture. When we do appear, it is in specialized forms—from charity telethons to plays about an individual struck down by tragedy—which impose the non-disabled world's definitions on us and our experience. (Morris 1991:85)

However, this initial focus on disability alone has given way to more complex analyses in which the representation of disabled people is mediated by other social factors, such as gender, ethnicity, class, and age. The most detailed studies have focused on the "gendering" of disability in literary texts:

> In many instances, the disabled woman is little more than a metaphor through which the writer hopes to address some broader theme. . . . Disability seems to undermine the very roots of her womanhood. Not surprisingly, therefore, the disabled women in these works frequently feel inferior to others and regard themselves with loathing. (Kent 1987:60, 63)

Studies have also explored the interaction between definitions of masculinity and disability. Thus, in films such as *Born on the Fourth of July* and *Waterdance,* individuals are portrayed as desperately trying to cope with the onset of impairment. The polarization of masculine potency and disabled impotency accentuates the presumption that if it is hurtful to feel unloved, it is much more damaging to be incapable of making love. In contrast, women are typically represented as vulnerable, passive, and dependent, so that the artistic interest in portraying disabled women is more focused on their role as tragic or saintly figures who may perhaps be "saved" by an "able-bodied" man. This reluctance to depict disabled women as sexual beings or in traditional female roles as wives and mothers is explored by two Australian writers, Helen Meekosha and Leanne Dowse (1997). They point to the contradiction between the general support by the disabled people's movement for images of disabled people in "normal" roles and the desire of feminists to challenge gender stereotypes.

The increasing breadth of the cultural studies literature is demonstrated in its engagement with specific artworks, texts, and performances. Lennard Davis (1995) traces the development of the "lexicon of disability," along with the social construction of "normalcy." "The implications of the hegemony of normalcy are profound and extend into the very heart of cultural production (Davis 1995:49). Indeed, he suggests that "one can find in almost any novel . . . a kind of surveying of the terrain of the body, an attention to difference . . . physical, mental and national" (p. 41). Another significant contributor to the analysis of disability representation in American culture is Rosemarie Garland Thomson (1997). Her sources include the traditional freak show, sentimental novels such as *Uncle Tom's Cabin,* and contemporary African American fiction. She also draws heavily on diverse theoretical traditions, including contemporary literary, feminist, and social theory, particularly its postmodern versions, to examine how "corporeal deviance" is a "product of cultural rules" about "able-bodiedness."

> Constructed as the embodiment of corporeal insufficiency and deviance, the physically disabled body becomes a repository for social anxieties about such troubling concerns as vulnerability, control and identity. (Thomson 1997:6)

Unlike so much of the cultural studies literature, Thomson also explores the appearance of an "active" counterrepresentation. For example, in the novels of Toni Morrison, "physically disabled or anomalous black women triumph," and the novels "repudiate stigmatization itself" (Thomson 1997).

Martin Norden (1994) also advances the understanding of disability representation in his comprehensive history of cinema. He shows how, going back to Thomas Edison's 1898 short film, *Fake Beggar,* stereotypical and distorted representations of disability were standard fare. As a visual medium, cinema used pictures to reveal character, and emotional and physical "cripples" were routinely equated. The cinema also inherited the entrepreneurial traditions of the freak show, or as Cecil B. De Mille remarked, "Affliction is much more saleable" (quoted in Norden 1994:71).

Norden (1994) traces the development of a range of stereotypes—Elderly Dupe, Saintly Sage, Obsessive Avenger, Sweet Innocent, Comic Misadventurer, Tragic Victim, Noble Warrior—which are used to oppress disabled people. However, he does detect positive changes of this imagery as it evolved from the early exploitative phase (1890s-1930s) through the explorative phase (1930s-1970s) to the incidental phase (1970s to present). Nevertheless, even in contemporary films, the negative stereotypes still appear.

Similar themes are stressed by Paul Darke in his examination of the representation of disability in films such as *The Elephant Man* (Darke 1994) and *When Billy Broke His Head and Other Tales of Wonder* (Darke 1995). He categorizes the latter as a *rite de passage* movie in which Billy Golfus, himself newly impaired after a motorcycle accident, explores the meaning of disability in America with its strong emphasis on individualistic (and capitalistic) values. Darke (1998) also explores the concept of "normality drama," which refers to a genre that uses abnormal or impaired characters to represent a perceived threat to the dominant view of normality. As such, it encompasses the cultural rationalization of the social disablement of the person with a perceived impairment.

One of the most widely cited attempts to locate an aesthetic and theoretical analysis of bodily representation with a broader concern toward social and political context is advanced by David Hevey (1992) in his study of charity advertising, *The Creatures That Time Forgot.* Hevey examines how British charities "market" particular impairments in ways that parallel the "branding" of commercial products in their search for public support. A hallmark of the early charity approach is the stark image of a person with impairment, usually in black and white, which centers on their physical "flaw." Its purpose is to evoke fear and sympathy in the viewer. Charity advertising is described as "the visual flagship for the myth of the tragedy of impairment" (Hevey 1992:51) and a highly significant component in the cultural construction of disability.

> It represents the highest public validation of the isolation of disabled people. It presents a solution to the "problem" of disablement by a disguised blaming of the victim. It fails to find a solution because it is itself the problem. (Hevey 1992:51)

The role of charity imagery in the lives of disabled people has been further linked to the role of pornography in women's oppression. In both cases, the focus is on the body, particularly on parts of the body (the breasts/the impairment). Moreover, the conditions in which the image is produced and interpreted are outside the control of the subject and involve wider meanings and power relationships (Shakespeare 1994). The aim is to stimulate an emotional reaction from the viewer that turns the subject into an object of desire or fear. This has particularly threatening consequences for many disabled women.

> There are also dangers here of the advertising industry moving from selling the beautiful and sculptured non-disabled body to selling the beautiful and sculptured disabled body. For women with degenerative or acquired disabilities, or illnesses not amenable to physical body sculpting, these images can further demoralize and undermine their sense of self-worth. (Meekosha and Dowse 1997:97-98)

Nevertheless, there have been recent moves by some charities away from the use of traditional images of disability to generate public donations. This approach has been categorized as "look at the ability, not the disability." Recent campaigns in Britain by SCOPE (formally known as the Spastics Society) have focused on prejudice and discrimination as constitutive of disability, although they have not dispensed entirely with a personal tragedy approach. The Leonard Cheshire Foundation followed suit as it shifted its emphasis from residential homes to other support services by developing a national advertising campaign that focused on the word *enabled*. The charity for people with learning difficulties, Mencap, has also sought a new and more "radical" image. Its tearful "Little Stephen" logo gave way to a more positive representation that embraced citizenship and social rights, although its advertising images are still dominated by the "desire to market attractive pictures" (Corbett and Ralph 1994:11).

More generally, through the last quarter of the twentieth century, there has been a discernible rise in more "positive" cultural and media images of disabled people. Through the 1980s in America, disabled characters began to appear in advertisements for Levi jeans, McDonalds, and Kodak films (Longmore 1987). There are also more "disabled" characters (although not all are played by actors with impairment) and disability story lines in British and American soap operas and dramas. A notable shift in British TV programming was signaled by the showing in 1994 of Skallagrigg, a mythical hero in stories told by disabled inmates of institutions. Such examples demonstrate how the media have begun to take "legitimate and conscious account of the film maker's or artist's encounter with and progress through the experience of disability" (Pointon 1997:237).

On a theoretical level, there remain contrasting emphases, with postmodernist, cultural studies approaches to disability representation relatively more evident in the American literature, compared with the more sociological studies of disabling imagery provided by British writers. The latter have been particularly influenced by the social model distinction between impairment as a property of the body and disability as a social relationship. Moreover, the American literature stresses linguistic and textual analysis and the link between corporeal diversity, unequal status and power, and cultural meanings, while its British counterparts have mostly concentrated on media representation to provide an ideological pretext for social exclusion.

Media Effects

As the media have grown in importance throughout the twentieth century as mechanisms for communicating ideas and information, their significance as a terrain of cultural politics has also increased. There has been a widespread presumption, in both the American and British literature on disability, that cultural and media imagery has a potent if not direct effect on its audience. This remains an empirical question, but it sits uneasily with recent characterizations of late-twentieth-century society and culture, which stresses the significance of social and cultural diversity rather than homogeneity. This raises doubts about the impact of the media in disseminating specific views, including disabling messages.

Hitherto, a straightforward "hypodermic syringe" model has prevailed in which the "naturalness" of disability is promoted or reinforced through the range of cultural forms. Against this, a "uses and gratifications" approach claimed that people are not simply inert or passive but actively interpret media materials in accordance with their own needs and interests (McQuail 1972). Others have used Gramsci's notion of hegemony to explore how the media "manufacture consent" to the dominant order while acknowledging that the media may be "read" in contrary ways so that audiences may negotiate or reject the intended messages (Hall 1980, 1997).

The possibility of an active audience is yet to be fully explored in the context of the media and disability. Certainly, media audiences will have already been socialized in a variety of ways and have developed firm views about particular subjects. There is a widespread presumption that negative cultural and media stereotypes of disability and disabled people reinforce and extend disability stereotypes held by the general public. This is evident in studies of mental illness (Philo 1996) and of HIV/AIDS (Kitzinger 1993), which demonstrate the media's pivotal role in the dissemination of information, images, and opinions. However, what is less certain is the extent to which the disabled population at large, as opposed to disability activists, interprets media representation.

Models tend to be static and do not necessarily reflect contradictory representations and change over time. They help us "fit" media stories into boxes, but do not necessarily aid in a more complex analysis of the processes involved in disability construction. Thus overall, the variety of elements of media analysis necessary to understand disability cannot be reduced to a simple categorization of content, but require a complex sensitivity to multiple dimensions of the process. (Meekosha and Dowse 1997:95)

DISABILITY CULTURE

Disability culture presumes a sense of common identity and interests that unite disabled people and separate them from their nondisabled counterparts. The exact bases for group cohesion and consciousness will vary, as will the level and form of any engagement in social and political action. The potential for disability consciousness is enhanced when there is agreement on the source of their collective social exclusion. This division between "insiders" and "outsiders" is developed and maintained by specific cultural styles, customs, and social interaction, such as in segregated, residential schooling, or from a distinctive language (as with Deaf culture). There is a further presumption that a disability culture rejects the notion of impairment-difference as a symbol of shame or self-pity and stresses instead solidarity and a positive identification. However, the transition from a medicalized, impairment-based self to a disabled identity and consciousness is not necessarily one-directional or one-dimensional.

A key issue is whether the disabled community is based on those with the range of impairments or restricted to a specific or limited impairment range. This might be the basis for differentiating a general disability culture from disability subcultures that are located around specific groups of disabled people. However, one immediate snag is that adherents to Deaf subculture would reject such a designation on the grounds that they are not a subgroup within the disabled population but a separate linguistic community. In contrast, organizations of people with learning difficulties have argued that they are effectively ignored or excluded by other disabled people.

From a postmodern perspective, the emphasis is on multiple and fluid identities. The notion of cultural politics has been layered with different subjectivities. The dominant (nondisabled) discourse regards difference as a technical or essential category, whereas postmodernists view it as a social construction. Equally, solidarity is not regarded as undermined by "difference"; in contrast, it accepts and thrives on diversity. For postmodernists, disability politics must move away from a concentration on single-issue politics, in which disability alone is the concern. In practice, this deflects attention away from the multiple and simultaneous sources of oppression based, for example, on age, class, race, gender, and sexuality. While the notion of internal differences within the disabled population is now broadly accepted, it remains a contentious issue in terms of political strategy. Whereas postmodernists stress diversity and fragmentation and the diminished relevance of broad political projects, more "traditional" disability theorists argue that this leads to political inaction. Can disabled people have it both ways, stressing their diversity while seeking unified political action?

Traditionally, the responses of the dominant culture to the prospect of a disability culture have questioned its legitimacy, being variously hostile, dismissive, and patronizing. Hence, disability culture has been built out of political struggle and with few resources. It is also important to note that within the disabled population, most people will have acquired their impairment later in life, and this means that their embrace of disability culture is inhibited by their immersion hitherto in a nondisabled environment.

Historically, embryonic disability communities have emerged most often from those segregated on the basis of their perceived impairment. With the growth of industrialization and urbanism, the resort to specialized institutions for the most severely impaired or "threatening" individuals has expanded significantly across North America and Britain. Their early religious character has increasingly been overtaken by a more secularized and professional medical regime (Parker 1988). For the disabled inmates, the shared experiences in areas such as schooling and rehabilitation agencies have raised the potential for development of a shared, albeit "defensive," consciousness. There are several sociological studies of this phenomenon. The most well known is Erving Goffman's (1961) picture of in-patient psychiatric life in *Asylums*. This work stresses the regulation of social deviance, but it also documents the possibility for individual and group subversion and the development of an alternative, shared culture of resistance. The seeds of a more critical and proactive disability culture are contained in the writings of Paul Hunt, who himself was a long-term inmate of residential institutions.

> Maybe we have to remind people of a side of life they would sooner forget. We do this primarily by what we are. But we can intensify it and make it more productive if we are fully conscious of the tragedy of our situation, yet show by our lives that we believe this is not the final tragedy. (Hunt 1966:156)

From the 1960s, with gathering forms of social protest spurred initially by the black civil rights movement in America, residential institutions provided a fertile seedbed for disabled activism. The emergence of the independent living movement in America gained a further significant stimulus with the return of disabled veterans from the Vietnam War. In Britain, disabled people's campaigns can be traced to action by a group of disabled residents at the *Le Court* Cheshire Home in Hampshire. These early years were taken up with identifying common interests and a policy focus for political grievances. As the disabled activist Elspeth Morrison explains,

> In the early days, if you take the personal as political argument, then meetings were deeply political in that it was very much personal experience which was getting people up and talking; about what it was like to have their particular impairment, what things dis-

abled them, how the world saw them and what it felt to be like that. (Quoted in Campbell and Oliver 1996:108-9)

The crucial divide in developing a disability consciousness has been to move away from the view that disability is an individual problem that requires equivalent individual (mainly medical) solutions—hence the significance of reading or hearing about other disabled people's experiences in books and journals and watching specialist disability TV programs. Since the 1970s, there has been a steady growth of disabled people's writings on their experiences, including the appearance of an "alternative" disability press, such as *Disability Rag* and *Mouth* in the United States. A significant proportion of disabled people have become sensitized to the shared experience of disability, although diagnoses of its sources and appropriate action are less agreed on.

Increased political activism also confronts the images of passivity and dependence that are so widely disseminated in the media. This has led to new representations of disabled people as active participants in protest action against inaccessible buildings and transport, charity events such as telethons, welfare benefit cuts, and a broad range of campaigns for civil rights. In the United Kingdom, for example, the media started to provide images of disabled people chaining themselves to buses and trains, blocking roads, and crawling along the streets (Pointon 1999). This, in turn, threw the spotlight on competing views among disabled people and contrasts between established organizations *for* disabled people and those organizations *of* disabled people that are controlled by disabled people themselves. A whole new realm of disability politics impressed itself on the media.

How the news media have responded is revealing. There was an overwhelming consensus that ensured the portrayal of disabled people as embroiled within a personal tragedy, a burden, surrounded by devoted caregivers, and, in the "best" cases, demonstrating the quality of courageous battlers. Initially, newspapers and TV were bemused and uncertain how to present these contrary images. References to the "last civil rights battle" were mixed with concerns that disability protest threatened to alienate their supporters or that acceding to the protesters' demands for an accessible environment was simply too expensive to contemplate. Although the political climate was changing toward disabled people, there was ample evidence that traditional prejudices had not been eliminated. Thus, editorial space was granted by the respected British broadsheet, *Sunday Telegraph,* to a condemnation of "the furious Quasimodos" who had engaged in a "red paint" demonstration in Downing Street. According to the writer, "They seemed not merely visually revolting, but completely horrible, embittered people" (Wilson 1997).

Years of campaigning eventually led to the 1996 Disability Discrimination Act, but it failed to go far enough for significant sections of the disabled people's movement. As Ann Pointon (1999) notes, "The press was playing to a largely sympathetic but relatively uninformed readership" (p. 232). Stories about the inclusion of people with HIV/AIDS with the "disabled" category and fears of the cost and impact of destroying historic sites to make them accessible dominated, rather than continuing concerns among disabled people that the act was little more than symbolic. Specialist disability radio and TV programs gave this subject fuller attention but failed to reach a mass audience, particularly among nondisabled people. There were also splits in the alliance of disability organizations. In sum, the wider disabled audience has started to openly reevaluate its own circumstances and experiences, leading to increased political activity, without overturning dominant media images.

IDENTITY POLITICS

Over the past decade, social theorists on both sides of the Atlantic have become engrossed with theories of the body and the ways in which it has become a key site for struggles around identity. Attention to self-improving and healthy "body projects" is regarded as a central theme in contemporary consumerist culture. This has given added significance to and exacerbated the existing representation of many disabled people in terms of their "flawed" bodies and as "dustbins for disavowal." Nondisabled people's anxieties about loss of control and incapacity are projected onto disabled people through artistic and media imagery (Hevey 1992; Shakespeare 1994; Thomson 1997; Wendell 1996).

> What we fear, we often stigmatize and shun and sometimes seek to destroy. Popular entertainments depicting disabled characters allude to these fears and prejudices or address them obliquely or fragmentarily, seeking to reassure us about ourselves. (Longmore 1987:66)

In contrast, identity politics is based on membership of an oppressed or marginalized group and extolling its virtues. According to survey evidence, Fine and Asch (1988) report that 74 percent of disabled Americans report a sense of common identity. This sense of "commonality" is not necessarily based on adherence to a social model of disability, nor does it necessarily lead to political activism. The transition to a disabled identity is often slow and uncertain, rather than a dramatic conversion "on the road to Damascus." Moreover, the character and the extent of this identification are not fixed but open to reformulation. This uncertainty is compounded because disability interacts within other major sources of identity or difference. Hence, what it means to be a young, disabled white woman, as opposed to an older, disabled black man, for example, defies easy categorization.

The generation of a separate cultural identity has divided disabled people. While some groups, such as deaf people, have long regarded themselves as having a distinctive culture, the most disabled people have been less enthusiastic. As Vic Finkelstein has noted,

> Firstly, there is a great deal of uncertainty amongst disabled people whether we do want "our own culture." After all, we all have had the experiences of resisting being treated as different, as inferior to the rest of society. So why now, when there is much greater awareness of our desire to be fully integrated into society do we suddenly want to go off at a tangent and start trying to promote our differences, our separate identity? Secondly, at this time, even if we do want to promote our own identity, our own culture, there has been precious little opportunity for us to develop a cultural life. Certainly few of us would regard the endless hours that disabled people used to spend basket weaving under the direction of occupational therapists in day centres as an artistic contribution that disabled people made to the cultural life of humankind. (Finkelstein, quoted in Campbell and Oliver 1996:111)

Yet as Simi Linton (1998) notes, from her American vantage point of the end of the century, disabled people have "solidified" as a group, although this still encompasses considerable individual variation.

> The cultural narrative of this community incorporates a fair share of adversity and struggle, but it is also, and significantly, an account of the world negotiated *from the vantage point of the atypical*. Although the dominant culture describes that atypical experience as deficit and loss, the disabled community's narrative recounts it in more complex ways. The cultural stuff of the community is the creative response to atypical experience, the adaptive maneuvers through a world configured for non-disabled people. The material that binds is the art of finding one another, of identifying and naming disability in a world reluctant to discuss it, and of unearthing historically and culturally significant material that relates to our experience. (Linton 1998:5)

The process has been likened to the experience of black people or gays and lesbians, insofar as attitudes and emotions hitherto confined to the "private" sphere have been translated into a public affirmation.

"Coming out" has become a favoured phrase among disabled people to signify moving toward an open identification as a disabled person. The personal is political, as shame and fear are personal burdens that are challenged by being made public. (Linton 1998:22)

This emphasis on identities, which have been "hidden from history" or submerged by "master" identities such as social class, "whiteness", or heterosexuality, is very much a feature of recent social protest movements (Weeks 1994). What had been a source of exclusion and marginalization is translated into a source of pride (as in "glad to be gay"). Yet this application to people with impairment is typically regarded as more contentious, with the notion of "glad to be impaired" far less accepted as a unifying theme for disabled people, and the calls for people with impairment to "come out of the closet" are meaningless for so many disabled people.

Hence, the emphasis on "multiple identities" focuses on what differentiates one disabled person from another disabled person. This is illustrated by the ways in which "disabled dykes" are excluded in "every sphere of lesbian cultural production" (Tremain 1996:16) because they expose

the white heterosexualism that dominates the disability rights movement, a movement which seldom aligns itself with queer struggles for justice in the institutional, symbolic-discursive, and social realms. (Tremain 1996:21)

The ambition of "consciousness raising" was to build on what was regarded as the common experience of social oppression among disabled people. This would lead to the growth of a general disability culture. However, this prospect has been increasingly criticized on the grounds that it reflects a white, middle-class, male perspective on the social world (Barnes, Mercer, and Shakespeare 1999). With the acknowledgment of social divisions within the disabled population, the presumed homogeneity of disability culture was replaced by cohesive subgroups identified (e.g., on the basis of gender, race, and age) or by impairment. Most recently, social theorizing has been preoccupied with the fluidity of social identity and its continuing re-creation and representation, through practice and discourse, across "multiple identities." This stressed the shifting boundaries of a disabled identity and the dissolution of the category of "disabled person."

An often overlooked issue in this deconstructionist approach, as Iris Young (1990) argues, is that it ignores power differences and conflicts of interest, both within and between these communities, while "contingent identities" are themselves reified in social policy and social protest.

DEAF CULTURE

The process of exclusion has been fundamental to the development of Deaf culture. There are references to hearing impairment stretching back at least to ancient Greece and the Old Testament in Western history. In the case of contemporary Deaf culture, it has its roots in the eighteenth century and the discovery of "deafness" and the development of schools for deaf children. Indeed, this was a period when countries across Europe began to develop education and training for specific groups of people with impairment, with a dozen schools for children with severe hearing impairment established by the end of the eighteenth century (Davis 1995).

Until that time, deaf people had little shared experience. They were typically isolated from other deaf people and lacked a shared, complex means of communication. The only exceptions were those who lived in families or areas where there were other deaf people. Given their effective exclusion from an oral culture, regular social interaction with other deaf people encouraged the growth of sign language as a means of communication. Restricted finger signs were supplanted by sign language (as is illustrated in its use by an established Deaf community in Paris in the second half of the eighteenth century) (Lane 1984). In North America, this potential is vividly illustrated in Nora Groce's (1985) study, *Everyone Here Speaks Sign Language: Heredi-*

tary Deafness in Martha's Vineyard. An inherited trait was brought to this island off Cape Cod, Massachusetts, in the early seventeenth century, which led to deafness in a relatively high proportion of the island's population. The ratio is estimated at 1 per 150 nondeaf people. Of particular significance is the general use of sign language by the islanders that led to the integration of the deaf minority into the "normal" life of the community. Groce quotes the comments of a *Boston Sunday Herald* reporter in 1895:

> The kindly and well-informed people whom I saw, strange to say, seem to be proud of the affliction—to regard it as a kind of plume in the hat of the stock. Elsewhere the afflicted are screened as much as possible from public notoriety. But these people gave me a lot of photographs, extending back four generations. (Groce 1985:51)

As Linton states (1998:66), "The reporter presaged the deaf pride movement by almost one hundred years," in his amazed comments that "the mutes are not uncomfortable in their deprivation" (quoted in Groce 1985:52-53). In short, the "knowledge of Deaf people is not simply a camaraderie with others who have a physical condition, but is . . . historically created and actively transmitted across generations" (Padden and Humphries 1988:2).

However, in understanding the cultural experience of deafness, it is necessary to distinguish between the following:

- people with a hearing impairment who may be described as deaf or hard of hearing,
- people who have often acquired or developed hearing loss and are not native users of British Sign Language (BSL) or American Sign Language (ASL),
- people with congenital hearing impairment who have been immersed in a BSL or ASL environment (whether at home with deaf parents or by attending a deaf school) and who then define themselves as deaf.

It is the latter group who provides the members of a Deaf culture that is located in a distinctive, shared language. (Here, the use of the capital "D" denotes membership and recognition of Deaf culture.) In addition, the community may also comprise certain hearing people, such as the children of deaf adults (CODA) who have grown up with sign language and other aspects of Deaf culture (Davis 1995).

Many deaf people explicitly refer to themselves as a linguistic and cultural minority, making the analogy with minority ethnic groups who are similarly likely to be excluded because they lack fluency in the dominant language. This goes with a resistance to being identified as disabled people or people with impairment (Lane 1995). This has been accompanied by considerable resistance to cochlea implants, which have the capacity to restore some hearing function, and to genetic screening to identify for termination a fetus with a likely hearing impairment.

In their struggles to avoid assimilation within an "oralist" culture and retain their separate cultural identity, deaf people have opposed wider campaigns by disabled people's organizations for inclusive schools. Instead, the Deaf community supports special deaf schools as the bastions of Deaf culture generally and, more specifically, for its emphasis on teaching and learning through the media of BSL and ASL. As British deaf activist Paddy Ladd affirms,

> Basically deaf people whose first language is BSL should be seen as a linguistic minority . . . our schools go back to the 1790s and our clubs to the 1820s. Our language is much older. Deaf people marry each other 90% of the time, 10% have deaf children. Our customs and traditions have been passed down the ages and these, together with our values and beliefs, constitute our culture. . . . The whole definition of culture is so much wider than the one the disability movement is espousing. (Ladd, quoted in Campbell and Oliver 1996:120)

Here, separate schooling for deaf children is regarded as central to maintaining deaf identity and consciousness:

All this has been achieved despite the disgusting work of oralists, our schools are where we are socialised into the culture. Integration threatens to destroy these centres of achievement, quite apart from the damage caused by thrusting lone deaf kids into mainstream schools with no access to what teachers are saying, no easy access to the rest of the school's activities, no deaf adults, the total lack of a peer group etc., etc. (Ladd, quoted in Campbell and Oliver 1996:121)

While there are those with a hearing impairment who do not identify in the same way with Deaf culture but see themselves as part of the broader disabled population and disability culture (Corker 1998), they are in a minority. As a result, there has been an uneasy "standoff" between deaf people and organizations of disabled people that has inhibited a political alliance with other groups of disabled people.

BEYOND "WESTERN" VIEWS OF DISABILITY

While the growth of the disabled people's movement has progressed significantly on a worldwide basis, the Euro-American literature on disability has been slow to acknowledge and review non-Western approaches to disability, including the form and character of disability culture(s). While there has been increased recognition that impairment and disability have different meanings, this is too often a preliminary to describing cultural differences at a superficial level. It encourages a particular form of academic voyeurism in which there is an opportunity to contrast approaches to disability, focusing on the "more exotic" differences, and variously condemn or celebrate one side of the "cultural divide" (Stone 1999).

Comparative studies are a valuable support in arguments for the social construction and contrasting meanings attached to disability, particularly when they attempt to provide an explanation that incorporates material as well as cultural factors (Ingstad and Whyte 1995). Such studies reveal the contingent character of disability over time and between cultures. Religion—over time and across societies—has been a particularly potent force in separating people regarded as "abnormal" (Miles 1995). There is a belief in Western societies that Eastern religions such as Hinduism, Buddhism, and Shintoism represent impairment as a divine judgment and retribution for past sins. This Eurocentric tendency to categorize notions of disability in other parts of the world, where most people (disabled and nondisabled) are thought of as "primitive" or variants on a "personal tragedy," is an approach that has not been seriously addressed by disability writers.

The predominant tone of discussions on disability in non-Western societies is that their approaches and cultures represent traditional life-worlds. These are viewed as inferior or anachronistic, rather than contrary and enduring, with their own strengths, contradictions, and relevance for the present day. The problems in bridging this divide are illustrated in debates within the World Health Organization over the international adoption of a Western, biomedical classification and terminology. There have also been attempts by Disabled Peoples' International to agree on a social model of disability, with its specific terminology. This has been hampered by considerable difficulties in translating the key terms.

DISABILITY ARTS

The emergence of a disability arts movement marks a significant stage in the transition to a positive portrayal of disabled people that builds on the social model of disability. Its focus is on cultural and media representation, and it represents the further self-identification of disabled people while drawing on and contributing to wider political campaigns.

> Disability arts would not have been possible without disability politics coming along first. It's what makes a disability artist different from an artist with a disability. (Sutherland 1997:159)

The disability arts movement encompasses several reinforcing dimensions. First, it argues for disabled people to have access to the mainstream of artistic consumption and production. Second, it includes impaired-focused art that explores the experience of living with impairment. Third, and most crucially, disability arts offers a critical response to the experience of social exclusion and marginalization. It involves the development of shared cultural meanings and the collective expression of the experience of disability and struggle. It entails using culture and media to expose the discrimination and prejudice disabled people face and to generate a positive group consciousness and identity (Barnes et al. 1999). This schema importantly retains the crucial distinction between "disabled people doing art" and "disability arts." It is important that disabled people have the right to paint, create, and write about anything, in any way; it does not have to be overtly "political."

Disability arts is potentially educative, transformative, expressive, and participative. It is a conception of cultural action that owes much to playwrights such as German dramatist Berthold Brecht and educationalists such as Brazilian Paolo Freire. They emphasized the potential of disability arts as a progressive, emancipatory force at both individual and social levels. Brecht wrote plays and songs that focus on oppression and injustice, while Freire viewed education as a means of unleashing people's political consciousness. Such accounts have their parallels in feminist analyses, which celebrate a "politics of signification" in which subversive representations or performances illuminate and confront discriminatory barriers and attitudes.

In contrast, traditional approaches to disabled people and the arts have been based on paternalism. It is where disabled people are viewed as incapable of productive work, filled with negative thoughts or unable to communicate their thoughts and feelings with others through normal conversation, that art is offered as a means of therapy or as part of the process of "rehabilitation." This is particularly a feature of the activities promoted within special schools, day centers, and segregated institutions. Such initiatives have tended to individualize and depoliticize creativity, but they have also been exploited for commercial purposes, such as charity Christmas cards. While there is obviously a place for art therapy, disabled people have increasingly developed a more active orientation, which goes beyond conveying a sense of their psychological state of adjustment to their impairment. Too often, art therapy is based on the assumption that disabled people have "nothing to communicate" (Sutherland 1997:159). Disability arts argues exactly the opposite (Vasey 1992). Since its emergence, disability arts has made a distinctive contribution to the growing politicization of disabled people:

> Arts practice should also be viewed as much as a tool for change as attending meetings about orange badge provision. . . . Only by ensuring an integrated role for disability arts and culture in the struggle can we develop the vision to challenge narrow thinking, elitism and dependency on others for our emancipation. To encourage the growth of a disability culture is no less than to begin the radical task of transforming ourselves from passive and dependent beings into active and creative agents for social change. (Finkelstein and Morrison 1992:20, 22)

Far from being a sideshow to the "real" political action, disability arts and culture have an important role to play in advancing the interests of disabled people. From the mid-1980s, there has been a substantial increase in work by disabled poets, musicians, artists, and entertainers that articulates the experience and value of a "disabled" lifestyle. These developments represent a gathering self-confidence among disabled people. Given their widespread exclusion from or disempowerment by mainstream arts training, it has been necessary to start from scratch. It is for this reason that the disabled people's movement has supported and nurtured its own artists (Cribb 1993; Morrison and Finkelstein 1993). Indeed, the involvement of significant numbers in the disability arts is one indicator of the maturity of the disabled people's movement.

Early initiatives in Britain include the first production of a television program in 1975 specifically for (and increasingly produced by) disabled people titled *Link* and the production of a range of newsletters and magazines by disabled people and groups. *In From the Cold,* is another magazine produced between 1981 and 1987 by Britain's Liberation Network of Disabled People. *Coalition,* the magazine of the Greater Manchester Coalition of Disabled People (GMCDP), first appeared in 1986 and is still going strong. In addition, *DAIL* (*Disability Arts in London*) magazine first appeared in 1987 and has a national circulation of 3,000 with an estimated 8,000 readers. These magazines include articles, features, reviews, and commentary on disability issues, culture, and arts. Further illustrations of this gathering trend include the establishment of the London Disability Arts Forum in 1986, the Disability Arts Conference in Manchester in 1987, and an upsurge of disability arts in conferences, exhibitions, workshops, cabaret, and performance throughout Britain (Keith 1994; Pointon and Davies 1997). Indeed, by the late 1980s, and in line with the general shift toward programming for minorities, other "specialist" disability programs appeared on British television, including *Same Difference, See Hear,* and *One in Four.* In 1993, the British Broadcasting Corporation (BBC) set up the Disability Programmes Unit staffed in the main by disabled people, many of whom had learned the skills of media presentation with *Link.* This promoted a critical awareness of the rights of disabled people and their growing militancy, which in turn stimulated others to adopt a "disabled" identity.

Parallel trends in North America led to a flourishing disability press, including *The Disability Rag,* the unofficial newspaper of the American independent living movement that began publication in 1980 (Brown 1997; Davis 1995). Frank Bowe (1978) offers one early view of the beginnings of a disability consciousness in America in the 1960s and 1970s. Autobiographical accounts flourished, and if most concentrated on the routine "living with my impairment" approach and individualistic adjustments (Brown 1997; Kleinfield 1977; Orlansky and Heward 1981), there were notable exceptions, such as Irving Zola's (1982) account of his personal and intellectual journey in rethinking disability and identity. This literature was complemented by a gathering production of novels, comedy, songs, poetry, drama, paintings, and sculpture that increasingly conveyed an emerging sense of group identity and interests (Brown 1997; Davis 1995; Hirsch 1995; Saxton and Howe 1989; Tremain 1996). The conclusion of American commentators is that disability culture flowered through the 1980s as a complement to disability rights protests. It helped to cement a group consciousness so that by the early 1990s, a "disability culture movement" was firmly established (Brown 1997; Hirsch 1995; Longmore 1995; Shapiro 1993).

Recognition of the importance of involving disabled people in mainstream culture has also taken off. In the United States, the Americans with Disabilities Act (ADA), for example, forced suppliers of television sets to build in a decoder chip so deaf people could receive a "closed-caption" (a type of subtitling) system for viewers with hearing impairment. In the United Kingdom, National Lottery funding was awarded to the Royal School for the Deaf to help build Europe's sign language video library, the first phase of a £1 million National Sign Language Video Centre.

Yet despite all these developments, notions such as "disability culture," "disability pride," and the "celebration of difference" remain problematic for many disabled people. This is particularly the case for those whose impairment is debilitating and painful or often results in premature death. While other oppressed groups may proclaim that "black is beautiful" or pronounce themselves "glad to be gay," it is harder for many disabled people to offer similar accolades to their impairment. While agreeing about the significant sociopolitical origins of many of the disabling barriers facing disabled people, many feel uneasy with assertions such as, "We can celebrate, and take pride in, our physical and intellectual differences" (Morris 1991:189).

Disabled people are more likely to develop an attitude of ambivalence toward impairment, insisting that people with perceived impairment should be allowed to lead valued lives while also refusing to glorify impairment.

The potential of disability arts is that it provides a vital component in the construction of an accessible route to empowerment. As Morrison and Finkelstein (1993) argue, disability arts, as well as the disabled people's movement, provides space for critical reflection on the variety of experiences among disabled people. However, the impact of disability culture and art will itself be exclusionary if it loses touch with its disabled constituencies. There is also the constant concern that it will be assimilated into mainstream culture with the result that its political significance is neutralized. Yet the potential contribution of disability arts to challenging the social exclusion of disabled people remains crucial.

> We are a long way . . . from emancipation, but to help us to get there I think committed disabled activists have the job of producing work of real clarity which truly describes our situation, so there can be no misunderstanding by anyone of the fact that we are oppressed and that there must be no recreation of that oppression in millennia to come. (Vasey 1992:13)

CONCLUSION

Historically, nondisabled people have produced representations of disability. This has resulted in a pervasive disabling imagery that has reinforced social and cultural divisions between disabled and nondisabled people. With the recent politicization of disabled people, a stimulus has been given to the formation of a disability culture. The aim has been to counter the individualization and medicalization of disability, the essentialist and determinist definitions of disability, the moral-laden character of "normalcy" and negative stereotyping of disabled people as well as disability as a metaphor for social exclusion, and the lack of subjectivity and agency among disabled people.

By highlighting difference and multiple identities, the spotlight immediately focuses on its political implications. Whereas some see renewed solidarity born out of recognizing multiple identities and differences, others fear that this, coupled with loss of a clearly defined goal, undercuts both a disability culture and a serious political project. An emphasis on fluid identities undermines political cohesion. It is a disability culture that helps generate and sustain those meanings, identities, and the consciousness that take a political movement forward.

The "new cultural politics of difference" seeks to resist the dominant representations of disability and establish a new disability identity (or identities). This is cast as a struggle over cultural hegemony, which entails shifting the balance of power relations. The search for new political strategies by disabled people has led to the development of a vibrant disability arts movement that is contesting a Gramscian-style cultural "war of position" in which dominant perspectives are being openly challenged (Hall 1992). The dilemma for those engaged with a broad disability culture is that it is constructing from new, where disabled people are themselves drawn in several directions by their own internal "differences." A further concern is that the exclusive focus on cultural representation is that it is disconnected from the wider processes of social exclusion and material disadvantage.

The potential of disability culture is revealed in its reinforcement of an "essential" similarity that makes political intervention possible; the dilemma is that disabled people, like other oppressed groups, have to constantly negotiate several kinds of difference, such as gender, race, class, and age, in their lives. Canadian writer Susan Wendell (1996) contends that "it would be hard to claim that disabled people as a whole have an alternative culture or even the seeds of one" (p. 273). As we have tried to show, many disabled people would strongly dispute her conclusion. They would also recognize that the impact of disability consciousness and culture has not been evenly felt across the disabled population. It offers new possibilities but also presents new contradictions. Nevertheless, the generation of a vibrant disability culture is central to confronting the social exclusion of disabled people.

REFERENCES

Barnes, C. 1992. *Disabling Imagery and the Media: An Exploration of Media Representations of Disabled People.* Belper: British Council of Organisations of Disabled People.

Barnes, C., G. Mercer, and T. Shakespeare. 1999. *Exploring Disability: A Sociological Introduction.* Oxford, UK: Polity.

Battye, L. 1966. "The Chatterley Syndrome." Pp. 3-17 in *Stigma,* edited by P. Hunt. London: Chapman.

Biklen, D. and R. Bogdan. 1977. "Media Portrayals of Disabled People: A Study of Stereotypes." *Interracial Books for Children Bulletin* 8:6-7.

Bogdan, R. 1996. "The Social Construction of Freaks." Pp. 23-38 in *Freakery: Culture Spectacles of the Extraordinary Body,* edited by R. G. Thomson. New York: New York University Press.

Bowe, F. 1978. *Handicapping America.* New York: Harper & Row.

Brown, S. E. 1997. " 'Oh, Don't You Envy Us Our Privileged Lives?' A Review of the Disability Culture Movement." *Disability and Rehabilitation* 19 (8): 339-49.

Campbell, J. and M. Oliver. 1996. *Disability Politics: Understanding Our Past, Changing Our Future.* London: Routledge Kegan Paul.

Campling, J., ed. 1981. *Images of Ourselves: Women with Disabilities Talking.* London: Routledge Kegan Paul.

Clogson, J. 1990. *Disability Coverage in Sixteen Newspapers.* Louisville: Avocado.

Corbett, J. and S. Ralph. 1994. "Empowering Adults: The Changing Imagery of Charity Advertising." *Australian Disability Review* 1:5-14.

Corker, M. 1998. *Deaf and Disabled, or Deafness Disabled.* Milton Keynes, UK: Open University Press.

Cribb, S. 1993. "Are Disabled Artists Cotton-Wooled?" *Disability Arts Magazine* 3 (2): 10-11.

Cumberbatch, G. and R. Negrine. 1992. *Images of Disability on Television.* London: Routledge Kegan Paul.

Darke, P. 1994. "*The Elephant Man* (David Lynch, EMI Films, 1980): An Analysis from a Disabled Perspective." *Disability and Society* 9 (3): 327-42.

———. 1995. "Autobiographies of Discovery." *Disability Arts Magazine* 5 (2): 11-13.

———. 1998. "Understanding Cinematic Representations of Disability." Pp. 181-97 in *The Disability Reader,* edited by T. Shakespeare. London: Cassell.

Davis, L. J. 1995. *Enforcing Normalcy: Disability, Deafness, and the Body.* London: Verso.

Fine, M. and A. Asch. 1988. *Women with Disabilities: Essays in Psychology, Culture, and Politics.* Philadelphia: Temple University Press.

Finkelstein, V. 1980. *Attitudes and Disabled People.* New York: World Rehabilitation Fund.

Finkelstein, V. and K. Morrison. 1992. "Culture as Struggle: Access to Power." In *Disability Arts in London,* edited by S. Lees. London: Shape.

Garland, R. 1995. *The Eye of the Beholder: Deformity and Disability in the Graeco-Roman World.* London: Duckworth.

Gartner, A. and T. Joe, eds. 1987. *Images of the Disabled, Disabling Images.* New York: Praeger.

Gerber, D. 1996. "The Careers of People Exhibited in Freak Shows: The Problem of Volition and Valorisation." Pp. 38-53 in *Freakery: Culture Spectacles of the Extraordinary Body,* edited by R. G. Thomson. New York: New York University Press.

Giddens, A. 1989. *Sociology.* Cambridge, UK: Polity.

Goffman, E. 1961. *Asylums.* Harmondsworth, UK: Penguin.

Gramsci, A. 1971. *Selections from the Prison Notebooks of Antonio Gramsci.* Edited and translated by Q. Hoare and G. Nowell Smith. London: Lawrence and Wishart.

———. 1985. *Selections from the Cultural Writings.* Edited and translated by D. Forgacs and G. Nowell-Smith. London: Lawrence and Wishart.

Groce, N. E. 1985. *Everyone Here Speaks Sign Language: Hereditary Deafness in Martha's Vineyard.* Cambridge, MA: Harvard University Press.

Hall, S. 1980. "Encoding/Decoding." Pp. 128-30 in *Culture, Media, Language: Working Papers in Cultural Studies, 1972-79,* edited by D. Hobson and S. Hall. London: Hutchinson.

———. 1988. "New Ethnicities." Pp. 27-31 in *Black Film, British Cinema*, edited by K. Mercer. London: Institute of Contemporary Arts.

———. 1992. "What is This 'Black' in Black Popular Culture?" Pp. 21-33 in *Black Popular Culture*, edited by G. Dent. Seattle, WA: Bay.

———, ed. 1997. *Representation: Cultural Representations and Signifying Practices*. London: Sage.

Hall, S. and T. Jefferson, eds. 1976. *Resistance through Rituals*. London: Hutchinson.

Haller, B. 1995. "Rethinking Models of Media Representations of Disability." *Disability Studies Quarterly* 15 (2): 26-30.

Hevey, D. 1992. *The Creatures That Time Forgot: Photography and Disability Imagery*. London: Routledge Kegan Paul.

Hirsch, K. 1995. "Culture and Disability: The Role of Oral History." *Oral History Review* 22 (1): 1-27.

Hughes, B. and K. Paterson. 1997. "The Social Model of Disability and the Disappearing Body: Towards a Sociology of Impairment." *Disability and Society* 12 (3): 325-40.

Hunt, P., ed. 1966. *Stigma: The Experience of Disability*. London: Chapman.

Inglis, F. 1993. *Cultural Studies*. Oxford, UK: Blackwell.

Ingstad, B. and S. R. Whyte, eds. 1995. *Disability and Culture*. Berkeley: University of California Press.

Karpf, A. 1988. *Doctoring the Media*. London: Routledge Kegan Paul.

Keith, L. 1994. *Mustn't Grumble*. London: The Women's Press.

Kellner, D. 1989. *Critical Theory, Marxism and Modernity*. Cambridge, UK: Polity.

Kent, D. 1987. "Disabled Women: Portraits in Fiction and Drama." Pp. 47-63 in *Images of the Disabled, Disabling Images*, edited by A. Gartner and T. Joe. New York: Praeger.

Kitzinger, J. 1993. "Media Messages and What People Know about Acquired Immune Deficiency Syndrome." Pp. 271-304 in *Getting the Message*, edited by Glasgow University Media Group. London: Routledge Kegan Paul.

Kleinfield, S. 1977. *The Hidden Minority: A Profile of Handicapped Americans*. Boston: Little, Brown.

Klobas, L. E. 1988. *Disability Drama in Television and Film*. Jefferson, NC: McFarland.

Kriegel, L. 1987. "The Cripple in Literature." Pp. 31-46 in *Images of the Disabled, Disabling Images*, edited by A. Gartner and T. Joe. New York: Praeger.

Kurtz, R. 1981. "The Sociological Approach to Mental Retardation." Pp. 14-23 in *Handicap in a Social World*, edited by A. Brechin, P. Liddiard, and J. Swain. London: Hodder and Stoughton.

Lane, H. 1984. *When the Mind Hears: A History of the Deaf*. New York: Random House.

———. 1995. "Constructions of Deafness." *Disability and Society* 10 (2): 171-89.

Linton, S. 1998. *Claiming Disability: Knowledge and Identity*. New York: New York University Press.

Longmore, P. 1987. "Screening Stereotypes: Images of Disabled People in Television and Motion Pictures." Pp. 65-78 in *Images of the Disabled, Disabling Images*, edited by A. Gartner and T. Joe. New York: Praeger.

———. 1995. "The Second Phase: From Disability Rights to Disability Culture." *Disability Rag and Resource* 16:4-11.

McQuail, D., ed. 1972. *Sociology of Mass Communications: Selected Readings*. Harmondsworth, UK: Penguin.

Meekosha, H. and L. Dowse. 1997. "Distorting Images, Invisible Images: Gender, Disability and the Media." *Media International Australia* 84 (May): 91-101.

Miles, M. 1995. "Disability in an Eastern Religious Context: Historical Perspectives." *Disability and Society* 10 (1): 49-70.

Morris, J. 1991. *Pride against Prejudice*. London: The Women's Press.

Morrison, K. and V. Finkelstein. 1993. "Broken Arts and Cultural Repair: The Role of Culture in the Empowerment of Disabled People." Pp. 122-27 in *Disabling Barriers—Enabling Environments*, edited by J. Swain, V. Finkelstein, S. French, and M. Oliver. London: Sage.

Murphy, R. 1987. *The Body Silent*. London: Phoenix House.

Norden, M. 1994. *The Cinema of Isolation: A History of Disability in the Movies*. New Brunswick, NJ: Rutgers University Press.

Oliver, M. 1983. *Social Work with Disabled People*. Basingstoke, UK: Macmillan.

———. 1990. *The Politics of Disablement*. Basingstoke, UK: Macmillan.

Orlansky, M. and W. Heward. 1981. *Voices: Interviews with Handicapped People*. Columbus, OH: Merrill.

Padden, C. and T. Humphries. 1988. *Deaf in America: Voices from a Culture*. Cambridge, MA: Harvard University Press.

Parker, R. A. 1988. "An Historical Background." Pp. 1-38 in *Residential Care: The Research Reviewed*, edited by National Institute for Social Work/I. Sinclair. London: Her Majesty's Stationery Office.

Philo, G., ed. 1996. *Media and Mental Distress*. Harlow, UK: Addison-Wesley.

Pointon, A. 1997. "Rights of Access." Pp. 234-40 in *Framed: Interrogating Disability in the Media*, edited by A. Pointon and C. Davies. London: British Film Institute.

———. 1999. "Out of the Closet: New Images of Disability in the Civil Rights Campaign." Pp. 222-37 in *Social Policy, the Media and Misrepresentation*, edited by B. Franklin. London: Routledge Kegan Paul.

Pointon, A. and C. Davies, eds. 1997. *Framed: Interrogating Disability in the Media*. London: British Film Institute.

Ross, K. 1997. *Disability and Broadcasting: A View from the Margins*. Cheltenham, UK: Cheltenham and Gloucester College of Higher Education.

Saxton, M. and F. Howe. 1989. *With Wings: An Anthology of Literature of Women with Disabilities*. London: Virago.

Schuchman, J. 1988. *Hollywood Speaks: Deafness and the Film Entertainment Industry*. Urbana: University of Illinois Press.

Shakespeare, T. 1994. "Cultural Representations of Disabled People: Dustbins for Disavowal." *Disability and Society* 9 (3): 283-301.

Shapiro, J. P. 1993. *No Pity: People with Disabilities Forging a New Civil Rights Movement*. New York: Times Books.

Shearer, A. 1981. *Disability, Whose Handicap?* Oxford, UK: Blackwell.

Smith, S. and A. Jordan. 1991. *What the Papers Say and Don't Say about Disability*. London: Spastics Society.

Sontag, S. 1991. *Illness as Metaphor: AIDS and Its Metaphors*. London: Penguin.

Stone, E., ed. 1999. *Disability and Development*. Leeds, UK: The Disability Press.

Sutherland, D. 1997. "Disability Arts and Disability Politics." P. 159 in *Framed: Interrogating Disability in the Media*, edited by A. Pointon and C. Davies. London: British Film Institute.

Thomson, R. G. 1997. *Extraordinary Bodies: Figuring Physical Disability in American Culture and Literature*. New York: Columbia University Press.

Tremain, S. 1996. *Pushing the Limits: Disabled Dykes Produce Culture*. Toronto: The Women's Press.

Vasey, S. 1992. "Disability Arts and Culture: An Introduction to Key Issues and Questions." In *Disability Arts Culture Papers*, edited by S. Lees. London: Shape.

Weeks, J. 1994. *The Lesser Evil and the Greater Good: The Theory and Politics of Social Diversity*. London: Rivers Oram.

Wells, H. G. 1979. *The Complete Short Stories of H. G. Wells*. London: Ernest Benn.

Wendell, S. 1996. *The Rejected Body: Feminist and Philosophical Reflections on Disability*. London: Routledge Kegan Paul.

Williams, R. 1958. *Culture and Society 1780-1950*. London: Chatto and Windus.

———. 1980. *Problems in Materialism and Culture*. London: New Left.

———. 1981. *Culture*. Glasgow, UK: Fontana.

———. 1989. *Resources of Hope*. London: Verso.

Wilson, A. N. 1997. "How Not to Win Friends." *Sunday Telegraph*, December 28.

Woodward, K., ed. 1997. *Identity and Difference*. London: Sage.

Young, I. M. 1990. *Justice and the Politics of Difference*. Princeton, NJ: Princeton University Press.

Zola, I. K. 1982. *Missing Pieces: A Chronicle of Living with a Disability*. Philadelphia: Temple University Press.

———. 1985. "Depictions of Disability—Metaphor, Message, and Medium in the Media: A Research and Political Agenda." *The Social Science Journal* 22 (4): 5-17.

Identity Politics, Disability, and Culture

22

LENNARD J. DAVIS

I n recent years, disability activists and scholars have fought hard to get disability included in the race-class-gender triad. This chapter questions the relative wisdom of that approach since identity, while a useful category, might well turn out to be a confusing if, not itself, oppressive category. Thinking through this issue by concentrating on culture—particularly the novel as a form—might help to clarify how the issue of identity fits into a disability critique. One might begin to understand the current primacy of identity, particularly in the United States, as a function of the postmodern moment by historicizing it as a set of interests. Wendy Brown (1995) postulates that identity politics arose in coordination with the late-twentieth-century liberal state:

> On the one side, the state loses even its guise of universality as it becomes ever more transparently invested in particular economic interests, political ends, and social formations. . . . On the other side, the liberal subject is increasingly disinterred from substantive nation-state identification, not only by the individuating effects of liberal discourse itself but through the social effects of late-twentieth-century economic and political life: deterritorializing demographic flows; the disintegration from within and invasion from without of family and community as (relatively) autonomous sites of social production and identification; consumer capitalism's marketing discourse in which individual (and sub-individual) desires are produced, commodified, and mobilized as identities. (P. 58)

While identity politics is generally subsumed to a more material analysis in England and Europe, in the United States, identity politics is linked to a larger array of political movements, sometimes referred to as the Rainbow Coalition, to use Jesse Jackson's term for the coalition that supported his presidential bid. However, in reality, that coalition in the United States has been one in name only with the different identity groups clashing on tactics and agendas, offering a fantasy of cohesion without actually creating one. The one thing these groups have in common is the wish to have the full rights of any citizen. Indeed, in a bourgeois democracy, the issue of rights is often regarded as paramount. Yet a rights-based approach, connected with empowerment, will necessarily lead to quite a limited and conservative goal of making sure that each disenfranchised group has the rights of white middle-class males. This goal, according to Brown (1995), "only preserves capitalism from critique . . . [and] sustains the invisibility and inarticulateness of class" (p. 61). Although a truly just government should establish a parity of interests for all identity groups, the larger goal would be to place the bar rather higher than set for the projected fantasy of the "middle class" in bourgeois democracies. Indeed, one can argue that, historically, the emphasis on rights, as opposed to economic inequalities, was ideologically coterminous with the foundation of Western democracy.[1]

I do not wish to convey the idea that I am against identity politics, nor do I think the issues raised by such in regard to the novel are invalid. However, I think we need to recognize that identity politics is a stage through which we are going and only a stage. I think that an analysis of disability can help us interrogate the stage of identity and help point toward a future politics. Indeed, my own work for the past few years has involved the identity of disability. I have been an active proponent of the notion that the tribunal bench needs to be redesigned so that people using wheelchairs as well as the deaf, the blind, and other people with disabilities can be accommodated. My concern is that the model we have of identity politics has some fundamental problems, and my work with people with disabilities has shown me the shortcomings of such a praxis. One must ask the following question: Is identity analysis the sharpest instrument with which to allow analysis and understanding of various cultural phenomena?

To focus, let us pay attention to the demand that disability should be included in the roster of the disenfranchised. The tendency is to see disability as "another" identity to be added to a welter of identities. Thus, one simply adds to a list of outrages committed by a dominant majority. By this standard, if I want disability to be recognized as part of a general outrage against the excluded and marginalized, I must develop a body of knowledge elucidating those injuries. While one perspective might be to turn to social policy, it is my intention in this chapter to focus on some cultural form—in this case, the novel—and show how historically people with disabilities are constructed and, by and large, negatively depicted by the dominant culture. Looking at many characters in novels who are depicted as having disabilities, I intend to show that often they are seen as villains, bitter and warped, or as innocent victims, good and kindly, although desexualized and devitalized.[2] They range from Quilp to Tiny Tim, from Ahab to Esther Summerson, from Quasimodo to Clifford Chatterly.

Yet disability is somewhat different from other identities, and it subjects people to a kind of scrutiny. Disability is an identity that, while it may intersect with other identity categories, is still mainly divorced from rubrics such as family, nation, ethnicity, or gender. I do not mean that disability has nothing to do with these other identities, but rather that it is generally perceived as being independent of one's identity as a citizen, a woman, or a parent, for example. In other words, disability is perceived by the majority as a nonpolitical identity. Disability activists and theorists have worked hard to make people understand that there is a political history to the body and to the formation of concepts of normalcy.

However, disability confounds the neat borders of identity in that it is not a discrete but rather a porous category. Anyone can become disabled, and it is also possible for a person with disabilities to be "cured" and become "normal." Linked to this porosity, race, nationality, and ethnicity have been considered biological disabilities in a eugenic culture. Because the category of disability is a shifting one, its contingent nature is all the more challenging to other identities that seem fixed. In some sense, disability is more like class, which is constructed but is not biologically determined. It is also like sexual preference, which, while there may be genetic factors involved, is generally regarded as separated from biological determinants.[3] We might say that disability is a very postmodern identity because although one can somatize disability, it is impossible to essentialize it the way one can with the categories of gender or ethnicity. Add to this the fact that there is no unanimity on which impairment is a disability. Furthermore, although disability is "of" the body, it is much more "of" the environment, which can create barriers to access and communication.[4] Also, the category of disability casts quite a wide net. In consulting definitions provided by the Americans with Disabilities Act of 1990, we find in the same grouping obesity, carpal tunnel syndrome, AIDS, deafness, dyslexia, attention deficit disorder, Down syndrome, and many other diverse conditions. Given this continuum, it is hard to imagine that any one person can be a representative for this group or be a representative character in a novel. Moreover, this very fact leads to a deconstructive potential against any individual claiming to represent the totality of an identity.[5]

More tellingly and to my point, the identity community, if one can call it that, in the United States has been slow to recognize disability as a legitimate member. Perhaps because of the ambiguities I just related, disability is seen in some sense as "spoiling" the neatness of categories of oppression, or victim and victimizer. Anyone working in the field of disability studies will know that disability, despite its legislative accomplishments, is seen generally as having a less legitimate minority status than other more high-profile identities.[6] Indeed, in multicultural curriculum discussions, disability is often struck from the list of required alterities because it is seen as degrading or watering down the integrity of identities. While most faculty would vote for a requirement that African American, Latin American, or Asian American novels should be read in the university, few would, at this point in history, mandate the reading of novels about people with disabilities. A cursory glance at books on diversity and identity shows that disability issues are rarely addressed. The extent to which people with disabilities are excluded from the progressive academic agenda is sobering. In addition, the use of ableist language on the part of critics and scholars who routinely turn a "deaf ear" or find a point "lame" or a political act "crippling" is shocking to anyone who is even vaguely aware of the way language is implicated in discrimination and exclusion.

These acts of omission and commission are all the more scandalous when one realizes that people with disabilities make up 12 to 15 percent of the population—a greater proportion than that of any other minority. This statistic can be increased for people in poorer countries. Likewise, about 15 percent of the population has a hearing loss and another 15 percent has impaired vision. With an aging baby boom population, the number of people with disabilities will only increase. In the Third World, poor nutrition, land mines, war, and disease increase the numbers of people with disabilities. Indeed, it is probably true that there is no one more oppressed in the world than a Third World disabled woman of color. Also, let us not forget children, particularly those of the Third World, who are the primary victims of discrimination, with 90 percent dying before they reach age 20, and 90 percent of children with mental disabilities die before they reach age 5. In the United States, 66 percent of people with disabilities are unemployed, while half the people with disabilities live on or near the poverty line. A recent Modern Language of America survey showed that there were twice as many members with disabilities as there were African American members. Yet, by and large, there is scant attention paid to disability in the identity political market, particularly in regard to novel studies. Certainly, this trend is beginning to reverse with the rise of disability studies, but the latter is about as recognized, at this point, as African American studies was in the early 1960s.

The lack of attention paid to disability by those in the forefront of identity and multicultural studies dramatically shows that the Occam's razor, used to evaluate critical works ("Does it focus on race, gender, or sexual orientation?") is a dull razor indeed. Rather, one can say that identity politics, as a method of literary analysis, will necessarily reflect the biases of its own time. While our consciousness of some selected and canonized identities has certainly been raised, the biases of those within the confines of the canon remain confirmed by their invisibility. Identity studies is no more perfect, value free, and objective than hermeneutics, structuralism, or any other applied discourse. Perhaps people of the future will be astounded, puzzled, and disturbed that works by scholars such as Eve Sedgewick, Judith Butler, Henry Louis Gates, bell hooks, and others managed to steer so completely away from any discussion of disability.

I should make clear that my solution to the problem of identity is not inclusion of disability to the roster of favored identities. Rather, the point is that identity studies itself is limited in our time by the necessarily taxonomic peculiarity of its endeavor. Inclusiveness will not solve the problem. The list of identities will only grow larger, tied to an ever-expanding idea of inclusiveness. After all, when all identities are finally included in the roster, how can there be this particular kind of identity? If alterity is subsumed under the rubric of identity, then what can identity mean, particularly if this kind of cultural identity is somehow actually based on a binary opposition between self and other? Identity becomes so broad a category that it cannot contain identity. In other words, identity politics, while useful during the latter part of the twentieth century in securing civil rights for some disenfranchised groups, has by the twenty-first century reached a paradoxical resolution to a problem that started as a logical extension of a discussion about rights. It is Wendy Brown's (1995) point, citing Foucault, that "the universal juridical ideal of liberalism," combined with "the normalizing principle of disciplinary regimes and taken up within the discourse of politicized identity," yields a new kind of subject "reiterative of regulatory, disciplinary society," which "ceaselessly characterizes, classifies, and specializes," working through "surveillance, continuous registration, perpetual assessment, and classification" and through a social machinery "that is both immense and minute" (p. 65). In other words, the classificatory and judgmental system inherent in an identity critique of novels will necessarily end up surveilling texts through an ever-expanding and therefore increasingly imprecise grid. This framework will therefore yield less and less information about more and more works and will become a system that explains everything, thus ultimately explaining nothing.

For example, if the function of identity criticism has been to point out the sexism, racism, ableism, homophobia, and so on in canonical texts, then this policing action will eventually turn in on itself. In this case, the ever-increasing trolling for missed identities or stereotypical characters will have to, by its own logic, begin to critique itself. Critics will then point to other critics who have failed to notice incidents of particular "isms." And so on. Likewise, identity critics can point favorably at other texts that exhibit positive images of oppressed identities. Finally, there is also the possibility of locating "resistant" texts that appeared in more oppressive periods but that managed to tactically and strategically pass muster of the dominant culture while offering transgressive and elusive readings that allowed certain collusive readers to find resistance to that dominant paradigm. That seems to be the extent of identity critique, and this kind of work seems to have a built-in half-life. How long can any particular critic perform this particular activity? What will be perpetually needed are new identities on the block to keep the process going, although methodologically not much new will be happening in that street game.

To complicate this already complicated critique further, I want to point to the inability of identity politics to include disability under its tent in some way other than with second-class status. My point is to question the following: How effective is an antidiscriminatory stance, based on identity politics, when the watchman always needs to be watched? Another way of putting this point is that no coalition of identity-based activists or scholars will ever be able to avoid marginalizing and minoritizing *some* group. Bosnian mothers, East Timorese Christians, or Ethiopian Jews will always be out of favor and, if not them, then tribal peoples of northern India or indigenous rebels in Sri Lanka. The point is that an inherent limitation of permitted or favored identities is precisely built into the definition of the project. Furthermore, the contradiction becomes more acute when we realize that much of identity politics in the United States is a reaction to a rights-based model rather than an economically egalitarian, political one, as it is in the United Kingdom. In the former case, then, the necessity for identity is actually a compromise formation in theory tailored to a largely middle-class—precisely, First World—audience seeking reassurance about the parameters of liberal thought and politics. Likewise, the interest in identity in novel criticism is a ratification of this reassurance. If one can say, for example, that women are depicted in a binary way in novels to be either the madwoman or the angel, an alternative to either of these roles is held out as a norm. What is that alternative but some superscription of the ideal of white middle-class men with full rights? Likewise, the benchmark for people of color is the depiction of the middle class or gentry as full-fledged members of society. As Brown (1995) writes, "Without recourse to the white masculine middle-class idea, politicized identities would forfeit a good deal of their claims to injury and exclusion, their claims to the political significance of their difference" (p. 61).

What, then, could the relevance of this discussion have to a cultural form such as the novel? I now wish to perform a paradoxical proof of the points I have been making by attempting to develop a theory of the novel that is solely based on the concept of disability. In other words, I want to prove that I can justify a disability-centered identity politics the way that others have done, for example, in establishing feminist-, ethnic-, or class-based models. In doing so, my aim is twofold: I want to show that disability is a viable identity, and, paradoxically, I want to demonstrate the limitation of an identity-based explanation for the novel. In other words, I want to show that disability can and should sit on the tribunal of identity politics, but I also want to show that including disability will not solve the problems inherent in the tribunal in the first place.

What are the possibilities for a disability-centered discussion of the novel? Initially, one would want to rethink the nature of the novel. An early definition of the novel, by Clara Reeve in 1785, states that

> the novel is a picture of real life and manners, and of the times in which it is written. . . . The novel gives a familiar relation of such things, as pass every day before our eyes, such as may happen to our friend, or to ourselves; and the perfection of it, is to represent every scene, in so easy and natural a manner, and to make them appear so probable, as to deceive us into a persuasion (at least while we reading) that all is real. (Reeve 1930:111)

Some 40 years later, John Dunlop (1845) defined novels as

> agreeable and fictitious productions, whose province it is to bring about natural events by natural means, and which preserve curiosity alive without the help of wonder—in which human life is exhibited in its true state, diversified only by accidents that daily happen in the world. (P. 362)

According to these relatively contemporary accounts, a new literary form with links to previous fictions, such as the romance, tales, the epic, and so on, had appeared on the scene in England and France. What characterizes this form is some notion that it treats "real" life in a "familiar" way that appears to be "true" without the intrusion of the elements that do not appear "natural." This technique, most familiarly called "realism," is so much a part of our critical vocabulary that perhaps we have reified it somewhat. What is realism, in fact? If novelists tried to create a real effect, does that mean that writers before them did not attempt to portray the real? The implication is that earlier writers of the romance and epic wrote imaginary tales or at least tales involving the supernatural—the realm of gods, witches, monsters, and so on. However, is realism any more "real" than other types of narrative? Is a representation of the real any more real than "the real"? Is the concept of what is real absolute? Why should realism have arisen in this particular period? Did novelists and readers just decide to get real?

Ian Watt (1967), as one of the early exponents of the origin-of-the-novel paradigm, explains rather glibly that "modern realism, of course, begins from the position that truth can be discovered by the individual through his senses: it has its origins in Descartes and Locke" (p. 12). Watt further explains realism as part of the middle-class interest in the individual and his or her perceptions of reality. His notion of "formal realism" is defined as such "because the term realism does not here refer to any special literary doctrine or purpose, but only to a set of narrative procedures which are commonly found together in the novel" (p. 32). This definition owes much to the time Watt's book was written, and his debt to formalism and new criticism is obvious. So for Watt, realism is not about the subject matter of the novel but more about the way the story is told and the consciousness that apprehends the story. Yet why does interest in the individual have to take the form of realism? Why couldn't the same interest take the form of rampant egocentric fantasy or one-sided, biased memoir (which seems to be the form realism takes in our own time)? Indeed, individual perception should lead more to individualist, sensory-based texts, more like twentieth-century literature, and not necessarily toward narratives about groups, social classes, and communities.

Instead of looking toward this explanation of realism, why not look elsewhere? The growing body of literature on disability indicates to us that part of the formation of the modern subject was tied up with the creation of the disabled object. Characteristic of the split between the "normal" and the "abnormal," which arose during the formative period of the novel (as we know it), is a distinction between normal bodies and abnormal bodies, between normal minds and abnormal minds, between normal environments and abnormal environments, and so on. The normal-abnormal dichotomy displaced an earlier paradigm based on a notion of the ideal. This notion of the ideal seems to have been the general rule in Western society and was linked ideologically to structures of kingship and feudal society. In this paradigm, an ideal (ruler, form, palace, god) occupied the pinnacle of a social-cultural triangle, and all other instantiations were by definition below the ideal. The transition to ideological forms of government that would legitimate the change from feudalism and mercantilism to capitalism required new forms of subjectivity and symbolic production. Since the fundamental paradox of bourgeois society, as it evolved, was one between the concentration of power and money in the hands of a relatively few and the ideological notion that all "men" were created equal, forms of symbolic production that glorified the ideal and placed all citizens below that ideal person would no longer be appropriate. Yet, at the same time, a truly equal, in the economic sense, citizenry depicted in literature would be equally prohibited. To bridge the gap between the obvious social and economic inequality in bourgeois democracies and the notion that all citizens are equal, one had to create that most perfect of subjects—the average citizen, *l'homme moyen,* performed by Adolphe Quetelet, at the beginning of the nineteenth century. Quetelet took physical measures of bodily dimensions to come up with the proportions of the average man, of whom Quetelet writes, "If one seeks to establish, in some way, the basis of a social physics, it is he whom one should consider" (Porter 1986:24).

The necessity for the average citizen in social thought was paralleled by the need for the average citizen in ideological thought. How do we think this average citizen? The answer would be symbolically. Thus, symbolic production on the ideological level should aim at the creation of average—that is, nonheroic, middle-class, "real"—citizens. In this sense, real means average. It is no coincidence that for the next hundred years or more, bourgeois society spent much of its culturally productive time trying to find what exactly *average* meant. This attempt was done largely with the aid of the new science of statistics, initiated by Quetelet and others, and in conjunction with the new science of eugenics.[7] This was when the word and concept of *normal* entered the English and French languages. Novels were novel precisely because they were a form engaged in depicting this average or normal life, as Reeve and Dunlop noted in their own time. Indeed, the project of creating "realistic" heroes and heroines was the aim of novel writing from the mid-eighteenth century to the end of the nineteenth century.

The word used repeatedly and regularly in conjunction with character in eighteenth-century discussions of the novel was *virtue.* Novels were judged to be good depending on the extent to which the story inspired virtue and the extent to which the protagonists were virtuous. *Virtue* implied that there was a specific and knowable moral path and stance that a character could and should take. In other words, a normative set of behaviors was demanded of characters in novels. Characters had to be "exemplary" (Reeve 1930:139). We can see in works such as *The Progress of Romance* that novels are judged mainly on two criteria—their realism or probability and their attitude toward virtue, which "should always be represented in the most beautiful and amiable light" (Reeve 1930:27). Both of these criteria, as we can see, are really discussions about normativity. If readers disagreed about the worth of a novel during this period, the argument revolved around whether an author depicted "human nature as *it is,* rather than as *it ought to be*" (Reeve 1930:141), and it revolved around whether the events of the story were "probable" or "improbable." Thus, the question for the eighteenth century was the extent to which the novelist conformed to a cultural norm and not, as Watt suggested, the formal aspects of writing or the perception of truth on an individual.[8] In fact, it is virtually impossible to find a discussion about the "formal" aspects of novel writing in this period.

Furthermore, the main characters of novels, in their virtuous incarnations, were national types. The requirements for their being realistic and virtuous was in effect a requirement for them to be typical. There are few novels from 1720 to 1870 whose main characters, the ones with whom we identify and sympathize, are not national stereotypes. Moreover, as such, these characters also have bodies and minds that signify this averageness. Protagonists of British novels are British, look typical, and embody the virtues that England values.[9] Love stories may offer a cross-national or class liaison but usually end up ratifying the norm.

This project of cultural typicality has to be seen for what it is—the incipient impulse of a tendency that would later be called eugenics. It is instructive that one of the founders of eugenics was Sir Francis Galton, cousin to Charles Darwin. Galton embarked on a project similar to that of the novel when he began photographing different racial and ethnic peoples to create composite photographs of the physiognomies of each type. So, for example, he photographed Jewish citizens of England and overlaid the photographic images to create the composite or, in some sense, typical Jew. He also photographed mental and tubercular patients to see if he could arrive at the physiognomies of the diseased (Booth, Phillips, and Squires 1998). This attempt to create typical images of racial and disabled "others" in photography must be seen as linked to the novelistic attempt to do likewise. The investigations of race and nationality in nineteenth-century novels demonstrate this linked interest.

There is virtually no major protagonist in a novel created during the eighteenth and nineteenth centuries who is in some way physically marked with a disability.[10] Indeed, realism, with its emphasis on probability, is linked to presenting normative characters and situations. This is so much the case that E. M. Forster (1968), in the course of *Aspects of the Novel*, sees the inclusion in a novel of a character with disability as unrealistic when he says that readers will protest deviations from a norm. "One knows a book isn't real, they say, still one does it expect it to be natural, and this angel or midget or ghost . . . no, it is too much" (Forster 1968:114). The midget is "too much" because midgets do not walk into one's bourgeois house any more than do Africans or angels.[11]

So, on some profound level, the novel emerges as an ideological form of symbolic production whose central binary is normal-abnormal. This dialectic works in a fundamental way to produce plots. Often, a "normal" character is made "abnormal" by circumstance. The most familiar of these has to do with depriving that character of social class, social milieu, family lineage, or money. So, the very normal Robinson Crusoe is made abnormal by unusual circumstance. The very normal Tom Jones is made abnormal by a ruse that deprives him of his noble birth. The very normal Pamela or Clarissa is made abnormal by abduction and the threat or act rape. Ironically, these rather unusual abnormalities in the life of a character are seen as "probable," given the novel's own rules of realism, when, in fact, it is rather unlikely that very many bourgeois people will lose all their money, social status, or personal freedom. Indeed, social class is defined by its persistence and interlocking guarantees. Another variation on this theme is that the protagonist is made "abnormal" by a certain trait or habit that, while not a disability, acts as a disability in contrast to the expectations of readers concerning the conventions of character in the novel. So, Jane Eyre is plain, which is quite normal, but it is rendered abnormal by the convention of novels, which insists that heroes and heroines be physically attractive, presumably since the national type is projected to be well proportioned in face and limb. Someone such as Evelina is made abnormal by her lack of proper parenting, which renders her socially maladroit.

In the realm of social class, the norm is typically not the mean but the ideological fantasy of a mean. This fantasy was an ideological necessity on the part of bourgeois capitalism to project a positive vision of its operative world as free, prosperous, and coherent. Not so strangely, the "average" novel hero of the mid-eighteenth to the mid-nineteenth century more often than not moves through the world not of the bourgeoisie but of the upper gentry and lower nobility. This netherworld of upper gentry and lower nobility elevated the tone and vision of bourgeois existence much in the way that contemporary television shows present upper-middle-class interiors as the norm, while most viewers are much less privileged.[12] Thus, the a deprivation of this fantasy norm is considered a disabling event for someone such as Oliver Twist, Jane Eyre, David Copperfield, or Gwendolyn Harleth. Even for someone such as Jude Fawley, the realistic norm of rural peasantry becomes a disabling situation, although, unlike many of the earlier heroes, he will never achieve the desired state of comfort.

So for the national norm to be consolidated, the major characters in novels must confront the disabling of their character in some way. For the norm to be created, the abnormal must also appear. The abnormal appears in all kinds of ways, from the social and financial, as I have indicated, to the unvirtuous, the mentally ill, the racial "other," and the appearance of characters with physical disabilities. In the eighteenth century, for the most part, normal characters with virtues are set off by abnormal characters with vices. Most often, the vice is sexual license in the form of a debauched, upper-class libertine or seductress or, in rarer cases, greedy and unprincipled parvenus. A simple Manichean battle ensues, and ultimately either the virtuous character triumphs or, in some cases, dies. Later, as a culture of the norm becomes fully operative in the nineteenth century, the immoral or negative is often depicted as having a physical disability. Here begins the novel with a recognizable villain who is often one-eyed, one-legged, walks with difficulty, stutters, manifests compulsive tics, and so on. The flip side of this character is the utterly innocent character with a disability, most often a child, a childlike person, a woman, or an aged character. Interestingly, this dichotomy can work in many other multicultural analyses because race, gender, and class were also integral parts of the eugenic analysis. In other words, moral characteristics become increasingly somatized, particularly as eugenics begins to codify physical, mental, and ethnic traits. Under this imperative, Zola and the neorealists are able to formulate a theory of the novel in which inheritable family traits determine character and behavior, thus institutionalizing the "scientific" work of eugenics in the very fabric of novel making.[13]

Plot, in the novel, is really more a device to turn what is perceived as the average, ordinary milieu into an abnormal one. Plot functions in the novel, especially during the eighteenth and nineteenth centuries, by temporarily deforming or disabling the fantasy of nation, social class, and gender behaviors that are constructed as norms. The *telos* of plot aims then to return the protagonists to this norm by the end of the novel. The end of the novel represents a cure, a fixing of the disability, a nostalgic return to a preexisting normal time. René Girard (1965) points to Stepan Trofimovitch's quotation of the New Testament at the end of Dostoyevsky's *The Possessed*: "But the sick man will be healed and 'will sit at the feet of Jesus,' and all will look upon him with astonishment." Girard says Stepan "is this sick man who is healed in death and whom death heals" (p. 290). This notion of cure as closure is the rule in novels in which the end represents the plot as strategic abnormality overcome or, as Girard puts it, "an obsession that has been transcended" (p. 300).

In this sense, the identity of the novel, if we can see the novel as having an identity, revolves around a simple plot. The situation had been normal, it became abnormal, and by the end of the novel, the normality, or some variant on it, was restored. We can put this simplistic paradigm into the language that Wendy Brown (1995) uses and say that the identity of the novel is therefore a "wounded identity." Like Philoctetes, the novel must have a wound. And like that of Philoctetes, the wound is necessary because without it, the novel would not be able to perform its function. Yet, also like that of the mythical character, the wound must be healed or cured.

I return to the notion of identity because I want to tie the novel, disability, and identity politics together around the issue of cure. The novel as a form relies on cure as a narrative technique. Protagonists must "change," we are told, for their character to be believable. Interestingly, this aspect of believability flies in the face of probability since most "real" people do not change easily, if at all. When characters change, they undergo a kind of moral or perceptual transformation that cures them of their problem. So, Emma is cured of her self-centeredness or Darcy is cured of his pride. Likewise, the plot is cured of its abnormal initiating events. The narrative, at its end, is no longer disabled by its lack of conformity to imagined social norms. The process of narrative, then, serves to wound identity—whether individual, bourgeois, national, gendered, racialized, or cultural. Readers read so that they can experience this wound vicariously, so they can imagine the dissolution of the norms under which they are expected to labor. As a temporarily wounded person, the reader can see the way that society oppresses various categories of being. At the same time, the reader can rejoice in the inevitable return to the comfort of bourgeois norms, despite the onus that these norms place on its beneficiaries as well as those excluded from the benefits of bourgeois identity.[14]

Yet the desire for a cure is also the desire for a quick fix. The alterity presented by disability is shocking to the liberal, ableist sensibility, and so narratives involving disability always yearn toward the cure, the neutralizing of the disability. This desire to neutralize is ironic because in a dialectic sense, the fantasy of normality needs the abjection of disability to maintain a homeostatic system of binaries. However, since this desire is premised on the denigration of disability, it will of course be invisible to the normate[15] readers who prefer the kindly notion of cure to the more dramatic notion of eradication. Likewise, the quick fix presented by issues concerning race, class, and gender is equally characteristic of the bourgeois imagination. The conflict between classes can be nicely reconciled in novels, so that in *North and South,* a kind of utopian factory emerges that bypasses labor unions and is achieved by rerouting surplus value through the benevolence of a female captain of industry in the form of Margaret Hale, or, in *Hard Times,* the working class struggle is seen as a "muddle" only soluble by Christian charity toward the poor who "will always be with you."

All of these cures are placebos for the basic problem presented to capitalism and its ideological productions in the form of modern subjectivity, which dons the form of the normal, average, citizen protagonist—that bell curve–generated fantastic being who reconciles the promise of equal rights with the reality of unequal distribution of wealth. However, the quick fix, the cure, has to be repeated endlessly, like a patent medicine, because it cures nothing. Novels have to tell the story over and over again, as do films and television, because the patient never stays cured, and the disabled, cured individually, refuse to stop reappearing as a group. Indeed, modern subjectivity is a wounded identity that cannot cure itself without recourse to cure narratives, which means that it cannot cure itself at all since the disability of modern subjectivity is inherent in the environment, not in the subject.

The problem with the notion of wounded identities, as Brown (1995) postulates, is that the ontology of their coming into being is best characterized by Nietzsche's notion of resentment as an "effect of domination [that] reiterates impotence, a substitute for action, for power, for self-affirmation that reinscribes incapacity, powerlessness, and rejection" (Brown 1995:69). Thus, identity is dependent for its motivation and existence on remembering and reinvoking the pain caused by oppression. Politicized identity "installs its pain . . . in the very foundation of its political claim, in its demand for recognition as identity . . . by entrenching, restating, dramatizing, and inscribing its pain in politics" (Brown 1995:74). Like the novel, identity is rooted in its wounds, and plot is a form of pain control. Thus, its solution must be to heal the wound and end the pain. However, like the novel that offers a cure to the oppressions of modernity, the cure offered to wounded identity spells the end of identity because identity is created by the initializing wound, just as the cure offered in novels spells closure for that novel. The answer to novels is more novels, not a cure offered to the actual ills of society. Likewise, the proliferation of politicized identities is symptomatic of the problem, and the addition of more identities will no more solve the problem of oppression than the proliferation of novels will solve the same problem. I want to add that we have needed the idea of identity to help combat racism, sexism, ageism, and so on. However, the limits of this kind of politics are now becoming increasingly evident. The solution is not to do without identity or to denigrate the identities involved. Rather, a reconsideration of oppression based around other parameters that can, at this point, create solidarity while maintaining difference is essential.

I have tried to make the case briefly that disability, as an identity, can legitimately be seen as the foundational model on which to argue the origin and theory of the novel. As a foundational origin, I can then say that all other identities—class, race, gender, sexual preference—should be subsumed under the hegemonic identity category of disability. In other words, I contend that the novel belongs to a history of ableist domination (while it has also tried to resist that domination). If I do that, I place myself in a line of critics who have argued for the centrality of their identity as foundational for the creation of modern subjectivity. By doing so, I can now make two observations. First, I clearly have not solved the problem of identity politics. Second, by adding my identity to the roster and even by claiming the greater adequacy of my identity (which can be seen as including and therefore superceding other identities), I have only rearranged the chessboard without creating a strategy for winning the battle. Neither will scholarship, like this chapter, propel disability into the forefront of identity politics for the simple reason that the other identity groups will not cede their place of priority. The reason for this reluctance is also relatively simple—to acknowledge truly that the existence of another identity dilutes the general category of identity, as well as to create a priority of identities, places some identities further down the line as significant. As an amplification of this point, disability will have difficulty being seen as having a primary place in identity politics because most academics are deeply implicated in ableism without, of course, realizing it. Disability is still routinely ignored, marginalized, or patronized by the very people most active in identity politics.

The answer is not to keep creating newer and newer categories of identity or to claim that cultural institutions are uniquely created by the oppression of one or other identity. The advantage that disability studies gives us in this regard is that it is an identity that interrogates and can help transform the very idea of identity. Disability, by the unstable nature of its category, asks us to redefine the very nature of identity and of "belonging" to an identity group. Only when identity is stripped of its exclusive nature and becomes part of the larger reformation of oppression can we all safely feel that we have truly regained our identity.

In this sense, culture will have to change as well. We need cultural forms that will promote a concept of the subject, of character and personality, that derives its strength from knowledge of where identity has been but more where it is going. The challenge for future novelists, filmmakers, and others involved in narrative is to find a way of describing subjectivity, the human body, and the social body that will not rely on the old stereotypes. It is not simply a question of rewriting the old formulas, plugging in plucky characters using wheelchairs or deaf characters who triumph over their condition. Rather, the whole way we think of the normal-abnormal paradigm will have to shift. It is hard to say what this kind of art will be like because in culture things cannot be formulated proscriptively, but it will signal a wide range of changes across the arts. In this sense, disability is not another plug-in. It becomes the way the whole system operates. In the ways that major reconceptualizations have created paradigm shifts, it seems inevitable that disability will force such a change.

NOTES

1. See my article "The Rule of Normalcy: Politics and Disability in the U.S.A. United States of Disability" (Davis 1999), which argues that the disabled citizen was created concomitantly with a rights-based political system in Europe during the eighteenth century.

2. Such work has been done by many disability scholars, including Rosemarie Thomson (1997), Leonard Kriegel (1987), and Paul Longmore (1987).

3. This is a disputed area of knowledge, so I do not want to make an absolute statement here. However, as deaf activists have pointed out, being gay or lesbian is like being deaf in that the child is "different" from the parents. So there is not the continuity of ethnicity, gender, nationality, and so on.

4. The notion of disability as created by barriers rather than inherent inabilities is the hallmark of recent thinking about the subject. For further information, see Chapter 1 of my *Enforcing Normalcy: Disability, Deafness and the Body* (Davis 1995).

5. Indeed, the universal sign symbol for disability—the wheelchair—is the most profound example of the difficulty of categorizing disability because only a small minority of people with disabilities use that aid.

6. We saw this denigration of disability's minority status in the 1996 U.S. presidential election when Bob Dole tried to use his status as a person with disabilities to forge a connection with African Americans and Latinos. Many in these groups doubted his genuine minority status and thought of his claims as mere politicking, which they no doubt were. However, the rapidity with which his claims were dismissed by the media and the public was telling. Clearly, having lost the use of an arm is downplayed in an ableist culture, although becoming a quadriplegic, as Christopher Reeve did, is a more acceptable way to claim disability.

7. For more on the conjunction of statistics and eugenics, see Chapter 2 of my *Enforcing Normalcy* (Davis 1995).

8. Clearly, as the culture moved from one of the ideal to one of the norm, this question concerning character became moot in novel criticism. No one in the late nineteenth century expected a character such as Jude or Verloc to be the embodiment of "human nature *as it should be.*"

9. In the most egregious examples, such as those of Kim or Tarzan, Britishness is so firmly a part of the character that it is indelible to cultural assimilation. And this indelible quality is also inscribed in terms of social class as well. Consider the likes of Tom Jones or Oliver Twist.

10. Statements such as this one cry out for readers to provide exceptions. I am willing to concede that readers may find exceptions to my statement but that the rule in general holds. For example, to find one exception myself, Esther Summerson in *Bleak House* is facially marked by smallpox. However, the exception of this case is so jarring that by the end of the book, Dickens has virtually erased the markings. In contrast, a character such as Captain Ahab in *Moby*

Dick is so marked, he becomes his disability and is not in the proper sense a hero like Ismael, who is unmarked. Indeed, like many disabled characters, he is seen in negative terms and is ultimately punished by the mechanism of the novel. Far fewer main characters can be found who are born disabled, although the literature is rife with minor disabled characters whose disability serves various moral or comic purposes.

11. Presumably, he felt the same way about homosexuals, considered to be a medical disability during this period, since he refused to publish *Maurice* in his own lifetime.

12. Because, in fact, the mean annual income of a family of four in the United States hovers around $37,000, the spacious suburban and urban interiors of most sitcoms are hardly the interiors from which most of America watches these shows.

13. David Mitchell and Sharon Snyder (1997) refer to the use of disability in novels as "narrative prosthesis." For them,

> a narrative issues to resolve or correct—to "prostheticize" in David Wills' sense of the term—a deviance marked as abnormal or improper within a social context. A simple schematic of narrative structure might run: first, a deviance or marked difference is exposed to a reader; second, a narrative consolidates the need for its own existence by calling for an explanation of the deviation's origins and formative consequences; third, the deviance is brought from the periphery of concerns to the centerpiece of the story to come; and fourth, the remainder of the story seeks to rehabilitate or fix the deviance in some manner, shape, or form. This fourth step of the repair of deviance may involve an obliteration of the difference through a "cure," the rescue of the despised object from social censure, the extermination of the deviant as a purification of the social body, or the revaluation of an alternative mode of being.

14. Obviously, I am speaking about middle-class readers, who traditionally make up the bulk of the reading public. Yet, within this category, various identities, most notably female, had the complex task of seeing their social setting as residing both within and outside of the norm. This dialectic is explored in many studies—notably, in the work of Nancy Armstrong, Mary Poovey, Catherine Gallagher, Janet Todd, and Ruth Perry, among others.

15. To use the term coined by Rosemarie Thomson (1997) in *Extraordinary Bodies*.

REFERENCES

Booth, Mark, Sandra Phillips, and Carol Squires. 1998. *Police Pictures: Photography as Evidence*. San Francisco: Chronicle.

Brown, Wendy. 1995. *States of Injury: Power and Freedom in Late Modernity*. Princeton, NJ: Princeton University Press.

Davis, Lennard. 1995. *Enforcing Normalcy: Disability, Deafness and the Body*. London: Verso.

———. 1999. "The Rule of Normalcy: Politics and Disability in the U.S.A. United States of Disability." Pp. 35-47 in *Disability, Divers-ability, and Legal Change*, edited by M. Jones and Lee Ann Marks. London: Kluwer.

Dunlop, John. 1845. *The History of Fiction*. 3d ed. London: Longman, Brown.

Forster, E. M. 1968. *Aspects of the Novel*. Harmondsworth, UK: Penguin.

Girard, René. 1965. *Deceit, Desire, and the Novel: Self and Other in Literary Structure*. Translated by Yvonne Freccero. Baltimore: Johns Hopkins University Press.

Kriegel, Leonard. 1987. "The Cripple in Literature." Pp. 31-46 in *Images of the Disabled, Disabling Images*, edited by A. Gartner and T. Joe. New York: Praeger.

Longmore, Paul. 1987. "Screening Stereotypes: Images of Disabled People in Television and Motion Pictures." Pp. 65-78 in *Images of the Disabled, Disabling Images*, edited by A. Gartner and T. Joe. New York: Praeger.

Mitchell, David and Sharon Snyder. 1997. "Narrative Prosthesis: The Materialty of Metaphor." Paper presented at the Disability Studies Conference, June, Oakland, CA.

Porter, Theodore M. 1986. *The Rise of Statistical Thinking, 1820-1900*. Princeton, NJ: Princeton University Press.

Reeve, Clara. 1930. *The Progress of Romance*. New York: Facsimile Text Society.

Thomson, Rosemarie Garland. 1997. *Extraordinary Bodies: Figuring Physical Disability in American Culture and Literature*. New York: Columbia University Press.

Watt, Ian. 1967. *The Rise of the Novel: Studies in Defoe, Richardson and Fielding*. Berkeley: University of California Press.

Making the Difference

23

Disability, Politics, and Recognition

TOM SHAKESPEARE

NICK WATSON

This chapter surveys the development of global disability politics and analyzes some of the key dimensions of the political activity of disabled people. This first section will introduce some of the concepts and levels of analysis that enable us to understand the scope and evaluate the impact of disability politics. The second section will give an overview of the way different areas of the globe have witnessed disabled people mobilizing as a political force since the late twentieth century. While space limits our discussion, we hope to give a flavor of the extent of disability politics and some of the distinctive features of the different global political arenas. In the third section, we begin to analyze the various forms of representation and involvement that are characteristic of the diverse disability groups and structures that have developed. Finally, in the fourth part of the chapter, we discuss what all this activity means. How can we judge the success of disability politics? Will the movement continue to flow, or has the tide of political mobilization begun to ebb? And, most important, what impact has disability politics had on the lives of the planet's estimated 450 million disabled people?

The late twentieth century brought radically new forms of political protest (Boggs 1986). Historically, mobilization around the claims of religion, class, and nationalism has been dominant. Politics has been, on one hand, a matter of violent social upheaval and, on the other hand, a matter of governments and parliaments. However, since the second half of the twentieth century, new social movements have arisen from hitherto invisible constituencies such as African Americans, women, lesbians and gay men, and, most recently, disabled people. Each wave of political protest has self-consciously modeled itself on those movements that have come before it. The new social movements have challenged the structural exclusion and disempowerment of their constituencies within both the state and the economy but have also served to create positive political identities on a local level. That is, as Alberto Melucci (1989) has written, the new politics operates both instrumentally and symbolically to achieve an improved social role for minority communities. In feminist terms, the personal is political.

Part of the newness of this identity politics is the use of different tactics to achieve change. Mainstream politics has relied historically on three strategies: electoral and parliamentary activity, forms of oppositional violence and terrorism, and workplace strikes, occupations, and other economic actions. The new identity politics, along with the new environmental and peace politics, has, in the main, developed nonviolent direct action as a response to exclusion from the processes of parliamentary democracy and lack of economic leverage. Direct-action protests have been a way of bringing the minority group message to public attention, particularly through publicity in the mass media. In the case of disabled people, direct action has enabled the movement to expose very directly the cause of disability oppression—for example, inaccessible buildings and transport systems or patronizing charity events. It has also challenged the prevailing view of disabled people as incapable, as lacking power and agency, and as pathetic victims of dysfunctional bodies and minds (Morris 1991).

In a sense, disability politics has been about establishing that disability is a political issue at all. Disability has never been on the agenda of mainstream political parties. Disabled people have not been seen as a collective group but merely as a series of individuals suffering impairments. Disability has not been considered as a matter of political power and oppression but as the outcome of physical incapacity and as the domain of medical and welfare professionals. Nancy Fraser (1989) has distinguished three political stages that correspond to the emerging disability politics. First, there comes the struggle over the political status of a given need. Second comes the debate over the interpretation and definition of the need. Third comes the struggle for the satisfaction of that need. So, for example, there was considerable opposition in the United States and in Britain to the idea of civil rights for disabled people: American politicians found it difficult to move away from the philanthropic attitude toward disability, while for a long time, British politicians could not accept that disabled people faced discrimination (Doyle 1996). While in Britain and America, disability politics has moved to the second and especially the third of Fraser's areas, in other parts of the world, the battle is still to establish the political status of disability.

Building on Fraser's (1989) approach, we would argue that three elements in considering the politicization of disability clarify what sort of a political claim is being made. First, there is the basic argument that disabled people are a disadvantaged or marginalized constituency. The evidence for this is overwhelming. A report for the United Nations states,

> [Disabled people] frequently live in deplorable conditions, owing to the presence of physical and social barriers which prevent their integration and full participation in the community. As a result millions of disabled people throughout the world are segregated and deprived of virtually all their rights, and lead a wretched, marginal life. (Despouy 1993:1)

Now, political elites usually accept this sense of disability as a political issue. Second, there is the claim that disabled people comprise a distinct minority and that disabled people themselves should initiate and lead social change for this group. In other words, disability is the sort of political issue that revolves around identity politics. Because nondisabled people, including professionals, families, and charity workers, have dominated the disability field, this second meaning of *political* involves a more radical challenge for the mainstream. Third, there is the social model of disability. This approach redefines disability. Rather than identifying disabled people in medical or individual terms, disability is defined as the way societies deal with people who have impairments. That is, people are disabled by society, not by their bodies. Disability is about discrimination and prejudice, not physical or mental incapacity or limitations (Oliver 1990).

This chapter will deal with these different dimensions of disability politics, conceived of as the challenge issued by the disability constituency to traditional political structures and values. The backdrop to the discussion are the stages outlined by Nancy Fraser (1989), supplemented by our threefold distinction in terms of what *disability politics* implies, and finally the three levels of political change that disabled activist James Charlton (1998) has identified. These levels comprise social change that occurs at the level of meaning (labels), changes to relations of daily practice (e.g., the response of professionals and caregivers to impaired bodies), and changes at a macro level (e.g., new legislation, policy, etc.). Like other new social movements, disability politics is about changing governmental responses, changing relations at an interpersonal level, and changing identities at an individual level.

Political identity is the crucial element of the new politics. The mobilization of disabled people themselves creates the distinction between traditional philanthropic or social democratic approaches to solving the problem of disability and the modern acceptance that disabled people have to be recognized both as a minority group and as the experts on their own lives. Identity often arises out of a consciousness raising—what Paolo Freire (1972) calls conscienticization —in which disabled people come to understand that their difficulties arise not primarily from their own bodies or minds but from the way society has treated them. As Charlton (1998) states,

> The critical consciousness that emerges from this position may lead some people to adopt the disability activist subject position which can involve street level political action or challenging and transforming the organisations for the disabled to become organisations of disabled people and so on. In this sense, to name disability as social oppression is not the defeated wailings of victims, but the clarion call of social change agents. (P. 192)

The Deaf community provides one example of this mobilization. During the 1970s, deaf people began organizing as a social movement, challenging the idea that they were impaired and defining themselves increasingly as a linguistic minority, using the model of ethnicity. In this period, slogans such as Deaf Pride and Deaf Power became popular. One of the culminations of this new deaf identity and political consciousness came with the successful 1988 Deaf President Now protest at Gallaudet University. After the appointment of a hearing president at this university for the deaf, students exploded into political action, closing down the college to demand that the Board of Trustees appoint the first deaf president in the school's history. As two analysts commented,

> The transformation involved deaf persons: (a) identifying themselves as members of a community sharing common values and traits (e.g., sign language) and (b) evaluating the group and its values and traits in a positive light. Ironically, as a group's members come to value themselves after a long period of self deprecation, the consciousness-raising can lead to anger, resentment, and political action over the perceived injustices. (Rose and Kiger 1995:522)

The same anger can be seen in the direct action of disabled people in many countries (which is well documented in Charlton 1998).

Yet the stress on identity raises questions, which we will also address in this chapter. How far does the disability movement represent all disabled people? To what extent are differences between different groups of disabled people—for example, deaf people and people with physical impairments—potentially undermining of the idea of a disabled minority group? Does the development of identity politics threaten to reinforce disabled people's status as different rather than truly to open up the mainstream to the inclusion of people with impairments?

One example of the problems of political identity comes in the field of learning difficulty. Social psychologists have found that people with learning difficulties are not always prepared to identify with that label (Finlay and Lyons 1998). Self-advocacy can either involve trying to change the perception of the group to which one belongs or trying to secure change for oneself as an individual. Collective action depends on identification with the wider group. The strategy of political movements such as People First, which are based on acknowledgment of the learning difficulty identity, and a challenge to its stigmatization may be limited because of the unwillingness of others to identify as having learning difficulties. The same problem applies to other groups of disabled people. For example, many disabled children do not identify themselves as disabled but see themselves as "just the same as everyone else" (Priestley, Corker, and Watson 1999). Many disabled adults do not want to identify themselves as disabled or to be part of disability politics, perhaps because other parts of their identities (race, gender, class) are more salient or perhaps because they prefer to win acceptance as individuals who happen to have but are not defined by their impairments.

This chapter, then, will raise questions and survey the field. We will address the relative importance of broader political goals versus the personal empowerment of individuals. We will explore the extent to which disability demands a rethinking of conventional political concepts such as equality, justice and citizenship, and democracy. Finally, we will assess whether the changing experience of disability is attributable to the demands of the disability movements or to changes in macro-political and economic relations.

MOBILIZING

One of the most important findings from interviews with more than fifty disability rights activists in ten countries is the similarity of lived disability experiences across cultures and political-economic zones. It is also clear that in the most disparate places, the disability rights movement approaches and resists the particularities of the disability experience in very similar ways. (Charlton 1998:4)

The disability movement is a global phenomenon. In the fourth quarter of the twentieth century, disabled people mobilized to demand social change in almost every country. In 1998, the Fifth World Assembly of Disabled Peoples' International was held in Mexico City. Nearly 2,000 delegates attended, representing some 78 countries. A network of international disability activists, sharing insights and strategies throughout the world, accounts for the similarities identified by Charlton (1998). Yet there is another dimension that his overview does not capture. The status of disabled people and the ways in which different societies deal with disability have to be related to the particular structures and traditions of different countries. Key determinants of disabled people's experience will be the level of economic development of a society and the strength of its economy, the extent of the welfare state and the residual role of family support, and the role of religious organizations and charities. The radical social approach to disability has been exported across the globe, and because of this, particularly the impact of United Nations' (1993) *Standard Rules on Equalization of Opportunities for Disabled Persons,* many countries have introduced civil rights legislation in response to pressure from disability groups. Yet no law is a panacea, and the effects of mobilization and legislation will be different in each country.

This discussion cannot do justice to the diversity of responses and experiences internationally, due to limitations of space and the availability of data to the authors. However, we will start by outlining the key dimensions of disability politics in the United Kingdom, United States, and Australia before discussing the salient differences between various European situations, as well as the role of European Union politics. Finally, there will be a brief discussion of disability politics in the "majority world" before a concluding summary of politics at a United Nations level.

The earliest social mobilization of disabled people in Britain dates from the interwar period, when the National League of the Blind and Disabled marched in protest at the poverty experienced by disabled people. However, it was the formation of the Disablement Income Group (DIG) by two disabled women in the late 1960s that marks the first stirrings of the disability movement. Yet, DIG included nondisabled people as well as disabled people and had limited objectives centering on improvements to welfare benefits. A more radical network arose from a letter written by Paul Hunt, a resident of a charitable institution, to *The Guardian* newspaper, suggesting that disabled people organize a consumer group. By 1974, this had led to the formation of the Union of Physically Impaired against Segregation (UPIAS), a radical grassroots network that formulated what Oliver (1983) later termed the "social model of disability" in its key publication, *Fundamental Principles of Disability* (UPIAS 1976). At the same time, other groups such as Sisters against Disablement and the Liberation Network of People with Disabilities were developing the idea of disability as a social oppression. In 1981, the various self-organized groups came together to form the British Council of Organisations of Disabled People (Campbell and Oliver 1996).

During the 1980s, coalitions of disabled people and centers for integrated living developed across the country. Campaigning on a range of issues to do with access and representation and using direct-action tactics brought disability politics to national attention. The new groups challenged the right of traditional unrepresentative charities to speak on behalf of disabled people. The introduction of community care enabled self-organized groups to start delivering a range of independent living services funded by the local state. However, the major political demand was the introduction of a civil rights law, a campaign that brought together both the traditional disability charities and the radical groups under the Rights Now umbrella. During the Conservative governments of 1979 to 1997, there was a reluctance to concede that disabled people experienced discrimination, and successive attempts to introduce legislation failed. Eventually, in 1996, the Disability Discrimination Act was passed, although this did not deliver comprehensive and enforceable civil rights. Extensions of the law by the new Labour government were also accompanied by attacks on disabled people's benefit entitlements in an attempt to control government spending. Meanwhile, the target of the radical Direct Action Network changed from an emphasis on winning accessible transport to a "Free Our People" campaign inspired by American struggles to liberate disabled people from nursing homes and other institutions.

The United States has a different tradition of protest and social reform than does Britain and much of Western Europe. Factors explaining the different developments of disability politics include the absence of a developed welfare state, strong trade unions, and socialist parties; the strong emphasis on rights, expressed in a written constitution; and the fullest development of the free market and competitive values (Oliver 1990:121ff). This political environment shaped the development of American disability politics, which has incorporated the philosophy of self-determination, equal opportunities, and self-respect for disabled people. Located within the American tradition of self-reliance and individualism, the U.S. disability movement followed the example of the civil rights movement, the women's movement, and the lesbian and gay liberation movements that preceded it (DeJong 1983:11). Whereas their European counterparts have laid more emphasis on collective mobilization to challenge the status quo and the structure of society, these American movements have been concerned with winning access to the mainstream for excluded sections of the population. Another key feature of the U.S. disability movement has been the origins among the young male disabled veterans of the Vietnam War. The main organizational advance came with the first formation of independent living centers, run by disabled people for disabled people, initially on the campus of the University of California, Berkeley.

Due to the lobbying of disability organizations, campaigners managed to secure the passage of the 1973 Rehabilitation Act, with its historic Section 504, the first example of anti-discrimination legislation (ADL). However, the greatest fight came after this victory, in trying to bring about the enactment of the clause that prohibits discrimination against disabled people in any federally funded program. When, in 1977, Secretary of Health, Education, and Welfare (HEW) Joseph Califano refused to sign Section 504, 300 activists organized a 30-day occupation of the HEW office, both highlighting the role of structural discrimination and challenging the stereotype of disabled people as powerless (Zola 1983:56). The same year, the White House Conference on Handicapped Individuals called for civil rights legislation for disabled people. A federal agency, the National Council on Disability, submitted draft legislation in 1988. After George Bush was elected president, the legislation was resubmitted and in 1990 became the Americans with Disabilities Act (ADA), extending discrimination protection to the private sector.

A large element of the movement in North America has stemmed from consumerism and self-help; for example, in the independent living centers, this emphasis plays a large part. This is a particularly American tradition of self-reliance and individual rights. Many writers focus on consumer involvement, whereas British approaches would stress political autonomy and democratic participation, not the market. Until recently, the social model has not been a part of U.S. disability discourse. Gareth Williams (1983) criticizes the market pluralist models of DeJong (1983) and others, seeing their faith in consumer sovereignty and self-reliance as being misplaced in the context of power imbalance. American disability campaigns focus on admitting disabled people to wider society, demanding the extension of existing social rights to them as a group. Pfeiffer (1996) suggests that American disabled people feel empowered as a result of the ADA and points to the evidence of barrier removal, although problems and hence frustration remain. Equally, it might be pointed out that more than half of disabled Americans live in poverty. Albrecht (1992) has highlighted the limitations of civil rights strategies:

> The problem with this approach is that it accomplishes little or nothing for poor and marginal Americans. Grass roots activism is confined principally to the educated middle class who are savvy about lobbying. The poor and marginal Americans do not represent themselves well and are not effectively represented by liberals. The result is that those most in need of services are least likely to receive help, especially in economic hard times. (P. 300)

As the African American experience also demonstrates, civil rights may bring formal equality but without the achievement of an improved standard of living or equality of outcome.

In Australia, as in many other countries, the 1981 United Nations Year of Disabled People provided the impetus around which disability politics coalesced. Like in Britain, the American model of independent living and civil rights was an important influence. A long period of Labour government facilitated moves toward normalization and independent living, and grassroots disabled people—especially networks of disabled women—mobilized to demand change. Organizations such as Disabled Peoples' International (Australia) and the National Federation of Blind Citizens Australia campaigned against the Miss Australia pageant and for better provision.

Legislative developments included the Disability Services Act of 1986, which recognized the need for advocacy services, and the Disability Discrimination Act of 1992. The latter law, like its later British equivalent, has little teeth, leaving it up to individuals to complain about discrimination. Unlike in America, the standards for implementation of such statutes are drawn up after it becomes law, and Australian disability rights groups were not fully involved in this process.

With the change to a Conservative coalition government after 1996, the high-water mark of disabled political influence in Australia has passed. The Human Rights and Equal Opportunity Commission was cut back, resulting in the abolition of the Disability Discrimination Act commissioner post. Cuts to budgets affected disabled people, and major disability rights groups were defunded. Newell (1996) traces a shift from the language of rights to the language of consumerism in recent Australian disability politics. So, for example, DPI (Australia) has collapsed, while the National Caucus of Disability Consumer Organizations has emerged, made up mainly of mono-impairment groups, not all of which are even controlled by disabled people. Women with Disabilities Australia is the only cross-impairment and disabled-controlled organization in the National Caucus. Part of the decline of disability politics has to do with the change of government and political culture. Another part has to do with the difficulty of organizing nationally in a country of Australia's vast scale. Yet Cooper (1999) argues that it is wrong to confuse the fate of particular organizations with that of the disability movement as a whole:

> While the political power of people with disabilities is most easily seen in national specific disability organisations debating issues with government policy makers a greater power is with the myriad of individuals and small groups, working mostly without funding, but armed with anti-discrimination legislation, and engaged in access battles. Maybe this is how our diverse society works best. (P. 225)

Returning to the European situation, Rachel Hurst (1995) has argued that there are three subregions within Europe. First, the Nordic countries and the Netherlands have a long tradition of human rights and equal opportunities. Together with economic stability, this has enabled a financial commitment to service provision, as well as the inclusion of consumers in the consultation process. The Scandinavian welfare state has been the most advanced in the world, and disabled people have benefited from good services, rehabilitation aids, integrated education, and a 20-year-old tradition of community rather than institutional housing. Yet, paradoxically, these benefits have resulted in a disabled population lacking radicalism and a positive identity. According to Hurst,

> This has bred a comparatively comfortable, passive body of disabled people whose organisations are well-funded and consulted by the state and who, because of their individual situation, do not have the impetus to demand change. (P. 530)

These countries are falling behind those nations in which the disability movement has had to fight for progress. For example, they lack equal rights legislation. Moreover, there is a lack of access to public buildings or transport, public attitudes remain largely negative, and there is little employment choice for disabled people.

Hurst's (1995) second group are what she calls the "colonizing countries," such as Britain, France, Germany, and Spain, which have been characterized by a paternalistic attitude to disability. Charities and religious organizations are important, and professionals tend to be in charge. Disabled people have experienced a lack of services, environmental barriers, and an absence of proper consultation. All these countries have antidiscrimination legislation, but none has mechanisms for enforcement. For example, Spain has had blanket laws against discrimination since the 1980s but has not been effective in delivering civil rights for disabled people.

Finally, Hurst (1995) aggregates the "poorer countries," such as Portugal, Italy, Ireland, and Greece, where a similar ethic and attitude predominates, but there is no meaningful social provision. Available resources tend to go to segregated projects run by professionals, the voice of disabled people is weak, and there has been no active grassroots disability politics. To Hurst's tripartite classification, we should add Central and Eastern Europe. In these areas, there is an ideology of egalitarianism and a strong welfare state. The collapse of communism has not brought major benefits to disabled people, who have been victims of the general economic dislocation, unemployment, and poverty. Except for Poland, religious organizations have been weak up to this point, although the legacy of state socialism is a lack of grassroots action and community politics. As with Hurst's third grouping, the family is a key element in support for disabled people. For the short term, the status of disabled people will be reduced. In the long term, international models of independent living and political identity may reduce dependency and improve the status of disabled people. For example, Hungary brought in a civil rights act in March 1998 after the National Federation of Disabled Persons Associations of Hungary (MEOSZ) organized street demonstrations and lobbying in response to government backtracking. The Rights and Equal Opportunities Act promotes disabled people's citizenship, educational inclusion, accessibility, and barrier removal.

These different European situations are likely to standardize in the future, as activists draw on the experience of other countries. This international networking has also operated at the scale of European institutions. The European Union (EU) has run the HELIOS and HELIOS 2 programs on disability. However, these have not been controlled by disabled people but instead have been dominated by civil servants, charities, and professionals. Disabled Peoples' International Europe has lobbied the European parliament for more consultation and for human rights work on disability. This has led to changes in structures such as the European Disability Forum and in the HELIOS 2 program. A key development occurred on December 3, 1993, the International Day of Disabled Persons. Despite initial opposition, a disabled people's parliament convened in the European Parliament building. The president of the parliament, commissioners, and other politicians listened to speeches from 81 of the 440 delegates telling their stories. This led to a major change in European political attitudes, acceptance of disability as a human rights issue, and support for the United Nations standard rules (Hurst 1998). While in the 1980s, the European Parliament and European Commission focused on the issue of quotas for employment, in the 1990s, there was a move toward the issue of disability discrimination (Waddington 1997:475).

Finally, we need to make some general observations about the majority world, which will be covered more extensively in other contributions to this volume. While in Europe, America, and Australia, we have noted campaigns for independence and integration, in much of the rest of the world, disability movements have to settle for whatever provision they can get. Yet, as Coleridge (1993) points out, self-organized campaigning and services have been a feature of many developing countries (e.g., Zimbabwe, Nicaragua, and India). Such countries, such as Uganda, Zambia, Madagascar, and many other nations, have passed civil rights statutes for disabled people during the past decade (Charlton 1998). International networking has played a major part in spreading disability politics into different countries. For instance, Narong Patibatsorakit attended the first DPI World Congress in Singapore, returning home to found the national Thai disability organization. In 1996, he became the first disabled person in Thailand to be elected to the country's senate.

While poverty and underdevelopment negatively affect disabled people in particular, transition to urban industrialized status offers threats as well as opportunities for disabled people. If assumptions and attitudes about disabled people are negative, then economic development may be based on their exclusion from public life and will be more disabling. Examples from Malaysia illustrate this problem. Disability activist Thanasayan suggests that the Malaysian public believes that "the disabled do not need access to public buildings facilities because they remain at home or in specialised institutions" (Jayasooria, Krishnan, and Ooi 1997:459). Second, the new light rail transit system in the Klang valley will be inaccessible to disabled people, evidence that leads authors to conclude that "Malaysia has missed a unique opportunity as a newly industrialising country to develop infrastructure that is accessible for all its people" (Jayasooria et al. 1997:459). Third, while traditionally the family has provided for its disabled members, largely through the work of women, industrialization will undermine this. With the transition from rural to urban living and the employment of women, disabled people are left without support. These Malaysian problems may well be replicated in other recently developing countries.

Finally, the impact of international politics cannot be ignored. United Nations activity started in 1975, when the UN General Assembly adopted the *Declaration on the Rights of Disabled Persons.* The 1981 International Year for Disabled Persons was the impetus for disability movements in many countries. It was followed by the UN Decade of Disabled Persons 1982-1992, which brought the *World Programme of Action* that focused on prevention of impairment, rehabilitation, and the participation and equal opportunities of disabled people. The period saw a shift toward an enablement and empowerment approach, rather than one based on narrowly medical and individual issues. Reflecting the increased stress on human rights, the United Nations adopted the *Standard Rules on the Equalization of Opportunities for Persons with Disabilities* in 1993. While this instrument takes the form of legal recommendations rather than binding statutes and tries to balance a medical and social model approach, it has been highly influential in levering change throughout the world. Whether the many new laws it has inspired represent merely formal equality of opportunity or will result in significant improvements in quality of life and status for disabled people remains to be seen.

REPRESENTING

While most countries of the world have witnessed the development of political groups of disabled people, organization has taken multiple forms. Traditionally, responses to the problem of disability have been based on a medical approach. This means that different impairments have been catered for by different charities or self-help groups. While the former may have developed from religious impulses, the latter may have been initiated by doctors specializing in a particular condition, often in alliance with the parents or families of people affected. So, the political landscape of disability is often already occupied by groups that are not only not controlled by disabled people but also fail to see that different impairment groups may have many issues in common.

In fact, Oliver and Zarb (1989) suggest that the separation of different impairment groups is not accidental. They point out that the British state delivers services in ways that foster divisions in the disabled population:

> Hence it gives tax allowances to blind people but not to other categories of disability, mobility allowances to those who cannot walk but not for those who can, and higher pensions and benefits for those injured at work or in the [armed] services than for those with congenital disabilities or those who have had accidents. This is not an unintended consequence of State provision but a deliberate tactic which the State has developed in its dealings with other groups and can be summed up as "divide and rule." (P. 222)

Whereas cross-impairment groups, on a local and national basis, are now a common feature of many European countries, in other parts of the world, the dominant groupings are still based on specific medical diagnoses.

The distinction between mono-impairment and multi-impairment groups is not the only division in the disability constituency. As noted earlier in this chapter, another major cleavage runs between those groups that are controlled by disabled people (and often allow only disabled people into full membership) and the more traditional groups, which are dominated by nondisabled people (whether they are the families of disabled people, professionals, or people inspired by philanthropic motives). Historically, it is the latter groups that have had access to power in the political arena and to most of the funding available from governments. A considerable proportion of disabled political mobilization has been directed toward either winning control of these organizations or challenging their right to speak on behalf of disabled people.

But these distinctions do not exhaust the differences within the disability constituency. Rights-based disability groups themselves come in different shapes and sizes. For example, Charlton (1998:136) distinguishes 10 different types of disability rights organizations:

1. Local self-help groups (e.g., Self-Help Association of Paraplegics/Soweto)
2. Local advocacy and program centers (e.g., Centres for Integrated Living)
3. Local single-issue advocacy groups (e.g., Acesso Libre in Mexico City)
4. Public policy groups (e.g., World Institute on Disability, Oakland, USA)
5. Single-issue national advocacy groups (ADAPT—USA)
6. National membership organizations (Organisation of Disabled Revolutionaries, Nicaragua; National Council of Disabled Persons Zimbabwe; Women with Disabilities Australia).
7. National coalitions/federations of groups (British Council of Disabled People)
8. National single-impairment organizations (National Association of the Blind—India; British Deaf Association)
9. Regional organizations (Southern African Federation of the Disabled; Disabled Peoples' International Europe)
10. International organizations (Disabled Peoples' International)

However, these different forms of representation and involvement are not necessarily all competing. Many structures are needed to play complementary roles and take on different tasks. For example, some groups, such as ADAPT or Britain's Direct Action Network (DAN), are involved in direct political action. Often, these groups involve a small number of individuals (approximately 500 members of ADAPT and nearly 100 members of DAN). Other groups may be prevented from such overt campaigning due to the legal restrictions placed on charities in countries such as Britain. Again, some groups are involved in consciousness raising and community development, either in a particular locality or among a particular impairment group.

Distinguished from these activist networks are the organizations, often set up in the second wave of disabled political activity, which are involved in service delivery. For example, many countries and regions of the world now have centers for integrated living, which provide advice, support, and services for disabled people at a practical level. Other groups may be involved in delivering training or developing access initiatives. Sometimes, these groups may lose the political edge or impetus that was the hallmark of their early life. Paid employees replace committed activists. Groups may become incorporated into mainstream public policy and welfare provision. There may even be a danger of complacency—of thinking that the battles have been won or failing to develop new generations of politicized disabled people. Charlton (1998) notes that there is a distinction between those militants who continue to take to the streets and the many organizations and individuals in the independent living and disability rights community who are not radical or are only narrowly political.

These changes may undermine the dualism that was the core of early disability politics between those organizations that were "for" disabled people—the traditional charities and paternalistic groups—and those organizations that were "of" disabled people—the radical rights-based groups. Due to the very success of the disability politics, the model must now embrace at least two other variants: (1) those traditional "for" organizations, which have moved to take onboard the disability rights approach and have become more responsive to and representative of disabled people and their priorities, and (2) those "of" organizations, as discussed above, which have become consolidated into the mainstream and have perhaps lost their radical edge.

Rather than the triumphalism, which is a characteristic of many discussions of disability politics, perhaps a note of caution is needed in analyzing the phenomenal explosion of the disability movement in recent decades. Questions need to be raised about the extent to which groups truly represent the majority of disabled people, particularly people in more excluded impairment categories or multiple minority groups. The intention is not to discredit disability organizations, and it should be noted that the criticism of the "unrepresentativeness" of political groups is often raised by their opponents. Instead, the analysis is intended to point to ways forward and to problems still to be addressed in the developing politics of disability.

The disability movement in many countries is dominated by a somewhat restricted section of the impaired population. For example, in Western countries, approximately half of all people with impairments are older than age 50. Yet most activists enter the movement at a much younger age, and older people who have impairments neither make up a significant proportion of the movement nor are as likely to identify with a civil rights perspective. Again, there have been persistent questions about the role and involvement of particular impairment groups. For example, people with learning difficulties may have been excluded because their particular access and language issues have not been properly understood or because they have not been welcomed. Some disabled people have sought to bolster their own status as people with physical impairments, at the expense of those with intellectual impairments. Another example is the Deaf community, which has resisted identification with the mainstream disability movement. Often, this is because deaf people see themselves as a linguistic minority, not as people defined by a medical condition. Of course, some disabled people themselves have rejected a medical identity, so perhaps the problem is less one of definition and more about separate cultures (Corker 1997). More of a problem is that dominant disability rights demands, such as inclusive education for all disabled children, are rejected by the Deaf community, which wants its children educated separately via the medium of sign language.

Aside from differences of impairment and age, other social cleavages are also evident in disability politics. Feminists have often criticized the disability movement for sexism and the exclusion of women's issues. Minority ethnic communities in some countries have felt ignored by disability groups dominated by the majority population. Lesbian and gay disabled people have experienced homophobia or have felt unwelcome in disability organizations that have taken on radical disabled perspectives but may be very conventional in terms of sexual politics. Finally, access to economic and social power is a strong determinant of the life experience of disabled people in general and also influences involvement in disability politics. Many leaders of the movement have come from privileged socioeconomic contexts.

Another set of questions relates to the relevance of ideologies such as the social model to different cultures. A graphic example of this is the problem of translating the difference between physical impairment and disability as a social relationship into languages other than English. Debates about terminology are ubiquitous in disability circles but are made more complex when languages such as French or Chinese or sign language may have trouble representing disability in nonmedical ways. Is an idea that was devised in developed Western countries straightforwardly applicable to very different cultural contexts? Do Western aid organizations such as Oxfam or the disability movement have the right to impose this model on other cultures? Emma Stone (1999) has demonstrated how developing new Chinese ideograms has connected with positive political change around disability in China, yet she also suggests that "only time will tell whether the transplant of Western-evolved disability discourses into non-Western contexts works for or against the lives of individual disabled people" (p. 146).

Again, how far should disability rights be balanced with the broader needs of developing countries and the majority population? As Potts (1998) asks in the context of education, "How far does the recognition of individual civil rights, including that to an appropriate education, get in the way of making economic progress?" (p. 121). The impetus for many countries' disability movements came when individuals attended world congresses of Disabled Peoples' International and brought back with them organizational and ideological ideas derived from other countries. This has been a great strength of disability politics, but perhaps it has also led to some inappropriate and possibly even ethnocentric developments. In Britain and America, nondisabled family members and allies are not usually welcome in the disability movement; however, in other cultures, a more inclusive model may be preferred.

There are also tensions and contradictions within the dominant ideology of disability rights. For example, there is a subtle but important difference between the minority group model and the social model. The former focuses on disabled people as a minority group, experiencing oppression and seeking social change. The latter focuses on disabling barriers and building an inclusive society but does not necessarily specify a constituency or change agent. Strategically, there may be a tension between a minority group approach, which rests on raising the status and situation of an identified constituency of disabled people, and a social model approach, which depends on removing barriers and changing society in general. This philosophical distinction is glossed over in practical disability politics because the minority group and social model perspective are so closely entwined in radical consciousness.

This distinction relates closely to another dilemma, which comes out most clearly in Helen Liggett's (1988) critique of minority group politics and draws on Foucauldian ideas. Disability politics, by its very nature, often rests on a fairly unreflexive acceptance of the disabled/nondisabled distinction. Disabled people are seen as those who identify as such. Disabled leadership is seen as vital. However, Liggett argues,

> From an interpretative point of view the minority group approach is double edged because it means enlarging the discursive practices which participate in the constitution of disability. . . . In order to participate in their own management disabled people have had to participate as disabled. Even among the politically active, the price of being heard is understanding that it is the disabled who are speaking. (Pp. 271ff)

Many disabled people do not want to see themselves as disabled, in terms of either the medical or the social model. They downplay the significance of their impairments and seek access to a mainstream identity. They do not have a political identity because they do not see themselves as part of the disability movement either. This refusal to define oneself by impairment or disability has sometimes been seen as "internalized oppression" or "false consciousness" by radicals in the disability movement. Yet this attitude itself can be patronizing and oppressive. After all, the denial of disability is implicitly based on the rejection of the idea of an exclusive "normality" and a refusal to be categorized. This approach may be rather individualist and may overlook the problems of discrimination and prejudice. However, surely it is a legitimate alternative to a minority group approach, which leaves the disabled-nondisabled dichotomy unchallenged and runs the risk of replacing an idea of disabled people as victims of their bodies by the idea of disabled people as victims of social relations.

These dilemmas point to the complexities and contradictions of disability politics. While the politics of gender, sexuality, and "race" can hardly be said to be straightforward, issues of representation and organization are perhaps most difficult in the field of disability. To conclude this discussion, we want to highlight a recent social development—namely, the self-organization of people with neurological differences. This example illustrates both the opportunities and difficulties posed by disability politics. Judy Singer (1999) writes about the development of a social movement of people with Asberger's syndrome (AS), a condition related to autism. This constituency of people whose impairment can undermine face-to-face interaction has the potential to be liberated by the Internet. An AS identity has developed, which is counterposed to the mainstream world of "neurotypicals" or NTs. Is this social group assimilable within the broader disability movement? Singer suggests,

> A challenge for the disability rights movement materializes: how do you include people who may need the benefits of inclusion, but cannot bear the physical and emotional presence of it? (P. 67)

Her conclusion is perhaps relevant to wider questions of disability identity and difference:

> Perhaps as the voices of the "neurologically different" are heard more loudly, a more ecological view of society will emerge: one that is more relaxed about different styles of being, that will be content to let each individual find his/her own niche, based on the kinds of mutual recognition that can only arise through an ever-developing sociological, psychological and now neurological, self-awareness. (P. 67)

THEORIZING

In this section, we will turn to an exploration of some mainstream concepts in political theory to begin to explore their relevance to the emerging politics of disability. *Justice, citizenship, democracy,* and *rights* are terms that are commonly deployed in the writings on disability politics. Oliver (1993), for example, points out that "to be disabled in Great Britain is to be denied the fundamental rights of citizenship to such an extent that most disabled people are denied their basic human rights" (p. 6). Yet is citizenship a robust concept? Can democracy deliver for minorities? Are civil rights the answer to the exclusion of disabled people? This section unpacks these concepts and situates them within disability politics.

Citizenship, as Ruth Lister (1997) in her monograph on the subject points out, is a contested subject. It is about both the relationship between individuals and the state and the relationships within a state between individuals. It incorporates notions of rights, responsibilities, obligations, needs, actions, virtues, and opinions. While approaches to citizenship include those of social liberalism, communitarianism, neoliberalism, and civic republicanism (Voet 1998), we will concentrate in this chapter on social-liberal and civic republic ideas.

Social liberalism is exemplified by the work of T. H. Marshall (1950), perhaps the most influential postwar writer on the subject. His notion of citizenship is contained within legal rights and legal obligations, and it is these concepts that lie at the heart of disability movement's demand for civil rights legislation for disabled people. According to Marshall, citizenship can be broken down into three elements: civil, political, and social. The civil element refers to individual freedom, the political to a right to participate in the exercise of political power, and the social to a right to economic welfare and security and access to resources through which the norms prevailing in that society can be achieved (Marshall 1950:10-11).

Oliver (1996) has used Marshall's (1950) tripartite formulation to argue that disabled people, in the United Kingdom at least, are denied full and active citizenship. He argues that disabled people are denied their full political rights, in that they are denied access to polling stations, information on which to base informed choices, and full inclusion in the political process. The underrepresentation of disabled people in the higher echelons of many of the political parties and at the higher levels of decision making throughout Europe and the rest of the world support these assertions. In addition, the glut of organizations for disabled people who speak on behalf of disabled people, as well as their relative wealth and subsequent power in comparison to organizations controlled by disabled people, further reduces disabled people's political rights.

There is also much evidence to support the assertion that disabled people are denied basic social rights. For example, Charlton (1998) documents how disabled people are abandoned or hidden by their families and are not allowed to enter the mainstream of social life. Further inaccessible environments can prevent disabled people from working, socializing, and conducting fully public lives (Barnes 1991). Disabled people are also often subjected to second-rate segregated education, thus denying them future employment opportunities (Oliver and Barnes 1998). Disabled people are also denied basic civil rights. For example, when in work they are often paid at a considerably lower rate for the same job as nondisabled people (Hyde 1996). Again, disabled children and adults are also more likely to be physically and sexually assaulted than their nondisabled peers (Westcott 1993).

These facts about the status of disabled people as second-class citizens and the struggle for full citizenship have been at the forefront of recent political campaigns by organizations of disabled people worldwide (Charlton 1998; Dreidger 1989). Under the influence of the civil rights movement in the United States and liberationist social movements throughout the world, disabled people have organized to demand their full inclusion as citizens. We could cite, for example, the independent living movement and its success in procuring social rights for disabled people, enabling many disabled people to live outside of institutions, and in reevaluating the notion of independence. However, despite recent successes, such as the Americans with Disabilities Act in the United States, the Disability Discrimination Act in the United Kingdom, and similar legislation in Australia, Canada, New Zealand, and throughout the rest of the world, the status of disabled people as second-class citizens has yet to be resolved. Similar legislation has failed to achieve significant improvements in the lives of many women, black people, and gays and lesbians and has led many writers to question the validity of approaches to citizenship founded on the notion of social liberalism.

Social liberalism, it is argued, downplays notions of difference, promoting the idea of a universal, abstract, disembodied individual. Lister (1997) suggests that in actuality, the citizen in social-liberal accounts is not disembodied but is, in essence, one who is male, white, heterosexual, and nondisabled. She argues that it is the standpoint of the privileged and powerful that has become the norm, and others are seen as deviant and inferior. Differences between disabled and nondisabled people are socially produced for a reason—to maintain dominance. If oppressed groups challenge the ideas of the powerful, their challenges are ignored because they are seen as the rantings of biased, partial, and selfish special interest groups that wish to seek favor for their own particular grouping at the expense of the mainstream (Young 1990:116).

This deficiency in social liberalism has led to a school of feminist thought drawing on, among others, the ideas of Arendt (1958), Sennet (1977), and Barber (1984). Rather than concentrating on citizenship, this school of thought argues for a new democracy, one that is based on participation associated with a pursuit of the common good. This is termed *civic republicanism*. Citizenship is about active political participation, a process that incorporates the views of women and minority groups within the public sphere, enabling the confrontation of difference and promoting inclusion. It is argued that democracy, as it currently exists, lets down people from minority groups. So, Iris Marian Young (1990) writes,

To promote a politics of inclusion, then participatory democracy must promote the ideal of a heterogeneous public, in which persons stand forth with their differences acknowledged and respected though perhaps not completely understood by others. (P. 119)

Young proposes that the ideal of participatory democracy can be achieved through what she describes as a "politics of group assertion" through which oppressed groups of people identify a positive sense of difference (Young 1990:167). While these groups may primarily emerge around single issues, Young suggests that coalitions will emerge as the groups unite to fight for a just society. However, she argues that oppressed groups need separate organizations to allow "group members to determine their specific needs and interests" (Young 1990:167).

Her argument, when applied to disabled people, suggests that democracy will be enhanced and the position of disabled people strengthened within a society if disabled people are brought into the political system as an interest group and that, through this presence, their demands will be legitimized. It further requires people with impairment to self-identify as disabled and through such a process reject the diminishing or displacing identities that others may wish to place on them. The implication is that disabled people must reject a notion of sameness. Disability rights and citizenship are not achieved through a claim founded on their equality with nondisabled people but through a particularistic claim based on their difference. While Young (1990) does not reject the benefits of the former approach—arguing that such an analysis exposes the arbitrary nature of what are thought to be natural group-based distinctions, presenting a clear standard of equality and maximizing choice—she contends that a society without group-based distinctions is neither possible nor desirable (Young 1990:163-64). Disabled people are one of many socially and culturally differentiated groups, and if democracy is to be achieved, all these groups must respect and affirm one another. Justice will only be achieved if disabled people's values are accorded the same worth as those of nondisabled people.

Yet perhaps Young's (1990) perspective has to be situated in the U.S. context. Group-based identities and identity politics have long been part of the American tradition of political representation and have acted as a bedrock of individual and collective rights in that country. For example, the women's movement, workers' movements, and ethnic movements all started in the late nineteenth century and are linked to the ideals of individualism and democracy prevalent in American society. It is in this way that much of the American disability rights movement differs from that of Europe and the rest of the world. In Europe and elsewhere, the disabled people's movement has challenged the state, the bureaucratization of society, capitalism, and consumerism and has aimed at social revolution. In America, in contrast, the aim has been less to challenge the legitimacy of such institutions but to demand that America live up to its ideals of equal rights for all individuals.

Another problem is that the difference approach demands that disabled people must self-identify as such, and, as we have already argued, many disabled people do not want to identify themselves as different. Indeed, disability politics has, in the past, tended to downplay notions of difference, seeing disability as a uniting factor based on social exclusion. There is a danger that if disabled people try to mobilize around an agenda driven by difference, then disabled people themselves will construct difference on the grounds of their different impairments, and the disabled people's movement will become disaggregated and fragmented. There will be no disabled people left. Furthermore, how can a politics of diversity exist alongside the necessary politics of solidarity without the need for solidarity appropriating diversity in the name of the common good? There is also the danger that calls for difference can lead to an essentializing of the category. That is, having to identify as disabled and different, differences can be perceived as naturally given.

Finally, further questions are raised about the stress placed on "independence" and "autonomy" as a goal. These ideals have to be understood in the context of the Enlightenment tradition of the individual liberal subject. Many people have criticized this idea as being a male-dominated perspective, which ignores the ways in which individuals are dependent on others. Carol Gilligan (1983) suggested that in addition to abstract political concepts such as rights and justice, there was an alternative set of ideals based on solidarity and care and relationships, which were not inferior but different. The feminist ethic of care philosophers such as Jean Tronto (1993) and Selma Sevenhuijsen (1998) offer an important correlative to the rhetoric of the independent living movement. For example, Sevenhuijsen criticizes autonomy and independence as a goal and the whole idea of "atomistic individualism":

The ideal of abstract autonomy in fact overlooks what it is that makes care an element of the human condition, i.e. the recognition that all people are vulnerable, dependent and finite, and that we all have to find ways of dealing with this in our daily existence and in the values which guide our individual and collective behaviour. (P. 28)

Because women have historically been the care providers, it is suggested that they are less likely to promote an unrealistic view of independence. They realize that a large proportion of people—babies and children, pregnant women, older people, and sick and disabled people—will rely on others in various ways and at various stages. Thus, Sevenhuijsen (1998) promotes the idea of "caring solidarity":

The feminist ethic of care points to forms of solidarity in which there is room for difference, and in which we find out what people in particular situations need in order for them to live with dignity. People must be able to count on solidarity because vulnerability and dependency, as we know, are a part of human existence; we need each other's disinterested support at expected and unexpected moments. (P. 147)

This notion of caring solidarity may perhaps offer some promise in trying to break down the dichotomy between disabled and nondisabled people, recognizing that everyone is variously dependent and that aspiring to independence reinforces rather than resolves a historic problem.

This brief discussion suggests that disabled people cannot necessarily just seek admission to existing political structures or draw on traditional political concepts. While at a rhetorical level, notions such as civil rights, democracy, and citizenship are powerful slogans, more complex responses are demanded to do justice to the complexities of the politics of disability. It may be that some of these responses challenge core assumptions within political theory itself.

CONCLUSION

What makes the disability rights movement subversive is paradoxically the extraordinary worldwide oppression of people with disabilities. The oppression is systematic. The principles, demands and goals of the disability rights movement cannot be accomodated by the present world system. (Charlton 1998:149)

In concluding this overview of disability politics, we want to raise two final questions, which in different ways are about the impact and ambitions of the disability movement. The first, raised by James Charlton's (1998) statement, is the extent to which disability politics is about reform or revolution. The discussion of political theory demonstrated that it is difficult to see the liberation of disabled people being delivered within existing structures or via mainstream concepts such as democracy and citizenship. Many commentators would see the liberal ambition of civil rights as being fundamentally doomed because of the broader systems of power and the underlying capitalist social relations. As the global market becomes more and more dominant, the scope for national-level social investment and egalitarian reform becomes more limited. Yet, equally, despite the revolutionary rhetoric of Charlton or Oliver (1990, 1996), global social transformation is not on the agenda either. It may be that the true empowerment of disabled people will only come about through a replacement of the dominant political and economic structures of the planet, but this does not seem an immediate or even medium-term possibility.

The second question is about the progress that has been achieved so far and about the extent to which the disability movement can take credit for this. We want to argue that, despite much of the hype, the impact of the disability movement may have been as much in personal and symbolic terms than in instrumental or structural terms. While thousands of people have developed positive senses of themselves through access to a political identity and, in the process, relationships between disabled and nondisabled people, and service users and professionals have undoubtedly begun to change, the broader political developments have not been fundamentally driven by disability activism. We are making a similar point to those who argue that the change in the social role of women in the postwar period has owed more to the changing requirements of capital and less to the militancy of the feminist movement. However, we add that the success or otherwise of disability politics is a factor of the broader political landscape, not the leverage of disabled people themselves.

Several examples may help substantiate our claim. In Australia, disabled protest and the growth of self-organized groups proceeded well during the period of Labour government. A Disability Discrimination Act was passed, which emulated the civil rights pattern of the United States and other countries, albeit as a gift of government, rather than as a concession to the movement. Yet, with change of government, the tide has flowed the other way. Organizations have been defunded, and now there is no DPI national affiliate structure in Australia. Activist groups are falling apart, and funding is only available for mono-impairment and consumer-type groups (Meekosha and Jakubowicz forthcoming).

Devolution or other political change may dilute commitment to equality and participation, as evidenced by the devolution of welfare funding from the federal to state level in the United States. This is also evident in the devolution of disability services from the federal to state level in Australia (Cooper 1999), as well as in Shakespeare's (1996) study of the impact of local government reorganization on disability groups in the United Kingdom. In the latter case, for example, disabled people's self-organization in the county of Avon developed very effectively through the 1980s. The presence of a core of disabled officers in the local authority, together with grassroots lobbying, led to funding for self-organized groups, the setting up of a center of integrated living, and other advances. This was enabled partly because no one political group had overall control of local government, and therefore considerable negotiation and strategy were involved in day-to-day running of Avon politics. Astute disabled advocates were able to play off different political parties, all of whom were concerned to be seen as supporting disabled people and therefore would promise funding and influence.

Two macro-political changes resulted in a different landscape. First, the advent of community care meant that local government grants were converted into contracts for services. In this climate, the Centre for Integrated Living flourished, but the Coalition of Disabled People withered because community development was a low priority. Second, local government reorganization meant that Avon was split into four unitary authorities. Disabled officers were divided among the different successor bodies, removing the strong core of allies within local council structures. Experience and expertise in equalities work were lost. Several of the new authorities had no interest in or understanding of disability. One authority supported a local consumer network of service users, rather than the political organization of disabled people. Bristol Council, now totally controlled by Labour, no longer needed to deliver benefits to disability groups to operate, and disabled voices were squeezed out of decision making, all of which now happens behind closed doors in the private meetings of the ruling group, rather than in open council debate.

What this suggests is that the tide of political success can flow both ways. In a democratic system, the party in control of government will dictate the role of disabled political groups and the policy toward disabled people. In general, parties of the left will favor intervention and action on equality; in general, parties of the right will favor cutting back state spending and leaving social outcomes to market forces. As well as ideology, the structures of local government are important. Higher-level authorities, serving a bigger population, are more likely to precipitate a critical mass of activists to mobilize for change. When no party is in overall control of a local or national government, disabled and other minority groups will be able to exert leverage. When there is a strongly dominant group, there is less need for leadership to take account of disabled constituencies.

These concluding comments are intended to highlight the importance of *realpolitik*, as opposed to idealism and rhetoric. Disability politics is a continuing project and will involve reversals as well as successes. There is no doubt that disabled people remain among the poorest of the poor, and this fundamental imperative makes disability a key item on the twenty-first-century political agenda. At the outset, we discussed the approaches of Fraser (1989) and Charlton (1998) and also proposed our own three-part typology of disability politics. Here we want to conclude by arguing that Fraser's first two stages of political reform have largely, but not entirely, been achieved. Disability is recognized as a political issue, and the mechanisms for achieving the liberation of disabled people as a minority group have been identified. There continues to be dispute over the extent to which this need has been satisfied, and there is evidence that some gains are vulnerable to reversal, given a change of government or a decline in national or global economic well-being. There has also been change in each of Charlton's three areas of political activity. The disability label has been increasingly seen in political and social, not medical terms, particularly in the Western world. The equation of disability with medical tragedy is very powerful and is by far from entirely displaced, but there is growing consciousness of the role of social forces in disabling people with impairment. It may be that the advent of genetic solutions to human problems goes some way to reversing this and reestablishing the connection of the disability experience to the impaired body. However, it would not be true to say that the social model of disability has been widely adopted. It is far more common, internationally, for disability to be conceived of as the outcome of social and bodily processes than it is for disability to be defined narrowly as social processes alone.

The development of disability as identity politics has been important in instrumental terms because it has led to campaigns for independent living and civil rights, which have made a material difference to the lives of millions of disabled people. Yet it has also been important in symbolic terms because it has redefined the meaning of disability for individuals and for societies. Disabled people do not have to identify in terms of impairment and deficit but can identify in terms of social oppression, resistance, solidarity, and pride. This conscienticization—or awareness of the role of social forces in disabling people—leads to renewed demands for change and political reform.

Here the work of Axel Honneth (1995) may be useful. He argues that it is important to reconcile the individual as well as the collective dimension of political struggles. Drawing on Mead and Hegel, he looks at the needs for recognition and self-respect, which impel minority communities to mobilize for change. Part of the effect of civil rights and citizenship is to enable individuals to have self-respect, knowing that they are valued and respected as equal citizens before the law. It is on the basis of this self-respect that rights can be won and lives changed. Therefore, we conclude that while there may be reversals in particular countries and certain battles may be lost, the course of politics is flowing inexorably and irreversibly toward a changed consciousness by disabled people and of disabled people. It is easy to look at Charlton's (1998) third area—the macro-political stage—and ignore the changed identities of disabled people and the changed relationships between disabled people and nondisabled people. The struggle for full equality and justice is hardly begun globally, but many people have begun to realize that they have a right to demand equality and justice and that they are worthy of equality and justice. A conservative might concur with Thomas Carlyle:

> To reform a world, to reform a nation, no wise man will undertake; and all but the most foolish of men know that the only true, though a far slower, revolution is that which each begins and perfects on himself.

Alternatively, we ourselves endorse the comment of Nelson Mandela, who said, "Those who are ready to join hands can overcome the greatest challenges."

REFERENCES

Albrecht, G. L. 1992. *The Disability Business: Rehabilitation in America.* London: Sage.
Arendt, H. 1958. *The Human Condition.* Chicago: University of Chicago Press.

Barber, B. 1984. *Strong Democracy, Participatory Democracy for a New Age.* Berkeley: University of California Press.

Barnes, C. 1991. *Disabled People in Britain and Discrimination: A Case for Anti-Discrimination Legislation.* London: Hurst.

Boggs, C. 1986. *Social Movements and Political Power.* Philadelphia: Temple University Press.

Campbell, J. and M. Oliver. 1996. *Disability Politics.* London: Routledge Kegan Paul.

Charlton, J. 1998. *Nothing about Us without Us: Disability, Oppression and Empowerment.* Berkeley: University of California Press.

Coleridge, P. 1993. *Disability, Discrimination and Development.* Oxford, UK: Oxfam.

Cooper, M. 1999. "The Australian Disability Rights Movement Lives." *Disability & Society* 14 (2): 217-26.

Corker, M. 1997. *Deaf and Disabled or Deafness Disabled.* Buckingham, UK: Open University Press.

DeJong, G. 1983. "Defining and Implementing the Independent Living Concept." In *Independent Living for Physically Disabled People,* edited by N. Crewe and I. Zola. London: Jossey-Bass.

Despouy, L. 1993. *Human Rights and Disability.* New York: United Nations Economic and Social Council.

Doyle, B. 1996. *Disability Discrimination: The New Law.* London: Jordans.

Dreidger, D. 1989. *The Last Civil Rights Movement.* London: Hurst.

Finlay, M. and E. Lyons. 1998. "Social Identity and People with Learning Difficulties: Implications for Self-Advocacy Groups." *Disability & Society* 13 (1): 37-52.

Fraser, N. 1989. *Unruly Practices: Power, Discourse and Gender in Contemporary Social Theory.* Minneapolis: University of Minnesota Press.

Freire, P. 1972. *The Pedagogy of the Oppressed.* Harmondsworth, UK: Penguin.

Gilligan, C. 1983. *In a Different Voice: Psychological Theory and Women's Development.* Cambridge, MA: Harvard University Press.

Honneth, A. 1995. *The Struggle for Recognition: The Moral Grammar of Social Conflicts.* Cambridge, UK: Polity.

Hurst, R. 1995. "Choice and Empowerment—Lessons from Europe." *Disability & Society* 10 (4): 529-34.

———, ed. 1998. *Are Disabled People Included?* London: Disability Awareness in Action.

Hyde, M. 1996. "Fifty Years of Failure: Employment Services for Disabled People in the UK." *Work, Employment and Society* 12 (3): 683-700.

Jayasooria, D., B. Krishnan, and G. Ooi. 1997. "Disabled People in a Newly Industrialising Economy: Opportunities and Challenges in Malaysia." *Disability & Society* 12 (3): 455-64.

Liggett, H. 1988. "Stars are Not Born: An Interpretative Approach to the Politics of Disability." *Disability, Handicap & Society* 3 (3): 263-76.

Lister, R. 1997. *Citizenship; Feminist Perspectives.* Basingstoke, UK: Macmillan.

Marshall, T. H. 1950. *Citizenship and Social Class.* Cambridge, UK: Cambridge University Press.

Meekosha, H. and A. Jakubowicz. Forthcoming. "Disability, Political Activism and Identity Making: A Critical Feminist Perspective on the Rise of Disability Movements in Australia, the USA and the UK." *Disability Studies Quarterly.*

Melucci, A. 1989. *Nomads of the Present.* London: Radius.

Morris, J. 1991. *Pride against Prejudice.* London: The Women's Press.

Newell, C. 1996. "The Disability Rights Movement in Australia: A Note from the Trenches." *Disability and Society* 11 (3): 429-32.

Oliver, M. 1983. *Social Work with Disabled People.* Basingstoke, UK: Macmillan.

———. 1990. *The Politics of Disablement.* Basingstoke, UK: Macmillan.

———. 1993. *Disability, Citizenship and Empowerment.* Milton Keynes, UK: Open University Press.

———. 1996. *Understanding Disability: From Theory to Practice.* Basingstoke, UK: Macmillan.

Oliver, M. and C. Barnes. 1998. *Disabled People and Social Policy.* London: Longman.

Oliver, M. and G. Zarb. 1989. "The Politics of Disability: A New Approach." *Disability, Handicap & Society* 4 (3): 221-40.

Pfeiffer, D. 1996. " 'We Won't Go Back': The ADA on the Grass Roots Level." *Disability & Society* 11 (2): 271-84.

Potts, P. 1998. "A Luxury for the First World: A Western Perception of Hong Kong Chinese Attitudes towards Inclusive Education." *Disability & Society* 13 (1): 113-24.

Priestley, M., M. Corker, and N. Watson. 1999. "Unfinished Business: Disabled Children and Disability Identity." *Disability Studies Quarterly* 19 (2): 87-98.

Rose, P. and G. Kiger. 1995. "Intergroup Relations: Political Action and Identity in the Deaf Community." *Disability & Society* 10 (4): 521-28.

Sennet, R. 1977. *The Fall of Public Man.* Cambridge, UK: Cambridge University Press.

Sevenhuijsen, S. 1998. *Citizenship and the Ethics of Care: Feminist Considerations on Justice, Morality and Politics.* London: Routledge Kegan Paul.

Shakespeare, T. 1996. "Current Issues in Disability and Social Work." Unpublished research report for BCODP and CCETSW.

Singer, J. 1999. " 'Why Can't You Be Normal for Once in Your Life?' From a 'Problem with No Name' to the Emergence of a New Category of Difference." Pp. 59-67 in *Disability Discourse,* edited by M. Corker and S. French. London: Sage.

Stone, E. 1999. "Modern Slogan, Ancient Script: Impairment and Disability in the Chinese Language." Pp. 136-47 in *Disability Discourse,* edited by M. Corker and S. French. London: Sage.

Tronto, J. C. 1993. *Moral Boundaries: A Political Argument for an Ethic of Care.* London: Routledge Kegan Paul.

Union of the Physically Impaired against Segregation (UPIAS). 1976. *Fundamental Principles of Disability.* London: Author.

United Nations. 1975. *Declaration on the Rights of Disabled Persons.* New York: Author.

———. 1993. *Standard Rules on Equalization of Opportunities for Disabled Persons.* New York: Author.

Voet, R. 1998. *Feminism and Citizenship.* London: Sage.

Waddington, L. 1997. "The European Community and Disability Discrimination: Time to Address the Deficit of Powers?" *Disability & Society* 12 (3): 465-80.

Westcott, H. 1993. *Abuse of Children and Adults with Disabilities.* London: National Society for the Protection and Care of Children.

Williams, G. 1983. "The Movement for Independent Living: An Evaluations and a Critique." *Social Science and Medicine* 17 (15): 1003-10.

Young, I. 1990. *Justice and the Politics of Difference.* Princeton, NJ: Princeton University Press.

Zola, I. 1983. *Socio-Medical Inquiries: Recollections, Reflections and Reconsiderations.* Philadelphia: Temple University Press.

Disability Human Rights, Law, and Policy

24

JEROME E. BICKENBACH

I t has been common for decades to identify the "human rights approach" to disability advocacy as the single most important political development in the struggle for equal participation by people with mental and physical disabilities. Although true enough, it is important to be clear what the human rights approach is, what it entails, and how it manifests itself in legal and policy terms. After a brief characterization of the approach, this chapter considers four models of the legal expression of human rights for persons with disabilities that can be found around the world. Given the variety, the question arises which is the best, or at least the better, approach. As this is an extremely difficult question to answer directly, two prior issues are considered instead: (1) the relative merits and drawbacks to a voluntary as opposed to an enforceable legal approach to human rights and (2) whether we should be content with the current antidiscrimination focus as a long-term strategy. It is suggested that a legal and policy approach, which emphasizes the universality of disability, rather than its special, minority status, has much to recommend itself as a basis for the theory and practice of disability human rights.

THE HUMAN RIGHTS APPROACH TO DISABILITY POLICY

International efforts to recognize basic human rights for individuals with physical and mental disabilities were the product of political action and lobbying, initially in the United States and throughout the world from the early 1960s on (Anspach 1979; Driedger 1989; Scotch 1984, 1989; Shapiro 1993). This call for a human rights approach to disability law and social policy was played out and continues to be played out against a background of specific entitlements and other social policy provisions found primarily in the areas of health, rehabilitation, transportation, education, and employment. Many of these provisions were originally overtly political responses to the needs of disabled veterans (Liachowitz 1988; Stone 1984). As a result, around the world, disability programs and policies have tended to be reactive and piecemeal responses to specific social conditions rather than fully coordinated and integrated into overall social policy. In addition, disability policies have been more responsive to the needs and ideologies of service providers and bureaucrats than to people with disabilities themselves.

The disability rights movement was rooted in the protest of those with disabilities who rejected this way of meeting their needs. Initially at least, what was demanded was not more programming or even specific entitlements but a reorientation of the very foundation of disability law and policy. What was needed, they argued, was an explicit recognition of the human rights of persons with disabilities. Evidence of international human rights abuse, although neither tracked by agencies such as Human Rights Watch or Amnesty International nor within the authority of the United Nations (UN) to monitor, was evident to those in the field. Change for the better, it was argued, would flow once it was acknowledged that people with disabilities are not given their rights as a matter of charity or the goodwill of others; they are entitled to them as equal members of society.

As most disability activists are aware, there is an extensive academic literature on rights, one that raises substantial controversies about the nature of rights and their strategic usefulness. The genesis, at least in the English-speaking world, of what is sometimes unkindly called "rights rhetoric" (Glendon 1991) are seventeenth- and eighteenth-century accounts of natural rights that formed part of the social contract account of the nature of the state and its relationship to its citizens (Strauss 1950). The rhetoric of natural rights, inalienable and absolute, suffuses the American Bill of Rights and the French Declaration of the Rights of Man and has also been be picked up by other countries, even when their historical and philosophical traditions are quite different. Philosophers agree that there are in fact four basic categories of rights—moral, legal, civil, and human—with different rationales and intellectual histories.

Of these, only legal rights (functionally defined as entitlements enforceable by courts or tribunals) are uncontroversial because, given their nature, it is a factual matter whether someone has or fails to have a legal right recognized by a court or other authoritative tribunal. An entitlement is a claim that an individual can make that is backed up, at least in principle, by the full weight and authority of a state's judicial system. An entitlement has actual, practical value; it is a key to resources or opportunities. Of course, we commonly speak of what we or others are "entitled to" even when we know or ought to know that there is no effective legal recourse that could be called on if we are denied what we believe we are owed. When we use the notion in this fashion, we are making a moral or political statement (roughly, our moral entitlement that there *ought* to be a legal entitlement). Moral entitlements are similar to the other kinds of rights that are, to the extent that they are not enforceable, normative constructs, whose existence depends not on some authoritative fiat or enforcement mechanism but on historical, cultural, and political consensus.

The traditional sociological distinction between civil rights and human rights is that the former, but not necessarily the latter, are inextricably bound to citizenship and so are bound to the existence of a state. On the highly influential account of T. H. Marshall (1950), indeed, the link between citizenship and civil rights is analytic: You cannot have one without the other (Barbalet 1988; Marshall 1950). The strategic virtue of this linkage, on which disability advocates relied heavily, was that one could demand civil rights by making the wholly unobjectionable demand that people with disabilities, despite their differences, are at least citizens and are owed the rights that are incidents of citizenship. At the same time, however, limitations on citizenship are commonplace, and it was tempting to seek a rhetorically stronger basis for rights—hence the appeal to universal human rights, those rights that are fundamental entitlements owed to humans as such, independent of cultural or political context. Rights such as those enumerated in the 1948 United Nations *Universal Declaration of Human Rights,* it was argued, were so utterly basic that their denial amounted to a travesty of justice. At the same time, since these rights were so general (and unenforceable), it was difficult to credit them with more than rhetorical significance (Nickel 1987).

Even in theory, especially for the political left, the notion of universal human rights was not an easy one to embrace unreservedly. Many saw that inasmuch as the modern notion of a right is historically and conceptually linked to private property, claims of universality entail an unshakeable commitment to some version of "possessive individualism," if not capitalism itself (Giddens 1982; Macpherson 1985). Some feminists worried about the patriarchal baggage of rights talk and advised theorists to look elsewhere (Smart 1989). Others on the left, however, argue that the only realistic prospect for social change is to embrace the entitlement-creating notion of a right, with all its dubious history (Taylor-Gooby 1991), or else to supplement sociological theory by adding an account of human rights to produce a more complete and consistent understanding of modern society (Turner 1993). For their part, disability advocates sometimes argued that rights discourse was simply too influential and powerful to ignore (Gooding 1994) or that the disability movement needed to concentrate on human rights issues, and "whether it's left-wing rights or right-wing rights doesn't matter" (advocate Stephen Bradshaw, quoted in Campbell and Oliver 1996:101).

This human rights approach, advocates realized immediately, required a very different conception of the notion of disability than was standardly used in the medical community. Turning to decades of work by sociologists and sociopsychologists, advocates adopted what is often called the "social model" of disability. On this model, disability is the outcome of an interaction between intrinsic features of the individual's body or mind (impairments) and the complete social and physical context or environment in which that the person carries out his or her life (Imrie 1997). To be disabled is to have limitations in the activities one can perform. Whether an activity can be performed, however, is a function of the presence or absence of environmental factors: physical or social obstacles that limit or prevent performance, on one hand, or resources that facilitate performance, on the other. Disability is not a feature of an individual's body or mind; in short, it is a socially constructed complex of relationships, some intrinsic to the individual and some part of the physical and social world.

Historically, disability policy was either a charitable response to perceived miseries (ad hoc responses to social emergencies or the needs of the medical profession) or, in more recent days, an attempt to cater to the economic doctrine of maximizing social output. Each of these approaches produces distinct and characteristic disability law and policy (Bickenbach 1993). However, underlying each approach is the assumption, rarely stated, that disability is entirely an attribute of a person: Disability is an abnormality, a lack, and a limitation of capacity. By contrast, disability advocates insisted that disability is a social phenomenon shaped by historical, cultural, linguistic, political, and economic forces—following some early work in social psychology (Wright 1983). Disability advocates were thus able to argue that disability law and policy should not be a matter of charity, professional need, compensation, or economic necessity but instead must be grounded in human rights.

The social model of disability plays a vital role in making the human rights approach plausible. On the social model, a person's inability to perform certain actions or to participate fully in social roles such as parent, student, or employee is, in part, a consequence of social attitudes and policies that create barriers. It makes little sense to say that one has a right, of any sort, not to have functional impairments because many impairments are outcomes of aging and other natural process that are unavoidable. It does makes sense to insist that one has a basic human right to be treated as an equal when one adds that social institutions and attitudes are responsible for creating disabling barriers that limit a person's participation in life activities. The social model and the human rights approach, in short, are mutually reinforcing.

As with all political movements, the disability rights movement was soon forced to confront the practical problem of translating theory and political slogans into a practical agenda for achieving the goals of equal opportunity, full participation, and respect of difference. Mike Oliver (1990a, 1990b, 1996) has shown in his work both the promise and the tribulations of social movement dynamics for disability advocates. Realists argue that disability law and policy must be assessed, not by its theoretical foundations but by what it actually delivers. Others argue that however attractive specific reforms may be, they will be temporary and fleeting unless grounded in a solid commitment to human rights. The debate continues.

In any event, there remains a practical dilemma for reformers. Should one set one's sights on the incremental but practically vital improvements in medical, education, employment, personal assistance, transportation, and housing policies—the things that actually affect a person's day-to-day existence—or should one put one's efforts in an expressed legal statement of human rights with the expectation that specific policy reforms will follow in due course? In other words, what precise legal expression of the human rights approach stands the best change of moving from political rhetoric to concrete results?

The question is a difficult one, both theoretically and practically. Around the world, only a handful of approaches to giving disability human rights legal expression have been adopted, and it is useful to survey these before returning to this core question. To be sure, some countries do not explicitly recognize disability human rights at all, although their disability policies may in practice further the goals of these rights. Without extensive comparative work in disability policy and tools for assessing the effects of this policy, neither of which are currently available, it remains an open debate whether explicit legal recognition of human rights is essential for disability policy consistent with the values embodied in those human rights. Yet, it is possible, at least schematically, to survey existing models of legal recognition of disability human rights.

APPROACHES TO THE LEGAL EXPRESSION OF HUMAN RIGHTS

Underlying all forms of the legal expression of disability, human rights is a fundamental distinction between rights that are legally enforceable entitlements and those that are not. When a formalized enforcement mechanism is absent, a society's commitment to human rights becomes a matter of goodwill or moral suasion and so ultimately a self-imposed or voluntary commitment. Disability advocates, for their part, have long insisted that the recognition of human rights for persons with disabilities is empty and meaningless, if not insulting, without explicit mechanisms for enforcing these values. And for good reason.

The distinction between enforceable and voluntary is muddied somewhat by the very common reliance in all social policy on inducements and incentives (e.g., tax incentives), which are embedded in social welfare or other entitlement legislation. For an advocate of human rights, the prospect of voluntary but induced recognition could well be viewed as inadequate and insulting. Respecting other human beings as equal citizens should not be contingent on blunt self-interest. Although obviously true, this concern may be less worrisome when inducements or incentives augment negative enforcement mechanisms, such as fines or compensation. In the end, the underlying operational model of all social policy is compromise and adjustment. The ideals implicit in the human rights approach will always need to be blended with practical issues of public acceptance, whether or not there is an enforcement mechanism in place.

When human rights are enforceable, they can be enforced as a consequence of a complaint initiated and pursued by an individual or group, or the state or one of its agencies can be wholly in charge of identifying infringements of rights and remedying them. When the state is the enforcement and monitoring agent, two basic approaches may be taken. The state may, as an expressly political act, commit itself at the highest legal level to human rights and use this explicit commitment as a standard against which to assess its own laws and policies. Alternatively, the state may set specific goals in particular sectors that represent concrete, practical manifestations of human rights in those sectors. In what follows, these subtle distinctions will be ignored to focus on the major differences between fundamental approaches.

There are four basic types of legal expression of human rights for persons with disabilities:

1. enforceable antidiscrimination legislation,
2. constitutional guarantees of equality,
3. specific entitlement programs, and
4. voluntary human rights manifestos.

These are not mutually exclusive approaches since most countries around the world rely on a cluster of laws, policies, and programs that fit into more than one category. Nonetheless, they are distinct ways of putting human rights into law.

Antidiscrimination Legislation

As a general matter, antidiscrimination legislation identifies grounds for discrimination (race, gender, religion, or disability) and areas of protection (employment, education, housing, and transportation). Antidiscrimination also sets out complaint and adjudication procedures and provides some form of enforcement mechanism, usually financial compensation. A postwar development, many antidiscrimination laws around the world are modeled on the U.S. Civil Rights Act of 1964. An important premise of this approach to human rights is that a violation of rights is a form of discrimination, treating people unequally on grounds or for unjustifiable reasons. Not hiring an individual who does not have the required educational background is not discriminatory; not hiring that individual because he or she is a member of a particular racial group is. The clearest example of discrimination is overt prejudice, when a person is intentionally treated unequally because others view him or her as inferior or unequal. Yet the notion of discrimination has, over time, evolved to include unintentional unequal treatment (tactic discrimination) or unequal treatment that results from the operation of rules or policies that are not themselves discriminatory in intention (systemic or indirect discrimination).

The earliest example of antidiscrimination legislation explicitly directed at disability was Section 504 of the U.S. Rehabilitation Act of 1973, which states that "no otherwise qualified handicapped individual . . . shall, solely by reason of his handicap" be discriminated against in any program or activity receiving federal financial assistance.

Historically in the United States, Section 504 was the result of two trends. One trend extended civil rights protections to other marginalized groups; the other broadened the range of social programming to benefit people with disabilities (Scotch 1984:7-11). By 1990, a considerably more refined and extended antidiscrimination act came on the scene, the Americans with Disabilities Act (ADA) (Kanter 1999). The ADA prohibits discrimination on the basis of disability in employment, in access to and benefit of public services, and in access to public accommodations, transportation and services, and communications. Though it is the antidiscrimination law in the United States, the ADA works in conjunction with several others, at the federal and state levels, such as the Fair Housing Act and the Individuals with Disabilities Education Act.

Parallel pieces of legislation can be found in other common law countries around the world. These include the Disability Discrimination Act 1992 (Australia), Disability Discrimination Act 1995 (United Kingdom), Human Rights Act 1993 (New Zealand), Disabled Persons Act (India), Israel's Disabled Persons Act 1998, and Canada's Human Rights Acts, at the federal and provincial levels. Most of this legislation was passed in the 1990s and, though derivative from the U.S. approach, display important differences in coverage, methods of adjudication, and the level of compensation awarded. There are legally interesting differences between the U.S. approach and, as examples, the approach taken in Australia and the United Kingdom (Doyle 1999; Jones and Marks 1999), but there is no need to survey these differences because it is what they have in common that is more relevant here. There are, in particular, two structural features worth highlighting.

First, antidiscrimination legislation takes pains to identify the difference between discriminatory and nondiscriminatory unequal treatment. The key to this distinction resides in a formula that has gained acceptance wherever antidiscrimination law applicable to disability is in effect. If an individual with a disability is treated differently (denied employment, access to medical care, or the opportunity to watch a movie), for reasons that relate to the disability, that is discrimination if it can be argued that there is no reasonable way of accommodating the difference that the disability creates so as to allow equal participation. What constitutes "reasonable" accommodation is defined in various ways for various areas but amounts to an accommodation that could be provided to the person with the disability without creating "undue hardship" for the discriminator (employer, the hospital, or the movie theater).

Second, by its nature, antidiscrimination legislation is primary reactive and complaint driven. That is, the legislation seeks to protect human rights by giving people a legal tool to use when they feel that their rights to equal participation and equal respect are being infringed. Antidiscrimination is "individualistic" legislation since the onus is on the individual to take the initiative to use the power it provides. It is assumed that, if they are given the legal mechanism for doing so, people will identify discrimination and take the necessary steps to redress it. The complaint and adjudication process is, as a consequence, adversarial. The complainant is required to raise the issue and make a case for discrimination; the other side has the opportunity to respond. Given the formula just mentioned, this debate involves whether the complainant is a person with a disability in the required legal sense, whether the unequal treatment was associated with that disability, and whether the accommodations that are possible would constitute undue hardship on the alleged discriminator.

Because of these two features of antidiscrimination law, no matter what mechanism is put in place to facilitate the process, invariably the process of determining whether discrimination has occurred is a long and costly one that becomes entangled, very quickly, in complex and often subtle legal argumentation. When a great deal is at issue, as it is in class action suits in which a group of similarly situated people bring a single complaint against a discriminator, the process is far slower, more costly, and less likely to yield concrete benefits to the people who could use them. Often, to their own detriment, complainants find it necessary, in order to qualify for protection, to emphasize the differences that were used to disadvantage them (Minow 1990). These are some of the reasons why, despite the successes of the civil rights movement, some have argued that the antidiscrimination approach subtly works against the wider agenda of securing equality of participation (Michelman 1969).

In part, as a response to these concerns, a few antidiscrimination laws incorporate provisions that require state agencies to assist complainants by seeking educational or conciliatory solutions prior to adjudication. Canada's federal and provincial Human Rights Acts are a good example of this approach. Often too, the legislation will require proactive responses, usually on the part of the government, to prevent discrimination in the provision of goods and services. Although the jury is still out on this, some studies of the ADA suggest that the greatest benefit of the act is to motivate employers and service providers to anticipate discriminatory situations and deal with them before they become problems (Pfeiffer 1995).

The principal rationale of the antidiscrimination approach to disability human rights is that acts of discrimination are responsible for the inability of persons with disabilities to enjoy their human rights and achieve the goals of equal participation, opportunity, and respect for difference. Access to needed resources and full participation in social life, it is assumed, will result when artificial and irrational obstacles are removed. The state is obliged not only to remove barriers it creates but also to provide the mechanism for hearing and adjudicating complaints about other obstacles in social life. In the end, though, these are battles that individuals should wage and win, without the active participation of the states and its agenda.

Constitutional Guarantee of Equality

The constitution of a country describes its basic political and legal structures in provisions that are supreme over all other legislation or government action. If a piece of legislation or a policy is inconsistent with constitutional dictates, it is "void and without effect." Because constitutional amendment is invariably a long and difficult political process—sometimes revolutionary in effect—entrenching human rights into constitutional documents endows them with the strongest legal and political commitment possible. Yet constitutions are general, even abstract documents that must be interpreted to apply to specific cases, and, although they bind the state and its agencies, they rarely bind private citizens directly.

An example of a constitutional guarantee of equality that has had clear implications for persons with disabilities is Section 15(1) of Canada's Charter of Rights and Freedoms (1981). This section states,

> Every individual is equal before and under the law and has the right to equal protection and equal benefit of the law without discrimination and, in particular, without discrimination based on race, national or ethnic origin, colour, religion, sex, age or mental or physical disability.

Other constitutional provisions around the world have the same effect, without explicitly mentioning mental or physical disability as protected grounds. The Antidiscrimination Act of the

Polish Constitution and Article 1 of the Dutch Constitution prohibit discrimination on grounds of "religion, personal convictions, political opinion, race, sex" or "any other grounds"; the latter phrase is understood to include disability (Hendriks, 1999). The German Constitution more broadly stipulates that no one must suffer disadvantages because of disability.

In the case of Canada, several Supreme Court decisions have carefully interpreted the constitutional provision to create a strong protection for persons with disabilities (Rioux and Frazee 1999). Since successful adjudication using the charter has constitutional force, all levels of government are bound to act in accordance with court decisions. In theory as well, all other parallel provisions or programs that might be analogously offensive to the constitutional guarantee of equality should be reviewed and, if necessary, amended. Although individuals can initiate constitutional legal challenges, the federal government of Canada, as well as certain provinces, has found it in its interest to initiate constitutional reviews (or "references," as they are called) of their own acts or policies to avoid future litigation.

Ultimately, when human rights are guaranteed constitutionally, enforcement is not restricted to providing compensation to one or a handful of individuals whose rights have been violated. Indeed, courts in Canada have become exceedingly creative in devising ways of altering offensive legislative provisions, up to the point of excising certain wordings and substituting others. The most prominent enforcement tool for courts is a declaration that a law is null and void (*ultra vires*), but, in practice, Canadian courts have taken to issuing far more subtle and effective judicial orders and remedies. Naturally, judicial "legislation" of this sort is highly dependent on the membership of the court and its political views, facts that draw considerable academic criticism.

Even setting aside this objection, the constitutional enforcement of disability human rights is not without its own problems. The discourse of human rights becomes specialized and removed from common understanding. An individual or group who wants to bring a case against a law or policy has the onerous task of bringing before the courts complex constitutional argumentation, and the defendant is the government, which can call on formidable resources in its defense. Even at its fastest, the process can take years, is extremely expensive, and can be dismissed, without comment, by a court that does not think the issues significant. Because cases involving the equality provision of the constitution will form part of the body of law interpreting the highest law of the land, there is an understandable reluctance on the part of judges to move too quickly or too far. Change, therefore, is slow.

Specific Entitlement Programs

Many countries, whatever else they have in place to give legal expression to disability human rights, have programs that create entitlements for persons with disabilities. As entitlements, these benefits are enforceable. A person who is eligible to receive the benefits or opportunities a program delivers can call on a court, tribunal, or other adjudicating body to enforce his or her claim to those benefits or opportunities. The fundamental difference between this approach to disability human rights and the previous two is that here the focus is on positive provision of resources and other facilitators to full participation rather than on the removal of discriminatory obstacles. The distinction between these two is often imperceptible in practice; nonetheless, there is an important difference in the form that the legal expression takes.

There is a considerable range and variety of entitlement programs. Income maintenance policies provide subsistence income; educational and preemployment development grants help to assist persons with disabilities into the workplace. Many countries provide subsidized or free transportation for persons with mobility or related disabilities or give financial supplements to purchase or repair assistive devices. The tax system has long been used to create entitlements that persons with disabilities can use to partially offset disability-related costs. In addition, most countries have social security programs in entitlement form, including permanent and temporary disability benefits, disability pensions, and work-related injury benefits.

Often, a state will indirectly create entitlements for persons with disabilities by providing incentives for private agencies to, for example, hire or train them. The German Severely Disabled Persons Act requires all public or private employers with 16 or more employees to fill 6 percent of open posts with disabled persons or else pay a compensatory levy for every unfilled compulsory place. France has had similar system, but with a wider scope, for several decades. Also in the employment sector, Israel's Employment (equal opportunities) Law 5748 (1988) provides for a subsidy for employers in industry who hire at least 20 extra new workers with moderate disabilities. Many states have followed the United States in using the tax credit approach to encourage employers to hire more persons with disabilities. The technique of requiring employers of a specified size to provide "action plans" for including more persons with disabilities into the workforce has been proposed in Australia and elsewhere. The worldwide variety in these entitlements is considerable.

The characteristic feature of all disability entitlements is their transitory nature. All entitlement programs arise from legislation that is subject to political and ideological trends, sometimes shifting the focus of the program radically. Governments are elected, and new or expanded entitlements are created. Then economic conditions are perceived to alter, or new governments with a different mandate are elected, and entitlements are wound down, restricted in coverage or in some other way revised to offer less tangible or useful benefits to persons with disabilities.

Another way to put this point is that disability entitlement programs answer to the same overall political and economic demands as all social policy. For governments, policymakers, and legislators, persons with disabilities are usually viewed as one of many constituencies and often one of the least politically influential. Recently, some welfare economists argue, in part as a response to the current neoconservative retrenchment from the welfare state, that the most efficient use of entitlements is to support supply side labor market trends, which in effect treat people with disabilities as means to larger economic ends. During periods of low unemployment, persons with disabilities should be entitled to generous income support packages to encourage them to leave the labor market. When the economy grows and more low-skilled employees are urgently required, these entitlements should be limited or removed to force persons with disabilities back into the labor market again (Culpitt 1992; Rothstein 1998).

Voluntary Human Rights Manifestos

The last legal expression of disability rights builds on a social commitment that is not enforced by any mechanism of the state, legal or administrative. One might say that these legal commitments are really manifestos or public statements of the moral entitlement that people with disabilities have to human rights. Manifestos serve the important function of bringing legitimate claims to public attention, and, in this sense, they do express a commitment. Voluntary manifestos are expressions of a sense of duty among members of society to ensure the independence of persons with disabilities and their full participation.

An example of this technique is Japan's Disabled Persons' Fundamental Law (1994). The purpose of this law was to lay out basic principles the state felt ought to govern all measures, public and private, for the benefit of persons with disabilities. Article 3 states that

> the dignity of all disabled persons shall be respected and they shall have the right to be treated in such a manner. All disabled persons shall, as members of society, be provided with opportunities to fully participate in social, economic, cultural and other areas of activity.

Although the Disabled Persons' Fundamental Law also contains entitlements that are enforceable, the core rights provisions, such as Article 3, are not. The intent is to express societal values, to make these known and declare that all citizens have the obligation to put these values into practice. Similarly, Hong Kong's Disability Discrimination Ordinance of 1996 identifies discrimination as a social problem and "prohibits" it but on a voluntary basis. Finally, China's Disabled Persons Act is a public statement that all aspects of social life should be open to persons with disabilities, though it also does not specify a complaint or enforcement mechanism.

It would be very easy to dismiss these examples as political window dressing or worse. However, that would be a mistake. If nothing else, cultural differences have to be taken in account. We in the West are comfortable with the notion that the obligation to respect human rights requires more than moral suasion. We tend to believe that the complex apparatus of legal enforcement must be part of the public affirmation of the values that support disability human rights. Yet this need not be true in other cultural contexts where social responsibilities are more quickly taken on by individuals. In such cultures, turning commonly held social values into enforceable obligations might appear unnecessary, if not disrespectful, of the citizenry. That a wholly voluntary scheme for preventing discrimination or ensuring equal opportunity is probably not a viable option in the West does not mean that it cannot be a more appropriate mode of legal expression of human rights elsewhere in the world.

In this light, it is relevant to consider the development of disability human rights at the international level, particularly as it occurred in the area of what might be called "transnational law" and as it has been shaped by the United Nations (Cooper and Whittle 1998; Whittle forthcoming; Whittle and Cooper 1999). This evolution reflects both the strengths and the weaknesses of international political organizations, which perforce rely on the voluntary approach. Although the United Nations has been a significant and persuasive force in the recognition and development of human rights in general and disability rights in particular, the prospect of enforcement has never been a viable possibility. Instead, the United Nations has used its moral authority in a public forum to generate momentum in several countries. This has resulted in domestic legal expression of rights, especially in the developing world. In addition, the United Nations is in the process of constructing what may turn out to be a new version of the voluntary model. This version concentrates on the standards by which all legislation and state action can be assessed for its tendency to obstruct or facilitate the cause of disability human rights.

The evolution of recognizing human rights for persons with disabilities by the United Nations exemplifies a different development of disability rights. After World War II, the United Nations sought to promote the rights of persons with disabilities by assisting governments in improving social welfare programs, particularly rehabilitation and training. Then, in direct response to initiatives from within the community of persons with disabilities in the 1960s, the United Nations initiatives embraced the notion of human rights for persons with disabilities, their full participation in all areas of society through an equalization of opportunities. In 1971, the General Assembly adopted the *Declaration on the Rights on Mental Retarded Persons* (United Nations 1971) as the first international statement of disability human rights. This was followed in 1975 by the more inclusive rights document, the *Declaration on the Rights of Disabled Persons* (United Nations 1975). This proclaims the equal civil and political rights of persons with disabilities around the world and sets the standard for equal treatment and access to services to further social integration.

In that year, steps were also taken to proclaim 1981 the International Year of Disabled Persons, with the theme of "full participation and equality." The principal outcome of this event was the formulation of the *World Programme of Action Concerning Disabled Persons*, adopted by the General Assembly in December 1982 (United Nations 1982). The *World Programme of Action* was a global strategy to enhance disability prevention, rehabilitation, and equalization of opportunities. On the heels of this was the proclamation of the United Nations Decade of Disabled Persons, 1983-1992.

These public events and manifestos, perhaps because of the very restricted enforcement capabilities of the United Nations, led to the development of an alternative version of the voluntary model. This model can be found in the *Standard Rules on the Equalization of Opportunities for Persons with Disabilities* (United Nations 1994). The *Standard Rules* set out explicit standards of law and policy for member states, standards that, if adhered to in practice, are designed to achieve equalization of opportunities and equal participation for persons with disabilities in all major areas of social life. It outlines, in detail, what policies and practices serve to guarantee rights to education, work, social security, and protection from inhuman or degrading treatment. Rule 15, in particular, mandates that all states have the responsibility to create the legal bases for all measures required to achieve the objectives of full participation and equality for persons with disabilities.

The *Standard Rules* is not a legally binding instrument, which is rare in international law in any event. Though a vitally important document for the recognition of disability human rights, it remains a manifesto that expresses moral and political values, rather than explicit legal protections and guarantees (Michailakis 1999). Work is now being done around the world, under the direction of the United Nations special rapporteur on disability, Bengt Lindqvist, to operationalize the rules more concretely so that countries around the world can have a tool for assessing their laws, policies, and practices. Yet, when this work is completed, the result will remain a recommendation to member states, not an enforceable demand. (It is perhaps for this reason that, parallel to the work done on the *Standard Rules,* proposals are now ahead for a general and legally more effective treaty on the rights of persons with disabilities.)

Looking over these four approaches, it is possible to see yet another dilemma for the disability policy reformer. It is safe to say that entitlement programs can be designed and launched to provide the resources and other requirements that stand a good chance of improving the lives of persons with disabilities. Yet the relationship these programs have to an underlying social commitment to human rights is tenuous and liable to be displaced by other social demands, real or perceived. Explicit antidiscrimination legislation or constitutionally entrenched disability rights are solidly imbued with a commitment to human rights but, in practice, because of their abstractness and the administrative costs they incur in both time and money, are less likely to result in practical and concrete benefits to persons with disabilities. On the other hand, voluntary manifestos, either nationally or internationally, are by far the most explicit affirmations of human rights for persons with disabilities; yet, these documents are not enforceable.

WHAT IS THE BEST APPROACH TO DISABILITY HUMAN RIGHTS?

These, then, are the predominant models of the legal expression of disability human rights. In time, it is hoped that multidisciplinary research into disability human rights will give us strong empirical reasons for favoring one model over another. Yet, before that kind of research can even begin, work needs to be done on ways to identify and measure the outcomes that are desirable. We need to be clear about the objectives of the human rights approach to disability policy that society is committed to and how we can measure when a society is getting closer or further away from those objectives. The grand goals of equal opportunity, full participation, and respect for difference are not controversial, but because they are so abstract, it is not always clear what, in concrete terms, they require.

Is there a best model of securing human rights for persons with disabilities? This large question needs to be divided into more manageable parts. We first need to ask whether it is plausible that human rights could be secured without relying on some form of legal enforcement. Then we should consider more closely the strengths and weakness of the antidiscrimination approach, which is the dominant model around the world. Finally, we should look at what underlies the entitlement approach and ask whether it is plausible that this approach, grounded in distributive justice, is a contender.

Enforceable or Voluntary?

It is arguable that manifesto statements of human rights are not only useless but also are counterproductive. When a state, the United Nations, or other international organization issues such a proclamation, the impression may be given that a genuine commitment has been secured and nothing more needs to be done. No doubt, when manifestos are released with public fanfare and political speeches, attention is directed to the social condition of persons with disabilities, and that alone is valuable. However, if nothing further follows, if the world programs of action and international years and decades pass without notable change, then the manifesto may have actually pushed the real issues into the background and away from public scrutiny.

Yet is it really inconceivable that a purely voluntary manifesto of the rights of persons with disabilities could, at least in some cultural contexts, be an effective way of securing these rights? One of the frustrating features of this area of disability studies is that we do not know the answer to this question. We can surmise that voluntary provisions, especially at the national level, are probably political techniques for raising public awareness—and, perhaps as well, for defusing potential protest—without having to commit public resources. We might also suspect that there is no cultural setting in which individuals will readily take on obligations to accommodate people with disabilities and ensure that differences are respected and equality is achieved without some form of legal incentive or coercion. Still, we cannot say for sure. There are some recent anthropological investigations into cultural perceptions of social obligations toward individuals with disabilities (Ingstad and Whyte 1995), but it is far too early to be confident about any hypothesis.

Nonetheless, from the perspective of those countries that have developed disability policies and have expressed a commitment to human rights for persons with disabilities, there is little reason to believe that the voluntary approach has much to offer. It is not an inconceivable approach to human rights recognition; it is rather, on the best of our evidence, an approach that in current circumstances is unlikely to be successful.

Antidiscrimination as a Human Rights Objective

If the voluntary approach to human rights can be set aside as inadequate, the real controversy is among models of enforceable law, specifically between the antidiscrimination approach and the entitlement approach. Around the world, it is clear that the antidiscrimination approach is gaining popularity. Some countries, notably France, believe that such legislation is unnecessary, but even in France, there is a growing interest in the ADA and in following the lead of other members of the European Community (Waddington 1999). There are subtle and legally significant differences between the Canadian constitutional approach and the U.S. approach, but these differences do not cut to the heart of a basic political and legal distinction between antidiscrimination and positive entitlement that needs to be explored in some detail.

Nearly every jurisdiction that has or is planning to have an explicit protection against discrimination on the basis of disability also has a range of specific entitlement provisions. The debate is not over whether there should be entitlement provisions but whether the antidiscrimination law should be the primary focus of the political aim of protecting human rights. For some advocates of the antidiscrimination approach, it is often thought that concrete entitlements will be forthcoming, almost automatically, if a strong protection against discrimination is in place.

Are there problems with the antidiscrimination approach or inherent weaknesses that argue against this unexpressed preference for this mode of expressing the human rights approach? What is at stake, and what is the alternative? Should we be confident that a sustained, enforced, and successful public policy of antidiscrimination really is the most important human rights objective for people with disabilities?

There are certainly those who have claimed this. Some years ago, disability scholar Harlan Hahn (1993) argued that

all facets of the environment are moulded by public policy and . . . government policies reflect widespread social attitudes or values; as a result, existing features of architectural design, job requirements, and daily life that have a discriminatory impact on disabled citizens cannot be viewed merely as happenstance or coincidence. On the contrary, they seem to signify conscious or unconscious sentiments supporting a hierarchy of dominance and subordination between nondisabled and disabled segments of the population that is fundamentally incompatible with legal principles of freedom and equality. (Pp. 46-47)

In this passage, Hahn (1993) ably identifies the core sentiment underlying the antidiscrimination approach to disability rights. Because of their minority group status, persons with disabilities are denied the full enjoyment of their rights primarily because of institutional or systemic discrimination brought about by prevailing attitudes that suffuse all civic and social institutions. For Hahn (1987), "the primary problems confronting citizens with disabilities are bias, prejudice, segregation, and discrimination that can be eradicated thorough policies designed to guarantee them equal rights" (p. 182).

Hahn and others put their faith in the express legal protection of rights found in antidiscrimination law such as the ADA. Hahn, in particular, appreciates that courts and judges are not immune to the effects of precisely those prevailing "disabling images" and attitudes that lead to the denial of human rights. Yet he believes that, more than any other political or social mechanism, legally enforceable prohibitions against discrimination based on disability stand the best chance of guaranteeing disability human rights. Guaranteeing these rights will make possible, if not guarantee, the availability of the concrete resources and opportunities that people with disabilities require for full participation.

From the beginning of the movement, disability advocates in the United States adopted and made their own the culture of individualism, and Hahn reflects that stance. To reject stereotypes of infirmity and childlike dependency, they believed it essential that people with disabilities strive for independence and self-sufficiency. In this environment of individual rights and the rejection of paternalistic state agencies, human rights advocates have tended to be highly suspicious of entitlement programming, especially income support and welfare policies, and have argued instead for economic self-sufficiency, usually in the form of remunerative employment. The aim was to make people with disabilities competitive in the open labor market and to give them a fair and equal opportunity to get and keep a job.

This employment-focused political strategy and the need to encourage people with disabilities to make demands for full inclusion into existing economic structures led quite naturally to the view that full employment for persons with disability should have long-range economic advantages for the society at large. This suggested that what prevented the employment of persons with disabilities could not be the labor market itself but economically irrational stigma and prejudice of the sort that antidiscrimination legislation is well designed to remedy. Without intending to, American disability advocates sent messages that clearly resonated with the growth of neoconservatism that went on to dominate the political landscape during the 1980s and 1990s.

The antidiscrimination approach, in real terms, has shown itself to be a proven success. Yet at least two inherent weaknesses in this approach are relevant to the larger issue of which is the best long-range strategy for recognizing the human rights of persons with disabilities (Bickenbach et al. 1999).

First, the approach entails that people with disabilities see themselves and be seen by others as a minority group that has historically suffered discriminatory treatment of a fundamentally irrational and prejudicial nature. Unfortunately, the required analogy between disability and, say, race, gender, or religion, has always been forced and awkward. The social stigma and stereotyping that undoubtedly exist in the case of disability vary widely between mental and physical impairments. People with disabilities do not have common experiences, nor, the Deaf community notwithstanding, is there a unifying culture or language that people with disabilities can point to for establishing transdisability solidarity. One does not have to be an anthropologist to observe that the leaders of the disability movement have tended to be highly educated, white middle-class males with late-onset physical disabilities and minimal medical needs, a group that is hardly representative of the population of people with disabilities around the world.

Second, even if the minority model fit the facts and people with disabilities do constitute a "discrete and insular minority" (in the words of the preamble of the ADA), there is, as was already noted, both a practical and a psychological problem in the implementation of the model. Any observer of the operation of the ADA would be concerned about the inordinate amount of time and energy being spent determining whether the individual complainant actually qualified as a member of the minority for whom antidiscrimination protection is sought. In addition, the adjudication process demands that one embrace an adverse label to qualify for protection. What could be more demeaning than having to earn one's human rights by showing that one is eligible to "special treatment" by virtue of being a member of a socially discredited group?

More problematic yet, legislative definitions of *disability* tend to combine in a confusing way the social phenomena of disability with the medical determinants of impairment. The ADA defines disability as a "physical or mental impairment that substantially limits one or more of the individual's major life activities" (Sec. 3(2)). (Antidiscrimination acts around the world use similar definitions. For example, the U.K. Disability Discrimination Act of 1995, Section 1(1), defines disability as "a physical or mental impairment, which has a substantial and long-term adverse effect on his ability to carry out normal day-to-day activities.") Although the legislative history of the ADA makes it clear that what was intended is a social conception of disability, nonetheless some ADA plaintiffs lose their complaints because they cannot provide sufficient or sufficiently unambiguous medical evidence about their impairments. This is particularly true for persistent pain, learning disabilities, and other forms of "medically hidden" impairments.

The problem here is not just a matter of the clarity or inclusiveness of legislative definitions of disability. It is rather that a potential complainant must also claim membership in the disability minority group and, to prove membership, is forced to rely on medical or rehabilitative conceptions of disability, thereby falling back on precisely the models of disability the human rights approach rejected. There is no choice but to medicalize disability because, in an adversarial context, self-identification would be immediately dismissed as self-serving, and a functional but nonmedical definition would be opened to the charge that the complainant was malingering.

There is another consideration. Antidiscrimination legislation is invariably the product of a political compromise in which irrelevant ideological positions can leave their imprint. This has yielded the peculiar result that some classes of persons with disabilities are excluded, not because they do not have or are believed to have medically ascertained impairments but rather because their condition is perceived to be a sign of moral fault. Thus, antidiscrimination legislation around the world follows closely the ADA practice of limiting coverage for persons who use illegal drugs and persons who are homosexual, bisexual, or transvestite. In addition, the ADA excludes mental conditions, such as compulsive gambling, kleptomania, and pyromania, from its list of legitimate impairments. The U.S. Supreme Court has gone on record affirming that outright discrimination against a recovered alcoholic is not a violation of antidiscrimination laws since the alcoholism was a "voluntary" disability, an indication of moral weakness and self-abuse (*Traynor v. Turnage* 1988). We have also seen a denial of ADA protection for a student with learning disabilities on the grounds that his functional need for more time and a quiet exam room is compatible with the unworthy disability of lack of motivation or the inability to overcome stress and nervousness (*Argen v. State Board of Law Examiners* 1994).

These results are well known and inevitable when the condition of inequality of people with disabilities is conceptualized solely as a matter of discrimination. Antidiscrimination legislation envisages a situation in which an individual is prevented from achieving goals by artificial barriers, founded on irrational beliefs, stereotypes, or prejudice about disability. While there is no doubt that these social evils exist, the real issue is whether they are the only or even the most important obstacles to equal opportunity and respect for difference. The antidiscrimination approach presumes that each individual has the motivational and other merit-creating abilities required for full participation in all areas of social life and can plausibly argue that he or she would succeed but for these artificial and irrational obstacles. Those with "moral failings" such as homosexuality, alcoholism, or lack of motivation would not succeed in any event, so discrimination is not an issue with them.

If nothing else, this presumption in practice clearly favors intelligent people with late-onset mobility or sensory impairments. Available statistics on complaints bear this out. The largest class of complainants under the ADA employment provisions has been people with lower back pain, and any redress for discrimination in employment on grounds of mental illness has been conspicuously absent (Baldwin 1997; Campbell and Kaufman 1997).

In short, antidiscrimination legislation tends to have little time for compulsive gamblers, alcoholics, or people who have mental or psychiatric problems and behave strangely, although all of these people have obvious impairment-related needs. It might even be argued that the antidiscrimination approach tends to produce another class of "inferior" people—namely, those people with disabilities for whom the absence of discrimination offers no benefit and for whom the kind of equality of opportunity that antidiscrimination legislation protects affords no relief. Their impairment-related needs go unmet, and they remain unemployed, uneducated, and powerless.

Finally, even if antidiscrimination law could be made to work effectively and without these drawbacks, the advocacy strategy that sets its sights entirely on antidiscrimination protection must, in the end, be judged to be of limited, ongoing value to people with disabilities. Undoubtedly, people with disabilities do face discrimination, and for that reason, antidiscrimination legislation is justifiable and important. Yet is that all there is to a recognition of human rights? Arguably not, especially when neutral forces such as economic factors create real disadvantages for persons with disabilities, because there is no insult and no insulter. There is a social evil; there is injustice and inequality. But of a different sort. Around the world, people with disabilities face nonaccommodating physical and organizational environments, lack of educational or training programming, impoverished or nonexistent employment prospects, confused and inadequate income support programs, underfinanced research for assistive device technologies, lack of resources to meet impairment-related needs, and policy neglect and minimal political influence. These are all social ills brought about by a maldistribution of power and resources. However, they are not forms of discrimination.

In the end, the underlying strengths and weaknesses of the antidiscrimination approach to securing human rights flow from the same source—namely, its implicit understanding of the root cause of inequality. That discrimination in private action and public policy creates obstacles is undeniable, although there have been surprisingly few empirical studies of the nature of such discrimination (Neufeldt and Mathieson 1995). Yet besides discrimination, there is another and arguably more fundamental cause of the inequality, one that also violates the human rights of people of disabilities. It is this cause that, however inadequate in practice, entitlement provisions seek to address—namely, distributive injustice.

Distributive Justice as a Human Rights Objective

What—at least ideally—is the objective of an entitlement program for which persons with disabilities can benefit, be it a training program for employment, a mandate for accessible public transportation, a voucher for vocational rehabilitation, or a subsidy to purchase an assistive device? The objective is to remedy an existing situation of inequality, in some particular arena or context, brought about by a failure to distribute resources in a way that meets needs. If opportunities do not exist or if resources are not available, this is an issue not necessarily of discrimination but of distributive injustice: an unfair or irrational distribution of resources and opportunities that has resulted in limitations of participation in social life for some.

Distributional injustice may be intentionally created but usually is an institutional or structural consequence of political and economic forces far too complex to be credited to the behaviors of any particular person or group. To be sure, we are currently witnessing the emergence of single individuals and corporations that are highly influential on their own in the world economy. Yet even these powerful entities are affected by background and impersonal economic forces. For people with disabilities, these forces can produce distributional injustice in part because of the variation, among people in general, in impairment-related needs and disability accommodations. As a rule, the higher the level of impairment need, the smaller the population cohort. This means that the economic marketplace tends to cater to the more trivial and common impairment needs (such as glasses for mild visual impairment or antidepressants for mild depression), while ignoring the more complex and less common needs (e.g., those for spina bifida or autism). In addition, there are far more disadvantages associated with mental and psychiatric impairments than the actual needs linked to those impairments would predict.

These distributional inequalities directly impinge on the lives and opportunities of people with disabilities around the world. Inequality in resource and opportunity allocation fundamentally violates basic human rights, insofar as inequality undermines the realistic achievement, within a social context, of equality of opportunity, respect for difference, and full participation. The concrete value of human rights, it can be argued, lies in the resources and opportunities that flow from a viable and enforceable social commitment to these rights. The range of particular entitlements is intended to address resource and opportunity inequality directly and, as such (at least in theory), can be argued to further human rights for persons with disabilities more directly and more concretely.

Unfortunately, the reality of the entitlement approach, as currently conceived, is not without its problems. The successes and failures of entitlement programs are very much a function of the kind of resource or opportunity involved, the overall costs of the entitlement, the number of people who benefit from them (and their relative political power), and how the program is perceived within each cultural and political environment. More important, entitlement programming for people with disabilities often falls victim to similar kinds of problems that limit the effectiveness of antidiscrimination law. As is widely known, a not inconsiderable portion of the costs of these programs is spent on determinations of eligibility that involve medical experts. Beneficiaries of these programs are stigmatized because, to qualify, they have to emphasize their inabilities rather than their strengths. Determinations of need are often made, for well-documented reasons (Stone 1984), by medical professionals who do not always understand nonmedical needs, such as for accommodation in the workplace. The resources that people with disabilities require are very often needed to overcome socially created obstacles that have little to do with their own functional limitations. Finally, as has already been noted, disability policy is notoriously volatile and reactive. Programs come and go, are extended or retrenched, and are always at the mercy of perceived demands on the state from other sectors.

These problems are well known, and many attempts have been made to isolate the underlying causes of what amounts to a persistent impasse in disability policy (Albrecht 1992; Barnes 1991; Bickenbach 1993; Oliver 1990a, 1990b, 1996; Stone 1984). It is undoubtedly true that disability policy in general has not received the attention it is due because of the relative lack of political power of persons with disabilities. At the same time, when people with disabilities organize to further their interests, governments treat them as "special interest groups," which have to be discounted as self-serving or else played off against other groups. Ultimately, the problem with entitlement programs for persons with disabilities is that they are perceived to be for a minority, a special group with special needs and, as such, not part of the mainstream. This has not served the interests of human rights. And this indeed may be the underlying problem that needs to be addressed.

Universal Disability Policy: Integrated Entitlements

Is there an alternative way of grounding entitlement programs, one that can further the human rights agenda of persons with disabilities? One alternative has been suggested, although the ramifications for the human rights approach and its actual effect on social policy design have yet to be worked out. It uses the entitlement approach but abandons the minority model and integrates entitlements into overall social policy. The theory behind this "universalistic" approach can be found in some remarks made by the late American sociologist Irving Zola.

In an influential article, Zola (1989) argued that "an exclusively special needs approach to disability is inevitably a short-run approach" (pp. 405-6). What is needed for a more mature and enduring approach "are more universal policies that recognize that the entire population is 'at risk' for the concomitants of chronic illness and disability." We need a political strategy that, as Zola put it, "demystifies the specialness of disability" because "by seeing people with a disability as 'different' with 'special' needs, wants, and rights in this currently perceived world of finite resources, they are pitted against the needs, wants, and rights of the rest of the population." We must turn to a more durable strategy for expressing the human rights of persons with disability, a strategy he dubbed "universalization." We need to acknowledge, he wrote, "the near universality of disability and that all its dimensions (including the biomedical) are part of the social process by which the meanings of disability are negotiated," only then "will it be possible fully to appreciate how general public policy can affect this issue" (Zola 1989:406).

In some of his last published works, Zola commented on the demographic commonplace that around the world, as people live longer, the incidence of disability will increase. He argued that as a consequence, the aged and people with disabilities have a unifying political agenda that ought to be exploited (Zola 1988). Yet, at a deeper level, and independent of population figures, disability is not at all a distinguishing feature of a group of individuals, let alone a defining characteristic of a minority group. It is rather an essential feature of the human condition. For complex sociopsychological reasons, disability has been treated as if it were not a normal feature of what it means to be a human being but rather as an aberration or abnormality. This is the source of the problem with disability policy and the pursuit of human rights.

Supporting Zola's universalistic strategy is his analysis of disability, not as dichotomous but as fluid, continuous, and entirely contextual. In this, Zola was in full agreement with the social model of disability that supports and is supported by the human rights approach. Moreover, as an advocate for the universalization of disability, Zola argued for the need to respect human difference and variation by widening the range of the normal, creating, so to speak, an inclusive sense of normality. Disability is a constant in human experience, a fundamental feature of the human condition, in the sense that no human being can be said to have a perfect repertoire of abilities suitable for all contexts. It would follow, then, that there are no immutable boundaries to the range of variation in human abilities. In other words, the ability-disability distinction is not so much a contrast as a continuum, and the complete absence of disability, like the complete absence of ability, is of theoretic interest only.

Disability is ubiquitous, Zola (1993) argued, in the obvious sense that human existence without disability is unimaginable: "The issue of disability for individuals . . . is not whether but when, not so much which one, but how many and in what combination" (p. 18).

In policy terms, this means that disability is not a "special" or exceptional condition that must be catered to or receive special treatment by the majority. It would be nonsensical to say that social policy has to be adapted to take care of the special case of people who need to breathe, eat, or seek the company of others. By the same token, Zola (1993) argued, it should be nonsense to say that social policy has to be especially adapted to deal with the fact that people have disabilities or that disability is an attribute of a person that qualifies him or her for special treatment or consideration. To universalize entitlement programming, we must first demystify the "specialness" of disability. Rather than identifying special needs that require specific legislation implemented by special agencies and served by specialists, we must begin with the premise that all people have needs that vary in roughly predictable ways over the course of their life spans.

In short, Zola's (1993) vision was for a universal disability policy (which, ironically, would cease to be a *disability* policy) that provides a realistic grounding in human rights by fully integrating entitlement programs into the overall social policy of a society. Universal disability policy expands the range of the human normality to more realistically include human variation as its actually exists. Closest perhaps to the theory of universal design in the built environment (Mace, Hardie, and Place 1991; Story, Mueller, and Mace 1998), Zola's vision was of social policy that can successfully benefit all human beings, given the full range of human variation.

Instead of catering to people who happen to fit within a relatively narrow range of the normal, we ensure that all environments, resources, and opportunities are suitable to as many as possible.

The core strategic issue of a universal disability policy would be that of democratically negotiating the range of normal human variation as the basis for an across-the-board universal design in social policy. There are predictable pressures to restrict the range of the normal, in favor of those who are powerful, and these pressures should be challenged. The more restrictive the range of normal human variation is conceived to be, the less likely that resources and opportunities will be equally distributed. The value of equality demands that no group should monopolize resources without justification, including those whose set of abilities happen to fall within some artificially restricted range of "normal" human variation.

The issues facing a person with a disability, Zola (1989) wrote, involve "the fit of [one's mental and physical] impairments with the social, attitudinal, architectural, medical, economic, and political environment" (p. 406). Of those aspects of the environment over which humans have a measure of control, the "fit" is determined by how society distributes resources and opportunities. Some distributions are inherently unfair because they disproportionally benefit some people at the expense of others. Unequal or irrational distribution of resources and opportunities can be the result of discriminatory behaviors and social practices. However, when discrimination is not involved, the injustice may well remain, should the distribution of society's resources and opportunities ignore the full range of human variation in need and cater instead to some frozen and arbitrary conception of the normal.

Universalism in disability policy, if the details can be worked out, represents a shift in the center of gravity for social policy. But more important, it may well be the key to the full and practically realizable expression of human rights for persons with disabilities. Fully integrated entitlement programs will serve the interests of all people, in relation to their impairment needs and in the areas of life in which those needs make the difference between limited and full participation. This is putting human rights into practice.

CONCLUSION

There are many descriptions of what constitutes a basic human right, but in the context of disability, proponents have usually argued that the human rights worth having embody the values of the respect for difference, equality of opportunity, and full participation in all aspects of social life. These values, though distinct, are also complementary. A respect for difference entails the recognition that although human beings come in different shapes and sizes, with varying degrees of talents, skills, and abilities, everyone deserves respect as a human being. To be respected, though, means to be respected for the person that one is, with all the intrinsic attributes and features that make up each individual's differences. At the same time, however, when differences make a difference in how one gets on with one's life and participates in social activities, equality as a political value demands that, at a minimum, no one be excluded from opportunities or prevented from participation for reasons that are not relevant to their capacity to participate.

Respecting difference entails that sometimes one's capacity to participate requires assistance or accommodation of some sort, the absence of which is a barrier to opportunities. Because equality demands that social roles and positions be open to everyone, where full participation is limited by artificial social barriers, including the failure to assist or accommodate difference, these must be addressed to fulfill the mandate of human rights. To thereby put the human rights agenda on a firmer footing, one must give considerable thought to identifying the attitudinal, social, and political obstacles to the goals of disability advocacy, as well as to developing the tools needed to move the debate from the piecemeal reaction to inequality to a sustained development of equality in all areas of human participation. Sound social scientific understanding of the historical and economic forces that have created our understanding of human rights and our current legal and policy techniques for securing these rights is urgently required. In addition, good empirical work is needed to identify objectives and ways of measuring success and failure in reaching those objectives. On all of this work, the future of disability advocacy and the dream of human rights depend.

REFERENCES

Argen v. State Board of Law Examiners, 860 F. Supp. 84 (1994).

Albrecht, Gary L. 1992. *The Disability Business: Rehabilitation in America.* Newbury Park, CA: Sage.

Anspach, Renee R. 1979. "From Stigma to Identity Politics: Political Activism among the Physically Disabled and Former Mental Patients." *Social Science and Medicine* 13:765-72.

Baldwin, Margorie. 1997. "Can the ADA Achieve Its Employment Goals?" *The Annuals of the American Academy* 549:37-83.

Barbalet, J. M. 1988. *Citizenship.* Minneapolis: University of Minnesota Press.

Barnes, Colin. 1991. *Disabled People in Britain and Discrimination.* London: Hurst.

Bickenbach, J. E. 1993. *Physical Disability and Social Policy.* Toronto, Ontario: University of Toronto Press.

Bickenbach, J. E., S. Chatterji, E. M. Badley, and T. B. Üstün. 1999. "Models of Disablement, Universalism and the ICIDH." *Social Science and Medicine* 48:1173-87.

Campbell, Jane and Mike Oliver. 1996. *Disability Politics.* London: Routledge Kegan Paul.

Campbell, Jean and Caroline L. Kaufman. 1997. "Equality and Difference in the ADA: Unintended Consequences for Employment of People with Mental Health Disabilities." Pp. 221-39 in *Mental Disorder, Work Disability, and the Law,* edited by Richard J. Bonnie and John Monahan. Chicago: University of Chicago Press.

Cooper, Jeremy and Richard Whittle. 1998. "Enforcing the Rights and Freedoms of Disabled People: The Role of Transnational Law. Part I." *Mountbatten Journal of Legal Studies* 2 (2) [Online]. Available: www.solent.ac.uk/law/silrd.html.

Culpitt, Ian. 1992. *Welfare and Citizenship: Beyond the Crisis of the Welfare State?* London: Sage.

Doyle, Brian. 1999. "From Welfare to Rights? Disability and Legal Change in the United Kingdom in the Late 1990s." Pp. 209-26 in *Disability, Divers-ability and Legal Change,* edited by Melinda Jones and Lee Ann Basser Marks. The Hague, the Netherlands: Nijhoff.

Driedger, D. 1989. *The Last Civil Rights Movement.* London: Hurst.

Giddens, A. 1982. "Class Division, Class Conflict and Citizenship Rights." Pp. 23-53 in *Profiles and Critiques and Social Theory,* edited by A. Giddens. London: Macmillan.

Glendon, Mary Ann. 1991. *Rights Talk.* New York: Free Press.

Gooding, Caroline. 1994. *Disabling Law, Enabling Acts.* London: Pluto.

Hahn, Harlan. 1987. "Civil Rights for Disabled Americans: The Foundations of a Political Agenda." Pp. 181-93 in *Images of Disabilities, Disabling Images,* edited by A. Gartner and T. Joe. New York: Praeger.

———. 1993. "The Political Implications of Disability Definitions and Data." *Journal of Disability Policy Studies* 4:41-50.

Hendriks, Aart. 1999. "From Social (In)security to Equal Employment Opportunities—A Report from the Netherlands." Pp. 153-70 in *Disability, Divers-ability and Legal Change,* edited by Melinda Jones and Lee Ann Basser Marks. The Hague, the Netherlands: Nijhoff.

Imrie, Rob. 1997. "Rethinking the Relationships between Disability, Rehabilitation, and Society." *Disability and Rehabilitation* 19:263-71.

Ingstad, B. and S. R. Whyte. 1995. *Disability and Culture.* Berkeley: University of California Press.

Jones, Melinda and Lee Ann Basser Marks. 1999. "Disability, Rights and Law in Australia." Pp. 189-208 in *Disability, Divers-ability and Legal Change,* edited by Melinda Jones and Lee Ann Basser Marks. The Hague, the Netherlands: Nijhoff.

Kanter, Arlene S. 1999. "Toward Equality: The ADA's Accommodation of Differences." Pp. 227-49 in *Disability, Divers-ability and Legal Change,* edited by Melinda Jones and Lee Ann Basser Marks. The Hague, the Netherlands: Nijhoff.

Liachowitz, Claire H. 1988. *Disability as a Social Construct: Legislative Roots.* Philadelphia: University of Pennsylvania Press.

Mace, Ronald L., Graeme J. Hardie, and Jaine P. Place. 1991. "Accessible Environments: Toward Universal Design." Pp. 155-75 in *Design Intervention: Toward a More Humane Architecture,* edited by W. E. Preiser, J. C. Vischer, and E. T. White. New York: Van Nostrand Reinhold.

Macpherson, C. B. 1985. *The Rise and Fall of Economic Justice.* Oxford, UK: Oxford University Press.

Marshall, T. H. 1950. *Citizenship and Social Class and Other Essays.* Cambridge, UK: Cambridge University Press.

Michailakis, Dimitris. 1999. "The Standard Rules: A Weak Instrument and a Strong Commitment." Pp. 117-30 in *Disability, Divers-ability and Legal Change,* edited by Melinda Jones and Lee Ann Basser Marks. The Hague, the Netherlands: Nijhoff.

Michelman, Frank. 1969. "On Protecting the Poor through the Fourteenth Amendment." *Harvard Law Review* 89:7-88.

Minow, Martha. 1990. *Making All the Difference.* Ithaca, NY: Cornell University Press.

Neufeldt, Alfred H. and Ruth Mathieson. 1995. "Empirical Dimensions of Discrimination against Disabled People." *Health and Human Rights* 1:1-34.

Nickel, James W. 1987. *Making Sense of Human Rights.* Berkeley: University of California Press.

Oliver, Michael. 1990a. *The Politics of Disablement.* London: Macmillan.

———. 1990b. *Disablement in Society: A Socio-Political Approach.* London: Thames Polytechnic.

———. 1996. *Understanding Disability: From Theory to Practice.* London: Macmillan.

Pfeiffer, D. 1995. "Survey Shows State, Territorial, Local Public Officials Implementing ADA." *Mental and Physical Disability Law Reporter* 19:537-42.

Rioux, Marcia H. and Catherine L. Frazee. 1999. "The Canadian Framework for Disability Equality Rights." Pp. 171-88 in *Disability, Divers-ability and Legal Change,* edited by Melinda Jones and Lee Ann Basser Marks. The Hague, the Netherlands: Nijhoff.

Rothstein, Bo. 1998. *Just Institutions Matter: The Moral and Political Logic of the Universal Welfare State.* Cambridge, UK: Cambridge University Press.

Scotch, Richard K. 1984. *From Goodwill to Civil Rights.* Philadelphia: Temple University Press.

———. 1989. "Politics and Policy in the History of the Disability Rights Movement." *The Milbank Quarterly* 67:380-98.

Shapiro, J. P. 1993. *No Pity: People with Disabilities Forging a New Civil Rights Movement.* New York: Times Books.

Smart, Carol. 1989. *Feminism and the Power of Law.* London: Routledge Kegan Paul.

Stone, Deborah A. 1984. *The Disabled State.* Philadelphia: Temple University Press.

Story, F. S., J. L. Mueller, and R. L. Mace. 1998. *The Universal Design File: Designing for People of All Ages and Abilities.* Raleigh: North Carolina State University, Center for Universal Design.

Strauss, Leo. 1950. *Natural Right and History.* Chicago: University of Chicago Press.

Taylor-Gooby, Peter. 1991. *Social Change, Social Welfare and Social Science.* Toronto, Ontario: University of Toronto Press.

Traynor v. Turnage, 485 U.S. 535 (1988).

Turner, Bryan S. 1993. "Outline of the Theory of Human Rights." Pp. 162-90 in *Citizenship and Social Theory,* edited by B. S. Turner. London: Sage.

United Nations. 1948. *Universal Declaration of Human Rights.* New York: Author.

———. 1971. *Declaration on the Rights of Mentally Retarded Persons.* Resolution 2856 (XXVI), 21.12.71. New York: Author.

———. 1975. *Declaration on the Rights of Disabled Persons.* Resolution 3447 (XXX), 9.12.75. New York: Author.

———. 1982. *World Programme of Action Concerning Disabled Persons: United Nations Decade of Disabled Persons, 1983-1992.* Resolution 37/52, Document A/37/51, Supplement No. 51. New York: Author.

———. 1994. *Standard Rules on the Equalization of Opportunities for Persons with Disabilities.* A/RES/48/96. New York: Author.

Waddington, Lisa. 1999. "The European Community's Response to Disability." Pp. 139-52 in *Disability, Divers-ability and Legal Change,* edited by Melinda Jones and Lee Ann Basser Marks. The Hague, the Netherlands: Nijhoff.

Whittle, Richard. Forthcoming. "Disability Rights after Amsterdam: The Way Forward." *European Human Rights Law Review.*

Whittle, Richard and Jeremy Cooper. 1999. "Enforcing the Rights and Freedoms of Disabled People: The Role of Transnational Law. Part II." *Mountbatten Journal of Legal Studies* 3 (1) [Online]. Available: www.solent.ac.uk/law.

Wright, Beatrice A. 1983. *Physical Disability—A Psychosocial Approach.* 2d ed. New York: Harper & Row.

Zola, Irving K. 1988. "Aging and Disability: Toward a Unifying Agenda." *Educational Gerontology* 14:365-87.

———. 1989. "Toward the Necessary Universalizing of a Disability Policy." *The Milbank Quarterly* 67:401-8.

———. 1993. "Disability Statistics: What We Count and What It Tells Us." *Journal of Disability Policy Studies* 4:9-20.

The Political Economy of the Disability Marketplace

25

GARY L. ALBRECHT

MICHAEL BURY

We've been there before but didn't get anywhere. The real problem is not with me nor with curb cuts, elevators and accessible bathrooms nor even with the medical establishment. The real problems are with managed care, access to education and jobs, raw capitalism in the workplace, emphasis on rugged individualism, social values favoring "good looking," young, productive, high-energy, nondisabled persons and a bunch of politicians who want things to continue just like they are.

—A disillusioned student with a spinal cord injury commenting on American social policy

The global emergence of disability is important because the absolute numbers of disabled people are increasing in every country of the world. This phenomenon is due to numerous factors: general population longevity related to improved diet, public health measures, and more effective medical care; ongoing wars involving the bombing of civilians and the use of land mines; the catastrophic consequences of HIV/AIDS, especially in developing countries; the rise of new infectious diseases; the return of old scourges such as tuberculosis; and longer lives among people with disabilities. Even in developing countries, chronic illnesses such as heart disease, cancer, stroke, and bipolar depression are affecting larger portions of the population. These dynamics have multiple implications. More of our friends, family members, and individuals will likely have the personal experience of disability. As Zola (1989, 1994) realized, disability is a universal experience. If we are not disabled now, we probably will be if we live long enough. Neither our families nor the rest of world is immune from the problem.

When we seek to understand complex problems such as disability and possible social responses, we often oversimplify the issues to render the problems seemingly manageable or apply our favorite models to make new and potentially threatening conditions comfortably familiar. These analytical simplifications are frequently compounded by an inattention to his-

AUTHORS' NOTE: Preparation of this chapter was supported in part by a Mary E. Switzer Distinguished Research Fellowship, National Institute on Disability and Rehabilitation, U.S. Department of Education, awarded to Gary L. Albrecht.

torical and cultural contexts. By decontextualizing problems and forcing evidence into established paradigms, we gain the semblance of control but are often lost in an illusion. In these instances, personal experiences, ideologies, values, and tradition are more likely to shape understanding and policy than the analysis of evidence. As the student in disability studies points out above, such is the case with many analyses of disability and related social policy (Albrecht and Verbrugge 2000). They often miss the mark.

To better understand disability within nations and around the world, we will focus on the political economy of disability. Much historical and contemporary thinking about disability has drawn attention to limitations in the individual or to the constraints of the physical and social environment. More recent conceptual work considers both the individual and the environment in an interactive model such as the new *ICIDH-2* (Bickenbach et al. 1999; World Health Organization 1997) and variants such as Verbrugge and Jette's (1994) model conceptualizing disability as the gap between the individual's capacity and environmental constraints (Bury 2000a, 2000b). This running discourse is enriched by consideration of the political economy of disability, which analytically focuses on the social structure within which disability is produced, defined, and addressed and on the forces that drive these processes. A political economic approach, sensitive to historical and cultural context, shifts the unit of analysis from individuals and their environments to institutions and the social structure and responds to a demand offer made in the sociological literature (Bloom and McIntyre 1998). This is critically important if we are to understand where and why disabled people act the way that they do and the physical and social environments that frame their activities.

We begin this chapter by presenting the political economic perspective used in our analysis of disability. Second, we describe and analyze the nature and growth of the disability business. Third, we examine the emergence of interlocked disability markets in an international context. Fourth, we explore the environmental forces that shape the disability marketplace and address the related issues of risk and accountability. Fifth, we examine the moral and ethical choices posed in the marketplace. Finally, we look at where we are headed and how a political economic perspective can help us understand the past and prepare us for future choices.

THE POLITICAL ECONOMY OF DISABILITY

Interest in political economic analysis has historical roots in the work of the classical economists Adam Smith (1723-1790), David Ricardo (1772-1823), Thomas Malthus (1766-1834), John Stuart Mill (1806-1873), and Karl Marx (1818-1883) (Schumpeter 1975). These classical political economists were principally concerned with expanding resources and in allocating them to stimulate growth and with the consequences, intended or unintended, that these processes produced. This work coincided with and was part of the context of the Industrial Revolution. For example, in *An Inquiry into the Nature and Causes of the Wealth of Nations,* Smith ([1776] 1976) attacked "mercantilism" and argued for "the system of natural liberty," which he postulated would open foreign markets, better use the division of labor, and stimulate economic growth. These political economists, however, were not dogmatic laissez-faire theorists. Rather, they were, apart from Marx, essentially utilitarians who supported government intervention when the public good was at stake. Yet, one could argue over who constituted the "public" and what was its "good." These scholars examined the interaction of economic and political forces in analyses of issues such as expanding markets, population growth, free trade, the well-being of the poor and working classes, and social revolutions. While this work has been aptly characterized as "a statesman's guide to economic growth" (O'Brien 1975:34), it also laid the theoretical foundations for political economic analyses of health and later for conjoint considerations of morality, values, and economics (see especially the insightful work of Sen 1992, 1995, 1999a, 1999b).

With the expansion of markets and growth in economies during the Industrial Revolution, population growth, and the emergence of a global economy in the twentieth century, neoclassical economists turned their attention to considering the most efficient allocation of given, scarce resources between competing consumer preferences.

> During this time, political economists constructed theory and initiated research which addressed two central, inter-related questions: 1) How do institutions evolve in response to individual incentives, strategies, and choices? and, 2) How do institutions affect the performance of political and economic systems? (Alt and Alesina 1996:645)

They sought to explain the initiation and dynamics of political processes and the development and implementation of public policy. Then, by focusing on how institutions limit and direct individual behavior, political economists turned their attention to investigating how institutions act in the marketplace to develop products and shape and stimulate demand. These activities are influenced by knowledge of consumer needs and desires, available technology, anticipated profits, benefit to the institution, and existing public policy. This approach emphasizes economic behavior in the political process and political behavior in the marketplace.

Disability is an important arena for political economic analysis because the numbers of people with disability are expanding as the world's population increases. Also, new types of disabilities are emerging, existing disabilities are more recognized, and people with chronic illnesses and disabilities are living longer and are more likely to bring their problems public. The demand for rehabilitation, social support, a health insurance safety net, and a hospitable environment is present. In the United Kingdom in 1998, for example, £133 billion were spent by the government on social protection, the vast bulk of which went to the elderly and disabled (Office of National Statistics 2000). This is important economically because most of these recipients immediately return their benefits to the marketplace through living expenses and the purchase of goods and services. Furthermore, numerous businesses and governmental, nongovernmental, and not-for-profit institutions are in place to define and respond to disability through the delivery of health, medical and social services, and activities to prevent disability. These forces and institutions not only raise political and economic issues but also raise questions of values, morality, and human rights in a society. The stakes are high because of the size of the marketplace and the amount of money involved in dealing with the problem. The strong feelings that surround these issues can directly influence national elections and indirectly influence social policy. Decisions about disability issues presage how a society values human life and citizenship.

Systematic political economic analyses of disability and rehabilitation are relatively recent (Albrecht 1997). The earlier theoretical work on disability and chronic illness concentrated on disabled individuals, their problems, socialization, identity, and rehabilitation (Albrecht 1973; Blaxter 1976; Bury 1982; Safilios-Rothschild 1970); disability in the context of the welfare state (Stone 1984); building and maintenance of client pools through manipulating disability definitions (Scott 1969); the social construction of disability (Albrecht 1981; Bury 1986, 1996); discrimination (Barnes 1991); the independent living movement (DeJong 1979; Zola 1981); the disability movement and civil rights (Percy 1989; Scotch 1985); domestic social policy and cross-national rehabilitation policies (Albrecht 1981; Bickenback 1993); and the history (Berkowitz 1987) and economics of disability (Arno, Levine, and Memmott 1999; Carrasquillo et al. 1999; Haveman, Halberstadt, and Burkhauser 1984). Later work developed the theoretical importance of the disabling environment (Barnes 1998; Imrie 1996) and more complex models encompassing the concepts of impairment, disability, activity, participation, and handicap (Bury 2000a, 2000b; Pfeiffer 1999; Üstün et al. 1999).

It was not until the 1990s that scholars began to focus their analytical lenses sharply on the political economy of disability and rehabilitation. Finkelstein (1980) made such an attempt when he located his discussion of attitudes and disabled people in the theoretical context of historical materialism. However, this fell short of undertaking a full and systematic political economic analysis. Stone (1984) had earlier made a significant advance when she conceptualized disability as an administrative category, subject to considerable interpretation, that entitles disabled people to privileges in the form of social aid. In her political economic analysis, Stone points out that specific definitions of disability in welfare states produce heated battles between the proponents of need-based and work-based systems of distributive justice. Yet, these approaches needed further elaboration. Oliver (1990:25-42) began such an analysis in his discussion of disability in the context of the rise of capitalist society. He suggests that "economic development, the changing nature of ideas and the need to maintain order, have all influenced social responses to and the experience of it [disability]." He concludes, "What needs to be considered next is the way the individualisation of life under capitalism has contributed to the individualisation of disability and the role of powerful groups, notably, the medical profession, in this process" (Oliver 1990:42). Here Oliver sounds a clear call to study the political economy of disability, though a tendency toward an "over socialized" view of disability (Bury 1997) leads him away from analyzing the actual health and social needs that disabled people face.

In *The Disability Business: Rehabilitation in America,* Albrecht (1992) undertook a full political economic analysis of the institutions that socially construct disability and organize the rehabilitation response. In the first instance, Albrecht, anticipating the later analysis of Alt and Alesina (1996), examined how institutions evolve in response to disabled people and their perceived needs, incentives, strategies, and choices. Second, he explored how institutions operate within and affect the existing political economic system. In these ways, institutions shape and fuel the disability marketplace.

Albrecht (1992) illustrated that an interaction of historical, organizational, cultural, and professional factors work within the American form of democracy and values and through an American version of capitalism to build and maintain disability as a multi-billion-dollar business. Businesses, such as coal mines and steel mills, and government activities, such as wars and nuclear and biological weapons, produced disability. Specific types of disabled people, such as veterans of foreign wars, merchant seamen, and railroad workers, received special benefits due to their historical importance to the nation's political economy. During the course of a nation's history, then, laws such as the Merchant Seamen's Act of 1776 and those enacting veteran's benefits and institutions such as the Veterans Administration (VA), Occupational Safety and Health Administration (OSHA), and Social Security Administration (SSA) in the United States and Social Security System in the United Kingdom were developed or modified to socially construct disability and define it as a social problem. This flurry of legislation and programs was instituted principally after the end of World War II to expand rehabilitation services in the United Kingdom, the United States, and Canada and to address the needs of veterans and those occupationally disabled in the war effort. The intent of these initiatives was to return people to work.

An essential aspect of the analysis undertaken by Albrecht (1992) identified the stakeholder groups in the political economy of disability and rehabilitation, illustrated their size and operations as well as market niche activities in the division of disability labor, and demonstrated how they worked in concert to constitute the disability business. These stakeholder groups included health care and medical professionals; hospitals, therapy businesses, and home care agencies; assisted care living facilities; the pharmaceutical, medical supply, and technology industries and insurance companies; law practices, banks, and accounting firms specializing in disability; government and lobby groups; politicians; and, finally, the consumer.

Stakeholder groups were analyzed in terms of their relative power and mutual interdependency in the disability business. Not surprisingly, the least powerful group, the vulnerable consumers in need, fueled the entire system. While the analysis was undertaken in the context of the United States, its general outline pertains to all nations. This is especially true today, in which the American model of managed care, delivery of technical medicine, definitional processes, and social policies are being exported around the world through multinational firms and government policies. This is also true where there is an interpenetration of policies, such as the adoption of welfare-to-work policies and notions of a stakeholder economy in countries such as the United Kingdom and the United States. There is a genuine fear on the part of many nations that American economics, cultural imperialism, health, and business practices will overwhelm their cultural institutions. From a distance, the distortions and abuses in the American system seem all too clear; therefore, people in other nations are reluctant to accept what they perceive to be a deeply flawed system that favors the rich and offers little in the way of a safety net to the truly needy. For them, a form of a disability and rehabilitation system based on private insurance exemplifies the excesses of rugged individualism, survival of the fittest, power politics, and raw capitalism. On the other hand, they marvel at the high quality of care and services available to those that have the means to purchase them.

On a theoretical level, Albrecht (1992:13-32) analyzed the transformation of rehabilitation goods and services into commodities. He argued that the very nature of disability and the rehabilitation response changed as disability became reified, defined as a social problem embedded in individuals and their social relationships, and proposed solutions became commodities to be bought and sold in the marketplace. This transition is in marked contrast to earlier traditions of caring for disabled people in families, communities, and charitable institutions where profit was not of primary concern in the health and human welfare sector (Castel 1995). In political economic terms, the rehabilitation industry became a response to disability defined as a social problem. "By definition, if rehabilitation constitutes an industry comprised of different businesses, then rehabilitation goods and services are commodities that are marketed, sold, and purchased. In such a market, consumers, providers, investors, and regulators profit and/or lose in the transactions" (Albrecht 1992:27).

Charlton (1998) broadened the discussion of political economy based on personal experiences in international settings. He recognized that the political economy of disability is concerned with social class, pertains around the world, and raises curious anomalies. Although most disabled people are poor and have little power, those who have good insurance coverage or adequate financial resources are able to access high-quality medical services and purchase the best in assistive technologies, such as high-tech wheelchairs and prosthetics, voice-activated computers and personal assistants, drivers, and exercise therapists. These differences in resources can mark the difference between those who can live independently and those who may have to live in institutions. Charlton points out that even within disability populations, there are stratification systems within and between countries. He further illustrates that inclusion in society is compounded by issues of culture, gender, race/ethnicity, age, and type of disability. For example, in Africa the disability consequences of HIV/AIDS place enormous burdens on families in which there are few resources and a crippled or nonexistent infrastructure. In South Africa, prevalence rates for HIV/AIDS are being established at between 25 and 70 percent of the population, depending on the local area or study population. The impact of this condition on the lives of individuals and the whole economies is incalculable (Campbell 2000). As a consequence of limited or no resources, disabled people with conditions such as HIV/AIDS or spinal cord injury in Africa, India, and some Middle Eastern countries usually die in a few years. Often, there is not enough to feed the family, let alone care for members with chronic illnesses and serious and persistent disabilities. Charlton quotes one interviewee from the Philippines, Danilo Delfin: "Nevertheless, the overriding issue for almost all people with disabilities in the entire region is just survival" (Charlton 1998:42).

In addition to these dynamics affecting individuals, families, and communities, the political economy of disability is at work among institutions even in developing countries. The governments of developing countries rarely have the interests of disabled people high on their political agenda, and if they do, they cannot afford to tackle their problems effectively. These people can be cared for at home, and out of sight is out of mind. As is evidenced in Chechnya, Kosovo, Cambodia, Sri Lanka, Rwanda, Peru, and East Timor, interest in disabled people generally comes from nongovernment agencies such as the International Red Cross and Red Crescent, churches, Doctors without Borders, and other humanitarian nongovernmental agencies. History demonstrates that strong racial, ethnic, and nationalistic sentiments often make their work well neigh impossible. Furthermore, rather than coordinate activities and enjoy governmental cooperation, these diverse groups frequently compete for clients, villages, and particular problems in an attempt to further their own agendas of "save the children," convert the peasants, or establish a neocolonial beachhead, particularly in those areas that have high numbers of inexpensively trained labor or scarce natural resources (Bennett, McPake, and Mills 1997a). While much good is accomplished by many of these humanitarian agencies, more often than not, interventions and policies are dictated by political economic self-interest. Having underscored how political economic forces operate around the world, let us now return our analytical lenses to the disability business in industrial and information-age countries.

THE NATURE AND GROWTH OF THE DISABILITY BUSINESS

In the United States, total health care spending is expected to rise from $1.15 trillion in 1998 to $2.13 trillion in 2007 (Gold 1999). Depending on how one calculates, the disability-rehabilitation business will increase from a $200 billion-a-year enterprise to nearly a $400 billion enterprise during the same time period. Similar projections of substantial increases in expenditures are true for the United Kingdom, France, Sweden, Italy, Japan, and other industrial countries. These national populations are aging dramatically with chronic conditions, increasing the numbers of disabled and frail elderly. Consequently, dependency ratios are rising and presenting serious threats to the viability of national social welfare systems. Although analysts often suggest the desire and capacity of advanced industrial countries to meet the needs of disabled and elderly people (Jefferys 1989), the constraints in doing so are real.

The growth in the disability and rehabilitation business is reflected in the number and sizes of major corporations that are uniquely targeted to those with chronic illnesses and disabilities. Among health care facilities, there is market segmentation among those corporations that deliver a full complement of health care services, including rehabilitation, those that concentrate on long-term care, and those that focus only on rehabilitation. Some of the latter two also offer community-based, home health care services. The financial size and health of some representative corporations are presented in Tables 25.1a to 25.1c.

These tables present the operating revenue, net income compound growth rate, and return on equity for the hospital management firms of Columbia/HCA, Health Management Associates, and Tenet Healthcare Corporation in the United States. It also presents the same information for the long-term care company, Beverly Enterprises, and the rehabilitation services company, HealthSouth Corporation. By any standard, these corporations are big business. They are all for-profit firms, listed on the New York Stock Exchange, and have captured the interest of investors because of their profit potential. For many of these companies, their stock price has doubled in the past five years. Currently, they are all billion-dollar companies; indeed, Columbia/HCA is a $19 billion company. The data show that these health care–rehabilitation businesses experienced remarkable growth during the 1990s when measured by operating revenue. The compound growth rate over a 10-year period was also extraordinary for the industry as a whole. Return on equity again reflects the dynamism and profitability of this marketplace. It should be noted, however, that there is intense competition in this business, forcing many corporations to struggle to maintain the past growth and profit levels, and some will probably be fighting for survival in the managed care marketplace. This will set the stage for more mergers and acquisitions that will raise questions about the relationship between the financial health of the corporation and the needs of those being served, as well as the quality of service delivered.

As a piece of this business, medical rehabilitation has enjoyed a tremendous growth spurt. From 1985 to 1994, the number of freestanding rehabilitation hospitals in the United States increased 175 percent from 68 to 187 hospitals. During the same period, the number of rehabilitation units based in acute-care hospitals grew from 386 to 804 units (DeJong 1996). The vitality of this market is rapidly changing because in the United States, inpatient rehabilitation facilities depend on Medicare for 70 percent of their revenues. As a consequence, hospitals and rehabilitation companies have merged to form chains such as the Continental Medical Systems group and the Allina System. To keep profits up, traditional medical rehabilitation providers are integrating vertically and horizontally, slashing costs, offering subacute care, providing niche marketing around problems such as wound care and HIV/AIDS, reorganizing therapy teams, and moving facilities into the community. The Rehabilitation Institute of Chicago, for

Table 25.1a Operating Revenue for Selected Heath Care Facility Corporations, 1992-1997

	Operating Revenue (in millions of dollars)					
	1992	1993	1994	1995	1996	1997
Columbia/HCA	807	10,252	11,132	17,695	19,909	18,819
Health Management Association	278	346	438	531	714	895
Tenet Healthcare Group	3,762	2,967	3,318	5,559	8,691	9,895
Beverly Enterprise	2,596	2,870	2,969	3,228	3,267	3,217
HealthSouth Corporation	407	482	1,127	1,556	2,433	3,017

SOURCE: Gold (1998a:28-30).
NOTE: Operating revenues refer to net sales and other operating revenues. Excludes interest income if such income is "nonoperating." Includes franchised/leased department income for retailers.

Table 25.1b Net Income Compound Growth Rate for Selected Heath Care Facility Corporations, 1992-1997 (in percentages)

	1 Year	5 Years	10 Years
Columbia/HCA	-5.5	87.7	NA
Health Management Association	24.4	26.4	27.3
Tenet Healthcare Group	13.9	21.3	12.0
Beverly Enterprise	-1.5	4.4	4.4
HealthSouth Corporation	23.8	49.3	52.3

SOURCE: Gold (1998a:28-30).
NOTE: Net income compound growth rate is the compounded growth rate over a specified time period. NA = not applicable.

Table 25.1c Return on Equity for Selected Heath Care Facility Corporations, 1992-1997 (in percentages)

	1993	1994	1995	1996	1997
Columbia/HCA	30.8	17.5	17.5	19.1	2.3
Health Management Association	19.7	22.0	22.2	22.9	22.2
Tenet Healthcare Group	14.1	11.7	17.2	NA	11.1
Beverly Enterprise	6.5	10.8	NA	6.2	6.8
HealthSouth Corporation	2.3	14.8	11.7	18.1	14.1

SOURCE: Gold (1998:28-30).
NOTE: Return of equity is composed of the net income, less preferred dividend requirements, divided by average common shareholder's equity. Generally used to measure performance and to make industry comparisons. NA = not applicable.

example, has increased outpatient services, has home visit programs, and has built satellite facilities in the wealthier suburbs where patients have better insurance coverage and can afford more out-of-pocket treatment.

The same patterns in corporate growth and return on equity hold true for health care product and supply companies that cater to the rehabilitation and long-term care industry (Gold 1999). Stryker/Physiotherapy Associates, Summit Care, RehabCare Group, U.S. Surgical Corporation, Abbott Laboratories, and Beckman Coulter, Inc. are major corporations also listed on the New York Stock Exchange that make wheelchairs, prosthetic devices, surgical instruments, dressings, and assistive devices for disabled people. Their stock price increases, capitalization, profits, and problems mirrored those of the rehabilitation facilities discussed above.

The pharmaceutical industry is another major player in the disability business. Some pharmaceutical companies just make drugs; others produce a broad range of drugs and other diversified goods that fit within a coherent product line. The data in Tables 25.2a to 25.2c indicate the operating revenue, net income compound growth rate, and return on equity for some representative pharmaceutical companies listed on the New York Stock Exchange.

The pharmaceutical industry enjoyed extraordinary growth and profits in the 1990s. An examination of some representative firms such as Merck & Co., Pfizer, Abbott Laboratories, Bristol Meyers Squibb, and Johnson & Johnson discloses that these companies increased their operating revenues between 45 and 155 percent over a five-year period. Their net income compound growth rate over the same period ranges from 11.1 to 15.8 percent. The return on equity is equally impressive, varying between 15.3 and 46.5 percent. The projections are that most leading drug makers will continue to report double-digit earnings for the foreseeable future (Saftlas 1999:1).

New but costly drugs are soon to emerge from the developmental pipeline for arthritis, heart disease, Alzheimer's disease, cancer, stroke, and depression. While disabled people do not account for the total sales of these pharmaceutical companies, they do constitute a disproportionate share of the market. Disabilities are often treated with combinations of drugs such as zalcitabine and AZT for HIV and copaxone, methylprednisolone, and oral prednisone for multiple sclerosis. These drugs are often necessary to control the underlying conditions, but they are very expensive, especially for poorer disabled people. The newer pharmaceuticals are even dearer because the purchaser is paying for significant research and development costs. This business is fueled by the changes in population dynamics that, with health and medical interventions, are allowing people to live longer with disabilities. These corporations are profiting not only from the sale of pharmaceuticals but also from the sale of related products such as dressings for wounds and diapers for people who are incontinent.

Managed care companies are a relatively recent addition to the disability marketplace but are having an enormous effect on access to care, the delivery of care, and the profit potential of the professionals, companies, and facilities that deliver care (DeJong and O'Day 1999). Again, in the United States, insurance companies are the organizations most often managing care (Enthoven 1988). They do this by using health maintenance organizations (HMOs), preferred provider organizations (PPOs), and in-house aggressive review of health care provider charges to control costs. They control costs by contracting with providers for a certain menu of care for a given medical condition at a fixed price. These actions limit the amount that providers can charge for a service and the amount of service that an individual can consume without paying out of pocket. These cost control interventions are one aspect of the concept of managed competition. The theory is that increased competition in the health care marketplace will lower costs. While this may be true, there is tremendous debate over the details (Ginsberg 1999). Critics argue that consumers cannot play this game well because they do not have, nor are they likely to have, the information necessary to make informed decisions. Critics also contend that the heavy-handed enforcement of managed care by powerful, for-profit insurance companies has limited access to care for those who most need it (many disabled people and the poor). They add that it is driving down the quality of care and destroying personal relationships and trust between providers (doctors, nurses, and hospitals) and the consumer (Priestly 1999; Reinhardt

Table 25.2a Operating Revenue for Selected Pharmaceutical Corporations, 1992-1997

| | Operating Revenue (in millions of dollars) | | | | | |
	1992	1993	1994	1995	1996	1997
Merck & Co	9,662	10,498	14,969	16,681	19,828	23,636
Pfizer	7,230	7,477	8,281	10,021	11,306	12,504
Abbott Laboratories	7,851	8,407	9,156	10,012	11,013	11,883
Bristol Meyers Squibb	11,156	11,413	11,984	13,767	15,065	16,701
Johnson & Johnson	13,753	14,138	15,734	18,842	21,620	22,629

SOURCE: Saftlas (1999:33-37).

NOTE: Operating revenues refer to net sales and other operating revenues. Excludes interest income if such income is "nonoperating." Includes franchised/leased department income for retailers.

Table 25.2b Net Income Compound Growth Rate for Selected Pharmaceutical Corporations, 1992-1997 (in percentages)

	1 Year	5 Years	10 Years
Merck & Co	18.9	13.5	17.7
Pfizer	14.7	15.1	12.4
Abbott Laboratories	11.3	11.1	12.7
Bristol Meyers Squibb	12.5	15.8	16.3
Johnson & Johnson	14.4	15.2	14.8

SOURCE: Saftlas (1999:33-37).

NOTE: Net income compound growth rate is the compounded growth rate over a specified time period.

Table 25.2c Return on Equity for Selected Pharmaceutical Corporations, 1992-1997 (in percentages)

	1993	1994	1995	1996	1997
Merck & Co	28.8	28.3	29.2	32.7	37.5
Pfizer	15.3	31.7	31.6	31.0	29.7
Abbott Laboratories	39.8	39.3	40.0	40.8	42.7
Bristol Meyers Squibb	32.8	31.6	31.4	46.0	46.5
Johnson & Johnson	33.3	31.6	29.7	29.0	28.5

SOURCE: Saftlas (1999:33-37).

NOTE: Return of equity is composed of the net income, less preferred dividend requirements, divided by average common shareholder's equity. Generally used to measure performance and to make industry comparisons.

1996). Whether the critics are correct is debatable; one has to ask to whose good, *cui bono*, the insurance companies are acting. The irony is that insurance companies, who most often manage care in the United States, are increasing their profits by controlling the sales and profits of other venders in the marketplace, limiting access to care, and forcing consumers to pay out of their own pockets (Robinson 1999).

The data in Tables 25.3a to 25.3c detail the operating revenue, net income compound growth rate, and return on equity for five representative managed care companies listed on the New York Stock Exchange: Aetna, Coventry Health Care, Humana, Oxford Health Plans, and United Healthcare Corporation.

The vitality of the managed care industry is apparent when measured in terms of operating revenue, net income compound growth rate, and return on equity. Aetna and United Healthcare Corporation are huge companies by any measure. The compound growth rate was inconsistent for Aetna but consistently high for the four other companies. In general, the return on equity has been quite good, although recently experiencing pressures. The amount of money generated by the managed care business is stunning when one realizes that these insurance companies do not deliver any direct health care services but mainly regulate and control those institutions that do (Pear 2000).

In addition to the traditional health care expenditures related to disability and rehabilitation, which are generally counted in national health and statistics and stock market analyses, there is an explosion of nontraditional therapies that are not typically included in the discussion. Patients frustrated with the costs and efficacy of many standard medical treatments for arthritis, for example, are turning to and finding satisfaction in shark cartilage supplements or glucosamine and chondroitin to alleviate discomfort with arthritis and increase mobility. Others are employing bee sting therapy to control neurological function for multiple sclerosis. Colostrum, the premilk fluid produced from the mother's breasts during the first 24 to 48 hours after birth and now derived from sheep and cows for medicinal purposes, is being used by millions in New Zealand, Australia, and North America to alleviate arthritis symptoms, improve chronic fatigue syndrome, control irritable bowel syndrome, and bolster the immune system (Vital Health News 1998). In the United Kingdom, trials are under way on the efficacy of cannabis for the treatment of multiple sclerosis. In the United States, between 1990 and 1997, there was a 50 percent increase in the use of alternative medicine therapies, such as biofeedback for headaches, chiropractics for orthopedic problems and pain, herbal medicine, exercise, and stress management techniques to control anxiety and depression. Every pharmacy in developed countries now displays a wide range of alternative medicine for the relief of symptoms in a variety of disabling disorders.

The competition for this disability-related business is heating up. Recognizing the growth potential of this market, Rush-Prudential is expanding its insurance coverage to include many of these alternative therapies, and Aetna and Humana are experimenting with pilot programs (Japsen 1999a). Not-for-profit hospitals in the United States are opening rehabilitative fitness centers that have drawn the wrath of commercial health club operators who take exception with their tax-exempt status (Japsen 1999b). This competition is interesting because it was commercial health clubs that first saw the market develop for outpatient rehabilitation services and responded by offering exercise and physical and occupational therapies in health clubs located in the community. Now hospitals are fighting back for their share of the market.

In developing countries where Western pharmaceuticals and high-tech medical treatments are unavailable or prohibitively expensive, folk remedies and the use of herbal medicine have historically been used, effectively or otherwise, for thousands of years. Dismissed as quackery by critics, drug companies have rather recently realized the potential of naturally based healing products and have established research programs in these areas that are delivering a range of efficacious drugs, often with fewer side effects than those based on synthetic compounds. In related actions, the National Institutes of Health in the United States and the Medical Research Council in the United Kingdom for the first time are now funding clinical trials of alternative therapies.

Table 25.3a Operating Revenue for Selected Managed Care Companies, 1992-1997

| | Operating Revenue (in millions of dollars) | | | | | |
	1992	1993	1994	1995	1996	1997
Aetna	17,497	17,117	17,524	12,978	15,163	18,540
Coventry Health Care	429	583	747	852	1,057	1,228
Humana	2,811	3,195	3,654	4,702	6,788	8,036
Oxford Health Plans	155	311	720	1,765	3,075	4,240
United Healthcare Corporation	1,441	2,527	3,768	5,670	10,073	11,794

SOURCE: Arege (1999:29-33).

NOTE: Operating revenues refer to net sales and other operating revenues. Excludes interest income if such income is "nonoperating." Includes franchised/leased department income for retailers.

Table 25.3b Net Income Compound Growth Rate for Selected Managed Care Companies, 1992-1997 (in percentages)

	1 Year	5 Years	10 Years
Aetna	22.3	1.2	–1.7
Coventry Health Care	16.2	23.4	NA
Humana	18.4	23.4	NA
Oxford Health Plans	37.9	93.6	NA
United Healthcare Corporation	17.1	52.2	38.9

SOURCE: Arege (1999:29-33).

NOTE: Net income compound growth rate is the compounded growth rate over a specified time period. NA = not applicable.

Table 25.3c Return on Equity for Selected Managed Care Companies, 1992-1997 (in percentages)

	1993	1994	1995	1996	1997
Aetna	NA	7.5	7.4	2.1	8.3
Coventry Health Care	27.0	25.7	0.0	NA	10.9
Humana	14.2	18.1	16.2	0.9	12.4
Oxford Health Plans	19.0	25.6	30.2	24.4	NA
United Healthcare Corporation	24.1	15.3	9.3	9.3	10.3

SOURCE: Arege (1999:29-33).

NOTE: Return of equity is composed of the net income, less preferred dividend requirements, divided by average common shareholder's equity. Generally used to measure performance and to make industry comparisons. NA = not applicable.

INTERNATIONAL DISABILITY MARKETS

The industries, corporations, and dynamics discussed in the preceding section are also operating forcefully in the international disability marketplace. Indeed, the disability marketplace is global ("The Americas Shift" 1999; Freudenheim and Krauss 1999). In classical health economics, disability market analysis is based on the supply and demand for rehabilitation and other goods and services related to disability. The market is the sum of the actual and potential constituents who are capable of purchasing the available products and services and can be encouraged to do so. Those in the market for rehabilitation goods and services ideally share interest, information, and ability to transact the exchange between provider and consumer and have access to these goods, services, and care.

In a free-market sense, the marketplace would be self-regulating because providers would seek to maximize profits, and informed consumers would shop for the best price, quality, and access mix. As Rice (1998) and Light (1986, 1997, 2000), among others, point out, however, the health care market has serious deficiencies that do not permit it to operate efficiently. Light (2000:396) argues that the basic premises of open competition necessary to form an efficient health care and, by implication, disability market are not met because of the following:

1. Often, a few or even just one hospital or provider group dominates a local market, and often a few or even one purchasing unit is buying.
2. These parties almost always have long, entangled relationships, obligations, or rivalries that deeply compromise rational purchasing.
3. A major goal of competition in health care is to restrict and channel choice, and often political pressures limit what services can be purchased or provided from whom.
4. There are high barriers to entry and exit in health care.
5. Market information about quality, service, and price is often incomplete, inaccurate, and fragmented.
6. Market information is very costly, asymmetrical, and largely controlled by the provider; access to it is often blocked (Saltman and Figueras 1996:26).
7. Buyers, even with good information, do not make choices that maximize their preferences and utilities (Rice 1997).
8. Market signals are slow or hidden, and markets can take months to "clear," if at all.
9. Prices are constructed realities that do not convey all a buyer needs to know.
10. There are significant externalities, especially through cost shifting and selection.

As a consequence and by extension, disability markets do not operate efficiently (McGinnis 1997). Therefore, it is not surprising that costs are high, services are not well integrated, access is limited, and customers are often dissatisfied.

Lane (1991) adds theoretically to this discussion when he says, "The market should be judged by the satisfaction people receive as a consequence of their market experience and by what they learn from them" (p. 3). Lane reasons that income and goods and services are only intermediate goals. Satisfaction or happiness and human development are the final goals. This approach to markets is compatible with Amartya Sen's (1999b) position that economics is a moral science and that development or enrichment of those in need should be seen as providing freedom. By these norms, the present disability market does not serve disabled people well.

Now, let us turn to the interlocked, international form of the market. The disability and rehabilitation market is interlocked because disabled people must purchase an interrelated market basket of goods and services to live a high quality of life. Second, the industries and firms that sell disability-related products are vertically and horizontally integrated so that disabled people must deal with the same limited number of actors to bargain for the goods and services they need. These factors put the consumer at a considerable disadvantage (Bates 1999; Bron 1999).

The disability market is also global. Many of the firms discussed in the previous section operate on most of the world's continents. In fact, due to the ongoing spate of mergers and acquisitions, it is difficult to know what the "nationality" of a company is. The major pharmaceutical and medical supply companies sell in Europe, Australasia, Africa, and Latin America as well as in North America. Recently, a number of these businesses have been making more profits outside than within the United States. Columbia/HCA, for example, owns and manages facilities in Switzerland, England, and Spain (*Moody's Handbook of Common Stocks* 1999). When they expanded to other countries, they took their corporate culture with them. After they acquired a mental health treatment facility in Switzerland, they told long-term residents, for example, that all patients would have to increase their monthly payments dramatically to remain in the institution or leave. Since most of the residents were on welfare or pensions, they were literally put out on the street. The Swiss and other Europeans used to a more benign welfare state and treatment of its citizens are not too keen on American corporate culture and fear the incursion of such American culture in their societies.

HealthSouth has expanded to the United Kingdom and Australia, where consumers are having the same experiences and voicing identical concerns as the Swiss (Standard and Poor's 1999). There is a current debate about the prices that major pharmaceutical and medical supply companies are charging for drugs and equipment in the developing world (McPake 1997). Many millions of Africans, for instance, are going relatively untreated for HIV/AIDS because the drug companies are charging the same prices in Africa as they are in North America, making treatment impossible for these people. This is especially important where the disabling consequences of HIV/AIDS may cause untold personal and social levels of distress as well as economic distortion on a continent where up to 40 percent of entire national populations may have the condition (Campbell 2000). Because the profit margins on these and similar drugs are high, there is a fundamental moral dimension to the argument. A similar situation exists among those in developing countries such as Bosnia, Cambodia, Thailand, Rwanda, Guatemala, Iran, and Iraq, where hundreds of thousands of innocent civilians lost limbs due to land mines. These people cannot afford prosthetic devices and assistive equipment at the prices being charged by large international firms. At the same time, chronic depression is a worldwide problem, frequently related to poverty and war, but psychotropic drugs remain unaffordable in many of the countries where they are needed (Simon et al. 1999).

The concept and practice of managed care are also being exported to many countries of the world. In Brazil, for example, Aetna owns half of Sul America Seguros, a corporation that generated $1.2 billion in revenues in 1996 (Stocker, Waitzkin, and Iriart 1999). During the same year, Galeno Life TIM (Technología Integral Médica), a managed care organization owned by the multinational EXXEL investment group, reported revenues of $181 million. Cigna has entered the managed care market in Mexico, Brazil, Argentina, and Chile. There is little doubt that multinational corporations in the disability-rehabilitation business are selling their ideas and products to whomever will buy them (Cook and Kirkpatrick 1988). It is not at all apparent, however, that the needs of disabled people are being met. Nor is it apparent that the cultures of other countries are respected (White and Collyer 1997, 1998). Potential profits, market share, return on investment, and shareholder value are the forces that drive the system (Evans 1997; Morgan et al. 1997).

RISK AND ACCOUNTABILITY

The political economy of disability and rehabilitation raises five critical questions about risk and accountability for disability on the societal, institutional, group, and individual levels. The five questions that pervade these different levels of analysis are the following: What is risk? Who is at risk? How are they at risk? What or who is responsible for the risk? What are the consequences? These questions are the source of numerous debates about theory and define the battleground for proposed policy initiatives. The present discussion will frame these issues in the disability context. Disability is an interesting example for an analysis of risk and accountability because disabled people generally are thought to be at risk and constitute a vulnerable population. In addition, most epidemiological and social analyses of disability are underpinned by assumptions about and theories of risk (Douglas 1986, 1992).

Risk can be conceptualized as the statistical probability that an event may occur or, more commonly, as the likelihood of a danger, injury, or event with adverse consequences (Freudenburg 1988; Gabe 1995). In this sense, disability is by definition a negative experience and implicitly leads to the individual or group, with the disability being labeled as vulnerable or disadvantaged. Not only does risk analysis of disability usually imply a set of negative consequences but also that disability is something to be avoided or kept at a social and physical distance. Researchers and policy analysts often point out how disability is associated with increased morbidity and mortality, increased dependency indices, and a growing social burden requiring expensive social programs. They also infer that it is a problem to be prevented or avoided (Pear 2000). Social model, environmental, minority group, and human rights theorists vigorously challenge such assumptions and arguments. These arguments and positions are eloquently presented and also criticized elsewhere in this book.

In reviewing such contentious debates, Douglas and Ney (1998) draw attention to the fact that risk of disability is not merely a statistical likelihood with certain consequences or a neutral event, but it is situated in a cultural context where it is embedded with deep-set social meanings and values. "Risk has become a way of talking about justice when the parties to the debate, not sharing the same history or institutions, have different ways of articulating their ideas of right and wrong" (Douglas and Ney 1998:136). They assert that a balanced analysis of risk must take into account the potentially "dangerous" event as well as observers and their viewpoints. "A risk perception is a perception of danger, and it cannot make sense to isolate it from the perceiver's life project or from the other ideas the person has of good and bad and the way to live" (p. 136). Disability risk is by implication a socially constructed concept.

According to one's perspective, theory, or ideology, disability risk can be conceived as rooted in the individual, in the environment, or in the interaction between individuals and their environments (Lupton 1995; Verbrugge and Jette 1994). One's position on these issues will shape one's definitions, measurement, and responses to disability. From our perspective, disability can be related to organically based impairments (being analyzed in depth now in the extended genome project) and socially produced in the environment (Bury 2000a). Molecular biologists and geneticists are leading the way in identifying the organic basis of impairments, while political economists explore the social production and responses to disability. A more complete theory of impairment and disability will occur when these two analytical streams are integrated. Unfortunately, current debates in this area are characterized more by heat than light because of strong ideological commitments to preestablished positions, a myopia with one's own position, and the propensity to react immediately to seemingly distasteful arguments. The field will make more theoretical and social policy progress when these differing positions can be clarified, more thoroughly analyzed, and potentially integrated.

Who is at risk? How are they at risk? What or who is responsible for the risk? What are consequences? These questions will be answered differently, then, based on one's explanatory model, value orientation, and ideology. Traditionally, risk has been addressed in Western societies as a problem of the individual and according to the Parsonian conception of the "sick role" and "impaired role"; rights and responsibilities follow from the adoption of a "functional" mode of behavior (Parsons 1978). As John Knowles (1977), a prominent physician, wrote,

> The individual has the power—indeed, the moral responsibility to maintain his own health by the observance of simple, prudent rules of behavior relating to sleep, exercise, diet and weight, alcohol, and smoking. . . . He should submit to selective medical examination and screening procedures. . . But the costs of individual irresponsibility in health

have now become prohibitive. The choice is individual responsibility or social failure. Responsibility and duty must gain some degree of parity with right and freedom. (P. 386)

From this viewpoint, disability would be a problem of the individual. The person would be at risk due to his or her genetic background or, more especially, to his or her "irresponsible behavior." Individuals are responsible for their disabling condition or at least for seeking to avoid disability-causing events and environments. They are also responsible to seek appropriate medical care and follow the prescriptions of the doctor. The disabled individual is potentially a deviant—a risk to the economy and social order, as a Parsonian view would suggest.

In responding to this theoretical position based on the medical model, Crawford (1979) shifted the unit of analysis from the individual to society and institutions where he used a political economic framework to argue that "medical services and health have always been objects of intense ideological activity. . . . Dominant economic and political interests are threatened by the failure to find a solution in the routine processes of health politics" (pp. 247-49). He objected to the proposition that living a long life or being disability free is a "do it yourself activity. These assertions perform the function of blaming the victim." A more useful analysis, Crawford asserts, is to attack health problems and, by implication, disability issues on the societal, institutional, and structural levels. Crawford argues that by focusing on the individual, attention is diverted from the influence of class structure, lack of control over working conditions, and the nature of environmental impact. In Crawford's analysis, it is the disenfranchised, poor, and minorities who are at risk for poor health and its outcomes. They are at risk due to the socioeconomic conditions under which they live and work rather than as a result of good or poor "individual" role performance.

McKinlay (1974) extended this type of political economic analysis by arguing that deep-seated change in health outcomes and, implicitly, the disability world will be best achieved by "focusing upstream" on the root causes of disability and illness:

Such a reorientation would minimally involve an analysis of the means by which various individuals, interest groups, and large-scale, profit-oriented corporations are "pushing people in," and how they subsequently erect, at some point downstream, a health care structure to service the needs which they have had a hand in creating, and for which moral responsibility ought to be assumed. (P. 503)

McKinlay reasons that improvement in health conditions will ultimately be best served by aiming at prevention activities and changes in the institutional and social structure to reduce the transferal of risk from the "haves" to the "have-nots."

Ulrich Beck (1992) contributed a new perspective to the risk discourse when he pointed out that we face a new generation of hazards that arise from the interaction of global forces we now experience as regional and civil wars, ethnic cleansing, destruction of the environment, the exportation of high-risk jobs to developing countries, and proliferation of weapons of mass destruction. He argues that with the global transparency of business and travel, we have moved into an uncertain and precarious condition called the "risk society." Paradoxically, as society becomes more scientifically accomplished, potential risks resulting from genetically modified food, growth hormone–fed animals, antibiotic-resistant known diseases, and newly discovered diseases such as the hanta virus and different forms of HIV/AIDS are rapidly diffused around the world. There is growing concern, for example, that scientific experimentation with cloning, bacteriophages, anthrax vaccinations, and targeted genetic interventions are not well controlled (Zimmerman 2000). The experience with conditions such as chronic fatigue syndrome and Lyme's disease, in which medical diagnosis and treatment were openly contested by lay groups, reflects public insecurity over matters such as food sources, work conditions, and the environment. Under these conditions, we all are at risk, and wealth is not necessarily protective. We are at risk from within through our food sources, genetic modification, and accumulated drug resistance, as well as from the environment, unknown hazards in the workplace, and unregulated proliferation of weapons of mass destruction. Responsibility is not so easy to assign, and, in some senses, we are the enemy of ourselves. The consequences are potentially enormous because the door is open for new health disorders and genetically modified human stock that could fundamentally alter evolutionary forces. While all of these theoretical approaches are important for considering disability risk, none was specifically targeted to do so.

In *The Disability Business: Rehabilitation in America*, Albrecht (1992) examined risk and accountability, specifically in relation to disability, and argued that disability risk is not transparent in society or globally, and the public is often not well informed of risk and appropriate responses. Despite access to more and more information about potential environmental risks, this equation may be changing to some extent. However, evidence about risk is still often difficult to ascertain and is frequently "chronically contested." This is in part due to the contradictory nature of scientific information and accepted decision rules and also because the types, nature, and severity of threats are so uncertain. Interventions are often in experimental stages, and long-term consequences are unknown. Judicious decisions may be extremely difficult to achieve. The consequences are sobering. While a great deal is known in some areas, we are left with the following question: Who is to look out for and protect the public good and the health and well-being of citizens?

MORAL AND ETHICAL CHOICES

Disability raises fundamental questions about the value of individuals and distribution of resources in a society because disabled people are a barometer of the moral health of a society. Nations are judged by how they treat their women, children, elderly, war veterans, *and* disabled people. In organized societies, there are a variety of social contracts between the state and its citizens. The state has an obligation to provide a social order, security, minimum standards of living, and a certain quality of life. The individual, in turn, is expected to be loyal to the state, pay taxes, and be economically productive. This contract plays out in different ways, depending on history, culture, and context. Uncertainties about the form and terms of this social contract in today's global community have prompted a renewed interest in the concept of citizenship (Gray 1995; Healtherington 1998). Social observers are asking, What does it mean to be a citizen? We are citizens of what community? What are our mutual duties and obligations to each other?

Many commentators are concerned that the realignment of strategic interests and worldwide proliferation of American values are producing a myopic view of citizenship. As an example, Guéhenno (1993) points out that degradation in democratic values such as respect, civility, loyalty, and commitment to legal redress are threats to citizenship and ultimately to social order. Countries such as the Soviet Union, Yugoslavia, Czechoslovakia, South Vietnam, and East Germany no longer exist. Other nations such as Kosovo, Rwanda, Cambodia, and the Congo have been fractured by civil war, and protectorates such as Panama and Hong Kong have been reassigned to other leaderships. Conservative groups in France, Austria, Germany, and the United States are railing against open immigration policies so that they can preserve what they believe to be their national identity and way of life. The effect of these political economic events is to destabilize existing national identities, attack culture, rock the social order, and undermine loyalty to established institutions. To adapt to such events, individuals must exercise a range of psychological and social coping mechanisms daily.

On the institutional level, Richard Sennett (1998) observes that similarly, the culture of the new workplace has a profound effect on individual and social values. He argues that it is difficult for individuals to be loyal to firms that do not offer stability or return loyalty. The "hot" firms on the world's stock market often exhibit short-term and self-centered behaviors. They are concerned about the next quarter's profit report and how it will affect their stock price. Long-term planning is usually only a few years because by that time, the industry will have changed, or the company will have merged or have been acquired by someone else, often across international boundaries. Employees are then "downsized" or reassigned to new jobs in reorganized companies under different rules. In this political economic environment, it is difficult, if not impossible, to promote loyalty and develop character because "character requires the prolonged nurturing of personal traits which we value in ourselves and for which we seek to be valued by others" (Sennett 1998:10). In this context, the contemporary strategic political alliances between governments and industry and the dynamics of the marketplace seem antithetical to the development of character and maintenance of persistent community values (Kramer 1999).

Employing a contemporary sports analogy, everyone has to be a "free agent" to survive. These sorts of values in the business world are captured by Fallows's (1999) comments on the career of Jim Clark, an American entrepreneur in his mid-50s. Clark is distinguished by his accomplishment of starting three firms (Silicon Graphics, Netscape, and Healtheon), each reaching a market value of more than $1 billion. Fallows notes in a book review of Michael Lewis's (1999) *The New New Thing: A Silicon Valley Story* and Charles Ferguson's (1999) *High Stakes, No Prisoners: A Winner's Tale of Greed and Glory in the Internet Wars* the following:

> A more important pattern is the ever-receding target high-tech officials set for how much money it would take to make them happy. People do this in all walks of life, but the scale is different in the boom economy. Before he started Silicon Graphics, Clark had told a friend that he'd be satisfied if he made $10 million. Before he founded Netscape, he told a different friend that his dream was to have $100 million. When his holdings were worth $600 million, he told Lewis that he wanted to have a billion dollars, after taxes. "Then I'll be satisfied." Prompted by Lewis, he finally admits, "You know, just for one moment, I would like to have the most [in the world]. Just for one tiny moment. (P. 14)

In this environment, the basic social contract is under threat.

In the spirit of the earlier nineteenth-century "Robber Barons," these capitalists are establishing philanthropic foundations to support their favorite causes after they have accumulated their incredible wealth. The Packer Foundation at $10 billion of assets recently overtook the Ford Foundation in size, and the Bill and Melinda Gates Foundation is currently endowed at $17 billion. True, the globalization of world trade and explosion of the computer-driven information society have generated incredible new wealth. However, the benefits are not being spread evenly throughout society (Levy 1998). On the contrary, these new markets seem to be accentuating the disparities between the rich and the poor within and between nations (Nelson and Cooperman 1998).

What does this mean for disabled people? Government by public opinion polls, fickle commitments to institutions and communities, accentuation of rugged individualism on the world stage, and expanding gaps between the rich and the poor do not bode well for disabled people. Yet, many countries are in the process of developing and implementing revised social policies for disabled people. While rugged individualism prevails in the United States and entrepreneurial values are propounded in countries such as the United Kingdom, there is increasing recognition that disability is a universal experience that requires more attention from the electorate as well as coherent government policies. As the largest transfer of wealth is occurring between generations, children are discovering that they are pushed beyond reasonable limits to care for their elderly parents who are experiencing the disabilities associated with chronic illness in later life. They also are conscious that they too are likely to become disabled. In confronting the moral conundrums of determining what is best for them and their parents, how much medical intervention is enough, where to put our parents, how to pay for services, and how much voice to give their parents in the decisions, they are caught with the disturbing questions. Such questions include the following: How would I like to be treated when my time comes? Who will I be able to count on? How will I preserve their dignity and my own? Do they like the way they are being treated? What can we expect from family, government, and institutions? These same questions apply to those that have a disabled person in their family or who personally experience disability. The painful answers to these questions are forcing citizens to reexamine their own personal values and behavior, as are institutions and governments participating in the "social contract" that holds society together. The responses differ by culture, resources, and values (Mechanic 1998).

In the United States, sobering discussions on the last years of life and living with disability raise the specter of being left alone in pain, of losing one's dignity, of having unacceptable quality of life, or even of being subjected to euthanasia. Nuland's (1994) *How We Die* underlines that most us will die from a disability-related chronic illness, not from a fatal accident or instantaneous myocardial infarction, and discusses how we might prepare for that eventuality. Barbour's (1995) *Caring for Patients* acknowledges that medically attending to pathophysiologies does not always deliver care for the person, nor does it address the "disabling capacity of many organic diseases" (p. vii). Spiro, Curnen, and Wandel's (1996) *Facing Death* provides perspectives on how to use one's values and enhanced spirituality to give meaning to disability and death. And in *How Will They Know if I'm Dead: Transcending Disability and Terminal Illness,* Horn (1997) offers insights on how to live a full life with a disability (amyotrophic lateral sclerosis, or ALS). It is clear from each of these discussions that disability and death are social events reflecting the value systems and political economy of the society in which people live. In the United States, as in many other countries, disability is easier to deal with if the individual or family is privileged. However, in the United States, there is no effective safety net for those who are most at risk. This fact raises serious questions about the nature of the social contract between citizens and the nation in which they live (Quadagno 1999). Individualistic values and the political economy of the American form of capitalism have their costs (Kuttner 1999a, 1999b; Madrick 1999; Miller and Sage 1999). The remedies to mitigate substantial risks for disabled people in the United States encompass increased pressures for human rights, which would underpin an incrementally developed safety net system. It also encompasses access to technology such as the Internet, self-help groups to empower disabled people, the encouragement of more participatory and informed decision making in a disabled person's health care and life choices, and tax and government incentives to assist families to better care for their disabled members. Yet even more radical is a suggested moderation of the values of "rugged individualism."

The tradition of the European welfare state presents a different approach to the problem (Barr 1998). European nations are democracies and capitalist societies of a different stripe. They provide a stronger and more comprehensive safety net for their citizens who may become disabled or unemployed (Drake 1999). Their social contract emphasizes the good of the community and groups over that of the individual. As a consequence of taxes, legislation, and welfare benefits, there is less disparity between the income, wealth, and resources of the rich and the poor in these countries, even though income inequalities have increased substantially over the past 20 years in countries such as the United Kingdom (Wilkinson 1996). In general, more people vote in Europe; they support these social programs and expect the government to provide a minimum standard of living, including generous educational, health, and welfare benefits. In many senses desirable, there are costs to these systems. Businesses and governments in these nations are less flexible to respond to the rapidly changing global economy. Their unemployment rates are relatively high, tax revenues are constrained, and the numbers of retirees and elderly are increasing at rates unsustainable for the traditional level of benefits. The choices are tough. Taxes must increase, thereby damaging the economy; benefits must be cut, or the economy must be moved toward a more American model. None of these solutions is attractive to Europeans. The likely outcome is some combination that preserves traditional European community values, limits benefits, and introduces more competition in the marketplace (Watson and Webster 1999). There are even trade-offs to be made on the micro level. For example, disabled people have embraced a minority rights perspective in the United States, resulting in increased accessibility in public places and even to education and jobs. This has occurred even though they live without well-defined safety nets. In continental Europe, by contrast, disabled people are likely to have less physical access to public places, but they have better levels of income support and health services. The internationalization of the disability community is likely to reduce some of these differences.

The British approach to the welfare state and disabled people is a hybrid between that of the United States and that of continental Europe (Drake 1999). Like other nations, Britain is feeling the effects of an aging population with disabilities, competitive pressures from global competition, and, at the same time, a responsibility to care for its citizens. The mantra of Tony Blair, leading a "New" Labour government, is to launch a "third way," a platform intended to renew social democracy (Giddens 1998). In one form or another, this approach is advertised as responsible labor or a compassionate conservatism. The compromise political position acknowledges that the state has a social contract with its citizens to provide a safety net and basic standards of living; yet, at the same time, it is cognizant that the state must generate revenues to pay for these promises in the context of the competitive world economy. The American and European welfare state and British approaches toward social welfare and disability policy are representative of their related but unique political economies, values, and traditions (Inglehart 1999). It is unlikely, then, that they will eventually converge, even though they will borrow solutions from each other.

None of these approaches, however, pertains well to developing countries. The trade-off decisions for leaders and disabled people in developing countries are even more complex and draconian than those in the rest of the world. For a start, 80 percent of disabled people live in nonindustrialized countries, yet only 20 percent of the world's health care dollars are spent in these nations. Many of these countries are caught in dictatorships, autocracies, gerontocracies, and the combined chaos of civil war and ethnic strife. In countries displaying more stability, there are still very limited infrastructures and resources. In fact, many of these countries spend substantial portions of their gross national product (GNP) just to serve their national debt. By circumstance, then, families and communities are forced to deal with disability at the local level (Bennett, McPake, and Mills 1997b). Medicines are often unavailable; medical care is remote, or, at best, oriented toward primary care; prosthetics are made at home from local materials. Many people under these circumstances will prematurely die or live longer lives dependent on their families for support. As the populations in developing countries are aging, the burden will become greater. The only viable structural interventions are to control regional strife, encourage latent democracies, help build infrastructure, and promote public health and prevention efforts. In an analogous situation, Jonathan Mann, former director of the World Health Organization's Global Programme on AIDS, reflecting on years of dealing with the AIDS epidemic in the developing word, said, "The ultimate answer to controlling the problem is through education; particularly the education of women for women bear a disproportionate share of the risk and the caretaker burden" (Mann 1991). A similar argument can be made for disability. Education will permit people in developing countries to prevent impairment where possible and better deal with consequences when they occur. What is clear from this political economic analysis is that the principles of analysis remain the same, but that they must be applied in creative ways to divergent contexts, cultures, and traditions.

THE FUTURE OF POLITICAL ECONOMIC ANALYSIS IN UNDERSTANDING DISABILITY POLICY

Our political economic analysis of disability leads us to make the following observations. First, further political economic research is needed if we are to better understand the social production, multiple definitions, and responses to disability. Such analyses are essential to understand the social structure, value systems, environment, allocation of resources, stakeholder interests, power dynamics, and institutional forces that impinge on the daily lives of disabled people (Hogan 1998). Such research produces the concepts and theories that make the practice of politics and art of policy development possible. Many innovative architects of strategic disability policies understand well the political economy of their world and acknowledge and involve the key powerbrokers in their vision. Yet, we have been struck at how little is known in countries outside the United States about the overall shape of disability economics and its links with key social and political institutions.

In this tradition, Mancur Olson (1999) organizes his most recent book, *Power and Prosperity: Outgrowing Communist and Capitalist Dictatorships,* around the metaphor that rulers are robbers. Based on this assumption, he convincingly argues that political stability is preferable to anarchy and that democracy, even in poor nations, has an advantage over tyranny because governments are more accountable to a wider set of constituencies. Therefore, the rulers have powerful incentives to redistribute wealth. He also points out that stable markets, which guarantee contract and property rights, are necessary conditions for the efficient exchange of goods and services. His arguments have crucial implications for disability policy and rehabilitation efforts around the world. Regardless of the abuses of "free" markets and democratic forms of government, Olson argues that they are preferable to anarchy and unpredictable markets. We advocate the extension of such theoretical analyses to the disability arena so that we can better understand the forces at work and the likelihood of introducing more informed and workable approaches to disability policy and practice.

Second, while there are common themes and structural forces at work within and between nations, there are also considerable differences that have gone unappreciated in most disability analysis. This implies that we do not assume that what works in one situation will apply in another. One of the core principles of disability studies is to appreciate differences while discovering commonalities. In a political sense, this means using a political economic perspective to understand differences within and among different disability groups before rushing to impose dominant models and popular solutions on social and cultural contexts when they may not fit well. Cultural imperialism exists in the disability world, as it does in international politics (Bennett et al. 1997a; Krugman 1998; Zukerman 1998).

Third, political economic analysis can help to explain the frictions between disability groups. A persistent question in disability studies has been the following: Why do disability groups compete with each other for scare resources rather than cooperate to accomplish overarching goals, such as passage of the 1990 Americans with Disabilities Act and subsequent legislation in Britain, Australia, Canada, and New Zealand? The answer to this question will help to explain the history of the disability movement, politics, and programs. An irony of disability studies is that while leaders preach inclusion, they often act in their own self-interests and practice exclusion. In fact, ideologically and geographically disparate groups often do not even talk to one another. For example, there are fault lines in the disability landscape between those interested in physical and intellectual disabilities, rehabilitation sciences and disability studies, organically based versus social and environmental models of disability, and disabilities found in the industrial world and those experienced in developing countries. These dynamics have emasculated the potential power of the disability movement and credibility of the field. The point is that the field will not mature until these different factions listen to one another and aim at building less contentious and more integrative positions.

Fourth, disability is a global phenomenon but typically is only acknowledged by scholars and studied in the industrial world. We know very little about disability in developing countries where 80 percent of the problem lies (Beresford 1996). In the Global Burden of Disease project, Murray and Lopez (1996a, 1996b, 1997) point out in a comparative analysis of eight areas of the world that the distribution of disabling conditions is distinguished by different geographical and political economic conditions. Disabilities resulting from malaria, diarrheal diseases, tuberculosis, and anemia are more prevalent in less developed nations, while disabilities related to heart disease, road traffic accidents, and chronic obstructive pulmonary disease are more typical of industrial countries. Also, the disabilities due to land mines and wars are to be found in the remnants of the old Soviet Union, the Balkans, Sri Lanka, sub-Sahara, and other parts of Africa. Disabilities associated with HIV/AIDS are disproportionately found in Africa and Southeast Asia. These patterns are also changing over time as political destabilization, industrialization, global warming, and population densities are altered. Because of international, interlocked markets and global travel, the political economy and health conditions in developing nations will have an increasing impact on the health and well-being of residents of postindustrial societies.

Fifth, disability and rehabilitation are businesses with markets, goods, and services. A political economic perspective compels us to recognize and deal with these realities. Disability is a significant part of the economy in industrialized countries and a drain in less developed countries. For medical and health businesses, disability and rehabilitation constitute a remarkable opportunity for growth. Many of the drugs, prosthetic and orthotic devices, rehabilitation, and home health care services are essential, and the profit margins are attractive for capital investors. It is important to situate the discussion of for-profit and not-for-profit disability and rehabilitation organizations. Every organization has to generate more funds than it consumes or it will not survive. In the for-profit environment, this is called profit, tax-favorable capital, and other investments. In the not-for-profit environment, this residual between income and expenses is referred to as retained earnings. While the quest for institutional survival is strong in both instances, and the environments are similar for organizations in the disability marketplace, one critical piece of the environment differs—tax status. All business organizations seek to minimize their taxes and maximize their profits, give dividends back to stockholders and profits to owners in the for-profit world, and invest in delivering more services or reaching a larger population for the not-for-profit organizations. Political economic analyses permit us to understand the rationale and dynamics of these marketplaces and their probable impact on disabled people.

Sixth, institutional analysis is important to comprehend the stakeholders in the marketplace and their behavioral incentives. Institutions are strongly driven to survive and flourish in the marketplace. Questions that arise are the following: Does the survival and health of institutions in the disability business translate directly into improved goods, services, and quality of life for disabled people? At what points do the interests of institutions and consumers converge, and where do they differ? Moreover, there is a strong argument in organizational theory that institutions in a similar marketplace will begin to look and behave in similar ways to compete and survive; they will become increasingly isomorphic (Wheatley, DeJong, and Sutton 1997, 1999). If this is true, and there is evidence to bear this out, what will be the impact on disabled consumers? What choices will they have?

Seventh, the consumer is central to the disability business. Political economic analysis leads us to ask, Who are the consumers? Are they individuals, families, rehabilitation facilities, employers, government agencies, HMOs, the National Health Service, and insurers? If so, who looks out for the interests of disabled people? How can disabled people be rational, informed consumers if they have incomplete information, have limited power, are emotionally pulled in divergent directions, and are making purchase decisions in a nontransparent marketplace? Consumers cannot play the game and hope to win if they do not know the rules.

Eighth, human rights and citizenship are critical concepts in the political economic analysis of disability because they provide the theories and value sets on which disabled people can build their raison d'être and bases for action. In a deep cultural sense, what happens to disabled people can happen to every citizen, and the way that disabled people are treated reflects the history, values, and traditions of the larger society. Disability is a morally defining issue that bears on issues such as euthanasia, right to life, right to die, and treatment of pain. Who has the right to make and who is responsible for these decisions, especially when rights have to be enforced through legal redress? The force of these arguments is played out in this volume in chapters by Wasserman (Chapter 8), Asch (Chapter 11), and Bickenbach (Chapter 24).

This chapter is a clarion call to look at the big picture, study history and culture to appreciate our past, employ theory to help understand what is, and use political economic analyses to construct and advocate for culturally sensitive, effective social policies for disabled people. We argue that disability is not a single, isolated issue in a larger society but a marker by which a society can be understood and judged. We have concluded by pointing the way to future research and policy initiatives.

REFERENCES

Albrecht, G. L. 1973. *The Sociology of Physical Disability and Rehabilitation.* Pittsburgh, PA: University of Pittsburgh Press.

———, ed. 1981. *Cross National Rehabilitation Policies: A Sociological Perspective.* London: Sage.

———. 1992. *The Disability Business: Rehabilitation in America.* Newbury Park, CA: Sage.

———. 1997. "The Health Politics of Disability." Pp. 367-89 in *Health Politics and Policy,* edited by T. J. Litman and L. S. Robbins. Albany, NY: Delmar.

Albrecht, G. L. and L. Verbrugge. 2000. "The Global Emergence of Disability." Pp. 293-307 in *The Handbook of Social Studies in Health and Medicine,* edited by G. L. Albrecht, R. Fitzpatrick, and S. C. Scrimshaw. London: Sage.

Alt, J. E. and A. Alesina. 1996. "Political Economy: An Overview." Pp. 645-74 in *A New Handbook of Political Science,* edited by R. E. Goodin and H.-D. Klingemann. New York: Oxford University Press.

"The Americas Shift toward Private Health Care." 1999. *The Economist,* May 8, pp. 27-28.

Arege, J. J. 1999. "Healthcare: Managed Care." *Standard & Poor's Industry Surveys.* New York: McGraw-Hill.

Arno, P. S., C. Levine, and M. M. Memmott. 1999. "The Economic Value of Informal Caregiving." *Health Affairs* 18:182-88.

Barbour, A. B. 1995. *Caring for Patients.* Stanford, CA: Stanford University Press.

Barnes, C. 1991. *Disabled People in Britain and Discrimination.* London: Hurst.

———. 1998. "The Social Model of Disability: A Sociological Phenomenon Ignored by Sociologist?" Pp. 65-78 in *The Disability Reader: Social Science Perspectives,* edited by T. Shakespeare. London: Cassell.

Barr, N. 1998. *The Economics of the Welfare State.* 3d ed. Oxford, UK: Oxford University Press.

Bates, E. 1999. "The Shame of Our Nursing Homes: Millions for Investors, Misery for the Elderly." *The Nation* 268:11-19.

Beck, U. 1992. *Risk Society: Towards a New Modernity.* London: Sage.

Bennett, S., B. McPake, and A. Mills, eds. 1997a. *Private Health Providers in Developing Countries: Serving the Public Interest?* London: Zed.

———. 1997b. "The Public/Private Mix Debate in Health Care." Pp. 1-18 in *Private Health Providers in Developing Countries: Serving the Public Interest?* edited by S. Bennett, B. McPake, and A. Mills. London: Zed.

Beresford, P. 1996. "Poverty and Disabled People: Challenging Dominant Debates and Policies." *Disability & Society* 4:553-67.

Berkowitz, E. O. 1987. *Disabled Policy: America's Programs for the Handicapped.* Cambridge, UK: Cambridge University Press.

Bickenback, J. E. 1993. *Physical Disability and Social Policy.* Toronto: University of Toronto Press.

Bickenbach, J. E., S. Chatterji, E. M. Badley, and T. B. Üstün. 1999. "Models of Disablement, Universalism and the International Classification of Impairments, Disabilities and Handicaps." *Social Science and Medicine* 48:1173-87.

Blaxter, M. 1976. *The Meaning of Disability: A Sociological Study of Impairment.* London: Heinemann.

Bloom, G. and D. McIntyre. 1998. "Toward Equity in Health in an Unequal Society." *Social Science and Medicine* 47:1529-38.

Bron, A. 1999. "Comment les caises maladie tiennent les médicins à l'oeil." *Tribune de Genève,* June 28, p. 2.

Bury, M. R. 1982. "Chronic Illness as Biographical Disruption." *Sociology of Health and Illness* 4:167-82.

———. 1986. "Social Constructionism and the Development of Medical Sociology." *Sociology of Health and Illness* 8:137-69.

———. 1996. "Defining and Researching Disability: Challenges and Responses." Pp. 17-45 in *Exploring the Divide: Illness and Disability,* edited by C. Barnes and G. Mercer. Leeds, UK: The Disability Press.

———. 1997. *Health and Illness in a Changing Society.* London: Routledge Kegan Paul.

———. 2000a. "On Chronic Illness and Disability." pp. 173-83 in *Handbook of Medical Sociology,* 5th ed., edited by C. Bird, P. Conrad, and A. Fremont. Upper Saddle River, NJ: Prentice Hall.

———. 2000b. "Health, Ageing and the Lifecourse." Pp. 87-105 in *Health, Medicine and Society: Key Theories, Futures Agendas,* edited by S. J. Williams, J. Gabe, and M. Calnan. London: Routledge Kegan Paul.

Campbell, C. 2000. "Selling Sex in the Time of AIDS: The Psycho-Social Context of Condom Use by Sex Workers on a Southern African Mine." *Social Science and Medicine* 50:479-94.

Carrasquillo, O., D. U. Himmelstein, S. Woolhandler, and D. H. Bor. 1999. "A Reappraisal of Private Employers' Role in Providing Health Insurance." *New England Journal of Medicine* 340:109-14.

Castel, R. 1995. *Les Métaphorphoses de la Question Sociale.* Paris: Fayard.

Charlton, J. I. 1998. *Nothing about Us without Us.* Berkeley: University of California Press.

Cook, P. and C. Kirkpatrick. 1988. *Privitisation in Less Developed Countries.* New York: Harvester and Wheatsheaf.

Crawford, R. 1979. "Individual Responsibility and Health Politics in the 1970s." Pp. 247-68 in *Health Care in America: Essays in Social History,* edited by S. Reverby and D. Rosner. Philadelphia: Temple University Press.

DeJong, G. 1979. "Independent Living: From Social Movement to Analytic Paradigm." *Archives of Physical Medicine and Rehabilitation* 60:438-47.

———. 1996. "Medical Rehabilitation Undergoing Major Shakeup in Advanced Managed Care Markets." *Eli Rehab Report* 3:3527-30.

DeJong, G. and B. O'Day. 1999. "Cross-Cutting Issues in Disability Policy and Services and Their Implications for Disability Research." Unpublished paper, NRH Research Center, Medlantic Research Institute, Washington, DC.

Douglas, M. 1986. *Risk Acceptability According to the Social Sciences.* London: Routledge Kegan Paul.

———. 1992. *Risk and Blame: Essays in Cultural Theory.* London: Routledge Kegan Paul.

Douglas, M. and S. Ney. 1998. *Missing Persons: A Critique of Personhood in the Social Sciences.* Berkeley: University of California Press.

Drake, R. 1999. *Understanding Disability Policy.* London: Macmillan.

Enthoven, A. C. 1988. "Managed Competition: An Agenda for Action." *Health Affairs* 7:25-47.

Evans, R. G. 1997. "Going for the Gold: The Redistributive Agenda behind Market-Based Health Care Reform." *Journal of Health Politics, Policy and Law* 22:427-66.

Fallows, J. 1999. "Billion-Dollar Babies." *New York Review of Books* 46:9-16.

Ferguson, C. 1999. *High Stakes, No Prisoners: A Winner's Tale of Greed and Glory in the Internet Wars.* New York: Times Books.

Finkelstein, V. 1980. *Attitudes and Disabled People: Issues for Discussion.* New York: World Rehabilitation Fund.

Freudenburg, W. R. 1988. "Perceived Risk, Real Risk: Social Science and the Art of Probabilistic Risk Assessment." *Science* 242:44-49.

Freudenheim, M. and C. Krauss. 1999. "Latin America Imports US Style Health Plans—Now Called 'Coordinated' Care-Prove Popular." *International Herald Tribune,* June 17, p. 13.

Gabe, J., ed. 1995. *Medicine, Health and Risk: Sociological Approaches.* Oxford, UK: Blackwell.

Giddens, A. 1998. *The Third Way: The Renewal of Social Democracy* Cambridge, UK: Polity.

Ginsberg, E. 1999. "The Uncertain Future of Managed Care." *New England Journal of Medicine* 340:144-46.

Gold, R. 1999. "Healthcare: Facilities." *Standard & Poor's Industry Surveys.* New York: McGraw-Hill.

Gray, J. 1995. *Enlightenment's Wake: Politics and Culture at the Close of the Modern Age.* London: Routledge Kegan Paul.

Guéhenno, J.-M. 1993. *La Fin de la Démocratie.* Paris: Flammarion.

Haveman, R. H., V. Halberstadt, and R. V. Burkhauser. 1984. *Public Policy toward Disabled Workers.* Ithaca, NY: Cornell University Press.

Healtherington, M. J. 1998. "The Political Relevance of Political Trust." *American Political Science Review* 92:791-808.

Hogan, A. 1998. "The Business of Hearing." *Health* 2:485-501.

Horn, R. C. 1997. *How Will They Know if I'm Dead: Transcending Disability and Terminal Illness.* Delray Beach, FL: GR/St. Lucie.

Imrie, R. 1996. *Disability and the City.* New York: St. Martin's.

Inglehart, J. K. 1999. "The American Health Care System." *New England Journal of Medicine* 340:70-76.

Japsen, B. 1999a. "New Prescription; in a Nod to a Growing Trend, Rush-Prudential Will Offer Partial Coverage for Alternative Therapies." *Chicago Tribune,* November 12, pp. B1, B3.

———. 1999b. "Clubs Medi Give Rivals a Headache." *Chicago Tribune,* August 20, pp. B1, B4.

Jefferys, M. 1989. *Growing Old in the Twentieth Century.* London: Routledge Kegan Paul.

Knowles, J. 1977. "The Responsibility of the Individual." *Daedalus* 106:376-86.

Kramer, R. M. 1999. "Trust and Distrust in Organizations: Emerging Perspectives, Enduring Questions." *Annual Review of Psychology* 50:569-98.

Krugman, P. 1998. "America the Boastful." *Foreign Affairs* 77:32-45.

Kuttner, R. 1999a. "The American Health Care System: Wall Street and Health Care." *New England Journal of Medicine* 340:664-68.

———. 1999b. "The American Health Care System: Health Care Insurance." *New England Journal of Medicine* 340:163-68.

Lane, R. 1991. *The Market Experience.* Cambridge, UK: Cambridge University Press.

Levy, F. 1998. *The New Dollars and Dreams: American Incomes and Economic Change.* New York: Russell Sage.

Lewis, M. 1999. *The New New Thing: A Silicon Valley Story.* New York: Norton.

Liem, H. N. 1998. *La facture sociale: Sommes-nous condamnés au libéralisme?* Paris: Arléa.

Light, D. W. 1986. "Corporate Medicine for Profit." *Scientific American* 225:38-45.

———. 1997. "From Managed Competition to Managed Cooperation: Theory and Lessons from the British Experience." *The Milbank Quarterly* 75:297-341.

———. 2000. "The Sociological Character of Health Care Markets." Pp. 394-408 in *Handbook of Social Studies In Health and Medicine,* edited by G. L. Albrecht, R. Fitzpatrick, and S. C. Scrimshaw. London: Sage.

Lupton, D. 1995. *The Imperative of Health: Public Health and the Regulated Body.* London: Sage.

Madrick, J. 1999. "How New Is the New Economy?" *New York Review of Books* 46:42-50.

Mann, J. 1991. "Education, AIDS and Human Rights." Paper presented at a seminar at Cook County Hospital to research staff, November, Chicago.

McGinnis, M. J. 1997. "What Do We Pay for Good Health?" *Journal of Public Health Management & Practice* 3:124-36.

McKinlay, J. 1974. "A Case for Refocusing Upstream: The Political Economy of Illness." Pp. 87-96 in *Applying Behavioral Science to Cardiovascular Risk,* edited by the American Heart Association. Dallas, TX: American Heart Association.

McPake, B. 1997. "The Role of the Private Sector in Health Service Provision." Pp. 21-39 in *Private Health Providers in Developing Countries: Serving the Public Interest?* edited by S. Bennett, B. McPake, and A. Mills. London: Zed.

Mechanic, D. 1998. "Public Trust Initiatives for New Health Care Partnerships." *The Milbank Quarterly* 76:281-302.

Miller, T. E. and W. M. Sage. 1999. "Disclosing Physician Financial Incentives." *Journal of the American Medical Association* 281:1424-30.

Moody's Handbook of Common Stocks. 1999. New York: Financial Communications.

Morgan, R. O., B. A. Virnig, C. A. DeVito, and N. A. Persely. 1997. "The Medicare-HMO Revolving Door: The Healthy Go In and the Sick Go Out." *New England Journal of Medicine* 337:169-75.

Murray, C. J. and A. M. Lopez, eds. 1996a. *The Global Burden of Disease.* Boston: Harvard University Press.

———. 1996b. "Evidence-Based Health Policy-Lessons from the Global Burden of Disease Study." *Science* 274:740-43.

———. 1997. "Regional Patterns of Disability-Free Life Expectancy and Disability-Adjusted: Global Burden of Disease Study." *Lancet* 349:1347-52.

Nelson, J. I. and D. Cooperman. 1998. "Out of Utopia: The Paradox of Postindustrialization." *The Sociological Quarterly* 39:583-96.

Nuland, S. B. 1994. *How We Die: Reflections on Life's Final Chapter.* New York: Knopf.

O'Brien, D. P. 1975. *The Classical Economists.* Oxford, UK: Oxford University Press.

Office of National Statistics. 2000. *Social Trends, No. 30.* London: Author.

Oliver, M. 1990. *The Politics of Disablement.* New York: St. Martin's.

Olson, M. 1999. *Power and Prosperity: Outgrowing Communist and Capitalist Dictatorships.* New York: Basic Books.

Parsons, T. 1978. "The Sick Role and the Role of the Physician Reconsidered." Pp. 132-53 in *Action Theory and the Human Condition,* edited by T. Parsons. New York: Free Press.

Pear, R. 1998. "Americans Lacking Health Care Insurance Put at 16 Per Cent." *New York Times,* September 26, p. A1.

———. 2000. "U.S. Seeks More Care for Disabled outside Institutions." *New York Times,* February 13, p. 20.

Percy, S. L. 1989. *Disability, Civil Rights, and Public Policy: The Politics of Implementation.* Tuscaloosa: University of Alabama Press.

Pfeiffer, D. 1999. "The IDIDH and the Need for Its Revision." *Disability & Society* 13:503-23.

Priestly, M. 1999. *Disability Politics and Community Care.* London: Jessica Kingsley.

Quadagno, J. 1999. "Creating a Capital Investment Welfare State: The New American Exceptionalism." *American Sociological Review* 64:1-11.

Reinhardt, U. 1996. "A Social Contract for 21st Century Health Care: Three-Tier Health Care with Bounty Hunting." *Health Economics* 5:479-99.

Rice, T. 1997. "Can Market Forces Give Us the Health Care System We Want?" *Journal of Health Politics, Policy and Law* 22:383-426.

————. 1998. *The Economics of Health Reconsidered*. Chicago: Health Administration Press.

Robinson, J. C. 1999. "The Future of Managed Care Organization." *Health Affairs* 18:7-24.

Safilios-Rothschild, C. 1970. *The Sociology and Social Psychology of Disability and Rehabilitation*. New York: Random House.

Saftlas, H. 1999. "Healthcare: Pharmaceuticals." *Standard & Poor's Industry Surveys*. New York: McGraw-Hill.

Saltman, R. and J. Figueras. 1996. *European Health Care Reforms: Analysis of Current Strategies, Summary*. Copenhagen: World Health Organization, Regional Office for Europe.

Schumpeter, J. A. 1975. *History of Economic Analysis*. New York: Oxford University Press.

Scotch, R. 1985. "Disability as a Basis for a Social Movement: Advocacy and the Politics of Definition." *Journal of Social Issues* 44:159-72.

Scott, R. A. 1969. *The Making of Blind Men*. New York: Russell Sage.

Sen, A. 1992. *Inequality Reexamined*. Cambridge, MA: Harvard University Press.

————. 1995. "Rationality and Social Choice." *American Economic Review* 85:1-19.

————. 1999a. "The Possibility of Social Choice." *American Economic Review* 89:1-21.

————. 1999b. *Development as Freedom*. New York: Knopf.

Sennett, Richard. 1998. *The Corrosion of Character*. New York: Norton.

Simon, G. E., M. VonKorff, M. Piccinelli, C. Fullerton, and J. Ormel. 1999. "An International Study of the Relation between Somatic Symptoms and Depression." *New England Journal of Medicine* 341: 1329-35.

Smith, A. [1776] 1976. *An Inquiry in the Nature and Causes of the Wealth of Nations*. Reprint, Oxford, UK: Clarendon.

Spiro, H. M., M. G. Curnen, and L. P. Wandel. 1996. *Facing Death: Where Culture, Religion and Medicine Meet*. New Haven, CT: Yale University Press.

Standard and Poor's. 1999. *Standard Corporation Description*. New York: Author.

Stocker, K., H. Waitzkin, and C. Iriart. 1999. "The Exportation of Managed Care to Latin America." *New England Journal of Medicine* 340:1131-36.

Stone, D. 1984. *The Disabled State*. Philadelphia: Temple University Press.

Üstün, T. B., J. E. Bickenbach, E. Badley, and S. Chatterji. 1999. "A Reply to David Pfeiffer: The ICIDH and the Need for Its Revision." *Disability & Society* 13:829-31.

Verbrugge, L. M. and A. M. Jette. 1994. "The Disablement Process." *Social Science and Medicine* 38:1-14.

Watson, R. and P. Webster. 1999. "MPs Defy Blair in Benefits Vote." *The Times*, May 21, p. 1.

Wheatley, B., G. DeJong, and J.b Sutton. 1997. "Managed Care and Transformation of the Medical Rehabilitation Industry." *Health Care Management Review* 22:25-39.

————. 1999. "Consolidation of the Inpatient Medical Rehabilitation Industry." *Health Affairs* 17:209-15.

White, K. and F. Collyer. 1997. "To Market, to Market: Corporatisation, Privitisation, and Hospital Costs." *Australian Health Review* 20:13-25.

————. 1998. "Health Care Markets in Australia: Ownership of the Private Hospital Sector." *International Journal of Health Services* 28:487-510.

Wilkinson, R. 1996. *Unhealthy Societies: From Inequality to Well-Being*. London: Routledge Kegan Paul.

World Health Organization. 1997. *International Classification of Impairments, Activities, and Participation: A Manual of Dimensions of Disablement and Functioning*. Beta draft. Geneva: Author.

Zimmerman, L. 2000. "A Stalinist Antibiotic Alternative." *The New York Times Magazine*, February 6, pp. 50-55.

Zola, I. K. 1981. *Missing Pieces: A Chronicle of Living with a Disability*. Philadelphia: Temple University Press.

————. 1989. "Toward the Necessary Universalizing of a Disability Policy." *The Milbank Quarterly* 67:401-14.

————. 1994. "Disability Statistics, What Counts and What It Tells Us: A Personal and Political Analysis." *Journal of Disability Policy Studies* 4:9-39.

Zukerman, M. B. 1998. "A Second American Century." *Foreign Affairs* 77:18-31.

Disability and Health Policy

26

The Role of Markets in the Delivery of Health Services

GERBEN DEJONG

IAN BASNETT

Those in the vanguard of disability movements in many countries bring conflicting views about the role of health care in lives of people with disabilities. On one hand, individuals with disabilities need more health care and thus have a greater stake in their respective health systems. They want to make sure that their health care system will be there for them when they need it. On the other hand, those who share the values of the disability movement have an aversion to the baggage that often accompanies the delivery of health care services. They particularly resent the way in which traditional health care delivery often entails paternalistic markings of the medical model and the sick role that echo their second-class citizenship from times past.

Societies have equally ambivalent views about the delivery of health care services—albeit along somewhat different lines. Many societies view health care as a public good that should be reasonably accessible, publicly accountable, and regulated to ensure key social policy goals. At the same time, many policy elites and governments view health care as potentially inefficient and expensive and thus want to introduce market-based mechanisms to induce competition, control costs, and foster greater consumer responsiveness. Every society has answered this conflict differently, consistent with its own values and the ideologies of the political parties in power.

This societal-level ambivalence presents a special challenge for individuals with disabilities. They understand their greater stake in the health care system, and they want the protections of the state, knowing that markets will perceive them as high-cost users and thus stint on the services they need. Yet they also want a more responsive system and perceive that market-based so-

AUTHORS' NOTE: Research for this chapter was made possible in part by the National Institute on Disability and Rehabilitation Research (NIDRR) in the form of two grants to the NRH Center for Health & Disability Research: (1) a research and training center on managed care and disability (H133B70003) and (2) a study on disability and risk adjustment (H133G70072). The views expressed in this chapter are solely those of the authors and not of the sponsoring organizations.

lutions may foster greater innovation and consumer empowerment—features that are less likely to occur in state-administered systems in which provider paternalism is more likely to prevail.

PURPOSE AND SCOPE

In many countries, the contrasts sketched here are not always stark or clear-cut. Nonetheless, we believe that they have heuristic value in understanding the difficult choices that people with disabilities face in many countries, especially today when the use of markets for the delivery of public services has gained increased favor among policy elites. Markets are seen by some as a better mechanism by which to allocate resources than government. The purpose of this chapter is to obtain some understanding about the ability or inability of health care markets to adequately address the needs, values, and concerns of individuals with disabilities—especially among those most closely associated with the disability movements in their respective countries.

To evaluate whether market mechanisms can be made responsive to the needs of individuals with disabilities, one must first ascertain what those needs in fact are. Thus, we begin by characterizing the health care needs of individuals with disabilities and the enormous stake that people with disabilities have in their respective health care systems. We then contrast this enormous stake with the longstanding aversion that disability advocates have had in dealing with health policy issues—at least in the United States and to some extent in the United Kingdom. We follow by identifying the events that helped to make health care a major policy issue for the disability movements in both the United States and the United Kingdom.

This chapter identifies four cross-national phenomena that have given new impetus and legitimacy to the use of markets as a means of allocating health care resources:

1. the demise of the Soviet Union,
2. globalization,
3. economic stagnation in parts of Western Europe, and
4. the intellectual ascendancy of "managed competition" as a key concept in the discussion of health care changes in many Western countries.

We outline managed competition's preconditions and its influence on the thinking about health policy changes in the United States and the United Kingdom. We juxtapose managed competition theory with the experiences of the United States and United Kingdom. This juxtaposition provides a useful framework for understanding key health policy choices in terms of their responsiveness to the needs and concerns of individuals with disabilities.

Managed competition should not be confused with managed care. *Managed competition* is how countries and their subjurisdictions organize and manage the competition between health plans or providers in the marketplace. *Managed care* is how health plans and providers organize and manage the delivery of health services in a more coordinated fashion, often at a fixed price. This chapter is more about the former and less about the latter. Managed competition is often confused with managed care because both concepts achieved currency, at least in the United States, at about the same time and because these terms were sometimes used interchangeably, although inaccurately, during the 1993 to 1994 health care reform debate in the United States.

Because of our firsthand familiarity with American and British health systems, we bring a distinct Anglo-American view of health care with all its inherent limitations. Yet American and British systems are very different in the degree to which they have embraced government and market-oriented mechanisms in the delivery of health services. We believe that these differences provide a sufficient degree of contrast and thus provide sufficient analytic space within our proposed framework for many other countries to locate their own systems and proposed reforms. We hope that our analyses here, while they spring from particular contexts and experiences, will have utility for others in understanding the role of markets in their own health care systems and the extent to which market mechanisms can or cannot respond to the needs of people with disabilities.

We want to make clear what this chapter is not about. It is not about how a nation finances its health care system via general taxes, payroll taxes, social insurance, or premiums. It is not about the relative merits of governments, employers, and trade associations as the vehicle for collecting the funds with which to pay for health services. It is not about the need for universal health care coverage or the lack thereof in some countries. All of these issues are worthy in their own right. They are more deeply rooted in a society's political history and social culture, which sometimes makes cross-national comparisons more difficult. This chapter is about the role of markets and nonmarket mechanisms in distributing health care resources and how market mechanisms may or may not accommodate the needs and concerns of individuals with disabilities. A society may be deeply committed to social solidarity and universal health insurance but may still choose to use market mechanisms to allocate its health care resources. In fact, as we will show, market concepts have gained acceptance in many countries that are deeply committed to social solidarity and that exhibit strong communitarian values.

In saying what this chapter is not about, we do not want to diminish the importance of universal health care coverage as a key social policy objective, especially if one considers access to adequate and quality health care to be a fundamental human right. Universal coverage greatly simplifies other health policy choices. Without universal coverage, a country's health care system must wrangle with the problem of cross-subsidies because uncovered populations will eventually present their needs to some part of the health care system. And without *mandatory* universal coverage, the financial risks of illness and disability are not adequately distributed and thus make health care expensive for potential new entrants and undermine political support for other health care reforms. To those who champion market-based mechanisms, we want to underscore that the need for cross-subsidies can make market pricing unduly complicated, introduce undesirable financial incentives, and lead to unintended behaviors by consumers, providers, and payers alike.[1]

HEALTH CARE NEEDS OF INDIVIDUALS WITH DISABILITIES

Any discussion about disability and health policy needs to start with a baseline characterization of how the health care needs and experiences of individuals with disabilities are similar to or different from those without disabilities. We cannot evaluate the adequacy of any one approach without first knowing what needs are to be met. Apart from broad public health measures that benefit the entire population (e.g., potable water, sanitation, immunizations), the test of any health care system is not how it addresses the needs of the majority who are fairly healthy and well but how it meets the needs of the minority who need it most.

It is difficult to generalize about the ongoing health care needs of people with disabilities, in part, because different disabling conditions have widely varying etiologies, pathophysiologies, comorbidities, and functional consequences. These differences often obscure the fact that people with disabilities experience most of the same health conditions experienced by people without disabilities. People with disabilities are, however, at greater risk for certain common health conditions than those in the general population. They often experience these conditions differently, and they may require a somewhat different and extended therapeutic regime that takes into account both their underlying impairment and their functional limitations.

There are many ways one can characterize the ongoing health care needs of people with disabilities relative to those of people without disabilities. At the risk of overgeneralization, we note eight ways in which the ongoing health care needs of people with disabilities can be different from those in the general population (American Congress of Rehabilitation Medicine 1993; Bockeneck et al. 1998; DeJong 1997).

First, people with disabilities generally have a *thinner margin of health* that must be guarded carefully if medical problems are to be averted (Pope and Tarlov 1991). This observation applies to health conditions that people with disabilities share with the nondisabled population (e.g., upper respiratory infection, pneumonia) as well as conditions more likely to appear among people with disabilities (e.g., urinary tract infections, pressure sores). It should be emphasized that people with disabilities are not "sick"; instead, most are generally very healthy. Their impairments and functional limitations, however, often render them more vulnerable to certain health problems.

Second, people with disabilities often do not have the same opportunities for *health maintenance and preventive health care* as those without disabilities. For example, people with mobility limitations usually have fewer opportunities to participate in aerobic activity needed for good cardiovascular health (Pope and Tarlov 1991).

Third, people with disabilities who acquired their impairment early in life may experience an *earlier onset of chronic health conditions* than those without disabilities. For example, people with longstanding mobility limitations are believed to experience an earlier onset of coronary heart disease than those without disabilities. Likewise, people with mobility limitations may experience an earlier onset of adult diabetes (Bauman 1993) because of obesity, and they may experience an earlier onset of renal disease (e.g., pyelonephritis) because of a neurogenic bladder.

Fourth, people with disabilities who acquire a new health condition, apart from their original impairment, are likely to experience *secondary functional losses.* For example, an individual with spinal cord injury who acquires arthritis in his or her upper extremity may have to migrate from a manual wheelchair to a powered wheelchair and from an automobile to a ramped van. Thus, the functional consequences of a new chronic health condition are usually more significant for a person who already has a disabling impairment.

Fifth, people with disabilities may require *more complicated and prolonged treatment* for a given health problem than people without disabilities. Likewise, a person with a disability may require a longer recovery period following an acute episode of illness or injury because of pre-existing functional limitations that limit a person's participation in various therapies (e.g., using a treadmill or exercise bicycle following an acute myocardial infarct).

Sixth, some individuals with disabilities may require *sustained pharmacologic support,* as in the case of long-term mental illness.

Seventh, people with disabilities may *need durable medical equipment and other assistive technologies.*

Finally, individuals with disabilities *may require long-term services,* such as personal assistance and ongoing medical supervision.

Even these eight characterizations cannot fully capture the health care needs of individuals with disabilities. Individuals may have health care needs that are very specific to their underlying impairments or health conditions, whether they are spinal cord injury, cerebral palsy, arthritis, sickle cell anemia, bipolar depression, or any number of other conditions.

Our characterizations have several implications for the design of any health care system. For example, the benefits available must be sufficiently broad and elastic to capture the diversity of needs represented in the disabled population and to allow for the substitution of services when needed. This may include home visits, which otherwise might not be available, and the ability to provide assistive technologies that are customized to the individual's functional needs. Likewise, provider networks must be sufficiently broad to obtain the scope and depth of expertise needed to address the health care needs of individuals with disabilities. More important, individuals with disabilities need ready access to specialists and others who understand their constellation of needs. Similarly, the provider network needs to include principal care providers who understand the primary care needs of individuals with disabilities and who can channel individuals to downstream providers in a timely and appropriate manner.

Less clear is whether the provision of long-term services, such as personal assistance, should fall under the aegis of a health care or a social service system. On one hand, funding everything under the aegis of the health care system allows for the funding of everything from one pot and thus may induce effective substitution and mixing of services that otherwise might not be possible. On the other hand, moving long-term services from under the health care system to a social service system minimizes the risk of medicalization deemed abhorrent to many disability advocates.

Our eight characterizations also indicate that individuals with disabilities are likely to use more health care services in any given year. Data from both the United States and United Kingdom clearly indicate that individuals with disabilities do in fact have more health care encounters than individuals without disabilities. Consider, for example, health care utilization among working-age individuals. In the United States, data from the Disability Supplement to the 1994 National Health Interview Survey indicate that working-age persons who are limited in one or more activities of daily living (ADLs) comprise only 1.1 percent of the working-age population (National Center for Health Statistics 1994). Yet they account for 7.5 percent of all physician visits, 9.1 percent of all hospitalizations, and 15.8 percent of all hospital days within their age group (see Figure 26.1). Likewise, if we liberalize the definition of disability to include those with activity limitations due to a health condition, we see a more dramatic impact on the overall health care system. Individuals with some activity limitation comprise 14.2 percent of the working-age population. Yet they account for 41.6 percent of all physician visits, 50.8 percent of all hospitalizations, and 63.7 percent of all hospital days within their age group (see Figure 26.2).

In the United Kingdom, using a somewhat different definition of disability, data from the 1994 General Household Survey indicate that working-age persons who have a longstanding illness, disability, or infirmity comprise 17.2 percent of the working-age population (Office of National Statistics 1994). Yet they account for 34.7 percent of all visits to general practitioners (GPs) and account for 45.4 percent of all hospitalizations (see Figure 26.3). Utilization rates are more dramatic among men with disabilities. Working-age men who have a longstanding illness, disability, or infirmity comprise 17.8 percent of the working-age population but account for 39.8 percent of GP visits and 55.7 percent of all hospital stays.

From the standpoint of health system design, these utilization data indicate that individuals with disabilities, as high users of health care services, risk potential discrimination in market-based systems and in systems in which providers may be capitated. Thus, payment systems need to be adjusted or weighted for the risk profiles or case mix differences that individuals with disabilities present. The issue of risk selection and payment, as we will underscore later, represents a major challenge in market-based health care systems.

FROM AVERSION TO ENGAGEMENT IN HEALTH CARE ISSUES

Despite their large stake in the health care system, those in the vanguard of the disability rights and independent living movements in the United States did not become seriously engaged in health policy issues until the 1990s. Movement adherents saw organized health care as a source of their social oppression. The role of patient was antithetical to the notion of an empowered consumer. They rejected the assumptions of the sick role and the medical model (DeJong 1979; Oliver 1985; Zola 1977) that rendered the individual with a disability a passive recipient of services over which they had little control. They viewed the health care system as intrinsically paternalistic and as a system that devalued them especially when they were expected to take on the sick role indefinitely.

This aversion, however justified, also blinded the disability leadership to their enormous stake in the health care system. Their arm's-length relationship with formal health care led to a reluctance to address health policy issues and kept health policy a dormant issue for the disability community for many years. Several key events served to move health care up the disability agenda in the United States. The first event was in 1992, when the state of Oregon requested a waiver from the federal government to reallocate its Medicaid dollars in keeping with a prioritized list of services and conditions. The list was based on community ratings of various health

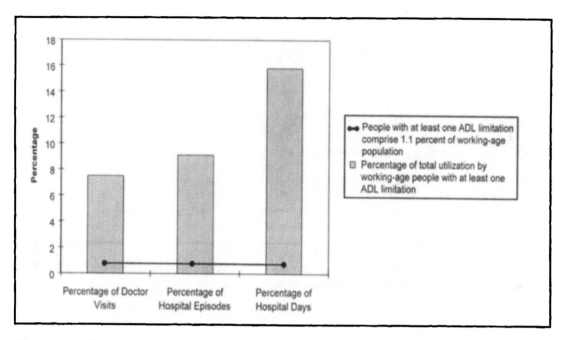

Figure 26.1. Percentage of Health Care Use by Working-Age Population with at Least One Activities of Daily Living (ADL) Limitation

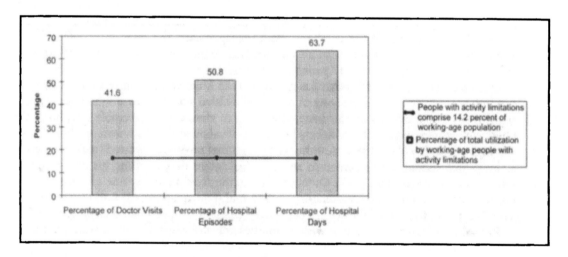

Figure 26.2. Percentage of Health Care Use by Working-Age People with Activity Limitations

and functional states. Disability advocates argued vigorously that the list reflected the negative values held by the community and thus faced undue discrimination (Menzel 1992).

The momentum of the Oregon waiver debate was sustained into the 1993 to 1994 national health care reform debate, which focused on the Clinton health care reform proposal and several other reform proposals introduced in the 103rd Congress. The disability community was very divided during the debate, mainly between those who supported the president's managed competition approach and those who supported a single-payer system because they distrusted the capacity of a market approach, even a well-regulated one, to meet their health care needs.

Since 1995, the disability community in the United States has been deeply disturbed by the rapid rise of managed care (not to be confused with managed competition), especially those forms of managed care that involve capitation payment to health care providers and require the

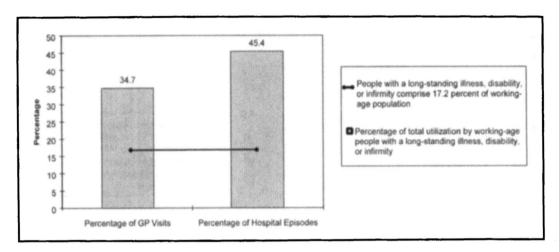

Figure 26.3. Percentage of Health Care Use in the United Kingdom by Working-Age People with a Longstanding Illness, Disability, or Infirmity, 1994

use of primary care gatekeepers to guard access to more costly specialty care. Capitation payment systems contain powerful financial incentives—mitigated only by the patient (first values of many individual health care providers)—to underserve individuals with high health care needs such as individuals with disabilities. Likewise, gatekeeping requirements may significantly limit a person's access to the specialists believed by many individuals with disabilities to be better equipped to meet their more complex health care needs (Sutton and DeJong 1998). Since 1998, in response to the concerns about managed care, the disability community has joined the debate on how best to regulate managed health plans, and it has supported proposed federal and state legislation for a "patients' bill of rights."

One other issue of the 1990s that has galvanized the American disability community in addressing health care issues is the issue of physician-assisted suicide. The disability community remains somewhat divided on this issue. One point of view, the more visible one, holds that physician-assisted suicide reflects deeply held societal values about the worth of a life of a person with a disability (Asch 1998). Another view holds that physician-assisted suicide represents a choice that should not be denied to an individual intent on exercising his or her right of self-determination (Batavia 1997). Others argue that the decision to take one's life is sometimes borne of desperation in a discriminatory society, and if adequate services and supports were available, the individual might not choose suicide (Basnett, Koperski, and Grumbach 2000).

Regardless of where individuals with disabilities fall with respect to these issues, the 1990s have placed health policy on a footing with other longstanding policy issues such as transportation, housing, and personal assistance issues. The hands-off attitude of previous decades has given way to a fuller engagement on health policy issues.

Individuals with disabilities in the United Kingdom have had less ambivalence about health care and their participation in health policy issues. Like their counterparts in the United States, disability leaders in the United Kingdom share much of the same apprehension about the medical model and the sick role that is sometimes conferred on individuals with disabilities. In the United Kingdom, however, individuals with disabilities are more politically vested in their health care and social service systems because they see their systems as more indispensable to their daily well-being. Impairment-specific disability groups have been very active on health care issues.

More recently, people with disabilities in the United Kingdom have become alarmed by the potential risks of the United Kingdom's emerging "internal market" approach to health care, which we will discuss later in this chapter. They fear becoming victims of rationing as decisions about resource allocation become more explicit. Their fear mirrors some of the angst of their American counterparts with respect to managed care. Generally speaking, however, individuals with disabilities in the United Kingdom continue to have a more favorable view of government beneficence than their American counterparts, who have a more mixed view of government—a view that alternates between government as ally and protector and government as inept and unresponsive.

An emerging health care issue in the United Kingdom, which is currently less prominent in the United States, is the challenge of the human genome project, which presents an enormous potential for new interventions that can prevent, eliminate, or ameliorate fatal or disabling illnesses and diseases. It also presents the potential to bar code each individual with a genetic risk profile. If misused, as disability advocates fear, such profiles can discriminate against individuals with disabilities as potential high-cost users to be averted in the health care system, especially among providers who may be capitated and at financial risk for the populations they serve. Advances in human genetics may also someday present the potential to alter one's genetic heritage and produce offspring deemed more physically and mentally superior (i.e., eugenics). The main concern to individuals with disabilities is that individuals without these socially valued characteristics will be devalued with enormous consequences for both health and social policy.

In one sense, individuals with disabilities have always had a major stake in their respective health care systems because they need and use disproportionately more health care services than do those without disabilities. However, with increased awareness and organization, individuals with disabilities are gradually also becoming stakeholders in the political processes that shape their health care systems. Still, their participation in health policymaking circles remains below the level expected of a group with so much at stake.

FOUR CROSS-NATIONAL PHENOMENA

During the last decades of the twentieth century, four phenomena raised anew some of the difficult health policy choices that societies and their respective citizens with disabilities face. The first event was the demise of the Soviet Union and its grip on Central Europe. This event caused the countries of Central Europe in particular to address anew the extent to which their health systems should rely on state-based or market-based mechanisms to ensure access and accountability. More important, this event has given new legitimacy to entertaining market-based solutions throughout the world. Following the Soviet Union's dissolution, some even argue that liberal (in the traditional sense of the term), market-based democratic systems represent the highest point of historic development (e.g., Fukuyama 1992).

The demise of the Soviet Union also helped to create the conditions for the second phenomenon—namely, the emergence of a new international system to replace the bipolar world created by the cold war. Friedman (1999) refers to this system as "globalization" and argues that it entails "the inexorable integration of markets, nation-states, and technologies." To survive and thrive in the new international system, nations must let market forces rule their economies. Friedman argues that as international markets become more integrated—as they already are in capital markets—nation-states will have to harmonize their economic and social policies. Nations, he argues, will have to

make the private sector the primary engine of growth, maintain a low rate of inflation . . . shrink the size of their state bureaucracies, maintain as close to a balanced budget as possible . . . lower tariffs . . . make their currencies convertible . . . open their industries, stock and bond markets to direct foreign ownership and investment . . . and allow their citizens to choose from an array of competing pension options and foreign-run pension and mutual funds. (Friedman 1999:86-87)

In short, nations will find themselves in a "straitjacket" that narrows their economic and social policy options. No nation can be too far out of line with respect to wages and tax rates if it wants to succeed in the new system (Friedman 1999; Thurow 1996). In terms of health care, the new system also increases pressures to dampen health care expenditures and legitimizes the use of market forces to curtail the growth of health care services.

The third phenomenon is the economic stagnation and high levels of unemployment in many Western European countries that date back to the early 1980s and persist in most countries, with such notable exceptions as the United Kingdom and the Netherlands (Delaney and Gossing 1999). This phenomenon has caused Western European nations to reexamine their high labor costs and social welfare expenditures to become more competitive within both the European and global economies. This reexamination dovetails with what has been a growing antitax mood within the electorates of some Western European countries. Moreover, Western European nations are attempting to pare down their persistently high national deficits to meet the deficit targets set forth in the Maastricht agreement, pursuant to the establishment of a single European monetary system. In the face of these economic pressures, Western European governments have become more willing to entertain market-based solutions as a way of bringing greater fiscal discipline to the delivery of health services while retaining their longstanding commitment to "social solidarity" as a key societal value (Jacobs 1998). The conditions of participation in Europe's new monetary system represent a microcosm of Friedman's (1999) new world order.

The fourth phenomenon is an intellectual one—namely, the concept of *managed competition* made popular by Alain Enthoven in the 1970s, 1980s, and 1990s. The concept of managed competition—again, not to be confused with *managed care*—responded to the inherent propensity of American health care markets to fail by competing on prestige and risk and not on price and quality. The theory of managed competition basically maintains that for competition to serve key health policy goals, it must be managed by the state or quasi-state bodies ("sponsors") that will set the rules for a more level playing field. The theory of managed competition appeals to market advocates because it tries to more nearly approximate the conditions required in the economic theory of "perfect competition." It also appeals to state advocates because it provides a clear role for the state as rule maker and referee. The theory of managed competition also resonates with the advocates of a "third way," championed by the Tony Blairs and Bill Clintons of this world who reject traditional left-right political dichotomies.

Today, elements of the theory of managed competition have made their way into the health care reforms and health care reform proposals of many Western nations (Jacobs 1998; Le Grand 1999). Other nations have not necessarily embraced the theory of managed competition in its American forms but have found ways in which to inject elements of competition to foster greater price and cost discipline in their respective systems. Health care reforms in the United Kingdom, Holland, and Germany are replete with references to managed competition (Jacobs 1998).

THEORY OF MANAGED COMPETITION

The theory of managed competition responds to the difficulty of attaining the basic conditions needed to make health care markets compete effectively on price and quality. Health care markets typically violate nearly all the conditions required in the theory of "perfect competition." Markets rarely, if ever, meet all the conditions of perfect competition, but to the extent that conditions are reasonably attained, markets are said to be competitive. An example of failure is the absence of a "homogeneous product" or, in the parlance of health care, the lack of a reasonably standardized benefit package that would enable Americans to make price and quality comparisons across health plans. Another failure is the lack of information about health care quality that purchasers and consumers can use to evaluate health care providers and health plans in terms of access to preventive services, consumer satisfaction, and health outcomes. Yet another failure is the presence of "externalities" in which costs are externalized or shifted to parties' external transactions. American health care, in particular, is replete with cost shifting.

Perhaps the most notorious failure in the American system—and one most relevant to the concerns of individuals with disabilities—is the problem of risk selection in which health plans and capitated providers avoid enrolling and serving high-cost patients to achieve a healthy bottom line. Health plans resort to a variety of strategies to enroll low-risk subscribers. Also, health plans that provide excellent services to subscribers with disabilities and chronic illnesses risk attracting higher risk populations.

The theory of managed competition seeks to redress these kinds of market failure by creating new rules that approximate more nearly the conditions of perfect competition, recognizing that perfect competition is never fully attainable. In short, the competition, if it is to be effective, needs to be managed and not left unfettered. Enthoven's (1993) theory of managed competition begins with the concept of a "sponsor" that sponsors an insured population and sets the rules by which health plans enroll and serve the population being sponsored. Sponsors may include, for example, large employers, government agencies, or health alliances of sufficient size to exercise clout in the marketplace.

In managed competition, sponsors invite proposals from health plans, specify the services to be included in a standardized benefit package, identify the indicators of health plan quality that each health plan must provide, manage the enrollment process, and risk-adjust health plan payment to help neutralize risk competition. For competition to work effectively, consumers must have a choice of health plans and be able to switch health plans at periodic intervals. In managed competition theory, competition needs to take place principally at the health plan level, not at the provider level, mainly because demand is much less price elastic when consumers seek out a provider to address an existing health condition. In other words, consumers are not in a good bargaining position with providers when they are already ill and desperately need a particular health care service. Instead, they have the most leverage as members of a larger group that can represent them and negotiate prices with health plans.

The Theory's Impact in the United States

The theory of managed competition shaped many of the health care reform proposals that surfaced in the United States in the early 1990s. Its features not only found their way into the Clinton health plan but also in many of the proposals sponsored by Republicans. Indeed, there were differences about the extent of universal health care coverage, the scope of proposed benefit packages, voluntary versus mandatory enrollment in health alliances (sponsors), the use of the federal tax code, and the extent of government oversight. However, these differences are minor compared to their common elements, such as the greater standardization of benefits, the use of health alliances to organize the demand side of the market, and the need for some degree of oversight.

The theory of managed competition remains the intellectual point of departure in the United States even today, when less than full-scale health reform ideas are proposed, debated, and implemented. For example, the Medicare + Choice program, authorized under the Balanced Budget Act of 1997, contains many managed competition theory features. Likewise, the report of the President's Advisory Commission on Consumer Protection and Quality in the Health Care Industry (1998) is replete with managed competition concepts. Though seldom invoked by name—probably because of its resemblance to the tarnished reputation of managed care—managed competition theory and its preconditions remain the benchmarks by which American policy analysts and elites evaluate market performance and evaluate public programs such as Medicaid managed care. In short, it remains the dominant paradigm that continues to shape policy alternatives at both the federal and state levels: Most proposals for reform seek to strengthen one or more key assumptions in the theory of managed competition.

The Theory's Impact in the United Kingdom

Enthoven's (1985) theory springs largely from an American experience, and its principal features address market failures that are peculiar to the American system of competing private health plans. While grounded in the American experience, Enthoven's theory has had a profound impact on the thinking of health policy analysts and economists in other parts of the world (Jacobs 1998; Le Grand 1999). In the United Kingdom, the impact has been more direct. In 1985, Enthoven wrote a paper in which he proposed an "internal market" for the National Health Service (NHS) (Enthoven 1985). More specifically, he proposed that each district health authority (DHA) be viewed as a health maintenance organization (HMO) that would receive a risk-adjusted payment to provide or purchase care for all district inhabitants. It could purchase care from providers within or outside the district and thus create competitive markets internal to the NHS. There would be a distinct split between purchasers and providers. The competition would not be at the health plan level because there would be only one DHA in a given geographic area, but it would be at the provider level. Providers would be made to compete on both price and quality.

In 1991, the Thatcher government reformed the NHS by creating "internal markets" as envisioned by Enthoven, except that the Thatcher reforms created two types of purchasers—namely, DHAs and large physician practices or "general practice (GP) fundholders." The success of these reforms is widely debated, in part, because there were few independent studies to evaluate their effects (Basnett et al. 2000; Dixon 1998; Koperski, Basnett, and Grumbach 1999; Le Grand 1999; Le Grand, Mays, and Mulligan 1998; Light 1997). Overall, the reforms appear to have had minimal success, in part, because the preconditions for competition were limited. For example, most districts already had a limited hospital capacity—unlike the excess capacity in American hospitals—and the system provided major barriers to market entry. Many larger hospitals occupied oligopolistic or monopolistic positions within their respective districts.

The creation of internal markets reflected the Thatcher government's broader interest in privitization of functions that were previously managed by the public sector (Mechanic 1995). Private health care was made more accessible through tax incentives, and public-private partnerships were encouraged to fund capital developments such as new hospitals.

After it came to power in 1997, the Blair government claimed to have eliminated internal markets but in fact retained several key features. Under the Blair government, all GPs have become members of primary care groups (PCGs) consisting of 20 to 50 GPs serving populations of about 100,000. PCGs can choose to assume greater autonomy from DHAs and take on greater responsibility for activities previously assigned to DHAs (e.g., budgeting) or assumed by GP fundholders. Thus, PCGs can choose to take on a wide range of roles—from those that are largely advisory in nature to those that are more administrative in nature. In the latter case, it can become a freestanding entity known as a primary care trust (PCT) and can take on the purchasing functions previously assigned to DHAs and GP fundholders. PCTs can also take the responsibility for providing some community services.

With increased role delegation to PCGs and PCTs, DHAs' most important role is a strategic planning one, under the auspices of what is known as the Health Improvement Program (HImP). Under the program, DHAs' responsibilities are to foster collaboration among providers, encourage the development of centers of excellence, and set standards for accountability. PCGs and hospitals can still retain their financial surpluses, but there is a more collaborative approach with DHAs as to their use in keeping with the HImP than with self-determined priorities. Thus, under the Blair reforms, cooperation replaces competition between providers and replaces the strained relationships between purchasers and providers. PCGs can, nonetheless, exercise its ultimate sanction by not purchasing from an institutional provider—although most hospitals are often deemed too large and too few to allow failure. In short, the purchaser-provider split introduced by the Thatcher government is retained.

The introduction of "internal markets" in the United Kingdom needs to be considered within a larger public health context. Britain has always had a much stronger geographic- and population-based health-planning tradition than has the United States, and that tradition is retained, if not strengthened, with the local DHAs' focus on strategic planning and collaboration. Market forces, to the extent that they exist in the United Kingdom, are intended to service specific population-based public health objectives. This is in marked contrast to the United States, which has a weaker health-planning tradition and where market forces are not steered by larger, agreed-on, public health objectives. Contrary to its promise, managed care in the United States has not achieved this level of public health planning. There are several excellent examples in which managed care has introduced selected population-level interventions in the form of immunizations, cancer screenings, and diabetes management but only for the population enrolled in the managed care plan.

The Larger Message

In looking at the different ways in which managed competition theory has affected thinking and policy in the United States and in the United Kingdom, one should not lose sight of the larger message for other nations implicit in the U.K. experience. The U.K. experience signals that it may be politically safe to at least test market-based approaches in nations that historically have relied on state-administered systems. While managed competition theory may have its origins in an American context, the theory's influence has washed onto other shores. Yet one should be cautious in extrapolating from the U.K. experience because the concept of "internal markets" and its successors were never meant to replace health care as a public good or to convert health care into a private commodity. Even under the Thatcher government, the incentives for individual gain via the market were almost absent.

Some observe that there has been a "North Atlantic convergence on managed competition" (Organization for Economic Cooperation and Development [OECD] 1994). Others dispute this observation, underscoring the enormous differences between nations and their respective health care systems (Jacobs 1998). Again, the larger point is sometimes lost in this debate. There is a greater willingness across nations to test market concepts, however limited in their respective health care systems, in the search for a more efficient and a more nimble health care system that can respond better to changing conditions and consumer preferences.

The U.K. experience also underscores that state-administered and market-driven approaches often coexist, sometimes uncomfortably, and that the boundaries between public and private sectors are often blurred as they also are in the United States. We want to make clear that we are not attempting to contrast "free-market" and "socialized" health systems and that such contrasts are analytically misleading and distort the choices that societies are trying to make. Managed competition means the introduction of rules that govern those segments of health care that have been "marketized" to induce greater efficiencies and greater responsiveness to individual health needs.

Managed Competition and Individuals with Disabilities

The issue at hand is whether managed competition can work for individuals with disabilities. More generally, can market-based features serve the interests of individuals with disabilities, or are they inherently incompatible with the interests of individuals with disabilities whose needs, on average, are well above the needs of those without disabilities? To answer these questions, we identify 10 features or conditions of managed competition and evaluate these features in terms of their compatibility with the needs, interests, and values of individuals with disabilities. We will attempt to show that the various features of managed competition, when implemented *collectively and rigorously,* are mutually reinforcing and hold considerable promise for individuals with disabilities. We also argue that halfway measures, often seen in today's managed care systems in the United States, can make things worse for individuals with disabilities.

The theory of managed competition argues that certain assumptions or conditions must be obtained if health care markets are to work effectively. Many of these conditions, as noted earlier, derive from the neoclassical theory of "perfect competition" and address the structural weaknesses of the American system. In short, in the absence of perfect competition, what rules or conditions must be in place to make health care markets work? In Figure 26.4 we outline 10 conditions—many of which have been proposed in one form or another by others (Enthoven 1993). Collectively, if all 10 conditions are met, the system would, theoretically, be prone to compete on price and quality as in other types of markets—not on risk selection, which remains a great concern to individuals with disabilities. Nearly all health care reform proposals seek to introduce or strengthen one or more of these conditions. Very few, if any, markets have been able to meet all of these conditions.

These conditions derive from the American experience and could, at least theoretically, be adapted to the U.K. health system in a number of ways given its new structure under the Blair government. For example, if the American brand of managed competition theory were rigorously and fully applied to the U.K. system, each DHA would act as a sponsor or purchaser by issuing requests for proposal (RFPs) to competing PCGs within a geographic area for a standardized benefit package, make price and quality information about each PCG network available to the district population, and conduct the enrollment. Once a year, or at some other interval, consumers would choose among competing PCG networks, and the DHA would allocate risk-adjusted or weighted capitated funds based on the risk profile of each PCG's enrolled membership. Such a system would bring competition at the consumer level as well as the provider level, where downstream providers now compete or contract with individual PCGs. Currently, quality information is largely designed for consumption by entities other than individual consumers. Naturally, such a system would reallocate existing responsibilities among DHAs, PCGs, and individual providers. DHAs would, nonetheless, retain their planning and needs assessment functions or could delegate some of the health screening and data collection tasks to PCGs as a condition for participation.

The conditions of managed competition are meant to be mutually reinforcing. In fact, individual conditions implemented in isolation are not nearly as effective as when they are implemented concurrently. Consider, for example, an issue of great concern to individuals with disabilities (i.e., risk competition or creaming). We can reduce risk competition by adjusting health plan or PCG payment for risk or case mix differences (Condition 7). We can reduce risk competition even further if one or more of the following conditions are also met: Condition 1d, in which sponsors create and enforce marketing and enrollment rules; Condition 3, in which health plans use standardized benefit packages and thus are unable to attract low-risk groups by tweaking their benefit packages; and Condition 8, in which health care quality and disenrollment rates are adjusted for risk. Moreover, conditions designed to stimulate quality competition will help to neutralize risk competition as well. Fortunately, there are few unpleasant policy trade-offs among these 10 conditions.

From a health systems perspective, individuals with disabilities are concerned mainly about five issues: access, price, quality, risk selection, and choice. To facilitate our discussion here, we have grouped these concerns into three sets of issues or dimensions:

access,

price-and-quality competition versus risk competition,

medical paternalism versus consumer choice and self-determination.

All are interrelated. The issue at hand is the extent to which the 10 conditions of managed competition adequately address these three sets of concerns that individuals with disabilities have about the nature of their health care system and how these 10 conditions can be used to evaluate the responsiveness of existing U.S. and U.K. systems. We believe that these conditions, in turn, can become a framework in which to evaluate the adequacy and responsiveness of other health care systems to the needs and concerns of individuals with disabilities.

1. **Sponsorship.** There is an entity that is capable of organizing the demand side of the market into sufficiently large groups. The entity

   a. issues requests for proposals (RFPs),
   b. negotiates with health plans or provider networks,
   c. makes price and quality information available to subscribers, and
   d. creates and enforces the rules for marketing and enrollment during open enrollment periods.

   Sponsors may include employers, government agencies, and health alliances.

2. **Price taking.** No health plan or provider network is dominant enough to set the price. They are price takers, not price makers.

3. **Standardization.** Health plans or provider networks have (a) one or more *standardized benefit packages* that will enable sponsors and individual consumers to compare price and quality differences among plans and networks. All plans and networks use (b) *standardized definitions of medical necessity* to help create predictability and minimize transaction costs.

4. **Consumer choice.** Consumers have a choice of health plans or provider networks and can switch plans and networks during designated open enrollment periods. Once in a plan, a consumer is limited to the provider network unless willing to pay an additional amount to obtain services from a nonnetwork provider.

5. **Accessible information.** Both sponsors and consumers must have accessible information about price and quality across health plans and provider networks to make informed choices.

6. **Financial risks.** Health plans and providers accept financial risk to encourage efficiency and financial discipline.

7. **Risk adjustment for payment.** Health plans and provider networks receive risk-adjusted payments or other adjustments for "cost outliers" to minimize risk selection and risk competition.

8. **Risk adjustment for quality.** Health plans and provider networks receive risk-adjusted quality scores to neutralize the impact of case mix on quality indictors (e.g., consumer satisfaction, outcomes, disenrollment rates). Disenrollment rates are risk-adjusted to encourage health plans and networks to retain more costly subscribers and optimize interventions over the long run.

9. **Rule-making body.** A public or quasi-public organization sets the rules for the competition to create a level playing field, encourage price and quality competition, and discourage risk competition.

10. **Governance.** The overall system should be governed predominantly by individuals representing the consumer side of the market. The health plan and provider sides of the market should be represented in the governance structure but should never dominate.

Figure 26.4. The Conditions of Managed Competition

Access

A paramount issue for individuals with disabilities is whether they have access to the services, the equipment they need, and providers who understand their particular constellation of health care need. Such needs include primary care needs and needs specific to the nature of their impairment and functional abilities outlined earlier in this chapter. Moreover, individuals with disabilities want physical, clinical, and financial accessibility, that is, facilities and clinical programs that are barrier free and affordable. Access will depend on a sponsor (Condition 1) that includes these concerns in its RFPs and on the health plan benefit package (Condition 3a). Moreover, standardized definitions of medical necessity (Condition 3b) that address the functional needs of disabled persons are required. Ultimately, access depends, in large part, on the degree to which risk competition is effectively neutralized. Access will always be limited if sponsors, health plans, or providers view people with disabilities as high-risk groups to be avoided.

Risk Competition versus Price-and-Quality Competition

We have already noted how risk competition can be minimized and perhaps eliminated by the mutually reinforcing nature of several managed competition conditions. Yet if risk competition is to be adequately neutralized, there must be effective price-and-quality (PQ) competition to replace it. PQ competition is typical of most product and service markets (e.g., automobiles, home appliances, lodging, and food services). The absence of effective PQ competition in health care is one of the reasons why health care markets fail or remain in arrested states of development. The difficulty in attaining genuine PQ competition in health care is also one of the reasons why some countries have chosen not to use a market-based approach to health care delivery.

PQ competition depends on nearly all of the conditions outlined in Figure 26.4. It depends on Condition 1 because without a sponsor, there is no entity to make price and quality information uniformly available to consumers and purchasers. It depends on Condition 2 because without price taking, health plans or provider networks do not have to present bids that are lower than those of their competitors. It depends on Condition 3 because without standardization, consumers and purchasers cannot make price and quality comparisons across health plans and providers. It depends on Condition 4 because without choice, there is no PQ competition. It depends on Condition 5 because without accessible information about price and quality, purchasers and consumers cannot make informed choices. It depends on Condition 6 because without financial risk, health plans and providers are not financially motivated to make the trade-offs in resource allocation. It depends on Condition 8 because without risk adjustment for quality, sponsors and consumers cannot make sound quality comparisons across health plans and providers. It depends on Condition 9 because without a rule-making body, there cannot be clear rules for price and quality outcome disclosures that lead to standardization. It depends on Condition 10 because without consumer governance, the information needs of consumers are less likely to be met.

Medical Paternalism versus Consumer Choice and Self-Determination

Historically, the culture of health care had a strong element of paternalism, where the provider was presumed to know what was best for the patient. As noted at the beginning of this chapter, one hallmark of the disability rights and independent living movements has been their aversion to this cultural trait in health care. Much of this paternalism has dissipated as a more assertive consumer population, both inside and outside the disability community, has learned to take greater control over its own health care and well-being.

Medical paternalism has been more a function of the culture of health care and less a function of market conditions. Nonetheless, medical paternalism is more strongly associated with select market characteristics. Interestingly, opposite ends of the market continuum are more likely to have vestiges of medical paternalism. Top-down, command-and-control health care systems such as the United Kingdom's old NHS prior to internal markets, as well as its opposite, less fettered market of American fee-for-service health care, are both more prone to have significant dollops of medical paternalism. The culture of top-down organizations simply does not permit much consumer choice and self-determination. While one would expect the opposite in a more unfettered market-based system, the old American fee-for-service system was a provider-dominated one. Patients acquired health care services largely on provider terms, in part, because providers also had most of the information—or what economists call information asymmetry in the marketplace.

The antidote to the information asymmetry problem in health care is to arm the consumer with as much information as possible about health plan and provider quality (Conditions 5 and

8) and then further arm the consumer with meaningful choices (Condition 4). Informed choice is strengthened in a system that favors standardization of health plan benefits (Condition 2) and is governed ultimately by the consumer side of the market (Condition 10).

The consumer choice condition (Condition 4) of managed competition remains, however, a difficult issue for individuals with disabilities mainly because the choice is principally at the health plan level and less at the provider level. In the United States, once in a health plan, the consumer is expected to use providers within the health plan's network. For individuals with disabilities, this can be problematic because they may not find a provider or physician they believe is adequately informed and equipped to address their particular constellation of health care needs—although they may have the option to obtain an out-of-plan provider at some additional cost. Yet, by neutralizing risk competition and making individuals with disabilities an attractive market segment, health plans theoretically would be encouraged to include providers who are knowledgeable about the needs of individuals with disabilities.

Framework for Assessment

The theory of managed competition and our knowledge of the issues that are important to individuals with disabilities present us with a framework that enables us to assess American and British systems. It also allows us to generalize, to some extent, beyond the American and British experiences to other health care systems.

The American and British systems provide sufficient levels of contrast that allow one to postulate the existence of a continuum of health systems in terms of the extent to which they rely on state-controlled mechanisms versus the unfettered market. This continuum is depicted as the horizontal axis in both Figures 26.5 and 26.6. Along this continuum, we can depict five different systems:

(A) the United Kingdom's NHS prior to the introduction of "internal markets,"

(B) the United Kingdom's NHS under the Blair reforms,

(C) an ideal managed competition system that includes all 10 features,

(D) U.S. managed care (not managed competition) as we know it today, and

(E) an unfettered (i.e., no government rules) fee-for-service market system.

This last system, System E, never fully existed but represents one end of our continuum. Although it had a fair amount of government regulation, the rapidly fading American fee-for-service health care system came reasonably close to such a system. The distance between each system type in Figures 26.5 and 26.6 is arbitrary. We place System C, managed competition, in the very center of the horizontal axis for convenience only. One could make an argument for shifting managed competition more to one end or the other end of the continuum. The relationships depicted in Figures 26.5 and 26.6 are meant to be neuristic, not exact.

Figures 26.5 and 26.6 have different continua on their vertical axes. In Figure 26.5, we contrast price-and-risk competition with price-and-quality competition. In Figure 26.6, we contrast medical paternalism with consumer choice and self-determination. Both of these contrasts can be considered continua.

Our proposed framework does not necessarily address all the dimensions of a good health care system. One might argue, for example, that the U.K. system is better at identifying the health care needs of an entire population within a given geographic area. It is thus better at prioritizing public health measures such as immunizations that benefit the entire population, including people with disabilities, than a pure managed competition system that caters to individual preferences in which the needs of people with disabilities might not be fully addressed. Others might argue that a risk-adjusted managed competition system would be better incent-

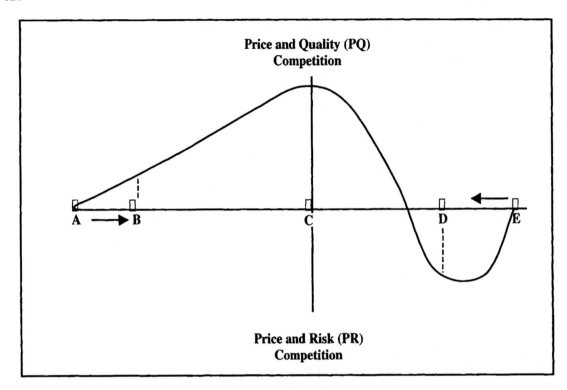

Figure 26.5.   Price and Quality Competition versus Price and Risk Competition

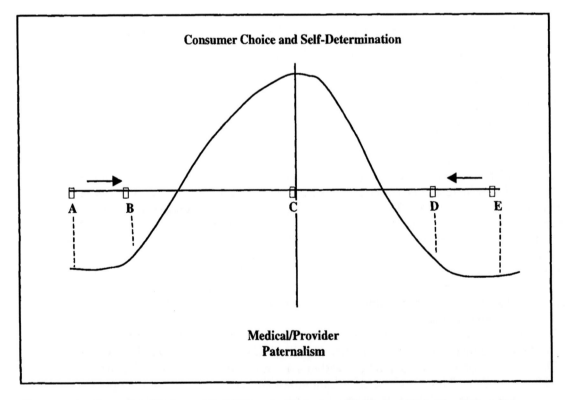

Figure 26.6.   Consumer Choice and Self-Determination versus Medical and Provider Paternalism

ivized to address the specific needs of individuals with disabilities that might be overlooked in broad public health measures.

Responsiveness of U.S. and U.K. Systems

U.S. System (Systems D and E)

Experiences of Individuals with Disabilities under Fee-for-Service Health Care (System E). Individuals with disabilities had very mixed experiences with the fading American fee-for-service system. They had relatively good access to providers of their choice—if they could find providers who were knowledgeable about their particular array of health care needs. Moreover, there was reasonable access to specialists and other downstream providers. On the downside, there was little coordination between primary care providers and specialists.

In the fee-for-service system, the individual provider was king, and the system overall could be described as a provider-driven system (DeJong and Sutton 1995). The system was replete with medical paternalism and all the baggage that came with it. Consumers had little access to information (Condition 5) that would enable them to make informed choices about either health plans or providers. As noted earlier, there was considerable asymmetry of information between the provider and consumer sides of the market, with providers holding most of the cards.

The fee-for-service system competed on risk at the health plan level; that is, health plans wanted to ensure a lower-risk population to attain a profitable bottom line—just as they do now. Risk competition at the health plan level, however, was mitigated at the provider level since providers were not at financial risk and were paid on a fee-for-service, not on a capitation basis. There was no financial incentive for stinting. In fact, there were powerful incentives to provide too much. Providers instead competed on prestige—namely, their use of the latest technology, the academic credentials of their medical staffs, their academic affiliations, the bed size of their health care facilities, and their acquisition of research grants. The system, particularly academic health centers, was willing to take on more complex and costly cases such as individuals with disabilities, although acute care medicine commanded greater prestige than chronic care medicine. The problem with prestige competition is that it led to a lack of financial discipline, a technological arms race among institutional providers, tremendous excess capacity, and runaway health care costs.

In terms of our 10 features of managed competition, providers tended to be price makers rather than price takers (Condition 2) under fee-for-service health care. While government price setting is quite common today in American health care—particularly in the Medicare program for hospital and physician services—providers balked at length about becoming price takers rather than price makers. Few other pro-consumer features were present in the system, in part, because the regulatory apparatus was underdeveloped and could not compel the system to behave differently. Moreover, in a largely private system, the government did not have near the leverage as it does now to shape system behavior.

Experiences of Individuals with Disabilities under Today's Managed Care System (System D). The problem with the American system today is that it has introduced financial risk (Condition 6) in the form of capitated managed care, but it has not introduced other conditions needed to mitigate the downside effects of financial risk such as the incentives to stint on services. Nor have federal and state governments been willing to establish the conditions needed to foster effective price-and-quality competition. More specifically, the American health care system has failed to introduce standardization (Condition 3), provide accessible information about price and quality (Condition 5), risk-adjust health plan payment (Condition 7) and quality indicators (Condition 8), or provide for adequate rule making (Condition 9) and governance (Condition 10). Some of these conditions are being met in somewhat embryonic form as in the case of health plan report cards (Condition 5), and several of these conditions are being introduced in the Medicare + Choice and Medicaid managed care programs. In short, the American system has yet to attain the conditions needed for an effective market-based health care system and remains stuck in its transition to real managed competition.

The arrested state of development in American health care may also account for the widespread disenchantment with managed care. Because it is partially stuck in the transition toward a real managed competition system, it now has the worst features of both the old and the current system. Americans remain unwilling to introduce all the features of managed competition because these features require new rules and regulations—something anathema to the American creed of the "free" market and American ambivalence about, if not outright hostility toward, government. Americans have moved toward managed competition but have not yet fully embraced it.

In the American system, the needs of individuals with disabilities have never been well served, even under the fading fee-for-service system. Under managed care—again, not to be confused with managed competition—many individuals with disabilities believe that their access to and the management of health care services have become worse. The empirical evidence for the efficacy of managed care among higher-need populations remains very mixed (Luft 1998; Ware 1996). Beatty, Burden, and DeJong (1999) find that individuals with disabilities are generally more satisfied with their access to primary care but are less satisfied with their access to specialists, prescription drugs, and assistive technology. It is difficult to determine if the expressed disenchantment of many disabled individuals with managed care arrangements reflects grievances with managed care per se or reflects a new awareness of disabled individuals with the shortcomings of the overall American health care system. In short, would individuals with disabilities be any less vocal today if they had to put up with the shortcomings of yesterday's fee-for-service system?

Theoretically, at least, managed care offers great promise for a more coordinated delivery of health care services for Americans with disabilities. Some providers have seized the opportunity to provide better-organized health care for working-age individuals with disabilities. Three examples include the Community Medical Alliance in the Boston area, the Shepherd Care Network in Atlanta, Georgia, and the Community Living Alliance in Wisconsin. All three programs are Medicaid-sponsored delivery systems, and all three serve limited numbers of disabled individuals carved out from the larger Medicaid population. Consumer satisfaction within these programs appears high. Similar experiences have been reported in the PACE (Program for All-Inclusive Care for the Elderly) programs targeted to older Americans with disabilities. PACE projects include long-term services and provide effective integration between acute and long-term care.

These programs are the exceptions; they tend to be customized to very narrowly defined subsets of the population and rely heavily on the federal-state Medicaid program, which, unlike Medicare or private health plans, also includes funding for long-term care services. Another common feature of these programs is the presence of one or more individuals or physicians who have made accessible and adequate health care for people with disabilities their special cause. These programs illustrate how the upheaval fomented by managed care has created a willingness to develop and test new delivery systems. This observation is in marked contrast to the United Kingdom, where decentralized innovation and experimentation are less likely to occur, even though the flexibility given to PCGs may spawn new systems to accommodate the needs of individuals with disabilities.

If anything, the disaffection that many Americans, including Americans with disabilities, have with managed care, in general, reflects a larger reality—namely, the arrested transition to real managed competition. It may also explain the demands for "patient bill-of-rights" legislation. Consumers believe that under managed care, providers are forced to pay more attention to the financial concerns of health plans and less attention to the health needs of individual patients. In addition, individuals with disabilities believe they are unattractive patients in a system that competes on price and risk. Under effective PQ competition, providers are, at least theoretically, more prone to balance their fiduciary responsibility to the patient with their financial accountability to the payer.

Responsiveness of the U.K. System (Systems A and B)

Despite the changes that have occurred during the Thatcher and Blair governments, they have not had a material effect on how consumers experience and perceive their interactions with their health care system. Most of the changes have occurred at the "wholesale level" rather than the "retail level." Consumers remain largely oblivious to the differences between GP fundholders or PCGs and their contractual arrangements with specialists, hospitals, and postacute providers. Their principal concern is the selection of a GP, not the PCG or its larger network of providers—and even that selection remains extremely limited. Individual consumers still obtain their primary care from a local GP within the catchment area in which they live. Consumer choice with respect to GP remains limited. Compared with the United States, the number of GPs available within a catchment area can be quite limited and even more so when GPs close their already busy practices to new patients. This state of affairs can be problematic for individuals with disabilities who have the added task of locating GPs who have the knowledge and skills needed to address their particular array of health care needs.

Still, consumers with disabilities look to their local GP as their principal gateway into the rest of the health care system, and many receive a service they consider excellent. As in some other European countries (e.g., the Netherlands), the local primary care physician has had a strong gatekeeping role that is more institutionally entrenched than it is in the United States. To some extent, this is a cultural difference. Americans with disabilities chafe at the gatekeeping role that managed care organizations have established for primary care physicians. Americans with disabilities often perceive gatekeepers as unnecessary barriers to more the specialized services they need. Moreover, gatekeeping flies in the face of American individualism—Americans do not want people telling them what they can or cannot do.

Although financial incentives for risk competition did exist for GP fundholders during the Thatcher regime and do exist for PCGs and individual GPs under the Blair regime, empirical evidence of significant risk competition has yet to be uncovered. Thus, in the United Kingdom, people with disabilities do not face the same barriers accessing health care that Americans with disabilities do as a result of risk competition. As in the United States, individuals with disabilities in the United Kingdom are not, for the most part, represented in health system governance at the national, regional, or district level. There is a fair amount of discussion about the involvement of individuals with disabilities; however, to date, little has happened.

In comparing the relative responsiveness of American and British systems, we need to bear in mind that the United Kingdom spends only 6.8 percent of its gross domestic product for health care, while the United States spends 13.9 percent, with only marginal differences in key health indicators such as life expectancy. On a per capita basis, the United Kingdom annually spends only one-third ($1,391) of what the United States spends ($4,095) on health care (Koperski et al. 1999; OECD 1999). People with disabilities in the United Kingdom participate in a system that is inherently more paternalistic but one that is also financially more efficient. Moreover, it is a system that provides for population-based needs assessment, health care planning, and public health interventions, such as screening and health promotion. It is also a system that provides a stronger linkage between health care and social services (Leutz 1999).

OVERALL ASSESSMENT

In writing this chapter, we have brought different perspectives about the role of markets and their ability to adequately address the needs of individuals with disabilities. Regardless of one's beliefs about the efficacy of market mechanisms, the conditions of managed competition serve as a useful checklist by which to evaluate the performance of different health systems. The conditions of managed competition contain many features of great interest to individuals with disabilities as consumers of health services. People with disabilities want, for example, clarity about the benefits available through their health plan (Condition 3), they want choice (Condition 4), they want useful information about quality (Condition 5), they want no adverse financial incentives (Condition 7), they want to make sure that their government is keeping a watchful eye on the system (Condition 9), and they want to be represented in the governance of the overall system (Condition 10).

We have used managed competition theory as a filter by which to evaluate the strengths and weaknesses of various health care systems. This chapter is not meant to be an endorsement of managed competition as the sole basis for organizing a health care system, although it does address, at least in theory, many of the weaknesses of other systems. The Achilles heel of a market-based system is its ability, or inability, to neutralize risk competition through risk adjustment—probably the single most important issue to individuals with disabilities. The art and science of risk adjustment remains problematic because many risk adjustment systems still permit some level of gaming and because it depends very much on the integrity and completeness of data from the very health plans and providers whose payments and quality indicators are to be risk adjusted. Untying the Gordian knot of risk adjustment is essential to an effective market-based health care system.

As noted, managed competition theory has served as the analytic point of departure for health care reforms both in the United States and elsewhere. It has served this role, directly or indirectly, for more than 20 years. The theory faces a new challenge that may strengthen some of its key assumptions but may also alter how health care is delivered and practiced in many countries. This challenge is coming from the Internet, which provides consumers remarkable access to information about specific health conditions, their management, and the providers who address these conditions. The Internet promises to strengthen the accessible information condition of managed competition (Condition 5) and reduce the longstanding asymmetry of information between the demand and supply sides of the market. It will also induce consumers to reach out to providers whom they perceive as the most knowledgeable about their health conditions—even if that means going well outside their usual sources of care. This more fractured utilization of health services may make performance and quality measurements more difficult in the short run but will enhance health system performance in the long run. Equally significant, we believe, is the manner in which this information will be available across national boundaries and lead to a greater "consumerization" of health care not only in the United States but also in more state-administered systems, such as the United Kingdom.

Managed competition, as a system of health care organization, finance, and delivery, cannot succeed fully unless a society is willing to adopt nearly all of its features, not just some of them—with due regard for the strengths and traditions of a society's existing system. This is what makes comprehensive health care reform so difficult in places such as the United States. Standing in the way of each precondition is a vested interest with a major stake in the current system or another system more to its liking. For example, health plans that benefit from risk competition are reluctant to give up their financial advantages. Providers who currently benefit from prestige competition are reluctant to participate in genuine-quality competition by disclosing their outcomes for fear of undermining the advantages that prestige competition has conferred on them. Since the demise of the Clinton health care reform initiative in 1993 and 1994, there has been little political stomach for comprehensive approaches in the United States. Nonetheless, we do believe that managed competition's principal features are congruent with many of the health care issues that are important to individuals with disabilities. The challenge for nations today, especially among Western nations, is how to achieve meaningful incremental reforms without incurring their downsides for higher users of health care services, such as individuals with disabilities.

NOTE

1. For those who need an example and are already familiar with the American Medicare and Medicaid programs, we direct attention to the use of "disproportionate share payments" made to hospitals to cover the costs of hospitals that serve disproportionately large shares of low-income and uninsured populations. One will recall how some state

governments exploited this feature of the Medicaid program and cynically converted disproportionate share payments into a backdoor form of revenue, sharing from the federal government to state governments that amounted to hundreds of millions of dollars. Ironically, those who exploited this feature the most included state governors most opposed to a strong federal role in American governance.

REFERENCES

American Congress of Rehabilitation Medicine. 1993. "Addressing the Post-Rehabilitation Health Care Needs of Persons with Disabilities." *Archives of Physical Medicine and Rehabilitation* 74 (12): S8-12.

Asch, Adrian. 1998. "Distracted by Disability: The 'Difference' of Disability in the Medical Setting." *Cambridge Quarterly of Healthcare Ethics* 7 (1): 77-87.

Basnett, Ian, Marek Koperski, and Kevin Grumbach. 2000. "British Managed Care from Thatcher to Blair: Lessons for the US, Part II." Unpublished paper.

Batavia, Andrew I. 1997. "Disability and Physician-Assisted Suicide." *New England Journal of Medicine* 336 (23): 1671-73.

Bauman, William. 1993. "The Endocrine System." Pp. 139-57 in *Aging with Spinal Cord Injury*, edited by Gale G. Whiteneck. New York: Demos.

Beatty, Phillip, Kelly Burden, and Gerben DeJong. 1999. *NRH-RC Analysts Explore the Opportunities of Managed Care for People with Functional Limitations.* Washington, DC: National Rehabilitation Hospital Research Center.

Bockeneck, William, Nancy Mann, Indira S. Lanig, Gerben DeJong, and Lee A. Beatty. 1998. "Primary Care for People with Disabilities." Pp. 905-28 in *Rehabilitation Medicine: Principles & Practice*, 3d ed., edited by Joel DeLisa and Bruce Gans. Philadelphia: Lippincott-Raven.

DeJong, Gerben. 1979. "Independent Living: From Social Movement to Analytic Paradigm." *Archives of Physical Medicine & Rehabilitation* 60 (October): 435-46.

———. 1997. "Primary Care for People with Disabilities: An Overview of the Problem and Opportunities." *American Journal of Physical Medicine and Rehabilitation* 76 (3): 1-7.

DeJong, Gerben and Janet Sutton. 1995. "Rehab 2000: The Evolution of Medical Rehabilitation in American Health Care." Pp. 3-42 in *Outcome Oriented Rehabilitation: Principles, Strategies, and Tools for Effective Program Management*, edited by Pat Kitchell Landrum, Nancy D. Schmidt, and Alvin McLean, Jr. Gaithersburg, MD: Aspen.

Delaney, Sara and Timm Gossing. 1999. "Finding Work Is Bust in Europe's Boom." *Washington Post*, September 28, pp. A1, A20.

Dixon, Jennifer. 1998. "The Context." Pp. 1-16 in *Learning from the NHS Internal Market: A Review of the Literature*, edited by Julian Le Grand, Nicholas Mays, and Jo-Ann Mulligan. London: King's Fund.

Enthoven, Alain C. 1985. *Reflections on the Management of the National Health Service.* London: Nuffield Provincial Trust.

———. 1993. "The History and Principals of Managed Competition." *Health Affairs* 12 (Suppl.): 24-48.

Friedman, Thomas L. 1999. *The Lexus and the Olive Tree.* New York: Farrar Straus Giroux.

Fukuyama, Francis. 1992. *The End of History and the Last Man.* New York: Free Press.

Jacobs, Alan. 1998. "Seeing Difference: Market Reforms in Europe." *Journal of Health Politics, Policy and Law* 23 (1): 1-32.

Koperski, Marek, Ian Basnett, and Kevin Grumbach. 1999. "British Managed Care from Thatcher to Blair: Lessons for the US, Part I." Unpublished manuscript.

Le Grand, Julian. 1999. "Competition, Cooperation, or Control? Tales from the British Health Service." *Health Affairs* 18 (3): 27-39.

Le Grand, Julian, Nicholas Mays, and Jo-Ann Mulligan, eds. 1998. *Learning from the NHS Internal Market: A Review of the Literature.* London: King's Fund.

Leutz, Walter N. 1999. "Five Laws for Integrating Medical and Social Services: Lessons from the United States and the United Kingdom." *The Milbank Quarterly* 77 (1): 77-110.

Light, Donald W. 1997. "From Managed Competition to Managed Cooperation: Theory and Lessons from the British Experience." *The Milbank Quarterly* 75 (3): 297-341.

Luft, Harold S. 1998. "The Impact of Financial Incentives on Quality of Health Care." *The Milbank Quarterly* 76 (4): 649-86.

Mechanic, David. 1995. "The Americanization of the British National Health Service." *Health Affairs* 14 (2): 51-67.

Menzel, Paul T. 1992. "Oregon's Denial: Disabilities and Quality of Life." *Hastings Center Report* 22 (6): 21-25.

National Center for Health Statistics. 1994. *1994 National Health Interview Survey* [Database on CD-ROM]. CD-ROM Series 10, No. 9. SETS Version 1.21a. Washington, DC: Government Printing Office.

Office of National Statistics. 1994. *General Household Survey.* London: Author.

Oliver, Michael. 1985. *Understanding Disability: From Theory to Practice.* Basingstoke, UK: Macmillan.

Organization for Economic Cooperation and Development (OECD). 1994. *The Reform of Health Care Systems: A Review of Seventeen OECD Countries.* Paris: Author.

———. 1999. *OCED Health Data '99.* Paris: Author.

Pope, Andrew M. and Alvin R. Tarlov, eds. 1991. *Disability in America: Toward a National Agenda for Prevention.* Washington, DC: National Academy Press.

President's Advisory Commission on Consumer Protection and Quality in the Health Care Industry. 1998. *Final Report: Quality First: Better Health Care for All Americans.* Columbia, MD: Consumer Bill of Rights.

Sutton, Janet and Gerben DeJong. 1998. "Managed Care and People with Disabilities: Framing the Issues." *Archives of Physical Medicine and Rehabilitation* 79:1312-16.

Thurow, Lester. 1996. *The Future of Capitalism: How Today's Economic Forces Will Shape Tomorrow's World.* New York: Morrow.

Ware, John E. 1996. "Differences in 4-Year Health Outcomes for Elderly and Poor, Chronically Ill Patients Treated in HMO and Fee-for-Service System: Results from the Medical Outcomes Study." *Journal of the American Medical Association* 276 (13): 1039-47.

Zola, Irving. 1977. "Healthism and Disabling Medicalization." In *Disabling Professions,* edited by Ivan Illich, Irving K. Zola, John McKnight, Jonathan Caplan, and Harley Shaiken. London: Calder & Boyars.

Disability Benefit Programs

27

Can We Improve the Return-to-Work Record?

BONNIE O'DAY
MONROE BERKOWITZ

THE PROBLEM AND ITS SETTING

Most developed countries throughout the world have a set of disability benefit programs as part of their social safety net (Social Security Administration 1997). The United States, like European countries such as England, Germany, the Netherlands, Sweden, and Denmark, has several such benefit programs, including those aimed at persons injured at work, those that pay benefits to persons who are disabled and poor, and general disability programs that pay benefits to those who are enrolled or "insured" in the program.

For the most part, these programs pay benefits to persons who are called on to demonstrate that they are unable to work or are limited in their ability to work. As discussed below, some common complaints in the developed nations are that these programs are growing too fast, that they have become too expensive, and that they do a less than adequate job in returning persons to work once they are on the benefit rolls.

We first examine the background of these various programs, the advantages some of the European countries apparently have in the transition to work, and how the United States is coping with its return-to-work issues. We then examine the implications of the most recent federal legislation in the return-to-work area and propose some radical experimental changes in how the federal disability benefit programs might operate.

THE DISABILITY PROGRAMS AND THEIR BACKGROUND

The work injury programs that pay benefits to persons who become injured or ill at work were, historically, the first programs to develop (Berkowitz 1987). In addition to these work injury programs, there are programs that pay benefits to veterans of the armed forces and programs

633

that pay benefits to government employees. Typically, each country has two other benefit programs. One pays benefits to disabled persons with a work history who are insured under the program, and the other pays benefits to disabled who are poor and can meet some means test (Hogelund 1999). Essentially, applicants for the means-tested disability program must not only show some evidence that they are disabled but must also demonstrate that they have limited financial assets and are unable to earn more than a minimum amount. Applicants for the insured program must show that they have been covered by the program for the requisite period of time and that they meet the disability tests.

In Europe, these programs date back to the early efforts of Prussia's Iron Chancellor, Bismarck, who pioneered a work injury program in the late nineteenth century, possibly to counteract those political parties with socialist leanings (Somers and Somers 1954). In the United States, the work injury programs that go by the name of workers' compensation began in Wisconsin and New Jersey in 1911. They began during the Progressive Era, when the federal government had no role to play in any of the social welfare programs. They spread to each state and remain today as state programs with no federal involvement.

In the United States, the general disability programs, both the insurance and the means-tested programs, can be traced to the 1930s. In an effort to lift the country out of the depression, Congress, at the urging of President Franklin D. Roosevelt, passed the Social Security Act of 1935, providing benefits for retirees and individuals who were blind. In 1956, the Social Security Disability Insurance (SSDI), Title II, was created to provide cash benefits to individuals who could show that they were disabled. Supplemental Security Income (SSI), Title XVI, was created in 1974 to provide income assistance for persons with disabilities, persons who are blind, and aged persons who have limited income and resources regardless of prior participation in the labor force.

DIFFERENCES BETWEEN THE U.S. AND THE EUROPEAN PROGRAMS

The U.S. disability programs differ from the Western European programs in several significant ways. Unlike the European programs (Hogelund 1999), SSDI and SSI, which we will refer to collectively as the U.S. disability programs, have no provisions for sick leave, partial disability, or short-term disability. Five states do have temporary disability programs, and many companies provide sick leave and short-term disability benefits, but there are no federal programs in this area, except those for federal civil service employees. The European programs all provide for *partial* disability payments (Thornton and Lunt 1997), whereas the U.S. programs do not.

Thus, in Europe, a person might become ill and unable to work and begin to receive sick pay from the governmental program. The details differ in each country (Cuelenaere et al. 1999), but just as the Europeans would expect to receive health care and medical benefits from a governmental program, the disabled European would also receive sick pay for some period of time from a government-administered program. After the sick pay period ended, if still disabled, the person might become eligible for cash benefits from one of the government disability programs.

At this point, another major difference between the U.S. disability programs and that of other countries emerges. Under the U.S. programs, either the person would be found to meet the disability test or not—there is no middle ground. The U.S. test is a severe one, with disability being defined in the context of work. Under SSDI and SSI, disability is defined as

an inability to engage in any substantial gainful activity by reason of any medically determinable physical or mental impairment which can be expected to result in death or which has lasted or (is) expected to last for a continuous period of not less than twelve months. (Social Security Act 1935, Section 223 [42 U.S.C. 423] c (1))

The European situation is different in that the programs allow for partial benefits. Thus, a person in the Netherlands, after examination by an occupational physician and perhaps by a vocational expert, might be adjudged to be 40 percent disabled and may receive partial benefits (Cuelenaere et al. 1999). Such an outcome would not be possible under SSDI or SSI. The person in the United States would have to be judged disabled and eligible for cash benefits or not disabled and ineligible for any benefits. In the United States, it is a go/no-go decision. In other countries, there are shades and degrees of gradation of disability.

It is unclear whether being allowed to make partial disability decisions makes the life of the decision maker easier or more difficult. One would think that the ability to compromise a claim would make life simpler for the adjudicator, but that may not be so. In the one program in the United States in which partial benefits are common, the state workers' compensation programs that pay benefits to those injured at work and with partial disability have turned out to be the most expensive and most controversial part of the program (Berkowitz and Burton 1987).

However, whatever its effects on the task of the decision makers, the effects on rehabilitation and return to work are simpler to discern. In the SSDI and SSI programs, there is no way to ease a worker into benefit status. It is true that under the so-called trial work provisions, a person could collect benefits for a limited period of time while working. However, there are no provisions for paying partial benefits for a period of time as the worker tests the labor market.

Neither is there any way to ease beneficiaries onto or off the rolls by paying temporary benefits when they are off work for a short period of time. The applicants cannot be told that they will receive temporary benefits until they recover from the ailment that is causing their job difficulties. Either they receive permanent benefits or they receive nothing. Either they meet the tests or they fail them and receive nothing. All of this, the lack of temporary and partial benefits, has implications for rehabilitation and return to work and may have affected the development and growth of the programs.

THE GROWTH IN THE PROGRAMS

There are no objective measures or yardsticks to determine when a benefit program is growing too fast. The record in the United States shows a rather steady increase in the number of DI and SSI beneficiaries since the programs began. Between 1989 and 1995, the number of SSDI beneficiaries grew from 2.1 to 3.4 million, an increase of 62 percent. The number of SSI recipients has doubled since its inception in 1974 (6.6 million beneficiaries in 1998), and payments in 1997 were five times higher than in 1974 (Rupp and Stapleton 1998).

The U.S. General Accounting Office (GAO) has issued report after report criticizing the U.S. programs for not doing enough to stem the growth in these programs by returning a greater number of beneficiaries to work (Sim 1999; U.S. GAO 1994, 1996, 1997, 1998). The European programs, despite their more flexible eligibility rules, have not been immune to the complaint that the programs are growing too rapidly and that they have become too expensive.

The Netherlands has become the symbol of excessive growth of disability programs, and its ministers have gone so far as to call this growth phenomena the "Dutch Disease" (Aarts, Burkhauser, and DeJong 1996). To follow the medical analogy, if it is a disease, there may well be a cure. The Dutch found a cure and have succeeded in slowing the growth in the numbers coming onto the disability rolls. They simply have taken the government out of the business of paying the first two weeks of sickness benefits and placed this responsibility on employers. Because the employers must now pay these benefits from their own resources, they police the program with more attention than when it was a government benefit. The Swedes and the Germans have also responded to the growth in the programs by cutting benefits and tightening eligibility rules (Hogelund 1999). Even in the United States, we see evidence of this draconian "meat axe" approach. Congress responded to criticisms of payment of benefits to persons with alcohol and drug problems by simply eliminating benefits and Medicare and Medicaid eligibility, effective January 1, 1997, for persons for whom drug addiction or alcoholism was a contributing material factor to their disability (PL 104-121).

IS THERE A BETTER WAY?

Can the return-to-work record be improved without cutting benefits or depriving those on the rolls of their legitimately earned benefits? It will not be easy—there are no magic cures on the horizon. Yet the importance of making the necessary reforms and improving the return-to-work effort is underlined when we realize that if we can just increase the number of persons coming off the rolls by 1 percent, the resultant lifetime savings is estimated at $3 billion (U.S. GAO 1997).

What needs to be done to keep more persons with disabilities at work and off the beneficiary rolls? The GAO's prescription (Sim 1999), borrowed largely from Germany and Sweden, is as follows:

- intervene as soon as possible after an actual or potential disabling event to promote and facilitate return to work,
- identify and provide necessary return-to-work assistance and manage cases to achieve return-to-work goals,
- structure cash and health benefits to encourage people with disabilities to work.

In each of these areas—early intervention, return-to-work assistance, and restructuring of health and cash benefits—there is good and bad news to report. The bad news is that given the way that SSDI and SSI are now organized and administered, it is difficult, if not impossible, to carry out these recommendations. The good news is that Congress has passed and the president has signed new legislation, the Ticket to Work and the Work Incentives Improvement Act (PL 106-70), which gives SSA the demonstration authority to test the feasibility of these recommendations.

EARLY INTERVENTION AND GRADUAL RETURN TO WORK

There is widespread agreement that early intervention is desirable (Sim 1999), but the Social Security Administration is faced with a dilemma. It never sees the potential beneficiary until the person applies for benefits, and it is not authorized to spend trust fund money that finances SSDI benefits until a person is actually admitted to the rolls and payments begin. At that point, but not before, SSA can make a convincing case that it is spending money to save money. If the money buys rehabilitation services that get the worker back on the job and off the rolls, then future benefits will not have to be paid out of the trust fund.

If, at the point of being granted benefits, the applicant is approached by a rehabilitation counselor eager to provide services to help the beneficiary get back to work, it is understandable that the counselor's efforts may be fruitless. The optimal time to intervene would have been much earlier. How much earlier is difficult to say. There are tales, probably apocryphal of the pioneering rehabilitation physicians, such as Henry Kessler and Howard Rusk, proclaiming that rehabilitation ought to begin, "Before the blood is dry on the wound." Certainly, the process ought to begin before the person leaves work, undergoes a regimen of medical care, begins to collect some sick benefits, finally applies to SSA for disability insurance benefits, and then spends months or possibly years proving to physicians, vocational experts, and hearing officers that work is not even a possibility. If there are services, be they medical, technological, or vocational, that can return the person to work, they need to be brought to bear before the applicant is thoroughly demoralized and persuaded that the only feasible life is one on benefits.

In contrast, under Sweden's General Insurance Act, employers are required to report to the social insurance office any employee receiving more than four weeks of consecutive sickness benefits. The employer, employee, and the social insurance office share responsibility for beginning a rehabilitation plan (Hogelund 1999). Once selected for rehabilitation services, the Swedish Social Insurance Board and its local and regional offices may purchase services from any approved training agency.

In Germany, workers are referred for services at the time they apply for sickness insurance. A wide variety of programs are designed to reintegrate workers back into the labor force when they are ready, including wage subsidies, job modifications, technical aids, transportation allowances, and a variety of others (Sim 1999).

In the United States, where there are no sickness benefit programs administered by the federal government, the first difficulty is that the SSA sees persons too late to provide meaningful and useful services. Moreover, there is a second difficulty that is equally troublesome. Just as in Germany and Sweden, the agency that pays the benefits (which in the United States is the Social Security Administration) is not now, nor has it ever been, a rehabilitation agency—a fact that was recognized from the very beginning of the agency.

From the outset, the program was to pay benefits to persons with disabilities. The responsibility for rehabilitation rested not with the paying agency but with the joint federal-state program of rehabilitation (Berkowitz 1987), which we will refer to as vocational rehabilitation, or simply VR.

When the disability programs were started, clients were to be referred to VR without special arrangements. Later, incentives were provided to VR by having SSA pay the costs of rehabilitation for those beneficiaries who left the rolls. Over the years, various changes were made to make these arrangements work better. For the most part, these efforts centered on changes in the ways that the vocational rehabilitation agencies were reimbursed for their services by SSA (Rubin and LaPorte 1982). Nothing seemed to work to the satisfaction of both agencies. Sim (1999) cites the evidence showing that few disabled workers left the rolls to resume work activities. Congress finally enacted legislation allowing private-sector rehabilitation agencies to enter this field and compete with the VR program (Sim 1999).

The more fundamental changes were enacted by Congress and signed into law by President Clinton on December 17, 1999. Several sections of the new act, the Ticket to Work and the Work Incentives Improvement Act of 1999 (PL 106-170), are designed to meet the GAO objections to SSA's return-to-work policies. The act is new, and several of its relevant provisions for return to work did not go into effect until the end of the year 2000, and then only in the form of demonstration authority. Nonetheless, the promise is there. For example, in Section 303, it does allow the SSA to mount a demonstration project in which they are given the opportunity to demonstrate the advantages of early intervention. Under this authority, SSA could refer workers for return-to-work services while they were still receiving sick leave pay or short-term disability benefits. For the first time, SSA will have the authority to spend funds on return-to-work services for persons who are not yet on SSA benefits.

This is brand-new exciting territory. No one knows how to select such persons. The task is to select persons with a high probability of ending up on disability benefits unless they receive appropriate services. The second task, of course, is to supply such services. If the implementation methods can be worked out, it will solve one of the outstanding problems faced by SSA in rehabilitating workers. It will place the U.S. program on a level playing field with the programs in other countries, where short-term benefits are part of the same program that pays long-term benefits and, consequently, where early intervention can take place.

In addition to the early intervention demonstrations, the new act also provides for a demonstration of graduated return-to-work benefits. Under the current law, as we stress above, a worker applies for DI and either receives full benefits or none at all, in contrast to European plans that allow partial benefits. Nothing in the new act disturbs this provision for workers coming onto the rolls. Yet interestingly enough, there are changes proposed for persons leaving the rolls. As matters stand now, workers who return to their jobs have all of their benefits cut off. They fall off the cliff, as it were. Now, under the contemplated demonstrations, a worker who is receiving SSDI benefits and returns to work will lose $1 in benefits for every $2 earned.

Such a provision is comparable to the provisions in the Supplemental Security Income Program, in which the amount of benefits received depends on the worker's family income and assets.

If this demonstration shows positive results, one can expect it to be carried further. Logic may dictate that the tests for getting onto the rolls be comparable to the tests for leaving the rolls. If that happens, the graduated return-to-work benefits may be the back door through which we introduce a partial disability benefit program in the United States.

THE TICKETS TO WORK

As its title provides, one of the provisions of the new act provides for tickets to work. The basic idea stems from a recommendation of a disability panel convened by the National Academy of Social Insurance (Mashaw and Reno 1996). Under the new legislation, newly admitted beneficiaries to the SSA disability rolls will be given a ticket. They need do nothing with the ticket since the entire process is meant to be voluntary. However, should they choose, they could deposit this ticket with a provider of services designed to return the person to work. The provider could be a traditional VR agency, a private-sector provider, or other nontraditional provider of services designed to return persons on benefits to the job.

The novel feature of the ticket proposal is the way that providers are to be reimbursed for their services. Instead of paying them on the basis of their costs or expenditures, they are to be paid a portion of the benefits that would have been given to the person on the rolls, once the person left the benefit rolls.

Currently, the rules and regulations for the ticket proposal are just being formulated, and many questions remain undecided. As originally proposed, the idea was to place much of the power and the trust in the hands of the person with the disability who was empowered to negotiate with the provider. It was thought that, if appropriate, persons with a disability might become their own providers. Also, the notion was that the market ought to be broadened to include a wide variety of providers, including those who have never been involved in rehabilitation endeavors. The whole idea was that SSA had nothing to lose because no payments would be made unless and until the person was working for a sufficiently long time so as to exit the beneficiary rolls. Even then, the provider would be paid only a portion of what SSA was paying in benefits.

THE HEALTH INSURANCE ISSUE

Persons with disabilities obviously face more than normal health care expenditures. Once on the SSDI rolls, a beneficiary becomes eligible for Medicare coverage after 24 months. A person on SSI is eligible for enrollment in the Medicaid program. The fear of losing these medical benefits is often cited as a more powerful disincentive to persons leaving the rolls than is the loss of cash payments (Friedland and Evans 1996; Leonard 1986; Oi 1996).

It is easy enough to see how a person on benefits would be reluctant to try a new job if there were any doubt about health insurance coverage. It would be trying enough to substitute an uncertain wage income for the security of assured benefit payments, but it might be much more devastating to face the uncertain prospects of a period without health insurance coverage that would pay for what is obviously a preexisting condition. Congress has responded to these concerns, and, under Section 1619 (b) of the Social Security Act, Medicaid coverage can be extended indefinitely to lower-income SSI workers, and Medicare coverage can continue for 39 months after successful completion of the trial work period. Under the Ticket to Work Act, Medicare coverage would be continued for a longer period of time, and states are given authority to expand Medicaid options.

ARE THE CURRENT AND PROPOSED REFORMS ENOUGH?

One's optimism that such provisions—early intervention, graduated return to work, tickets to work, and extending health insurance—will be the panacea is tempered by an examination of the European experience. Sweden, Germany, Denmark, and the Netherlands, like other European countries, have these provisions in their law. Each of these countries has partial benefits, temporary benefits, and universal health insurance. Yet each of these countries has faced crises in its programs that have resulted, in some cases, in fairly drastic remedies.

The Dutch experience was the most obvious because the expansion in the disability programs gave rise to a number of fairly drastic remedies. Although less dramatic, reforms were also instituted in the Swedish and German systems (Hogelund 1999) that slowed their rate of growth but did little to improve the return-to-work record for those persons on long-term disability benefits. The public expenditures for disability benefits and labor market measures for persons with disabilities were substantially higher in Germany and Sweden than in the United States (Aarts and DeJong 1996).

European countries are faced with the same problems of persuading persons on the rolls to return to work. In these countries, health insurance coverage for workers on benefit rolls is simply not an issue. These workers have health insurance coverage that is independent of their benefit status. In these countries, administrators have a great deal of flexibility with temporary and partial benefits available as options. Perhaps further reforms are necessary if the return-to-work record is to be improved.

A MORE RADICAL REFORM

In considering what can be done to improve the return-to-work record, one can think of a baseball analogy. Whenever the New York baseball team wins too many World Series in succession, the cry is raised, "Break up the Yankees." Perhaps, the time has come to break up the largest disability insurance organization in the world. The SSA disability programs were paying benefits to 5.7 million beneficiaries as of September 1999, 12.9 percent of all Social Security beneficiaries, including seniors on retirement (www.ssa.gov). Such a huge organization has all that it can do to mail the checks in time. Of necessity, it must process cases on the basis of case files. Of necessity, it must decide the bulk of its cases on the basis of "medical listings," regardless of what the new paradigm might tell us about disability being the result of an interaction between a person and the environment. Of necessity, the sheer volume of applications dictates that it can strive only for what Mashaw (1983) has called "bureaucratic justice." It cannot spare the time and attention that a clinical approach to return-to-work demands.

If we break up the disability insurance program, what can be put in its place? The radical changes in the welfare system in the past several years might serve as an example of what might be done in the disability programs. In 1966, the federal government ended more than 60 years of guaranteed assistance to the needy and replaced it with a system of block grants to the states that could use the funds to enact their own welfare programs. The Temporary Assistance to Needy Families (TANF) block grant replaced the Aid to Families with Dependent Children that had been part of the Social Security Act of 1935. Under TANF, states were given broad discretion to determine eligibility and benefit levels subject to certain conditions requiring benefit recipients to do community service or to work at jobs (Wright 1999).

In April 1999, President Clinton announced that the reforms had succeeded in reducing the number of persons on welfare to its lowest level in 30 years (Wright 1999). Although not all of this decline could be attributed to these reforms, since the economy remained strong during this period, a portion of the credit must be given to the change in philosophy. The basic idea behind the TANF reforms was that welfare mothers should work. If middle-class mothers with children were entering the labor market in unprecedented numbers, then persons on welfare with children should also be expected to find jobs.

A comparably radical change in philosophy was embodied in the Americans with Disabilities Act (DeJong and Batavia 1990). That act was intended to make the labor market a less hostile environment for persons with disabilities who now could be expected to work if they had the appropriate accommodations, but the problems are not simple ones. What a person needs to work depends very much on that person and the immediate environment. It might be an accommodation at work, more flexible working hours, or transportation to the job or some individual health care device available on the job.

Given the sheer size of the task, the SSA has difficulty adopting this case-by-case approach to handling cases. Perhaps a smaller state program with the incentive of a block grant and the freedom to explore new paths might be the answer. Given the demonstration authority under Public Law 106-70, block grants might be given to one or more states to determine if the return-to-work record could be improved while still preserving the equity considerations under the current law.

The rewards would be great if such a program could be made to work. The savings would not be in money alone. The European experience is convincing that if the record does not improve, lawmakers stand ready with drastic remedies in which the cure may be worse than the disease.

REFERENCES

Aarts, L. J. M., R. V. Burkhauser, and P. R. DeJong. 1996. *Curing the Dutch Disease: An International Perspective on Disability Policy Reform.* Aldershot, UK: Avebury.

Aarts, L. J. M. and P. R. DeJong. 1996. "European Experiences with Disability Policy." Pp. 129-66 in *Disability, Work and Cash Benefits,* edited by J. L. Mashaw, V. P. Reno, R. V. Burkhauser, and M. Berkowitz. Kalamazoo, MI: Upjohn Institute for Employment Research.

Berkowitz, E. 1987. *Disabled Policy: America's Programs for the Disabled.* Cambridge, UK: Cambridge University Press.

Berkowitz, M. and J. F. Burton. 1987. *Permanent Disability Benefits in Workers' Compensation.* Kalamazoo, MI: Upjohn Institute for Employment Research.

Cuelenaere, B., T. J. Veerman, R. Prins, and A. M. van der Giezen. 1999. "In Distant Mirrors: Work Incapacity and Return to Work." Unpublished manuscript, College van toezicht sociale verzekeringen, Zoetermeer, Holland.

DeJong, G. and A. Batavia. 1990. "The Americans with Disabilities Act and the Current State of U.S. Disability Policy." *Journal of Disability Policy Studies* 1 (3): 65-74.

Friedland, R. B. and A. Evans. 1996. "People with Disabilities: Access to Health Care and Related Benefits." Pp. 357-88 in *Disability, Work and Cash Benefits,* edited by J. L. Mashaw, V. P. Reno, R. V. Burkhauser, and M. Berkowitz. Kalamazoo, MI: Upjohn Institute for Employment Research.

Hogelund, J. 1999. "Bringing the Sick Back to Work." Ph.D. dissertation, Roskilde University, Denmark.

Leonard, J. S. 1986. "Labor Supply Incentives and Disincentives for Disabled Persons." Pp. 64-94 in *Disability and the Labor Market,* edited by M. Berkowitz and M. A. Hill. Ithaca, NY: Industrial and Labor Relations Press.

Mashaw, J. L. 1983. *Bureaucratic Justice: Managing the Social Security Disability Claims.* New Haven, CT: Yale University Press.

Mashaw, J. L. and V. P. Reno. 1996. "Overview." Pp. 1-32 in *Disability, Work and Cash Benefits,* edited by J. L. Mashaw, V. P. Reno, R. V. Burkhauser, and M. Berkowitz. Kalamazoo, MI: Upjohn Institute for Employment Research.

Oi, W. 1996. "Employment and Benefits for People with Diverse Disabilities." Pp. 103-25 in *Disability, Work and Cash Benefits,* edited by J. L. Mashaw, V. P. Reno, R. V. Burkhauser, and M. Berkowitz. Kalamazoo, MI: Upjohn Institute for Employment Research.

Rubin, J. and V. LaPorte, eds. 1982. *Alternatives in Rehabilitating the Handicapped.* New York: Human Sciences Press.

Rupp, K. and D. C. Stapleton, eds. 1998. *Growth in Disability Benefits: Explanations and Policy Implications.* Kalamazoo, MI: Upjohn Institute for Employment Research.

Sim, J. 1999. "Improving Return-to-Work Strategies in the United States Disability Programs, with Analysis of Program Practices in Germany and Sweden." *Social Security Bulletin* 62 (3): 41-50.

Social Security Administration. 1997. *Social Security Programs throughout the World—1997.* Research Report No. 65, SSA Pub. No. 13-11805. Washington, DC: Government Printing Office.

Somers, H. M. and A. R. Somers. 1954. *Workmen's Compensation.* New York: John Wiley.

Thornton, P. and N. Lunt. 1997. *Employment Policies for Disabled People in Eighteen Countries: A Review.* York, UK: University of York, Social Policy Research Unit.

U.S. General Accounting Office (GAO). 1994. *Social Security: Disability Rolls Keep Growing, While Explanations Remain Elusive.* Document No. GAO/HEHS-94-34. Washington, DC: Government Printing Office.

———. 1996. *SSA Disability: Program Redesign Necessary to Encourage Return to Work.* Document No. GAO/HEHS-96-62. Washington, DC: Government Printing Office.

———. 1997. *Social Security Disability Programs Lag in Promoting Return to Work.* Document No. GAO/HEHS 97-46. Washington, DC: Government Printing Office.

———. 1998. *Social Security Disability Insurance: Multiple Factors Affect Beneficiaries' Ability to Return to Work.* Document No. GAO/HEHS-98-39. Washington, DC: Government Printing Office.

Wright, J. W., ed. 1999. *The New York Times Almanac 2000.* New York: Penguin.

A Disability Studies Perspective on Employment Issues and Policies for Disabled People

28

An International View

KAY SCHRINER

Employment concerns are of paramount importance to disabled individuals around the world.[1] How will they get the opportunities, training, and experience necessary to engage in farming or fishing, get a job, or start their own businesses? How will negative attitudes affect their abilities to support themselves or their families? How can they be appreciated for what they *can* do rather than become objects of pity and subjects of charity? How can their communities become more accessible and responsive to their desires for true integration and equality in all of society? The ability and opportunity to participate in the economic life of their communities are indeed central to the quality of life lived by disabled people.

The purpose of this chapter is to provide an overview of employment issues facing people with disabilities internationally; place these issues in the context of major political, economic, and social circumstances and trends; and analyze employment policies designed to improve conditions for people with disabilities. Special attention will be paid to the majority world because of estimates that 80 percent of people with disabilities live in those countries (United Nations 1986).[2] I will discuss the approaches that appear to offer the most promise and argue for solutions that respect the integrity of disabled individuals and their families, demonstrate cultural competence, recognize the importance of promoting the economic independence of individuals with disabilities and their communities, and promote social justice. Finally, I will emphasize the centrality of putting disabled individuals at the center of the problem-solving process as societies struggle to improve conditions for them and their families.

WHO IS DISABLED?

Definitional issues are among the thorniest questions in any discussion of employment because of the practical and policy relevance of such definitions. The debate about how to define *disability* has been raging for many years and has not been resolved. Scholars and policymakers *are* beginning to agree that definitional schemes must incorporate interactions between individuals and their environments (defined broadly to include architectural, programmatic, and attitudinal variables), but as yet, there is no agreement on how to operationalize this concept of disability.

In an emerging paradigm, disability is viewed as the end result of the lack of societal institutions and practices to accommodate the full range of individual differences (Higgins 1992; Scotch and Schriner 1997). This *human variation* paradigm defines disability as the result of institutions "having been constructed to deal with a narrower range of human variation than is in fact present in any given population" (Scotch and Schriner 1997:155). While still in the nascent stage of development, the human variation model offers an alternative to analyzing all disability-related problems as medical, economic, or discrimination problems.

The issue of contextualizing definitions of disability arises when estimating the number of people who are disabled *with respect to work*. The Canadian Health and Activity Limitation Survey, for example, asks whether an individual is restricted in hearing, seeing, moving, working, and so on, as would any "normal" person (Crichton and Jongbloed 1998:230), which yields the estimate that about 10 percent of the population has a disability. In the United States, estimates are that about 10 percent of people ages 16 to 64 have such a disability. Disability is defined as "a limitation in the amount or kind of work they are able to perform, due to a chronic condition or impairment" (LaPlante et al. 1996:1).

The contextual challenges of defining disability become clear on closer examination of U.S. work disability data.[3] One such instance is the finding that there are "weak correlations between individual *physical or mental attributes* and work *disability* at the empirical level" (McDonough 1997:78, emphasis added). Future research will be directed to sorting out the causal relationship between environmental variables such as the availability of work (e.g., Yelin 1992) and the pull of family roles (McDonough 1997) on individuals' perceived and actual ability to obtain and maintain employment.

These observations have been noted for the data being generated in developed nations, but what about the information on work disability as it applies to developing countries? Researchers have noted that the economies of many countries in the developing world are agriculturally based and have very high rates of unemployment in the formal sector. Also, many people (with and without disabilities) may not be participating in the formal economy (Barnartt 1992), which speaks to the need to consider adaptations to U.S.-style questions when estimating the prevalence of work disability in another culture. (Devlieger [1998] refers to a Zimbabwe survey that identified some 250,000 individuals with disabilities in that country, about 40,000 of whom "have lost skills and productive capacity" [p. 25].) Furthermore, there are no good data on the incidence or prevalence of *impairments* in most countries (Barnartt 1992; Coleridge 1993).

These facts illustrate the difficulty in arriving at reliable and valid estimates of the number of people who have work disabilities in any given country. Each set of national data would need to reflect how individual differences interact with environmental conditions to affect the ability to participate in the economic sphere, and this interaction will no doubt vary from country to country. The interactions between social context and impairments will be vitally important, for as Groce (1995) explains,

A spinal cord injury resulting in paraplegia may prove far more disabling, both socially and economically, to an impoverished sugar cane cutter than to a college professor. The loss of sight for an impoverished washerwoman living in a shanty town might place significant burdens on her family and friends. Unable to work at her former trade and needing assistance to work within the house, watch children or negotiate in the world outside, her standing and status within the family and community might be significantly altered. A wealthy woman with an identical loss of sight, may find the disability far less incapacitating. Her loss of vision may place her at no real disadvantage in terms of socio-economic survival, nor might the well being of her family be substantially compromised. Indeed her need for assistance to maintain a household or career may create jobs for one or several additional individuals. (P. 1136)

Another complication is that national work disability rates are not static. Demographic changes are reverberating through the population, resulting in new incidence and prevalence rates in various age groups and new patterns of etiology within those groups. Especially in the developed world, improved health care and socioeconomic conditions are "aging" the population, which increases the number of individuals with disabilities since disability is more likely to occur as one ages.

Other factors also are contributing to changes in the size and characteristics of the group of people who are disabled. Current military conflicts are an especially important concern in Africa and parts of Eastern Europe, and the aftermath of war in Asia also continues to produce disability because of the many remaining land mines. Nonmilitary violence is also an issue. In the United States, for example, there have been questions raised about possible implications of the high rate of injuries caused by firearm violence and the ability of the vocational rehabilitation program to respond to the victims (Groce 1999).

The socially constructed nature of disabilities, as well as the variations in the way disability is produced through demographic and cultural forces, supports Barnartt's (1992) contention that "one definition [of disability] which fits all countries or situations will not be found" (pp. 47-48), but perhaps this is less problematic than it appears, for as Coleridge (1993) concludes, "No matter what the actual number of disabled people in the world, the case for civil rights is the same" (p. 103).

EMPLOYMENT ISSUES FACING PEOPLE WITH DISABILITIES

No matter whether they live in the most prosperous nations of the world or the least, people with disabilities are among the most economically disadvantaged groups in society. In developing nations, there are few data from government sources regarding the socioeconomic status of individuals with disabilities. There are indications, however, that many people with disabilities occupy a marginalized status in those nations. For example, one African service provider indicates that in urban areas, the unemployment rates for people with disabilities are "five times more than for others" (Campos 1995:71).

In many developing nations, conditions for women with disabilities are worse than for disabled men—both generally and specifically with regard to economic self-sufficiency. Many of these women have very limited or no access to health care, putting their very survival at stake (Groce 1998). Because of legal and cultural limitations on their right and ability to participate in the labor force, such women also have much less earning power throughout their life span (Groce 1998). When they do work outside the home, they are more likely to toil in dangerous occupations with few opportunities for improvement in their economic circumstances. And rates of "unemployment" for women with disabilities may not reflect the significant contributions they make to their families' well-being by engaging in homemaking, child care, and other home-based activities—whether or not these contributions are noticed or appreciated by governments, neighbors, or their own family members (Groce 1998).

A fact that complicates the question of the employment status of disabled people is that the nature of work in developing nations is very different than in postindustrial economies where the information age is in full swing. Many people around the world work at subsistence activities such as farming or fishing or are self-employed as merchants or artisans, so estimates of work disability in those economies should reflect these primary economic roles.

The data concerning the employment conditions for people with disabilities in the developed world are generally more available, though no more encouraging. In Western countries, people with disabilities are chronically underemployed and unemployed. In Britain, two-thirds of people with disabilities do not work, though a government survey found that one-half of these individuals expressed an interest in working (Gooding 1994). Also, people with disabilities were more likely to be employed in manual or unskilled occupations and less likely to hold professional or managerial positions. Only about one-third of workers who become disabled as adults retain their jobs. A survey conducted by the Association of Disabled Professions found that one-third of those responding believed that their "intellectual abilities and professional training" were not being fully used (Gooding 1994:6).

Figures from the United States and Canada are similar. In the United States, unemployment rates among working-age persons with disabilities continue to be very high, despite advancements in assistive technology, rehabilitation practices, and the antidiscrimination provisions of the Americans with Disabilities Act. A recent national survey indicates that while more than 80 percent of the general population is employed, only 3 in 10 working-age adults with disabilities are employed (Louis Harris and Associates 1998). In Canada, while nearly 70 percent of nondisabled individuals have jobs, only 40 percent of persons with disabilities are employed (Crichton and Jongbloed 1998).

Unemployment rates vary among subgroups of people with disabilities. A report from the United States shows much lower employment rates for people with severe disabilities and African American and Hispanic individuals with disabilities (McNeil 1997).

A consistent finding is that women with disabilities are less likely to be employed than are other subgroups of disabled people or nondisabled individuals. In Canada, fewer than 31 percent of working-age women with disabilities are employed, compared with almost one-half of men with disabilities, while 60 percent of nondisabled women and almost 80 percent of nondisabled men have jobs (Crichton and Jongbloed 1998). In one study, Canadian women were found more likely to report they were unable to engage in paid work if they "were not living with children and [were] structurally disadvantaged according to low levels of education" (McDonough 1997:89). In the United States, disabled women from minority groups are particularly disadvantaged (National Institute on Disability and Rehabilitation Research 1992).

Furthermore, having a disability is also associated with lower earnings for those persons with disabilities who do work. English studies show that people with disabilities who work earn only about two-thirds the wages of nondisabled persons (Gooding 1994). In the United States, while the median monthly income among nondisabled men ages 21 to 64 in 1994 and 1995 was $2,190, those with a nonsevere disability earned only $1,857, and those with a severe disability earned only $1,262. Similarly, nondisabled women in the same age group earned a median monthly income of $1,470, while women with nonsevere disabilities earned $1,200. Women with severe disabilities earned only $1,000 per month (McNeil 1997).

Even when disabled individuals are working, they are often apt to be working fewer hours than others. This is true in Canada, where almost 81 percent of women with disabilities (as compared to about 61 percent of nondisabled women) and about 60 percent of disabled men (as compared to 31 percent of nondisabled men) work part-time, that is, less than 30 hours per week (Crichton and Jongbloed 1998:246).

In sum, it does not seem to overstate the case to say that people with disabilities are almost universally on the bottom rung of the socioeconomic ladder. The combination of empirical and anecdotal evidence clearly indicates that throughout the world, disabled people are less likely to be employed in valued roles in their nations' economic activity than are their nondisabled counterparts. The agendas of governments, private relief organizations, and disability rights groups will rightly focus on questions of economic independence and interdependence in the years to come.

WHY ARE PEOPLE WITH DISABILITIES SO LIKELY TO BE UNEMPLOYED?

Developing effective strategies for improving the employment circumstances of people with disabilities requires an appreciation of the social, economic, and political factors that conspire to keep them marginalized. In this regard, the most important contribution of recent years is the now-flourishing scholarly pursuit of a contextualized understanding of disability. In stark contrast to the knowledge bases of the disability professions, such as special education and rehabilitation—which threaten to become moribund soon without an infusion of significant new ideas and strategies—disability studies has yielded important and fresh perspectives on disability *in society.*

These insights begin with the fundamental notion that disability is socially created. In the past, we rarely questioned the designation of impairment as a disability. We *knew* that mental retardation, mental illness, deafness and blindness, and physical impairments were "problems." We drew from this analysis the faulty conclusion that if we corrected the individual's limitations through medical treatment and rehabilitation, the "disability problem" would be solved. The devaluation of particular forms of individual differences was easily explained and almost as easily justified; after all, who would question that these differences were problematic? It seemed to be the natural order of things to mark individuals with such differences for different treatment, good and bad.

Now, we know that disability is not located exclusively in the individual. Rather, some individual differences are marked as disabilities through a complex interchange of social, economic, and political processes (Corker 1998; Oliver 1996; Priestley 1999; Rioux and Bach 1994). Disability is *created.* Furthermore, the disability category can be *contested* (e.g., as it is in the case of learning disabilities) in ways that clarify these processes. The old truism of disability, then, is an illusion. If societal conditions produce disability by attaching to some impairments architectural, programmatic, and attitudinal disadvantage, we must know more about these structural impediments, where they came from, and how they can be removed. Such an understanding is imperative if the employment issues facing disable people are to be meaningfully addressed.

Culture

A primary concern must be to develop a culturally informed perspective on disability and culturally competent employment programs and policies. Cultural factors are bedrock to disability studies by virtue of their importance in illuminating the social bases for the disadvantages associated with individual differences. By developing culturally specific knowledge about disability, we can reflect on and assess our successes and difficulties in addressing employment issues and improve on promising approaches.

One mechanism for developing such a knowledge base is the historical and critical analysis of disability portrayals in media, literature, and other carriers of culture. Represented in important recent works, such as the collections by Mitchell and Snyder (1997) and Thomson (1996) (and also addressed in other chapters in this volume), this scholarship promises to unveil the social processes that support the stigmatization and marginalization of people with disabilities.

Understanding cultural influences is also important for understanding societies' definitions of disability and the circumstances in which disabled people live. Cultural factors not only dictate how the cause of an impairment will be understood but also whether the impaired individual will even survive—and will survive until adulthood—the social roles designated as appropriate for that person (Groce 1993). Groce (1993) describes some particular cultural responses to impairment:

In societies where belief in reincarnation is strong, such as among Southeast Asian groups or in Indian society, a disability is frequently seen as direct evidence of a transgression in a previous life, either on the part of the parents or the child. Those who are disabled are frequently avoided or discounted because of their past lives, while they are simultaneously urged to lead particularly virtuous lives this time around. Answerable both to the past and the future, too little time and energy are often devoted to improving life in the present. (P. 1049)

Even within a cultural group, class membership may produce very different experiences. As Groce (1998) notes,

A woman's social and economic class, her marital status, her family's social networks, her level of education, and her specific type of disability will make a dramatic difference in her quality of life and her ability to make choices. For example, even within the same community, the quality of life for a rural peasant woman with multiple sclerosis will usually be dramatically different than that of the wife of a prominent politician. A daughter with mild mental retardation born into a wealthy family may be well cared for and even put under the supervision of a full-time companion (whether she wants this or not) to ensure her comfort and safety. A daughter of a family living in a nearby shanty town with a comparable degree of mental retardation may well find herself on the streets and at risk of abuse and prostitution by her early teenage years. (P. 179)

Similar observations may be made about men with disabilities. A man who is disabled may be considered a shame to his family, even when his impairment is acquired in war (Barnartt 1992).

It must be said, however, that not all understandings of disability are negative. Some explanations for impairments (especially what we today label as "mental illness" or "mental retardation") describe them as gifts from a divine source. Ingstad (1990) describes the reaction of an African mother to the birth of her disabled daughter:

When African people talk about God's will they seem to place a much more positive emphasis on it than do Europeans. God's will is not seen as a punishment, but more as God's trust in the parents' ability to take care of a special child. Thus a Botswana mother who gave birth to a child with very deformed feet called her "Mpho ya modimo," a gift from God. (P. 191)

Public Policy

Governments play an important role in affecting the likelihood that people with disabilities will be active participants in the economic lives of their communities. They may recognize people with disabilities as a category of citizens and develop strategies for addressing their needs and concerns, or they may largely or completely ignore the population of disabled individuals within their national boundaries. In either event, governments help determine what happens to people with disabilities.

Many Western nations have established elaborate disability policy systems that directly (in the case of income maintenance and rehabilitation programs) and indirectly (in the case of health care, transportation, housing, and education programs) affect the employment circumstances of people with disabilities. These systems are characterized by their histories of incremental policy development over decades in a patchwork fashion by bureaucrats and professionals with little influence from individuals with disabilities. As Berkowitz (1987) notes,

In disability, as in social welfare in general, the only avenue of fundamental reform [has been] to add another program to existing programs and to cope with the resulting confusion. . . . Because of these tendencies, our disability policy, viewed in historical context, consists of layers of outdated programs. (P. 227)

As will be discussed in more detail later, the disability policy in many Western countries now poses significant challenges to policymakers, service providers, and people with disabilities who wish for more coordination and consistency between and within publicly funded programs. In countries such as Sweden, Germany, and the United States, there are significant disincentives to work in public policy. Social insurance programs that provide income support conflict with rehabilitation programs. In some instances, income maintenance is tied to the receipt of health care. These conflicts in purpose and function result in significant disincentives to workforce participation, particularly when access to health insurance is tied to receipt of disability-related income benefits.

The situation in developing nations is quite different. On one hand, they may have the comparative "luxury" (if it can be called that) of not facing the problem of stagnant public policies. On the other hand, these countries have significantly fewer economic resources to spend on national programs dedicated to people with disabilities. They tend to be much more concerned with economic development, education, and basic health care than with the "special" needs of people with disabilities (Barnartt 1992; Metts and Metts 1998). In fact, funds for disability programs in these countries come primarily from the donations of nongovernmental organizations (NGOs) such as international aid groups, missionaries, and government programs sponsored by developed nations (Barnartt 1992). Because the developing nation typically has little or no control over the activities of NGOs, their ability to be proactive is limited.

Still, it is by no means the case that countries in the majority world do not demonstrate concern and commitment to disabled people. Developing countries are establishing publicly funded programs for disabled people (which, although representing a growing awareness, are apparently reflecting some of the "unintended and unfortunate consequences" of specialized services in Western nations) (Ingstad 1990). It is equally important to realize that, as Devlieger (1998) notes with respect to Zimbabwe, in many countries, the provision of assistance and support is an inherent part of the survival strategies of native people. This cultural resource, when viewed as a part of a nation's informal disability policy, becomes a potent force in meeting the needs of disabled people.

Impairments

Whether impairments are important is the subject of some debate. Some scholars argue that the primary determinants of employment outcomes are prejudicial attitudes and discriminatory behavior directed at individuals with disabilities. From this perspective, the removal of discrimination barriers through policy and other tools is a necessary and, some would say, sufficient step to making it possible for disabled persons to get and keep jobs.

Alternatively, others argue that impairments are indeed important (though they acknowledge the very detrimental effects of disability discrimination). This point of view holds that the individual differences that we typically label as disabilities (e.g., cognitive impairments, physical disabilities, psychiatric impairments, communication disorders) do in fact matter, and there is some evidence that people with disabilities themselves believe this to be the case. Walter Oi (1991), for example, who is blind, argues that "disability steals time" (p. 31). A Canadian report cautions that "most Canadians who are not in the labour force regard themselves as being completely unable to work, while others are involved in activities which makes it unlikely that they would or could take a job if one was offered to them" (cited in Crichton and Jongbloed 1998:247). Surveys conducted in the United States add support to this notion; the latest Harris survey reports that "an overwhelming majority (85 per cent) of people with disabilities who are not working say that an important reason why they are not working or looking for work is that their disability or health problem severely limits what they can do" (Louis Harris and Associates 1998:43).

The question of whether impairments matter, requiring us to choose between societal-level factors such as discrimination and individual-level factors, sets up a false dichotomy, however. It is not necessary, nor is it a good idea, to pose the question in this way. Rather, we should be searching for some resolution to the broader question of why some impairments seem to matter for some people in some circumstances and what this understanding implies for developing solutions to the employment problems people with disabilities experience.

We know, for example, that in industrialized countries in the West, the disability category serves an important economic and political function by demarcating those individuals who will be freed from the obligation to participate in the workforce as part of the "deserving poor" (Stone 1984). People with certain impairments that are inconsistent with the production needs of society are thus excused from the work-based system of reward and allowed to participate in the need-based system of social welfare programs (most notably, disability insurance schemes). The disability category collects and sorts the cognitive, communication, physical, and emotional differences that "matter" in the economic arrangements of a nation.

Once these impairments are assembled (and an administrative structure put in place to "objectively" document them), governments may provide these individuals with an exit from the workforce and services designed to help some of them reenter the workforce. The political responses objectify in public policy what the processes and institutions of production have already made real—the devaluation of some forms of individual difference based on their economic implications. It should be no surprise, then, that people with disabilities in these countries are more likely to be unemployed or underemployed. Indeed, it is the very *purpose* of the disability category to separate them out of the workforce—at least in industrialized economies (Stone 1984).

Furthermore, production methods influence the degree to which individual differences can be accommodated in a society's workplaces. Ingstad (1990), reflecting on the simple technologies used in earlier times in Europe, characterizes the situation of disabled people in these "close knit rural communities" as "natural integration" (p. 188). In regard to industrialized economies, Ryan and Thomas have argued that the organization of work in the new factories was less accommodating than the less rigid ways of agrarian life:

> The speed of factory work, the enforced discipline, the time keeping and production norms—all these were a highly unfavourable change from the slower, more self-determined and flexible methods of work into which many handicapped people had been integrated. (Quoted in Gooding 1994:13-14)

What is less clear is how and why the disability category has evolved in the way it has or what these histories imply for current policies in other countries whose economic structures have been subjected to less interpretation by disability studies scholars. As Gooding (1994) notes, "There have been no detailed historical studies of the effects of changes in the modes and relations of economic production upon the integration of disabled people into the labour market" (p. 13). Clearly, this is an important topic for future research.

PUBLIC POLICIES AFFECTING
EMPLOYMENT OF PEOPLE WITH DISABILITIES

Commonalities in European and American Approaches

Employment has been on the center stage of disability policy in industrialized nations for a very long time.[4] With the exception of veterans' benefits, no other focus has been more prominent or longstanding than employment. Western societies use several strategies to address this issue, including social insurance, vocational rehabilitation programs, hiring quotas, tax credits for employers or individuals with disabilities, and antidiscrimination protections. Yet underemployment and unemployment persist as serious problems for most people with disabilities.

The approach taken by Western nations to dealing with the employment participation of workers with disabilities typically consists of a combination of ameliorative and corrective strategies (Haveman, Halberstadt, and Burkhauser 1984). Ameliorative responses include workers' compensation, disability insurance programs, and health care coverage. These provide workers with disabilities partial replacement of lost income and medical services on either a temporary or permanent basis. Also included in the ameliorative category are welfare programs such as the U.S. means-tested Supplemental Security Income.[5]

Corrective programs are those intended to rehabilitate workers who become disabled during their adult years or to habilitate individuals whose disabilities are congenital or acquired at an early age. The most important of such efforts are the national rehabilitation programs that provide counseling, restoration services, education or vocational training, and placement services to eligible individuals with disabilities. A complementary strategy is to institute legal protections against disability-based discrimination in the workplace in an effort to promote the use of accommodations; perhaps the most notable example of this approach is the U.S. Americans with Disabilities Act.

This general outline of disability policy with respect to employment obscures important differences in the particulars of these various programs. A comparison of approaches in Sweden, Great Britain, Holland, West Germany, and the United States illustrates the range of policies. Each of these countries includes social insurance and welfare programs in the mix, but the emphases differ.[6]

Historically, Holland and Sweden have had more generous income replacement policies for people with disabilities who have participated in the labor force. Their benefit levels (i.e., percentage of predisability income replaced by disability insurance payments) are higher than in West Germany, Great Britain, or the United States. By contrast, Germany and England both place more emphasis on rehabilitation, although Germany's program is generally regarded as more effective (Aarts and DeJong 1996).

While it is not possible to discuss in any detail the intricacies of Western-style disability policy, it is useful to briefly identify the major points of the criticisms leveled against these approaches in recent years. In the United States, where health care benefits are tied to participation in income maintenance and disability insurance programs, politicians and the disability community have focused on removing the disincentives to workforce participation. Restructuring incentives is also a major concern in Sweden and the Netherlands. In Germany and in the United Kingdom, where workforce participation rates are higher, the question of incentives has been less important. The Swedish and Dutch programs are concerned with improving the efficiency and fairness of their administrative structures (Aarts and DeJong 1996). In commenting on the complexities of managing disability programs, Aarts and DeJong (1996) remind us that

> good social policy and practice . . . not only require able administrators, using appropriate policy tools, but an intelligent design of the incentive structures implied both by the programs and by their management. This may seem obvious, but it took about three decades before this insight finally broke through among European [and U.S.] supporters of the welfare state. (P. 159)

Disability Policy in the Majority World

Unlike the wealthier nations of the world, most countries do not dedicate significant funds to programs targeted to people with disabilities. Many African nations are simply unable (and perhaps unwilling) to spend national resources on programs specifically for individuals with disabilities (Barnartt 1992; Metts and Metts 1998). In these countries, nongovernment organizations (NGOs) are active in meeting the needs of disabled people and their families. Much of this activity occurs in the context of economic development initiatives (Metts and Metts 1998). For example, NGOs (such as the United Nations and its various component programs) and the U.S. Agency for International Development (USAID) provide funds, technical assistance, and personnel to countries throughout Africa to help promote the establishment of economic infrastructures and programs. Increasingly, these programs are being pressured to include people with disabilities in their governance and as targets of programmatic activities (Metts and Metts 1998), but there remains considerable prejudice and misunderstanding regarding disabled people. Peter Coleridge (1993), who has worked in international disability programs for a decade, reports the following:

> In many developing countries disability is often perceived by governments and aid agencies as a problem, but not as a priority. Income, access to land and/or jobs, basic health care, the infant mortality rate, and the provision of sanitation and clean water are all seen as greater and absolute priorities. These are the pressing problems, and disabled people can be attended to later. . . . Even people who are "progressive," "gender-aware," and in all other respects "developmentally minded" perceive disabled people as belonging to a category marked "social welfare," which is the new term for "charity." The implication is that disabled people can be ignored altogether in the development debate. (P. 5)

The problem is compounded by the fact that economic aid is often focused on large-scale projects, but the needs of disabled people are considered a local problem. Metts and Metts (1998) quote a U.S. government source who draws the conclusion that USAID officials believe that the focus on "helping the population of developing countries by improving their overall economic condition . . . may work against the inclusion of the disabled where the primary focus is on the grassroots level" (p. 32). At any rate, the lack of understanding of aid officials remains a problem in these countries.

The majority world's primary approach to rehabilitation is changing. Having seen the difficulties produced by over-professionalization and specialized services in the Western world, a community-based rehabilitation (CBR) strategy is slowly replacing older practices. In this model, the communities in which disabled people live are provided technical assistance by rehabilitation professionals, who help "ordinary people" such as family members, neighbors, and teachers, develop the skills necessary to accommodate the disabled person (McConkey and O'Toole 1995). The rehabilitation professional focuses more on the community through consultation, building relationships, developing and using training skills, nurturing the family's and community's capacity to cope, and promoting community "ownership" of the person with a disability (McConkey and O'Toole 1995). Supported by international aid agencies, CBR is moving the majority world away from the tradition of "rehabilitation palaces" (Werner 1995:18) to a greater reliance on localized, consumer-driven strategies.

REMAKING "REHABILITATION": A CALL FOR TRANSFORMATIVE REHABILITATION PRACTICE

Rehabilitation Past and Present

The disability policies of nations around the world have been affected by a long pattern of international relations between disability professionals and organizations representing people with disabilities. In fact, Groce (1992) argues that rehabilitation is in actuality an invention of these international connections:

The historical distinction between national and international rehabilitation activity is somewhat artificial. For many years ideas flowed from one arena to the other and back again. . . . Ideas, approaches and concerns that American leaders were instrumental in developing within the United States, were carried on into their work abroad. Likewise, ideas and innovations to which United States leaders were exposed in international rehabilitation programs were often quickly incorporated into programs in the United States . . . it should [also] be noted that [there has been a] shift over the past century within the field of disability and rehabilitation from a group of fragmented programs, disciplines and experts, to an increasingly unified disability rights movement. (P. 5)

As a field of theory and practice, though, it seems apparent that around the world, rehabilitation has been overly influenced by Western ideals and ideas. The medical model of disability, the development of professions in health and disability services, and the prominent role of the state in providing services and benefits to disabled persons are largely Western creations. However, majority countries have had mixed experiences when they attempt to adopt the rehabilitation approaches of the United States, England, and other developed nations. Often they find that the establishment of a professional class of rehabilitation workers is financially impossible (Barnartt 1992; McConkey and O'Toole 1995). In some instances, when funds are expended to train rehabilitation professionals, countries find that the professionals become dissatisfied with the relative lack of attention and status associated with their roles or are enticed to take jobs in other countries because of better pay and better working conditions (McConkey and O'Toole 1995).

Developing nations have also struggled with decisions about where to establish rehabilitation programs and their relationship to broader education and social service efforts. In many countries, most or all rehabilitation centers are located in urban areas that are not easily reached by disabled people because of their geographic and cultural distance from urban areas (Barnartt 1992; Groce 1998).

Another question is whether to employ a "specialized services" approach or to incorporate rehabilitation into more general education and social service programs. There are different approaches and mixes of approaches, used in both developing and developed countries. Belgium, Finland, and France, for example, all provide vocational guidance in "ordinary" programs, although Finland provides specialized services for persons with severe disabilities (International Labour Conference 1998:25). Many scholars and activists, however, claim that establishing special services for disabled people is a flawed approach in that it perpetuates the stigma attached to disability and provides an excuse for mainstream programs not to make the adaptations necessary to provide services and activities to *every* citizen (Schriner, Rumrill, and Parlin 1995).

Gender is another important concern. Women with disabilities in developing and developed countries have different experiences with rehabilitation. When cultural practices discourage or prevent women from traveling by themselves or living without male supervision and protection, they are less likely to access rehabilitation services (Groce 1998).

More fundamental to the analysis of international rehabilitation is the general critique of professionalism. Expressed persuasively by scholars such as John McKnight (1995) and Ivan Illich (1976, 1987), part of this critique focuses on the possible (and actual) iatrogenic effects of professions' helping behavior—effects that may occur at both the individual and societal levels. One source of iatrogenic effects is an overemphasis on the individual as the source (and solution) of the "disability problem." Professionals engage in clinical reasoning, which, as Stone (1993) warns,

profoundly changes the way social problems are defined, the political instruments used to resolve them, and the relative power of social groups. . . . [Clinical reason] accords with the liberal tradition of justifying differences in status and rewards by differences in individual achievement, merit, and even need. Clinical reason seems to give an independent source of knowledge to social and political authorities, rendering them less vulnerable to the (manipulative) desires of individuals. (P. 64)

This emphasis on individual-level change is caused, in part, by the training professionals receive, which tends to focus on disability as a characteristic of individuals and overstates the importance of diagnostic testing and assessment procedures. A case in point are the licensing criteria of the U.S. National Council on Rehabilitation Education that require no training in community development, systems consulting, or other strategies that have proved useful in furthering social change. This individual focus is a politically conservative approach to disability—one that first stops short of confronting and challenging the structural and attitudinal barriers that keep disabled people and other disadvantaged groups from being fully integrated into society and, second, attracts budding professionals who are more interested in producing individual change than social change.

The clinical approach is reinforced by the state's role in funding training programs for rehabilitation professionals and employing them. The result is "profoundly antidemocratic"; by transforming social problems into "clinical syndromes," the state

elevates a particular type of expert knowledge and denigrates or even ignores the knowledge, perceptions, and interpretations of ordinary citizens in their relationships with other individuals and with social institutions. . . . Ultimately, the most profound consequence of the rise of clinical authority is that it disguises or displaces conflict in the first place. Once a situation is defined as a matter of health and disease, or normality and pathology, both the problem and its treatment appear to be dictated by nature and no longer a matter of value choice and political resolution. (Stone 1993:65)

In addition to these concerns, a practical matter with serious implications for the future of rehabilitation is the fact that *very few individuals with disabilities* participate in rehabilitation programs. Helender (1993, cited in Groce 1998:182) estimates that only about 3 percent of people with disabilities receive services from such programs, an estimate that is roughly consistent with the 2 percent figure cited for "conventional rehabilitation centers" in Zimbabwe (Devlieger 1998:26) and the 7 percent figure cited by the U.S. General Accounting Office (1993). It seems safe to say that rehabilitation services would not be funded at levels necessary to expand services to the entire eligible population.

Given this critique of rehabilitation services, the time is ripe for a thorough evaluation of rehabilitation theory and practice, as well as the possibility for a *transformative rehabilitation practice* that focuses on the societal conditions that create disadvantage for people whose individual characteristics are outside the societal norm. In the subsequent sections, we will draw the outlines of such an approach and discuss its advantages. We will also suggest some broad measures for evaluating a transformative rehabilitation practice and briefly acknowledge the obstacles to its development.

What Should a Transformative Rehabilitation Practice Be?

The most important question is the following: What should a new transformative "rehabilitation" practice be? This is the central query arising from this many-faceted debate about employment issues and the traditional rehabilitation profession that is supposed to address them. Traditional programs, especially in developed countries, seem to exist in isolation from basic institutional structures such as families, neighborhoods, employers, religious groups, and other voluntary associations. Professionals are housed in offices, are largely invisible in their communities, and spend little time consulting with employers or other community members and institutions about making accommodations or improving attitudes toward people with disabilities.

Table 28.1   A Comparison of Traditional Rehabilitation Profession and Transformative Rehabilitation Practice

	Traditional Rehabilitation Profession	Transformative Rehabilitation Practice
Construct of disability	Disability as an individual phenomenon. Recognizes role of discrimination but falls short of critical analysis of societal structures and practices.	Assumes that social structures and practices produce disability from impairment. Uses systems-level interventions to address disabling conditions.
Target of intervention	Primarily individual, with limited emphasis on families, schools, and employers. One person at a time.	Community; social and political systems; attitudes.
Purpose of intervention	To increase levels of individual functioning.	To produce fundamental change in social, economic, and political structures.
Intervention strategies	Training, education, and support of person with a disability. Limited consultation with employers. Almost always focused on accommodating one individual.	Systems analysis and consultation, inclusive community and economic development, political action. Practitioner works with elected officials, educators, community planners and activists, employers, and so on.
Disciplinary traditions	Medicine, psychology, education.	Community development, political science, sociology, economics.

Instead, professionals confer with one-after-another "consumer" and a generally small number of community providers from whom services are purchased.

At the societal level, professionals rarely engage in the larger political dialogue regarding the status of people with disabilities. While professionals may take part in political debates to protect professional turf or integrity, they are less likely to weigh in on the side of creating fundamental changes in the political and economic relations of a society.

Thus, the professional dominance in disability policy is costly, has iatrogenic effects, and is incompatible with fundamental social change. If we believe that society itself is, metaphorically speaking, throwing disabled people into the river of unemployment, then why are we picking them out of the river one at a time rather than running upstream to stop them from being thrown in in the first place?

A new transformative rehabilitation would involve societal and community-level efforts to make the built and attitudinal environment more hospitable to disabled people. Although this is, obviously, a much different usage of the word *rehabilitation* than has historically been the case, it may be an appropriate application in that it denotes the remaking of society. Furthermore, the term *rehabilitation profession* is replaced by the term *rehabilitation practice* in the hope of overcoming the artificial elevation of expert knowledge over the knowledge possessed by ordinary people (see Table 28.1 for a comparison of the traditional rehabilitation profession with a transformative rehabilitation practice).

The "What" of Transformative Rehabilitation Practice. Professional knowledge about the individual-level aspects of disability should not be the only strategy—or even the primary strategy—in a transformative rehabilitation tool chest. Fundamental social change is the key to the doors of acceptance and opportunity that must be opened for disabled people. Fundamental change is necessary to transform the social, economic, and political structures of a society so that disabled people are viewed as normal and offered parallel opportunities to influence and benefit from those systems. This change must occur at all levels of a society, from the loftiest centers of political and economic power to the relations between and within families, workplaces, and neighborhoods. To produce such reforms, we propose that a transformative rehabilitation practice take what is known about the individual aspects of impairment and disability and apply this perspective within the context of a social change strategy. This transformation would permit the application of this knowledge to the situations of many more disabled people than can be helped by any number of traditional rehabilitation professionals.

The most promising possibility for meaningful progress, then, would be to move toward the development and implementation of a transformative rehabilitation practice. By this, we mean a rehabilitation practice that would focus on producing fundamental social change—and would measure its success in those terms—rather than focusing on the individual and individual-level change. The practice of rehabilitation would become driven by the circumstances of the *society* (not the individual), would recognize and take advantage of the strengths of the *society,* and would work throughout the *society* to address the needs and concerns of disabled people. In short, the society would become the unit of analysis rather than the individual.

The implications of taking such an approach are significant to the extent that the CBR approach has recognized the strengths of the community and the potential of the community to solve the problems experienced by disabled people. It has anticipated this "transformative rehabilitation." What is now required is a transformation of the conversation. Rather than beginning with the needs of the individual and going from there to the community-based changes that are required to accommodate that individual, let us begin by asking how accommodating the *society* is—at all levels and in all areas—and go from there to the individual implications of societal-level change to improve its accommodative stance.

This conversation will be based on a thorough understanding of how societies work and how they may be worked *with*. It will be grounded in theories of power and influence, community and social change, and economic and community development. The inquiry will focus on the structural characteristics of the society, the attitudinal features of the society, and the components of the society that can be called into action through the promotion of enlightened, indigenous leadership with whom a rehabilitation practitioner consults and produces change. The activities of the rehabilitation practitioner will be focused on the society. The practitioner will apply knowledge about systems, social change, culture, and community to the problem of moving the society as a whole from where it *is* to where it *might be*. The rehabilitation profession is remade into a social change process founded in hope and faith.

This transformative rehabilitation practice also makes use of the tremendous amount of knowledge we have acquired concerning the adaptations that may be made in society to accommodate individual differences. The rehabilitation practitioner will know what accommodations are required and how to promote a more accommodative stance in political, economic, and social structures at all levels. Policymakers, educators, business owners, and leaders of voluntary associations will have access to the practitioner's knowledge about these strategies.

However, there are notable differences between the traditional rehabilitation profession and this transformative rehabilitation practice. A transformative rehabilitation practice would be grounded in a substantially different theoretical understanding than is the traditional rehabilitation profession. The primary theoretical orientation would be derived from those fields that are systems—and change—oriented, such as political science, sociology, community psychology, community and economic development, and systems theory. These theories would permit practitioners to adopt a conceptual framework that is more consistent with the widely recognized need to produce societal-level change.

Thus, the practitioner's primary mode of operation would be dictated not by an individual-by-individual analysis of problems and solutions but rather by an analysis of the societal systems through which fundamental change may be achieved to improve the accommodation and acceptance of disabled people. When analysis verifies that parts of the political or economic structures are inaccessible, the practitioner may support people with disabilities as they together engage the larger system in a change process. The outcomes of this approach would most certainly affect *individuals* with disabilities, and those effects will be direct and observable. However, the practitioner's work will begin not with the individual (indeed, practitioners may not even know the eventual beneficiaries of their work) but with the society as a whole and with its discrete parts. The practitioner's efforts would involve working with policymakers, the private sector, and other institutions and actors to ensure that barriers are *systematically* addressed and reduced.

The "Who" of a Transformative Rehabilitation Practice. A transformative rehabilitation practice will require a practitioner who is prepared to engage a wide range of individuals and groups operating in the political, economic, and social spheres. Such work will demand an understanding of power and economic relations, the ability to identify and establish collaborations with leaders in those spheres, and a sophisticated approach to supporting and promoting the change process.

This reinterpretation of the rehabilitation process and its reassignment to the societal level offers a greater opportunity to empower people with disabilities than does the weakened version of empowerment envisioned by the traditional rehabilitation profession. In the weakened version, power must be wrested away from the professional (or granted by the professional) and is typically thought of as a characteristic of the individual that does not depend on—and, in fact, is irrespective of—objective conditions of power in the social, economic, and political spheres. Empowerment used in this way is almost a misnomer. In the alternative model of transformative rehabilitation practice, empowerment is a natural by-product of the process, although it occurs not because of professional intervention with disabled individuals but rather because of intervention at the societal level. Through transforming the systems of society, the objective conditions in which disabled people live may also be transformed, resulting in true empowerment for the individual who has a disability. Empowerment results not from the benevolence of a professional but from change in the attitudinal and built structures of the society in which the disabled person lives.

Transformative rehabilitation practice will focus on change in the political, economic, and social spheres of society. Because of space limitations, it is impossible to address in any great detail what this practice would look like in each of these spheres or what would be the results of such a practice. However, we will touch on a few general themes in the context of the political and economic spheres.

TRANSFORMATIVE REHABILITATION PRACTICE IN THE POLITICAL SPHERE

Practitioners of transformative rehabilitation and their allies will naturally want to focus on political issues. These may include the development or reform of policies affecting people with disabilities, the representation of disabled people in elected governments, or any myriad other political concerns. This connection to the political sphere is one that is largely overlooked in the traditional theories and profession of rehabilitation and sorely deserves attention. In the United States, for example, rehabilitation training programs focus almost exclusively on individual-level phenomena, and thus a traditional rehabilitation professional is ill equipped to analyze or affect the political process. This is a startling omission given the widespread acknowledgment that politics plays a significant role in the quality of life of disabled people.

A transformative rehabilitation practitioner will have the theoretical understanding of political issues required to act strategically within the political system to produce fundamental change. For example, when candidates and political parties within a representative democracy fail to address the concerns of disabled people accurately or adequately, the practitioner and his or her partners (which would include local disability groups or other indigenous partners) may conduct voter education campaigns, which provide information to the disability community about candidates' positions on disability issues, thus producing more well-informed voters and more attentive candidates. Similarly, if U.S. courts were to misinterpret the Americans with Disabilities Act's definition of a covered individual (thereby restricting the breadth of coverage), the transformative rehabilitation practitioner might assist in crafting remedying legislation. Or, the transformative rehabilitation practitioner might promote the adoption of treaties banning the use of land mines and participate in negotiations to improve working conditions for all disadvantaged groups.

This proposed political role for the rehabilitation practitioner is reminiscent of the systems-level advocacy often engaged in by centers for independent living in the United States. The infusion of an overtly political focus into a transformative rehabilitation practice acknowledges and emphasizes the significance of public policy in the lives of disabled individuals. The traditions of rehabilitation theory and professionalism have ignored the dynamics of the policymaking process at the peril of persons with disabilities, and the inclusion of policymaking issues here is designed to remedy this omission.

TRANSFORMATIVE REHABILITATION PRACTICE IN COMMUNITY AND ECONOMIC DEVELOPMENT

A vital part of a transformative rehabilitation practice is the purposeful integration with broader community and economic development activities. Efforts in this direction are already a strong focus in the developing world (see Harper and Momm 1989; Metts and Metts 1996), where so many decisions about resource allocation are driven by economic development needs but should also be a focus in the developed world as well.

An illustration of the way rehabilitation services can be part of a larger economic development effort is the example of microenterprise programs. Established first in Bangladesh, the microenterprise movement began with the provision of small loans to poor individuals (many of whom were women) who had almost no access to banks or other traditional sources of capital. The first such programs established small lending groups that were given a relatively small pool of money from which to make loans to group members. Group members worked with staff to develop individual business plans, and then groups made the decision to loan money to individuals when those individuals had demonstrated that they had taken the necessary steps to succeed in their businesses. These programs have been established in some locales in the United States and are showing considerable promise (Metts and Metts 1996).

Self-employment can also occur outside of a microenterprise program, of course. Harper and Momm (1989) describe the experiences of more than 50 disabled entrepreneurs in Gambia, India, Indonesia, Kenya, the Philippines, and Zimbabwe and argue that self-employment may have the "potential for remoulding traditional rehabilitation approaches, at least in developing countries" (p. 5), because of the nature of the economies there. While self-employment would not be an appropriate choice for every individual with a disability, it should not be dismissed as an option.

A critical characteristic of the self-employment model is its contribution to economic and community development. In general, these enterprises are small and require little capital investment, perhaps only a basket in which to display goods for sale. There is typically little infrastructure required because the entrepreneurs use the roadsides or public urban spaces for their activities. These small businesses are labor intensive, and unused labor is common. Self-employed people often operate in their own communities, thus making little demand on limited transportation capacity. They tend to produce goods that poor people need and can afford to purchase (Harper and Momm 1989).

Self-employment, defined broadly as including not only small business but also larger enterprises owned by one or more disabled individuals, has another significant advantage. It provides a true economic stake for people with disabilities, one that will inevitably lead to empowerment in both the economic and political spheres. In this respect, self-employment (though still largely an individual-level effort) is consistent with a transformative rehabilitation practice by emphasizing the importance of ownership of economic resources. When the numbers of disabled business owners reach some critical mass, it is at least possible that they will become a political power base within their communities or larger society.

EVALUATING A TRANSFORMATIVE
REHABILITATION PRACTICE

Evaluating the effectiveness of a transformative rehabilitation practice (and other aspects of disability policy such as income maintenance and health care programs) is a pressing concern. Perhaps because of its colonial past, writers from Africa seem especially sensitive to the need to evaluate such efforts in terms of fundamental social change. David Werner (1995), for example, states that

> the long-term value of any rehabilitation or development effort must be evaluated in terms of how much it empowers marginalised groups and moves us toward fairer, more fully democratic social structures. (P. 25)

Thus, a significant emphasis in the evaluation process should be the degree to which oppressive conditions for all people with disabilities are relieved in all spheres of society. While it is by no means clear how such achievements would be measured, it does seem reasonable to suggest that broad measures of political, economic, and social equality might be identified and used to evaluate the effectiveness of a transformative rehabilitation practice.

The circumstances of minority individuals with disabilities and women with disabilities must be given significant attention in evaluating such efforts. Inquiries that are limited to simple demographic and outcome measures at the program level (e.g., the number of minorities and women who participate, the kinds of disabling conditions they have, the services they receive, and their employment outcomes) are myopic. Evaluating a transformative rehabilitation practice will require attention to the systemic exclusionary policies and environmental and attitudinal barriers that have kept minorities of all kinds in marginalized circumstances. A transformative rehabilitation practice must cast a wide net with respect both to the strategies employed and the outcomes to be achieved.

MAKING CHANGE: THE CHALLENGES
OF POLITICS AND CULTURE

Creating a transformative rehabilitation practice will require overcoming several major challenges. First among these are the institutions and practices they engage in to develop and run traditional rehabilitation programs around the world. In the developed nations, these take the form of well-established professions whose position and role in society are generally supported by both politicians and the general public. In the majority world,

> There is an enormous industry based on disability, in which charitable institutions vie with "community-based programmes" for major funding; vested interests are well entrenched among rehabilitation professionals; [and] UN agencies and NGOs debate disability at their conferences. (Coleridge 1993:5)

The habits of professionals and their supporters will be difficult to change, but it is by no means impossible.

A related problem is that rehabilitation programs are controlled by nondisabled individuals, who, according to Coleridge (1993), dislike the "militancy exhibited by disabled people—who, it is assumed, should keep quiet and accept their situation as unfortunate but unchangeable" (p. 5). The disability rights movement must be an integral part—indeed, the foundation—of change efforts. Because it is fundamentally about changing the social construction of disability, the movement has the intellectual prowess to analyze the impairment-environment interaction from the basis of its members' personal experience and to apply this analysis to the question of a new paradigm for rehabilitation.

The disability rights movement is actively engaged in developing the breadth of leadership necessary to enunciate all variations of the impairment-environment interaction. The movement continues to focus on improving its capability to attract and represent the interests of women with disabilities, minority individuals with disabilities, and other parts of the disability community whose experiences and concerns historically have not found expression in the movement. Because disability organizations historically have been headed by men and have concentrated on men's issues, women's experiences and interests have not been fully explicated or represented in the movement's agenda. Recent advances, made through the efforts of the United Nations International Decade, Rehabilitation International, the World Institute on Disability, Mobility International USA, and other national and international organizations promise to remedy this situation, but much more work is necessary.

CONCLUSION

In this chapter, we have evaluated the conditions in which people with disabilities live and have argued that the economic status of people with disabilities is intimately connected to a nation's ability to accommodate and value individual differences. Furthermore, we have suggested that many current policies and practices—particularly traditional rehabilitation theories and professions—have the unintended consequence of impeding the fundamental social change that appears necessary to produce true empowerment for disabled people. We have proposed that a new approach, which we call transformative rehabilitation practice, be taken to address the societal-level conditions that act as barriers to true equality for disabled individuals, and we have briefly described examples of how such practice might work in the context of the political and economic spheres. We have also recognized that there are many impediments to the establishment of this new transformative rehabilitation practice.

Given the continuing disadvantaged status of individuals with disabilities, it seems apparent that programs and policies targeted to employment concerns are in need of a critical reexamination, which asks the most basic questions about the level of analysis and intervention for such efforts. Why is it that we continue to operate primarily at the individual level of analysis and intervention, even when the evidence continues to indicate that people with some kinds of difference are disabled by societal-level policies and practices? Why do we persist in emphasizing the evaluation and labeling the individual—as well as the provision of specialized treatment, education, and training to the disabled individual—despite the continued resistance of mainstream settings that could and should provide such supports and services as part of their routine functioning? Perhaps the answer lies in the continued reliance on theories and professions that operate from the perspective of the individual to the almost complete exclusion of the society. We would propose that individual differences could be accommodated and valued only when societies themselves change. This is hardly a new observation, but the application of this perspective to a transformation of the rehabilitation profession may be.

In many countries, attitudes and policies have relegated disabled people to the margins of the economy. The steps taken to remedy this isolation and stigma are usually politically conservative measures that, often inadvertently, contribute to the continued disadvantage of disabled people by identifying their differences and issues as "special" and "unique." Traditional rehabilitation theories and professions are such strategies. By labeling disabled people as different, abnormal, and wanting—albeit deserving—the rehabilitation profession and its intellectual justifications largely ignore the many ways the attitudinal and built environment identifies and devalues the forms of individual difference called disability.

The development and implementation of a transformative rehabilitation practice will require different emphases in research and policy. With respect to the research agenda regarding employment issues, we will need to expand our attention to questions about the structure of economies and their consequences for the production and management of individual difference. We will need to ask more questions about the creation and use of technologies to expand opportunities for disabled people, and these inquiries will need to include examination of the resource flow between developed and developing nations. Other research efforts consistent with a societal-level analytical and intervention strategy include, for example, comparative analysis of strategies for enforcing antidiscrimination measures in the workplace. It also includes evaluation of political efforts taken to reduce the presence of land mines around the world; the development and validation of measures for evaluating change in political, economic, and social systems; and the evaluation of methods for engaging advocacy groups in producing such change.

Social policy may also require reform. One can imagine (though not necessarily predict), for example, the rewriting of the U.S. Rehabilitation Act to "turn it on its head" and create a federal-state partnership for producing fundamental social change. The act might define its purpose in terms of creating such change and might fund transformative rehabilitation practitioners to analyze societal conditions and forge relationships with local, state, and national groups to improve the accessibility of society at all levels and in all respects. Funded activities might include working with local governments to ensure the accessibility of housing and transportation, investigating claims that local banks discriminate against disabled business loan applicants, promoting parity for mental health treatment in health insurance plans, and advocating with the state chamber of commerce to require that its members commit to hiring more disabled people. Practitioners might be evaluated on the amount and effectiveness of such engagements. Agency ombudsmen might be employed to ensure that such evaluations are not affected by the influence of economic and political entities.

These are but a few thoughts on the research and policy implications of our musings about a transformative rehabilitation practice. Further consideration of the many issues and questions surrounding the future of employment-related programs, policies, and practices should involve the entire international disability community. We conclude this chapter by emphasizing that it *is* possible to create new programs and policies that are culturally competent and that contribute to economic and social justice. This imperative creates a powerful claim on the world's intellectual and political resources. Disabled people and those who live with and care about them can shape a changing universe to make it more accepting and accommodating to people whose individual differences have historically been marginalized and stigmatized. To do so will take courage, creativity, and great perseverance, but the potential benefits are so significant that we must accept the challenge.

NOTES

1. The terms *disabled person* and *person with a disability* (and their variations) will be used interchangeably in this chapter in recognition of the preferences of people with disabilities in different countries (and sometimes within the same country) for different terms.

2. The terms *developing countries* and *majority world* both refer to those non-Western nations that have less economic development than in the West. However, it is important to note that the term *developing country* is *not* used to imply that these nations have fewer cultural resources than industrialized nations or have nothing to teach "developed" countries. In that sense, it is unsatisfactory but is still employed to relieve the monotony of using only one term.

3. This chapter will address issues affecting only disabled adults. It is recognized, though, that the cultural variables determining how and to what extent children with disabilities will be educated and otherwise prepared to assume adult roles are very important in predicting the employment status of adults. The reader is referred to Groce (1993) for an excellent discussion of this topic.

4. People with disabilities often access services through programs that are not specifically targeted to them, such as Temporary Aid to Needy Families (the U.S. general welfare program). These programs are not addressed in this chapter. Nor will this chapter discuss transportation, technology access, education, and other programs that target people with disabilities but are not specific to employment.

5. Fair and efficient administration of these programs is difficult, as many scholars have noted (e.g., Stone 1984). It also leads to some interesting evaluation procedures. In Israel, women who are not in the competitive labor market may nonetheless be provided income maintenance benefits; some disabled women have been required to demonstrate to government officials, in "housewife tests" conducted by the National Insurance Institute, that they are unable to perform 18 household chores such as making beds, doing laundry, mopping floors, and cleaning closets ("Can't Clean?" 1999).

6. The policies of only a few Western nations are highlighted here. For more detailed information, the reader is referred to Thornton and Lunt (1997).

REFERENCES

Aarts, Leo J. M. and Phillip R. DeJong. 1996. "European Experiences with Disabilty Policy." Pp. 129-66 in *Disability, Work, and Cash Benefits*, edited by Jerry L. Mashaw, Virginia Reno, Richard V. Burkhauser, and Monroe Berkowitz. Kalamazoo, MI: Upjohn Institute for Employment Research.

Barnartt, Sharon N. 1992. "Disability Policy Issues in Developing Countries." *Journal of Disability Policy Studies* 3 (1): 45-65.

Berkowitz, Edward D. 1987. *Disabled Policy: America's Programs for the Handicapped*. Cambridge, UK: Cambridge University Press.

Campos, Mavis. 1995. "Developing Livelihoods." Pp. 71-84 in *Innovations in Developing Countries for People with Disabilities*, edited by Brian O'Toole and Roy McConkey. Lancashire, UK: Lisieux Hall.

"Can't Clean? Prove It, Officials Tell Housewives." 1999. *Arkansas Democrat-Gazette*, February 25, p. 3A.

Coleridge, Peter. 1993. *Disability, Liberation, and Development*. Oxford, UK: Oxfam.

Corker, Mairian. 1998. *Deaf and Disable, or Deafness Disabled?* Buckingham, UK: Open University Press.

Crichton, Anne and Lyn Jongbloed. 1998. *Disability and Social Policy in Canada*. North York, Ontario: Captus.

Devlieger, Patrick J. 1998. "Vocational Rehabilitation in Zimbabwe: A Socio-Historical Analysis." *Journal of Vocational Rehabilitation* 11 (1): 21-31.

Gooding, Carolyn. 1994. *Disabling Laws, Enabling Acts*. London: Pluto.

Groce, Nora. 1992. *The U.S. Role in International Disability Activities: A History and a Look towards the Future*. New York: Rehabilitation International.

———. 1993. "Cultural and Chronic Illness: Raising Children with Disabling Conditions in the Culturally Diverse World." *Pediatrics* 91 (5, Pt. 2): 1049.

———. 1995. "Quantifying the Quality of Life: A Social Scientist's Perspective on the World Bank's Disability-Adjusted Life Years." *Bulletin of the International Statistical Institute* 3:1131-41.

———. 1998. "Women with Disabilities in the Developing World." *Journal of Disability Policy Studies* 8 (2): 177-93.

———. 1999. "Firearm Violence, Disability Rights, and Rehabilitation: Policy Revision in Light of Shifting Demographics." *Journal of Disability Policy Studies* 9 (2): 93-110.

Harper, Malcolm and Willi Momm. 1989. *Self-Employment for Disabled People: Experiences from Africa and Asia*. Geneva: International Labour Office.

Haveman, R. H., V. Halberstadt, and R. V. Burkhauser. 1984. *Public Policy toward Disabled Workers*. Ithaca, NY: Cornell University Press.

Higgins, Paul C. 1992. *Making Disability: Exploring the Social Transformation of Human Variation*. Springfield, IL: Charles C Thomas.

Illich, Ivan. 1976. *Medical Nemesis: The Expropriation of Health*. New York: Pantheon.

———. 1987. "Disabling Professions." Pp. 11-40 in *Disabling Professions*, edited by I. Illich, I. K. Zola, J. McKnight, J. Caplan, and H. Shaiken. New York: Marion Boyars.

Ingstad, Benedicte. 1990. "The Disabled Person in the Community: Social and Cultural Aspects." *International Journal of Rehabilitation Research* 13:187-94.

International Labour Conference. 1998. *Vocational Rehabilitation and Employment of Disabled Persons*. Geneva: Author.

LaPlante, Mitchell P., Jae Kennedy, H. Stephen Kaye, and Barbara L. Wenger. 1996. *Disability and Employment*. Disability Statistics Abstract No. 11. San Francisco: Disability Statistics Rehabilitation Research and Training Center, University of California.

Louis Harris and Associates 1998. *1998 N.O.D./Harris Survey of Americans with Disabilities*. Washington, DC: National Organization on Disability.

McConkey, Roy and Brian O'Toole. 1995. "Towards the New Millennium." Pp. 3-14 in *Innovations in Developing Countries for People with Disabilities*, edited by Brian O'Toole and Roy McConkey. Lancashire, UK: Lisieux Hall.

McDonough, Peggy A. 1997. "The Social Patterning of Work Disability among Women in Canada." *Journal of Disability Policy Studies* 8 (1/2): 75-98.

McKnight, John. 1995. *The Careless Society: Community and Its Counterparts*. New York: Basic Books.

McNeil, J. M. 1997. *Americans with Disabilities: 1994-95 (P70-61)*. Washington, DC: U.S. Bureau of the Census.

Metts, Robert L. and Nansea Metts. 1996. "Self-Employment Strategies for People with Disabilities in Kenya and the United States." Pp. 22-34 in *The Entrepreneur with a Disability: Self-Employment as a Vocational Goal*, edited by Leonard G. Perlman and Carol E. Hansen. Alexandria, VA: National Rehabilitation Association.

———. 1998. "USAID, Disability and Development in Ghana." *Journal of Disability Policy Studies* 9 (1): 31-57.

Mitchell, D. T. and S. L. Snyder, eds. 1997. *The Body and Physical Difference: Discourses of Disability*. Ann Arbor: University of Michigan Press.

National Institute on Disability and Rehabilitation Research. 1992. *Digest of Data on Persons with Disabilities: 1992*. Washington, DC: Author.

Oi, Walter Y. 1991. *Disability and Work: Incentives, Rights, and Opportunities*. Washington, DC: The Enterprise Institute.

Oliver, Michael. 1996. *Understanding Disability: From Theory to Practice*. New York: St. Martin's.

Priestley, Mark. 1999. *Disability Politics and Community Care*. London: Jessica Kingsley.

Rioux, Marcia H. and Michael Bach, eds. 1994. *Disability Is Not Measles: New Research Paradigms in Disability*. North York, Ontario: Roeher Institute.

Schriner, K., P. Rumrill, and R. Parlin. 1995. "Rethinking Disability Policy: Equity in the ADA and the Meaning of Specialized Services for People with Disabilities." *Journal of Health and Human Services Administration* 17 (4): 478-500.

Scotch, R. K. and K. Schriner. 1997. "Disability as Human Variation: Implications for Policy." *The Annals of the American Academy of Political and Social Science* 549:148-59.

Stone, Deborah A. 1984. *The Disabled State*. Philadelphia: Temple University Press.

———. 1993. "Clinical Authority in the Construction of Citizenship." Pp. 45-67 in *Public Policy for Democracy*, edited by Helen Ingram and Steven Rathgab Smith. Washington, DC: Brookings Institution.

Thomson, Rosemarie Garland, ed. 1996. *Freakery: Cultural Spectacles of the Extraordinary Body*. New York: New York University Press.

Thornton, Patricia and Neil Lunt. 1997. *Employment Policies for Disabled People in Eighteen Countries: A Review*. York, UK: University of York.

United Nations. 1986. *Manual on the Equalization of Opportunities for Disabled Persons*. New York: Author.

U.S. General Accounting Office. 1993. *Vocational Rehabilitation: Evidence for Federal Program's Effectiveness Is Mixed*. Washington, DC: Author.

Werner, David. 1995. "Strengthening the Role of Disabled People in Community Based Rehabilitation Programmes." Pp. 15-28 in *Innovations in Developing Countries for People with Disabilities*, edited by Brian O'Toole and Roy McConkey. Lancashire, UK: Lisieux Hall.

Yelin, Edward H. 1992. *Disability and the Displaced Worker*. New Brunswick, NJ: Rutgers University Press.

Science and Technology Policy

29

Is Disability a Missing Factor?

KATHERINE D. SEELMAN

> The National Science and Technology Policy, Organization and Priorities Act of 1976 has just about everything in it that would be useful, except the word "handicapped" ... add a focus on the special needs of the handicapped to be served by new scientific and engineering technological developments.
>
> —Schloss (1976:283)

I n this quotation, Irving P. Schloss, on behalf of the American Foundation of the Blind in 1976, made a plea to have the newly adopted U.S. science and technology policy framework serve disabled people. Disabled people want to move beyond the confines of health and benefits policy, in which their interests have been segregated, to policy that can allocate research and development resources for assistive technology, accessible consumer products, built environments, telecommunications, and transportation.

The focus of this chapter is to show that the nature of science and technology, as well as its relative autonomy and self-governance, has had a limiting effect on participation by disabled people in government decisions about investments in technology. This effect may be similar to the experience of women, people of color, and poor people. Disabled people have traditionally faced barriers to active citizenship because of stigma, and their interests have been sequestered in health and benefits policies. Ironically, policymakers continue to sequester the needs of disabled people in health policy, despite the possibilities for applying cutting-edge science and technology—materials science and microelectronics—to accessible infrastructures and assistive technology as well as to medical rehabilitation. Consequently, disabled people have pursued their science and technology objectives through alternative policy channels, especially those of international human rights and national civil rights policy.

This chapter places the special case of the demands for participation in assistive technology decisions in the larger context of public participation in science and technology policy in the

AUTHOR'S NOTE: Many people from around the globe have reviewed this chapter. I want to thank them. Special thanks to Dr. Dawn Carlson and Ms. Mary Darnell at the National Institute on Disability and Rehabilitation Research who spent many hours working on this chapter.

United States and, to a lesser extent, in the European Union and Japan. Although the science and technology interests of disabled people have been largely relegated to health issues, disabled people have been further stymied by the lack of participation within these governments. These democracies have few institutions through which citizens can become critically engaged in choosing or designing technology (Sclove 1995). For example, for most of the post–World War II period, U.S. science and technology investments have been focused on the big missions of national security, space, energy, and health (Smith and Barfield 1996). In Europe, too, research and development for social needs such as assistive technology did not have the economic and industrial weight of other sectors (E. Ballabio, personal communication, 1999). Direct communications with policymakers, researchers, and advocates in Europe and Japan have allowed for a more candid discussion about allocations of resources such as applied research, regulatory behavior, and international issues. There is, of course, a great need to address the assistive technology demands of developing countries in which most disabled people live.

Clearly, disabled people have a fundamental interest in decisions about allocation of science and technology resources because these decisions involve issues of survival, freedom, and independence. However, both Europe and the United States have had difficulty separating health policy from that which encourages research for the development and deployment of technology that supports higher-level functioning and accessibility (E. Ballabio, personal communication, 1999). Ultimately, decisions about investments in research and development are decisions that can support or deter independent living, community integration, and learning and working in the community. For example, national science and technology policies could incorporate the principal of universal design and could make research and development investments in universal design applications for transportation, the built environment, telecommunications, and consumer products as well as in research to support medical rehabilitation and health and wellness for disabled people. A well-known U.S. architect, Ron Mace, defined universal design as "design[ing] all products and environments to be usable to the greatest extent possible by people of all ages and abilities" (Mace, Hardie, and Plaice 1991:2). However, diversity of function—diversity based on differences in hearing, seeing, moving, and processing information—is a new concept. Diversity of function, unlike gender, ethnic, and racial diversity, is not yet a widely recognized principal for understanding discrimination in science and engineering career paths and in the technological marketplace. The assistive technology marketplace is composed of many disability subgroups based on function. National science and technology policy could also compensate for the small, fragmented niche-assistive technology marketplace that is widely acknowledged to exist in Europe and the United States (Lane 1997). Users of assistive technologies are diverse in their functional characteristics. For example, the market for hearing aids is different from the market for augmentative communication devices.

Definitions

Many terms in this chapter are open to definitional interpretation. For the most part, we adopt a position of a common understanding of these terms. *Assistive technology* refers to any item, piece of equipment, or product system—off the shelf, customized, or modified—that is used to increase, maintain, or improve functional capabilities of disabled individuals. *Assistive technology* is a broad term that may include individual medical devices such as implantable pumps for diabetes, chronic pain, spasticity, and Parkinson's disease; social devices for individuals, such as augmentative communications boards for nonvocal people; and systems technology to give people access to transportation and to the built and information technology environments. For example, disability accessibility features have been built into the operating system for Microsoft Windows 95 and 98. The markets for medical and social devices for individuals and for systems technology can be quite different. There may be large markets for certain medical devices, but devices that support higher social function, such as augmentative communication boards, are usually small because of marketplace fragmentation. For example, the assistive technology user marketplace is composed of different disability subgroups (e.g., nonspeaking people) purchasing assistive technology appropriate to their functional needs. Assistive technology companies are often small companies with domestic rather than global marketing strategies. While third-party payers may fund devices for individuals, the devices must usually meet medical, not social use, criteria. Because of the fragmentation of the assistive technology marketplace and the small user populations, assistive technology is sometimes labeled orphan technology. Problems of small marketplaces and inadequate public funding support have driven the disability community to support the notion of universally designed buildings, information and transportation systems, and consumer products. At the design stage, these systems and products would have the capability to be used by a broad range of users, including those with diverse functional capability. Very different market forces operate for information technology and other large systems. Large companies, such as Microsoft and IBM, with global marketplaces, make choices about add-on features that might stimulate increased sales.

The terms *science* and *technology* are themselves the subject of considerable definitional discussions. For the purpose of this chapter, a somewhat crude line is drawn between basic science, on one hand, and applied science and technology, on the other. Rehabilitation science and rehabilitation engineering are subsets of applied science. Applied science and technology are used relatively interchangeably. According to policy analyst Bruce Smith (1990), science and technology policy is a subset of policy studies that involves allocations of research and development of science resources such as basic and applied research, commercialization, regulatory behavior, and international issues. The science and technology enterprise involves research, technology development, and training.

Academic Fields

The disability movement, the establishment of disability studies and rehabilitation science in universities, and the allocation of research funds to support independent living–related research in the United States, Europe, and Japan are generating a body of knowledge framed in a social paradigm of disability. The social paradigm is an evolving framework that is characterized by a unit of analysis on the group level, interdisciplinary orientation, and an expanded range of disciplines, including disability studies, business and management, and information science. The literature on social movements is vast, as is the literature on participation in governmental decision making. A special issue of the *Journal of Disability Studies* on political participation by disabled people identifies major factors in participation resources, recruitment networks, and psychological engagement, including interest in issues and membership in groups that have common values or interests (Schur 1998). The international debate about the nature of science and technology has been the energizing intellectual force behind the establishment of new academic fields such as the social study of science and science and technology policy. Although academics from these new fields have paid scant attention to the activities of disabled people, they have made invaluable contributions to the historical, ideological, social, and policy implications of science and technology. Social studies of science, for example, have shown that demands for participation in decision making about science and technology are anchored in a historical debate between those who argue for the autonomy of science and those who argue for a linkage between science and technology and social goals. There are many nuances to this debate, not the least of which is whether power and values can be isolated from the process of doing science.

Three Approaches: Ideology, History, and Public Policy

We will use three different approaches to examine representation and participation of disabled people in science and technology policy and research. These include the following:

1. an ideological approach to probe the assumptions about the nature of science and technology,
2. a historical approach to identify the consensus about science and technology and government in succeeding stages after World War II,
3. a public policy approach to describe the past and present bases for distribution of science and technology resources.

For the ideological approach, it is appropriate to ask if something in the assumptions about the nature of science and technology creates barriers to involvement by disabled people beyond being the subjects of scientific study. For example, do assumptions about normalcy and what is natural predispose the enterprise to exclude certain groups? If, as some believe, science must be self-governing to be innovative, and disability is a deviation from the norm, how can disabled people become legitimate participants in science and technology? As we shall see, thinkers who have disabilities have waded into this debate with great energy, arguing that discriminatory values are built into the science and technology enterprise.

The historical approach also tells a story about the development of consensus regarding the role of science, technology, and government and the corresponding influence and activities of disabled people in science and technology policy development. History provides a panorama of events that have implications for incorporation of the interests of disabled people in science and technology policy. Events such as war, the end of the cold war, scientific inventions of antibiotics and the transistor, and leaders with disabilities, such as Franklin Delano Roosevelt, may be factors in shaping the dominant views about participation in science and technology and in shaping decisions about allocation of resources. Following World War II, the great infrastructure of a global economy, driven by innovations in science and technology, has been built with competitive and dynamic marketplaces and a highly trained technical class. Different models for the authority and legitimacy of science and technology have characterized successive historical periods. These include the expert model, in which the scientist is the authority over decisions about allocations of science and technology resources; the civic model, in which citizens participate in decision making; and the economic model, in which economic factors drive allocation of resources. These models vary in responsiveness to various interests, including participation of laypeople. History has provided an interesting report of how disabled people have used advocacy and public policy tools to move their agenda.

The public policy approach identifies strategies used by disabled people and their technically trained allies to introduce non-health-related issues, such as universal design and orphan technology, onto the science and technology agenda. For example, democratic institutions, such as the European Parliament, and policy tools, such as standards development, have been useful in the implementation of science and technology objectives. A universal standard for wheelchairs, for example, makes it possible to market wheelchairs in a global marketplace. As with environmentalists and antimilitarist protesters, disabled people throughout the world have tried to use their social movement and more formal democratic institutions to further their policy goals. The importance of democratic institutions in scientific decision making and participation for disabled people is one of the most important themes in the chapter. Of course, research and development budgets are the best indicators of science and technology program commitments. They show over time who gets allocations of precious science and technology dollars and for what. A lengthy budgetary analysis is not within the purview of this chapter. There is a dearth of research on allocations of science and technology resources for rehabilitation science. The Institute on Medicine report, *Enabling America,* came up with a figure of less than $300 million (Brandt and Pope 1997).

Equity Issues

Equity issues pervade the science and technology policy discussion as it applies to disabled people. At present, U.S. private and public research and development (R&D) is approximately

40 percent or more of the world R&D (Sarewitz 1996). The science and technology infrastructure that has developed since World War II does not extend to the poorest countries of Latin America, sub-Saharan Africa, and South Asia. On the disability and rehabilitation level, there are great inequities in the distribution of science and technology resources. On one hand, increases in the population of disabled and elderly people in the industrialized countries are generating interest and investment in assistive technology. Indeed, attention to these demographic trends addresses a major equity issue. On the other hand, because investments appear to be concentrated in industrialized countries, there is inequity in the distribution of resources because most disabled people live in Third World countries. Unquestionably, even in the industrialized countries, disabled people as a group are poor. However, disability movement activities, over time, have been effective in advocating for R&D investments for social purposes, such as accessibility in telecommunications that may have implications for global accessibility. A final section will set out a future agenda for research; this is no small matter for a world with an increasing population of people with diversity of function, especially older people. Public policy will be very much a part of that future agenda.

THE GREAT DEBATE: SCIENCE AND TECHNOLOGY FOR WHOM? WHO DECIDES?

The question of whether the inner content of basic science is socially constructed involves ancient philosophical positions that may never be resolved. However, these positions will be explored because they inform the dialogue about the social construction of applied science and engineering. The great and complex debate that continues today in the United Kingdom, Europe, the United States, and other parts of the world involves the nature of science and technology and the implications for public life and scientific training. Japan, as we will see, may have a different ideological basis for its science and technology activities than that of Western industrialized countries but, nonetheless, may face similar issues. In the West, two distinct approaches to the controversy have emerged. They can be reduced to one question: Is science a social phenomenon or not?

Positivism and Mechanism versus a Social Approach

Applying the notion of two approaches to science and technology studies, David Edge (1995) summarizes the debate well. He refers to the first approach as the "received view." This approach assumes that science and technology are "asocial, impersonal activities—a positivistic, even mechanistic, picture of an endeavor that defines its own logic and momentum. The authority of nature is independent of, and prior to, the authority of society." The other approach views science and technology "as essentially and irredeemably human (and hence social) both in the context that nourishes, supports, and directs them and in their inner character" (Edge 1995:3-23). According to Edge, the first approach found a particularly sympathetic audience in the East European and Soviet countries and in China, which at the time had centralized bureaucracies struggling to base decisions about investments in science and technology on expertise. The second approach, which assumes that science is a social system, is rooted in the sociology of science and the works of Robert Merton (1973), Thomas Kuhn (1970), J. D. Bernal (1939), and Michael Polanyi (1962). The debate also involved the education of scientists. Charles Percy Snow (1964) sparked the so-called two cultures debate in a lecture at Cambridge in the 1960s. Subsequently, there has been considerable discussion about whether to train scientists in a scientific specialized culture or a broad humane culture that would prepare scientists to act with social responsibility. The debate became particularly hot in the 1960s, a period of intense questioning about military spending, civilian nuclear power, and the impact of science on the environment.

The Expert Model and the Social Model

English physicist John D. Bernal and Hungarian-born physical chemist Michael Polanyi are often cast in history in the roles of protagonist for each of the two approaches to science. In his now-classic article, "The Republic of Science," which appeared in the journal *Minerva,* Polanyi (1962) explains why he believes science must be an autonomous enterprise. Polanyi argues,

> What I have said here about the highest possible coordination of individual scientific efforts by a process of self-coordination may recall the self-coordination achieved by producers and consumers operating in a market. It was, indeed, with this in mind that I spoke of "the invisible hand" guiding the coordination of independent initiatives to a maximum advancement of science, just as Adam Smith invoked "the invisible hand" to describe the achievement of the greatest joint material satisfaction when independent producers and consumers are guided by the prices of goods in a market. (P. 56)

Polanyi's position exalts the lone scientist, the expert whose activity must be uncurtailed to innovate and whose social context, guided by an invisible hand, inevitably coordinates and links these creative people, resulting in even more innovation. Bernal's position is clearly that of a socialist who had a deep empathy for the scientific orientation of the Soviet Union. In his *Social Function of Science,* first published in 1939, Bernal praised the qualitative characteristics of Soviet science and its originality, particularly in the choice of problems, and attributed this to the trend toward choosing problems connected with experience. He attributed the insufficiently critical attitude of Soviet science to youthful enthusiasm that would be corrected over time. His position on the social nature of science is reflected in the following quote:

> Induction and proof remain as they were . . . dialectical materialism can . . . do two things: suggest the direction of thought which are likely to be particularly fruitful in results and integrate and organize different branches of scientific research in relation to one another and to the social processes of which they form a part. (Bernal 1939:231)

An excellent summary of the Bernal-Polanyi debates is found in Christoper Freeman's (1993) *The Economics of Hope.* The works of Bernal (1939) and Polanyi (1962) have had important implications for disabled people. Polanyi's position, which may be more representative of science and technology policy in the industrialized countries, argues for the autonomy of science and its separation from social goals. Bernal believed that some method of determining government priorities for science and technology must be established and argued in support of debating these priorities and encouraging new initiatives. In doing so, as Freeman points out, Bernal laid the foundation for science and technology policy. Freeman observes that there are at least three areas of government involvement in science and technology. They are governmental provision for basic research, decisions about subdivisions of the global science budget (e.g., cell biology, chemistry, and medieval history), and responsibility for the health and efficiency of parts of the system (e.g., national laboratories, libraries, and patent offices). Freeman, of course, could have provided examples of research decisions of interest to disabled people such as a universal design program funded by national research and development budgets and conducted in national laboratories as well as support for training disabled personnel. Indeed, if governments allocate public resources for support for training scientists and engineers, then political and cultural factors may be introduced into the training.

Cultural Differences in the Training of Scientists and Engineers

The United States, Europe, and Japan have had a historical interest in maintaining cultural values as part of training in the sciences and in engineering. In personal correspondence with Dr. Shigeru Yamauchi of the National Rehabilitation Center for the Disabled in Japan, Yamauchi provided his interpretation of Japanese understanding of the nature of science and technology. He observes that there is not a tradition of truth in traditional Japanese and Chinese culture. By truth, he means activity to find out basic principles of nature. Yamauchi traces the current Japanese understanding of science and technology to Confucianism and to the notion of *bushido,* which insisted on absolute loyalty to the lords, continued as a robust concept in the modern period, and was understood as loyalty to support a rich and strong nation. Japan established its first engineering school, the Imperial College of Engineering, in 1873. The country has clearly enjoyed a lively dialogue on engineering training and curricula. In a 1877 article in the journal *Nature,* it was clear that the Japanese were critical of the engineering education in England, which was deemed too practical and training oriented, and education on the continent was deemed too theoretical ("Letter to the Editor" 1877:44). In a 1904 letter to the editor of *Nature,* Henry Dyer, said to be the father of Japanese engineering, stated the following on technical education in Japan:

> Many of the men who are supposed to have had a complete technical education are very poor specimens of humanity, wanting in individuality and character, devoid of all originality and with a very narrow view of the world. Some of them may manage to pile up fortunes for themselves, but they will do little to make their country great. . . . The outcome of it all is that the national consciousness is directed to the attainment of national objects by men whose individual powers have been trained to make effective use of western science, and the results have been simply wonderful. (Dyer 1904:150-51)

According to U.S. rehabilitation engineer Dudley Childress, engineering schools in the United States have also had a historical concern about how to train engineers to be well-rounded individuals in society as well as persons of great technical ability and creativity (D. Childress, personal communication, 1999). The incorporation of cultural and civic values into technical training courses is seen as an important strategy for supporting a country's traditional values and governmental philosophy. The academic study of science and technology has been highly sensitive to these and other subjective influences.

Gender, Culture, and Class

As the social study of science has developed, scholars have been critical of science and technology. For example, on the individual level, both feminists and disabled people have argued that discrimination on the basis of being different from the norm has excluded them from science. In the tradition of Bernal, they have also addressed the social system, arguing that limited control of the means of doing science has served a narrow band of economic interests. Writing from a feminist perspective, Evelyn Fox Keller (1999) notes the following:

> Women were caught on the horns of an impossible dilemma—a dilemma that was unresolvable as long as the goal of science was seen as the unequivocal mirroring of nature, and its success as admitting of only a single standard of measurement. It was only with the introduction of an alternative view of science—one admitting of a multiplicity of goals and standards—that the condition arose for some feminists, in the late 1970s and early 1980s, to begin to argue for the inclusion of difference. (P. 236)

She describes the dilemma, in part, as women having to repudiate their gender, disavowing their difference from men to be productive in science. Keller (1999) argues that there are two power bases for the epistemological authority of scientists: exclusion on the basis of differences such as gender and exclusion on the basis of the nature of scientific knowledge as either objective or relative. This critique, of course, is very useful to disabled people who also have had to deny their identities as disabled people and, in fact, are labeled impaired and diseased and the subject of scientific study, which is objectified.

The literature also addresses the implications of assumptions about science and technology for minorities and Third World cultures, language, and religion. Citing disability research experience in China, Emma Stone (1997) counseled as follows:

> Research into indigenous concepts of and responses to disability is a vital but frequently neglected part of researching disability in developing countries. To do this properly, the researcher should not be a slave to outsider theories or socio-political movements. Definitions need to begin with individuals, families and communities at the grassroots and not with outsiders. (P. 222)

Stone (1997) argues that academicians should not be spokespeople for the disability movement. She argues against disability researchers following on the heels of feminists and gay and lesbian researchers who have been proponents of identity politics, which often excludes as legitimate those who have not experienced the particular identity.

In the *New Politics of Science,* David Dickson (1984) presents a view that develops the Bernal orientation to a modern stage of science and technology policy in which economic objectives are paramount. Dickson recognizes the political nature of scientific decisions and issues related to allocation of resources. He explains, "I intend to . . . look at how the patterns of control over science reinforce and reproduce basic patterns of political control that operate in society. For the increasingly *economic* importance of science gives it political significance" (p. 5).

Dickson (1984) believes that science is the single most important factor molding the lives of others, replacing an individual, group, or social class with access to superior civilian or military force. Insofar as decision making about science and technology relies on "market forces to determine research and development priorities, it can skew priorities away from where the social needs are pressing and the economic incentives to tackle these needs is weak" (Dickson 1984:52). He cites, as an example, microelectronics applications for the disabled. Dickson's analysis is supported by the inequities in the U.S. and European assistive technology marketplace referred to earlier. The assistive technology marketplace is fragmented, small, and weak. It lacks capital for research, development, and purchase. In the tradition of Polanyi and Bernal, Dickson posits two approaches to the social impacts of science and technology. He describes them as follows:

> The first, favored by those who seek a "rational" approach to the problems by the imposition of solutions reached through a consensus of experts, can be characterized as the technocratic approach. Even when encouraging participation in the process of reaching consensus, this approach leaves unquestioned the basic political structures through which the solutions, usually expressed in technical terms, are to be put into effect. In contrast, the second approach stresses the importance of procedures as much as goals, arguing that the rationality of solutions offered by the experts is often illusory, and that the best protection against this is to exploit to the full the opportunities for wide participation in making decisions, not merely talking about which decisions should be made. This approach acknowledges greater confidence in the opportunities for participation offered by federal and state legislative bodies, by the courts and by broader political movements such as public interest groups and labor union, and bases its strategies on the assumption that the solutions to the problems caused by the applications of science requires a redistribution of political power as much as the insight of technical expertise. (P. 219)

In this quote, Dickson (1984) introduces into the debate the very important issue of the role of democratic institutions and people's movements in participation in science and technology decisions.

The Disability Movement and Participation in Science and Technology

The disability movements in various countries have become more involved in the research process as well as in the legislative process. The intense anger expressed below from the book, *No Pity,* illustrates the motivation behind involvement of the disability movements:

> Faith in technology can play into the hated image of cure and pity that the disability rights movement has sought to erase. No two devices have held the public more in awe than the Functional Electronic Stimulator (FES) and the cochlear implant. . . . To some, cochlear implants are a miracle. To others, they are an instrument of cultural murder. (Shapiro 1993:223)

Perhaps similar to feminists, low-income communities, and communities of color, disabled intellectuals view research as exploitative. Fed by dashed hopes and unintended impacts of technology suggested by the excerpt from *No Pity,* many disabled people have taken radical positions on the research process and on guidelines for policy. Some have also supported identity politics that would exclude from disability research researchers who have not had the experience of disability. These more radical critiques appear to be directed at applied social research rather than biological and engineering research. In England, for example, issues arose about the use of research to support professional power to control the everyday lives of disabled people and keep them institutionalized. Criticism was also leveled at the World Health Organization's *International Classification of Impairment, Disability, and Handicap (ICIDH)* and researchers for not breaking the implied causal relationship between disability and impairment by recognizing the importance of environmental factors to the ability to function (World Health Organization 1980).

Emancipatory Research

In England, a group of researchers developed an approach to research called emancipatory research (Barnes and Mercer 1997). Emancipatory approach assumes the need to transform the social and material relationship of research production. Barnes and Mercer (1997) describe the emancipatory paradigm as follows:

> The emancipatory paradigm rejects the notion of researcher-experts moving between projects like "academic tourists," and using disability as a commodity to exchange for advancing their own status and interests. The response of disabled people is quite simple: "no participation without representation." (P. 6)

The significance attached to people's subjective experience of disability and impairment is similar to that attached to the subjective experience of women. In much the same way as feminism, the respected English disability theorist Mike Oliver (1997) contextualized emancipatory research. He explains it in the following passage:

> The development of such a paradigm stems from the gradual rejection of the positivist view of social research as the pursuit of absolute knowledge through the scientific method and the gradual disillusionment with the interpretive view of such research as the generation of socially useful knowledge within particular historical and social contexts. The

emancipatory paradigm, as the name implies is about the facilitating of a politics of the possible by confronting social oppression at whatever levels it occurs. (P. 16)

Oliver (1997) argues that the emancipatory paradigm highlights reciprocity, gain, and empowerment. The emancipatory approach addresses not only the research process but also control of resources needed to undertake research. The resources needed to undertake research include funding but also power to establish the content and method of research priorities. Control over both process and resources, of course, implies social change potential.

Participatory Action Research

Proponents of the emancipatory approach are critical of the participatory action research approach (PAR) that has been emphasized by researchers in the United States. They argue that PAR reinforces power structures rather than developing or confronting them. Indeed, PAR is more oriented toward problem solving in particular situations than in social transformation. In a conference sponsored by the U.S. National Institute on Disability and Rehabilitation Research (NIDRR), PAR was defined as follows:

Participatory Action Research (PAR) is an approach to research designed to place individuals being studied at the center of the decision-making process. PAR has developed in a broader social context that has moved toward recognition of the personal expertise and particular needs and rights of individuals in society. It has emerged in a research context that is moving toward increasing use of qualitative inquiry strategies. The role and value of this approach in disability and rehabilitation research has been an ongoing topic of interest in the decade of the 1990s. (Tewey 1997:iv)

Researchers and Participation

The research community has been interested in the question of end-user involvement in research, particularly PAR. At a meeting of the NIDRR directors in January 1995, Dr. John Whyte, an American physician and researcher, presented a paper that described the complexity of objectives, roles, and function in research projects (Whyte 1995). He suggested that the social context of research and the nature of that which is studied are often confused. Whyte believes that PAR is most useful in studying and changing sociotechnical systems and promoting social change. PAR assumes that participants in sociotechnical systems have knowledge and information that are not possessed by "outsiders" (i.e., most researchers) and that this knowledge is needed not only to answer research questions but also to ask them. Using the transit system as an example, he notes that disabled people can identify the problem areas and therefore the research problems in using subways. Whyte is referring to the generation of research problems based on the experience of the disabled user of the public transit system. For Whyte, PAR really has nothing to say about nonsocial systems, such as the study of nuclear physics, except possibly for a role in the study of the social system in the lab, as well as development of training curriculum and how it is presented and taught.

In an e-mail dialogue with Professor Alan Newell, Department of Applied Computing, University of Dundee in Scotland, Newell clarified some of his recent comments on participation in the process of doing applied computing research (Newell 1998). Newell has been researching computer-based systems for people with disabilities for 30 years. He has addressed a number of controversies, including the role of the researcher, the defining characteristics of the research process, intergenerational equity, user participation, and ethical implications of user involvement. Newell argues that assistive technology research priorities and characteristics are different from those of health research and that the medical model is seldom appropriate for researchers in this field. He believes that such researchers should focus on the needs and the wants of users, and this is achieved by a user-centered design methodology. The involvement of clinicians and potential and actual users is very important, but this must be done with care; otherwise, it will compromise the very process that user participation is supposed to serve (Newell 1998).

Newell (1998) believes that assistive technology research is a long-term activity, and although the researcher should be sensitive to the needs and wants of the current generation of disabled people, the responsibility of the research community is to the next generation. He expresses his position in the following:

> Particularly in this field, there is a tendency to avoid leading edge issues, because these are thought to be of little practical value, or involve new expensive and/or untried technology. We do a great disservice to disabled citizens of the future by not giving priority to such work. (Pp. xlviii-liii)

He argues that people with disabilities have as much right to eventually reap the benefits of "Blue Sky research" as able-bodied people. The research process must thus allow researchers to use their imaginations and try out ideas that are either not understood by the users or are not popular with them. As support of his position on an effective research process, he describes useful research findings and products that were not initially supported by users and clinicians. Within the research paradigm, disabled users must realize that they personally may not benefit from the outcomes of the research and that some research may show that certain techniques are not successful. An aspect that is not common to mainstream research, however, is the problem of informed consent. This can raise ethical issues of which the researcher needs to be fully aware. Newell (1998) says that at Dundee University, there are and have been both able-bodied and disabled researchers, and their research has been enriched by the perceptions of individual disabled users who are attached to the research group and by specifically constituted panels of users with disabilities. However, the input from these users is modified by the researcher's vision of what can be achieved. As would be expected in a user-centered design paradigm, users have made tremendous contributions to the research over many years and to the commercial products that have grown from the research. The primary rewards for the individual users with disabilities within the research team come from their being internationally known in the field, attending international conferences, and giving lecture tours. They are truly members of the research team, and the group is very fortunate to have their input to the research.

When asked about ideas that are less than popular with the majority of clinicians and users at the early stage of research, Newell responded as follows:

> I was referring to a number of products which we have produced over the years. The one which stands out was the overall idea behind our work on the original CHAT (Conversation Helped by Automatic Talk) system, and other systems we developed from this, such as Talksback. The idea was that it was more important for non-speaking people to say something than have complete control over what they would say. This idea was originally completely rejected by many therapists on the grounds that we were removing control of what they said from users. This antagonism lasted a number of years, but now is accepted by the majority in the field and many AAC devices contain features of this nature. (A. F. Newell, personal communication, 1999)

Clearly, the question of the degree of freedom and choice designed into devices is an issue for all users, but it may have particular significance for disabled users who use it as a substitute for basic human activities and thus may present more human rights and human freedom issues.

Technically Trained People Who Are Disabled

People such as Rolf Hotchkiss and Lars Augustsson, who have experience with disability and technical training, have described some of the dilemma of disabled people's participation in research and development. In 1976, Hotchkiss stated the following:

Unless there's a group of people who understand both the disabilities and the technical things at the same time, then it'll be basically as it has been. It'll be the technocrats misleading the disabled people, and vice versa in a way, and not a good deal of press. . . . It seems you need to really hunt and find people with a combination of abilities—and there are enough around—but most of the good, disabled engineers I know are in industry, and they're not about to join the civil rights movement on a voluntary basis. (P. 217)

Lars Augustsson, an engineer, was in charge of R&D in the field of motor impairments at the Swedish Handicap Institute from 1978 to 1988. Similar to Hotchkiss, Augustsson described the problem of being unable to have the best-informed consumers working in key technical spots as follows:

In Sweden, consumer organizations usually do not have access to the best-informed consumers to send to advisory boards. Those disabled consumers who have enough expertise in an area such as telecommunications are usually already employed in a company and the disability organization cannot compete. If for some reason they can afford to hire someone as "their expert on assistive technology," as the larger organizations can, that person cannot be expected to be an expert on a large part of the field of assistive technology. (L. Augustsson, personal communication, 1999)

These comments by Hotchkiss and Augustsson further illustrate the barriers to decision making and participation and suggest the need for some compensatory activity in the policy arena. The characteristics of the policy arena, much like the ideological basis for participation in science and technology, are determined by prevalent historical factors.

SCIENCE AND TECHNOLOGY POLICY: THE HISTORICAL CONTEXT

Assumptions about the nature of science and technology, the role of the citizen, and the objectives of science and technology policy as well as the development of an institutional framework for science and technology are evolving and are very much conditioned by opinion and attitude during recent historical periods. Bruce L. R. Smith (1990) has created a useful three-stage developmental framework for U.S. science and technology policy, beginning in the post–World War II period. The framework arranges science and technology policy within three periods: the age of the professional or expert, the age of dissent, and a pluralistic period. Time frameworks, such as Smith's, are not universal but rough estimations. His three-stage framework will be adjusted to provide a description of general trends in Europe and Japan and also to provide a description of the activity in the disability movement. Smith uses the framework to organize consensus about the role of science and technology and government within three post–World War II periods. His framework is applied in the history section to serve three purposes. First, the framework is used to organize general trends in science and technology within post–World War II stages, especially as they relate to participation. Important factors include consensus around whom should make scientific decisions, the goals of science policy, and the emerging governmental framework. Second, the time framework is used and modified to accommodate the consensus of disabled people, about who should decide their policy issues and objectives and the means used to accomplish these objectives. Third, we will explore relationships between the general level and the level of disabled people. Finally, in each chronological stage, relevant policy tools are identified. Budgets, regulation, tax policy, and standards, for example, can be used either to benefit or deprive disabled people. They are very important to the next section on public policy.

1945-1965: The Age of the Scientist and the Professional

General Trends

During this period, the expert model dominated the basis for authority in science and technology policy rather than models that are based on economics or popular democratic institutions and movements. This is a period of restoration of industry and economic growth in Europe and Japan, where vast areas of infrastructures were destroyed during World War II. Japan, in particular, went through a period of technology transfer to be followed by economic growth and rapid industrialization. The industrialized countries, especially the United States, expanded its resource base to support industrial innovation with large investments in basic research. It was also the beginning of the cold war and the launching of *Sputnik* by the USSR.

In the United States, federal investments in research and development were in defense, space, and atomic energy—all essentially derived from the cold war. Although some believed that the relationship between universities and business was too close and that the public would be better served if the nonspecialist controlled the scientific effort, this position did not prevail. In the United States, a consensus about science was more or less guided by Vannevar Bush's (1990) report, *Science—The Endless Frontier*. The report seemed to suggest a linear line from basic research to commercialization. Reminiscent of Adam Smith and Michael Polanyi, commercialization, according to Bruce L. R. Smith (1990), was assumed to come almost automatically as a result of the government's support of basic and applied research. The authority of the expert and the professional was reflected in rehabilitation.

Disability and Rehabilitation

One of the great influences on future allocations of science and technology resources for disabled people was launched during the 1945 to 1965 period. The United Nations (1948) adopted the *Universal Declaration of Human Rights* as the framework for the rights of many groups. Disability groups would draw on human rights to substantiate their need for assistive technology for social integration.

However, most rehabilitation activity in the United States, Europe, and Japan was mobilized to address the medical needs of those injured in World War II, especially veterans. Health and benefits programs were established. This was a period of development of the fields of medical rehabilitation and rehabilitation engineering. For U.S. rehabilitation engineer Dudley Childress (1977), who wrote *Historical Sketch Concerning Federal Support of Research to Aid the Handicapped*, World War II marked the beginning of U.S. science and technology in rehabilitation (Childress 1976; see also Brandt and Pope 1997). In the field of assistive technology, research and development focused on advancements in the more medically related technology of prosthetics and orthotics. Early identification of assistive technology within medical technology may be the basis of seemingly intractable perception within policy that links the technology needs of disabled people with the health domain. Recognition of the need for social technology would wait for another period. Individual countries, such as the United Kingdom and the United States, were active in building professional capacity, not only in medical rehabilitation and rehabilitation engineering but also in vocational rehabilitation.

United States

In the United States, Mary Switzer, who was named head of the U.S. Office of Vocational Rehabilitation in 1950, was instrumental in the development of vocational rehabilitation training to support employment rather than dependency for disabled people (Obermann 1965). She broadened disabled policy to include employment objectives. She also brought the United States into international rehabilitation. The Office of Vocational Rehabilitation supported projects in Israel, India, Pakistan, Egypt, Poland, Yugoslavia, Brazil, Burma, and Syria. Research included development in the design and manufacture of prosthetics and orthotics that would be made available to U.S. manufacturers. During this period, the United States supported exchange of international experts in rehabilitation, especially medical rehabilitation.

Big Science and the Third World

Western aid to developing countries during this period has been described by Nora Groce (1992) as follows:

> Until recently, Western professionals were considered . . . the final arbiters of needs of people with disabilities and international aid was directed toward the building of rehabilitation centers and projects, and the training and support of professional groups. In the Developing World, state of the art hospitals, institutions and clinics were the equivalent of enormous hydroelectric dams and highways through the jungles. While often effective in their own right, these programs were simply not reaching many who need[ed] them most. (P. 97)

According to Groce (1992), a new approach, known as community-based rehabilitation (CBR), was introduced at the 1969 meeting of Rehabilitation International in Ireland. CBR emphasizes essential services, economic development, and the importance of training disabled people, family members, and local health personnel in rehabilitation techniques that make a difference in an individual's ability to do everyday tasks. CBR has much resemblance to an empowerment or independent living approach.

Europe and Japan

The European Union countries have had a long history of involvement in disability. Some of that history is captured in the country-by-country descriptions in the 1994 European Union study, titled *European Service Delivery Systems in Rehabilitation Technology* (Commission of the European Communities 1994). The following description of the immediate post–World War II period for the Netherlands is particularly interesting:

> The multi-disciplinary approach in rehabilitation was designed. Rehabilitation centers were established to concentrate professionals and expertise in specialized centres. Areas such as technical aids, mobility, transport and accessibility, however, were not identified as rehabilitation. Progress was made on medical aspects of prosthetics and orthotics. (Commission of the European Communities 1994)

According to Dr. Yamauchi, the post–World War II period and the occupation of Japan by forces under General Douglas MacArthur was a most difficult time in modern Japanese history. Yamauchi notes that new dealers in MacArthur's headquarters established the basic structure of legislation for disabled persons and tried to establish a social welfare system. In rehabilitation, the main measure was to provide prostheses to war casualties. There was no participation of disabled people in R&D (S. Yamauchi, personal communication, 1999).

In general, in the early post–World War II period of 1945 to 1965, an expert model prevailed as the basis for science and technology authority. Governments directed their resources to reconstruction of industry, revitalization of the economy, and rehabilitation of those injured by war throughout the world. The United States, in the enviable position of emerging from the war without major destruction of its industrial capacity, took an early lead in science and technology investments in basic research that would be maintained throughout the cold war. There was a consensus around the importance of the Western scientific model, the establishment of a large scientific infrastructure, and the authority of the expert to decide about investments to support economic activity and technological development. However, the international human rights effort was launched, and the rights approach would eventually be a countervailing force to the approach based on the sole authority of experts.

These characteristics were also evident in disability and rehabilitation. Although representatives from veterans organizations began to articulate their needs, the voice of the disabled consumer was not yet heard. Disciplines, such as medical rehabilitation and rehabilitation engineering, were established, and a cadre of personnel was trained to meet the needs of those injured in war. Much like the larger research and development field, rehabilitation became medicalized and professionalized. The range of technology, like rehabilitation itself, was associated with medical needs, especially prosthetics and orthotics. In the early stage of this period, rehabilitation research and development investments flowed into medical fields and later into the new field of vocational rehabilitation. Again, a professional cadre developed. In the developing world, while community-based rehabilitation was launched, large-scale Western science was the dominant model. Even in this period, there were signs of broadening the rehabilitation horizon beyond medical technology to access to the built environment. Canada issued a national building code supplement in 1965 on building standards for the handicapped.

1966-1980: The Age of Dissent

General Trends

People's movements challenged the basis of authority for science and technology decisions and demanded more participation into decisions. This period is characterized by protests. As science and technology were increasingly associated with political and economic power, a civic culture emerged. The consensus around the authority of experts and professionals that marked the previous period broke down. In Japan, students revolted against authoritarianism of universities and criticized scientific research. Thalidomide babies attracted people's attention. Lawsuits were initiated against pollution. The antiwar movement in the United States and the environmental movement that swept the United States and Europe were examples of protest against leaving science to the scientists (Organization of Economic Cooperation and Development [OECD] 1979). The objectives of science and technology policy and R&D investments were questioned insofar as they seemed to support a vast military complex and generate environmental damage.

Countries further institutionalized their science and technology practices. In the United States, the law that was the source of Schloss's (1976) lament (see the beginning of this chapter) was adopted. However, very tenuous attempts were made to create democratic structures for decisions about science and technology. Community-based research projects were supported in some of the European countries (Sclove 1995). The U.S. Congress established institutions, such as the Congress Office of Technology Assessment (U.S. PL 92-484), to address the social implications of technology. U.S. President Jimmy Carter, by Executive Order 12044, directed all agencies to ensure that opportunity existed for early public participation in the development of federal agency regulations. The OECD (1979) issued a report titled *Technology on Trial: Public Participation in Decision-Making, Related to Science and Technology*. Dorothy Nelkin, editor of *Politics of Technical Decisions*, observed that the political protests might have been less against specific technological decisions than against the declining capacity of citizens to shape politics that affect their interests and less against science than against scientific rationality to mask political choices (Nelkin 1992). Questions about the appropriate level and mode of participation of nonscientists, as well as the role of the politically accountable generalist policymakers in the design and evaluation of research programs, were asked by environmentalists, antimilitarists, and disabled people.

Disability and Rehabilitation: Human Rights

The movement for human rights continued forward and began to associate human rights with access to technology. The *Declaration on the Rights of Disabled Persons* (United Nations 1975) was proclaimed by the United Nations General Assembly on December 9, 1975. (For a collection of pertinent international documents, especially those by the United Nations, go to www.independentliving.org.) This document included the right to prosthetics and orthotics, indicative of the kinds of injuries that veterans had experienced in World War II. However, future international declarations would cite assistive technology more broadly as aids and devices. According to Dr. Yamauchi, the 1981 International Year of the Disabled brought a concept of normalization into Japan. From then on, *normalization, full participation,* and *quality of life* have been key words in disability policy.

The civil rights approach was further advanced during this period. The United States adopted the Rehabilitation Act of 1973 (PL 93-112) that provided for the statutory basis for rehabilitation services, including assistive technology, but also prohibited discrimination against people with disabilities in federal employment and related activities. U.S. courts would interpret the obligation to desist from discriminating as an obligation to provide reasonable accommodations in employment.

People in various countries expressed the need for research to support the development of accessible infrastructures and assistive technology for social integration. In 1976, the U.S. Congress held hearings on research for disabled people. The hearings were inspired by various professionals and advocates such as William A. Spencer and Lex Frieden (1976), who later would become instrumental to the development of the Americans with Disabilities Act (ADA, PL 101-336) (U.S. House of Representatives, Committee on Science and Technology 1976). Incidentally, these hearings led to the establishment of the National Institute on Disability and Rehabilitation Research (NIDRR) in 1978.

Social Model of Disability

The 1976 testimony of Andre Dessertine from the World Veterans Federation in Paris set forth a comprehensive social framework for the policy issues and objectives of disability research and the authority of the disabled person in the rehabilitation process—inadvertently providing support for a link between science and social goals. Implying that applied science through medicine is not objective, Dessertine argued that from the beginning of medical care, the physician should take a holistic approach so that the disabled individual is not an object of medical care but an individual with his or her own personality and social group. Dessertine observed that the environment is manmade and that barriers are designed by human beings. He described the difficulty getting around on the streets, finding housing, and carrying out activities of daily living. He introduced the notion of universal design of the social environment. He also argued that devices for individuals must be integrated in that individual's functional and social needs and that the individual should choose whether to accept the device. He also addressed the Third World and the need for cultural sensitivity to their needs (U.S. House of Representatives, Committee on Science and Technology 1976).

Independent Living, Participation, and Freedom

In their testimony during the 1976 congressional hearings, U.S. independent living representatives delivered a stinging criticism of rehabilitation practices. They testified to the legitimacy of their need to shape politics that affect their interests by recommending modes of participation in decisions about the design and evaluation of research programs. Spokespersons, such as Penny Styles and Judy Heumann, claimed that disabled people had been shut out of the process of research and development of products to meet their needs (U.S. House of Representatives, Committee on Science and Technology 1976). Reminiscent of Michael Oliver in England, they suggested that research projects be chosen more on the basis of the researcher's interest in the problem than on the basis of the need of the disabled person. Able-bodied individuals make decisions about which devices to invest in and test the technologies under development. They questioned the effectiveness of assistive technology research that limited trials to clinical settings rather than settings in the community. If disabled individuals use technology to live effectively in the world, then it must be tested in the world, not only in clinical settings. They recommended a participatory mechanism to alleviate the problem. Panels of disabled people should be set up to recommend which federal grants would be funded. Disabled people could also help guide the development of concepts, based on experience as well as whatever training they bring to the job. Some of these recommendations would be incorporated in a 1982 U.S. Congress Office of Technology Assessment (OTA) report, *Technology and the Handicapped* (U.S. Congress Office of Technology Assessment 1982). The OTA report identified a number of reasons for inadequate consumer involvement, such as attitudes and willingness to interact with disabled people. The OTA noted that a very critical reason for the inadequacy of consumer involvement is a lack of knowledge about how to design the advisory mechanisms that consumers would fit into to ensure effective involvement.

Independent living representatives also brought up issues about the role of disabled people vis-à-vis professionals and the contribution of disabled people to bridge gaps and talk with professional associations about what is available and what should be provided. Heumann, for one, emphasized the need to establish standards for technology and have government support these standards (U.S. House of Representatives, Committee on Science and Technology 1976). Both professionals and advocates regarded standards as an important public policy tool.

The problem with protection of research subjects, potential liability, and who decides about risk is another area of concern and contention for researchers and consumers. Reminiscent of Alan Newell's (1998) observation about risk factors (discussed earlier in this chapter), independent living advocates took a very clear position on the relationship between risk and freedom. Penny Styles of the Westside Community for Independent Living in Los Angeles testified as follows:

There are those individuals and groups who hesitate to accept the handicapped in positions regarding research and development of new products not because they doubt the intelligence of the handicapped, but rather they fear the risks involved. Manufacturers call it "potential liability." We call it: limiting the freedom of each individual who is disabled, and who wants to be a part of the answer to his problems of mobility and lifestyle. (U.S. House of Representatives, Committee on Science and Technology 1976:200)

International Issues

International issues were also addressed at the 1976 congressional hearings on disability research. Certain countries were identified as models for technology research and deployment. Judy Heumann, among others, seemed to envy activity going on abroad, especially in Sweden. Sweden seemed to have incorporated disabled people in the evaluation of equipment and decisions about where the government money was being spent. There was also testimony about the need for more investment in and international coordination among research and deployment entities. Jack M. Hofkosh, from the American Physical Therapy Association, reminisced about the development of the field of rehabilitation, noting the medical imperative in getting the wounded back to duty and later the social imperative for social reintegration. In a stinging criticism of practice as it was conducted in 1976, Hofkosh said that today, more than 35 years later, a wheelchair, crutches, arm and leg prostheses, canes, and braces were only slightly more tolerable than in earlier times. A system must be found that uses the myriad adaptations—which to date have been designed and used in countries such as Sweden, Great Britain, Denmark, and the United States—that have tried to meet unresolved needs. Hofkosh argued for designs specifically for the disabled rather than remade able-bodied equipment. Hofkosh defended the need for orphan technology as Dessertine defended the need for universal design (U.S. House of Representatives, Committee on Science and Technology 1976).

Indeed, like the United States in the period from 1966 to 1980, European countries, such as the Netherlands and Sweden, were also transitioning from a research and development period characterized by medicalization and caregiving to a more emancipatory period in which consumers were more in charge. A decade before the United States established NIDRR, Sweden established the Handicap Institute in 1968, later hiring Lars Augustsson as the director of technical services.

In general, the 1966 to 1980 period was characterized by the activities of citizens who became more conscious of the fact that science and technology involved extraordinary political power and that decisions about allocations of these resources were narrowly controlled. The global economy, driven by the great engines of science and technology, was on the horizon. Questions were asked about the role of government, the goals of science and technology policy, the use of research and development investments, and the emerging science and technology framework within governments. A tenuous democratic response emerged in the form of an institutional role for technology assessment, community-based research, and open universities. A short-lived People's Science movement was launched. This civic culture introduced into mainstream attitudes and scholarly literature the notion of the social nature of science and technology.

For disability and rehabilitation during this period, parallel activities occurred. Dessertine and others articulated a social, rather than a medical, approach to meet the needs of disabled people. Heumann and others went to the heart of the nature of the science controversy by arguing for a change in the power relationship between consumers and researchers. She suggested that legitimacy should be based on the needs of the user and that the experience of the disabled person was a basis for scientific authority (U.S. House of Representatives, Committee on Science and Technology 1976). Furthermore, disabled people should have the right to decide about the risks that they are willing to take. Disabled people used public hearings in a democratic representative institution—the U.S. Congress—to argue for the establishment of participatory mechanisms, such as panels with authority to decide about research funding projects. They saw standards as a very important policy tool for accomplishing their technological goals. Finally, consumers, researchers, providers, and industry in the United States formed a consensus around the need to devote research and development resources to solve problems in social integration. In 1978, Congress established the National Institute on Disability and Rehabilitation Research. Thus, the United States joined some European countries in the recognition that R&D funds should be directed to applied research.

1981-1999: A Period of Economic Hegemony

General Trends

The period from 1981 to the middle of 1999 was characterized by the alignment of research and development with economic objectives. The earlier model of a semiautonomous scientific enterprise that characterized U.S. science and technology policy and perhaps that of other industrialized countries was no longer dominant. The expert model became insufficient to a world dominated by economic institutions and a global marketplace. A new model had emerged in which science and technology were strongly associated with the economy. Technocratic optimism had reemerged in the 1980s with the resurgence of innovation in biotechnology, microelectronics, and new industrial materials. Even in the 1980s, globalization and shifting geopolitical relationships were evident. The European Union established a research and development framework that became the principle driving force behind science and technology cooperation in Europe (Commission of the European Communities 1997). With the signing of the Treaty of Maastricht in 1992 and the establishment of a common currency in 1998, Europe became more capable of binding member states to its decisions.

The fall of the Berlin Wall in 1989 and the dissolution of the USSR closed an era in science and technology policy and opened another. Europe and the United States sought new markets in East Europe and in the new countries that were the former USSR. However, a European document on science and technology (S&T) indicators expressed concern that the less-developed south remained largely excluded from the international science arena (Commission of the European Communities 1997). A U.S. report on S&T indicators does not even refer to these countries, most of which are located in Latin America, South Asia, and sub-Saharan Africa (U.S. House of Representatives, Committee on Science 1998).

Free from the rationale that the cold war required huge military budget subsidies, science and technology decision makers were now open to questions about the social objectives of science and technology in the context of basic policy directions. There is no doubt that Europe and Japan were also driven by demographic trends that showed a bumper crop of older people. To some extent, the industrialized countries began to relate science and technology resources to human and social purposes. In a 1998 paper for the European Parliament and Council on the Fifth Framework Programme of the European Community for Research, Technological Development and Demonstration, the European Commission argued that research efforts should address issues of public concern such as employment, quality of life, and competitiveness (Commission of the European Communities 1998). These funds have supported disability projects. Like the other industrialized countries, science and technology in Japan were tools for serving the economy but also emerged as tools for the welfare of the people. Japan adopted a Science and Technology Basic Law in 1995 and a Science and Technology Basic Plan in 1996. Dr. Yamauchi interprets this plan as using science and technology to build a strong nation but also to serve the welfare of the people (S. Yamauchi, personal communication, 1999).

In the United States, there were signs of support for more participation in science and signs of disregard of participation. On one hand, in 1995 after the election, a new Congress voted to eliminate the U.S. Congress Office of Technology Assessment. On the other hand, a 1989 National Academy of Sciences report, *Federal Science and Technology Budget Priorities,* lists among four categories of science and technology research systems, a category that links science and technology to major national priorities of democratic institutions of the Congress and the presidency. The category also names issues such as environmental change and research on AIDS. In a *New England Journal of Medicine* editorial, Dr. Harold Varmus, director of the National Institutes of Health (NIH), announced the implementation of two important recommendations from a recent National Academy of Sciences Institute on Medicine report. NIH had established an office of public liaison, offices in each institute and center, and a Director's Council of Public Representatives (Varmus 1999). Harvey Brooks (1996), a distinguished U.S. science and technology scholar, spoke of a new paradigm for science and technology introduced by the Clinton administration. The new paradigm speaks not only to the creation of new knowledge but also the integration of old knowledge with new knowledge and enlistment of it in the betterment of the human condition. Perhaps as an expression of the new paradigm, on January 13, 1999, President Clinton announced support for assistive technology budget items related to accessibility in telecommunications (White House, Office of the Press Secretary 1999).

Human Rights

As in the past, global human and civil rights activity has been relentless in advocating accessible infrastructures and the availability of devices to live, learn, and work in the community. In 1983, the *World Programme of Action Concerning Disabled Persons* stated that efforts should be increased to develop rehabilitation services and to transfer technology that addresses disabling conditions (United Nations 1983). A briefing document prepared for a U.S.–European Union transatlantic conference held in 1998 in Spain points to the importance of the rights-based perspective on disability worldwide and the role of the United Nations and its various specialized agencies in promulgating this perspective (US/UE Conference 1998). In 1993, the General Assembly of the United Nations adopted the *Standard Rules of the United Nations on the Equality of Opportunities for People with Disabilities.*[1]

This document is the main reference for the universal rights for people with disabilities and operates as a framework for reflection of the policies of member states. The *Standard Rules* addresses accessibility in the physical environment and access to information and communication. The landmark Americans with Disabilities Act (ADA) was enacted by the U.S. Congress in 1990. The ADA provides for civil rights protections in employment, public goods, and services, including transportation, private goods and services, and telecommunications. Availability of assistive technology as a reasonable accommodation and accessible infrastructures are central to the provision of civil rights protection. In 1997, the European Union adopted the Treaty of Amsterdam that addresses discrimination based on disability (European Commission 1997). In 1993, Japan adopted the Basic Law for the Disabled Person, using the ADA as one model for the law (S. Yamauchi, personal communication, 1999). After the United States and the European Union signed the Science and Technology Agreement in 1998, both delegations included representatives of disability agencies committed to an independent living model.[2]

Applied Research and Development in the United States

In the United States, investments in R&D began to divide between those directed specifically at medical rehabilitation and those with broader objectives. In 1990, the National Center for Medical Rehabilitation Research was established within the National Institutes of Health (PL 101-613) to conduct and support rehabilitation research, training, and dissemination of health information. The nation's scientific establishment began to recognize disabled people as a minority that must be incorporated in its efforts to train future scientists and engineers. In 1999, the congressionally mandated Commission on the Advancement of Women and Minorities in Science, Engineering, and Technology Development added disability to the groups represented on the steering committee (U.S. House of Representatives 1998). During this period, the National Science Foundation and the National Institutes of Health (NIH) had already targeted some support for disabled students and researchers. The NIH, for example, had established a research supplement for disabled individuals and a predoctoral fellowship award.

The National Institute on Disability and Rehabilitation Research

The National Institute on Disability and Rehabilitation Research (NIDRR), founded in 1978, had established itself as a leader in assistive technology policy and research and development. Reflecting the U.S. bias for investments in basic research and in big mission-oriented research rather than applied research and diffusion of knowledge, NIDRR has been constrained by a relatively flat budget. NIDRR is a comprehensive research institute with programs in medical rehabilitation, rehabilitation engineering, and the social sciences. NIDRR supports 14 rehabilitation engineering research centers and administers a technology deployment program under the Assistive Technology Act, originally adopted in 1988 (PL 100-407). Initially, NIDRR's research investments were more medically oriented but also included rehabilitation engineering research on devices for individuals, including prosthetics and orthotics, wheelchairs, hearing aids, and Braille printers. Eventually, research in universal design in the built environment became part of NIDRR's research investments as well. Recently, NIDRR has increased its investments in systems-level, information-age technology, including telecommunications, telerehabilitation, and universal design. In the tradition of Mary Switzer and the first historical period in U.S. rehabilitation, NIDRR has also increased its support for international rehabilitation with projects for consumers, professional exchange, and land mine survivors. NIDRR provides research support to individual scholars through the New Scholar's Program for undergraduate disabled students and the Switzer Fellowship Program, open to all scholars at the doctoral and postdoctoral levels. These programs have enabled a number of disabled students to enter the field of rehabilitation science and disability studies.

Professional Associations

Appropriate to the international nature of science and technology, NIDRR has had a partnership relationship with the Rehabilitation Engineering Society of North America (RESNA), which has an international network. Established in 1979, RESNA was conceived as an interdisciplinary society to promote the transfer of science, engineering, and technology to meet the needs of disabled individuals. RESNA members provide a forum for discussion and professional development and have been instrumental in the development of international technical standards for assistive technology.

The incorporation of assistive technology into mainstream research and development increased. In 1997, the Association of Access Engineering Specialists (AAES) was formed as a specialty under the National Association of Radio and Television Engineers (NARTE) and in partnership with RESNA. The AAES's purpose and mission are to initiate, foster, and promote an ongoing dialogue between the disability community and industry. The AAES is but one indication that industry and mainstream research and development are beginning to respond to new regulations that require accessibility. Companies, such as Microsoft, have set up accessibility units and hired personnel trained in rehabilitation engineering and related fields.

Congressional Activity

During this period, the U.S. Congress has increasingly recognized the importance of technology for disabled people. In addition to the ADA and the Assistive Technology Act, Congress passed the Telecommunications Act of 1996 (PL 104-104), the country's basic communications law. Section 255 of the Telecommunications Act requires that telecommunication service and equipment be accessible where readily achievable. In 1998, in recognition of the influence federal procurement can have in the marketplace and the purchase of accessible equipment, Congress strengthened Section 508 of the Rehabilitation Act of 1973, which directs federal agencies to comply with electronic equipment accessibility (PL 105-220). The political process that brought about these accessibility features were indicative of a maturity in the relationship between disability community advocates and their technically trained colleagues in the research community. Gregg Vanderheiden, a principal investigator for a NIDRR engineering center and an internationally recognized engineer, was central to the effort.

Applied Research and Development in the European Union

With the establishment in the 1980s of a coordinated effort for research and development within five-year frameworks, Europe also invested in a coordinated research and development effort for disabled people beyond medical rehabilitation and health. In the 1980s, the European Union supported a number of studies in the area of telecommunications, such as COST219 Future Telecommunications and Teleinformatics Facilities for Disabled People in 1986 (Ballabio and Moran 1998). With support from the European Parliament, they became convinced of the necessity for a distinct research and development program in the field of disability. The parliament allocated funds for a program called Technology for the Integration of Disabled and Elderly People, popularly referred to as TIDE.[3]

The TIDE program was initiated in 1991. Unlike NIDRR in the United States, which had a broader constituent base, TIDE's origins are more limited to the demands of European researchers in the assistive technology field.

Technology for the Integration of
Disabled and Elderly People (TIDE)

TIDE had a long and difficult birth, according to Egidio Ballabio, a former TIDE disability and elderly unit director. In personal correspondence, Ballabio indicated that the program has always been a matter of political maneuvering between those who would have it under a health and medicine program and those who would have it independent of that program. He emphasized the importance of members of the European Parliament in supporting TIDE. In the Fifth Framework Program (1998-2002) for research, technological development, and demonstration activities, the European Parliament again set aside a plan to merge disabled and elderly activities with health activities and supported a separate program (Commission of the European Communities 1998).

TIDE was initiated to meet the needs for advanced technologies to improve the capacity for elderly and disabled people to deal with ordinary life situations. The rise of the elderly population was a major factor. In addition, markets for research and technology were highly fragmented by national regulation, culture, sector, and even impairment. Because of its origins within the European Union's market-oriented research and development effort, TIDE, far more than NIDRR, has been sensitive to economic forces. The TIDE model involves supporting collaborative research and development projects through collaborative ventures from different sectors in the member states of the European Union. TIDE is helping to develop a supportive infrastructure and market conditions for a successful European assistive technology (AT) industry. Although not R&D, certain support actions are important to the success of TIDE, including analysis of market initiatives that encourages standardization, regulation, and rationalization.

Ballabio notes that there are a number of challenges, including the following:

1. Assistive technology is still considered a medical matter.
2. Europe lacks policy and legislation that would correspond to the ADA and the Rehabilitation Act.
3. The AT sector is competing with R&D funding with sectors of much higher industrial and economic weight.
4. User involvement needs to be stimulated.

Ballabio strongly recommends that these challenges are addressed and that continued support is directed to product development and standardization activities as well as to ethical and human rights issues (E. Ballabio, personal communication, 1999). In this way, the Europeans have emphasized the very important role of public policy tools to support assistive technology for independent living. In Europe, like RESNA in the United States, an association of technical people was formed. In 1995, the Association for the Advancement of Assistive Technology (AAATE) in Europe was established to stimulate the advancement of assistive technology for the benefit of persons with disabilities, including elderly people. AAATE looked to TIDE as RESNA does to NIDRR for a complementary relationship in research and development.

Applied Research and Development in Japan

Japan also was developing a broader range of research and development support for its disabled and elderly. The elderly population became a major social issue in Japan. According to Dr. Yamauchi, people began to pay attention to assistive technology, especially personal care and household appliances. Prostheses were not the representative assistive devices anymore. Social participation and independent living of disabled people became a main issue (S. Yamauchi, personal communication, 1999). As indicated earlier, Japan passed the Basic Law for Disabled Persons in 1993 under the influence of the ADA. The country also enacted the Technical Aids Law in 1993, which aims at R&D and service delivery of assistive technologies. Users began to participate in decisions on research and development of assistive technology. Giant business enterprises such as Panasonic, Hitachi, and Mitsubishi are now taking part in the assistive technology market where the quality is nearly the same as that in Europe and the United States. Japan has also been working with Third World countries. The National Rehabilitation Center is engaged in training professionals from Asia, Africa, and South America. A program of user participation is run by the Japan Society for Rehabilitation of Persons with Disabilities (JSRD). It has a training course for rehabilitation experts and leaders of the organizations of persons with disabilities. JSRD also organizes the Rehabilitation Action Network for Asia and the Pacific.[4]

Between 1981 and 1999, science and technology were more closely aligned to economic objectives of the industrialized countries. Expertise diversified into areas of marketing, international finance, corporate management, and science. R&D was clearly tied to creation and support of rich and powerful nations.

After the end of the cold war, geopolitical consolidation, scientific innovation, and a global infrastructure emerged for many of the countries of the world, but not for the world's poorest countries. Science, engineering, and industry support the development of a technical cadre of trained engineers, scientists, and management specialists. However, it is unclear whether policymakers will direct science and technology resources beyond economic objectives to serve social welfare needs for food and shelter, education, housing, transportation, information technology, and the environment science and technology. Of the great emerging industrial areas of biotechnology, microelectronics, and material sciences, there is some indication that telecommunications and informatics may be incorporating policy interests beyond simple return on investment.

For disability and rehabilitation during the 1981 to 1999 period, the human rights agenda in the international arena and the civil rights approach adopted by many countries began to be integrated into laws pertaining to mainstream technology, such as the U.S. Telecommunications Act. Responding to the imperative of increases in the elderly population, as well as pressure from the disability movement, research and development programs were broadened beyond health to address technology issues for daily living and for universal design. However, many countries have not yet adopted the political infrastructure to support these programs.

In the United States, in particular, advocates and researchers had begun to work together on universal design problems such as access to telecommunications. With support of the new research and development agencies and professional associations, a technical cadre developed that was more identified with independent living. Some opportunities opened to support disabled students in science and engineering careers and disabled laypersons as participants in the research process. Public policy tools, such as regulations and standards, became increasingly useful in the joint pursuit by disabled people and technically trained allies for science and technology policy objectives. While these advancements pertain particularly to the industrialized world, some of them may have benefits for the Third World.

SCIENCE AND TECHNOLOGY POLICY

Trends in the allocation of science and technology resources since the end of the cold war seem modestly supportive of social objectives in targeted areas. However, R&D expenditures in one country—the United States—show the extraordinary disparities in the distribution of science and technology. In 1994, the U.S. federal R&D budget amounted to about $70 billion. Adjusted for inflation, the R&D was the same in 1995, when it accounted for about 1.2 percent of the gross domestic product. Nearly 55 percent went to military R&D, and even today, military R&D remains about 51 percent of total U.S. government R&D investment (Committee on Criteria for Federal Support on Research and Development 1995). According to Brandt and Pope's (1997) *Enabling America,* total federal spending on programs emphasizing rehabilitation-related research represented $147 million. This amounted to about 0.2 percent of the 1995 federal R&D budget.

However, the most recent period does show some promising trends both on the general level and the level of disabled people. Minority rights have become an important factor in the recruitment and training of scientists and engineers. The human rights umbrella is now also beginning to expand to use minority incentives to include disabled students and researchers. In addition, using democratic political institutions such as the U.S. Congress and the European Parliament, rather than the more expert-oriented process within scientific institutions, the disabled community has managed to achieve some support for universal design and orphan technology through legislation and programs. The U.S. Telecommunications Act and the TIDE initiative to support commercialization through integration of the assistive technology marketplace in Europe are but two examples. The United States, Europe, and Japan have also begun to distinguish between technology for health and technology for social integration by allocating modest budgets to programs such as NIDRR, TIDE, and the National Rehabilitation Center.

The end of the cold war seems to have freed up modest resources in money and political commitment that have benefited disabled people in areas of universal design and orphan technology. The development of international technical standards (stimulated by industry in the United States) and the establishment of the World Wide Web Accessibility Initiative for universal telecommunications design (stimulated by the U.S. government and a Canadian-based foundation) are interesting examples (R. Cooper, personal communication, 1999). Both are international in scope.

Technical Standards

In earlier sections of this chapter, researchers and users from a number of countries, including Judy Heumann, Rolf Hotchkiss, Lars Augustsson, Alan Newell, and Egidio Ballabio, expressed interest in technical standards development and related issues of market viability, user involvement, consumer choice and relationships, and roles of consumers with professionals. The development of standards for wheelchairs is an interesting use of a policy tool—standards to address an international need shared by consumers, researchers, providers, and industry.

According to Douglas Hobson of the NIDRR Rehabilitation Engineering Research Center on Wheeled Mobility at the University of Pittsburgh, the U.S. wheelchair industry became involved in the development of wheelchair standards in the 1970s (D. Hobson, personal communication, 1999). Industry wanted to be competitive with Europe but lacked the financial support for standards that would make them competitive in domestic and international markets. Early in the 1980s, at the request of industry, RESNA became involved and was designated by the American National Standards Institute (ANSI) as the official U.S. standards development body in the area of disability products. The ANSI/RESNA standards group serves on the delegation of the International Standards Organization. According to Hobson, standards were developed to meet the following purposes: safety, durability, standardized consumer product information, compatibility between products, and participatory forums. These standards also minimized border trade barriers for both imports and exports. Rory Cooper, an engineer at the Human Engineering Research Laboratories, also at the University of Pittsburgh, has often noted that the drive by users to improve sports performance through lighter-weight equipment continues to revolutionize the wheelchair industry and will lead to reduced costs and improved quality (Cooper et al. 1997).

Standards development provides an example of the role of government in partnership with and support of professionals and users to reach a shared goal. The U.S. effort has received indispensable government support initially from the Veterans Administration and later from NIDRR. Standards development illustrates the use of R&D funds to support social integration, albeit in a health product marketplace. Finally, the development of wheelchair standards shows the importance of involvement by disabled interests in domestic and international science and technology activities. According to Hobson, wheelchair technology has been at the leading edge of the standards development in assistive technology. Other areas of assistive technology are making significant progress. He cites computer access and telecommunication guidelines and standards, which serve as the final example in this section (D. Hobson, personal communication, 1999).

World Wide Web Accessibility Initiative

Exhibiting considerable political sophistication, the disability community enlisted both the White House and powerful nongovernmental agencies to discuss the need for an industry initiative in telecommunications. The U.S. National Economic Council and the Yuri Rubinsky Insight Foundation arranged for a meeting at the White House in January 1997. The intent was to bring together key players in the industry, academia, and government. Gregg Vanderheiden, a principal investigator of an NIDRR-funded engineering center, was again instrumental to a technical presentation of the need for an international effort. As a result, NIDRR and the National Science Foundation funded the World Wide Web Accessibility Initiative (WAI) concept through a grant-making process. The Worldwide Web Consortium, a consortia of the world's largest telecommunications companies, hired Judy Brewer, an NIDRR-funded director of the Massachusetts Technology Act project who is disabled, as the director of the International Program Office.

The WAI was established in 1997 with the support of the United States, Canada, and the European Union.[5] The WAI is an International Program Office of the World Wide Web Consortium (W3C). The W3C, housed in three internationally recognized research facilities, coordinates the evolution of the Web, and its mission is the realization of the full potential of the Web, including leadership to remove accessibility barriers. The purpose of the WAI is to coordinate five Web-related program activities: technology development, development of tools, guidelines for use of the technology, educational outreach and research, and advanced development. Recently, the W3C/WAI issued Web accessibility guidelines. In its grant proposal, the W3C acknowledged additional motivation to build accessibility into the Web's infrastructure, citing requirements in U.S. and potential European national laws that might extend into a pan-European framework and could be considered for adoption worldwide (National Science Foundation and Massachusetts Institute of Technology 1997). The ADA; Section 508 of the Rehabilitation Act; Sections 255, 256, and 305/713 of the Telecommunications Act; and the Television Decoder Circuitry Act were cited. The W3C argued that there was a "clear and compelling social argument" for undertaking this work, but it is also good business because it opens new markets and creates new products, including disability and those who cannot read.

FUTURE AGENDA AND CONCLUSIONS

Irving P. Schloss (1976), whose quote introduced this chapter, recognized the important role of government for one minority group—disabled people. He recognized that science and technology law would guide policy and decisions about research and development resource allocations. Perhaps he recognized that the science and technology enterprise was characterized by semiautonomous governance structure and decisions made by experts. He seemed to imply that law that does not specify disabled people might be law that would not incorporate their issues and enlist their participation. This chapter suggests that he was largely correct.

Schloss (1976), however, did not take the measure of a great countervailing force, the international human rights and domestic civil rights movements. As this chapter has documented, people's movements have strongly affected democratic legislatures, which, in turn, have legislated in areas that affect mainstream science and technology policy. Future policy research must further address the adequacy of national science and technology law and institutions to incorporate the interests of disabled people. Future policy research must also recognize that increasingly, R&D expenditure is shifting to the private sector and that the disability research community must be concerned with what is going on in the private sector. The nature of applied science and engineering will present continuing challenges within the global, nation-state, and economic frameworks.

The Nature of Science

The section on the nature of science suggests that assumptions about the basis for truth in the West, either objective or subjective, and the standard of normalcy create a predisposition for judgment that may adversely affect disabled people. Future research in the philosophy and sociology of science should probe the impact on the choice of research problems and design of widely accepted assumptions in applied science and engineering. What is the impact on applied research problems of assumptions in the basic sciences that knowledge precedes social construction or that the norm automatically informs understanding of any class of individuals and design features of their environments?

It is not widely recognized that R&D has a particularly intimate relationship to the lives of disabled people, especially their lives as citizens. For example, availability of technology for speech output within a universally designed information kiosk at the voting booth eliminates the intermediary that blind people must use to read ballots. Technology design may trade off choice or basic freedom for efficiency or a range of options. Engineering and sociological research on the design process in medical, social, and systems technology is long overdue.

The roles of the researcher and the end user deserve attention. At the research project level, for the technical researcher, scientific values are preeminent. The research process must be intergenerational and the hypothesis refutable. While the user is concerned about the reliability of the product, user concerns often relate to choice of relevant research problems and the design of technology that can be used in actual settings where they live, learn, and work. The power relationships between researchers and users are complex and cannot be solved ideologically. Risk analyses studies are needed to address the various factors involved in participation in research projects. Questions about who and how funding decisions are made deserve attention. They involve levels of analysis from local to international and units of analysis that include many institutions of government and the private sector. Power relationships might also be eased if career pathways are opened. There is a great need to probe the incentives and disincentives for disabled people to pursue science and engineering careers.

Clearly, support for the complex research characterized by most research and development could be diversified so that some funds could be committed to community-based research that shifts the power relationship more to the user. However, debate has been reignited in works such as the Donald E. Stokes's (1997) book, *Pasteur's Quadrant*, about whether there are real distinctions between basic and applied research. Applied research and often a problem-solving orientation are germane to people who have diverse functional characteristics (Stokes 1997).

Historical Approach

The historical perspective has provided a tale about the great forces of history, including wars and scientific innovation, that have generated a series of models on which the authority of science is based. History also provides a perspective on the significance of these models for disabled people. The expert or professional model was dominant throughout most of the cold war period. The citizen participation model made a brief entrée in the 1960s. The economic model appears to have become dominant and to hold promise for possible social investments. The economic model suggests the need for further research on incentives and disincentives for large corporations to incorporate design for all features in their products. Future research should explore the citizen participation model and tools developed by environmentalists, such as social impact assessment, to ascertain applicability to disability. The importance of social movements to science and technology policy is an important research item. History tells stories of mobilization of great investments of research and development resources to provide for defense and for veterans. In contrast, even in the post–cold war period, minimal resources have been invested in the infrastructure needs of civilians. Disabled citizens, in particular, are interested in research and development investments for universally designed transportation, buildings, telecommunications, and consumer products. Demographic trends should be researched as a possible rationale for identifying needs in the post–cold war period.

History has also told tales of lack of science and technology development in the world's poorest countries. The disability population in these countries does not have the benefit of big science. Research could address short-term and long-term science and technology needs for these countries. Necessarily, some of this research should profile health, education, and culture. While economic development models based in the resources and culture of these countries are very important, models may also be considered that guide these countries in the development of the complex infrastructure that supports modern science and technology.

Public Policy and Markets

The science and technology enterprise, like the human rights movement, is inherently international. Unlike international human rights, science and technology decisions are influenced by economic factors and made by the private sector. Yet, authoritative decisions about science and technology resources—support for research, commercialization, and training—also repose in governments. With the end of the cold war, there appeared to be a shift to an open information service model. The model has been eroded by the commercialization of the Internet. Nonetheless, the significance of the model as amended for disabled people should be the subject of research. Will it contribute to further differentiation between health policy and other policy that provides support for social integration? What are the appropriate incentives to stimulate markets? Large companies will be interested in "add-ons" for accessibility only insofar as tax credits and regulation inspire them to do so. Small companies require their own incentives to produce and upgrade orphan products. To what extent will international cooperation create robust markets and increase availability and variety of products? What funding mechanisms are available for individual consumers in the various countries to purchase technology for higher-level functioning?

Nongovernmental organizations (NGOs), especially international NGOs, must add science and technology to their social agenda and work with technical associations such as RESNA, AES, and AAATE. Studies of organizational behavior are needed both domestically and in the international arena. There is a need for research to develop models of culturally appropriate science and technology infrastructure for developing countries that will allow these countries to compete in the global marketplace and bring benefits to bear on independent living needs of their disabled and elderly populations.

As with indigenous peoples, science and technology take their toll on the disabled cultures. For example, culturally deaf people often oppose cochlear implants; hard-of-hearing and late-deafened people look to technology for relief from impending deafness. Studies might explore the conditions under which acceptance or rejection of an implant might empower disabled people.

Research and development figures are not easily extrapolated from domestic budgets. These figures must be analyzed to ascertain national and international investments in accessible transportation, telecommunications, built environments, and consumer products as well as in medical rehabilitation and health.

There is a critical need to identify incentives to enhance democratic representation and participation of people with diverse functional characteristics. As history unfolds and science and technology increasingly become the basis of political power, democracy is challenged to modernize institutions. As this chapter has shown, marginalized groups and citizens who may not have political power because their interests may be separate from, or incompletely shared by, the majority are at risk of being barred from citizen activities. Special resources should be made available to provide scientific expertise, incentives for career development, and institutional participatory mechanisms so that disabled people are motivated and enabled to participate. In market-driven economies, disabled people may lack a socioeconomic net that will allow them to pursue advanced education and acquire skills with which to compete in a technologically based society.

Discrimination against disabled people in science and engineering is deeply embedded in scientific values, infrastructure, career paths, and policy. The research efforts of many disciplines must be brought to bear on the multiple problems discrimination has bred.

NOTES

1. The *Standard Rules on the Equalization of Opportunities for Persons with Disabilities* was adopted by the United Nations General Assembly at its 48th regular session on December 20, 1993, by its resolution 48/96.

2. For information on the U.S.–European Union Agreement on Scientific and Technological Cooperation, please visit the Internet at www.state.gov/www/global/oes/science/.

3. For a review of TIDE projects, see Slater (1998).

4. For information about the Japanese Society for Rehabilitation of Persons with Disabilities, visit the Internet at www.jsrp.or.jp/index_e.html.

5. Information about the Web Accessibility Initiative can be found on the Internet at www.w3c.org/WAI/.

REFERENCES

Ballabio, E. and Rosalyn Moran. 1998. "Addressing the Need and Potential of Older People and People with Disabilities in the Information Society." Pp. 1-34 in *An RTD Approach for the European Union.* Luxembourg: Office for Official Publications of the European Communities.

Barnes, C. and Geof Mercer, eds. 1997. *Doing Disability Research.* Leeds, UK: The Disability Press.

Bernal, John D. 1939. *The Social Function of Science.* London: Routledge Kegan Paul.

Brandt, E. N., Jr. and Andrew M. Pope, eds. 1997. *Enabling America: Assessing the Role of Rehabilitation Science and Engineering.* Washington, DC: National Academy Press.

Brooks, H. 1996. "The Evolution of U.S. Science Policy." Pp. 15-48 in *Technology, R&D and the Economy*, edited by Bruce L. R. Smith and Claude E. Barfield. Washington, DC: Brookings Institution and American Enterprise Institute.

Bush, V. 1990. *Science—The Endless Frontier.* Washington, DC: National Science Foundation.

Childress, D. 1976. "Testimony before the U.S. House of Representatives, Committee on Science and Technology." In *Report of the Panel on Research Programs to Aid the Handicapped.* Washington, DC: Government Printing Office.

———. 1977. *Historical Sketch Concerning Federal Support of Research to Aid the Handicapped.* Pp. 29-32 in *Report of the Panel on Research Programs to Aid the Handicapped.* Washington, DC: Government Printing Office.

Commission of the European Communities. 1994. *HEART: Horizontal European Activities in Rehabilitation Technology: European Service Delivery Systems in Rehabilitation Technology.* Luxembourg: Office for Official Publications of the European Communities.

———190. 1997. *Directorate General XII, Science, Research and Development: Second European Report on S&T Indicators.* Luxembourg: Office for Official Publications of the European Communities.

———. 1998. *Second Modified Proposal for a European Parliament and Council Decision Concerning the 5th Framework Programme of the European Community for Research Technological Development and Demonstration Activities (1998-2002).* Luxembourg: Office for Official Publications of the European Communities.

Committee on Criteria for Federal Support on Research and Development. 1995. *Allocating Federal Funds for Science and Technology*. Washington, DC: National Academy Press.

Cooper, R. A., J. P. Gonzales, B. Lawrence, A. Rentschler, M. L. Boninger, and D. P. VanSickle. 1997. "Performance of Selected Lightweight Wheelchairs on ANSI/RESNA Tests." *Archives of Physical Medicine & Rehabilitation* 78:1138-44.

Dickson, D. 1984. *The New Politics of Science*. Chicago: University of Chicago Press.

Dyer, H. 1904. "Education and National Efficiency in Japan" [Letter to the editor]. *Nature* 71 (1833): 150-51.

Edge, D. 1995. "Reinventing the Wheel." Pp. 3-23 in *Handbook of Science and Technology Studies*, edited by Sheila Jasanoff, Gerald E. Markle, James C. Petersen, and Trevor Pinch. Thousand Oaks, CA: Sage.

European Commission. 1997. *Amsterdam: A New Treaty for Europe: Citizen's Guide*. Luxembourg: Office for Official Publications of the European Communities.

Freeman, C. 1993. *The Economics of Hope: Essays on Technical Change, Economic Growth and the Environment*. London: Pinter.

Groce, N. 1992. *The U.S. Role in International Disability Activities: A History and a Look towards the Future*. New York: Rehabilitation International.

Hotchkiss, R. 1976. "Testimony before the U.S. House of Representatives, Committee on Science and Technology." In *Report of the Panel on Research Programs to Aid the Handicapped*. Washington, DC: Government Printing Office.

Keller, E. Fox. 1999. "The Gender/Science System." Pp. 234-42 in *The Science Studies Reader*, edited by Mario Biagioli. New York: Routledge.

Kuhn, T. 1970. *The Structure of the Scientific Revolution*. Chicago: University of Chicago Press.

Lane, J. P. 1997. "Roles for the Technology Transfer Intermediary." Pp. 357-62 in *Advancement of Assistive Technology*, edited by G. Anogianakis, C. Buehler, and M. Soede. Amsterdam: IOS.

"Letter to the Editor." 1877. *Nature*, May 17, p. 44.

Mace, R., G. Hardie, and J. Plaice. 1991. "Accessible Environments: Toward Universal Design." Pp. 155-76 in *Design Interventions: Towards a More Humane Architecture*, edited by W. E. Preiser, J. C. Vischer, and E. T. White. New York: Van Nostrand Reinhold.

Merton, R. K. 1973. *The Sociology of Science: Theoretical and Empirical Investigations*. Chicago: University of Chicago Press.

National Academy of Sciences. 1989. *Federal Science and Technology Budget Priorities*. Washington, DC: Author.

National Science Foundation and Massachusetts Institute of Technology. 1997. *Web Accessibility Initiative: Cooperative Agreement No. IRI-971392*. Arlington, VA: National Science Foundation.

Nelkin, D., ed. 1992. *Controversy: Politics of Technical Decisions*. Newbury Park, CA: Sage.

Newell, A. F. 1998. "Assistive Technology Research and Technological Development." Pp. xlvii-liii in *Improving the Quality of Life for the European Citizen: Technology for Inclusive Design and Equality*, edited by Immaculada Placiencia Porrero and Edigio Ballabio. Amsterdam: IOS.

Obermann, E. 1965. *A History of Vocational Rehabilitation in America*. Minneapolis, MN: T. S. Denison.

Oliver, M. 1997. "Emancipatory Research: Realistic Goal or Impossible Dream?" Pp. 15-31 in *Doing Disability Research*, edited by Colin Barnes and Geof Mercer. Leeds, UK: The Disability Press.

Organization for Economic Cooperation and Development (OECD). 1979. *Technology on Trial: Public Participation in Decision Making Related to Science and Technology*. Paris: Author.

Polanyi, M. 1962. "The Republic of Science: Its Political and Economic Theory." *Minerva* 1:54-73.

Sarewitz, D. 1996. *Frontiers of Illusion: Science, Technology and the Politics of Progress*. Philadelphia: Temple University Press.

Schloss, I. P. 1976. *Report of the Panel on Research Programs to Aid the Handicapped*. Washington, DC: Government Printing Office.

Schur, L. L. 1998. "Disability and the Psychology of Participation." *Journal of Disability Policy Studies* 9 (2): 3-31.

Sclove, R. 1995. *Democracy and Technology*. New York: Guilford.

Shapiro, J. 1993. *No Pity*. New York: Random House.

Slater, J., ed. 1998. *High Tide*. Luxembourg: Office for Official Publications of the European Communities.

Smith, B. L. R. 1990. *American Science Policy since World War II*. Washington, DC: Brookings Institution.

Smith, B. L. R. and Claude E. Barfield. 1996. "Contributions of Research and Technical Advance to the Economy." Pp. 1-14 in *Technology, R&D and the Economy*, edited by Bruce L. R. Smith and Claude E. Barfield. Washington, DC: Brookings Institution and American Enterprise Institute.

Snow, C. P. 1964. "The Two Cultures." Pp. 1-21 in *The Two Cultures and A Second Look*. Cambridge, UK: Cambridge University Press.

Spencer, W. A. and L. Frieden. 1976. "Testimony before the U.S. House of Representatives, Committee on Science and Technology." In *Report of the Panel on Research Programs to Aid the Handicapped*. Washington, DC: Government Printing Office.

Stokes, D. E. 1997. *Pasteur's Quadrant*. Washington, DC: Brookings Institution.

Stone, E. 1997. "From the Research Notes of a Foreign Devil: Disability Research in China." Pp. 207-27 in *Doing Disability Research*, edited by Colin Barnes and Geof Mercer. Leeds, UK: The Disability Press.

Tewey, B. 1997. *Building Participatory Action Research Partnerships in Disability and Rehabilitation Research*. Washington, DC: U.S. Department of Education, National Institute on Disability and Rehabilitation Research.

United Nations. 1948. *Universal Declaration of Human Rights*. New York: Author.

———. 1975. *Declaration on the Rights of Disabled Persons*. New York: Author.

———. 1983. *World Programme of Action Concerning Disabled Persons*. New York: Author.

———. 1993. *Standard Rules of the United Nations on the Equality of Opportunities with Disabled People*. New York: Author.

U.S. Congress, Office of Technology Assessment. 1982. *Technology and Handicapped People*. Washington, DC: Government Printing Office.

U.S. House of Representatives. 1998. *Commission on the Advancement of Women in Science, Engineering and Technology Development Act (PL 105-255)*. Washington, DC: Government Printing Office.

U.S. House of Representatives, Committee on Science. 1998. *Unlocking Our Future: Toward a New National Science Policy* Washington, DC: Government Printing Office.

U.S. House of Representatives, Committee on Science and Technology. 1976. *Report of the Panel on Research Programs to Aid the Handicapped*. Washington, DC: Government Printing Office.

US/UE Conference. 1998. "Harnessing the Information Society to Raise Employment Levels for People with Disabilities: Scope and Employment for People with Disabilities within the Framework of the United States and the European Union." Papers developed at a Transatlantic Conference, October, Madrid, Spain.

Varmus, H. 1999. "Evaluating the Burden of Disease and Spending the Research Dollars of the National Institutes of Health." *New England Journal of Medicine* 340 (24): 1914-15.

White House, Office of the Press Secretary. 1999. Remarks by the President on Disability Initiative. Washington, DC, January 13.

Whyte, J. 1995. "Participatory Action Research." Unpublished presentation to the NIDRR Directors Meeting, April, Washington, DC.

World Health Organization. 1980. *International Classification of Impairments, Disabilities, and Handicaps: A Manual of Classification Relating to the Consequences of Disease*. Geneva: Author.

Disability, Education, and Inclusion

30

Cross-Cultural Issues and Dilemmas

LEN BARTON

FELICITY ARMSTRONG

The increasing struggle on the part of many disabled people and their organizations for participation, equity, and social justice in their lives is motivated by an informed recognition of the degree and stubbornness of disabling barriers within society. This chapter will examine the extent to which formal education contributes to or is critical of the disabling barriers within society. The issues involved are complex and contentious, and these become particularly acute when cross-cultural factors are introduced. Drawing on a range of insights from comparative research and analyses, the chapter examines the possibilities and limitations of cross-cultural work; the issue of globalization and points of commonality and difference in educational policy and practice; the question of democracy, disability, and the struggle for inclusive education; and the identification, challenge, and removal of disabling barriers.

We have attempted to highlight some of our values, priorities, and concerns, but it is crucial that this chapter is not viewed as the definitive statement on any of the topics considered. By critically engaging with our ideas, we hope that we can contribute to an increasingly informed cross-cultural dialogue. Complacency, arrogance, and dogmatism have no place in the struggle for an inclusive society.

In proposing the significance of inclusivity in relation to education, it is essential that the values, priorities, and desired outcomes informing existing policy and practice are carefully identified and critically examined. This examination will also provide us with some insights into the nature of exclusion within educational systems. The assumptions influencing our perspective in relation to this task include, first, that education must not be viewed in a vacuum. Educational institutions play a major role in social and cultural reproduction. This dynamic relationship between education and society is both complex and contradictory, providing spaces for alternative ideas and practices. Second, educational issues are contentious and thus involve struggles between different interest groups over purposes, meanings, and functions in relation to education. Thus, the degree to which schools should be run as a formal business and parents and

AUTHORS' NOTE: We are grateful for the constructive comments of the editors on an earlier draft of this chapter.

pupils viewed as customers, what form of management structure schools require, and what degree governments should intervene in schools represent points of conflict within and between different interested parties. The use of the term *inclusion,* therefore, can represent a range of meanings, and this is a particular issue that arises in relation to cross-cultural analysis. Finally, educational decision making is fundamentally political in that, for example, it involves governments making choices about resource allocation supported by a vision of desirable outcomes and of wider concerns such as the relationship between the individual and society. The extent to which such decisions reinforce or seek to redress existing inequalities, in terms of access and the quality of educational experience, is a perennial concern to those who are committed to the struggle for education for all. Thus, in an analysis of schooling in what they call "developing countries," Harber and Davies (1997) indicate the need for a political analysis of the function of mass schooling and contend that

> in most countries, formal schooling acts as a gate-keeping mechanism, controlling access to the elite, to higher education or to prestigious jobs. It legitimises the inevitable inequalities in a society by attributing a person's occupational low-status to failure in previous educational performance. (P. 32)

Thus, educational policy and practice are not a neutral, autonomous activity but are linked to wider socioeconomic and political forces and relations.

The notion of *social exclusion* is complex and contestable. In this chapter, we support the perspective articulated by Walker (1997), who maintains that it

> refers to the dynamic process of being shut out, fully or partially, from any of the social, economic, political and cultural systems which determine the social integration of a person in society. Social exclusion may, therefore be seen as the denial (or non-realisation) of the civil, political and social rights of citizenship. (P. 8)

The demands of inclusion raise questions concerning who is included and on what terms and, crucially, what are they included in (Levitas 1998). This chapter briefly explores the latter question and demonstrates the radical nature of the changes required.

CROSS-CULTURAL CONCERNS AND DILEMMAS

In attempting to address an international audience, it is extremely important that we outline some of our concerns in relation to the difficulties and challenges facing cross-cultural analysis generally and education particularly.

The world appears to have become both smaller, in that we think we "know" more about it (the coziness of the "global village"), and "larger" and more confusing in the sense that its diversity of cultures and practices places hitherto dominant Western "knowledge," values, and interests in a wider, more critical, and relative perspective. Knowledge and certainty are undermined, being relative, contingent, more complex, and less penetrable than researchers, advisers, and policymakers ever imagined. The implications of cross-cultural approaches for research in all areas of social science are exciting and frightening—exciting because they release us from old straitjackets that have controlled and limited the imagination and frightening because they challenge what we thought we knew and throw into turmoil research agendas and processes, as well as the underlying assumptions and power relations to which Western research communities have all contributed. It is disturbing, too, to realize that concepts such as *human rights, equality,* and *justice,* previously regarded as universal (and hence, in some sense, "safe"), are relative in that they are not conceptualized, interpreted in the same way, or commonly shared across cultures (Miles and Hossain 1999).

Comparative research in education has a long history as a systematic field of study, dating back to the nineteenth century. An often-quoted statement made by Michael Sadler in 1902 serves as a useful introduction to some of the issues surrounding the nature (and dilemmas) of "comparative" research:

> In studying foreign systems of education we should not forget that things outside the schools matter even more than the things inside the schools, and govern and interpret the things inside. . . . The practical values of studying in a right spirit and with scholarly accuracy the working of foreign systems of education [are] that it will result in our being better fitted to study and understand our own. (Sadler 1902:44)

Central to this view of comparative research are two main arguments. First, an understanding of the fundamental role of context is of the utmost importance in understanding differences and similarities between countries. Policies, practices, and values arise out of particular historical and social contexts and can only be explained in these terms. They cannot easily be exported and applied in other contexts, nor can generalizations made across countries on the basis that they appear to share some common characteristics or practices pass unquestioned.

Second, it is argued that a practical value of studying "foreign systems of education" is that it will help researchers understand *their own systems,* not that countries can borrow and apply policies from other countries uncritically in their own context. This view contrasts with "policy borrowing" of the kind that, argue Halpin and Troyna (1995), "rarely has much to do with the success, however defined, of the institutional realisation of particular policies in their countries of origin; rather, it has much more to do with legitimating other related policies" (p. 304).

The questions raised by comparative and cross-cultural research into education and disability illustrate clearly the difficulties associated with comparative research. These questions suggest that much can be learned from a cross-cultural approach that takes into account the cultural and political legacies of historical change and development, particularly cultural and national contexts, as well as the values and attitudes that underpin them.

The approaches adopted by research organizations and individuals to the study of education systems in different countries reflect fundamental differences in the way they understand the nature and purpose of research and the meanings they attach to the social relations and values that underpin the particular systems they are studying. Research is itself a social practice, embedded in complex social and cultural contexts within which certain assumptions and "ways of seeing" are important to determining research agendas, methodologies, and analytical frameworks. However, researchers are not conditioned in some deterministic way by the social worlds they inhabit, and research is itself an arena for struggle between values and ideologies that are fundamentally different.

Tony Booth and Mel Ainscow (1998) refer to two common features of comparative research in inclusion and exclusion in education. First, it is often assumed that there is "a single national perspective on inclusion or exclusion." The second assumption is that "practice can be generalised across countries without attention to local contexts and meanings" (p. 4).

They argue that what is presented as a "national perspective" is frequently an official version of policy. They cite, for example, the United Kingdom, where there are different education systems and legislative arrangements in Scotland, Northern Ireland, England, and Wales. It is also the case that in England, there are enormous differences in the way in which formal policies are interpreted in different local education authorities (LEAs) and that official "national" versions of policy in England do not usually acknowledge this.

> The tendency to present single national perspectives is often matched by a failure to describe the way practice is to be understood in its local and national context. . . . This lack is part of a positivist view of social science in which research in one country can be amalgamated and summed with that of another. . . . The problem is compounded by differences of meaning of concepts, which is of particular significance in relation to categories of inability and disability. (Booth and Ainscow 1998:4-5)

This problem is illustrated by large-scale research projects that attempt to make cross-national comparisons, such as the Organization for Economic Cooperation and Development (OECD 1995) study, *Integrating Students with Special Needs into Mainstream Schools.* In this study, a number of features were compared, including categories of disability in individual countries, the numbers of the school population classified as disabled in different countries, and the percentage of school populations receiving some form of special education. This study raises some interesting questions and difficulties relating to large-scale comparative research. In a study of this size, it would perhaps be regarded as too cumbersome to provide rich contextualizing background material against which the adoption of particular policies, structures, and practices have been adopted. While there is a quantity of data provided relating to the *surface structure* of the different educational systems such as classification of disability, legislation, and formal policy statements, we learn little about the nature and complexity of the cultures and populations concerned. We also learn little about the ways in which policies are made at different levels.

For example, in the figures given for the school-age population in special education in France, important differences such as cultural and economic background are hidden. The material presented in the study implies that the population is homogeneous. There is no possibility for exploring issues, such as the overrepresentation of young French North Africans in the special classes for students with learning difficulties in secondary education (Dumay 1994) or the effects of poverty and unemployment. Furthermore, the exclusion of many special institutions from the education system altogether is not discussed in any detail.

There are further problems associated with the collection of data provided by the individual countries concerned. It is not possible to ensure uniformity or rigor in the methods used to collect or analyze data or to verify that the data collected are of the same kind. Linked to this problem is the question of terminology. For example, different uses of terms such as *integration* or *learning difficulties* demonstrate that the data collected are not comparable. Meanings and values can be altered or become lost in the process of translation from one language to another.

Part of the data collected in the OECD (1995) study focused on the percentages of children in the school-age populations of different countries recorded as having a particular named disability. There are some very noticeable differences between countries in the categories adopted, the number of different categories, and the numbers of children and young people identified as belonging to particular categories.

Underlying the difficulties relating to categorization and terminology is an issue of far greater importance than the "technical" problem of making comparisons between countries; this concerns the confusion surrounding the meanings attached to the term *disability* and its frequent use to mean *impairment.* Thus, in the OECD (1995) study, a large variety of terms, derived from the material provided by different countries involved in the study, is used to describe "impairments" and "difficulties" of all sorts. These terms are usually based on the medical "within-child" model similar to that adopted by the World Health Organization (WHO). The authors of the report recognize this (OECD 1995) and point to what they perceive as a move away from the medical model in some countries in favor of the term *special educational needs* (SEN).

This analysis still includes an adherence to old assumptions that place difficulties "within the child" through a discourse of "having SEN" and fails to recognize that disability is not an "individual pathology" but a form of oppression and exclusion produced by and within particular social and political conditions and relationships.

Different societies construct disability in culturally specific ways, expressing their particular dominant social norms and practices. Far from being "scientific facts" based on objective, universally understood definitions of difference, the categories and labels assigned to different groups in different societies are contingent, temporary, and subjective. This analysis offers some insights into the reasons for the wide variations between countries in the ways they recognize and identify differences between people.

In the context of this debate, for a researcher to say he or she is adopting "a cross-cultural approach" could mean that the researcher positions himself or herself in ways that disrupt traditional models of research and assumptions about the world that underpin them. It does not follow that cross-cultural research recognizes and reflects on the possible (or inevitable?) ethnocentric assumptions that underpin the formulation of the research question or focus, the particular methodology, and the ways of seeing the social world implicit in the data analysis: "We do not invariably and unfailingly recognise and allow for any ethnocentric biases and assumptions in theoretical work" (Dale 1994:34).

Cross-cultural research can be helpful in understanding disability and difference in educational contexts in a number of ways.

1. It is powerful in revealing the specific, contingent, and culturally constructed nature of social phenomena, which are traditionally regarded as fixed or "natural."
2. It can powerfully counter the view that dominant values and practices and taken-for-granted power relationships in particular societies are universal, natural, rational, or inevitable.
3. It invites the researcher to look at the society to which he or she belongs from different angles and with greater critical awareness and sensitivity to heighten understanding of the overt and covert processes and values relating to inclusion and exclusion.
4. It offers greater possibilities for critical examination of the structures and practices that hold together different societies but recognizes the subjectivity of the language used to describe and analyze them. It acknowledges that what is "seen" and analyzed is mediated by the researcher's own values and assumptions.

These points raise particular issues in terms of the need for the researcher to acknowledge his or her responsibility in the research process in relation to language and representation.

In the context of these issues and debates surrounding cross-cultural research, the impact of colonialism and the domination of Western media and values must not be underestimated. As Miles and Hossain (1999) argue, for example,

[A] (graver) difficulty in providing Islamic inputs to international debate (on disability) lies in the western domination of language (i.e. English) and media (i.e. press, satellite TV, Internet and educational publishing) and the ideological imperialism that uses the media to obliterate or marginalise cultural and conceptual notions differing from the latest European-mezzo brow trends. . . . In the western world of disability, new terms are rapidly manufactured, consumed, discarded, and dumped in used condition on third world countries. Asian educational policy makers still trying to discover whether "normalisation" and "special needs" have any meaning for children in their cities and rural schools now meet western advisers nudging them onwards to "differentiation" and "inclusion." (P. 73)

Comparative research, then, is a minefield in terms of the nature of the work and the responsibilities for the researcher. The relationships between values and ideology, research questions and processes, policymaking at all levels, and context and representation all need to be understood within particular temporal or spatial and cultural settings.

A cross-cultural perspective attempts to take into account both the cultural and political legacies of historical change and the underlying processes and values within different contemporary national contexts. Such an approach is powerful in terms of the possibilities it opens—possibilities for trying to understand different societies, their complexities, and what we can learn from them.

GLOBALIZATION AND COMMONALITY
OF EDUCATIONAL POLICY AND PRACTICE

Within industrialized countries, the centrality of economic rationality, with regard to decision making in education at both a central and local level, has had an increasing influence on policy and practice. This has ushered in a series of significant changes in the values, priorities, purposes, outcomes, and governance of education. Part of this pressure for change is due to the influence of globalization and the interdependency of nations generating new economic conditions that challenge existing systems (Bauman 1998).

In a paper examining the changing nature of educational policy across some industrialized countries, Levin (1998) identifies emerging commonality of themes. These include the following:

the impact of economic rationality on change and competition in education nationally and internationally,

the demand for change is part of a wider set of criticisms of schools and teachers,

these changes are not supported by adequate financial support, and

underpinning these developments is a strong emphasis on standards, accountability, and testing, which contributes to a view of schooling as a market commodity.

A far-reaching reconstruction of social policy and welfare took place during the period of four successive conservative governments. The key assumptions informing their political agenda included the belief that a socialist welfare state created dependency and was morally disabling; welfare provision provided by the market, family, and self-help was viewed as superior to that of the state; and the centrality of the enterprise culture and the role of financial incentives were important in creating benefits for all. Inequality from this perspective was viewed as the driving force of the enterprise culture.

This relentless pressure for particular kinds of changes in education has been driven by powerful directives, such as the necessity of demonstrating value for money with regard to educational practices and outcomes, the fundamental importance of providing dependable assessment information, the value of competition between individuals and institutions as a spur to improvement, and the required changes to how education is managed, supported by a discourse of enhancing excellence in standards, quality, and performance of individuals and institutions. This is why we must not underestimate the significance of market-driven systems of provision and practice on, for example, our notions of success and failure, the rhetoric of exclusion and inclusion, how pupils' and teachers' identities as learners and people are being constructed and challenged, how education should be managed and judged, and our vision of education.

The demand for efficiency, quality that can be clearly demonstrated, and performativity have been powerfully inspired and shaped by external forces and measures. These find expression in what constitutes appropriate forms of assessment and its functions. One influential analyst has argued that institutions such as hospitals, prisons, and schools are characterized by what he calls "disciplinary technologies" (Foucault 1977). These involve dividing practices through which individuals are spatially isolated through manipulative forms of social control. Distinguishing individuals from other groups involves the use of classification and categories, and these institutional forms of action develop social and personal identities. Foucault (1977) is interested in the normalizing tendencies of these disciplinary techniques and how they affect identities, thoughts, behaviors, and gestures.

Using this and other theoretical frameworks in her research in schools in Ireland, in which the perspectives of pupils were of particular concern, Devine (1999) is able to powerfully demonstrate from her findings several key influences at work in the lives of pupils and teachers in their daily interactions. These factors are mediated by class, age, and gender and include a sense on the part of pupils of being judged and experiencing surveillance in both formal and informal ways by teachers. The perception that children had of themselves in both academic and social terms was significantly shaped by experiencing education as something that is "done to them" and, importantly, their ability and performance being judged in highly specific ways. The children contributed to this process through the exercise of abuse or admiration of their peers within a highly competitive ethos in which they were jostling for status.

Within these schools, many children expressed a significant worry about their work—*the fear of failure* and the desire of not wanting to be shown up in front of their peers. They experienced the importance of answer-centered learning and thus felt happy when they got their work correct and received some form of praise. The centrality and function of failure have been highlighted by many research projects and are also linked to various forms of exclusionary practices within schools based on ability, behavior, and attitude. In the official thinking of government in England and Wales, this label is now being applied to schools and is supported by the influence of an inspection process and procedures carried out on behalf of government that encourage a "shame-and-blame" mentality of the institutions involved. The tabloid press is quick to seize on such cases, adding to the demoralization and disempowerment of the staff involved.

In a study of quasi-markets in social policy, Le Grand and Bartlett (1993) contend that "cream-skimming" poses a major threat to the pursuit and realization of equity. Cream-skimming involves providers of services favoring those customers or clients who will provide the greatest return for the least investment. In this form of practice, providers will tend to discriminate against the more expensive users.

Within education, academically high-attaining pupils are the "cream" that increasing numbers of schools seek to attract. They stay in schools longer, perform well on tests and examinations, and enhance the attractiveness of the schools. In a study of such schools, Gerwitz, Ball, and Bowe (1995) found that "able," "gifted," "motivated," and "committed" pupils were seen as most desirable by schools and the "less able" and those with emotional and behavioral difficulties the least attractive.

One of the fundamental reasons why this form of differentiation takes place has been identified by Whitty (1997) in a comprehensive and detailed cross-national study of recent research on parental choice and school autonomy. He argues that

> as long as schools tend to be judged on a uni-dimensional scale of academic excellence, many commentators have predicted that, rather than choice leading to more diverse and responsive forms of provision as claimed by many of its advocates, it will reinforce the existing hierarchy of schools, based on academic test results and social class. (P. 12)

Schools are becoming more selective, and this is expressed internally through the establishment of greater streaming, setting, and tracking. Beane and Apple (1999) powerfully highlighted the challenge to the establishment of democracy within schools.

Social capital in the form of parental knowledge, material, and cultural resources is a powerful factor influencing children's access to, experience within, and outcomes from particular schools. Within many societies, it is a major means by which existing inequalities within society are generally reinforced and extended. Selection of children for unequal provision has been a powerful organizing principle shaping educational systems. The greater the emphasis on schools competing with one another for particular pupils (based on behavior and academic abilities), the more likely will schools exclude those pupils who may hinder the enhancement of school performance. If we are to understand and challenge the damaging differentials in terms of access and duration of school experience, we need to engage in a critical examination of structural, political, and historical constraints. How schools are organized is not a matter of chance or a form of neutral decision making and thus can be a means of sustaining existing inequalities that often remain hidden behind a plethora of facilitative rhetoric.

Developing countries have not escaped these forms of pressure. The legacy of colonial experience and the dependency on donors, such as the World Bank, have led to meeting policy obligations as a condition of receiving financial support. This necessitates structural adjustments informed by external sources resulting in significant tensions and dilemmas between human and economic developments and their effective realization. An outcome of this dependency has been the thoughtless cross-national transfer and imposition by powerful Western societies of educational planning and practice.

Far from redressing the existing inequalities and providing a more just society, the market-led approach to policy and welfare has contributed to socially divisive outcomes. In a book concerned with the growth of exclusion in Britain during the period of conservative governments, Walker and Walker (1997) conclude that the market-led approach provides a "depressing catalogue of increasing poverty and social exclusion, growing social divisions, individual misery, premature deaths and the massive waste of human potential" (p. 287).

It is against the realities of this background that the position and function of schools in relation to the issue of inclusion need to be understood. While government investment in education is fundamentally important, the extent to which education can reduce inequalities in a direct way is open to serious doubt (Giddens 1998).

DEMOCRACY, DISABILITY, AND EDUCATION

Integral to questions relating to inclusive education and the diverse ways in which different societies construct and respond to disability and difference are the notions of democracy and governance. What is the relationship between the values, discourses, and practices that permeate society and their realization in terms of the experience and opportunities available to children and young people? Are any groups particularly privileged, marginalized, or excluded in terms of educational opportunity, and, if so, what questions does this raise about how the notion of democracy is understood? More particularly, how are disabled people positioned in relation to policies and practices that claim to be concerned with enhancing equality and participation? Does the notion of democracy provide a meaningful conceptual and ideological framework within which exclusions and inclusion in society may be understood?

Although the terms *democracy* and *democratic* are attached to many different kinds of societies, they need to be critically examined in terms of the social relations and levels of participation that operate at different levels of social life. In general, the notion of "democracy" is used to signal a fundamental distinction in terms of *other* systems regarded as *un*democratic, that is, "totalitarianism" or "religious" or "single-party" states. While "democracy" is a highly contested notion, it is generally used to refer to the principle of government by the *majority* and the projection of *minority* rights (Davies 1999). It also refers to principles of *participation* and *equality of opportunity*. Struggles over how these principles are articulated and interpreted in different contexts take place at all levels and in every society, and they often reveal broader struggles about social justice.

The disjuncture between principles of democracy and equality and the control exercised over people's choices and opportunities by powerful groups in society opens up a vast space within which sections of communities are disadvantaged and marginalized. This is exemplified by the persistent exclusion of disabled children and young people from full participation in education in virtually all countries of the world, regardless of whether these countries are considered "democratic." There has been a systematic failure to link the democratic project of full and equal participation in social life to the treatment of disabled people. Perhaps the emphasis placed by dominant Western discourses on "democracy" as the servant of the majority and as "protecting" the interests of "minorities" serves to underwrite structures, attitudes, and practices that disempower and discriminate against disabled people. This argument could be extended to explain in part the persistence of the attachment of medicalized labels (or of the mega-category of "special educational needs") to some young people, which are then deployed as criteria for their exclusion from ordinary education.

At the same time, "democracy" is also closely associated with capitalism in which processes, referred to as economic "democratization," imply the promotion of privatization and "free markets" in which, argues Lynn Davies (1999),

> capitalism . . . tends to undermine democracy because it compels most people to transfer their natural powers of self-development to economic "overlords" who control capital and other resources. This "extractive" transfer to a minority results in social inequalities and political domination by the capitalist class (Macpherson, 1973). Democratic capitalism in the West has certainly not been "antithetical" to the acceptance of inequality. (P. 129)

Paradoxically, while "democracy" is traditionally conceived of as being concerned with majority rule, it is reinterpreted as a necessary component of capitalism in which the majority are denied full enjoyment—or a fair distribution—of the fruits of their labor and protection from want. This observation is borne out by the widespread policymaking in Western countries that any legislation favoring an increase of participation of disabled children in ordinary schools should be economically viable, not detrimental to the education of other children and, in some cases, judged to be "in the child's best interest." These restrictions on equal participation demonstrate that Western-style "democracy" is not about equality or about protecting the rights of minorities. Davies (1999) argues that in the United Kingdom, although an emphasis on the rights of the consumer and parental "choice" is part of the democratic society, "consumer power is not equally distributed across social and ethnic divisions." Inequalities in education, in terms of "choice" and opportunity, are even more deeply entrenched for disabled children or "children with special needs."

There has, however, been a recent movement at the level of international pronouncements and agreements in favor of increasing the participation of all children in ordinary education (i.e., United Nations 1992; United Nations Educational, Scientific, and Cultural Organization [UNESCO] 1994). The values and practices surrounding notions such as democracy, equality, and inclusion are highly complex and contradictory. Like the notion of "rights," they are rooted in particular cultures. As Miles and Hossain (1999) argue, what constitutes "rights" in terms of children's lives and opportunities in Western countries is very different from the ways children's rights are understood in other cultures.

In Pakistan, all children have "the right" to full participation in the social life of their usually large extended families in which mutual rights and obligations are paramount, as opposed to individual rights and entitlements. The family is seen as the principle place where education and socialization take place. In theory, all children in Pakistan have the right to education, regardless of difference and difficulty, but only half the population of children actually begins primary school. Only half of those complete their primary education. Girls and disabled children are less likely to go to school than boys, but as Miles and Hossain (1999) explain,

> Expectations, choices and opportunities vary greatly between all these children, sometimes as a result of disability or difference, sometimes through gender, social and economic class, urban or rural situation, regional location or other factors. Yet these wide variations are a traditional feature of life and not necessarily perceived as problematic or "unfair." (P. 74)

Data collected from government sources suggest that there has been a steady growth in special schools in Pakistan over the past 50 years, reaching 210 in 1996 with 12,476 children enrolled. Miles and Hossain (1999) estimate that of the 20 million children enrolled in ordinary schools, 200,000 (or 1 percent) will have noticeable impairment. Of the estimated 40 million children in Pakistan, there will be an estimated 2.2 percent who have a serious or noticeable impairment, the majority of whom do not attend school at all.

In Bangladesh—one of the economically poorest countries of the world, with a population of 130 to 150 million—there is limited educational provision for disabled children. There are only 13 government institutions with a collective enrollment of 820 students and only 27 institutions run by NGOs for disabled children and adults (Miles and Hossain 1999) that, unfortunately, reflect "Western" concerns and values rather than responding to those of the population of Bangladesh. Thus, demands for the "empowerment" or the "inclusion" of disabled people are not easily understood or digested in cultures in which disabled people very often participate in the social life of communities as a matter of course. This raises issues about the usefulness of Western "democratic" models of education, which themselves have a long way to go in terms of providing equal access and opportunities for all. Indeed, in many "developing" countries, disabled children are included in their local rural school areas as a matter of course (Ainscow 1999; Miles 1992). The danger of measuring development in terms of social responses to disabled children, as exemplified by the level of specialist provision (i.e., special schools and units), is that it ignores the importance of existing social and cultural practices, which are inclusive but do not figure in Western life.

In Western societies, the structures and purposes of different kinds of services and institutions are very clearly—often rigidly—defined. Particular images of difference and models of provision are imposed through formal policymaking, processes of assessment and identification, and bureaucratic control. "Special education" and medically based categories of impairment, although highly contestable, are the bastions that exclude many disabled children from ordinary social and learning environments.

In all societies, perceptions of disability and education are mediated by cultural values and practices as well as by economic and environmental contexts, which are themselves challenged by events and processes taking place domestically and worldwide.

In China, official support is given for "inclusive education," but this is interpreted both as improving the professional standards of special schools and as increasing participation of disabled children in ordinary schools.

> In the context of the exclusion of numbers of children from any sort of educational provision until recently, it could be argued that both kinds of development represent greater inclusion however inconsistent building up the segregated sector seems to be. (Potts 1999:61)

Since the adoption of compulsory schooling in China (1986), disabled children have been included in the goal of universal education. As in many Western countries, the barriers to greater participation in ordinary education occur both at an attitudinal level and at the level of structures and the processes of selection according to attainment. However, there appears to be a real concern to explore ways of transforming curricula and teaching practices in favor of achieving greater participation.

The massive social and political upheavals that have recently taken place in many countries have destabilized all aspects of those societies, including attitudes toward minority groups and disabled people. Processes of democratization have had paradoxical effects in Eastern Europe, with rapid inflation and unemployment producing greater poverty and social exclusion. Yet there have been attempts at policymaking levels to enhance opportunities and participation of disabled people in social life (Garguilo et al. 1997; Ursic 1996). In the case of the Czech republic, this has involved introducing change after 40 years of a highly selective system of education in which disabled children and young people attended segregated schools removed from the community.

> The basic change from a communist/socialist state to a democratic/capitalist structure, and from a bureaucratic hierarchical system to a collaborative one, necessitates a reversal of beliefs about personal empowerment and attitudes about life in general (Cerná, 1994b). There is a renaissance of the human spirit under way, a rebirth of human rights

and a renewed concern for the individual rights of *all* citizens. (Gargiulo, Cerná, and Hilton 1997:22-23)

The introduction of the National Plan of Measures to Reduce the Negative Impact of Disability (1993) by the government of the Czech republic recognized the need for a change in attitudes, as well as the need to make schools physically accessible, and introduced changes in teacher education. Importantly, the plan addresses issues relating to disabled people in all areas of their lives and across life spans, including independent living, vocational training, the elimination of barriers, and so on. Thus, reforms favoring greater participation in the ordinary education of disabled people are seen as part of a wider democratic project concerned with human rights (Gargiulo et al. 1997). Figures provided by the Czech republic government show a massive increase in special schools during the period of communist control. In 1960 and 1961, there were 42,247 students enrolled in 728 special schools. By 1990 to 1991, these figures had increased to 102,295 students placed in 1,355 special schools. However, by 1994 to 1995, reforms had gradually begun to have an effect, and these figures dropped to 73,243 students attending 1,049 special schools. Government policies link greater participation with the transformation of ordinary schools and in wider society (Gargiulo et al. 1997).

The situation in Romania is in sharp contrast to that of the Czech Republic, where all children are entitled to receive an education. The economic, social, and cultural histories of the two countries are profoundly different. Both emerged from communist governance at the end of the 1980s, but this is perhaps the only point that the two countries have in common. The situation of disabled Romanian children, which was revealed following the turbulent times of the late 1980s, caused shock and horror. Despite a commitment by professionals in Romania to reform (and some aid from outside), thousands of children still live in appalling conditions in vast segregated institutions that are—disturbingly—hidden from view (Moore and Dunn 1999).

It is too easy and far too crude to pin blame for such abuses of human rights on particular kinds of governance (e.g., "communism"). There is much to be learned from trying to understand the causes of oppression and exclusion of disabled people created by attitudes, practices, and conditions in so-called "advanced" capitalist democracies.

DISABLING BARRIERS

Barriers to inclusion in ordinary schools arise through the ways policy is made and interpreted at the levels of discourse, attitudes, assessment, curriculum and pedagogy, and the distribution of resources. Disabled children and young people are also excluded from common educational settings because of the physical access arrangements to buildings and the spatial organization of schools. While being perhaps the most visible and literal barriers to exclusion, physical-spatial factors in the built environment are rarely the focus of debate among the education research community. As Imrie (1999) remarks, "Writings concerning disabled people are, by and large, aspatial." Yet the literal, physical barriers to access to ordinary social settings are part of a whole set of disabling and excluding barriers in terms of educational structures, school cultures, discourses, curricula, and pedagogy reflecting and reproducing discrimination and exclusions in wider society.

The use of space, the designation of particular sites for particular purposes, the marking of boundaries, and the erection of frontiers are powerful processes in society and in education systems in defining social relations within and between different communities. In many societies, the spatial arrangements and distribution of children and young people among a highly differentiated set of educational structures curricula produce and reproduce values and meanings that hegemonically create and maintain differences and exclusions.

In some countries, the construction of these separations and exclusions are statutory (through legislation and ministerial directives), curricular (students are not "taught the same things"), cultural (the meanings associated with membership of particular institutions are different), and physical (separate buildings, different sites). These differences are seen as ordinary because of the familiarity of the practices and discourses that surround them.

In France, for example, some children and young people do not attend schools under the control of the Ministry of Education but are assigned to various medically oriented institutions, according to impairment, and they do not have access to a common curriculum. In England, despite statements by central and local government that purport to favor "inclusion," segregated special schools and classes continue to exist in most areas of the country, and the numbers of children receiving their education "outside" ordinary settings have scarcely decreased. Medical diagnosis still plays an important role in assessing and labeling children. These labels serve to explain and justify the continued exclusion of many disabled children from their local schools (Armstrong and Barton 1999).

Terms that implicitly involve making judgments and demarcations, such as *having special needs, excellence, raising standards, target setting, failing school,* and *school improvement,* have become a fundamental part of educational discourse in the United Kingdom. The routine language, which is part of the procedures and practices of education, are powerful mediators in the interpretation of policy (Marks 1994) and the creation of stereotypes. Discourse as social practice expresses literal exclusions that operate at many different levels of society and are often made natural or invisible through the discourses and practices that surround them. Discourses such as those referring to "*illegal* immigrants," "*single-parent* families," and "emotional and behaviorally disturbed kids" mask the actual oppression and marginalization of some groups in society on the basis that they transgress socially constructed ideas of "the normal." Paradoxically, while such discourses hide from view, they also mark out and make explicit exclusions in society. Discourses of exclusion are embedded in policymaking through formal and informal policies and practices (Armstrong 1999).

The social relationships created and fostered through the planning and division of physical and social space in the school through the organization of pupils for learning and the ways in which teaching and learning are conceptualized are important interlocking ways in which exclusions and inclusion are realized.

THE STRUGGLE FOR INCLUSIVE SCHOOLS

Children, young people, and adults experience exclusion when they are debarred entry to ordinary educational settings on the grounds of disability, learning difficulty, or difference. Settings that are described as being "provided for" or "especially for" particular groups hide their role in segregating groups and individuals from ordinary social experience behind a discourse of solicitousness and accommodation. Schools, centers, and institutions that are described as *for* particular groups occupy multiple roles and identities in both "protecting" and "providing for" those identified and categorized as different, removing them from public gaze, preventing participation in ordinary social life, and denying the wider community the opportunity of knowing them. These separating conditions and processes contribute to the creation of stereotypes, which, argues Sibley (1995),

> play an important part in the configuration of social space because of the importance of distanciation in the behaviour of social groups, that is, distancing from others who are represented negatively, and because of the way in which group images and place images combine to create landscapes of exclusion. (P. 14)

At the same time, exclusions can be experienced *within* ordinary schools and colleges through their curricula, cultures, and practices. These exclusions relate not just to the physical environment but also to teaching and learning, assessment, school organization, position and role in the local community, interpersonal relationships, and the discourses deployed in relation to all of these. This argument understands *curriculum* as being at the center of the procedures, processes, and cultures in schools and the views of the world they represent and transmit.

> Curriculum is concerned with the messages that institutions transmit about knowledge and culture through its rules and social practices, as well as with the formal content of lessons. This notion of curriculum implies that selections are made from existing cultures, values and "canons of knowledge" at all levels, thus involving the drawing of boundaries and the assigning of differential spaces to different groups. These boundaries and spaces are both literal (the particular school, institution, classroom) and symbolic (their culture and curriculum) and they sustain each other. Underpinning both are the processes and procedures involved in selection and demarcation in the curriculum. (Armstrong 1999:82)

The introduction of the National Curriculum (Education Reform Act 1998) in England and Wales has had profound effects in institutionalizing and regimenting the experience of teaching and learning and in imposing a particular "English" interpretation of what counts as knowledge. Far from reflecting the country's cultural diversity and richness, the National Curriculum has "asserted a particular strain of 'heritage culture,' which ignores or devalues other cultures and experience" (Armstrong 1998:158) and is thus instrumental in excluding many students from full recognition and participation in education.

Issues and debates surrounding inclusion and exclusion involve *all* members of the community, including any groups or individuals who may experience discrimination and exclusion on the grounds of race, gender, socioeconomic or political status, impairment, perceived academic attainment, or lifestyle. This view of inclusive education, far from being a diversion or dilution, greatly strengthens the arguments surrounding the exclusion of disabled students from ordinary educational settings because it connects those arguments to wider issues involving whole communities in a common struggle.

Part of the task of removing injustices in education involves

> a self-critical analysis of the role schools play in the production or reproduction of injustices such as disabling barriers of various forms. Schools need therefore to be welcoming institutions. It is more than mere access which is at stake here. It is a quest for the removal of policies and practices of exclusion and the realisation of effective participatory democracy. It also involves a wider concern, that of clarifying the role of schools in combating institutional discrimination in relation to, for example, the position of disabled people in society. (Barton 1997:234)

Interest in comparative research and cross-cultural issues has been part of a wider interest relating to processes of globalization and a repositioning and reinterpretation of relationships between and within countries and cultures. There is an emerging interest in questions about social exclusion, and demands for a more "inclusive society" are being articulated in different ways in a variety of contexts. Inclusion is a highly contested notion, made more complicated by the commonly paradoxical relationship between stated policies purporting to be concerned with equality and social justice (e.g., "care in the community," the U.K. Disability Discrimination Act of 1995) and enacted policies as they affect disabled people. Formal policies in education at national, LEA, or school levels relating to "integration" or "inclusion" may be reworked and reinterpreted in an infinite number of ways, through the mediation of particular agents and conditions. Policy, argues Fulcher (1999), is made through struggle between different actors in multiple arenas:

> In classrooms, the teacher's decision to call a child an integration child (or by one of the more obviously derogatory disability labels), to include or exclude a student, is clearly a struggle, sometimes easily won, sometimes not: whether that means changing the curricu-

lum to include a student, or persuading unwilling parents to agree to exclusion, or calling a psychologist to "assess" a student.

Implicit in seeing these different encounters and their products (reports, debates over means, exclusion, etc.) as policy is the idea that policy takes different forms. Thus government reports or law, a teacher's decision, or a style of pedagogy, can equally be called policy, as the exercise of power, that is, the capacity to make decisions and act on them. (Pp. 7-8)

It follows, then, that barriers to inclusion in ordinary schools arise through the ways policy is made and interpreted at the level of discourse, attitudes, assessment, curriculum, and pedagogy.

In 1994, Professor John Tomlinson was appointed to chair a committee that was set up to examine existing policies and practices for students with learning difficulties or disabilities in the Further Education sector in England. This was the first committee commissioned to examine the national situation. It worked for three years and published a report titled *Inclusive Learning* (Further Education Funding Council [FEFC] 1996).

The committee was critical of a series of unacceptable preconceptions that it maintained had dogged much of the provision for disabled students. It included the beliefs that

these students are different from their non-disabled peers in the way they learn or in the amount they are capable of learning, that these students are distinguished by experiencing greater difficulty in learning than all other students. (FEFC 1996:2-3)

However, what the committee found was a number of commonalities between disabled and nondisabled students. They both

use the same repertoire of processes for learning. They each bring different experiences of success and or failure to the learning task and as a consequence, have developed strategies which may assist or get in the way of learning. (FEFC 1996:33)

Indeed, they argued that when students experienced such difficulties and achieved less, it was because of an "insufficient match between how and what they need and what to learn and what is actually provided" (FEFC 1996:33).

Teachers as mediators of learning were particularly criticized for often not knowing about the variety of ways in which people learn. Also, the report identified low expectation on the part of many teachers as being another barrier to learning.

Pupils experience exclusion *within* school practices and interactions and as a result of being *removed from* schools. Others exclude themselves by refusing to attend school. Exclusion also applies to those who have never been allowed entrance into mainstream schools. Thus, segregated special education, according to two key proponents of inclusion in the United States, plays a major sorting role and has increasingly become a means by which the smooth running of the mainstream system can be maintained (Lipsky and Gartner 1996). For many disabled people, especially for their organizations, such provision is viewed as part of the disabling barriers that need to be challenged and removed. In relation to segregated provision, Morris (1990), a disabled feminist, argues that

this is one of the most important lessons I have learnt. People's expectations of us are formed by their previous experience of disabled people. If disabled people are segregated, are treated as alien, as different in a fundamental way, then we will never be accepted as full members of society. This is the strongest argument against special schools and against separate provision. (P. 59)

Parents, in their role as advocates for their disabled children, are often engaged in challenging deep-seated beliefs about disability. Cross-cultural research indicates that this is often a frustrating, stressful, and disempowering experience, especially as many professionals ignore or devalue the everyday knowledge that parents have about their children (Brown 1999; Ware 1999).

A group of parents in Sheffield, England, demanding that their disabled children be educated in ordinary schools, illustrates something of the passion and intensity of the commitment involved in the following statement:

> For us the concept of segregation is completely unjustifiable—it is morally offensive—it contradicts any notion of civil liberties and human rights. Whoever it is done to, wherever it appears, the discrimination is damaging for our children, for our families and for our communities. We do not want our children to be sent to segregated schools or any other form of segregated provision. We do not want our children and our families to be damaged in this way. Our communities should not be impoverished by the loss of our children. (Murray and Penman 1996:vii)

The existence of segregated provision, catering for "special" pupils taught by "special" teachers supported by "special" courses in teacher training, has all contributed to the legitimation of values, attitudes, and practices that are inimical to the realization of an inclusive society and educational system (Lipsky and Gartner 1997).

In presenting an argument in support of inclusive education, we are very aware that not all groups are in favor of such an approach. For example, there are differences of view within the Deaf community between people who have acquired or developed hearing loss and are not native users of sign language and those whose congenital hearing impairment has involved them in using sign language with their deaf parents. The latter define themselves as deaf. They perceive themselves as a linguistic minority and support segregated education and separate social existence. This has been a contributing factor in creating difficulties to relations between deaf people and the disability movement as a whole (see Barnes, this volume). Some examples of both the complexity and degree of challenge that this entails, in terms of struggling for a more inclusive encounter, are illustrated by Corker (2000) in her report of an ongoing research project involving deaf children in schools. She highlights the difficulties of bullying in the interaction between deaf and hearing pupils within the deaf social group. Some examples of progress are also evident in the ways in which the deaf and hearing pupils increasingly come together to negotiate tasks and to share goals in the pursuit of what it means to "include" in this context. We do not underestimate, therefore, the learning that has still to take place between all parties, the risk taking that such a project involves, or the forms of support that will be required for inclusion to become a reality within schools and society more generally.

CONCLUSION

The analysis we have offered in this chapter attempts to challenge some existing perspectives on the question of inclusion and exclusion. By focusing on the issue of inclusion into *what*, we have briefly highlighted some of the fundamental exclusionary policies and practices that are endemic to the existing educational system. These are both deeply rooted and multifaceted and are informed by inequalities and discriminations at work within the wider socioeconomic conditions and relations of society.

It is essential that the question of inclusion be viewed as a fundamentally political issue, which, as Slee (1999) maintains, "is about who is in and who is out, about which students are in the educational mainstream and who is consigned to the status of 'others' " (p. viii). This raises serious questions, including the following: What will it take to change this discriminatory structure? What are schools for and for whom? What do we most value about schools and why?

From the perspectives we have adopted, inclusion is not about placement into an unchanged system of provision and practice. Also, it is not merely about the participation of a specific group of formerly categorized individuals (Ainscow, Booth, and Dyson 1999). Thus, it goes well beyond the issue of disablement. It is about removing *all* forms of barriers to access and learning for *all* children who are experiencing disadvantage. This approach is rooted in conceptions of democracy, citizenship, and a vision of the "good" society.

For Oliver and Barnes (1998), their vision is of

> a world in which *all* human beings, regardless of impairment, age, gender, social class or minority ethnic status, can co-exist as equal members of the community, secure in the knowledge that their needs will be met and that their views will be recognised, respected and valued. It will be a very different world from the one in which we now live. (P. 102, emphasis added)

Thus, inclusive education is not an end in itself but a means to an end—that of the realization of an inclusive society. This necessitates schools adopting a critical stance both internally and externally toward all forms of injustice and discrimination.

REFERENCES

Ainscow, M, 1999. *Understanding the Development of Inclusive Schools.* London: Routledge Kegan Paul.

Ainscow, M., T. Booth, and A. Dyson. 1999. "Inclusion and Exclusion in Schools: Listening to Some Hidden Voices." Pp. 139-51 in *Inclusive Education: International Voices on Disability and Research,* edited by K. Ballard. London: Falmer.

Armstrong, F. 1998. "The Curriculum as Alchemy: School and the Struggle for Cultural Space." *Curriculum Studies* 6 (2): 145-60.

———. 1999. "Inclusion, Curriculum and the Struggle for Space in School." *International Journal of Inclusive Education* 3 (1): 75-87.

Armstrong, F. and L. Barton. 1999. "Is There Anyone There Concerned with Human Rights? Cross-Cultural Connections, Disability and the Struggle for Change in England." Pp. 210-29 in *Disability, Human Rights and Education: Cross Cultural Perspectives,* edited by F. Armstrong and L. Barton. Buckingham, UK: Open University Press.

Barton, L. 1997. "Inclusive Education: Romantic, Subversive or Realistic?" *International Journal of Inclusive Education* 1 (3): 231-42.

Bauman, Z. 1998. *Globalization: The Human Consequences.* Oxford, UK: Polity.

Beane, J. and M. Apple. 1999. "The Case for Democratic Schools." Pp. 1-29 in *Democratic Schools,* edited by M. Apple and J. Beane. Buckingham, UK: Open University Press.

Booth, T. and M. Ainscow. 1998. *From Them to Us: An International Study of Inclusion in Education.* London: Routledge Kegan Paul.

Brown, C. 1999. "Parent Voices on Advocacy, Education, Disability and Justice." Pp. 28-42 in *Inclusive Education: International Voices on Disability and Justice,* edited by K. Ballard. London: Falmer.

Corker, M. 2000. "Disability, Politics, Language Planning, and Inclusive Social Policy." *Disability and Society* 15 (3): 445-62.

Dale, R. 1994. "Applied Educational Politics or Political Sociology of Education?" Pp. 31-41 in *Researching Education Policy,* edited by D. Halpin and B. Troyna. London: Falmer.

Davies, L. 1999. "Comparing Definitions of Democracy." *Compare* 29 (2): 127-40.

Devine, R. D. 1999. "Structure, Agency and the Exercise of Power in Children's Experience of School." Ph.D. dissertation submitted to the National University of Ireland, Dublin.

Dumay, J. M. 1994. *L'école agressée* (School under Attack). Paris: Belfond.

Foucault, M. 1977. *Discipline and Punish: The Birth of the Prison.* London: Penguin.

Fulcher, G. 1999. *Disabling Policies? A Comparative Approach to Education and Disability.* Sheffield, UK: Philip Armstrong.

Further Education Funding Council (FEFC). 1996. *Inclusive Learning (Tomlinson Report).* Coventry, UK: Author.

Gargiulo, Richard M., M. Černá, and A. Hilton. 1997. "Special Education Reform in the Czech Republic." *European Journal of Special Needs Education* 12 (1): 21-29.

Gerwitz, S., S. Ball, and R. Bowe. 1995. *Markets, Choice and Equity.* Buckingham, UK: Open University Press.

Giddens, A. 1998. *The Third Way.* London: Polity.

Halpin, D. and B. Troyna. 1995. "The Politics of Education Borrowing." *Comparative Education* 31 (3): 303-10.

Harber, C. and L. Davies, eds. 1997. *School Management and Effectiveness in Developing Countries: The Post Bureaucratic School.* London: Cassell.

Imrie, B. 1999. "Disabling Environments and the Geography of Access Policies and Practices in the United Kingdom." Unpublished manuscript.

Le Grand, J. and W. Bartlett, eds. 1993. *Quasi-Markets and Social Policy.* London: Macmillan.

Levin, B. 1998. "An Epidemic of Education Policy: (What) Can We Learn from Each Other?" *Comparative Education* 34 (2): 131-42.

Levitas, R. 1998. *The Inclusive Society? Social Exclusion and New Labour.* Basingstoke, UK: Macmillan.

Lipsky, D. and A. Gartner. 1996. "Inclusion, School Restructuring, and the Remaking of American Society." *Harvard Educational Review* 66 (4): 762-96.

———. 1997. *Inclusion and School Reform: Transforming America's Classroom.* Baltimore: Brookes.

Macpherson, C. 1973. *Democratic Theory: Essays in Retrieval.* Oxford, UK: Clarendon.

Marks, G. 1994. "Armed Now with Hope: The Construction of the Subjectivity of Students within Integration." *Disability and Society* 9 (1): 71-84.

Miles, M. 1992. "Concepts of Mental Retardation in Pakistan: Towards Cross-Cultural and Historical Perspectives." *Disability, Handicap and Society* 7 (3): 235-55.

Miles, M. and F. Hossain. 1999. "Rights and Disabilities in Educational Provision in Pakistan and Bangladesh: Roots, Rhetoric, Realist." Pp. 67-86 in *Disability, Human Rights and Education: Cross Cultural Perspectives,* edited by F. Armstrong and L. Barton. Buckingham, UK: Open University Press.

Moore, M. and K. Dunn. 1999. "Disability, Human Rights and Education in Romania." Pp. 193-209 in *Disability, Human Rights and Education,* edited by F. Armstrong and L. Barton. Buckingham, UK: Open University Press.

Morris, J. 1990. "Progress with Humanity: The Experience of a Disabled Lecturer." Pp. 58-60 in *Disability Equality in the Classroom: A Human Rights Issue,* edited by R. Rieser and M. Mason. London: Inner London Education Authority.

Murray, P. and J. Penman, eds. 1996. *Let Our Children Be: A Collection of Stories.* Sheffield, UK: Parents with an Attitude.

National Plan of Measures to Reduce the Negative Impact of Disability. 1993. *Resolution of the Government of the Czech Republic, No. 493.* Prague: Board of Representatives from the Organisations of Disabled People.

Organization for Economic Cooperation and Development (OECD). 1995. *Integrating Students with Special Needs into Mainstream Schools.* Paris: Author.

Oliver, M. and C. Barnes. 1998. *Social Policy and Disabled People: From Exclusion to Inclusion.* London: Longman.

Potts, P. 1999. "Human Rights and Inclusive Education in China: A Western Perspective." Pp. 54-66 in *Disability, Human Rights and Education,* edited by F. Armstrong and L. Barton. Buckingham, UK: Open University Press.

Sadler, M. 1902. *The Unrest in Secondary Education in Germany and Elsewhere in Board of Education.* Education in Germany: Special Reports on Education Subjects, Vol. 9. London: Her Majesty's Stationery Office.

Sibley, D. 1995. *Geographies of Exclusion.* London: Routledge Kegan Paul.

Slee, R. 1999. "Series Editor's Preface." Pp. 119-31 in *Inclusive Education: International Voices on Disability and Justice,* edited by K. Ballard. London: Falmer.

United Nations. 1992. *United Nations Convention on the Rights of the Child.* London: Children's Rights Development Unit.

United Nations Educational, Scientific, and Cultural Organization (UNESCO). 1994. *The Salamanca Statement and Framework for Action on Special Needs Education: Access and Equality.* New York: Author.

Ursic, C. 1996. "Social (and Disability) Policy in the New Democracies of Europe (Slovenia by Way of Example)." *Disability and Society* 11 (1): 91-105.

Walker, A. 1997. "Introduction: The Strategy of Inequality." Pp. 1-13 in *Britain Divided: The Growth of Social Exclusion in the 1980s and 1990s,* edited by A. Walker and C. Walker. London: Child Poverty Action Group.

Walker, A. and C. Walker, eds. 1997. *Britain Divided: The Growth of Social Exclusion in the 1980s and 1990s.* London: Child Poverty Action Group.

Ware, L. 1999. "My Kid, and Kids Kinda Like Him." Pp. 43-66 in *Inclusive Education: International Voices on Disability and Justice,* edited by K. Ballard. London: Falmer.

Whitty, G. 1997. "Creating Quasi-Markets in England: A Review of Recent Research on Parental Choice and School Autonomy in Three Countries." *Review of Research in Education* 22:3-47.

Support Systems

31

The Interface between Individuals and Environments

SIMI LITVAK

ALEXANDRA ENDERS

raditionally, professional and clinical services for people with disabilities have used a curative or medical model focused on fixing and adjusting people. Since the 1970s, conceptual frameworks concerning the source of disability have been refined, and an ecological model is now emerging in which disability is seen as an interaction between an individual and an environment, not as something simply intrinsic to the person (Hahn 1984; U.S. Department of Education 2000).

Responding to this shift in emphasis, policymakers have spurred creation of accessible public physical and social environments, including buildings, transportation systems, telecommunications infrastructure, and medical, social, and income support programs. However, there are limits to the degree of environmental changes that can be made to accommodate the needs of every individual.

Our concern here is to focus on ways to decrease disability further by using supports to reduce the demand of an activity or increase a person's capacity to perform the activity (Verbrugge and Jette 1994). Supports include technology (ranging from sophisticated electronic-augmented communication to a simple one-handed jar opener), personal assistance from human beings or animals, and the strategies employed to carry out the task. Supports influence the degree of disability that an individual experiences. The role of supports is to reduce the impact of functional limitations on disability.

Supports make it possible for disabled people to carry out their daily lives, gain access to their world, and participate as citizens. More crucially, supports literally are a matter of survival for people who are significantly disabled. Presence or absence of supports can make the difference between dying, living in an institution or nursing home, being dependent on the good will and energy of relatives, or living as one chooses in the community.

The distinction between one's degree of disability with and without the use of supports has "strong implications for public health statistics, design and development of disability technology and for long term care policy" (Verbrugge and Jette 1994:9). The nature and breadth of supports will continue to increase in importance as our vision of the roles people with significant disabilities can play in society expands (e.g., parent, worker, executive, student, home-maker, athlete, public servant, dancer).

Support *systems,* not individual support services, are the primary focus of this chapter because integration and fluidity of various supports are necessary to serve individual needs. Supports move together. They overlap. They interact, depending on the friendliness of the environment (Enders and Leech 1996). For example, an individual in a wheelchair, cooking in an adapted kitchen, and using countertops, cupboards, and sinks that move up and down with the push of a button may not need the reacher and low table. Nor would he or she need the person to fetch utensils and food that he or she would need in an unmodified kitchen anywhere in the world.

Support systems bring together a full range of elements necessary to enable human beings to function in the world and community and to accomplish tasks. Individuals have limited control of the environment. However, humans do have control over the tools and people that enable us to live our lives. This is true for everyone, not just for people with disabilities. For example, if you want to eat dinner, there is a range of options, including going to a restaurant or eating at home. To eat at home, one can have cooking as an option; one can also have food delivered or hire a cook. These are supports everyone uses, but they get special labels when they are targeted to people with disabilities (i.e., meals-on-wheels and personal assistance). The act of obtaining dinner involves a complex interaction between people, tools, skills, resources, and choices available to accomplish everything from getting the food to the house to taking out the garbage at the end of the meal.

A personal support system, based on an individual's choices and resources, serves as the actual interface between the individual and all the different aspects and variations of his or her multiple environments. When personal support systems are an integral and well-functioning part of life, they are transparent; that is, we tend not to notice them, and they require little or no specific attention. Curb cuts and building ramps, along with electric wheelchairs and scooters, are so ubiquitous in many areas that they are not noticed by the general public. By and large, however, support systems for individuals with disabilities have not reached that stage of transparency.

In addition, the existence of supports cannot be taken for granted, nor are they necessarily adequate (i.e., qualitatively and quantitatively sufficient to enable the individual to carry out the desired task). The utopia does not yet exist where persons using a wheelchair or scooter may assume that they can easily get into every building in town, use all the facilities, and move from area to area. People without disabilities rightly make this assumption all the time. Similarly, the utopia does not exist, except in very special places, where an individual who is deaf can communicate with anyone.

There are wide variations in the nature of an appropriate support system. The adequacy and transparency of the support system both shape and are shaped by an individual's conceptual framework of self, role, and community. Yet within any given culture or society, there is likely to be agreement on how a support system should function and recognition of when it is not working for the individual. When support system adequacy or transparency is lost, the primary reasons tend to be related to resource allocation, choice, and self-determination and the controversies, disagreements, or policy conflicts surrounding resources and choice.[1]

Support systems, whatever their configuration, are intensely and intimately individual. Support systems are dynamic. The integration, fluidity, dynamism, and individuality of people's support systems may seem like an obvious and simple concept, particularly to the people who use them. Medical and rehabilitation professionals, policymakers, and the general public, more than people with disabilities, often do not recognize how important integration and individuation of supports are. Barriers between professions, differences in funding streams, and compartmentalization of disability services are major stumbling blocks to achieving integration and responding to changes in the circumstances of individual disabled people. Often, services and supports are pitted against each other, vying for funding, recognition, and respect (Enders 1995; U.S. Department of Education 2000). Achieving their integration is currently difficult unless one is independently wealthy. For example, in the United States, people in nursing homes are given manual wheelchairs. The federal health program for seniors will not pay for power chairs. So, instead of being able to come and go as they please, nursing home residents have to rely on scarce, overworked aides to push them where and when they want to go.

Consumer choice and control of one's supports help guarantee the best fit possible between the person and the environment, assuming that the supports needed are available and accessible. When resources are limited, when professionals have to be case or resource managers as well as service providers, and when people with disabilities are unaware of support possibilities or choices, "best fit" is an elusive goal.

To explore this subject more fully, we discuss supports in their particularity and in their interaction. This chapter is divided into several parts. We begin with defining and describing supports specific to people with disabilities, personal assistance services (PAS), assistive technology (AT), and assistive strategies (AS) for carrying out activities. We explore PAS and AT in more detail, including their varieties, history, political economy, and their availability throughout the world. Later, we define and discuss the interaction of these three components of a disability support system against the backdrop of universal support systems, which involve cooperation with others, tools, and people's skills and strategies for enhancing interaction with the environment. Finally, we analyze the role played by consumer control and choice in determining individual supports. This chapter concludes by raising outstanding policy and research issues and problems concerning support systems and individual supports, along with possible solutions and future direction for policy and research.

DISABILITY-SPECIFIC SUPPORTS

Personal Assistance Services

Personal assistants (PAs) are people who provide aid to people with disabilities so they can perform their daily tasks, tasks they would ordinarily perform for themselves if they were not disabled. The personal assistance services (PAS) provided may include hands-on, cuing, or stand-by assistance with tasks such as self-care and hygiene, including feeding, bathing, and dressing; ongoing paramedical needs, including catheter care and injections; household maintenance, such as shopping, cooking, and cleaning; sexual positioning; child rearing, such as positioning the baby to nurse; cognitive functions such as planning time, signing contracts, and judging social situations; and communication and transportation (Litvak, Heumann, and Zukas 1987).

Personal assistance services can be provided in a variety of settings ranging from institutions, nursing homes, and group homes to private homes, workplaces, schools, recreation sites, and other public venues. In this chapter, we are concerned with PAS provided to people in private homes and various community settings and the people (PAs) who provide these services.

PAs can be paid (formal) or unpaid (informal), family member or not, live-in, or independent provider or home care/home health agency employee. In some instances, such as sign language interpreters, telephone relay operators, or facilitators for people with cognitive disabilities, the PA may serve the person with a disability and persons who are not disabled. Personal assistants tend to be middle-aged, unskilled women (mostly minorities in the United States) or students who prefer erratic schedules. Those who work for home care or home health agencies may have some training in basic personal care such as bathing and transferring. Independent personal assistants may or may not have some training. Actually, many in the independent living movement prefer hiring personal assistants who are not trained. In this respect, the person with the disability can train the worker without having to discourage "bad habits" such as presuming to speak for the disabled employer.

As long as there have been people with disabilities, there have been PAs. Typically, these services have been provided informally in the home by the family or, more recently and more formally, in institutions and nursing homes. Institutional settings, mainly for poor people, developed with the rise in public welfare in the late nineteenth and the early twentieth centuries in developed countries and much later in developing countries (Jayasooria, Krishnan, and Ooi 1997).

In underdeveloped countries, people with significant disability receive PAS from family members or household servants. They often live shorter lives and face major cultural and architectural obstacles to leaving their homes and participating in community life as workers and citizens. The provision of publicly funded PAS has only just begun to be considered an issue by disabled people in these areas (World Institute on Disability [WID] 1999). Wealthy and sometimes middle-class families have the resources to hire servants. Poorer people rely on family, friends, and sometimes charity. Recently, disability activists from developing countries have charged that the sexism in their culture may dictate that women take care of disabled men and boys first and foremost, while disabled girls and women come last, if at all (WID 1999).

Publicly financed PAS in homes and in the community became a trend in the last part of the twentieth century in many developed countries worldwide, such as the United States, Canada, England, Australia, all the Scandinavian countries, and Germany. This was due to several factors. During this period, there was an increase in the number of significantly disabled young people and elders as a result of technological advances in medicine and rehabilitation. At the same time, there has been expansion in the proportion of working mothers and shrinkage in the size of the extended family, thus creating an increased need for assistance from people outside the immediate family.

Research is demonstrating, as disabled people have long maintained, that there is an increase in work and community engagement when one has PAS (Kimmick and Godfrey 1991; Nosek, Fuhrer, and Potter 1995; Richmond et al. 1998). Research on PAS shows outcomes of using PAS, population in need of PAS, efficacy of various models of PAS, and the value of consumer control. Studies of cost of various models, legal analyses of liability, consumer satisfaction, and demonstrations of consumer-driven models among people of all ages in several North American states and in Europe show that many consumers prefer PAS that allow them to be in control. These studies also show that such programs are legally and economically feasible (Beatty et al. 1998; Benjamin and Matthias 1998; Cameron and Firman 1995; Egley 1994; Litvak 1996; Reiff, Zawadski, and Hyde 1996; Sabatino and Litvak 1996). Consumer direction and control have become a viable option.

As the independent living and disability rights movements spread worldwide in the 1980s and 1990s, disability leaders in the European Union and in the United States asserted that PAS delivered in the home and the community is a civil right (European Union [EU] resolution, WID resolution). These disability leaders argued that the failure of society to provide PAS means that people with disabilities are disabled by society. In the landmark U.S. Supreme Court decision *L.C. v. Olmstead* (1999), the justices affirmed this logic when they agreed that people with disabilities can use the Americans with Disabilities Act, a civil rights act for disabled people, to require states to provide PAS to enable people to live in the community.

The transition to community-based PAS has not been easy. In many countries, the call for home-based PAS met the resistance of home care and nursing home industries, as well as labor organizations representing hands-on providers in institutions and nursing homes (Simon-Rusinowitz et al. 1999). In the United States, labor based in nursing homes and institutions has sometimes seen community-based PAS as threat to their future employment.

Government-financed PAS in the community is more widely available in some advanced capitalist countries than others. In Scandinavia, PAS is nearly universally available and grew out of society-wide services for disabled and nondisabled citizens alike, such as care for sick children or parents of working people (Doty, Kasper, and Litvak 1996). In Britain, the Netherlands, and some of the more advanced Eastern European countries, such as Russia, which built villages for disabled people, the provision of services in the community has been slower to develop. As the European Union becomes more structurally integrated, activists have called for a disability rights law that guarantees disabled individuals access to the services available in any one of the member states, regardless of one's nationality (Waddinton 1997). In the United States, where some states have been more interested in providing PAS in the home, there has been a slow, gradual increase in community-based PAS programs and numbers served since the 1960s (Litvak and Kennedy 1991). In contrast, Japan began providing PAS in selected areas in the 1980s (Kaiya 1998; WID International Conference 1999).

We consider PAS to be a cross-disability service, but this is not universally agreed on. The use of PAS by people with cognitive and emotional or psychiatric disabilities, which enables them to live in their own homes in the community, is only now being addressed and only in certain places such as Scandinavia and the United States (Stewart 1992; Vivona, Dresen, and Litvak 2000). Issues regarding differences in training and skill levels between those providing cueing or stand-by assistance with personal hygiene and maintenance versus those providing assistance with learning tasks (in or out of the classroom), participation at meetings, or making judgments in social situations have not been fully explored. For example, what should be the skill level and pay for people working with people who are not fully self-directed? In addition, in the United States, people with vision impairment have tended to maintain that they do not use PAS because they receive assistance on an informal or volunteer basis with driving, reading, shopping, and other tasks that are not necessarily tied to medical survival needs. In addition to the pressure for deinstitutionalization, the independent living movement, particularly in the United States and Scandinavian countries, has pushed for consumer-controlled and consumer-directed personal assistance services (National Council on Aging 1996; Ratzka 1993). This followed from their conviction that independence does not mean being able to do everything for oneself; rather, it means being in control of one's supports. In this way, the PAS user determines when, where, and how he or she receives PAS rather than this being the decision of professionals and providers. The personal assistant becomes, literally or in spirit, the employee of the disabled individual. Governments have responded to independent living demands by allowing people with disabilities more self-determination in directing their own services in a variety of ways. This change occurred as governments realized there was a consumer constituency wanting control, that consumer control would not lead to widespread abuse of people with disabilities, and that services provided in this way are less expensive because they do not require the enormous operating costs of government-monitored, -administered, and -managed services (Cameron and Firman 1995; Degener 1992; Glendinning 1991; Ratzka 1986; WID 1999; Zarb and Nadesh 1994).

For-profit home care agencies have seen the independent living call for control and direction of their PAs and PAS in the home and community as a threat to their way of doing business. They have argued that PAS, provided and supervised by qualified agencies, is safer and of higher quality. Benjamin, Matthias, and Franke (2000) have shown in their research in the United States that these differences do not exist, however. Similar results were found in examining the German PAS system, which allows for a choice of direct payment to the disabled individual or government-arranged PAS (Weiner and Cuellar 1999). Large-scale demonstrations, which parallel the German experiments, are currently taking place in three states in the United States: Florida, New Jersey, and Arkansas (Simon-Rusinowitz et al. 1999). Similarly, PAS has advanced in the United Kingdom, where deinstitutionalization and direct payments for the disabled have been government policy since 1996 (Weiner and Cuellar 1999).

Health and social service professionals have been slow to grasp the significance of PAS to the lives of disabled people. In contrast, there are volumes of research on the impact of "caregiving" on members of the disabled person's family. This lack of interest of professionals concerning the impact of PAS on the lives of disabled people stems from reasons such as paternalism, the tendency to overmedicalize tasks that require little professional expertise, the lack of connections professionals have to the day-to-day lives of disabled people with chronic functional disabilities, and the training professionals receive that emphasizes the notion that if one cannot accomplish a task without the help of another person, then one is dependent.

The provision of publicly funded PAS has been plagued by other controversies as well. The overlap between personal assistance services and domestic servants has been an arena of conflict in locations that lack a strong social welfare orientation. Is it the role of the state to provide all the PAS a person could use? In the United States in particular, the struggle over the true nature of these supports is occurring. Are PAS special services for disabled people that therefore require special service delivery mechanisms, or are they services easily deliverable by nonspecialized personnel or agencies, which are far less costly? This debate has crystallized in the United States around the nature of medical supervision required for these services (Sabatino and Litvak 1996; Wagner, Nadesh, and Sabatino 1997).

Another issue involves PAS at the work site. Who pays for PAS on the job, and who provides PAS at the job site? What is the difference between secretaries and personal assistants? Is it appropriate for employer and public accommodation policy to provide PAS for personal care, such as assistance with toileting functions and eating?

Service Animals

Service animals, a subset of PAS, are another support available to people with significant disabilities. These are animals, primarily dogs, trained to assist disabled people with their daily tasks. For example, animals hear alarms, telephones, and doorbells for deaf people. They guide people with vision impairments, pick up things for those with mobility limitations, or pull a wheelchair for manual chair users who experience fatigue at the end of a day or who do not have quite the strength necessary for hills. As in the case of other supports, using animals to extend human capabilities is an old idea. However, programs that train animals to assist those with disabilities are twentieth-century phenomena, mainly available in the wealthiest countries.

Blascovish (1996), in his research on the value of service dogs, found that dog users showed improvements in self-esteem, internal locus of control, psychological well-being, increase in school and work attendance, and a dramatic decrease in paid and unpaid personal assistance hours. Clearly, there is substitutability between use of dogs and hours of personal assistance. As a consequence, Blascovish concluded that "trained service dogs can be highly beneficial and potentially cost-effective components of physically disabled people's support systems" (p. 1006). One cannot conclude, however, that service animals should automatically substitute for people or that an individual can even maintain a dog without assistance of another person.

Assistive Technology and Tools

An assistive technology device is defined in one U.S. law as "any item, piece of equipment, or product system, whether acquired commercially off the shelf, modified, or customized, that is used to increase, maintain, or improve functional capabilities of individuals with disabilities" (PL 100-407, Technology-Related Assistance for Individuals with Disabilities Act). In other U.S. laws governing medical reimbursement for technology, however, the definition is considerably more restricted to items that are *medically necessary,* a term subject to interpretation by health insurers. In general, technology that is covered must be specifically designed for or distributed to disabled people. Similar distinctions exist in other developed countries, even those providing technology through universal health programs. In Australia and Canada, for example, it is the responsibility of individual provinces to define what technology will be covered. Some provinces define assistive technology very tightly. Others do not care if the technology is only aimed at disabled consumers, as long as the technology works. In some areas, medical necessity is not even a factor.

These definitional differences greatly affect what governments and private insurance will provide, and they are based on the vastly different interpretations of people with disabilities and policymakers. From a grassroots disabled person's perspective, it does not matter what the technology is, just that it fits, works, and is useful. From a disabled person's perspective, her or his speaker phone, abbreviation expansion software for the computer, and ergonomic office chair are as much assistive technology (AT) as are her or his powered scooter, van with a lift, hip replacement, and typing splints.

In other words, if the products selected require you to consider your disability issues first, then they are assistive technology—even if they are widely available, mundane, mass-market products. If you did not have a disability, you would not have to think about these product features when you make your choices. When your disability is defining or narrowing your product choices and options, you are buying assistive technology, whether you are calling it that and whether it was designed to be AT (Enders 1997). First, wheelchair riders shop for the cars in their price range that can accommodate the wheelchair (i.e., "Can I get in, get my chair in, and operate the controls?"). Then they select from that small pool of consumer features they like, such as performance and gas mileage—not the other way around. Similarly, a person with multiple chemical sensitivities must take into account irritants when selecting personal care and household products such as deodorant, lotion, and dish soap, often being forced to purchase less available, more costly, but safer products.

It does not matter what the technology is; the important aspect is who is using the tool and what he or she is trying to accomplish with it. That is grassroots commonsense. However, this is frequently not how professionals see the use of technological interventions. The arbitrary distinctions made in resource allocation decision making, especially in medical, model-based service systems, rarely use this broader perspective. For example, an augmentative communication device that is built into a general-purpose computer is less likely to be reimbursed than a special-purpose device that can be used only for communication—even if the computer-based system is less expensive and provides a greater range of function.

The focus narrows only to disability-specific applications, and the larger context is avoided. The U.S. Medicare definition of *durable medical equipment* is equipment that

> can withstand repeated use,
>
> is primarily and customarily used to serve a medical purpose,
>
> generally is not useful to an individual in the absence of an illness or injury, and
>
> is appropriate for use in the home. (42 CFR 414.202)

This distinction is driven by policymakers who want to ensure that public funds are expended on medically oriented products. Public and private policies discriminate against mass-market products that incorporate universal design features in favor of a "special" product targeted only and specifically to the disability market. The Center for Universal Design defines *universal design* as "the design of products and environments to be usable by all people, to the greatest extent possible, without the need for adaptation or specialized design" (Connell et al. 1997:1). As universal design becomes more prevalent and disabled people have more control over their technology choices, "specialness," as well as the stigma that often accompanies specialness, is dropping away, however. The vast increase in the older population in the more developed countries is triggering entrepreneurs to consider a broader range of human performance in their product design. For example, automobile manufacturers are beginning to design cars that will enable people with bending and squatting problems to enter and exit cars more easily (Hamilton 1999). Spurred by clever marketers, aging baby boomers are discovering the benefits of many specialized disability products. In the process, the stigma is dissolving, as the product is repackaged and repositioned in the marketplace. Like the eyeglasses that prevented a nearsighted woman from being hired as an airline stewardess a generation ago, disability products are now acceptable once boomers discover and redefine them. Eyeglasses are now fashion statements, and some restaurants in Los Angeles provide reading glasses to use when reading the bill. Therapy equipment has transformed into exercise gear and made its way into the home fitness market, and accessible exercise equipment is appearing in health clubs. Large-handled kitchen equipment is trendy. The Oxo Good Grips line of large, black-handled kitchen utensils has successfully straddled the fence—letting people with disabilities know that it would be useful without acquiring the traditional stigma of handicapped devices.

Technology, such as a mobilized wheelchair with custom seating, can serve one person or many people, such as a taxi or bus with a built-in lift. Public technology is generally built to incorporate standardized features deemed useful to a broad range of individuals. It tends to become a part of the environment and useful to disabled and nondisabled people as well. Accessible taxis, such as those in Vancouver, British Columbia, are used by artists to move large art pieces because the taxis have a tall open space in the back and a lift. Curb cuts probably see more delivery handcarts, baby strollers, and skateboard use than wheelchair tires.

Personal technology may be selected or built with more individualized characteristics. Housing modifications can be public technology, for example, building units may be constructed using U.S. standards, such as the Americans with Disabilities Act Accessibility Guidelines (ADAAG) or Uniform Federal Accessibility Standards (UFAS), which incorporate accessibility features (in the macro environment). They can also be personal (e.g., when modifications are made in an individual's housing unit configured to the specific requirements and measurements of the resident).

There have always been technological solutions to disabling conditions. However, the pace of innovation accelerated greatly in the last half of the twentieth century. Advances in materials, especially in computer technologies, have led to revolutionary discoveries not only in information processing and telecommunications but also in areas such as the design and fitting of artificial limbs, automobile adaptations, and functional electrical stimulation for sphincter control. Undoubtedly, the future will bring even more innovation. Prototypes for machine-produced, real-time sign language interpretation and brain wave–controlled computers are here today. The Rehabilitation Engineering Research Center on Telecommunications Access, sponsored by the National Institute on Disability and Rehabilitation Research (NIDRR), has already demonstrated the feasibility of using Internet II for real-time captioning and sign language interpretation. When wireless networks with enough bandwidth are available, this type of interface will make a remote sign language interpreter locally available on demand, anytime, anywhere. The captions or the interpreter could be viewed on a mobile laptop computer, allowing the person to carry the interpreter along. The system is designed to send audio over the network to the interpreter's site. A small camera built into the unit also allows the deaf person to sign to the interpreter.

Technological advances will also blur the line between specialized and generic products. Advances such as miniaturization may have unintended and sometimes undesirable side effects for access, unless universal design principles are uniformly and transparently incorporated into technological trends.

As the philosophy of the independent living and disability rights community has spread, and as people with disabilities have become designers, manufacturers, and marketers of assistive technology, we are seeing more acceptable, stylish, and noninstitutional equipment. Product design increasingly recognizes that people with disabilities are actively living in the community. Equipment has emerged that supports active lifestyles and roles. For example, wheelchairs, both manual and powered, have become sleeker and more maneuverable; activity-specific products for different competitive sports continue to evolve; and aesthetics are considered, as well as comfort and function.

Technology that is "medically necessary" may be available to disabled people who have personal resources or health insurance (either private or public) that will pay for the equipment. The newer, more community-oriented technology is not always covered, even in countries with universal health care. Technologically sophisticated devices such as complex powered mobility systems, augmentative communication systems, extensive workstations, and adapted vehicles (e.g., vans with lifts) can be very costly and beyond the reach of most people with disabilities.

The availability of assistive technology in developing countries and rural areas is much more limited. Frequently, people are quite literally "left to their own devices" because homemade equipment is the only technology available. According to Whirlwind Wheelchair International (WWI; www.whirlwind.sfsu.edu), equipment imported by developing countries has not been consistently available in all the types and sizes that are needed. It has been difficult or impossible to repair (imported parts are required but are often not available), and it has been ill suited to the rough urban and rural environments of developing countries.

By tapping into the ingenuity of local people with disabilities, Ralf Hotchkiss's WWI work is creating a worldwide network of wheelchair inventors and builders to address serious problems of wheeled mobility around the world. Collaborating with riders and inventors in developing countries, Hotchkiss has greatly increased his—and his peers'—likelihood of eventual success. There are other similar grassroots efforts internationally, some of them documented in *Nothing about Us: Developing Innovative Technologies for, by and with Disabled Persons* (Werner 1998), an idea book written for people with disabilities, their relatives, friends, and helpers, as well as for clinicians.

Will Technology Replace Assistance?

Many nondisabled professionals have the idea that technology and animals will eventually supplant the need for PAS. The belief in the eventual triumph of technology is rooted in a very long tradition going back to the dawn of the industrial revolution. It is a persistent fantasy. The 1950s French film *Mon Oncle,* in which all housework is performed with the push of a button, and the 2000 film *Bicentennial Man,* in which an increasingly anthropomorphic robot substitutes for any and all human assistance, are just two of a myriad of examples.

In fact, in the twentieth century, the use of PAS alone for people who are aging actually declined, the use of AT increased, and the use of AT and PAS together are increasing steadily and likely to increase further (Manton, Corde, and Stallard 1993; Longino 1994). Moreover, Agree (1999) concluded in her research that people who use only technology tend to be less significantly disabled, while those with higher levels of disability use both technology and PAS. This same relationship may or may not hold for people with cognitive or emotional disabilities.

It can be dangerous and destructive to pit PAS and AT against each other as competing resources, rather than as complementary components of a support system. It is not uncommon, for example, for professionals to write documentation for environmental control products, stating they will "reduce the need for attendant care." Technology is seen as a less expensive substitute for personal assistance services. Professionals also use the appealing argument of an increase in autonomy and independence with the use of technology. For instance, they may argue that a person can use an automatic leg bag opener rather than asking a person to do the chore. Yet who helps the individual put the device on, and who empties the leg bag on the day the automatic "widget" is broken or needs cleaning or replacement?

The idea of substituting one type of support for another may be seductive, but the one-size-fits-all approach this implies is not compatible with consumer responsiveness and control over one's life. It fails to acknowledge the wide range of variation among people with disabilities, due to resources and choices as well as size and shape. Because policy does not look at the relationship and connectedness of PAS and AT as support system elements, it encourages an absolute either-or alternative. In other words, choose a tool or a person, not a combination or the most appropriate at any given time or place. Just pick either the device or the person but rarely both. This is disastrous for people with significant disabilities but not an unfamiliar situation. In the words of a disabled activist, "We don't get what we need; if we are lucky, we may get what is gettable" (Enders and Heumann 1988:582).

People functioning as assistants conceptually become an element of a support system. However, people must never be considered as being interchangeable with the other elements. Utilitarians would argue that humans are interchangeable and can be measured as units with completely disregarding the less tangible benefits and skills humans bring to a support system. Interpersonal connection and interaction are major elements of being human. Collectivist cultures recognize and incorporate these values even more than cultures more focused on the individual (National Council on Disability [NCD] 1999). However, even in highly individualistic cultures, such as in the United States, human interaction is an essential value to most people. Even in the most consumer-controlled model of personal assistance, where the consumer acts

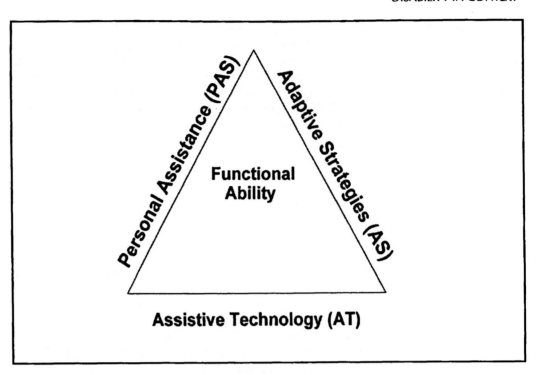

Figure 31.1.   Elements of a Functional Ability Support System

as the employer of the personal assistant, the nature of the human interaction has a large part in determining the quality of the personal assistance received (DeGraff 1988).

Finally, technology is not an alternative to personal interaction as when proponents of "care robots" speak of the value a talking machine brings to the caregiving role or a talking toy brings to child development. Technology such as telephones and e-mail can be a conduit for human contact. Technology may function as a substitute for companionship. Television noise in the background often plays this role; yet, technology should not be mistaken for human interaction. "High-touch, high-tech" advertising slogans cannot mitigate the risk of depersonalization stemming from the increasing loss of human interaction in a high-tech environment.

SUPPORT SYSTEMS

Having discussed personal assistance services and technology in their particularity and considered whether one is a substitute for the other, we now turn to the ways that technology and personal assistance interact to form a support system. What follows is a description of various characteristics of support systems for people with disabilities.

Interaction and Interrelatedness of Support System Elements

Assistive technology, personal assistance services, and adaptive strategies are the basic elements of a disability-specific support system. To aid in further discussion, we depict these elements as three sides of a triangle because they are interrelated and nonlinear (see Figure 31.1). The triangle focuses solely on the specialized or highly individualized elements in a disabled person's support system. The sides or legs of the triangle are labeled assistive technology (AT),

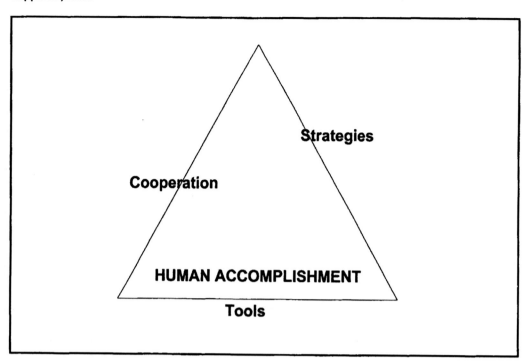

Figure 31.2.   Elements of Any Generic Support System

personal assistance services (PAS), and adaptive strategies (AS). The area within the triangle is labeled *functional ability*. It represents an individual's functional ability. The lengths of the sides of the triangle constantly change in response to environments and individual participatory roles. The triangle provides a framework for thinking about the dynamics of the relationship between PAS and technology and the options one has to achieve function and accomplish tasks. The triangle shape is meant to imply that if you remove one of the legs, the whole framework collapses.

A disabled person's ability to function is determined by the adequacy of her support system. How and where the elements are interrelated is dependent on factors such as an individual's culture, community, and interests. The elements can shift dramatically, depending on the environment within which the support is used.

Embedding of Disability-Specific Supports within the Support System for All Human Accomplishment

Not just people with disabilities but all human beings have a dynamic support system that links the individual to the physical environment. The basic elements of anyone's support system are tools, cooperation, and strategies. Tools include technology and physical objects. Cooperation encompasses people (and animals) and our interactions with them. Strategies are the ways we do things, as well as the techniques and skills we have or acquire.

These elements are represented as three sides of the human accomplishment triangle, which is larger than the functional ability triangle because it supports all people (see Figure 31.2). Figure 31.2 is labeled "Elements of Any Generic Support System" because it portrays the elements of any individual's support system. The sides are labeled tools, strategies, and cooperation. The area is labeled human accomplishment. It shape-shifts as a person's environmental situation changes. As environmental demands change, one uses more or less of each of the support elements. The shape also changes when the individual changes roles (e.g., parent, student, or pia-

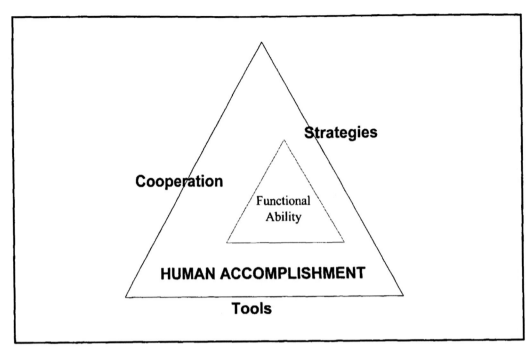

Figure 31.3.   Human Accomplishment Support System

nist) within the same environment. Individuals can find support for specialized needs within the human accomplishment triangle when generic tools, communities, and skill development opportunities are built flexibly enough to incorporate a range of experience and interests.

The "special" triangle of disability-specific supports is a subset of this larger support system that all humans use. Therefore, a more accurate picture of a support system for a person with a disability is achieved by placing the smaller functional ability triangle within the larger human accomplishment triangle (see Figure 31.3). In this way, the functional ability triangle is embedded in the larger human accomplishment triangle.

Neither the first nor second triangle (Figures 31.1 and 31.2) alone can accurately describe a support system because they never occur separately. The shapes must be "nested." The human accomplishment triangle is always larger than the functional ability triangle. (The only exception may be if one is very sick or very rich and can afford to have every support customized.) Both large and small triangles are dynamic, responding to changes in environment, individual circumstances, and participatory role.

Not just people with disabilities can be characterized in terms of these figures. The labels on the smaller triangle will vary for different people, depending on focused activities, role, and identification (e.g., a mountain climber has a specialized small triangle, with elements unique to her or his functional requirements in a hostile environment). The difference is that when a person has a disability, the disability usually takes precedence over any other label. For example, when the mountain climber has a disability, the focus is likely to be more on her disability than the mountain climbing, despite the fact that there are as likely to be as many support issues related to being a woman and a climber than specifically having a disability.

This embedding of specialized supports within generic supports, while often overlooked in traditional disability service systems as well as by the general public, is the rallying cry for many in the disability movement under the banner of universal design. Universal design changes the shape and possibly the size of the inner triangle. An individual may need the same amount of support overall, but it may come more cheaply, more easily, and with less stigma from the larger generic tools, cooperation, and strategies area that are universal to all. For example, people with visual or mobility impairments may get all the individualized service they need to match colors or find garments by using the assistance of personal shoppers in upscale department stores, a service useful to all.

A blending of specialized and universal can be seen in the policy changes in the U.S. education system from segregated special education to integrated and inclusive education for children with disabilities. Although after 25 years, compliance still lags behind legislation, even in the most exemplary programs, both disability-specific and broader supports are used to accomplish full inclusion (NCD 2000). Educators use a full spectrum of available supports, without making distinctions between them, and they are integrating special supports for children within the larger student context. Before the policy shift, educators only wanted to do the "normal" (big triangle), and they left the "special" (little embedded triangle) to the medical model. Now educators can no longer teach children in a different and segregated environment, even if the student requires "special" supports such as PAS and AT. Serendipitously, as these special accommodations are introduced into the general classroom, their utility for all children is being discovered. For example, technological, electronic curb cuts often function like sidewalk curb cuts and are equally useful to a range of people.

Universal design has and will continue to have an important influence on the lives of people with disabilities, especially as disabled people redesign the supports and boundaries, and it becomes more recognized that supports need to be addressed wherever possible within the larger human accomplishment triangle (see Figure 31.3).

When support systems for disabled people are described by professionals, the larger context of the human accomplishment triangle (see Figure 31.3) is sometimes forgotten or ignored. The focus turns primarily and sometimes solely on the more specialized elements of a support system (e.g., assistance to eat and use the bathroom at work, which is in fact only a small but essential aspect of a disabled person's total support system, including one's boss, supervisor, and coworkers). The words used to describe the aspects viewed as disability related can quickly degenerate into professional jargon (e.g., an *attendant*). Even when "politically correct" language (e.g., *personal assistant*) is used, the words still carry an aura of differentness and stigma.

Until people with disabilities forged a disability rights movement, some disabled people felt they had to forego disability-specific supports (i.e., not use the technology or personal assistance they needed if they wanted to operate effectively in an integrated setting). They did not want to draw attention to their disability. Understanding that we all use special and generic supports takes away some of the pressure to use supports that are as "normal" as possible—normal as externally defined—while still operating in an integrated environment. While individuals will want to maintain the same quantity of accomplishment, how they decide to design their own support system to facilitate that accomplishment has many more possibilities if both supports in the big triangle and the smaller embedded triangle are recognized and available. It may be possible for people to get assistance from a supervisor or a coworker through an informal arrangement, rather than from an outside provider.

One of the problems with focusing primarily on an individual's disability is that professionals can forget that everyone, including people with disabilities, lives in a larger generic support envelope. Too often, the focus gets restricted to the part related to the "special needs" relevant to disability. The bigger picture—the generic supports needed to exist in the community—either gets overlooked or taken for granted. Hence, contextual considerations—both the strengths and weaknesses of real life—are too often omitted from policy, planning, and practice in disability-related systems.

Isolated support systems for disabled people may produce de facto discrimination. Pushing all the supports into the disability-specific triangles results in solutions such as segregated housing only for the handicapped, sheltered workshops, and other separate, isolated, and inherently unequal supports. Supports for living within the bigger generic triangle will never be considered or developed if one does not recognize that the bigger triangle exists for disabled people too. Being able to describe how an element of a support system has to work dynamically in multiple environments, within a larger context, may help professionals, disabled people, their significant others, and the larger public not only to understand but also to aim for the balance and interaction needed in everyday life between all of these elements.

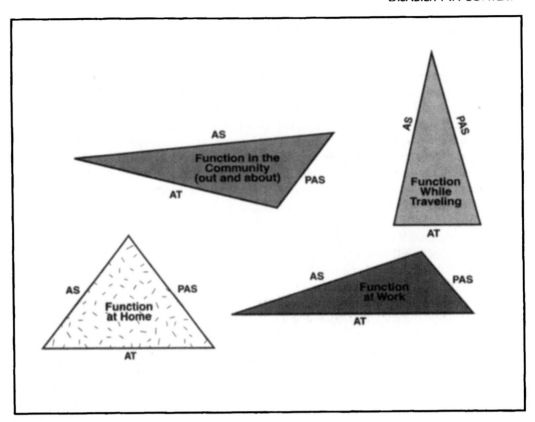

Figure 31.4. Support Systems Change

Dynamics of Support Systems

Support systems are dynamic because they vary depending on changing environmental (e.g., weather, terrain, built, physical and social) and situational demands (one's role), location (i.e., home, community, travel, work), strategies, and psychosocial orientation. Different circumstances call for different balances among elements of a personal support system (see Figure 31.4, "Support Systems Change)."

The four triangles pictured are differently shaped. The lengths of the sides are different because the quantity of the three types of support varies. Assistive technology, personal assistance services, and adaptive strategies vary—in this case, in different locations. When one travels, one may use far more PAS and AS because the situation changes all the time and requires lots of adaptation to unusual situations. But at work, one may use less PAS because one has more ability to maneuver using available technology and has worked out ways of accomplishing tasks that are fairly consistent. In the community, one may depend on AT and AS to maneuver from location to location but not require much PAS. Finally, at home, the functional ability triangle may be more equilateral because of the wide variety of tasks, roles, and situations one encounters.

Support systems are by their very nature dynamic. Different situations call for different balances among elements of a personal support system. Also, in each situation, the functional ability triangle is embedded in a larger human accomplishment triangle, which changes shapes as well in response to the individual's environment and participatory role.

Because environment and participatory role are dynamic contexts, motion is a better way to convey an individual's continuous dynamic interplay with the environment. Imagine a cartoon with a small anthropomorphic triangle: moving out the door of the house, changing shape to reflect the changing nature of the support system, and changing and morphing continuously throughout the day, as the environment, roles, activities, locations, and available supports shift.

It is easy to forget the continuously dynamic nature of supports, especially when policy and service delivery systems are focused primarily on a single environment (e.g., work or home) or a single role (e.g., student or employee). For example, professional services and policies may assist in developing and equipping an ideal environment at home, ignoring the fact that the person also needs to be able to go to the toilet at school or work and use the phone at the airport. While the computer at school may be appropriately accessible, the system at the neighborhood public library may not be.

Environmental demands require different sets of support elements. There is a strong correlation between the friendliness of both the micro and macro of the environment and the need for specialized support systems elements. The more hostile the environment becomes, the more individualized supports will be needed to venture out into it successfully. A climber at an indoor climbing wall at a health club requires very different technology, skills, and team members than a mountaineer attempting to summit Mount Everest. Both are climbers (role), and both are gaining elevation one step at a time (activity). However, Everest is far more hostile and much less forgiving than the protected environment in an urban gym. Climbing wall–specific tools and skills and companions, by themselves, will be inadequate preparation for a Himalayan climb. The parallels in disability might compare a person with a disability, learning skills, and the use of technology within a hospital environment with another individual with a mobility disability attempting to navigate a completely inaccessible city or living situation.

The more "friendliness" that can be built into the environment, the fewer specialized supports the person will need to carry along. While elevators are not likely to be installed on Everest, curb cuts on city streets and accessible buses reduce the "hostility" of the environment. Continuing to see the problem as being in the individual (the medical model), as opposed to seeing the environment or society as being disabling (the interactive or environmental model), leads to design priorities for building stair-climbing wheelchairs rather than building ramps and curb cuts.

Resource allocation decisions are frequently posed as this type of "either-or" alternative, rather than as complementary options. Operationalizing a set of options would allow choices in developing and maintaining individually appropriate support system. Either-or alternatives may appear to enable choices, but in reality they tend to offer untenable trade-offs (e.g., do you want to go to the bathroom at work or at home?).[2]

CONSUMER CONTROL IN CHOICE OF SUPPORTS

Independent living means self-determination. It means being in control of one's life, choosing one's own goals and activities, and ultimately defining one's own support system, including the tools, strategies, and people or animal supports necessary to accomplish any given task or objective in all the environments in which the support system is needed. (Collectivist cultures may frame this argument in language more consistent with their perspectives. However, the issue of having a voice is essential, whether the language used is independence or interdependence.)

The gap between professionals', families', and disabled persons' perceptions of the nature of supports is at the very heart of the independent living and consumer control debates. Unfortunately, the views of health and rehabilitation professionals also influence those of family members, people with disabilities, and society as a whole. Professionals are the gatekeepers who open the door to publicly funded supports, and they shape the views of those new to the world of disability and policymakers. Often, professionals do not understand, or they feel they have little ability to influence the interrelated nature of a support system, preferring to put their efforts into one or the other type of intervention. This is not so much a perceptual difference as a systems problem.

Likewise, the view of strategies is generally not as disparate between professionals and people with disabilities as is their view of tools and cooperation. Strategies are a combination of the ways we do things and the skills we acquire. Therapists are paid to teach strategies. All take it for granted that throughout life and situational changes, we will learn new skills and ways of doing things—whether through individual ingenuity from peer networks and family or from professionals. Yet the choice and flexible nature of strategies are the area of conflict.

Unfortunately, while most rehabilitationists and habilitationists understand that they are teaching individuals new strategies and different or adapted ways of doing things, some still feel that providing technology or encouraging use of personal assistance are options of last resort. In advanced industrial societies, health professionals fear that electric or motorized mobility technologies (power scooters) may result in less function due to disuse, thereby increasing dependence and restricting options. Yet, a person with a disability may prefer to have a powered scooter that can be driven to the gym where he or she can work out more effectively and maintain strength and flexibility with other health-conscious neighbors, rather than be exhausted from walking between locations, in an attempt to maintain mobility.

There is also a strong bias against using personal assistance services, as if they were some kind of last resort, "treatment failure," or low-level social welfare and family "problem" not requiring professional consideration or intervention. There is stigma attached to such assistance. In most societies, children and sick people need "help." Even disabled people resist using PAS. Yet PAS is an essential part of the support system for people with significant disabilities, particularly those who would otherwise be in institutions or incarcerated in their own homes.

Even after overcoming the above biases, professionals often decide the strategy for achieving a task and select the tools (technology) or the cooperation of others (PAS/service animals) with little regard for the disabled individual's unique circumstances. The independent living (IL) or self-determination position is that for disabled people to be able to function adequately in the world, the disabled individual, to the greatest extent possible, makes the choices regarding the preferred mix of strategies, tools, and cooperation.

The level of control and self-determination an individual achieves depends on a broad range of factors. The role of people with disabilities can vary from patient to consumer to inventor or manager in relationship to AT and PAS. However, the disabled individual determines the choice of roles in the IL paradigm. When he or her cannot be in full or partial control, his or her representative may be called on to make these choices or facilitate them being made according to the disabled individual's preferences.

Consumer control does not mean that there is no role for professionals in deciding the mix of supports needed. The role of professionals is to teach people to choose and use their tools and technology, manage the assistance received from a person or service animal, and foster problem-solving skills. In addition, the selection of appropriate services and devices is often enhanced by peer counseling from an individual who has a similar disability and has reached a higher level of independence—for example, learning to do a wheelie (balance on just the two rear wheels) or jump a curb in a wheelchair or simply sharing information about which equipment vendors are the most consumer responsive. Few publications have documented the expertise of experienced technology users. Beneficial Designs has recently developed a wheelchair training guide for manual wheelchair users, and a manual for powered wheelchair users is in progress (Axelson et al. 1998). Based on the experience of a wide range of wheelchair riders, these well-illustrated books can be used for "cross-training." Using these manuals, a wheelchair user can develop new skills. A therapist can use the same material to train new users. Increasingly, professionals, as well as peers, are teaching people to decide, advocate for themselves, make choices, and expand their options.

Criteria for Making Choices

Many factors influence the amount and types of tools or cooperation a disabled person might use. It is difficult to generalize about when technology, PAS, or a service animal is a better choice. The following is a list of criteria that individuals may consider in making decisions about their support needs. Due to a lack of research in this area, our list is not exhaustive and is not meant to imply any type of hierarchy.

1. Cost of the support and ability of the individual or family to pay (countries that publicly fund PAS, AT or service animals, and skills training make the acquisition of supports by all sectors of the disabled population more possible).
2. Time required to use one type of support versus another.
3. Availability of the support in one's society and area (this is influenced by labor shortages or gluts and the level of technological sophistication and economic development).
4. The degree of privacy and confidentiality versus companionship that a particular type of support affords.
5. Out-of-pocket cost of managing the support, including personnel, training, supervision and quality control issues, upkeep of equipment, maintenance of animals, and amount of training required to use the support well.
6. Physical and mental ease of use.
7. Visibility, intrusiveness, and degree of stigma attached to the support.

The choices are affected by many factors. *Culture* plays a role. There is a power dynamic involved in the choice of whether to use a PA. In the United States, being separate from one's family is admired. In other cultures, the individual would not even consider putting his or her individual needs above that of the family group.

Individual differences are a factor. There are people who would have difficulty training a PA. Some people prefer human contact, others enjoy using equipment and gadgets, and others dislike animals.

Age biases influence decisions as well. It is culturally expected that old people and children get hands-on care. So, powered wheelchairs, for example, may be seen as unnecessary for them, especially when there may be someone to push them in a manual wheelchair. Likewise, there are culturally motivated assumptions about the level of control young people and seniors want and can exercise over their services (Shaw forthcoming).

Temporal differences between technology and PAS also come into play. Certain things can be done quickly by a human being, but in the long run, using a service animal or inanimate technology may be more economical. The reverse is also true. The balance between short-term and long-term use of resources is decidedly a factor to consider.

Functional ability of the individual throughout the day and over days, months, and years affects support choices because PAS and technology and the trade-off between them have to adapt to changes in the individual's ability.

The cost of labor, which varies by country, is a factor. In a less-developed country, PAS are more readily available because unskilled labor is plentiful and not very costly. On the other hand, locally produced technology can also be less costly because wages are very low and local materials are less expensive.

Finally, as has been discussed at length, individuals may make different choices for different activities, in different situations and environments, or when they are filling different roles.

A good example of one of these trade-offs is the communication choices afforded to people who have speech impairments as a result of cerebral palsy: a PA/translator, an alphabet board, an augmented communication device, or their own voice. These choices involve low- and high-tech solutions as well as using a person as an alternative to or augmentation of technology. Though many people use voice synthesizers, others find them time-consuming and socially bizarre in particular situations. Can you imagine a room full of people communicating in the same voice? Imagine using an electronic communication aid in the shower or while making love? Others prefer the intimate contact and ease involved in using an alphabet board or a PA. For others, these supports are too slow. Still others prefer using their own voice, but this often requires the listener to master the speaker's personal speech patterns, which can be very energy intensive. Under these circumstances, who is the support system for—for other people or for the person with the speech impairment? Obviously, people with communication disabilities face a myriad of choices.

CONCLUSION

The issues of personal assistance services and assistive technology incorporate the much larger questions of power, resource distribution, stereotypes, barriers to employment, cross-cultural issues, and universal design. They call into question the sociology of impairment and the definition of disability, independence, accommodation, and technology.

Resource allocation, policy decisions, and bottom-line financing drive the nature of available supports that enable people with disabilities to live self-determined lives in the community. Because of scarce resources, as technology use increases, the tension between PAS and AT is likely to increase. Kate Seelman (1993) succinctly describes the emerging tension: "[In the United States] some members of the disability community perceive assistive technology as threatening their lobbying efforts on behalf of funding for Personal Assistance Services. Therefore, research is needed to determine the relationship between assistive technology and personal assistance" (p. 129).

As funding mechanisms for personal assistance services, assistive technology, and other supports are being developed and prioritized in policy and practice, clearer understanding is needed on how these supports can be blended so they act as complementary enhancers of functional ability. Before we debate how many resources should be allocated to each category, more clarity is needed on how supports can and should work together and then how they can be linked in policy, practice, and payment.

Recognition of the relationship between facets of a support system allows us to objectively discuss mutually effective systems change strategies that help an individual with a disability develop a support system that is effective in multiple environments (not just at home but at school, at work, in the community, and while traveling) while enabling the individual to pursue personal goals in life.

Several policy issues and questions beg for basic and applied research, theoretical clarity, and solutions to resolve the issue.

To begin with, cultural, behavioral, and sociopolitical forces shape the very foundations of an individual's support system. Research is needed on what supports people expect, how they determine the adequacy and appropriateness of the supports they have, how and when they recognize the need for support system change, and where they believe the change should occur (e.g., should there be curb cuts or curb-climbing wheelchairs?). This research needs to be done cross-culturally and cross-disability and age. For example, the development of technology to aid people with cognitive disabilities is a very new concept.

Another basic issue is the need for more clarity on the nature and interplay of supports. This has ramifications for research and for policy. To develop policy, we need to know how many people use assistive devices or technologies, how many use PAS, and how many use both. How does use in one country compare with another, and do these differences across nations affect outcomes? For example, in the United States, 29 to 38 percent of people with disabilities use PAS.[3] Approximately 32 to 45 percent of people with disabilities use assistive technology. Are there similar percentages in other countries? In the United States, only 20 percent of the people needing PAS receive some or all of it from public sources. Public and private third-party sources have offered complete or partial payment for 52 percent of users' assistive technology devices and for 23 percent of users' home adaptations. How does this differ in countries with national health plans and in less-developed countries? We need to look at the differences in the use of PAS and AT technology from country to country, in relationship to independent living and quality-of-life outcomes against the backdrop of the environmental factors in these countries.

Support systems are the interface between a person and the environment. We need careful theory building on what constitutes the elements of environment and how they can be differentiated. We also need to understand how they work together. Does the notion of a micro and macro environment help in our understanding? We need clear concepts and models to do research.

There is no agreed-on set of indicators that ties together the conceptual shifts in disability theory with the actual day-to-day impacts that are recognizable on an individual level. Unless there is tangible improvement in the daily life situation of individuals with disability, the framing concepts and social constructs remain academic. Developing measurements and indicators, which appropriately relate activities such as enhanced participation, functioning, and choice, to real-world observable events will almost by necessity need to be made in the arena of support system dynamics. However, currently available indices are linear and do not adequately represent the complexity of person-environment interaction. For example, many fall back on old notions of independence and assume that if one uses PAS, then one is dependent and therefore less independent than one who uses technology. Using both implies less independence than using neither. Schema such as these are not much more than thinly veiled measures of resource utilization, no matter how many politically correct words such as *independence* and *functional* are in their names.

Not only do measures of supports need greater refinement, but they also need to be viewed within the context of the environment. In addition, the questions and scales need to be developed within a strong participatory action research framework. Cultural considerations and variances need to be included to make the instruments more universal because concepts related to cultural heritage and social environment are extremely complex across nations and within nations (NCD 1999; Saxton et al. 1997).

The lack of availability of PAS and AT is a serious issue. There are not infinite resources available for these supports. Who should get these publicly funded supports? Should we provide a little bit to everyone, those with the most significant disabilities, those who can work successfully, or only people who are poor? The growing mobilization of people with disabilities to push for needed support to become integral parts of their societies will surely have an impact on these resource allocation questions. Possible solutions include reframing the social contract in each society so that PAS and technology are seen as civil or human rights, more equally spreading wealth and increasing the standard of living, and increasing equality of opportunity. These questions will have different answers in societies whose goal is equality of opportunity versus societies who believe in equality of outcome. Do we level the playing field, or do we make sure everyone can play?

We need research to help us provide supports efficiently. PAS and AT are integral parts of any effective support system. Yet, people may be forced to use equipment because that is the only reimbursable service available, or they are denied equipment and forced to use only PAS because equipment and environmental modifications or the right equipment and modifications are not a covered service. In many countries, people do not receive enough supports to allow them to function effectively. Policy research is needed to determine how these inefficiencies affect people's abilities to achieve their full potential and what their ultimate cost is to society in terms of money and values.

Governments are concerned about being able to hold recipients accountable for using supports efficiently and effectively. How do we decide what types of PA, AT, and skill training deserve public support? Where does the role of PA end and that of butler, maid, and secretary begin? What is the line between service animals and pets? When people with a psychiatric disability request an animal companion to calm them down in stressful situations, are they asking for a pet or a service animal? There needs to be much more theoretical clarification on the distinction between supports everyone uses and supports that are necessary to enhance the function of disabled people. How can we expand the definition of supports to include low- and high-tech (i.e., anything that works)? Does the inability of most delivery systems to do that now interfere with people's level of accomplishment?

The nature and availability of supports are changing rapidly at this time. Now that people with disabilities are participating more in deciding their own fates, new forms of PAS, assistive technology, and strategies for employing them will continue to appear. We have also begun to see the expanding role of service animals. As these developments occur, on an individual and collective level, delivery systems need to develop policies that enable constant reevaluation of the mix of supports that people need in light of new developments. Also, as people with disabilities become more and more crucial to choosing individually effective supports, disability policy must ensure that people with disabilities are part of the decision-making process and team.

The nature, remuneration, and training of PAs for people with intellectual and psychiatric disabilities, as well as for people who are deaf, need debate and policy development. Skills required for facilitators at meetings and in the learning situation in schools (not for personal care) remain uncharted. What is the distinction between training and PAS for people with intellectual disabilities? There is just beginning to be interest in the use of PAS by people with psychiatric disabilities (Stewart 1992; Vivona et al. 2000). Research needs to be done on ways to foster consumer control and direction in the home and community situation rather than remaking the home into an institution by using forced treatment. For example, the utility of advanced directives when an individual is in crisis needs exploration. Do advanced directives enable the personal assistant to know the disabled individual's preferences in such a situation? Does the person want to take drugs or be hospitalized? Are there other options that the consumer would like to try first? Do advanced directives shorten the crisis period as compared to other approaches to crisis management? PAS and AT at work raise cost and efficiency issues that continue to need attention. When support systems are an integral and well-functioning part of life, they are transparent. Support systems for individuals with disabilities have not universally reached that stage of transparency. Until people with disabilities forged a disability rights movement, some disabled people felt they had to forego disability-specific supports (i.e., not use the technology or personal assistance they needed if they wanted to be accepted in an integrated setting). It is hoped that as countries adopt disability rights legislation, this dilemma will disappear. However, if PAS and technology are transparent in the workplace, how does that differ from job sharing or role duplication (Litvak 1996)? Is a particular support a reasonable accommodation for one person that must be granted immediately, or is it a support that everyone in the workplace needs and therefore must wait for organization-wide distribution? These questions are currently being decided in the courts.

Of major concern to people with disabilities in the more developed countries is growing scarcity of people who want to work as personal assistants. Some projects are experimenting with a variety of new sources for PAs, including conscientious objectors in Germany and people with developmental disabilities and welfare recipients in various parts of the United States. A comparative study of the results of these efforts would be very useful.

The distinctions between AT and PAS will likely become more blurred in the future. We have already discussed the use of animals as assistants. They are not mechanical, and they can think, reason, and respond in a limited fashion. The development of smart technology with personality that learns and evolves and has greater dexterity and maneuverability starts to blur the distinctions between technological and animal and human assistants. As robotics become more sophisticated, will they be able to perform increasingly more complex tasks, such as bed making or child bathing? Is R2D2 soon to be a reality? If so, will that be a solution to the lack of PAS providers?

Finally, it appears that there is more to achieving independent living and self-determination than having available PAS and AT. For example, in the state of Massachusetts and in Sweden, there are no penalties for working built into their system. In Massachusetts, disabled people who work are able to buy health and PAS coverage from the Massachusetts Medicaid program at a very reasonable cost on a sliding scale basis. Sweden has universal health coverage and provides PAS. Both places provide technology. So, even though AT and PAS are available in Massachusetts and Sweden, people with disabilities are not working in these areas in significant numbers. In Massachusetts, only 30 percent of people with disabilities ages 18 to 65 are employed. We continue to manipulate the various supports in the system, but we need a much better understanding of the interaction between the elements and the whole.

Without an agreed-on concept of the nature of support systems, the role and interplay of their components, and the different views of that relationship existing between people with disabilities, rehabilitation and medical professionals, and policymakers, advocacy efforts for different kinds of supports may work at cross purposes. Advocates and policymakers will argue against each other and squander limited systems change resources on infighting and divisive competition. Recognition of common goals, development of common strategies, presentation of shared objectives, and insistence on integrated outcome measures are needed to develop a unified agenda for individualized or integrated support system development.

NOTES

1. Agreement of the nature of personal support systems could be an indicator that concurring individuals share a common culture. The discrepancy between how a disabled person views a support system and how a professional in the same society views it could itself be a strong indicator that there is indeed a distinct disability culture.

2. Judy Heumann once suggested that if toilets on airplanes could not be made accessible, then they should be removed, so all passengers would face the same inability to use the toilet on a five-hour flight (personal communication, March 1995)!

3. These figures are based on using the SIPP figure for 54 million disabled (McNeil 1997) and the NHIS figure of 38 million with activity limitations (LaPlante and Carlson 1996). The number of PAS users is 14.5 million according to Kennedy and LaPlante (1997), and the number of technology users is 17 million, according to the National Center for Health Statistics (1994).

REFERENCES

Agree, Emily M. 1999. "The Influence of Personal Care and Assistive Devices on the Measurement of Disability." *Social Science & Medicine* 48:427-43.

Axelson, P., D. Y. Chesney, J. Minkel, and A. Perr. 1998. *Manual Wheelchair Training Guide.* (Available from Beneficial Designs, P.O. Box 8317, Santa Cruz, CA 95060-8317)

Beatty, P. W., G. W. Richmond, S. Tepper, and G. DeJong. 1998. "Personal Assistance for People with Physical Disabilities: Consumer-Direction and Satisfaction with Services." *Archives of Physical Medicine and Rehabilitation* 79 (6): 674-77.

Benjamin, A. and R. E. Matthias. 1998. "Who's in Charge? Who Gets Paid? A Study of Models for Organizing Supportive Services at Home." Unpublished manuscript, UCLA, Department of Social Welfare, Los Angeles.

Benjamin, A., R. E. Matthias, and T. M. Franke. 2000. "Comparing Consumer-Directed and Agency Models for Providing Supportive Services at Home." *Health Services Research* 35 (1, Pt. 2): 351-66.

Blascovish, Allen K. 1996. "The Value of Service Dogs for People with Severe Ambulatory Disabilities: A Randomized Controlled Trial." *Journal of the American Medical Association* 275 (3): 1001-6.

Cameron, K. and J. Firman. 1995. *International and Domestic Programs Using Cash and Counseling Strategies to Pay for Long-Term Care.* Washington, DC: National Council on the Aging.

Connell, B. R., M. Jones, R. Mace, J. Mueller, A. Mullick, E. Ostroff, J. Sanford, E. Steinfeld, M. Story, and G. Vanderheiden. 1997. *The Principles of Universal Design.* Raleigh: Center for Universal Design, North Carolina State University.

Degener, T. 1992. *Personal Assistant Service Programs in Germany, Sweden and the USA: Differences and Similarities.* Oakland, CA: World Institute on Disability, and Rehabilitation International.

DeGraff, A. 1988. *Home Health Aides: How to Manage the People Who Help You.* Fort Collins, CO: Saratoga Access.

Doty, P., J. Kasper, and S. Litvak. 1996. "Consumer-Directed Models of Personal Care: Lessons from Medicaid." *The Milbank Quarterly* 74 (3): 377-409.

Egley, L. 1994. "The Cost of Program Models Providing Personal Assistance Services." Unpublished manuscript, World Institute on Disability, Rehabilitation Research and Training Center on Personal Assistance Services, Oakland, CA.

Enders, Alexandra. 1995. "Personal Assistance Services and Assistive Technology: Allies or Adversaries." Pp. 584-86 in *1995 RESNA Proceedings.* Arlington, VA: RESNA.

———. 1997. "Universal Design: Implications for Service Delivery." Handout for special session at the 1997 RESNA conference.

Enders, Alexandra and J. Heumann. 1988. "How Adults with Disabilities Get the Everyday Technology They Need." Paper presented at ICAART 88, the 1988 RESNA Conference, June, Montreal, Canada.

Enders, A. and P. Leech. 1996. "Low-Technology Aids for Daily Living and Do-It-Yourself (DIY) Devices." Pp. 27-60 in *Evaluating, Selecting, and Using Appropriate Assistive Technology,* edited by Jan C. Glavin and Marcia J. Scherer. Rockville, MD: Aspen.

Eustis, N. N. and L. R. Fischer. 1992. "Common Needs, Different Solutions? Younger and Older Homecare Clients." *Generations* 16 (1): 17-22.

Flanagan, S. 1994. *Consumer-Directed Attendant Services: How States Address Tax, Legal and Quality Assurance Issues.* Cambridge, UK: Systemetrics.

Glendinning, Caroline. 1991. "Losing Ground: Social Policy and Disabled People in Great Britain, 1980-90." *Disability, Handicap & Society* 6 (1): 3-20.

Gray, David, Louis Quatrano, and Morton Lieberman. 1998. *Designing and Using Assistive Technology.* Baltimore: Brookes.

Hahn, H. 1984. "Reconceptualizing Disability: A Political Science Perspective." *Rehabilitation Literature* 48:362-65.

Hamilton, W. L. 1999. "Week in Review Desk, the Nation: Stealth Design; You're Not Getting Older: Products Are Getting Better." *New York Times,* June 27.

Jayasooria, D., B. Krishnan, and G. Ooi. 1997. "Disabled People in a Newly Industrialized Economy: Opportunities and Challenges in Malaysia." *Disability and Society* 12 (3): 455-65.

Kaiya, Y. 1998. "Independent Living as a Superior Policy towards People with Severe Disabilities—Case in Tokyo." Unpublished manuscript.

Kennedy, J. and M. P. LaPlante. 1997. *A Profile of Adults Needing Assistance with Activities of Daily Living, 1991-1992.* Washington, DC: National Institute on Disability and Rehabilitation Research.

Kimmick, M. and T. Godfrey. 1991. *New Models for the Provision of Personal Assistance Services: Final Report.* Bethesda, MD: Human Services Research Institute.

LaPlante, M. P. and D. Carlson. 1996. *Disability in the United States: Prevalence and Causes.* Washington, DC: National Institute on Disability and Rehabilitation Research.

L.C. vs. Olmstead, No. 98-536 (11th Cir. June 22, 1999).

Litvak, S. 1996. "Personal Assistance Services and Public Policy: Issues and Options in the Post ADA World." Pp. 365-87 in *Implementing the Americans with Disabilities Act,* edited by Jane West. Oxford, UK: Blackwell.

———. 1998. *American Rehabilitation.* Washington, DC: Rehabilitation Services Administration.

Litvak, S., J. Heumann, and H. Zukas. 1987. *Attending to America.* Oakland, CA: World Institute on Disability.

Litvak, S. and J. Kennedy. 1991. *Policy Issues Affecting the Medicaid Personal Care Services Optional Benefits.* Oakland, CA: World Institute on Disability.

Longino, C. 1994. "Myths of an Aging America." *American Demographics,* August, 36-43.

Manton, K., L. Corde, and E. Stallard. 1993. "Changes in the Use of Personal Assistance and Special Equipment from 1982 to 1989: Results from the 1982 and 1989 NLTCS." *The Gerontologist* 33 (22): 168-76.

McNeil, J. M. 1997. *Americans with Disabilities, 1994-95: Household Economic Studies Current Population Reports P70-61.* Washington, DC: U.S. Bureau of the Census.

National Center for Health Statistics. 1994. *Trends and Differential Use of Assistive Technology Devices.* Hyattsville, MD: Author.

National Council on Aging. 1996. *Principles of Consumer-Directed Home and Community-Based Services.* Washington, DC: Author.

National Council on Disability (NCD). 1999. *Lift Every Voice: Modernizing Disability Policies and Programs to Serve a Diverse Nation.* Washington, DC: Author.

———. 2000. *Back to School on Civil Rights: Advancing the Federal Commitment to Leave No Child Behind.* Washington, DC: Author.

Nosek, M., M. Fuhrer, and C. Potter. 1995. "Life Satisfaction of People with Physical Disabilities: Relationship to Personal Assistance, Disability Status, and Handicap." *Rehabilitation Psychology* 40 (3): 191-202.

Ratzka, A. D. 1986. *Independent Living and Attendant Care in Sweden: A Consumer Perspective.* New York: World Rehabilitation Fund.

———. 1993. "The User Cooperative Model in Personal Assistance: The Example of STIL, the Stockholm Cooperative of Independent Living." Pp. 36-43 in *Personal Assistance Services in Europe and North America: Report of an International Symposium,* edited by Barbara Duncan and Susan T. Brown. New York: Rehabilitation International.

Reiff, L., R. Zawadski, and J. Hyde. 1996. *Bold Action for a Challenging Problem: Immediate Steps and Long-Term Solutions for Improving Services for Impaired Adults, Los Angeles County.* Los Angeles: Los Angeles In-Home Supportive Services Study.

Richmond, G., P. Beatty, S. Tepper, and G. DeJong. 1998. "The Effect of Consumer-Directed Personal Assistance Services on the Productivity Outcomes of People with Disabilities." *Journal of Rehabilitation Outcomes Measurement* 1 (4): 48-51.

Sabatino, C. P. and S. Litvak. 1996. "Liability Issues Affecting Consumer-Directed Personal Assistance Services: Report and Recommendations." *Elder Law Journal* 4 (2): 251-368.

Saxton, M., L. Yasumoto, K. Eckels, D. Katsnitz, M. Guillermo, and J. Mullins. 1997. "Cultural Diversity and Personal Assistance Services: Is the Independent Living Model Best Suited for All People with Disabilities?" Unpublished manuscript, World Institute on Disability, Rehabilitation Research and Training Center on Personal Assistance Services.

Seelman, K. 1993. "Assistive Technology Policy: A Road to Independence for Individuals with Disabilities." *Journal of Social Issues* 49 (2): 115-36.

Shaw, M. Forthcoming. "PAS and Youth and Transition." In *Semiotics of Disability,* edited by Linda Rogers and Beth Blue Swadener. New York: SUNY.

Simon-Rusinowitz, L., A. Bochniak, K. Mahoney, and D. Hecht. 1999. *Implementation Issues for Consumer-Directed Programs: Views from Policy Experts.* College Park: Center on Aging, University of Maryland.

Stewart, L. 1992. "PAS for People with Psychiatric Disabilities." Pp. 67-71 in *Personal Perspectives on Personal Assistance Services,* edited by J. Weissman, J. Kennedy, and S. Litvak. Oakland, CA: World Institute on Disability.

U.S. Department of Education, Office of Special Education and Rehabilitative Services, National Institute on Disability and Rehabilitation Research. 2000. *Long Range Plan 1999-2003, Executive Summary.* Washington, DC: Author.

Verbrugge, L. M. and A. M. Jette. 1994. "The Disablement Process." *Social Science Medicine* 38 (1): 1-14.

Vivona, V., J. Dresen, and S. Litvak. 2000. *Exemplary Consumer Directed Personal Assistance Services (PAS) Programs for People with Physical and/or Cognitive Disabilities.* Oakland, CA: World Institute on Disability.

Waddinton, Lisa. 1997. "The European Community and Disability Discrimination: Time to Address the Deficit?" *Disability & Society* 12 (3): 455-80.

Wagner, D., P. Nadesh, and C. Sabatino. 1997. *Autonomy or Abandonment: Changing Perspectives on Delegation.* Washington, DC: National Council on Aging.

Weiner, J. M. and A. E. Cuellar. 1999. "Public and Private Responsibilities: Home- and Community-Based Services in the United Kingdom and Germany." *Journal of Aging and Health* 11 (3): 417-44.

Werner, D. 1998. *Nothing about Us: Developing Innovative Technologies for, by and with Disabled Persons.* Palo Alto, CA: HealthWrights.

World Institute on Disability (WID). 1999. Unpublished data from the third wave of data on PAS programs in the United States.

WID International Conference. 1999. *Global Perspectives on Independent Living for the Next Millennium: The International Summit Conference on Independent Living* [Online]. Available: www.ilru.org/summit/index.htm.

Zarb, G. and P. Nadesh. 1994. *Cashing in on Independence: Comparing the Costs and Benefits of Cash and Services for Meeting Disabled Peoples' Support Needs.* Derbyshire: British Council of Organizations of Disabled People.

The Relationship between Disabled People and Health and Welfare Professionals

32

SALLY FRENCH

JOHN SWAIN

This chapter examines the development of the relationship between disabled people and professionals in the second half of the twentieth century from the perspectives of both professional and disabled people, concentrating primarily on the latter. The growth of the ideologies and organization of professionals are crucial to the social and historical context in which disability has been constructed in Western societies. We will trace the development of power structures and relations within the medical and social professions and the production of disability through institutional discrimination. Central to this analysis are the role of professionalization and the discourses of needs and assessment in the enforced dependency of disabled people and the pervasive ideology of normality. This provides the basis for a critical analysis of the development of professional models of professional expertise, professional-client partnerships, and consumer-led services.

We also examine the development of professional-disabled people relations from the viewpoint of disabled people. In particular, we will discuss the growth of the disabled people's movement and the establishment of the social model of disability in the reconstruction of power relations and structures in professional-disabled people relations. The emergence and redefinition of disability as a human and civil rights issue have underpinned fundamental challenges to professional ideologies and models. Particularly significant are the establishment of centers for independent living and the provision of services for disabled people by disabled people. The increasing popularity of "direct payment" for disabled people, which enables them to buy and organize their own care, will also be discussed.

All such analyses are necessarily circumscribed, and we develop a particular focus in a number of ways. First, we take orientation toward defining disability as a form of oppression and institutionalized discrimination. The social model of disability has historical roots in political action and struggles by disabled people in America (Zola 1994), Britain, and elsewhere (Barnes, Mercer, and Shakespeare 1999). Second, we concentrate on specific examples of the emergence and manifestations of disabled people's relations with professionals in Britain. In doing so, we recognize that there are clear differences between countries, for instance, in terms of the general policy context of such relations. Drake (1999) suggests that it is possible to recognize different models of policy, including the laissez-faire (or minimalist) model, the maximal welfare approach, a hybrid welfare–civil rights approach, the rights-based policy model exemplified by the United States, and the piecemeal approach in Britain. We would argue, however, that the general issue generated by unequal power relations between disabled people and professionals is relevant notwithstanding policy differences.

Third, the analysis is informed by qualitative research, particularly studies of the views and experiences of disabled people. Throughout the chapter, we illustrate the discussion by drawing on a number of qualitative research projects we have conducted. These include a case study of institutional discrimination in professional services, a case study of services provided by disabled people themselves, and a study of the views and experiences of disabled professionals. Such evidence seeks to illuminate and illustrate issues, particularly from the viewpoint and experiences of participants.

This analysis of professional-disabled people relations then examines the social and historical struggles in the construction of disability and the control of professional services. The aim of this chapter is to examine the relationship as constructed in the dialectic between professionals and disabled people. Critical questions can no longer focus on professionals, their skills, expertise, and interventions for "cure or care." The possibilities for moving forward are generated within changing power structures and relations between disabled people and professionals.

THE DEVELOPMENT OF PROFESSIONAL POWER

The relationship between disabled people and health and welfare professionals has never been an easy one, and an analysis of the relationship needs to take into account a broad and complex context. The relationship cannot be understood without reference to the social and historical development of professions; the structural elements, particularly the hierarchical nature of professions; the relationship between the state, professionals, and disabled people; the relationship between different professional groups; and the ideologies and discourses that underpin professionalism and professional-disabled people relations. The picture becomes more complex if an account is given to differences in the development, structures, and ideologies of different professions (such as those between physiotherapists and social workers) and differences among groups of disabled people, including disabled people from ethnic minority communities.

Notwithstanding the complexity of this context, notions of power have underpinned analyses of professional-disabled people relations and their social and historical context. Though he largely omits disability from his analysis, concentrating rather on sexism and racism, Hugman (1991) states, "Social power is an integral aspect of the daily working lives of professionals. The centrality of power in professional work has been increasingly recognized" (p. 1). Focusing specifically on disability, French (1994a) takes hierarchical power relations as her starting point:

> It is an unequal relationship with the professionals holding most of the power. Traditionally professional workers have defined, planned and delivered the services, while disabled people have been passive recipients with little if any opportunity to exercise control. (P. 103)

As Thompson (1998) argues, then, "an understanding of the workings of power is an essential part of challenging inequality, discrimination and oppression" (p. 43). He suggests that in relations between professionals and disabled people, power manifests itself in a number of ways, including control over the allocation of resources; the legitimization of knowledge, expertise, and skills; and statutory powers.

In this section, we outline possible elements in this unequal relationship and trace these within the history of health and welfare provisions for disabled people. In general terms, three associated elements of professional power can be analyzed within professional-disabled people relations, each justified and constructed within ideologies of professionalism (Harrison and Pollitt 1994). The first concerns the power of individual professionals to assess disabled people, define their problems and needs, specify solutions in terms of interventions, and evaluate the effectiveness of solutions. In McKnight's (1981) analysis of professional services, he states that

> we see the professions developing internal logistics and public marketing systems that assure use of tools and techniques by assuming that the client doesn't understand what he needs. Therefore, if the client is to have the benefit of the professional remedy, he must also understand that the professional not only knows what he needs but also how the need is to be met. (P. 83)

Professional dominance can be seen in assessment procedures where, for example, the therapist's or nurse's observations may be viewed as objective, whereas the patient's perceptions are viewed as subjective (Coates and King 1982), and where pseudo-scientific language serves to mystify and confuse service users (French 1993; Grieve 1988). Because of the specialization of the various professional groups, definitions of *need* tend to be narrow, their scope being dictated by specialized knowledge and interests (Ellis 1993). The needs of disabled people, on the other hand, tend to be multifaceted. As Marsh and Fisher (1992) point out,

> If the process of assessment becomes one of professional discovery of "need," rather than a negotiation of problems, then users tend to feel hemmed in by the definitions used to describe their circumstances and trapped by the choices they are faced with. (P. 50)

The second aspect of power involves professionals as powerful groups within society, essentially in pursuit of self-interest, with the mystification, defining, and control of expertise. This is seen in the establishment of occupations as professions controlling, quintessentially, the qualifications and credentials that define who is and who is not a nurse, physiotherapist, or other professional. As Hugman (1991) points out, this also serves as a "basis for defining the boundaries of the profession with other professions, and it provides the foundations for power exercised by the professionals in relation to the users of their services" (p. 83). Davis (1993a), a disabled writer and activist, traces professional self-interest to its most basic roots:

> It is a well-established form of parasitism, resting on bits of biblical dogma such as "the poor always ye have with you" (John, xii. 8). The updated version of the old Poor Law, which sustains most of today's welfare professionals, depends for its continuity on such counsels of despair. It has become, let's face it, a nice little earner. (P. 199)

The third aspect of professional power is seen in the agents or representatives of the state or, as in some models (Illich 1976), the economic and political elite. Of particular importance to professional-disabled people relations is the maintenance of the status quo by pathologizing and individualizing problems that have been socially and economically created. Oliver and Sapey (1999) developed a model of the relations between the state, professionals, and disabled people with particular reference to social work, although it can be generalized to all health and welfare professions. In this model, professions stand between the state and disabled people, acting as agents of the state, particularly as arbiters of need. Needs are defined within an individualized (medical, tragic) model that asserts the expertise and professionalism of the professions (Wilding 1982).

The growth of professional power in relation to disabled people, in each of the three aspects, has been traced by a number of writers to the changing nature of work and the associated mass segregation of disabled people in industrial nations in the nineteenth century (Finkelstein 1991; French 1994a; Oliver 1990; Ryan and Thomas 1987). The segregation of disabled people into specific institutions was influenced by the growing medical profession, which tended to view disabled people in terms of their individual impairments. As Barnes et al. (1999) state, "Most recent sociological writing now explains medicine's rise to dominance as a historically specific process which involved a power conflict with other interested groups. Crucially, state patronage established orthodox medicine in a dominant position" (p. 56). Segregation and institutionalization created dependency of disabled people and facilitated the development of the medical profession and a whole range of new professions, most of which were dominated by medicine. The domination of the medical profession in professional-disabled people relations contributed to the segregation of and discrimination against disabled people and produced arguments, usually biological in nature, to justify the exclusion of disabled people from mainstream social and economic life. This growth of professional power, particularly of the medical profession, in the lives of disabled people led to the medicalization of many areas of disabled people's lives. Doctors became involved in decisions and assessment procedures that had little to do with medicine, such as housing, education, and employment.

Perhaps the most intrusive, violating, and invalidating experiences for disabled people emanate from the policies, practices, and interventions that are justified and rationalized by a personal tragedy view of disability and impairment. The tragedy is to be avoided, eradicated, or nondisabled "normalized" by all possible means. Such negative presumptions about impairment and disability are so common that the abortion of impaired fetuses is barely challenged. There is considerable and growing pressure on women to undergo prenatal screening and to terminate pregnancies in which impairment has been detected. The use of genetic technology in its different forms in so-called preventative measures is, for many disabled people, an expression of the essence of the personal tragedy model. The erroneous idea that disabled people cannot be happy or enjoy an adequate quality of life lies at the heart of this response. The disabled person's problems are perceived to result from impairment rather than the failure of society to meet that person's needs in terms of appropriate human help and accessibility. There is an assumption that disabled people want to be "normal." However, disabled people who know themselves that disability is a major part of their identity rarely voice this. Disabled people are subjected to many disabling expectations, for example, to be "independent" and "normal," as well as to "adjust" and "accept" their situation. It is these expectations that are disabling, rather than the impairment itself (Swain and French 2000).

Any brief summary of professional power in relation to disabled people needs to recognize the complexity and often contradictory nature of professional-disabled people relationships. The medicalization of disability has produced some positive effects, including increased survival rates and increased life expectancy for some disabled people. For instance, one of the authors of this chapter has insulin-dependent diabetes and would not have survived without medical intervention. Furthermore, as French (1994b) suggests, most people would agree that it is sensible to strengthen muscles, move joints, and assist a person's balance following a spinal cord injury. Nevertheless, the medical profession has taken undue credit for the reduction of both disease and impairment. McKeown (1979) and Sagan (1987) provide a great deal of evidence to show that economic and social development improved housing and diet, and purification of water and the efficient disposal of sewage were far more important than medicine in reducing the incidence of infectious diseases such as poliomyelitis. It is still the case today that most disease and impairment can be found among those with limited material resources (Benzeval, Judge, and Whitehead 1995), and most "accidents" also occur within this group (Jacobson, Smith, and Whitehead 1991). Furthermore, professional power has played a crucial role in the maintenance and justification of the individual tragedy model of disability and the enforced dependency of disabled people. Oliver (1993) argues that there are a number of ways in which dependency is created through the delivery of professional services:

> The kinds of services that are available—notably residential and day care facilities with their institutionalized regimes, their failure to involve disabled people meaningfully in the running of such facilities, the transportation of users in specialized transport and the rigidity of the routine activities which take place therein—all serve to institutionalize disabled people and create dependency. (P. 54)

This notion of enforced dependency is a recurring theme in the accounts of disabled people's experiences with health and welfare services. Slack (1999) writes,

> The creation of dependency . . . has little to do with choice and much to do with how structures are organized. Disabled people variously become "clients," "patients" or "service users." They are then filed on computer (permission for this practice is rarely sought), and they "belong" to that department. (P. 34)

Specifically, in terms of professional-disabled people relationships, Oliver argues that the creation of dependency is two-way. Professionals are also dependent on disabled people for their jobs, salaries, status, quality of life, and so on. Furthermore, the construction of disability within the medical model has been contingent on the expanding production of medical and rehabilitative services. "The social meanings given to impairment and disability shape public and institutional responses to these conditions and lay the foundation for the construction of a rehabilitation industry" (Albrecht 1992:67). The power of professionals in controlling language, knowledge, and the social response to disability has defined professional-disabled people relations. It has also contributed to the dominant individual definition of disability, defined the identity of disabled people as service users, and, as discussed below, dominated the daily lives and experiences of many disabled people. It is in this light that Barnes (1991) judges rehabilitation services as "highly discriminatory" and "a major disservice to disabled people" (p. 132). He states, "With the removal of the economic and social barriers which confront disabled people, the need for rehabilitation in its present form would be greatly reduced or eliminated altogether" (p. 132).

In general terms, this basic analysis of the relationship between professionals and disabled people applies throughout the West, notwithstanding significant differences in the detail of their expression in different cultures. It seems too that there are similar issues in developing countries. Coleridge (1993), for instance, suggests that professional training in developing countries tends to follow Western models, and Western funding for disability projects is "directed at the medical model run by professionals wedded to it" (p. 73). Sanders (1985) states that the funds spent on constructing one teaching hospital in Zambia could have been used to build 250 health centers in the countryside where most people live. He concludes that the traditional practices and practitioners of Zambia have been discredited by the import of Western medicine.

PROFESSIONAL POWER: DISABLED PEOPLE'S EXPERIENCES

The evidence from research and the writings and recollections of disabled people suggests that professional-disabled people relationships are varied but can be experienced as dehumanizing and abusive by disabled people. Straughair and Fawcitt (1992) report that the young people with arthritis they interviewed were sometimes accused of being neurotic when their symptoms did not fit into neat diagnostic slots. Wendell (1996) refers to the power of professionals to undermine people's beliefs in the reality of their bodily experiences as "epistemic invalidation." Doubt can be cast on immediate experiences unless they are confirmed by authorized medical descriptions. One example she gives is of Gloria Murphy (from the work of Register 1987) who experienced acute dizziness, numbness in her legs, inability to walk at times, double vision, and bladder, kidney, and bowel problems.

> During most of the five years between the onset of her symptoms and her receiving a diagnosis of multiple sclerosis, she was told . . . that she had "housewife's syndrome" and needed only to get busy and to get away from her children to feel better. (Wendell 1996:124)

A further example she gives concerns the experiences of a small percentage of people with advanced multiple sclerosis who experience severe pain in their bones, muscles, or skin.

> Until recent studies confirmed that the disease processes of MS could indeed cause this pain, patients were told that the pain they reported was impossible. (Wendell 1996:125)

Lonsdale (1990), reporting her interviews with disabled women, relates many harmful experiences of hospital treatment and medical care. This particularly concerned doctors, who were often perceived by the women as being nothing more than "groups of anonymous men" (p. 89). An issue they repeatedly raised was how frightening their hospital experiences, especially as children, had been. They could recall being asked very personal and insensitive questions, photographed unclothed, and compelled to walk nude in front of medical students.

This "public stripping," which is now recognized as a form of institutional abuse, was also experienced by Merry, a disabled woman interviewed by Sutherland (1981). She recalls, "They paraded me up and down on the stage, and the surgeon was saying 'who can say what's wrong with this young lady?' " (p. 124). Michlene, another disabled woman interviewed by Sutherland, has similar unpleasant recollections. She states,

> My memory is basically of a whole series of experiences of being very coldly and formally mauled around. It's very alienating. It's as if you're a medical specimen . . . I was never told that I was nice to look at or nice to touch, there was never any feeling of being nice, just of being odd, peculiar. It's horrible. It's taken me years and years to get over it. (P. 123)

Lonsdale (1990) points out that incidents such as these were recalled by women of all ages and cannot be dismissed as belonging to "the bad old days." Coleridge (1993) believes that the self-image of many disabled people has been damaged by constant involvement with professionals, particularly during childhood when play, enjoyment, and discovery were replaced by stress, medical examinations, and developmental programs. He quotes Joshua Malinga, the secretary general of the Southern Africa Federation of the Disabled:

> The point is that they believe that they have solutions to our problems. They do not see us as belonging to society, they think we belong to them, they have to keep files on us throughout our lives, and decide when we should see a doctor and so on. (P. 74)

While this seems to convey experiences shared by many disabled people, "damaged self-image" does not seem to be a necessary consequence. Nasa Begum, for instance, is a black disabled activist and is "involved in the struggles and celebrations of many movements" (Keith 1994:216). She writes of her experiences of regular sessions of physiotherapy during her childhood:

> I couldn't see the point of all these agonizing exercises. I was never very good at accepting the fact that things I didn't like could be "good for me" and the physiotherapist managed to do a really good job of making me a conscientious objector for the rest of my life. (Begum 1994:48)

Four disabled people, interviewed by Johnson (1993), who had received physiotherapy had similar experiences to those of Begum and largely dismissed physiotherapy as having no importance in their lives. Such dismissal is not easy in unequal relationships. Ellis (1993) found that people with knowledge of their entitlements were frequently viewed as "grabbing," demanding, or fussy. Practitioners preferred disabled people who accepted with gratitude what was on offer and described those who challenged this as manipulative.

Morris (1989) interviewed women with spinal cord injuries. The most common compliant about health and welfare professionals was their lack of concern with emotional issues. One woman said, "There is no space allowed for us to express our grief. . . . There is often pressure put on us to 'cope' and if we fail to live up to the standard demanded of us we are categorized as a 'problem' " (p. 24). They reported receiving little or no help in coming to terms with paralysis and often felt compelled to be jolly and play a particular role. As one woman put it, "The staff expected you to have a smile on your face all the time" (Morris 1989:24). Some women experienced a need for counseling and said that the only thing that made life bearable for them in hospital was their relationships with other patients. Many of the women believed that the rehabilitation they received was unnecessarily competitive, sports orientated, and geared toward men. Some women believed that there was too much emphasis on walking and bladder training. Morris states that most women

> found that communication of the vital information about paralysis was poor, that their emotional experience was ignored, that their needs as women were not addressed, and finally they were given little help in planning for the future. This experience seemed to be as common in the 1980s, as it was during the 1950s, 1960s and 1970s. (P. 33)

Boazman (1999) had mixed responses from health professionals when she became aphasic following a brain hemorrhage:

> Their responses towards me varied greatly, some showed great compassion, while others showed complete indifference. I had no way of communicating the fact that I was a bright, intelligent, whole human being. That is what hurt the most. (Pp. 18-19)

People with aphasia, interviewed by Parr and Byng (1997), reported similar mixed experiences. One person, talking of doctors, said that

> when you can't communicate they treat you like a kid and that is just so frustrating—A handful of doctors were just awful. You just wanted to say, "Do you know what this is like?" (P. 74)

Begum (1996) reports many similar themes to those discussed above in her study of disabled women's experiences of general practitioners, although there seemed to be greater variation in experiences than in studies undertaken in institutions such as hospitals. This research was done by a postal questionnaire, 80 of which were completed and returned. She found, for instance, examples of general practitioners (GPs) refusing to believe physical symptoms:

> If I don't get well they say it's psychological (hypochondria, etc.). If it's psychological it's not real/"genuine" (apparently). If it's not real, it doesn't need treatment. If it doesn't need treatment, it's a sign I just need to "pull myself together." (Begum 1996:186)

Begum (1996) takes institutional discrimination as her basis for analyzing difficulties in the relationships between disabled women and their GPs. Her framework of physical, communication, and attitudinal barriers is similar to the analysis adopted for the case study in the next section of this chapter. Begum found that such barriers deny opportunities to people with impairments and can impede access to the services women require. Disabled women, for instance, often find that information is withheld from them. One of her respondents explained that she had not been told that multiple sclerosis had been diagnosed, yet her husband had been told two years before she was informed. It seems too that the flow of information from disabled people to their doctors is liable to distortion and failures. This is, at least in part, due to GPs' responses to impairment. One respondent in the research wrote, "Sometimes I find that a GP—particularly one who is only here for a short time and fairly new—is more interested in my sight problem, or my child's sight problem, than in what I've come to ask about" (Begum 1996:183-84).

CASE STUDY: A GP PRACTICE

This case study is based on a group interview with four staff members at a GP practice in the north of England. It takes institutional discrimination as the framework for analysis:

Unfair or unequal treatment of individuals or groups which is built into institutional organisations, policies and practices at personal, environmental and structural levels. (Swain, Gillman, and French 1998:5)

The notion of institutional discrimination has played an important role in the development of theories of disability. It is also a notion that links the experiences of people from minority or oppressed groups together (Thompson 1997). Disabled people face institutional discrimination in a social and physical world that is driven by and for nondisabled people. This prevents their full access to and participation within organizations and within society. Institutional discrimination can be understood in terms of attitudinal, environmental, and structural barriers. Attitudinal barriers are constructed on environmental barriers that, in turn, are founded on structural barriers. Essential to understanding discrimination as being institutionalized is to reject individualized or victim-blaming explanations of unjust treatment.

The GP practice is housed in a building that was erected in the early 1990s. The building contains various physical features that are essential to disabled people. For example, the building has an adapted toilet and automatic doors, but many limitations were highlighted. There is no lift to the upper floor, and although this does not affect patients and clients, it precludes the employment of disabled staff who cannot manage the stairs as well as disabled colleagues from other institutions. Pauline, the health visitor, recalled the following:

We once had a lady from the Community Health Council. She was in a wheelchair and she couldn't get up here. So disabled professionals are stuck I think.

No disabled staff are, or have been, employed in the practice.

The fire doors also create a problem. Tom, the GP, explained,

One thing we've got [are] fire doors on the consulting rooms which are quite heavy and that's quite difficult for people. I mean not just people in wheelchairs but people who are frail and elderly. But I don't think there's any way round that.

Many of the disabling features of the building adversely affect nondisabled patients and staff as well. Evelyn, the receptionist, explained,

The reception isn't very good even for able-bodied people because the desks are at a terrible height, with them standing on one side and us sitting on the other. There is a lower area for people who are in wheelchairs but it's completely out of the way, in the wrong place . . . so it doesn't get used. Also, it's a very noisy area and it's not very good for confidentiality.

The height of the couches also poses a problem. Angela, the practice nurse, said,

The difficulty that I have is if someone has to get from a wheelchair to a high couch, that it [is] quite difficult for them because I'm usually working by myself. . . . If they've got someone with them, a carer, they'll come in and help because they know how the person likes to be moved and what they can do.

The high couches also pose a problem for Tom and his patients, and it changes the way he works:

I think the difficulty is, people in wheelchairs particularly, unless there's a good reason we tend not to examine them on the couch. This is not necessarily the best thing but it is the most practical thing really.

These problems could be solved, in part, by having adjustable couches.

The building also poses problems for disabled parents with young children. Pauline explained,

We have a problem in the clinic area. I can think of one lady who has a disability with a young child and all of our changing mats are up at a height, the scales are on a table, it's all designed for able-bodied people. She has great problems lifting the baby, she has to bring a relative in to give her a hand.

The staff have available to them a list of interpreters to assist communication with deaf people. Pauline and Evelyn have both attended evening classes, which they financed themselves, to learn sign language. Unfortunately, they do not get sufficient practice. Evelyn said,

Anyone who came in who was deaf, I used to say, "Do you sign?" and they would say, "No." Then last week this deaf chap came in and I said, "Do you sign?" and he said "Yes" and he started to sign away at me and I said, "Stop, I've forgotten it all."

Angela highlighted particular ways in which deaf people might be denied full access to the service:

You might not pick up on the cues you get from people who are hearing. You know, how they come in with a sore throat and they want to talk about their marriage or whatever it is. With someone who is profoundly deaf you would just treat the sore throat. . . . You wouldn't pick up the subtleties.

Very little adaptation is made in the practice for visually disabled people, even though the practice leaflet has been transcribed into Braille. Angela mentioned the hazards of the car parking lot:

It's horrendous. If blind people are using a stick there is nothing to guide them across from the pavement. There's a small path but they've still got to get over the car parking area and cars are always coming and going. And there's the bollards.

People with learning difficulties are seen in the practice, but no specific provision is made for them. Tom said that no service would be knowingly denied and that every person would be treated as an individual. There is a Community Learning Disability Team in the area, and Angela, talking of routine health checks, felt that it might be better if people with learning difficulties received such services from the specialist team:

Personally I would find it quite difficult. I mean people who are trained in dealing with learning disability they know exactly what level to pitch their communication. I find that quite hard to do. They were suggesting a nurse to do smears, blood pressure and things like that, but if we've got a Community Learning Disability Team who are specialists, why not use them but perhaps bring them into the practice if we've got a room available.

Looked at in terms of institutional discrimination, this GP practice has numerous disabling features that preclude many disabled people from working there and cause great difficulty for disabled patients, clients, and staff, even though it was built in the 1990s. The building was designed without any consultation with the staff or with disabled people. Angela thinks it meets legal requirements but no more.

Some of the adaptations that have been made are useful, but they can be regarded, overall, as tokenistic. An example of this is the single leaflet translated in Braille. The practice has many other leaflets, regarding health education, which are not accessible to many visually disabled people or people with learning difficulties. There is no information in large print or on audiotape, even though only a fraction of visually disabled people read Braille. Evelyn said, "I've found this out—like most deaf people don't sign." This illustrates many environmental barriers in institutional discrimination.

Several examples of structural discrimination arose in this interview. Although the staff in the practice seem keen to provide disabled people with a quality service, they have not had the opportunity to attend disability equality training and are forced to rely on "intuition" and "common sense." Evelyn said,

We do a lot of training but we've never done that kind of training. I think the girls are very intuitive, most of them have been in the job a long time, they're very good about picking up on people who can't read, for example, or filling in their forms. It [disability equality training] has never come up and I've been here for 15 years. It's long overdue.

There is no user involvement in the management and running of the practice. Tom tentatively justified this in terms of the nonrepresentation of people who join committees:

It has been muted obviously but we decided it wasn't really. . . . I don't know how to put it. . . . They're not representative of the population really, the usual sort of thing, the same sort of patients all the time.

This argument for the exclusion of disabled people has been strongly rejected by disabled people. Oliver (1996) states,

In representative democracies, representation is always less than perfect, the Conservative Party does not represent all Conservative voters, nor does the British Medical Association represent all doctors. . . . And yet the right of the Disability Movement to represent disabled people is continually questioned by politicians, policy makers and professionals alike. . . . If the legitimate claims of the movement to represent disabled people is denied, who else will represent our interest—doctors, politicians, the Royal Institutes and Associations? (P. 150)

The issue of how far people with learning difficulties should be mainstreamed into health and social services is also a contentious one. Although there may be some advantages to specialist services, as outlined by Angela, the existence of specialist services has the potential to create feelings of inadequacy and deficiency in other workers and goes against the philosophy of inclusion of disabled people in society. Sperlinger (1997) states,

A significant number of GPs do not feel that they should have the lead responsibility for dealing with general medical problems of people with learning disabilities, but assert that it should be the role of medical staff from the specialist learning disability team. . . . Studies consistently show that primary health care team members acknowledge that they have only minimal education on the needs of this client group, yet only a minority welcome the possibility of further training. (P. 12)

Treating people at home, as a solution to an inaccessible environment, can also deny disabled people the opportunity to participate fully in society, and treating people "as individuals," as a substitute for dismantling disabling barriers, is unlikely to bring about equality of service or full accessibility for disabled people.

DISABLED PROFESSIONALS

Disabled professionals stand in an interesting position in an analysis of the relationship between professional and disabled people. As Zola (1994) points out, in the United States, "university training programs for physical and occupational therapists and rehabilitation counselors were being established and many had explicit, if not written, policies against accepting students with disabilities" (p. 55). Indeed, it can be argued that the acceptance of more than a few disabled people into professions could seriously challenge the traditional professional-disabled people relationship in which the professional is considered to be the expert and occupies a dominant position over the client (French 1995). The emergence of disabled professionals can be seen as particularly significant for marginalized groups such as ethnic minority deaf people (Ahmad et al. 1998). Studies have shown that disabled people are effective as professionals. The American Society of Handicapped Physicians found that approximately 75 percent of doctors with a wide variety of impairments remain successfully employed in clinical practice (Wainapel 1987; Wainapel and Bernbaum 1986). French (1990), in her interviews with physiotherapists, found various advantages in being visually impaired, including an increased knowledge of disability, the ability to empathize, and the breaking down of professional barriers.

Nevertheless, the available evidence suggests that the power of professionals in relation to disabled people is perpetuated through discrimination against disabled people in entering professions. In our research in the area of social work (French, Gillman, and Swain 1997), we found that disabled people have experienced institutional discrimination when attempting to gain entry to social work training (Baron, Phillips, and Stalker 1996; James and Thomas 1996). Once qualified, some disabled social workers have had to overcome significant barriers to employment and promotion (French 1988). Much has been written about the institutionalized racism and sexism that exclude women and blacks from the higher echelons of social work management. In contrast, very little has been written about the discrimination experienced by disabled professionals. In French et al. (1997), there is a case study of Alan Dudley, who is blind and a senior social worker. The barriers he faced began in gaining access to training when he received 10 rejections before he was offered a place on a course. Once qualified, he had similar difficulties finding a job. He said,

> I was told by many local authorities, "Well if you want to work with blind people we'll offer you a job, but if you don't, we're not prepared to." I can actually remember crying tears of frustration over this issue. (French et al. 1997:57)

This is compatible to the findings of French's (1988) study of the experiences of disabled health and welfare professionals. She concluded,

> A sizable minority . . . had experienced some degree of negative discrimination either as a result of their colleagues' attitudes or lack of understanding. Most of these problems occurred when attempting to gain access to training and during training. (P. 184)

Baron et al. (1996) found that there were many disabling barriers to recruitment and training on diploma in social work programs. They state that "a lack of experience of disability issues was evident as well as the absence of an active approach to arrange support at all levels of the programme" (p. 375). James and Thomas (1996) undertook a program to give greater prominence to work with disabled people on a social work diploma course and to attract more disabled students to social work training. They found that many practicing teachers in voluntary and statutory settings were reluctant to recruit disabled students and cited fire regulations or the fear that they would be vulnerable to violent or aggressive clients as justifications. It is clear that discrimination and oppression occur, albeit sometimes unintentionally or subconsciously, within professionals' own agencies. Such oppression and discrimination are embedded within everyday practices such as student recruitment and training.

DISABLED PEOPLE POWER

As we have seen, professional-disabled people relations are unequal and dominated by professionals. However, the danger of such an analysis is that it casts disabled people in a passive role, with no account given to active resistance. In this section, we turn to disabled people power in controlling the provision of services and professional help. Indeed, it can be argued that with the growth of the disabled people's movement, the greatest challenge to professional dominance has come from disabled people themselves.

Since the inception of the welfare state, disabled people have constituted, potentially, a powerful political force, yet because of the widespread discrimination against them, in terms of education, employment, transport, professional power, and so on, they have been rendered relatively powerless. This situation has, however, gradually changed, and disabled people have come together to campaign for change, and a strong disabled people's movement has emerged (Campbell and Oliver 1996). The movement consists of organizations of disabled people—that is, organizations that are controlled by disabled people themselves, even though many welcome nondisabled allies. In Britain, perhaps the most significant turning point for the disabled people's movement was the formation in 1974 of the Union of Physically Impaired against Segregation (UPIAS). Davis (1993b) explains how UPIAS fought to change the definition of disability from one of individual tragedy to one of social oppression. This paved the way for the development of the social model of disability. This model has arisen from the experiences of disabled people themselves. It is borne out of the collective experience of disabled people, challenging "the way they had been defined and controlled by the experts who manipulate disability policy" (Davis 1993b:289). It is no coincidence that the disabled people's movement and the social model of disability have developed together. The social model emanates from the pooled experiences and discussions of oppression. As Rachel Hurst of Disabled Peoples' International states,

> When you come together with other disabled people, you have the time and the opportunity to discuss what the situation really is—what oppression is, who is oppressing you; where oppression comes from; what discrimination is and where it comes from. (quoted in Coleridge 1993:54)

The growth of organizations run and controlled by disabled people has taken place in many countries when disabled people come together through choice. Khalfan, for example, was inspired to found the Association of Disabled People of Zanzibar after meeting disabled people from around the world at a conference in Singapore. On occasion, active associations have stemmed from the dissatisfaction of disabled people living in segregated institutions. This is how the disabled people's movement in Zimbabwe started. It is now one of the strongest in Africa. In Lebanon, the disabled people's movement was triggered by the large number of people disabled in the war, and it is now the strongest in the Middle East (Coleridge 1993; French and Swain 1997).

The political implications of the social model, often explicitly stated, are to promote the collective struggle by disabled people for social change. One measure of the effectiveness of the model has been the proliferation of the disabled people's movement and the burgeoning of not only many small organizations throughout the world but also national umbrella organizations, all of which are organized by disabled people—for example, the British Council of Organizations of Disabled People (BCODP) (founded in 1981), now called the British Council of Disabled People, and the international organization known as Disabled Peoples' International (DPI) (also founded in 1981). BCODP continues to expand and now represents some 112 organizations and more than 200,000 people, while the DPI represents more than 70 national assemblies of disabled people throughout the world.

The DPI grew out of conflict between disabled people and nondisabled professionals. Until 1981, the only international organization concerned with the needs of people with impairments was Rehabilitation International, which consisted almost entirely of rehabilitation professionals. A minority of disabled people was, however, involved. At the 1976 congress of Rehabilitation International, a group of disabled Swedish and Canadian delegates put forward the resolution that at least 50 percent of the delegation should consist of organizations of disabled people. The resolution was strongly defeated, providing the impetus for the 250 disabled

ments was   people present to form their own organization. Driedger (1989) describes the hostility this caused among the rehabilitation professionals, one of whom said,

> To me they are going through a developmental stage which resembles the adolescent or young adult in a family, who often becomes rebellious for a period of time. After this stage an excellent partnership and relationship with the "family" evolves and life goes on better than before. (P. 37)

A large number of BCODP's member organizations comprise coalitions of disabled people and centers for integrated living (CILs) or centers for independent living, as they are also known. The philosophy of integrated living, evolving as it has from the social model, and the CILs provide a clear challenge to the dominance of professionals in relation to disabled people. One assumption, for instance, is that "people who are disabled by society's reaction to physical, intellectual and sensory impairment and to emotional distress have the right to assert control over their lives" (Morris 1993a:7). The CILs, which employ many disabled people, gained much of their inspiration and impetus from the independent living movement in the United States, which developed in the 1960s and 1970s. There are important differences between CILs in the United States and those in Great Britain. The main difference is that in Great Britain, owing to the existence of the welfare state, CILs work, to a varying extent (Leaman 1996), in harness with health and local authorities to develop new approaches and to ensure that disabled people receive their rightful support (French 1994c). In the United States, CILs operate more independently. This difference is reflected in the naming of the centers; they are called "integrated" in Great Britain and "independent" in the United States.

The first CIL was established in Berkeley, California, in 1973, and within 10 years, more than 200 CILs had been established across the United States (Priestley 1999). Related projects also emerged in mainland Europe in the 1970s, including the Fokus projects in Sweden, Collectivehaus initiatives in Denmark, and Het Dorp in the Netherlands (Klapwijk 1981; Priestley 1999; Zola 1982). The Derbyshire Centre for Integrated Living (DCIL) (the subject of a detailed case study below) was the first to be established in Britain. This is now one of a few examples of organizations of disabled people that have successfully provided services promoting independent living (Morris 1993b). In relation to the power of professions, the growth of "consumerism," self-help, and the movement for independent or integrated living can be seen as an emerging countertendency (Zola 1987). Priestley (1999), in his research with DCIL, shows that "key value differences between the competing agendas of British disability policy and the disabled people's movement are both numerous and complex" (p. 77). The first, from an individual tragedy model, has been preoccupied with care, medicalization, and segregation, while the latter, from a social model viewpoint, has promoted participation, inclusion, and equality. He argues that while the implementation of community care policies has reinforced professional domination, the exploitation of "informal carers," and the individualization of disability, the disabled people's movement has advanced values of self-help, communalism, and citizenship. For Priestley, controlling evaluation of services is crucial, particularly the promotion of life quality issues rather than the technicalities of quality assurance systems. He states,

> Quality of life is hard to define and any attempt to do so is inherently value-led. The selection of measurement indicators is not only a technical process but also a political one. For this reason the ability of particular groups to define "quality," and the value base which they use to do it, will also determine the kinds of services which are thought to have "value." (P. 187)

It can be argued that the diminution of professional power allows disabled people more freedom to organize their own care. The introduction of direct payments to disabled people is one example. Oliver and Zarb (1992) found that disabled people who received direct payments had more freedom to participate in employment and leisure activities of their choice. They could arrange to receive the type of help they wanted at a time that would fit their requirements and schedules. The notion that personal assistance should be provided by trained and qualified personnel has also been challenged by disabled people:

> I'm not looking for professional qualifications, nurses are definitely out, I'm looking for people who are enthusiastic . . . I want to train them in my own way. (Morris 1993a:32)

Such flexibility allowed disabled people to follow the lifestyles of their choice. From their research in which 70 disabled people were interviewed, Zarb and Nadesh (1994) state,

> Findings from the research highlight that payments schemes are associated with higher quality support arrangements than direct service provision. In particular, the payments option clearly offers disabled people a greater degree of choice and control, and, consequently, leads to higher user satisfaction. Most importantly, support arrangements which are funded through the payments option are almost invariably more reliable (and, therefore, more efficient) than those supported by direct service provision. (P. ii)

From his research with the Derbyshire Centre for Integrated Living, however, Priestley (1999) suggests that some disabled people require help in managing their own package of financial support, such as the information, advocacy, and peer support provided by organizations of disabled people.

CASE STUDY: DERBYSHIRE CENTRE FOR INTEGRATED LIVING

The Derbyshire Centre for Integrated Living (DCIL) was founded in 1985 as an initiative of the Derbyshire Coalition of Disabled People working in collaboration with the Derbyshire County Council. The aim of the DCIL is to secure a full economic, public, and social life for disabled people in accordance with their own wishes and desired lifestyles. It exists to find ways of removing barriers that stand in the way of disabled people leading full and satisfying lives. The center is run jointly by disabled and nondisabled people working in partnership.

The aims of the center are based on seven basic needs, which have been identified by disabled people themselves. These needs, which all interact and must therefore be provided in an integrated way, are for information, technical aids, transport, counseling, housing, personal assistance, and access.

The DCIL maintains an up-to-date and comprehensive information base for disabled people, their assistants, and service providers. It is also available to researchers. This database of information is extensive, including, for example, information on holidays with more than 3,000 accessible venues. The first point of contact for inquirers is with a disabled person who has wide knowledge of disability issues as well as personal experience of disability. A minicom is provided so that hearing-impaired people can use the telephone, and the information is also available in Braille, large print, and on audiotape. A Braille, large-print, and computer consulting service is available commercially to other agencies.

The DCIL has a team of trained peer counselors who primarily are disabled themselves. This service provides support for disabled people who are feeling isolated or experiencing difficulties in areas such as sexuality or transition to independence. The counselors bring their own experience of disability to the situation and are not shocked by sensitive subjects or feelings such as grief and anger. The DCIL also provides training that, though tailored to specific requirements, is based on a thorough understanding of the social construction of disability. Training is provided for volunteers, counselors, information workers, and local access and transport groups. A range of courses is offered on a commercial basis.

The Derbyshire Centre of Integrated Living provides personal support services and personal assistance. It states that the

counselors, ii

> DCIL supports the right of all disabled people to determine, how, when, where and by whom the services they need are provided. (Derbyshire Centre for Integrated Living n.d.-a)

Personal assistance can be defined as help provided by other people to enable disabled people to live the life they choose. Support may be needed in returning to work, going to college, or coping with rehabilitation or the onset of impairment. Each package of personal assistance is designed to meet the individual wishes and needs of the disabled person and is managed by or comanaged with the disabled person.

The Derbyshire Centre of Integrated Living works in partnership with many other organizations, including SCOPE, the British Association for Counseling, and the Consortium on Opportunities for Volunteering. Its aim is to highlight disabling practices and to help develop more appropriate services for disabled people. DCIL participates in joint planning with health and social services, ensuring that the personnel of these services understand the priorities of disabled people.

Viewed in terms of institutional discrimination, it appears that many of the barriers disabled people routinely face have been removed within the organization. The building is accessible to people using wheelchairs, and Braille, audiotape, and large print are all provided. The people giving information have a broad knowledge of disability issues, not only in a professional sense but also in terms of personal experience. A counseling service is provided by qualified disabled counselors who have firsthand experience of encountering and removing barriers that stand in the way of a fulfilling lifestyle.

The Derbyshire Centre of Integrated Living provides disability equality training to its own staff and to volunteers and outside agencies. Disability equality training, in contrast to disability awareness training, does not focus solely on attitudes but also on every aspect of disabling barriers and institutionalized discrimination. This is to ensure that people, such as volunteers, understand the full extent of the barriers that disabled people face and that the attitudes are seen within a historical and cultural context.

The staff of DCIL works within the community, not simply to visit and help disabled people overcome problems but also to empower them to bring about changes themselves. DCIL helps disabled people to find appropriate personal assistance, which is not controlling or patronizing, to enable them to lead the lifestyle of their choice. DCIL states that

> in the past many disabled people have had services delivered to them which have not given them sufficient control over their lives, for example services which of necessity have had to conform to particular models of service provision into which disabled people had to fit. . . . We offer a different approach. Because we believe that disabled people have the right to determine their own lives in every aspect, we offer a service that reflects this approach. (Derbyshire Centre for Integrated Living n.d.-b)

In his research in Derbyshire, Priestley (1999) endorsed the findings of previous studies concerning indicators of process quality important to disabled people, including "increased flexibility, choice, control and reliability which self-management offered them" (p. 143). These criteria were apparent in "outcomes" identified by users of DCIL personal support service. Terry stated,

> I can go shopping when I want to. I can go out for a day if I want to, under the restraints that there are . . . and I could only do that sort of thing because I've got people to rely on. (Priestley 1999:174)

When services are provided to disabled people by large bureaucratic organizations, unacceptable delays are common. Carol states,

> They wouldn't let me keep changing my times . . . I felt as if I just couldn't organize my life in any way. I couldn't just say, have a lie in, because I'd got to ring social services just to have a lie in. (Priestley 1999:144)

There is often a lack of concern or understanding that disabled people are dependent on equipment, such as a wheelchair, a visual aid, or a car, to function adequately at work or to enjoy leisure pursuits. These delays are frequently underpinned by structural discrimination where disabled people are viewed as unimportant or where lack of resources makes delays inevitable. The repair and maintenance service at DCIL remove the anxiety and frustration when equipment breaks down and help disabled people remain active citizens on their own terms.

It is likely, then, that within the culture and ethos of DCIL, attitudes and behavior toward disabled people are good, illustrating that attitudes are shaped by organizational philosophies and practices. Decision making and working practices within the organization are controlled by disabled people who do not regard disability as an individualized tragedy but as a human and civil rights issue. Every aspect of the work is geared toward the fulfillment of disabled people on their own terms and in viewing disabled people as active, capable citizens who are restricted not by impairment but by a disabling society.

CHANGING PROFESSIONAL-DISABLED PEOPLE RELATIONS

Brisenden (1998) writes,

> I have a fantasy that in some future world people with disabilities will be able to insist on the right to interrogate doctors, rather than be interrogated by them. In this fantasy, a doctor is placed on stage in front of a large audience of people with disabilities, in order that we may come to understand the stigma of a career in medicine, and the effect this may have on family and friends . . . the feeling of power might prove too irresistible to be ignored. (P. 22)

Is this pure fantasy, or are professional-disabled people relations moving toward a shift of power? In this concluding section, we focus specifically on possibilities for a changing relationship between professionals and disabled people. As throughout the analysis in this chapter, various competing and contradictory factors need to be taken into account. Such factors include changing the discourse within professional-disabled people relations, such as reference to disabled people as clients, users, and customers and to notions of empowerment; changing the relations between professionals and the state, particularly with the crisis of the welfare state and the introduction of the market into welfare provision; changing legislation in fostering and limiting change; and growing the disabled people's movement.

The notion of changing professional-disabled people relations we are pursuing here, then, is founded on a shift of control to disabled people. As recognized by Finkelstein and Stuart (1996), there are two components to such a shift. The first is at the personal level of individual disabled people taking an active role in realizing their own goals. As French (1994d) states,

> Disabled people define independence, not in physical terms, but in terms of control. People who are almost totally dependent on others, in a physical sense, can still have independence of thought and action, enabling them to take full and active charge of their lives. (P. 49)

The term *empowerment,* though inconsistently used, is often invoked to convey the inherent changes in professional-disabled people relations. The second component is a collective control of policy and the organization of services that are best achieved, according to Finkelstein and Stuart (1996), through the supervision of the collective services by national and local representative organizations of disabled people. *Consultation* is the most widely applied term.

The implications that a social model of disability has for professional practice have been conceived and pursued under a number of guises, such as *partnership, empowerment,* and *emancipatory practice.* The starting point for the last of these is the recognition that professional practice can "either condone, reinforce or exacerbate existing inequalities or they can challenge, undermine or attenuate such oppressive forces" (Thompson 1998:38). Thompson argues that the development of emancipatory practice is a challenge that faces everyone in the human services and is founded on an understanding of the concept of power and its role in the relationship between professionals and disabled people.

To a certain extent, the parameters of a changing relationship are set out in legislation. In some countries, including Australia, the United States, Canada, and New Zealand, antidiscrimination legislation can provide a framework for confronting institutionalized discrimination. However, the effectiveness of such legislation is contentious. Certainly, the legislation itself needs to be founded on the social model of disability and effective mechanisms for enforcement. Thus, while the Americans with Disabilities Act of 1990 is viewed as comprehensive civil rights legislation, the more recent Disability Discrimination Act of 1995 in Britain is more piecemeal and reflects an individual model of disability. The act is piecemeal legislation since large areas of life, such as education, are only included to a very limited extent. All that colleges are required to do, for example, is to provide a statement of intent with regard to disabled students. New transport has to reach minimum standards, but this only applies to land-based transport. It is therefore legal to discriminate against disabled people, and discrimination can be justified, for example, by employers in ways it cannot be justified in the Sex Discrimination Act and Race Relations Act. In Britain, as in some other countries, however, community care policy has been underpinned by legislation that, at least at the policy level, sets the context for increased control by disabled people over the services they receive—for instance, with the passing of the National Health Service (NHS), the Community Care Act (1990), and the Direct Payments Bill (1995).

Despite the potential for a changing relationship, there is little evidence of any shift in power in relationships between professionals and disabled people. There has been recognition that empowerment is essentially a political activity addressing power and control, rather than the development of the capacities of disabled individuals by professional intervention. Williams (1993) conveys the following:

> To recognize clients' experiential knowledge as the foundation for learning, with the professional's expert knowledge at the service of the client. . . . It removes power from them and hands it over to the client; and locates their base of power with their clients rather than with their professional body. (P. 12)

Yet, reviews of the available evidence consistently suggest that "health and welfare organizations and the professionals who control them are unwilling or unable to surrender power to their users and thus meaningfully empower them" (Jack 1995:38). Professional claims of empowerment can be seen as protection of their own power by appearing to share it with disabled people (Gomm 1993:137).

Moves toward consultation have also been seen as limited rather than reflecting far-reaching change. In his overview of the changing scene across Europe, Daunt (1991:54) suggests that there are signs that service providers are paying more attention to organizations of disabled people. However, researchers such as Bewley and Glendinning (1994) show that disabled people face considerable barriers in their involvement in planning community care, particularly those disabled people historically marginalized in service provision such as ethnic minority communities and the Deaf community.

Ultimately, it can be argued, the relationship between professionals and disabled people is a reflection of the social structures, ideologies, and power relations that disable people with impairments. Disabled people are generating the impetus for fundamental change, but the focus for change is professional structures, policies, practices, and ideologies. Power relations and structures are, by their nature, deeply ingrained, and cosmetic changes mask lack of fundamental change. The challenge for professionals is that, from the experiences of disabled people, they have been part of the disablement of people with impairments. Central to a changing relationship is the changing paradigm from a medical to a social model of disability and, with this, possibilities for professionals to work for and with disabled people in confronting the barriers of institutional discrimination. Jack (1995) concluded that "true empowerment in community care is attainable only through self-help activity and user-led services" (p. 38). However, many disabled people would agree with Mike du Toit, a South African disabled activist, that

> the movement does not reject the role of the professionals. What we reject is the inappropriateness of so much of the work that is being done, and the inappropriateness of their attitudes, and the complete inappropriateness of their seeking to represent us. (Coleridge 1993:77)

As in this chapter, the critique of professional power is pursued as a foundation for relationships in which, as in Brisenden's fantasy, disabled people are in control rather than forced into dependency.

In this chapter, we have considered the relationship between disabled people and health and welfare professionals by tracing the development of professional power and examining the experiences of disabled people, including disabled health and welfare professionals. We have also provided two contrasting case studies of service provision and discussed the rise of the disabled people's movement. From this we conclude that the only way forward for health and welfare professionals is to relinquish their power and become allies of disabled people.

REFERENCES

Ahmad, W., A. Darr, L. Jones, and G. Nisar. 1998. *Deafness and Ethnicity: Services, Policy and Politics*. Bristol, UK: Policy.

Albrecht, G. 1992. *The Disability Business: Rehabilitation in America*. London: Sage.

Barnes, C. 1991. *Disabled People in Britain and Discrimination*. London: Hurst.

Barnes, C., G. Mercer, and T. Shakespeare. 1999. *Exploring Disability: A Sociological Introduction*. Cambridge, UK: Polity.

Baron, S., R. Phillips, and K. Stalker. 1996. "Barriers to Training for Disabled Social Work Students." *Disability and Society* 11 (3): 361-77.

Begum, N. 1994. "Snow White." Pp. 46-51 in *Mustn't Grumble: Writing by Disabled Women*, edited by L. Keith. London: The Women's Press.

———. 1996. "Doctor, Doctor. . . .: Disabled Women's Experience of General Practitioners." Pp. 168-93 in *Encounters with Strangers: Feminism and Disability*, edited by J. Morris. London: The Women's Press.

Benzeval, M., K. Judge, and M. Whitehead, eds. 1995. *Tackling Inequalities in Health: An Agenda for Change*. London: King's Fund.

Bewley, C. and C. Glendinning. 1994. *Involving Disabled People in Community Care Planning*. York, UK: Joseph Rowntree Foundation.

Boazman, S. 1999. "Inside Aphasia." Pp. 15-20 in *Disability Discourse*, edited by M. Corker and S. French. Buckingham, UK: Open University Press.

Brisenden, S. 1998. "Independent Living and the Medical Model of Disability." Pp. 20-27 in *The Disability Reader*, edited by T. Shakespeare. London: Cassell.

Campbell, J. and M. Oliver. 1996. *Disability Politics: Understanding Our Past, Changing Our Future*. London: Routledge Kegan Paul.

Coates, H. and A. King. 1982. *The Patient Assessment*. Edinburgh, UK: Churchill Livingstone.

Coleridge, P. 1993. *Disability, Liberation and Development.* Oxford, UK: Oxfam.

Daunt, P. 1991. *Meeting Disability: A European Response.* London: Cassell.

Davis, K. 1993a. "The Crafting of Good Clients." Pp. 197-200 in *Disabling Barriers—Enabling Environments,* edited by J. Swain, V. Finkelstein, S. French, and M. Oliver. London: Sage.

———. 1993b. "On the Movement." Pp. 285-92 in *Disabling Barriers—Enabling Environments,* edited by J. Swain, V. Finkelstein, S. French, and M. Oliver. London: Sage.

Derbyshire Centre for Integrated Living. n.d.-a. *Derbyshire Centre for Integrated Living: A Profile of an Organisation.* Ripley, UK: Derbyshire Centre for Integrated Living.

———. n.d.-b. *Personal Support Services.* Ripley, UK: Derbyshire Centre for Integrated Living.

Drake, R. 1999. *Understanding Disability Policies.* Houndmills, UK: Macmillan.

Driedger, D. 1989. *The Last Civil Rights Movement: Disabled People's International.* London: Hurst.

Ellis, K. 1993. *Squaring the Circle: User and Carer Participation in Needs Assessment.* London: Joseph Rowntree Foundation.

Finkelstein, V. 1991. "Disability: An Administrative Challenge?" Pp. 19-39 in *Social Work, Disabled People and Disabling Environments,* edited by M. Oliver. London: Jessica Kingsley.

Finkelstein, V. and O. Stuart. 1996. "Developing New Services." Pp. 170-87 in *Beyond Disability: Towards an Enabling Society,* edited by G. Hales. London: Sage.

French, S. 1988. "Experiences of Disabled Health and Welfare Professionals." *Sociology of Health and Illness* 10 (2): 170-88.

———. 1990. "The Advantages of Visual Impairment: Some Physiotherapists' Views." *New Beacon* 75 (872): 1-6.

———. 1993. "Setting a Record Straight." Pp. 227-32 in *Disabling Barriers—Enabling Environments,* edited by J. Swain, V. Finkelstein, S. French, and M. Oliver. London: Sage.

———. 1994a. "Disabled People and Professional Practice." Pp. 103-18 in *On Equal Terms: Working with Disabled People,* edited by S. French. Oxford, UK: Butterworth-Heinemann.

———. 1994b. "In Whose Service? A Review of the Development of Services for Disabled People in Great Britain." *Phsyiotherapy* 80 (4): 200-4.

———. 1994c. "The Disability Movement." Pp. 68-83 in *On Equal Terms: Working with Disabled People,* edited by S. French. Oxford, UK: Butterworth-Heinemann.

———. 1994d. "The Disabled Role." Pp. 47-60 in *On Equal Terms: Working with Disabled People,* edited by S. French. Oxford, UK: Butterworth-Heinemann.

———. 1995. "Visually Impaired Physiotherapists: Their Struggle for Acceptance and Survival." *Disability and Society* 10 (1): 3-20.

French, S., M. Gillman, and J. Swain. 1997. *Working with Visually Disabled People: Bridging Theory and Practice.* Birmingham, AL: Venture.

French, S. and J. Swain. 1997. *From a Different Viewpoint: The Lives and Experiences of Visually Impaired people.* London: Royal National Institute for the Blind.

Gomm, R. 1993. "Issues of Power in Health and Welfare." Pp. 131-38 in *Health, Welfare and Practice: Reflecting on Roles and Relationships,* edited by J. Walmsley, J. Reynolds, P. Shakespeare, and R. Woolfe. London: Sage.

Grieve, G. P. 1988. "Clinical Examination and the SOAP Mnemonic." *Physiotherapy* 74 (2): 97.

Harrison, S. and C. Pollitt. 1994. *Controlling Health Professionals: The Future of Work and Organization in the National Health Service.* Buckingham, UK: Open University Press.

Hugman, R. 1991. *Power in Caring Professions.* Basingstoke, UK: Macmillan.

Illich, I. 1976. *Limits to Medicine.* Harmondsworth, UK: Penguin.

Jack, R. 1995. "Empowerment in Community Care." Pp. 11-42 in *Empowerment in Community Care,* edited by R. Jack. London: Chapman & Hall.

Jacobson, B., A. Smith, and M. Whitehead. 1991. *The Nation's Health: A Strategy for the 1990s.* London: King's Fund.

James, P. and M. Thomas. 1996. "Deconstructing a Disabling Environment in Social Work Education." *Social Work Education* 15 (1): 34-45.

Johnson, R. 1993. " 'Attitudes Don't Just Hang in the Air. . .': Disabled People's Perceptions of Physiotherapists." *Physiotherapy* 79 (9): 619-26.

Keith, L., ed. 1994. *Mustn't Grumble: Writing by Disabled Women.* London: The Women's Press.

Klapwijk, A. 1981. "Het Dorp, an Adapted Part of the City of Arnhem (the Netherlands) for Severely Disabled People." In *Development Trust for the Young Disabled: An International Seminar on the Long-term Care of Disabled People.* London: Development Trust for the Young Disabled.

Leaman, D. 1996. "Four Camels of Disability." Pp. 164-69 in *Beyond Disability: Towards an Enabling Society,* edited by G. Hales. London: Sage.

Lonsdale, S. 1990. *Women and Disability.* London: Macmillan.

Marsh, P. and M. Fisher. 1992. *Good Intentions: Developing Partnership in Social Services.* London: Joseph Rowntree Foundation.

McKeown, T. 1979. *The Role of Medicine.* Oxford, UK: Basil Blackwell.

McKnight, J. 1981. "Professional Service and Disabling Help." Pp. 24-32 in *Handicap in a Social World,* edited by A. Brechin, P. Liddiard, and J. Swain. Sevenoaks: Hodder.

Morris, J. 1989. *Able Lives.* London: The Women's Press.

———. 1993a. *Community Care or Independent Living?* York, UK: Joseph Rowntree Foundation.

———. 1993b. *Independent Lives: Community Care and Disabled People.* Basingstoke, UK: Macmillan.

Oliver, M. 1990. *The Politics of Disablement.* Basingstoke, UK: Macmillan.

———. 1993. "Disability and Dependency: A Creation of Industrial Societies?" Pp. 49-60 in *Disabling Barriers—Enabling Environments,* edited by J. Swain, V. Finkelstein, S. French, and M. Oliver. London: Sage.

———. 1996. *Understanding Disability: From Theory to Practice.* London: Macmillan.

Oliver, M. and B. Sapey. 1999. *Social Work with Disabled People.* 2d ed. Basingstoke, UK: Macmillan.

Oliver, M. and G. Zarb. 1992. *Greenwich Personal Assistance Schemes: An Evaluation.* London: Greenwich Association of Disabled People.

Parr, S. and S. Byng. 1997. *Talking about Aphasia.* Buckingham, UK: Open University Press.

Priestley, M. 1999. *Disability Politics and Community Care.* London: Jessica Kingsley.

Register, C. 1987. *Living with Chronic Illness: Days of Patience and Passion.* New York: Bantam.

Ryan, J. and F. Thomas. 1987. *The Politics of Mental Handicap.* London: Free Association Books.

Sagan, A. 1987. *The Health of Nations.* New York: Basic Books.

Sanders, D. (with R. Carver). 1985. *The Struggle for Health: Medicine and the Politics of Underdevelopment.* London: Macmillan.

Slack, S. 1999. "I Am More Than My Wheels." Pp. 28-37 in *Disability Discourse,* edited by M. Corker and S. French. Buckingham, UK: Open University Press.

Sperlinger, A. 1997. "Introduction." Pp. 3-16 in *Adults with Learning Difficulties: A Practical Approach for Health Professionals,* edited by J. O'Hara and A. Sperlinger. Chichester, UK: Wiley.

Straughair, S. and S. Fawcitt. 1992. *The Road towards Independence: The Experiences of Young People with Arthritis in the 1990s.* London: Arthritis Care.

Sutherland, A. T. 1981. *Disabled We Stand.* London: Souvenir.

Swain, J. and S. French. 2000. "Towards an Affirmative Model of Disability." *Disability & Society* 15 (4): 569-82.

Swain, J., M. Gillman, and S. French. 1998. *Confronting Disabling Barriers: Towards Making Organisations Accessible.* Birmingham, UK: Venture.

Thompson, N. 1997. *Anti-Discriminatory Practice.* 2d ed. London: Macmillan.

———. 1998. *Promoting Equality: Challenging Discrimination and Oppression in the Human Services.* Houndmills, UK: Macmillan.

Wainapel, S. F. 1987. "The Physically Disabled Physician." *Journal of the American Medical Association* 257:2936-38.

Wainapel, S. F. and M. Bernbaum. 1986. "The Physician with Visual Impairment and Blindness." *Archives of Ophthalmology* 104:498-502.

Wendell, S. 1996. *The Rejected Body: Feminist Philosophical Reflections on Disability.* New York: Routledge.

Wilding, P. 1982. *Professional Power and Social Welfare.* London: Routledge Kegan Paul.

Williams, J. 1993. "What Is a Professional? Experience versus Expertise." Pp. 8-15 in *Health, Welfare and Practice: Reflecting on Roles and Relationships,* edited by J. Walmsley, J. Reynolds, P. Shakespeare, and R. Woolfe. London: Sage.

Zarb, G. and P. Nadesh. 1994. *Cashing in on Independence: Comparing the Costs and Benefits of Cash and Services for Meeting Disabled People's Support Needs.* Clay Cross: British Council of Organisations of Disabled People.

Zola, I. 1982. *Missing Pieces: A Chronicle of Living with a Disability.* Philadelphia: Temple University Press.

———. 1987. "The Politicization of the Self-Help Movement." *Social Policy* 18 (1): 32-33.

———. 1994. "Towards Inclusion: The Role of People with Disabilities in Policy and Research Issues in the United States: A Historical Political Analysis." Pp. 49-66 in *Disability Is Not Measles: New Research Paradigms in Disability,* edited by M. H. Rioux and M. Bach. North York, Ontario: Roeher Institute.

Public Health Trends in Disability

33

Past, Present, and Future

DONALD J. LOLLAR

Traditional public health approaches to disease prevention and health promotion have failed to take into account the concerns and needs of people with disabilities. As a result, public health messages have often depicted people with disabilities as the negative result of "unhealthy" actions. Acutely aware of this devaluation of their experience, people with disabilities have rejected public health as inimical to their very existence. However, a more positive relationship has begun to evolve over a period of time, but not without continued substantial tension. Developing a positive relationship will continue to require mutual understanding of the different factors that have brought initially disparate movements into contact.

As part of the divergent histories, the concepts and terms, which carry different nuances for public health professionals and persons with disabilities, need to be examined and clarified. For example, terms such as *disability* and *morbidity,* constructs such as *health* and *wellness*, and factors such as *technology* and *environment* have different meanings across communities and among countries (Linden, Me, and Vanek 1996; Madden and Hogan 1997). Forging common ground from substantially different beginnings, in light of medical and technological advances and with a growing disability empowerment movement, is a challenge of great global importance for the future of both communities.

This chapter defines areas where disability and public health can mutually inform one another to respond to the particular needs of people with disabilities. Public health has a long tradition in surveillance and primary prevention activities; both represent strategies that can be translated into methods to better respond to the circumstances of people who experience disabilities. While primary prevention messages are equally valid for people with and without disabilities, public health has an opportunity to focus efforts on preventing the onset of other health conditions (secondary conditions) that may be associated with disability. In addition, traditional public health surveillance activities highlight the magnitude of health problems and are equally applicable to people with disabilities. The major public health need in this area is the development of methods to capture information about disability status as a demographic characteristic of the population, just as gender and age can be captured. Moreover, using a conceptually rigorous framework of disability to describe and measure activity, participation, and environmental factors allows an appreciation of the complexity of an individual's experience in relationship to society. Understanding the complexity of disability may lead to more appropriate public health interventions and policies that have the capacity to enhance the lives of people with disabilities.

THE PUBLIC HEALTH MODEL

The public health movement developed over several hundred years, beginning with efforts to prevent diseases that, unchecked, could affect much of the population. Emphasis, naturally, has been on preventing diseases and conditions that take lives prematurely. In its simplest form, the public health process includes identifying a disease, isolating the mechanism by which the disease is transmitted, and intervening to stop its spread. Initially, public health professionals used whatever interventions were available (e.g., improving sanitation) to halt the transmission of a communicable disease. As science improved, public health used additional new tools, such as antibiotics, for intervention. This approach has been used throughout the world by public health agencies since their inception. To monitor the success of public health interventions, researchers collected mortality data, and surveillance—the procedure for tracking the course of the disease and its impact on human mortality—was used. (The term *surveillance* itself conjures images of intrusion and elicits feelings of invasion among the general population, including those with disabilities.) An equally important part of the disease prevention process was identification of population subgroups that were more vulnerable to a particular disease. This process of identification, intervention, and follow-up assessment became established as the public health process. Although the process is straightforward, the issues surrounding it are quite complex. In most countries, several agencies have mandates to address various aspects of the process, from conducting cellular research and social marketing surveys to addressing human behavior change. The strength of this scientific process for public good has long been used and accepted.

By the early 1970s, however, conditions other than communicable diseases began to receive considerable attention, and the role of public health changed, expanding to deal with emerging health issues. For example, the ferocity of the HIV epidemic challenged public health to find ways to influence human behavior. Moreover, once public health professionals added new interventions, other conditions and approaches were added. Injuries and chronic diseases, such as diabetes and arthritis, came within the purview of public health surveillance and interventions. In addition, social and behavioral science assumed a greater role in the public health process. As a result, over the past 10 years, numerous structural changes have been made to expand the science and programs to address this broadened public health agenda.

In 1988, the Centers for Disease Control and Prevention's (CDC's) National Center for Environmental Health (NCEH) initiated a program for disability prevention in the United States. This initiative was the first of its kind within the U.S. public health structure. Its primary responsibilities were the following:

1. to coordinate disability prevention activities,
2. to establish surveillance systems for disabilities,
3. to identify populations at risk and develop interventions, and
4. to provide states with assistance to build their own capacity (Houk and Thacker 1989).

The program initially focused on preventing conditions that contribute to disability, such as traumatic injuries, birth defects, developmental disabilities, or chronic illness. Simultaneously, specific emphasis was given to the specific "causes" of disabling conditions. CDC established two new centers, the National Center for Chronic Disease Prevention and Health Promotion (NCCDPHP) in 1989 and the National Center for Injury Prevention and Control (NCIPC) in

1991. In addition, the Division of Birth Defects and Developmental Disabilities within the NCEH continued to expand its activities, including work to prevent both fetal alcohol syndrome and autism.

These were important new public health initiatives in several ways. First, they focused attention on nondisease causes of death in the population. Second, they required public health to pay attention to outcomes beyond mortality. (In public health, this set of outcomes is referred to as *morbidity*—the medical outcomes, excluding death.) Morbidity is classified using the *International Classification of Diseases (ICD)* codes. These changes in public health opened the door for attention to be given to the health of people living with a disability—those who might be viewed in traditional public health terms as failures of the primary prevention model. Third, the initiatives pointed to the need for clearer concepts, constructs, terminology, and data to apply the public health model to people with disabilities. In fact, although morbidity has often been confused with disability (Chamie 1995), morbidity is but one factor that contributes to the disabling process, while environmental factors also contribute substantially to disability.

As primary prevention activities for conditions leading to disability increased, relatively little attention was paid to the health of people with disabilities. The attention that was given usually addressed the relative lack of information about the impact of disability on the quality of life or on a few secondary medical complications that affect independence (Houk 1991). In fact, public health professionals generally lacked an understanding of the factors affecting the lives of people with disabilities. It was natural, then, to spend ever more energy on the time-honored model of primary prevention—identifying the disease (in this case, disability), addressing the mechanisms for its cause (birth defect, developmental disability, injury, chronic illness), and intervening to reduce or prevent the primary condition from occurring. Modifying the model to address secondary problems of people already experiencing disability was difficult, to say the least. Changes included seeing disability not as a negative outcome such as illness and injury but rather as a health state experienced by the person and influenced by the environment, as well as accepting the premise that people with disabilities can be healthy.

People with disabilities have pressed for involvement in any areas affecting their lives. "Nothing about us without us," the disability community mantra, is now in the public domain. "Disability prevention" is viewed by many in the disability community as an attempt at least to devalue if not eliminate the lives of people with disabilities, and primary prevention activities are perceived as the implementation of this concept. The public health community, on the other hand, has tended to see disability as a purely medical issue. Contributing to the tension has been public health's failure to frame comments, survey questions, or presentations with sensitivity to the concerns of people with disabilities who increasingly identify themselves as a minority group. Although conceptually it may be possible to move seamlessly from the primary prevention of conditions creating disabilities to promoting the health and well-being of people with disabilities, practically, this shift has not occurred. Over time, it may be possible to integrate the best of public health science and practice into the advocacy and networks of people with disabilities to create a powerful force for improving the health of this segment of the public. Until that time, data, interventions, and programs may continue to seem somewhat artificial. Public health programs that view people with disabilities as a population to whom their primary prevention messages should be directed are the most helpful way to begin the integration. For example, programs should provide information to people with mobility limitations about preventing falls or provide cancer screens for people using catheters or bowel stimulation programs.

MAJOR WORKS: DATA

Data resulting from this emerging public health perspective have grown in their capacity to track conditions associated with disability. Four principal associations have been made with disability in the primary prevention public health model, regardless of the country where people with disabilities reside (Australian Institute of Health and Welfare 1997; Secretary of State for Health 1991). These associations include birth defects, developmental disabilities, injuries, and chronic diseases or conditions. As data are presented, it is important to understand that definitions of *disability* may differ across various "causes." For example, a diagnosis of cerebral palsy or spinal cord injury itself often defines a disability. At other times, disability may refer to the activity limitations experienced by a person with a particular diagnosis. Different approaches to data collection produce different statistics, often making comparisons impossible. The reasonable emphasis in primary prevention statistics is to make the connection between certain characteristics and certain outcomes. For example, motor vehicle crashes create the largest percentage of spinal cord injuries. Low birth weight is strongly related to developmental disabilities, such as cerebral palsy, sensory impairments, or mental retardation. It is clear that identifying such relationships is required to provide the basis for interventions if these conditions are to be reduced or prevented. Wearing seat belts and providing adequate prenatal care are examples of primary prevention activities within the public health model. Intervention approaches will be further explored later in this chapter.

Birth Defects Data

Birth defects have been the leading cause of infant mortality in the United States over the past few years (Erickson 1997). Currently, surveillance data are collected in nearly 40 states in the United States, and a National Birth Defects Prevention Network has been developed (Edmonds 1997). The International Clearinghouse for Birth Defects (1991) has chronicled the establishment of birth defects surveillance programs in European countries and the United States as a result of the thalidomide outbreak some 40 years ago. Because there are often no prevention strategies, the natural product of the known strategies focuses on preventing the condition and reducing costs to society. Particular attention has been given to research showing that folic acid use among women in childbearing years could reduce neural tube defects by at least 50 percent (Mulinare and Erickson 1997). Intervention strategies, therefore, emphasize increasing the number of women of childbearing age who have adequate amounts of folic acid in their daily diet. Other conditions are those associated with alcohol use during pregnancy but often not identified until much later (fetal alcohol syndrome [FAS]) or with a chromosomal anomaly (Down syndrome). The prevalence of FAS is estimated to be 1.4 per 1,000 live births, while Down syndrome is estimated at 1 per 1,000 live births. Intervention for FAS can clearly focus on women of childbearing age not drinking if pregnancy is a possibility or not getting pregnant if drinking is not eliminated. There is, as yet, no preventive activity for Down syndrome. Of course, numerous other conditions are monitored in birth defects surveillance systems, but likewise, no prevention strategies have been identified.

Developmental Disabilities Data

Population-based data on developmental disabilities are very difficult to collect. *Developmental disabilities* is the term used to describe a group of severe chronic conditions that affect basic areas of function during the childhood or adolescent period. The conditions usually include cognitive delay/deficit or sensory or motor impairments. The first population-based study of the prevalence of these conditions in the United States is the Metropolitan Atlanta Developmental Disabilities Study (MADDS). Among 10-year-old children, the multiple-source approach found the prevalence of various conditions per 1,000 children—mental retardation, 10.3; cerebral palsy, 2.0; hearing impairment, 1.0; and visual impairment, 0.6 (Yeargin-Allsop et al. 1992). For this study, most of the data were collected through school system identification. The Research and Training Center on Community Living at the University of Minnesota has analyzed the U.S. National Health Interview Survey, Disability Supplement (NHIS-D). The

1994 to 1995 family household survey produced a prevalence of 1.62 percent of the total population with mental retardation or other developmental disabilities (MR/DD Data Brief 1999). The definition of *developmental disabilities* explicitly requires substantial limitations in major life activities, such as self-care, receptive and expressive language, learning, mobility, self-direction, ability for independence, and economic self-sufficiency. For purposes of intervention, one study has shown the use of magnesium sulfate associated with decreasing cerebral palsy and mental retardation among very low birth weight infants (Schendel et al. 1996). Murphy et al. (1998) suggest that research addressing the relationship between socioeconomic and other factors for mental retardation, while challenging, is an important area for exploration.

Injury Data

Injuries are also closely associated with disabilities. Given the continuing acknowledgment of the need for primary prevention strategies to reduce mortality and disability associated with injuries, the NCIPC has developed guidelines for collecting information on central nervous system injuries (CDC 1996). This surveillance protocol allows continuity of data collection across states within the United States. Data show that there are 33 million injury-related emergency department visits each year in the United States, the most common causes being motor vehicle crashes, falls, and violence. Twenty-five percent of the injuries treated during emergency department visits are alcohol related. Traumatic brain injuries affect 2 million people, while spinal cord injuries hospitalize 10,000 people each year (CDC 1997b). Rehabilitation services are not available consistently across the country, and many that are geographically accessible are not financially accessible (CDC 1999b). Violence against women has also been a major public health concern. NCIPC estimates that 1.8 million women are assaulted each year.

Prevention activities have emphasized improved trauma care, improved counseling regarding alcohol use, and partnering with the National Institute of Justice to complete a national survey that could estimate partner violence and health outcomes. Results indicate that initiation of a trauma care system can decrease preventable deaths by 50 percent, as demonstrated in Orange County, California. Clinical preventive services focusing on alcohol use counseling can reduce consumption for 20 percent of patients with mild or even moderate drinking patterns (CDC 1999b). The violence survey will identify gaps in information about violence toward women and will provide the basis for a research program to address the problem. Women with disabilities would appear to be a particularly vulnerable group, given the results of research in Texas (Nosek et al. 1997) and Massachusetts (Myers et al. 1997).

Chronic Disease Data

Chronic disease is another major contributor to disability, creating major activity limitations for more than 1 of every 10 people in the United States—approximately 25 million people. Chronic disease also is responsible for 7 of 10 deaths each year. Cardiovascular disease causes about 40 percent (960,000) of all deaths in the United States each year (CDC 1998a). In addition, as the population ages, chronic conditions will increase. The NCCDPHP indicates that 16 percent of the population was older than age 60 in 1998, but by 2020, that percentage will increase to 25.

Preventive measures in the field of chronic diseases focus on four areas: promoting individual healthy behaviors, expanding early detection activities, providing intensive health education in schools and communities, and enhancing healthy communities. These public health activities clearly are relevant to all people, including people with disabilities. The individual behaviors related to extinguishing tobacco use, increasing physical activity, and encouraging good nutrition are extremely relevant for people with disabilities. For example, data from the Behavioral Risk Factor Surveillance System (BRFSS) indicate that people with disabilities are more likely to smoke than are people without disabilities (Wilber et al. 1998). Likewise, early screening for chronic diseases such as cancer, diabetes, and arthritis is crucial for people with disabilities, who may be more vulnerable but often do not receive adequate primary health care. Unfortunately, in many of the population-based surveys, there is no demographic-like variable identifying "people with disabilities" for purposes of comparing rates of cancer, diabetes, and arthritis. Rather, emphasis is on these conditions "creating" disability. Population-based data are not available to make that connection because people with disabilities are not identified, thereby eliminating the opportunity to place this group alongside other subgroups of the population, such as men and women, ethnic or racial groups, socioeconomic status, or education level. Children and adolescents in school may be exempt from physical and health education, and special education classes are often not included in health education curricula. Finally, communities encourage health for the population by establishing health promotion programs or walking trails, but these are not accessible to people with disabilities. The potential for public health primary prevention activities to include people with disabilities is substantial but not currently strong.

All the data sources previously described focus on a particular diagnostic group. The basis for this emphasis is twofold: the medical orientation of public health and the correlative use of the *ICD* as the basis for data collection and surveillance activities. As a result, public health stresses developing and implementing interventions on the basis of a diagnostic group. The emphasis, then, is on primary prevention, not on the people who already experience the condition. A recurring theme is the lack of public health emphasis on people who fall through the primary prevention net.

Even if public health attempts to address the health of people with disabilities, this approach can only focus on those conditions selected as most prevalent, most severe, or most costly. Although these are worthy criteria, they do not cover all individuals experiencing limitations, thereby excluding from public health interventions many people with disabilities. In view of this gap and in the context of the public health model, an alternative system for identifying people with disabilities is required. A public health framework for disability needs to include a conceptual system that encompasses all limitations, outlines the constructs, and provides a way to classify limitations for the purpose of surveillance.

Proposed Data Framework

The system that most nearly meets these needs is the World Health Organization's (1997) *International Classification of Impairments, Disabilities, and Handicaps (ICIDH-2)*. This conceptual model is the revision of the classification system begun in 1980 to elaborate the consequences of diseases, disorders, and injuries that are classified using the *ICD*. This system has been outlined previously in this volume. For these purposes, suffice it to say that the *ICIDH-2* provides a classification system addressing broader dimensions of a person's life beyond diagnosis. For public health use in disability, there needs to be the opportunity to focus on limitations in activities, regardless of diagnosis. A person's limitations in moving around, for example, because of cerebral palsy, spinal cord injury, or stroke present similar challenges. This cross-diagnosis approach is well illustrated by "seeing" limitations. Regardless of the reason for having poor vision, similar challenges for mobility, personal care, and domestic activities are present. "Activity limitations" is one of the four dimensions of the *ICIDH-2*. The *ICIDH-2* provides the system for crossing diagnostic groups to permit data collection. Additional important dimensions of the *ICIDH-2* include classifications of body functions and structures, such as mental functions or reproductive functions; participation in society, including work, self-determination, social relations, civic events, and so on; and environmental factors, including social attitudes, policies, and systems and physical, built, and communication environments.

This approach to conducting cross-diagnostic data analysis, however, is still in its infancy. Lollar and Fedeyko (1999) and Hough, Campbell, and Lollar (1999) have followed the lead of

Hogan et al. (1997) in using the disability supplement of the 1994 to 1995 National Health Interview Survey to generate data using activity limitations, rather than diagnoses, as the framework for classifying persons with disabilities. Data from these analyses allow national and state public health programs to focus on the actual limits experienced by people with disabilities, providing the basis for public health interventions regardless of diagnosis. Instruments to measure participation levels and environmental factors have been developed and are being piloted within the disability community and the general population.

Secondary Conditions

For public health to address the health of people with disabilities, the principal focus should be on preventing additional problems—called secondary conditions—and promoting healthy behaviors and a healthy environment. A *secondary condition* is defined as any condition to which a person with a primary diagnosis is more susceptible and may include medical, physical, emotional, family, or community problems. A second characteristic often associated with a secondary condition for public health purposes is that it does not have to occur; that is, it can be prevented. There is the need, then, to collect information about the various secondary conditions experienced by people with disabilities. Virtually no emphasis has been given to understanding these various conditions. The prime example of secondary conditions that cross diagnoses is that of skin sores, decubitus ulcers, and pressure sores. This breakdown of skin is not unusual for individuals who have poor sensation, regardless of cause. Skin sores are common for people who experience spina bifida or spinal cord injury. Public health should address this secondary condition across diagnoses. Of course, any medical facility or professional specializing in a particular medical condition, such as spinal cord injury, will treat pressure sores. It is only recently, however, that preventing secondary conditions has received attention as a public health concern.

The concept of prevention acquires a different meaning in the context of secondary conditions. Prevention addresses secondary conditions and is usually associated with health promotion. In this context, prevention loses its negative connotation of preventing the person with a disability from living. Instead, emphasizing the prevention of these conditions creates a positive message to maintain health, participate in societal activities, and increase quality of life. To prevent secondary conditions, we must first identify and count them. In rehabilitation, when a secondary condition appears to occur frequently in a group, programs are initiated to prevent its onset. In public health, however, the approach is broader, may involve medical personnel, but may also include advocacy groups, independent living centers, and community organizations, including fitness centers and churches. The key to public health intervention is the ability to monitor how often a condition is occurring, provide an intervention, and continue to track how many people are affected. Surveillance of secondary conditions is even more challenging than surveillance for limitations across diagnostic groups. An important part of the surveillance of secondary conditions is identifying environmental factors that may contribute to a person's medical status and general well-being. The lack of reliable transportation may lead to poor physical conditioning, creating vulnerability to respiratory problems as well as depression and social isolation. Appropriate surveillance for secondary conditions requires the capacity to monitor these factors in the environment.

Several instruments have been developed to measure secondary conditions among people with disabilities. Seekins et al. (1990) generated a 40-item surveillance tool for use across diagnostic groups. In fact, one of the most important findings of the early structural analysis was the lack of a relationship between specific impairments and secondary conditions—that is, specific diagnoses did not predict which secondary conditions would be found. Rather, certain secondary conditions clustered in a syndrome-like fashion, and others focused on severity of impairment, regardless of impairment (Ravesloot, Seekins, and Walsh 1997). The "common knowledge" that each medical diagnosis includes its own set of secondary conditions was not supported by the data. While it may be true that certain medical and physical conditions are more associated with particular activity limitations, specific diagnoses are not predictive of secondary conditions. White, Gutierrez, and Mace (1993) reported that 83 percent of independent living center consumers had experienced one or more secondary conditions within the past 6 months. Seekins et al. (1990) indicated that people with disabilities in Montana reported an average of 14 secondary conditions within the past 12 months, suggesting that secondary conditions are common.

Lollar (1997) modified the instrument for use with adolescents, including additional areas, such as social relationships, family conflicts, dependence, and behavior problems. Results indicated that secondary conditions among adolescents differed from those among adults in the Montana study. Also of interest were the results of a stepwise regression analysis indicating that behavior accounted for the largest portion of variance related to the number of secondary conditions. This finding indicates that behavioral, rather than medical or physical, factors contributed most to the presence of secondary conditions.

Krause (1998) developed a 50-item questionnaire to assess secondary conditions among persons with spinal cord injuries. The instrument included six general categories, five addressing body systems, such as cardiopulmonary or skin, plus psychosocial problems. Results suggest that muscle spasms, urinary tract infections, and muscle or joint pain are the three most prevalent physical secondary conditions during the previous 12 months for the sample.

Data on secondary conditions are just now emerging as instruments are developed. The need to collect population-based information on secondary conditions experienced by persons with disabilities is crucial for public health to generate health promotion programs and secondary condition prevention activities.

Data issues abound as public health scientists attempt to use the traditional public health model for addressing issues of disability. Particular interventions are much more clearly associated with specific causative factors related to conditions that contribute to disability. For example, substantial activity limitations can be associated with fetal alcohol syndrome, which leads logically to public health interventions focusing on drinking and pregnancy among women of childbearing age. While the risk behaviors of drinking and pregnancy may be difficult to address, there is clarity of data and science. To varying degrees, primary prevention activities have a clearer connection between the data and its collection and the interventions introduced to reduce the condition associated with disability. On the other hand, identifying secondary conditions among people with disabilities across the life span is neonatal by comparison. As surveillance instruments and data collection mechanisms are developed, secondary conditions will be understood more clearly, common patterns of secondary conditions perhaps related to activity limitations will be delineated, and intervention strategies will emerge with scientific and face validity.

INTERVENTION

In this section, intervention focusing on health promotion and prevention of secondary conditions among people with disabilities will be emphasized. Although each specific etiology associated with disability has substantial intervention activities, the chapter could not easily encompass them all. Particular interventions addressing prevention of secondary conditions and health promotion for specific conditions will be discussed.

Intervention levels can range from broad policy issues addressing poverty as it affects and is affected by disability, public health education, and the personal level associated with clinical or rehabilitation intervention. Public health intervention differs from clinical intervention, however, in that pubic health interventions usually are framed to influence a broad number of people—the public—rather than individually oriented clinical intervention. This does not mean that public health interventions cannot be implemented in a medical or rehabilitation setting. Instead, the aim is not deficit or medically focused but emphasizes health. Also, public health interventions are preventive in nature—that is, the activities attempt to keep a condition from oc-curring. Most countries, for example, have injury prevention programs in occupational settings, and many work sites provide health promotion activities, such as smoking cessation programs and fitness centers.

Primary Prevention Activities

Primary prevention activities attempt to keep conditions associated with disability from oc-curring so that the disabling condition is prevented. Moreover, primary prevention activities also try to target particularly vulnerable groups. For example, the Early Hearing Detection and Intervention (EHDI) program (CDC 1997a) is part of a national effort to improve early hearing screening, diagnosis, and intervention in the United States (CDC 1999a). This program focuses on identifying infants with hearing impairment to prevent communication limitations. Project Choices is an intervention targeting women at high risk for alcohol-exposed pregnancy, includ-ing women in jail, in alcohol treatment programs, in primary care settings, and women re-cruited though a media campaign (CDC 1999a). These are but two of the important intervention programs to reduce the incidence of FAS in children and to prevent the communi-cation problems associated with late diagnosis of hearing impairment.

Secondary Conditions Activities

Specific programs addressing the prevention of secondary conditions among people with disabilities are also being developed. The University of Illinois at Chicago has created a compre-hensive health promotion program with three major components (Rimmer and Hedman 1998). These components are exercise, nutrition, and health behavior. Individuals from several diagnostic categories, including stroke, diabetes, Down syndrome, and arthritis, are currently testing the program. Providing transportation for participants, culminating in a 90 percent at-tendance rate, has alleviated a major barrier to participation in such programs. It is important to replicate programs such as these so that health and wellness can become the focus of individuals with disabilities, rather than simply the absence of disease or illness.

Self-efficacy theory is the basis for another set of interventions. Lorig, Mazonson, and Homan (1993) have developed a self-management approach for individuals with chronic ill-nesses. Individuals are taught problem solving and decision making and how to tell their story to medical professionals. Lay leaders direct a four- to seven-week course using scripted material to help people know what to expect and to feel safe. Four-year follow-up has shown decreased pain and number of physician visits, with increased self-efficacy in the presence of increased ac-tivity limitations—a crucial finding. A parallel approach has been taken by Seekins et al. (1991), who developed *Living Well with a Disability*. This is a curriculum that has been shown to reduce secondary conditions by 37 percent and outpatient physician visits by 43 percent, when indi-viduals with disabilities who have completed the course are compared with other individuals with disabilities not experiencing the course. Currently, the curriculum is being used by eight independent living centers throughout the United States as a way of obtaining data about the potential cost-effectiveness of such an approach (Seekins and White 1997).

Groups who are at risk for a particular condition are usually identified by epidemiological studies; if people with disabilities were identified as at risk for the occurrence of a certain condi-tion, primary prevention efforts could be focused on them. For example, if cardiovascular dis-ease were associated with people with disabilities, hypothesized due to lack of opportunity to exercise, fitness programs for people with disabilities could be developed, implemented, and evaluated for effectiveness. Cardiac problems would be considered a secondary condition, a preventable condition associated with aspects of the primary disabling condition. Therefore, what is called primary prevention activities would be targeted to preventing secondary conditions among people with disabilities. This approach is more akin to the clinical end of the public health intervention spectrum.

Actually, clinical preventive services (CPS) are at the heart of public health interventions. The Institute of Medicine has defined *access* as "the timely use of personal health services to achieve the best possible health outcomes" (Millman 1993). Although access to clinical services is person oriented, the objective of providing them is prevention. Clinical preventive service guidelines were outlined in a 1989 report, revised in 1995 (U.S. Preventive Services Task Force 1996). The intent is to provide immunizations, screening tests, and counseling within a clinical setting to prevent disease and detect problems early when treatment is more effective. People with disabilities, again, are limited by the lack of available data to monitor whether they are receiving these services. Only two of the most common clinical preventive services address individuals with disabilities. Both focus on women older than age 55 with a disability and their use of Pap smear tests and mammograms. Data suggest that an equal percentage of women with and without limitations have had at least one Pap smear in their lives, but women with limitations of simple movements, such as reaching and grasping, more frequently do not return for regular exams. Older women and those with more severe limitations are less likely than others to adhere to the recommendations. Women with limitations are also less likely to receive mammograms (CDC 1998b).

Predictors of receiving clinical preventive services include having health insurance, higher income, and a primary care provider. To the extent that many people with disabilities are relatively poor, are therefore often on government plans that may not provide CPS, and may have specialty but not primary care, they are at risk for not having the services needed to prevent secondary conditions. In addition, the inaccessibility of clinical offices undermines access to the services.

Education

To the extent that an intervention, however, includes people with disabilities as another part of the "public," the issue is making sure that this select population has access and information, including materials in Braille or in acceptable formats to facilitate communication. Dissemination of information in various formats is a critical public health issue for people with communication limitations.

Education is another major public health intervention, particularly through the dissemination of community-based materials. The National Arthritis Action Plan (Arthritis Foundation 1999) places great emphasis on increasing awareness of arthritis, the importance of early diagnosis, appropriate management, and effective interventions. *Physical Activity and Health* (U.S. Department of Health and Human Services [DHHS] 1996) was a report of the U.S. Surgeon General. In that report, educational emphasis was placed on increasing the amount of time spent by elementary school students being physically active in physical education classes. However, children in special education classes often are not identified as being at risk for decreased physical activity, a problem that underscores the need for inclusion of individuals with disabilities in important public health messages and activities.

Societal Interventions

The broadest level of intervention is at the societal level. Fujiura (1999), LaPlante (1997), and Yelin (1998) report the significant relationship between disability and socioeconomic status. Disability may predispose one to lower socioeconomic status, and low-income status may predispose one to disability. While the exact nature of the relationship is unclear, the association is, nonetheless, strong. Hogan et al. (1997) and Bresloski et al. (1999), in addition, have shown that for families that have a child with an activity limitation(s) and adults with activity limitations, having less than a high school education accounts for much of the variance associated with racial or socioeconomic differences. While not directly the mandate of public health, it is clear that interventions to increase educational attainment or achievement and increase employment rates are extremely relevant to people with disabilities.

OUTCOMES

Given the breadth of data pursued and the range of interventions, public health outcomes are also in the eye of the beholder. Outcomes in primary prevention, for example, are the presence of a spinal cord injury or a particular birth defect, such as spina bifida. The reduction of these events is the desired outcome of a public health intervention. This approach to outcomes is relatively straightforward on the surface. Count the number of children born with spina bifida, for example, before and after an intervention to increase the consumption of folic acid by women of childbearing age, and the outcome is apparent. Of course, at each step of the process, there are substantial barriers. "Counting the number" requires having personnel who will be diligent in reporting each case—whether in a relatively small geographical area, such as metropolitan Atlanta, or progressively larger areas, such as a state, region, or nationally. Consistent counting is much more difficult than it appears. "With spina bifida" requires consistent identification. While spina bifida is usually identifiable at birth, there is no consistent reporting from hospitals. Moreover, in some conditions, such as FAS or autism, identification does not come at birth but later. Criteria for deciding if a child has the condition are often difficult to identify reliably. "Before and after intervention" on a national scale assumes good condition identification and reliable reporting across time, and it assumes the intervention is going to be evenly implemented across whatever population is being targeted. In the case of folic acid consumption, even when the target group is women of childbearing age—not a small group in any country—outcomes are complicated. A second intervention-related level of outcome is added, usually the percentage of women who report taking sufficient folic acid in their normal eating regimen or by supplement. Outcomes become nested, one relating to another.

Spinal cord injury is another example of an outcome targeted by public health interventions. The approach is to use hospital data as a method for tracking the number of individuals coming to hospitals and diagnosed with a spinal cord injury. Information about the cause of the injury and circumstances surrounding the injury and demographic information is collected. Analysis of these data allows public health staff to establish factors most related to the injury (e.g., 18- to 35-year-old men) and develop intervention strategies at this group. This might include media campaigns to increase seat belt use or to discourage diving into unknown bodies of water. As the interventions begin, the outcome sought is a decrease in spinal cord injuries related to these causes in this age group.

Public health outcomes related to secondary conditions are much more difficult to put into effect. For people with disabilities, the outcomes are actually the opportunity to participate in life activities on a par with everyone else in the society. Traditionally presented, public health would focus only on physical or medical outcomes that undermine participation. The World Health Organization, however, has conceived health as not just the absence of disease but as the presence of vitality, and the goals include physical, social, and spiritual well-being. This, of course, substantially broadens the potential outcomes to be addressed by public health professionals. Outcomes could then not only include the actual levels of participation in activities and the negative physical conditions that contribute to that loss of participation but could also address issues of access to health care from both a physical perspective ("Can I get to the physician's office?" or "Can I get into the physician's office?") to systems access ("Are assistive devices covered by my medical plan?"). Environmental barriers can be as toxic to the health of people with disabilities as water or air pollution.

In the broad area of public health outcomes, numerous summary measures of health status have been developed, including years of healthy life and quality-adjusted life years (QALYs).

QALYs have been the accepted U.S. Public Health Service metric for summary health. This measure combines costs with quality-of-life assessment so that economic and person-centered factors are included. Years of healthy life makes the assumption that "healthy" life includes those without a disability. This assumption again equates disability with lack of health, interpreted as illness. WHO, along with the World Bank, has sponsored a project to develop and implement the Global Burden of Disease Study at Harvard University (Murray and Lopez 1996). The basis for the project is to attempt to measure the impact of various conditions on the overall health status of people around the world. The outcome measure generated is called disability-adjusted life years (DALYs). Unfortunately, the developers have chosen to equate any "nonfatal health outcome" with disability (Hough 1999). Actually, the better term for this construct would be *morbidity*, as described earlier. While the goal of the project is an important one, equating morbidity with disability continues the tension between public health and disability communities. The actual conceptual, methodological, and statistical problems with the approach have been covered elsewhere in this volume; suffice it to say that DALYs represent an additional element to increase suspicion of the public health community by the disability community.

RESEARCH ISSUES

As with every area of endeavor, public health surveillance and research activities should be grounded by the participation of persons with disabilities from the questions asked to the design, implementation, analysis, and dissemination of scientific information. This approach is not the traditional one taken by public health to any scientific study, but communities are beginning to be involved in public health activities. *Community* in the usual public health approach is defined geographically. When there has been, for example, a concern that an environmental hazard threatens the lives and health of a community, public health staff have become sensitized to the need to involve the community in planning and implementing its assessment and intervention strategies. The concept of community was expanded during the HIV/AIDS epidemic when public health activities targeted the community of homosexual men. The disability "community" again requires expansion of the concept, beyond geography and lifestyle. Diversity is present in the disability community, but the disability perspective must be represented throughout public activity activities.

Given the broad range of public health data, interventions, and outcomes, numerous issues arise. Surveillance issues first emphasize the need for a case definition. That is, if one is to count the number of persons with a condition, that condition must be defined. In primary prevention activities, the case definition is usually associated with a diagnosis (e.g., cerebral palsy or traumatic brain injury) often made by a medical staff member. If, on the other hand, one is striving to identify "people with disabilities" to assess whether their level of participation in school or work or community activities parallels everyone else in the society, defining "people with disabilities" can be enormously challenging. Medical personnel may equate a diagnosis with disability. People with a diagnosis, however, may not identify themselves as having a disability or even a limitation, except that created by environmental barriers. In addition, certain groups of individuals with limitations may be excluded from surveys. For example, people with hearing impairments may not be able to respond to telephone surveys. Individuals with mobility limitations may not be able to get to a telephone before the survey staff hangs up. Persons with learning limitations may be viewed as unreliable in their responses. Research to close these gaps should continue until all gaps are filled.

Problems also arise when research projects are designed to address the needs of people with disabilities. Again, environmental barriers can reduce involvement among those interested in participating (Rimmer and Hedman 1998). Transportation, for example, may also affect retention in the studies (White 1998). In the United States, an additional research issue is framed by emphasis on costs of intervention and the effectiveness of interventions from a cost perspective. As presented earlier, QALYs are an attempt to integrate cost and quality-of-life measures into a summary measure. For people with disabilities, developing a case for interventions to prevent secondary conditions and promote health is a particularly challenging one. Data such as that presented by Kinsman and Doehring (1996) reported that 47 percent of hospital admissions of adults with spina bifida over an 11-year period were due to secondary conditions, which were potentially preventable. These types of data are needed to highlight the need for appropriate interventions. Work by Seekins et al. (1996) has provided evidence that self-help groups targeting preventing and managing secondary conditions have decreased secondary conditions by 37 percent and have decreased physician visits by 45 percent over a six-month follow-up period. A comparison group not receiving the intervention did not show similar results.

In those instances when financial issues may not be as pertinent, other research issues may arise. The Royal College of Physicians (1998) in the United Kingdom published a charter and guidelines, titled *Disabled People Using Hospitals*. This document grew out of a 1992 charter that outlined the needs of people with disabilities in hospitals and by the 1995 Disability Discrimination Act. This document is important for several reasons, including the cooperative efforts of physicians and consumers in the project, the community-based approach, and the potential for more services for people with disabilities. Research is now needed to evaluate the degree to which the guidelines are being implemented and the impact of this effort on the health of people with disabilities.

MAJOR DIRECTIONS

Public Health and Disability Communication

A new sense of opportunity is emerging across the world as well as a developing convergence of new and focused direction for the disability community. The disability movement continues to be strengthened through organizations such as Disabled Peoples' International (DPI) (Hurst 1999) and Rehabilitation International. Public health disability researchers are as likely themselves to have a disability as not. Also, many of those who do not currently experience a disability are in close collaboration with those who do. Disability advocates are intimately involved with public health directions and issues, demonstrated most clearly in DPI's executive director chairing the World Health Organization's Environmental Task Force for revising the *ICIDH-2*. Public health's awareness of issues related to people with disabilities is growing. Public health history, then, is being changed by this participatory action in both research and policy. The glow of positive change, however, cannot overshadow substantial issues that still exist. Still, the first major direction is the conversation that is developing between public health professionals and the disability community.

Unifying Framework

Domzal (1995) has presented the 50 or so different definitions of disability included in U.S. statutes. The United Nations (1996) has also indicated the varied and diagnostically oriented definitions of disability in countries responding to United Nations questions about disability surveillance. For the purpose of clarifying policy and program issues, more consistent constructs must be used to identify people who experience disabilities. Definitions have tended to emphasize medically related information as a proxy for disability. A second major public health emphasis is clarifying definitions and a framework for disability.

With collaboration from advocates in the disability community, public health is drawing closer to establishing a common framework from which surveillance, policy, and programmatic activities can emerge. The *ICIDH-2*, providing a broad framework in which "disability" refers to the overarching construct, can provide that unifying approach. For public health purposes, it is crucial to distinguish among body functions, the person's activities or limits in those activities, and the person's participation in the society, as well as to acknowledge the influence of the environment at each of these levels of experience. Otherwise, if these various dimensions are mixed together for counting purposes, there will always be confusion about which factors affect which. Public health historically has used a linear model focusing exclusively on the body functions or dysfunctions of the person, and that assumes the person's body dysfunctions and activity limitations are totally responsible for the individual's lack of involvement in the society (e.g., not working). Environmental factors were excluded because of the difficulty in measuring them. *ICIDH-2* provides the opportunity to clarify the conceptual framework, differentiate the varied constructs, and provide clearer definitions of dimensions and a classification system. In the coming years, such a unifying effort across public health and disability communities should continue to be strengthened.

The most important reason to address definitional and conceptual questions is to increase awareness of the needs and concerns of people with disabilities around the world. A second reason, however, specifically relates to another major public health issue outlined in this chapter. Primary prevention activities, using the *ICIDH-2* perspective, address preventing conditions that can create "impairments" at the body function or structure level. Public health professionals may be concerned about the morbidity associated with these impairments, but they are generally less or not at all concerned with the person-level activity limitations, restrictions in societal participation, or environmental factors that affect health and well-being. The nuances are less important than the actual impairment. Rather than continuing to confound public health data, policy, and programs, awareness of the different constructs related to disability can provide the basis for integration of public health efforts.

Public Health Perceptions

A third basic issue emerges from this discussion—using people who have disabilities in media campaigns as examples of the negative results of "risk behaviors" by the general population. Public health must move beyond its tendency to devalue the lives of people with disabilities in the name of preventing disability. Impairments, even personal limitations, should not be portrayed as inimical to the human condition. This tendency builds mistrust among people with disabilities for anything associated with public health and also is a barrier to public health professionals seeing people with disabilities as a population at risk for other health concerns.

At the heart of this issue is the human tendency to find ways to categorize and place value and to stereotype on the basis of imputed inferiority. Public health, truth be told, is but one part of the global society that fears the loss of perceived physical, mental, or emotional perfection sufficiently to place less value on the lives and experiences of those with limitations. If, indeed, there is still survival of the fittest, then people with disabilities must be the fittest, given the physical, social, and policy barriers to be overcome. The public health community, however, must acknowledge that portraying images of people with disabilities in primary prevention media campaigns demeans the life experience of people with disabilities. This is no way to make a case for encouraging or discouraging targeted behaviors, whether wearing seat belts to reduce spinal cord injuries or taking folic acid to reduce the incidence of neural tube defects.

The public health sector is a part of those mapping the human genome (Khoury 1997). People with disabilities are concerned that this activity will lead to public health decisions that once again devalue the experience of disability to the extent of trying to eliminate those people who have certain genetic makeups that are associated with impairments or limitations. The need for including people with disabilities in the decision-making processes about the use of genome mapping is crucial. In addition, people with disabilities in the United States cannot separate this discussion from the current assisted-suicide debate, in which some medical doctors are moving the line between "death with dignity" for those with terminal illness closer to assisted suicide for people with varied disabilities (Hahn 1998). Those in the fields of public health and disability must use every mechanism at their disposal to discuss these gravely important issues.

Healthy People with Disabilities

A fourth significant and positive contribution, which public health is making to people with disabilities, is the development of health objectives for the year 2010. Healthy People is the national public health agenda, begun for 1990, continued for 2000, and moving into the new millennium (U.S. DHHS 1998). While several countries, including the United Kingdom (1993) have long-term health objectives, these objectives have dealt mostly with primary prevention activities. For the public health objectives for the year 2010, the U.S. Department of Health and Human Services began an initiative to include objectives for people with disabilities. These objectives have provided an opportunity to frame important issues of health and well-being for people with disabilities. Dr. Gro Brundtland (1999), the current World Health Organization director general, has stated that "health is a basic human right." She described health as "physical, mental and social well-being which includes participation in the full range of personal and social activities" (p. 57). The *Healthy People 2010* chapter, "Disability and Secondary Conditions," outlines basic directions for the future, encompassing the elements of well-being outlined by Dr. Brundtland.

The objectives in this chapter have been to address major health and well-being concerns for people with disabilities. These include standard data items to identify people with disabilities across health surveys in the United States, a demographic-like variable. This will allow the opportunity to describe people with disabilities along with other select populations, such as sex, race, ethnicity, and socioeconomic status. Sufficient emotional support and assistance will be an objective for both children and adults with disabilities. Emphasis on increasing social participation and life satisfaction is included. Objectives emphasize increasing employment rates of people with disabilities to those without disabilities and increasing regular education time for students with disabilities. Reducing the negative impact of environmental barriers for people with disabilities is also discussed, with additional emphasis on ensuring that, consistent with the Americans with Disabilities Act (ADA), health and wellness facilities and treatment programs be fully accessible to people with disabilities. Other objectives are increasing the use of appropriate assistive technology and devices. Eliminating institutions for children with developmental disabilities and reducing by half the number of adults with developmental disabilities living in institutions are another objective. Finally, the last of the 13 objectives focuses on implementing disability and health programs in each state, territory, and tribal unit in the United States. Surveillance activities and health promotion programs are needed both for people with disabilities and for caregivers.

The history of public health and disability has been long and often filled with tension. There is still tension, but the outlines of a new relationship around the world can be seen. Several public health directions are beginning and will require considerable attention in the coming years to further strengthen the growing commitment to improving the health of people with disabilities.

Developing a public health framework, which can be used throughout the world, will be a first and major step. While this activity may seem of little importance, global acceptance of a mutually acceptable set of concepts and terms by public health and the disability community will provide the atmosphere for significant growth. The World Health Organization's inclusion of people with disabilities in the revision of its *ICIDH-2* is a major step forward. In addition, the United Nations' disability statistics activity to standardize questions about disability for census and surveys globally using the WHO framework will provide further continuity and direction. The development of a disability-friendly summary health measure is also critical. This, however, will require continued challenging of measures, such as DALYs, which maintain an antiquated notion of disability. Finally, instruments that assess the role of environmental factors on health and well-being will be crucial if data are to influence policy.

From the standpoint of policy development, there will need to be continued efforts to eliminate the disparities in access to medical and other health services. The sources may be as diverse as medical staff's negative attitudes, poor or no transportation to health care facilities, or equipment that does not accommodate the needs of people with disabilities. In addition, public health mechanisms could be the conduit for evaluating environmental barriers that undermine the health of people with disabilities. Public health personnel are in a unique position to influence medical and health care policy, already possessing a population perspective. The implementation of universal design principles could be evaluated through public health mechanisms across these settings. Public health could lead in this venture to improve the health and well-being by eliminating the environmental barriers to medical and health care. Of course, as with other interventions, these would improve the lives of all people, not just those with disabilities. Public health now has the opportunity to be partners with the disability community, encouraging societal participation, eliminating environmental barriers, and improving health and well-being.

REFERENCES

Arthritis Foundation. 1999. *National Arthritis Action Plan: A Public Health Strategy*. Atlanta, GA: Author.

Australian Institute of Health and Welfare. 1997. *Australia's Welfare 1997: Services and Assistance*. Canberra, Australia: Author.

Bresloski, T., D. Hamel, J. Panarace, J. Park, D. Hogan, and R. C. Avery. 1999. *Functional Limitations among Rhode Island Adults, 1996*. Providence: Rhode Island Department of Public Health.

Brundtland, G. H. 1999. *World Disability Report: Disability '99*. Geneva: International Disability Foundation.

Centers for Disease Control and Prevention (CDC). 1996. *Guidelines for Surveillance of Central Nervous System Injury*. Atlanta, GA: National Center for Injury Prevention and Control.

———. 1997a. *Early Hearing Detection and Intervention Program*. Atlanta, GA: National Center for Environmental Health.

———. 1997b. *Program Briefing*. Atlanta, GA: National Center for Injury Control and Prevention.

———. 1998a. *Program Briefing*. Atlanta, GA: National Center for Chronic Disease Prevention and Health Promotion.

———. 1998b. "Utilization of Cervical and Breast Cancer Screening in the United States among Women with and without Functional Limitations." *Morbidity and Mortality Weekly* 47 (40): 853-56.

———. 1999a. *Program Briefing*. Atlanta, GA: National Center for Environmental Health.

———. 1999b. *Home Page* [Online]. Atlanta, GA: National Center for Injury Prevention and Control. Available: www.cdc.gov.

Chamie, M. 1995. "What Does Morbidity Have to Do with Disability?" *Disability and Rehabilitation* 17 (7): 323-37.

Domzal, C. 1995. *Federal Statutory Definitions of Disability*. Washington, DC: National Institute on Disability and Rehabilitation Research.

Edmonds, L. D. 1997. "Birth Defect Surveillance at the State and Local Level." *Teratology* 56 (1): 5-7.

Erickson, J. D. 1997. "Introduction: Birth Defects Surveillance in the United States." *Teratology* 56 (1): 1-4.

Fujiura, G. 1999. "Disability Trends among Minority Populations." Paper presented at the Secondary Conditions and Minorities Conference, March, Chicago.

Hahn, H. 1998. "No Need for Dr. Death." *Los Angeles Times,* November 26.

Hogan, D. P., M. E. Msall, M. L. Rogers, and R. C. Avery. 1997. "Improved Disability Population Estimates of Functional Limitation among American Children Aged 5-17." *Maternal and Child Health Journal* 1 (4): 203-16.

Hough, J. 1999. "Important Considerations about 'Disability-Adjusted Life Years' as Outcome Measurements for Disability Research Studies." Unpublished manuscript.

Hough, J., V. Campbell, and D. Lollar. 1999. "State Estimates of Activity Limitations Using NHIS-D Phase I Data." Paper presented at the National Data Users Conference, August, Washington, DC.

Houk, V. N. 1991. "Plenary: Opening Session." Paper presented at the National Conference on the Prevention of Primary and Secondary Disabilities, June, Atlanta, GA.

Houk, V. N. and S. B. Thacker. 1989. "The Centers for Disease Control Program to Prevent Primary and Secondary Disabilities in the United States." *Public Health Reports* 104 (3): 226-31.

Hurst, R. 1999. "Ways of Making you Talk." Pp. 48-50 in *World Disability Report: Disability '99*. Geneva: World Disability Foundation.

International Clearinghouse for Birth Defects. 1991. *Congenital Malformations*. Amsterdam: Elsevier.

Khoury, M. 1997. *Translating Advances in Human Genetics into Public Health Action: A Strategic Plan*. Atlanta, GA: National Center for Environmental Health/CDC.

Kinsman, S. L. and M. C. Doehring. 1996. "The Cost of Preventable Conditions in Adults with Spina Bifida." *European Journal of Pediatric Surgery* 6 (96, Suppl. 11): 17-20.

Krause, J. S. 1998. *The 20-Year Minnesota Longitudinal Study: Applications to Secondary Conditions after Spinal Cord Injury*. Atlanta, GA: Centers for Disease Control and Prevention.

LaPlante, M. 1997. "Trends in Disability Prevalence." Paper presented at the Fourth National Disability Statistics and Policy Forum, June, Washington, DC.

Linden, A., A. Me, and J. Vanek. 1996. "Improving Statistics on the Population with Disabilities: Work of the United Nations Statistics Division." Unpublished paper.

Lollar, D. J. 1997. "Secondary Conditions among Adolescents with Spina Bifida." *European Journal of Pediatric Surgery* 7 (Suppl. 1): 55.

Lollar, D. J. and H. Fedeyko. 1999. "Activity Limitation Scales Using NHIS-D Data." Paper presented at the National Data Users Conference, August, Washington, DC.

Lorig, K. R., P. D. Mazonson, and H. R. Homan. 1993. "Evidence Suggesting That Health Education for Self-Management in Patients with Chronic Arthritis Has Sustained Health Benefits While Reducing Health Care Costs." *Arthritis Rheum* 36 (4): 439-46.

Madden, R. and T. Hogan. 1997. *The Definition of Disability in Australia: Moving towards National Consistency*. Canberra, Australia: AIHW.

Millman, M., ed. 1993. *Access to Health Care in America*. Washington, DC: National Academy Press.

"MR/DD Data Brief." 1999. *1994 National Health Interview Survey: Disability Supplement* 1:1-7.

Mulinare, J. and J. D. Erickson. 1997. "Prevention of Neural Tube Defects." *Teratology* 56:17-18.

Murphy, C. C., C. Boyle, D. Schendel, P. Decoufle, and M. Yeargin-Allsop. 1998. "Epidemiology of Mental Retardation in Children." *Mental Retardation and Developmental Disabilities Research Review* 4:6-13.

Murray, C. J. L. and A. D. Lopez. 1996. *The Global Burden of Disease*. Geneva: World Health Organization.

Myers, A. R., D. S. Mitchell, A. Bisbee, S. Brody, S. Garman, T. Jessiman, K. Kronenberg, C. Leon, N. Lynn, K. Page, K. Spaulding, T. Taylor, and M. Valdes. 1997. *Referrals of Complaints for Investigation and Criminal Prosecution by the Commonwealth of Massachusetts's Disabled Persons Protection Commission, 1995-1997*. Boston: Boston University School of Public Health.

Nosek, M. A., D. H. Rintala, M. E. Young, C. C. Foley, C. Howland, G. F. Chanpong, D. Rossi, J. Bennett, and K. Meroney. 1997. *National Study of Women with Physical Disabilities*. Houston, TX: Baylor College of Medicine.

Ravesloot, C., T. Seekins, and J. Walsh. 1997. "A Structural Analysis of Secondary Conditions of Primary Physical Disabilities." *Rehabilitation Psychology* 42 (1): 3-16.

Rimmer, J. H. and G. Hedman. 1998. "A Health Promotion Program for Stroke Survivors." *Topics in Stroke Rehabilitation* 5 (2): 30-44.

Royal College of Physicians. 1998. *Disabled People Using Hospitals: A Charter and Guide*. London: Author.

Schendel, D. E., C. J. Berg, M. Yeargin-Allsop, C. A. Boyle, and P. Decoufle. 1996. "Prenatal Magnesium Sulfate Exposure and the Risk for Cerebral Palsy or Mental Retardation among Very Low-Birth-Weight Children Aged 3 to 5 Years." *Journal of the American Medical Association* 276:1805-10.

Secretary of State for Health. 1991. *The Health of the Nation: A Consultative Document for Health in England*. London: Her Majesty's Stationery Office.

Seekins, T., J. Clay, S. Kirchmyer, O. Ali, K. Murphy, and C. Ravesloot. 1991. *Developing and Implementing a Program for Preventing and Managing Secondary Conditions Experienced by Adults with Physical Disabilities*. Missoula, MT: RTC on Rural Rehabilitation.

Seekins, T., C. Ravesloot, K. Norris, A. Szalda-Petree, Q. R. Young, G. White, K. Golden, J. C. Lopez, and J. Steward. 1996. "Cost Containment through Disability Prevention: Preliminary Results of a Health Promotion Workshop for People with Physical Disabilities." CDC Project Report R04/CCR808519-03-1, University of Montana, Missoula.

Seekins, T., N. Smith, T. McCleary, J. Clary, and J. Walsh. 1990. "Secondary Disability Prevention: Involving Consumers in the Development of a Public Health Surveillance Instrument." *Journal of Disability Policy Studies* 1 (3): 21-35.

Seekins, T. and G. White. 1997. "Health Promotion for People with Disabilities and Prevention of Secondary Conditions." Request for Proposals, Centers for Disease Control and Prevention, Office on Disability and Health, Atlanta, GA.

United Nations. 1996. *Manual for the Development of Statistical Information for Disability Programmes and Policies.* New York: Author.

U.S. Department of Health and Human Services (DHHS). 1996. *Physical Activity and Health: A Report of the Surgeon General.* Atlanta, GA: U.S. DHHS, CDCP, National Center for Chronic Disease Prevention and Health Promotion.

———. 1998. *Healthy People 2010 Objectives: Draft for Public Comment.* Washington, DC: DHHS Office of Disease Prevention and Health Promotion.

U.S. Preventive Services Task Force. 1996. *Guide to Clinical Preventive Services.* 2d ed. Baltimore: Williams & Wilkins.

White, G. 1998. "Health Promotion and Reduction of Secondary Conditions for Women with Mobility Limitations: Lessons Learned and New Directions." Paper presented at the National Conference on Disability and Health, October, Dallas, TX.

White, G., R. Gutierrez, and M. Mace. 1993. "Using Community Organization's Information Systems to Reduce Risks of Secondary Medical Conditions for People with Disabilities." Paper presented at the Fourth Biennial Conference on Community Research and Action, June, Williamsburg, VA.

Wilber, N., D. Allen, A. Meyers, and K. MacDonald. 1998. "Findings on Smoking Behavior and Efforts to Address Tobacco Use among Individuals with Disabilities in Massachusetts." Poster presented at the National Conference on Disability and Health, October, Dallas, TX.

World Health Organization. 1997. *International Classification of Impairments, Activities, and Participation: A Manual of Dimensions of Disablement and Functioning.* Beta Draft. Geneva: Author.

Yeargin-Allsop, M., C. C. Murphy, G. P. Oakley, and R. K. Sikes. 1992. "A Multiple-Source Method for Studying the Prevalence of Developmental Disabilities in Children: The Metropolitan Atlanta Developmental Disabilities Study." *Pediatrics* 89 (4): 624-30.

Yelin, E. 1998. "Prevalence of Work among Persons with Disabilities." Paper presented at the Interagency Subcommittee on Disability Statistics, April, San Francisco.

Disability in the Developing World

34

BENEDICTE INGSTAD

During the past two decades, there has been a considerable increase in professional interest concerning disability and rehabilitation in what may be called the developing world—most countries outside Europe and North America. The International Year of Disabled Persons (IYDP) in 1981 played an important role in promoting such awareness, locally as well as internationally. The increased interest in programs related to disability is also due to the strengthened position of organizations of people with disabilities in the rich countries and their lobbying and influence on general aid programs. It is now becoming more acceptable to include people with disabilities as a target group for aid to developing countries.

In 1983, the United Nations General Assembly signed a *World Programme of Action Concerning Disabled Persons,* which was followed by the Decade for Disabled Persons 1983-1992. The overall objectives of the *World Programme of Action* were to "promote effective measures for prevention of disability, rehabilitation and the realization of the goals of 'full participation' of disabled persons in social life and development, and of 'equality' " (United Nations 1983:1). The program has developed 22 *Standard Rules on the Equalization of Opportunities for Persons with Disabilities* (United Nations 1994) that do not bind but rather serve as recommendations for the member states.

During the IYDP and the following decade, a large number of countries in the developing world developed official policies, laws, and action plans to ensure the rights of persons with special needs. Although action has not necessarily followed legislation and much still remains to be done, such documents are essential to ensure that services will be provided in the long run (Eleweke 1999).

This chapter will focus mainly on experiences and problems in implementing rehabilitation programs in developing countries. Most often, such programs are based on models developed by United Nations agencies or nongovernmental organizations originating in Europe or North America and need considerable adjustment to local conditions to succeed. However, before we go on to our main topic, we will touch on two issues that have strong bearing on the implementation of such programs: the problem of surveys and the question of attitudes.

Closely linked to this is the issue of *culture.* To what extent is it necessary and possible to take cultural considerations in planning and implementing rehabilitation programs, and to what extent are we able to do so? These questions will be addressed throughout the chapter.

AUTHOR'S NOTE: I am very grateful to Janine Stenehjem for help with language editing of this chapter.

THE PROBLEM OF SURVEYS

Intentions to do something for persons with disabilities worldwide soon raised new questions, such as "who are they," "where are they," "how many," "what are their needs," and so on, and it was realized that very little was known. The World Health Organization (WHO), in connection with the launching of its program for community-based rehabilitation (discussed later), stated that about 10 percent of any population could be considered disabled in one way or another. This was meant to serve as a guideline for other countries planning their services. However, it was initially unclear how these figures came about. In later years, these numbers tended to be modified due to lower survey result figures from several member countries. The reason given for the initial relatively high figures was that malnourished children had been included.[1]

This illustrates one of the problems with using surveys as a tool for the planning of services for people with disabilities—namely, finding and agreeing on a definition of what is and is not a disability. Which impairments and what degrees of severity should be included? The inclusion criteria have tended to vary in the extent to which surveys of people with disabilities from various developing countries have elaborated on these points (which they often have not), thus making global or regional comparisons very difficult.

Attempts have been made to classify disabilities through the *International Classification of Impairments, Disabilities, and Handicaps (ICIDH)* (developed by WHO 1980) and to estimate the costs involved though the disability-adjusted life years (DALY), launched by the World Bank (1993) in its *World Development Report. ICIDH* was developed in response to the need for a framework to describe the consequences of what we usually understand as chronic and nonfatal outcomes of disease. It describes three dimensions of consequences such as *impairment, disability* and *handicap. ICIDH* has served as a guide for community assessment and planning of (re)habilitation[2] programs and has underpinned national-level policies and practices that affect equal opportunities and social integration of people with disabilities (Goerdt et al. 1996). DALY aims at measuring the economic burden of both disability and mortality from more than 100 diseases in all regions of the world for the purpose of health care planning and policymaking.

According to the *ICIDH,* the statistical division of the United Nations Department of Social and Economic Development has established a disability statistics database that includes information on the prevalence of impairments and disabilities in more than 90 countries. A *Disability Statistics Compendium* (United Nations 1990) presented these data from 55 countries. It is interesting to note from this compendium that census questions that identify impairments produce lower reported rates than questions that identify disabilities. Among the 55 countries, impairment rates varied from 0.2 percent to around 6 percent, while disability rates varied from approximately 7 percent to 20.9 percent (Goerdt et al. 1996).

ICIDH and DALY, however, have been met with criticism from disabled people and their organizations as well as from social scientists concerned with the issue of culture and the problem of cross-cultural comparison. Pfeiffer (1998) argues that disability is not necessarily a burden and that time spent as a person with a disability is not time lost. Thus, he claims that classifications and measurements of the impact of disability are a treat to communities of people with disabilities. He points out that disability is not a health question but a political one.

> By making disability a health question or associating it with health problems, the WHO contributes to the oppression of persons with disabilities. It contributes to the oppression when people with disabilities are actually the victims of class-based standards and barriers. (Pfeiffer 1998:519)

Bickenbach et al. (1999), however, argue against what they call the disability group approach to models for the classification of disabilities on the basis of constraints caused by physical, social, and political barriers. They claim that such a model is provocative but blurs the facts that some barriers to functioning are also inherent in the impairment as such, and some barriers are not necessarily discriminatory in their intentions.

Keck (1999), in a study or the Yupno people of Papua New Guinea, demonstrates the problem of applying *ICIDH-1* and definitions of impairment, disability, and handicap to a society in which the explanation of illness and its consequences is totally different from that of biomedicine. She challenges the assumed objectivity and culture-independence of biomedical concepts by showing how Yupno ideas of "being different" are "closely tied up with, and only understandable, against the background of their theory of personhood and their medical system" (Keck 1999:275).

Kleinman and Kleinman (1996) criticize DALY for not giving a real picture of human suffering. They advocate that such an approach should be complemented by "narratives, ethnographies and social histories that speak to the complex, even contradictory human side of suffering. Absent this other side, the economistic measurement of suffering leaves out most of what is at stake for peoples globally" (p. 15). Bickenbach et al. (1999), however, argue in favor of the revised *ICIDH-2*, which they claim takes into account many of the complaints to the earlier version made by groups of people with disabilities. The *ICIDH-2* version also tries to meet the anthropological critiques in that it is developed by means of a process of consensus involving both developed and developing countries. The WHO has conducted at each of the steps an extensive social-anthropological exercise called cultural applicability research (CAR), designed by an anthropologist specializing in the applicability of epidemiological instruments cross-culturally.[3] Whether this meets the arguments made by Keck (1999) and Kleinman and Kleinman (1996), as discussed above, remains to be seen.

Despite the problems of definitions and criteria for inclusion, or perhaps because these problems have not often been raised locally, surveys are highly cherished tools by planners and politicians who usually see this type of information as mandatory before any discussion about action can be initiated. Thus, inclusion criteria become essential for political and economic reasons because results of a survey may indicate the standard of living or level of health care in a country as well as commit that country to future rehabilitation costs.

On the individual level, another more serious impact of surveys is that they raise expectations that often cannot be fulfilled. Clearly, a disabled person or family visited for the purpose of a survey will easily come to expect that something will be done to help them. However, only rarely will a rehabilitation program be able to help all those who are surveyed. A survey often exhausts most of the available donor money so that once the figures are completed, there is little more that can be done. For this reason, voices have been raised, especially from the organizations of people with disabilities themselves, to limit (or drop) the surveys and start to give help, on a small scale, to those in need and to expand help as needs arise. This has been a viable policy for many nongovernmental organizations (NGOs) but clearly not sufficient for government policymaking.

THE ISSUE OF ATTITUDES

In the field of cross-cultural disability and rehabilitation studies, a powerful "myth" stands out and influences much of what has been said and done, especially in connection with the IYDP. This is the myth that people in non-Western societies hide, abuse, and even kill their disabled family members. We saw this myth strongly emerging in connection with fund-raising during IYDP,[4] underlying the design and consequently often the conclusions of many knowledge, attitude, and practice (KAP) studies and appearing in official documents from the WHO:

> The survival of disabled people is even today threatened by attitudes, prejudices and beliefs common among non-disabled people. The resulting behavior has led to, and still leads to premature death caused by negligence. . . . Moral trespasses or "sins" and "evil thoughts" may remain hidden, but the appearance of disability in a family will make the

"sin" visible to all. In a close knit society, this may lead to rid oneself or one's family of such obvious proof of evil-doing. (Helander 1984:34-35)

Elsewhere, I have argued (Ingstad 1995, 1997) that there are several problems attached to such a "myth." First, it wrongly assumes that there is a direct link between what people say about their attitudes and beliefs and what they actually do. Second, such a "myth" breeds arrogance in the modern rehabilitation workers and blurs their vision to the fact that most families with disabled members try their best to care for their disabled family members; by underestimating their motivation for care, they may lose a valuable resource in rehabilitation. Third, it may also serve as an excuse for governments and hide the fact that premature deaths of disabled persons are more likely to be the result of general poverty and poor health care than the family's lack of will to care. I am *not* saying that abuse and neglect never take place. However, we do not make single cases of child abuse to be typical examples of child care in industrialized countries. So why should we do so when it comes to the developing part of the world? Instead of making assumptions about developing countries in general, we should base our actions on actual knowledge, not the least of the numerous other factors besides "beliefs" and "attitudes" that determine the quality of care.

What We Know About Beliefs, Attitudes, and Behavior[5]

If we turn to the past, our knowledge of beliefs, attitudes, and behavior toward people with disabilities is scarce indeed and originates mainly from legends, folktales, and scattered historical sources that only scratch the surface of the topic.

We find statements in the Bible about disabilities being negatively stigmatized when people with psychiatric symptoms are seen as possessed by unclean spirits and physical impairment seen as the consequence of sins. We also find many such statements in the classical literature of Hinduism, some of which advocates concern and care for persons with impairment, while others state the contrary (Miles 1999). From studying Old Irish and Icelandic manuscripts, Bragg (1997) concludes that these sources show a very different picture, where aberrancy is seen as the mark of an outstanding person, a hero, a seer, or a god. In the old Norwegian fairytales, we find stories of children born with impairment who were seen as the offspring of the small people living underground, exchanged at night for the normal human child. Such children should be beaten or in other ways abused so that the original parents would feel sorry for the child, take it back, and thus bring the human child back to its parents. On the other hand, these same folktales also include stories about people with "strange behavior" or mild mental retardation who went from farm to farm doing odd jobs and being what we today call "integrated" in the community. In a Tswana folktale from Southern Africa, we hear about an albino girl who was initially kept out of the family because of her deviant looks. But when she managed to show her capacity as a hard worker and contributor to her household, she was accepted and loved even more than her lazy sister who was not albino.

The interpretation of such fragments of history and folktales, of which there are many more examples, must take into account that they are just as much mythical and symbolic in their message as an account of what actually took place in the old days. Still, they may tell us something about what people valued most and what was needed to be accepted and "integrated," as in the story about the hardworking albino girl.

One of the first modern scientists to take an interest in the topic of disabilities cross-culturally was the anthropologist Robert Edgerton. With a special focus on mental retardation, he based his analysis on the anthropological database Human Relations Area File (HRAF), as well as fieldwork among American Indians and four different tribes in East Africa. He found large variations in both culturally prescribed attitudes as well as actual behavior. As an example, he mentions that among the Chagga of East Africa, where customs prescribed that even severely retarded people should be well treated, some fathers risked punishment by killing their severely retarded infants. In contrast, in societies where such killings were accepted and recommended, many severely retarded survived and were well cared for and loved by their families. Thus, Edgerton (1970) draws the following conclusion:

> So extreme is the dearth of existing data that most conclusions about the nature of mental retardation in these societies may remain quite speculative. Still, however inadequate these existing data may be, they are sufficient to call into question any notion that what is said or done about mental retardation in non-western societies is highly uniform from society to society. Quite the contrary is true. What is said and done is highly variable, so much that given the inadequacy of the present available data, it is difficult to generalize about this world at all . . . we must declare a moratorium upon facile assumptions, and upon programmatic polemics, and must engage in the collection of data that will answer our perennial and essential questions about mental retardation. (P. 555)

Whyte (1991a, 1991b) did a study of attitudes toward and management of a mental health program in two regions of Tanzania in connection with a baseline evaluation of a WHO/DANIDA program for mental health. She found that respondents showed a marked complexity in their attitudes toward different conditions. Different individuals had different feelings toward the same condition, and single individuals could show marked differences in attitudes toward various conditions. One of the most commonly expressed concerns was the inability to support oneself and to contribute to the family and the village. The practical burdens of care were seen to lie with the family and not with other members of the community, and large families were expected to be supportive and kind to their disabled members.

Goerdt (1984) studied persons with physical disabilities in Barbados. She found that they were not expected by others to fulfill normal adult roles, partly due to beliefs and concepts about disability and partly by their observations of what persons with a physical disability were actually able to do in that society.

From Nigeria, two different studies on attitudes of parents toward their disabled children show quite different results. Okunda (1981) found that among Yoruba parents of visually, auditory, and physically disabled children, the Western-educated elite were less favorably disposed to handicaps in children than those in traditional settings. Enwemeka and Adeghe (1982) found in their study that most fathers with physically disabled children were rather indifferent to their children. There were, however, highly significant differences between fathers with higher and low education; the fathers with high education were the most interested in their children. From Zimbabwe, a study by Jackson and Mupedziswa (1988) found that beliefs and attitudes expressed by informants toward persons with a disability often seemed to be in contradiction with how they acted toward them.

A collection of articles in *Culture and Disability* (Ingstad and Whyte 1995) discusses the concept of personhood as a central theme in understanding how impairments are perceived in a society and to what extent and on which conditions disabled people are included as full members of a society. From societies as different as the Maasai of Kenya, the Punan Ba of Sarawak, and those from Somalia, Botswana, Uganda, and Nicaragua, we are told how the acceptance of a person with a disability is not mainly a question of physical or mental condition but more of conforming to the defining characteristics of full personhood in the particular society. Such defining characteristics may be sociability or living together with other people and having a socially recognized father and thus rank and kinship identity, marriage, and children and the ability to contribute to the household economy. People with impairment may find it difficult to live up to such characteristics, but it is often seen as the responsibility of the family to make it possible. Thus, in many developing countries, personhood depends more on social identity and the fulfillment of family obligations than on individual ability.

The issue of personhood is followed up further in a collection on culture and intellectual disability (Jenkins 1998). In the introduction, Jenkins points out how capacities, potentials, and adequacies must be understood as socially constructed and ascribed and will thus vary between different local and cultural settings. The competence of a person is usually not doubted until it *is* in doubt. However, in all local settings, there are persons to whom the presumption of competence is not extended or has been withdrawn. Thus, assumptions of incompetence may be based on various types of otherness such as race, appearance, mental capacity, or any deviance from local perceptions of "fitness." Interestingly, though, childhood and old-age senility are not usually perceived as incompetence but rather as aspects of natural development and adequate humanness. Whyte (1998), in a case from eastern Uganda, demonstrates how in a society that values relatedness and mutual family support, the incompetence of mentally disabled persons lies primarily in their inability to extend and strengthen their families through social activities and relationships. As a result, a mental impairment may not be considered a problem if the person is able to behave in a socially acceptable manner and contribute somehow to his or her family. The modern school system, with a heavy emphasis on grading of children's performance, brings in something new by seeing intellectual capacity as the main criterion for competence and thereby risks labeling children as dull who might otherwise be considered competent. Nuttal (1998), in a case from western Greenland, shows how disabled children from remote villages are taken far away from their families to get special education in boarding schools, while the teachers and authorities keep alive a myth that they are "dumped" and neglected by their families. He tells a touching story about a boy, Nils, with a hearing impairment, who was being trained by his father to be a fully competent hunter until taken away by the school authorities and sent to boarding school far away. Nuttal concludes that "not only was Nils categorized as incompetent, but his family were also left feeling a sense of inadequacy and incompetence at being deprived of caring for him" (p. 192).

Few studies have seriously tried to document the issue of "hiding" and "abuse" of people with disabilities beyond mere statements. Weiss (1998) is one exception. In a study of families with what she calls "appearance-impaired" children, she found that nearly 50 percent of all families in Israel that gave birth to children with major physical or medical defects chose to leave them behind at the hospital. Going in-depth into four families that eventually brought their disabled children home, she reveals a picture of hiding, shame, and despair but does not give the deeper insight into their life situation that enables us to understand how such situations are generated. She largely blames it on parental "attitudes." Neither do we get an insight into characteristics of Israeli culture, society, and health care that may create a picture of abandonment that we recognize from European history but that fortunately seems to be exceptional these days.

This brief review of some studies on beliefs, attitudes, and behavior concerning disabilities and toward disabled persons shows us some of the global variety and the danger involved in drawing conclusions as in the WHO quotation that opened this section. It also shows us the need to understand the sociocultural context in which "attitudes" are acted out. Most of all, it shows us that we do not know enough, and more studies are needed on the life situation of people with disabilities in non-Western societies as a foundation for providing adequate rehabilitation services in developing countries.

REHABILITATION IN DEVELOPING COUNTRIES

We shall now turn to look at the development and implementation of programs for rehabilitation in developing countries. In doing so, I have chosen examples from Botswana, Zimbabwe, Palestine, and Eritrea, well aware that there are numerous other examples that could equally have represented the topic. Much-needed thorough analysis of rehabilitation experiences from (a large number of) developing countries remains (to my knowledge) yet to be written. In the meantime, I will use this chapter to give a contribution from the examples that I know best. What happens today, however, cannot be seen in isolation but must be understood on the background of a history, which, especially for the previously colonized countries, has strong links to the history of rehabilitation in Europe.

The Missionaries and the Colonial Powers

The first contact that people in developing countries had with what we today call rehabilitation came through missionaries and representatives of the colonial powers. These agencies, although seemingly quite different in their intentions, often walked hand in hand, and medical services, especially in the rural areas, were more often run by missionaries than by the colonial powers (Comaroff and Comaroff 1991; Vaughan 1991).

This was also the case for medical care regarding rehabilitation. Linked to education, also from the start a missionary concern, biomedical knowledge provided new options for treatment of conditions that previously seemed unchangeable. For missionaries preaching the gospel of love and mercy, the seemingly most disadvantaged members of a society would often become the focus of attention. Thus, many youngsters with physical or sensory impairment got their chance to health care and education by becoming the protégés of missionaries. Some missions would focus their activities only on people with a disability (e.g., the German-based Cristoffel Blinden mission, which for years has been running training facilities for people with hearing impairments in Africa). Another example is the Mission of Cyrene in Zimbabwe, where persons with a physical disability were taught to become artists (Devlieger 1998). Yet, for the most part, the mission's activities for people with disabilities have been part of their general setup of church, hospital, and educational services.

While missionaries were relatively few and often lived scattered throughout rural areas, the colonial powers brought a larger number of administrative personnel, often accompanied by family members. Settlers claiming land was a third category. These people brought with them their European standards and habits, and when some of their own children needed special medical care or special education, special schools and institutions were created after the model from the "mother country" at the time. These early services for people (mostly children) with disabilities were usually located in the capital or larger centers and catered to children of the newcomers and sometimes to the children of the local educated elite. While late eighteenth-century Europe recognized the benefits of special education for children with sensory impairments, those with a mental disability were usually sent away to large institutions or mental hospitals. This pattern, to some extent, has prevailed in developing countries. Lucky were those children with mental retardation whose parents could not afford or had not heard about such "help." In countries that developed a system based on (more or less official) segregation of races (e.g., South Africa and South Rhodesia, which is now Zimbabwe), the services developed for the "whites" clearly had much higher standards than those (if any) developed for the local nonwhites.

The colonial powers brought with them the principle that assistance to people with disabilities should be financed through fund-raising and private donations and organized by specially committed groups or private persons. This coincided with traditions of almsgiving in religions such as Islam and Hinduism (Miles 1999), as well as with tribal traditions of the rich sharing wealth with poorer segments of the population. Until today, such principles, which we may call the "spirit of charity," have stuck to the services for disabled persons in many developing countries and may have served as a reason for the failure of governments to commit to full responsibility for disabled citizens.

The Role of Wars

Wars have always been a major "producer" of impairment, and war victims have always held a highly regarded position—provided they were on the "right" side. Bruun (1995) has shown how both sides in the Nicaraguan conflicts used war victims for their propaganda purposes. The Sandinistas depicted them as "heroes" and "martyrs" of the revolution and thus brought together connotations of religion and machismo, two important values in Nicaragua, with the values of the revolution. The political opposition, on the other hand, presented the martyr aspect but not the heroism. As victims of the wrong policy, those who suffered for a lost case therefore were liable to pity and provided for charity (Bruun 1995:202).

Following the two world wars, the building of rehabilitation centers and the introduction of disability pensions for war victims took place in many European countries. For instance, in Norway, a war disability pension was introduced after World War II, and it is interesting to note that the payment from this source is higher than that from an ordinary disability pension, thus marking the special honored status of a war victim. The Norwegians who joined the Nazis and were impaired fighting on the East Front would not be considered for such a pension. Rehabilitation centers and pensions for wounded soldiers have also been introduced in a number of developing countries following their wars for independence (see the case of Zimbabwe below).

In recent wars, we have seen how the plight of land mine victims has come up as a new agenda, attracting considerable funds and new attention. This has occurred despite the fact that land mines have been around for a long time and are probably accountable for a relatively small proportion of physical impairment in the world.

The United Nations and Community-Based Rehabilitation

As mentioned in the introduction, the United Nations General Assembly in 1971 adopted a *Declaration on the Rights of Mentally Retarded Persons*[6] and a *Declaration on the Rights of Disabled Persons* in 1975.[7] Both these declarations established the same civil and political rights for a person with a disability as for other people.

In a resolution adopted on December 16, 1976, the United Nations General Assembly proclaimed 1981 to be the International Year of Disabled Persons (IYDP) with the theme "full participation" and "equality." In 1979, the Decade for Disabled Persons was proclaimed to be from 1983 to 1992[8] and later prolonged for another 10 years to 2002, with the objective of achieving "a society for all" by 2010.

In 1982, a *World Programme of Action Concerning Disabled Persons* was adopted by the General Assembly to provide for effective international and national measures to ensure the full participation of disabled persons in social life and the development of their societies.[9] It emphasizes prevention, rehabilitation, and the equalization of opportunities, and it encourages disabled persons to organize to make themselves heard. The coordination, implementation, and evaluation of this program are to be done by the United Nations Center for Social Development and Humanitarian Affairs in Vienna (International Labor Organization [ILO] 1998). A set of standard rules to be used as recommendations for member countries was developed on the basis of the *World Programme of Action* and adopted by the General Assembly in 1993.[10]

The IYDP in 1981 and the following decade, for the same purpose, were probably among the more successful ventures of this kind. Awareness was created globally about the needs of people with a disability and the promotion of *integration,* meaning that disabled people should participate in society on their own premises, and *normalization,* meaning that the various sectors of society should take part of the responsibility to see this happen.[11] Much of this discourse was strongly influenced by a debate that had been going on in the Scandinavian countries since the early 1960s, closely linked to the ideology of the welfare state and its concept of "equal rights" (Ingstad 1995).

The WHO had for some time been preparing itself for the IYDP. The idea of launching a program for community-based rehabilitation (CBR) was introduced in 1976 and was adopted by the World Health Assembly later that same year. The program was seen as part of the strategy toward "Health for All by the Year 2000." It was no coincidence that the CBR program that was consequently launched by the WHO had many similarities to the debate that had been going on in Scandinavia during the previous decade, launching concepts such as *integration* and *normalization*. The head of the WHO rehabilitation department, one of three coauthors of the first CBR manual, was a Swede (a medical doctor),[12] and so was one of the other authors (a physiotherapist). The program was planned especially for the developing countries and represented a first attempt to create a worldwide model that could be used cross-culturally. After field testing in nine different countries (1979-1982), it was recommended that governments should take urgent steps, in cooperation with the WHO and NGOs, to plan for an implementation of CBR within the context of primary health care (WHO 1982).

The WHO claimed that CBR represented a *new* approach, which in a sense was both right and wrong. As pointed out by one of its main critics (Miles 1985), it was wrong because the awareness for the need of decentralized rehabilitation measures building on local resources existed prior to 1976, and there had been scattered attempts at doing this in several developing countries. However, it was true in the sense that the CBR program was the first attempt at creating a rehabilitation model to be implemented on a worldwide scale.

The *model* of community-based rehabilitation, as seen by the WHO, is a low-cost way to reach out to persons with a disability by integrating rehabilitation services in already existing infrastructures. Four different levels of services have been identified, which correspond well to the organization of primary health care and its system of referral in most countries:

1. At the community level, the household is the main area for rehabilitation work and family and community members the important actors.
2. The county level is the first level of referral for rehabilitation problems that cannot be handled sufficiently at the community level. The person mainly responsible for CBR at this level should be the rehabilitation assistant, which corresponds to the village health worker found in many developing countries.
3. The provincial level is the second level of referral. Here we may find a provincial hospital with specialized health personnel (e.g., physiotherapist) as well as other rehabilitation facilities.
4. The national level is the third level of referral for rehabilitation problems that cannot be solved at lower levels. Here we find specialists such as orthopedic surgeon, cardiologist, and so on, as well as special institutions for rehabilitation. At this level, it is suggested that there should be a national coordinator of the CBR program who would often (but not necessarily) be located under the Ministry of Health (Helander 1993; Ingstad 1997).

The main *tool* of this CBR approach is a manual consisting of several different booklets with simple drawings and instructions to be used by family members and local supervisors in the training of persons with various types of disabilities. Thus, we recognize in the WHO-CBR approach the principles of *low-cost, community participation* and *simple technology* that were commonly found in discourses about "development" at the time.

The WHO's initiative in CBR was closely followed by the ILO with a CBR program for community-based vocational training. Actually, the initiative of the ILO in the field of vocational rehabilitation dates back as far as 1921, when it explored how the obligation to employ disabled ex-servicemen, as well as methods of placing disabled persons in employment, might be introduced in national legislation. As a result of the conclusions adopted by the experts consulted and the legislative measures that were proposed, the vocational needs of disabled workers gained international recognition for the first time in 1925 (ILO 1998). The ILO continued to play an active role in the process leading up to the *World Programme of Action Concerning Disabled Persons* and passed its own convention and recommendation concerning vocational rehabilitation and employment at an ILO conference in 1983.

The ILO-CBR involvement differs from the one by the WHO in that it seems to be more concerned with advocacy and policymaking than with implementing a particular model for how vocational rehabilitation should be done at the local level. While the ILO had previously given technical assistance to the establishment of vocational training centers and sheltered workshops, it now turned to establishing programs aimed at giving assistance for disabled individuals to start informal-sector, income-generating activities. The ILO also emphasizes the mainstreaming of training and employment opportunities for vocational skills. Thus, ministries have been assisted in adapting training facilities, curricula, and equipment for the inclusion of trainees with disabilities (ILO 1998).

The third United Nations organization directly involved in CBR is the United Nations Educational, Scientific, and Cultural Organization (UNESCO), with an emphasis on "education for all." It states that special-needs education should not be developed in isolation but be made to form part of an overall educational strategy and of new social and economic policies. This implies a shift in emphasis from special schools and institutions to the integration of children with disabilities in mainstream schools and classes. This clearly implies great challenges to all involved parties, especially when it comes to the integration of children with mental or sensory impairment. A World Conference on Special Needs Education in Salamanca, Spain, in 1994 (attended by 300 participants representing 92 governments and 25 international organizations) put down a statement and framework for action on special-needs education (UNESCO 1994). Judging from a collection of "success stories" published by UNESCO, it seems that the principle of CBR has been used quite differently in projects in different countries. While some countries have put the main emphasis on enabling teachers to integrate disabled pupils in local schools, others have used the WHO-CBR model as a starting point for early stimulation and school integration (UNESCO n.d.).

In the early days of CBR efforts, the communication between the WHO, the ILO, and UNESCO seems to have been rather limited, sometimes more of a competition. One of the problems seems to have been that the various United Nations organizations tended to have their separate projects in various developing countries, attached to different ministries (Ministry of Education, Ministry of Health, etc.). Consequently, instead of joining forces, they tended to compete for government funds and public attention.[13]

Realizing this problem, the three organizations held a meeting in 1994 and came up with a joint position paper. The purpose of their joint position was "to clarify for policy makers and program managers the objective of CBR and the methods for implementing it" (ILO/UNESCO/WHO 1994).

Thus, they also managed to agree on a definition:

Community-based rehabilitation is a strategy within community developed for the rehabilitation, equalization of opportunities and social integration of all people with disabilities. CBR implemented through the combined efforts of disabled people themselves, their families and communities, and the appropriate health, education and social services. (ILO/UNESCO/WHO 1994:2)

What is new in this definition is defining CBR as a *strategy within community development*. This opens various ways of applying the concept that are sensitive to local cultural, political, and socioeconomic conditions, not just the implementation of one model.

The Role of Nongovernmental Organizations

With all its good intentions of implementing CBR, the United Nations system was faced with one big problem: its shortage of funds. This was also the problem of most countries involved in implementation. Thus, help was sought in international NGOs (e.g., the Red Cross) and in NGOs based in the more developed countries.

NGOs from more developed countries had long been involved in rehabilitation in developing countries, implementing their own ideal models and according to their own definitions of need. Such models tended to be isolated islands of local projects, mostly small scale, and sometimes in collaboration with local NGOs. Sometimes the support took the form of large buildings intended to be rehabilitation centers. These easily ended up as so-called white elephants —nice for a government to show off to visitors as a proof of engagement in the cause of rehabilitation but difficult to sustain when donor money came to an end. The new challenge for the

NGOs was to become partners in a development process that involved local government, local NGO(s), and a United Nations organization providing morale and sometimes short-term technical support.

Other types of NGOs are the international organizations formed by the disabled people themselves (e.g., Disabled Peoples' International, International League of Societies for the Mentally Handicapped, etc.). These have come to play a vital role as partners of dialogue in the United Nations developments outlined above and in disseminating information about human rights issues to sister organizations in developing countries. We often see that organizations started by disabled persons come into being in developing countries when a close family member of a prominent person in society becomes disabled. We have seen this happen in China, Nicaragua, and Kenya, to name a few countries. The problem with such organizations in developing countries seems to be that they easily become a city or elite activity advocating for specialized and centralized services for their particular group. Also, in a situation when there is a shortage of funds and positions for persons with a disability, they easily end up in internal struggle and eventually may split instead of joining forces. This was the case in Botswana, where for many years, two organizations by the blind and physically handicapped went into what seemed like an endless power struggle, which kept them from presenting joint demands to the government.

The idea that disabled people should be active in creating and running a CBR program is a central theme in the book *Disabled Village Children: A Guide for Community Health Workers* by David Werner (1987)[14] and later in *Nothing about Us without Us: Developing Innovative Technologies for, by, and with Disabled Persons* (Werner 1998). The main difference between this model and the WHO-CBR approach is that it centers on the idea that the persons with disability should generate and sustain the activities that they perceive as necessary. Thus, this model is less than the one by the WHO, which is concerned with replicability but visualizes different forms of rehabilitation activities emerging from different sociocultural circumstances.

We can sum up a few of the main problems facing CBR in an early phase:

There are unclear definitions of what a "community" is and its potential for mobilization, and the potential of a "community" for volunteering is overestimated. Is community participation often lacking?

There is a lack of sufficiently trained people, which in combination with insufficient community mobilization, may lead to the program becoming an outreach program instead of community based.

CBR (especially by the WHO) is presented to governments in developing countries as "cheap," thus not sufficiently preparing them for the needs of future investment in training and infrastructure.

The attachment of CBR to one particular sector or one particular United Nations organization may easily become a barrier for collaboration with other sectors.

The Present

The outline of the development of modern rehabilitation services in developing countries given above reveals a dilemma that gradually emerges in most countries. Should one aim at giving community-based services for all people with a disability, or should high-quality specialized services that invariably reach only a limited number of those in need be the first priority?

Outreaching services combining the expertise of, for instance, a physiotherapist or speech therapist based in a center with regular home visits in the district(s) nearby is a middle solution. This is, however, often costly (because of need for transport) and cannot reach everyone in need.

In most countries, however, the developments are not steered by government decision making alone but are the result of complex processes in which history, influences from foreign agencies, and general socioeconomic development play important roles. We can illustrate this with two examples from the neighboring African countries Botswana and Zimbabwe.

The Case of Botswana

Botswana achieved its independence in 1965 as a result of political negotiations and without having to fight a war of independence. Being previously a British protectorate, the country had been seen mainly as a source of labor reserve to the mines of South Africa. This meant that few investments had been made, and few Europeans had come to stay for longer periods of time. The few activities that had taken place in rehabilitation had been mainly in terms of scattered and very limited NGO efforts. Since independence, as a result of large diamond finds, Botswana has had a blooming economy and is today one of the richest countries in Africa. It has also been blessed with political stability and a multiparty democracy.

In the launching of the WHO's CBR program, Botswana was chosen in 1979 as one of nine pilot countries for field testing and thus already had some experience by the start of IYDP in 1981. After holding several workshops with people from the WHO, it was decided to make the program nationwide from the start. One reason for this choice was the relatively small population.[15] What was forgotten was the long distances that field-workers had to cover between settlements. A pyramidal structure was created with a Commissioner for the Handicapped at the top, located in the Ministry of Health. Social welfare officers (SWO) for rehabilitation are located in each of the district health teams, which are part of the primary health care (PHC) structure. At the local level, the SWOs are supposed to refer to the family welfare educator (FWE), which is the Botswana version of the village health worker. However, this collaboration has never been much of a success. The FWEs have always felt that they have had enough other things to do in PHC and that they have not received sufficient training to carry out CBR. They also feel that their superiors, the clinic nurses, have resented the interference of the SWOs in clinic routines. The onset of HIV/AIDS, causing more than 40 percent of all pregnant women to be HIV positive in some places and adults and children to be dying from the epidemic, has in recent years pushed rehabilitation of disabled people even further down the list of priorities. Without the FWEs to rely on, the task of community mobilization for CBR has become impossible for the SWOs, and their activities have become mainly outreaching and, to a large extent, transporting disabled people who need referral to hospital or rehabilitation centers. The SWOs have been mostly social workers with little or no previous training in rehabilitation. With a low salary and a feeling of insufficiency, the turnover rates have been high and the vacancies many. The CBR manual is not regularly used, and local participation and mobilization have been minimal.

Another problem impairing the national CBR program from the beginning was the launching of a parallel CBR program by the Botswana Red Cross, which was heavily supported by a foreign donor. Instead of collaborating to make the government program more successful, these two programs soon became competitive, leaving the SWOs with a feeling of insufficiency because they were not as well equipped with cars and funds for workshops as were their Red Cross counterparts. However, as the mobilization of Red Cross volunteers for CBR failed and the donor money eventually came to an end, the Red Cross chose to withdraw from CBR and is now concentrating its efforts on running a rehabilitation center.

With the nationwide CBR program being largely a failure or at least having become a structure with very little content, the field has been left wide open for various NGOs to take over. Some of these were established shortly after independence, catering to special groups of impairments (the blind, the deaf, the mentally retarded), while others, which have come more recently, aim somewhat broader (the multihandicapped, various types of physical disabilities). Two large centers, one in the north and one in the south, run some outreach CBR services in addition to their institution-based activities. There are also special schools for deaf and blind children, respectively. The various activities of the centers remain largely uncoordinated. This has occurred despite the establishment of a Botswana Council for the Disabled (BCD), which is supposed to function as an umbrella organization and allocate government funding for rehabilitation. However, for long periods of time, the BCD has been paralyzed by weak leadership or internal disagreements between its member NGOs.

Following the launching of a long-awaited National Plan for Rehabilitation in 1996,[16] the Ministry of Health has allocated a fairly large sum of money to the BCD to distribute according to needs of its member organizations. Also, the Ministry of Education has provided funds for teachers' salaries at some of the special schools. Despite this, most special schools and centers still rely heavily on donor money and fund-raising through "charity walks" and private donations to sustain their activities (see Ingstad 1995, 1997, 1999 for further discussion of CBR in Botswana).

The Case of Zimbabwe

Zimbabwe, the former South Rhodesia, obtained its independence in 1980 after a civil war in which the black majority population succeeded in freeing itself from an apartheid system imposed by a white minority of settlers whose ancestors arrived from Europe around the turn of the century. Followed by some years of tribal power struggle, the political situation has, during the past decade, been seemingly calm (but increasingly tense) under the surface of a socialist one-party system. Although the reconciliation between the previous main opponents seems to have succeeded, one of the major political controversies has been the (still unresolved) issue of allocation of agricultural land from white farmers to the poor rural black majority. Despite being rich in agricultural and other natural resources, the economy of Zimbabwe has been deteriorating in recent years.

Although the white Rhodesians had established special schools and rehabilitation services according to European models for their own disabled children, very little had been done for those of the black majority. Following independence, these previously "white-only" schools were also opened for black children but were far from enough to meet the needs of the majority. However, these centers, with their well-trained staff, have become valuable resource and referral centers for more decentralized rehabilitation activities.

The civil war left Zimbabwe with many disabled war veterans, and one of the first rehabilitation activities of the new government was (with the help of donor money) to build a large rehabilitation center for people with a physical impairment, mainly war injuries. However, this center turned out to be exactly the "white elephant" that many people had feared and is today used more for multipurpose training activities.[17] A pension scheme was also introduced for disabled war veterans.

CBR was introduced to Zimbabwe in 1982 by the local Red Cross Society and supported by a foreign donor, the same as the one supporting the Red Cross program in Botswana.[18] However, contrary to Botswana's ambition of reaching the whole country right away, Zimbabwe decided to start small, in only one district. After three years of gaining experience and following a favorable evaluation, the Red Cross allowed the CBR activities in the first district to be run by government services and went into a second district, eventually to follow the same procedure there. After having gained experience from the Red Cross in these first two districts, the government felt secure enough to go on alone. In 1988, a policy was made giving the Ministry of Health and Child Welfare the responsibility for introducing CBR on a national scale (Chidyausiku et al. 1998). The process, however, has purposely been gradual, not only due to lack of funds but also because the danger of expanding too fast has been realized. Thus, by February 1999, about 55 percent of the country had been covered by CBR. Although the content and quality of the services vary somewhat between districts according to an evaluation report (Chidyausiku et al. 1998), the experience so far has been good. There has been a considerable amount of enthusiasm and participation locally, and the CBR manuals are regularly used and have been translated into the main local languages.[19]

Around the same time that CBR was introduced, the government of Zimbabwe[20] started a process of upgrading a large number of the district hospitals. Included in this upgrading were rehabilitation wards that were staffed with physiotherapists or occupational therapists. These have come to serve as important support and referral centers for the rehabilitation technicians responsible for CBR at the district level. As part of the decentralization and expansion of rehabilitation services, the government, in collaboration with the WHO and the Red Cross, opened a school for rehabilitation technicians in 1981. This new cadre of health workers is given a two-year course covering relevant fields of knowledge for the dissemination of CBR to persons with various types of impairment. In addition to this, the University of Zimbabwe has commenced occupational and physiotherapy training. Thus, we see that CBR in Zimbabwe is part of a comprehensive government program at all levels (institution based, outreached, and community based) that aims at giving "rehabilitation for all."

How is it then that Zimbabwe, despite a more difficult political and economic situation, seems to have been much more successful in its attempt at introducing CBR than Botswana? In Botswana, the dream of "rehabilitation for all" through CBR has been largely (although not officially) abandoned in favor of a model based on private initiatives, which may provide higher-quality services for some but can hardly reach persons with a disability living in the more remote areas. To the extent that these rural-based individuals are involved, it implies leaving their families to go far away to rehabilitation centers and special schools for a large part of the year. They may have problems maintaining contact with their family and home community, and when they return home, they often have a problem finding employment suitable to the training they have been given. One example is a primary school with boarding facilities for deaf children in Francistown in northern Botswana. Many of the children there come from remote villages and are transported to school by social workers. The children are taught sign language, but since the teachers hardly ever see the parents, the advantages of this type of communication are rather limited when they return home. Another example is that of two blind sisters I encountered in a very remote village in the Kalahari. One had been trained for two years at a craft center for the blind. The other sister had finished secondary school for the blind in one of the larger towns. She wanted to become a switchboard operator but had no options for further training. On her return to the home village, the first sister found that the material she had been trained to work with was not locally available. The other sister had but a few books in Braille on which to practice her skills. She became very depressed and eventually committed suicide. Fortunately, few stories end this sadly, but it clearly demonstrates the dilemma involved in choosing between the principles of giving less ambitious but perhaps more applicable training locally and more specialized higher-quality services. Ideally, one should not have to choose. Both options should be freely available for those in need. However, in developing countries, with limited economic resources and a shortage of trained manpower, options are very difficult to achieve.

In comparing the development of rehabilitation services in Botswana and Zimbabwe, we find that Zimbabwe has had certain advantages that are grounded partly in historical conditions and partly in political choices that have been made along the way.

❖ The need and motivation to do something were eminent as a result of the war, not mainly because of an International Year and Decade of Disabled Persons and pressure from the international community to "do something" (as in Botswana).

❖ When starting to plan the rehabilitation services at all levels, one could draw on local experts who had been trained by the institutions for the whites in the old South Rhodesia. This knowledge of what was needed must also have played a role in investing in the education of rehabilitation technicians and occupational and physiotherapists. (Botswana has no such training facilities.)

❖ The decision in Zimbabwe to start small and expand step by step was enforced by the size of the population as well as by the scarcity of economic resources available.

❖ Both countries established, under the Ministry of Health, an office in charge of planning, administration, and coordination of rehabilitation services in the country. Why the one in Zimbabwe seems to have been more efficient than the one in Botswana is difficult to say. It may have been a question of personality factors, most likely the result of differences in economic allocations and other support from government. It is, however, tempting (but probably controversial) to speculate whether a government based on socialistic principles is more likely to show willingness to promote equal opportunities for disadvantaged groups than one leaning more on ideologies of "private enterprise" and the "spirit of charity."

Thus, while the main future constraint in Zimbabwe is the economic developments in the country and the nation's possibility to realize its plans for rehabilitation at all levels, the problem in Botswana is more a lack of a sincere government commitment and a heavy reliance on the spirit of charity. Such commitment does not imply that all activities need to be government run and financed but takes overall planning, implementation, and coordination that demonstrate the willingness to promote equal rights for persons with a disability. Over the years, plenty of good intentions have manifested in Botswana's National Development Plans but not enough in real action.

The New Role of NGOs[21]

The role and importance of NGOs internationally have radically changed during the past 20 years. While NGOs used to base their finances mainly on their own resources, they are today, to a large extent, supported by donor governments.[22] Before, NGOs used to be involved in small-scale activities and only with local NGOs as partners. Today, they may be important actors in general aid policies in donor countries as well as in the policies of the World Bank and other United Nations agencies.

The role of international and local NGOs in rehabilitation has to some extent undergone the same change. Similarly, the concept and content of CBR have also changed. The emphasis is no longer mainly on the implementation of a model but more on a strategy based on community development and the promotion of equal rights. An international NGO may, in partnership with (a) local counterpart(s), serve as adviser to a government and focus on the following:

> integration of projects or programs for persons with disabilities into mainstream development activities;
>
> strengthening of ongoing rehabilitation activities in governmental and private sectors;
>
> support in development of governmental, national, and sector policies and guidelines;
>
> strengthening of interministerial collaborations and multisectorial approaches in rehabilitation.

In addition to financial support, in this new role, the NGOs will have to provide relevant technical input and accept more complex projects and programs with the need for macro-planning. This new role will emphasize the importance of technical and financial sustainability by promoting the development and strengthening of ongoing activities. The NGO has the advantage of being flexible, compared to the United Nations system. It is thus in a position to promote the necessary local collaboration between governmental and private initiatives and implementation, making sure that long-term responsibility will be in the hands of the different local players. This approach will need adaptation to the different local settings and thus will differ from country to country. Two programs by the Norwegian Association of the Disabled (NAD), in collaboration with other countries, may serve as examples.

Palestine

Thirty years of military occupation and being without governmental institutions resulted in a strong local NGO sector in Palestine. Therefore, the CBR program started in 1990 was an initiative of a consortium of 20 NGOs in different parts of the country. The implementation was done by the NGO through the existing structures and networks. The external input from NAD was financial and technical support for documentation, research, planning, and training. Gradually, the complexity and geographical coverage increased. By 1999, the program covered approximately 60 percent of the population and included most of the relevant sectors (health and medical rehabilitation, social welfare, vocational training and job placement, and general education). Without a government structure, macro-planning and national policies in disability were lacking. After the peace process started in 1993, this became possible through the establishment of the Palestine National Authority. The main challenge for the program was to integrate the different activities into mainstream development policies and establish a functional collaboration between governmental and private sectors. Today, the NGO sector is still mostly responsible for grassroots implementation, while the government is gradually taking over the role of policy development and national planning. The main objective in the program has been social integration of persons with disabilities in their local communities. The program in Palestine was supported by the Norwegian and Swedish organizations, NAD and Diakonia. The two organizations were also to some extent coordinating support for disability programs from other international organizations.

Eritrea

Eritrea, as Palestine, has passed through a long period of conflicts, occupation, and war. By the time the CBR program was established, the new government was in place and responsible for all renovation, rebuilding, and development. The NGO sector was weak or nonexistent, and the government approach was very centralized and politically controlled. This created less space and flexibility in the program design, and the approach had to be different from that in Palestine. Some of the main features and conditions for the CBR program in Eritrea were that it had to be developed at the central governmental level and integrated into governmental policies and institutions. Interministerial collaboration needs political authorization before being implemented, and government employees are the focal point at all levels, from central level to community level. International NGOs thus will have to accept a limited and restricted role.

An important question is whether a centralized regime such as this can develop an environment conducive for the implementation of a CBR program and for the promotion of rights and integration of persons with a disability. As in Palestine, one important factor was the change in awareness that had taken place during the time of conflict and war. Persons with disabilities who had been injured during wartime were considered heroes and martyrs. This had a general positive effect on people and promoted community responsibility and inclusion. In addition, community development is the general government policy. Thus, the use of limited governmental resources focuses on support of community development, promoting local initiatives and responsibilities. From the beginning, the CBR program concentrated on development of national policies and planning documents. Technical training of governmental rehabilitation employees at different levels was also given priority. This bureaucratic approach was necessary for the integration of the program in the government structure, political support to the program, ownership, and development of the necessary technical competence. Compared with a program based on a vital local NGO sector, this takes more time and resources before it can produce results. However, there are advantages when it comes to sustainability and local financial and political support. The CBR program in Eritrea today promotes an inclusive policy in different governmental institutions as education, health, and social welfare. The main focus of the program is to support persons with a disability, their family, and the local community. In the future, the program will need to increase its geographical coverage and include the persons targeted in the decision-making processes.

Some lessons learned by NAD from these experiences are the following:

> Programs for persons with a disability are low on the priority list in all developing countries. Local governmental and NGO partners have to take the main and long-term responsibility for the projects and programs.
>
> International NGOs should not be involved in implementation of activities.

Financial and technical sustainability can be maximized by external investments into already ongoing activities and activities with a local priority.

International NGOs should provide technical support to programs for persons with disabilities according to need defined by the local partners.

Persons with disabilities, their families, and the local communities should be included in planning and implementing CBR programs.

International NGOs should be clear in their role and in input to a CBR program and promote cooperation between nontraditional partners in the communities (local NGOs, farmers groups, religious groups, etc.).

THE FUTURE

If we look further into the twenty-first century, some global problems of relevance for persons with disabilities can already be foreseen. Medical science has not only brought about an increased infant survival rate for normal and healthy children but also for those born with impairment. People carrying genetic disorders survive to adult age and may eventually have a wish to bear children, thus contradicting the principle of "survival of the fittest." New reproductive technologies often lead to multiple and premature births. However, infants with a birth weight of less than 500 grams may survive today, although with increased risk of becoming disabled. Amniocentesis, genetic screening of fetuses, donor eggs and semen, and frozen embryos are not science fiction anymore but open up new possibilities for parents to create the "perfect child." Thus, medical technology raises numerous ethical questions that we have barely begun to debate but will be even more pressing in the future (Davis-Floyd and Dumit 1998).

What type of society do we want? Should parents in their wish for the perfect child be allowed to use modern technology to achieve this goal? Or should any child, even those who are most severely impaired, have the right to be born? What consequences will prenatal screening have for those who are born with or acquire impairment anyway? Will they be even more marginalized, or will there be more resources to support them? What about prenatal screening and selective abortions to obtain a child of the desired gender, which rumors say is already happening among middle- and upper-class people in some Asian countries? What about the right of parents and unimpaired siblings to choose away a life with a disabled child that will clearly place great strains on family life? What about the right to choose not to identify and abort an impaired fetus (Rapp 1998)? For most of these questions, there are no simple answers.

Wars are not likely to disappear in the future, and modern wars have the capacity to affect even the unborn through radiation, chemical weapons, and the like. Chernobyl, so far, has been the largest atomic disaster during a time of peace but may easily be followed by other manmade disasters, creating not only illness and death but also chronic impairments and disabilities. The victims of land mines are now starting to receive their due attention thanks to the 1997 Nobel Peace Prize, the late Princess Diana, and other less famous but equally dedicated promoters of their case. A special vertical program for land mine survivors has been established in the WHO. Also, the Ottawa Convention for the prohibition and use of land mines was signed by 135 countries in 1997.[23] Although land mines are important as a political issue, they represent a minor cause of disability globally. On the local level, the problems and needs of mine victims are not much different from that of polio victims, victims of traffic accidents, or other physically disabling conditions. There is concern that the sudden increase in interest for their cause and the large sums of money involved may create land mine victims as a category more "deserving" of help than other people with disabilities. We have seen this happen in many countries, with war "heroes" becoming more privileged than others with disabilities.

What then will happen to attitudes and behavior toward persons with disabilities in the future? Will we see integration and increased empowerment, or will demands of the modern, increasingly technological society lead to marginalization and increase the gap between people with or without the ability to stay on the "carousel" of modern living? We can only make a qualified guess. There is no doubt that the information technology (IT) revolution, with its new communication technology, opens new possibilities for persons with a disability. For instance, voice computers for people with cerebral palsy and access to the World Wide Web may also break the isolation experienced by some disabled persons and make them aware of the rights and activities of people with disabilities worldwide. However, such technology is not a good substitute for human contact and integration and, in a global perspective, will only be available to the economically (and educationally) more privileged in the foreseeable future.

The final but perhaps most important question concerns the family with a disabled member: Will it be able to cope with the demands of the future? We are already starting to see the consequences of demographic transition in the more (or perhaps overly) developed countries, with an increasing aging population and a decreasing or stagnant younger population to take care of them. These are the combined effects of improved health care and family planning, which are increasingly becoming evident in developing countries (Kalache 1994). People no longer die from their first stroke, necessarily, but may live for years with care-demanding handicaps. Longevity also gives rise to increased illnesses such as dementia, cancer, and diabetes. At the same time, families are producing fewer children, and the old family values of caring for the elderly are being challenged by new options for individual careers and consumer goods in the modern society (Ingstad et al. 1992).

New illnesses, such as AIDS, also create new problems in relation to disability, rehabilitation, and care by the family. With the younger generations diminishing in many countries, care for people with disabilities is left to the elderly, who are often also in need of care. The so-called home-based care for AIDS patients that is being introduced in many of the countries that are hit hardest by its effects tend to be little more than sending the dying patient home with a supply of gloves to be used by the caretaker. Faced with such an enormous challenge, the family, as a care unit, will inevitably have to make priorities in their caregiving, and members with a disability are quite likely to be the losers. If science eventually discovers medicines that can harness the HIV virus at a cost affordable to the hardest-hit developing countries, we may, at least for some time, be faced with large population segments that are chronically impaired and even disabled.

Yet AIDS is not the only threat to family care in developing countries. The process of what we call "development" itself causes changes that challenge old values and patterns of family life. The change from a subsistence-based to a money economy contributes to labor migration from rural to urban areas. It is mostly the young people who migrate, leaving the old and frail, persons with a disability, and sometimes also the small children behind. Ideally, the young people will contribute part of their salary to the village family, but sometimes all they find is unemployment. In addition, the salaries are often so low and the costs of living in the city so high that there is little left to contribute to the family.

Education, which is usually seen as having an indisputable positive value in development, also has its unintended consequences that affect people in need of care. The emphasis on personal achievement and career easily comes into conflict with traditional values of family support and caregiving. Young people no longer rate family obligations as their highest priority but are more concerned with achieving consumer goods and personal success (Ingstad et al. 1992). Education may also increase the gap between the able and the not-so-able but at the same time may give persons with a disability new possibilities for competence and a respected place in society.

In summary, the situation of people with a disability and their families in what we call the developing countries is one of both problems and hope. The struggle lies in poverty and the problematic life situations that many families face, whether or not they have a family member with a disability. A person with a disability will rarely fare better than the general standard of living of people around him or her and, in some cases, will fare worse. Thus, to improve the quality of life for people with disabilities does not only imply equalizing individual opportunities but also improving the life conditions of the whole *family* providing care to a disabled member. This again implies implementing rehabilitation programs that take people's total life situation into consideration—not only the physical, economic, and political constraints for achieving "normalization" and "equal rights" but also their values, knowledge and beliefs, and their perception of personhood—what we often call culture (Ingstad and Whyte 1995; Leavitt 1999; Miles 1996).

Another problem is the often lacking ability of governments at all levels to give priority to a group of the population that cannot normally be expected to contribute much to the national economy. The promises come easily during "International Years" and when donor money is flowing due to a sudden international fad. Sustaining such activities when the international attention turns to other matters is something else.

However, there is much hope. There is hope in the increased awareness of people with disabilities internationally and in the efforts that are being made to improve their quality of life through donor contributions and the continuous development of suitable models for rehabilitation at all levels. There is also hope in the increased global contact between disabled people's organizations, which increases the awareness of the rights of the disabled and the need for integration and normalization. Only by joining all these positive efforts and thereby empowering the developing countries to help themselves can we hope someday to approach the goal of "rehabilitation for all."

NOTES

1. Personal communication with Dr. Einar Helander, former head of WHO's Rehabilitation Department.

2. In medical terminology, a distinction is often made between *habilitation* for those who are born with an impairment and *rehabilitation* for those who have become impaired later in life. For the sake of simplicity, this chapter will use *rehabilitation* for both purposes.

3. I am grateful to an unknown reviewer for making me aware of this point.

4. At least in the Scandinavian countries.

5. Parts of this section are based on an overview of the literature previously given in Ingstad (1997).

6. Resolution No. 2856 adopted by the General Assembly on December 20, 1971.

7. Resolution No. 3447 adopted by the General Assembly on December 9, 1975.

8. Resolution No. 37/53 adopted by the General Assembly on December 3, 1982.

9. Resolution No. 37/52 adopted by the General Assembly on December 3, 1982.

10. Resolution No. 48/96 adopted by the General Assembly on December 20, 1993.

11. The education sector should take responsibility for educating disabled children; the transportation sector should make public transport available and accessible.

12. Dr. Einar Helander.

13. This was the case in Botswana in the mid-1980s.

14. Previously well known for the useful primary health care handbook *Where There Is No Doctor* (Werner 1993).

15. At the time, there were fewer than one million inhabitants.

16. The process of formulating such a policy was started in 1987.

17. Personal communication with Mrs. Chidyausiku, head of Rehabilitation Department, Ministry of Health and Child Welfare, Zimbabwe, December 1999.

18. The Norwegian Red Cross Society.

19. Personal communication with Mrs. Chidyausiku, December 1999.

20. Supported by loans from the World Bank and grants from Norway.

21. I am very grateful to the Norwegian Association of the Disabled, especially Jens Mjaugedal, for a valuable contribution to this section.

22. For instance, in Norway, 30 percent of the government aid budget (NORAD) is earmarked for the NGO sector.

23. Among the countries that did not sign were the United States, Russia, and China.

REFERENCES

Bickenbach, J. E., S. Chatteri, E. M. Badley, and T. B. Ustun. 1999. "Models of Disablement, Universalism and the International Classification of Impairments, Disability and Handicaps." *Social Science & Medicine* 48:1173-87.

Bragg, L. 1997. "Oedipus Borealis: The Aberrant Body in Barbarian Europe." *Disability Studies Quarterly* 17 (4): 258-73.

Bruun, Frank. 1995. "Hero, Beggar or Sports Star." Pp. 196-229 in *Disability and Culture*, edited by B. Ingstad and S. R. Whyte. Berkeley: University of California Press.

Chidyausiku, S., J. Munandi, M. Marasha, D. Mbadzo, F. Mhuri, H. Oppelstrup, and C. Nleya. 1998. *Community-Based Rehabilitation Programme in Zimbabwe*. Stockholm: Sida Evaluation.

Comaroff, Jean. 1991. *Of Revelation and Revolution: Christianity, Colonialism and Consciousness in South Africa*. Vol. 1. Chicago: University of Chicago Press.

Davis-Floyd, R. and J. Dumit. 1998. *Cyborg Babies: From Techno-Sex to Techno-Tots*. New York: Routledge.

Devlieger, Patrick J. 1998. "Representations of Physical Disability in Colonial Zimbabwe: The Film of Cyrene." *Disability & Society* 13 (5): 709-24.

Edgerton, Robert B. 1970. "Mental Retardation in Non-Western Societies: Towards a Cross-Cultural Perspective on Incompetence." Pp. 523-59 in *Social Cultural Aspects of Mental Retardation*, edited by H. C. Haywood. New York: Appleton-Century-Crofts.

Eleweke, Jonah C. 1999. "The Need for Mandatory Legislations to Enhance Services to People with Disabilities in Nigeria." *Disability & Society* 14 (2): 227-37.

Enwemeka, C. S. and N. U. Adeghe. 1982. "Some Family Problems Associated with the Presence of a Child with Handicap in Nigeria." *Child Care, Health and Development* 8:113-40.

Goerdt, Ann. 1984. *Physical Disability in Barbados: A Cultural Perspective*. Ann Arbor, MI: University Microfilms International.

Goerdt, Ann, J. P. Koplan, J. M. Robine, M. Thuriaux, and J. K. Van Ginneken. 1996. "Nonfatal Health Outcomes: Concepts, Instruments and Indicators." Pp. 99-116 in *The Global Burden of Disease*, edited by Christopher J. Murray and A. D. Lopez. Boston: Harvard University Press.

Helander, Einar. 1984. *Rehabilitation for All: A Guide to the Management of Community-Based Rehabilitation*, Vol. 1. *Policymaking and Planning*. RHB/84.1. Provisional version. Geneva: World Health Organization.

————. 1993. *Predjudice and Dignity: An Introduction to Community-Based Rehabilitation*. New York: United Nations Development Programme.

Ingstad, Benedicte. 1995. "Public Discourses on Rehabilitation: From Norway to Botswana." Pp. 174-95 in *Disability and Culture*, edited by Benedicte Ingstad and Susan R. Whyte. Berkeley: University of California Press.

————. 1997. *Community-Based Rehabilitation in Botswana: The Myth of the Hidden Disabled*. Lewiston: Edwin Mellen.

————. 1999. "Problems with Community-Mobilization and Participation in Community-Based Rehabilitation: A Case from Botswana." Pp. 207-16 in *Cross-Cultural Rehabilitation. An International Perspective*, edited by Ronnie L. Leavitt. London: W. B. Saunders.

Ingstad, Benedicte, Frank J. Bruun, Edwin A. Sandberg, and Sheila Tlou. 1992. "Care for the Elderly, Care by the Elderly: The Role of Elderly Women in a Changing Tswana Society." *Journal of Cross-Cultural Gerontology* 7:379-98.

Ingstad, Benedicte and Susan R. Whyte 1995. *Disability and Culture*. Berkeley: University of California Press.

International Labor Organization (ILO). 1998. *Vocational Rehabilitation and Employment of Disabled Persons*. Report No. III. Geneva: Author.

Jackson, H. and R. Mupedziswa. 1988. "Disability and Rehabilitation." *Journal of Social Development in Africa* 3 (1): 21-30.

Jenkins, Richard, ed. 1998. *Questions of Competence: Culture, Classification and Intellectual Disability*. Cambridge, UK: Cambridge University Press.

Kalache, Alex. 1994. "Ageing: The Global and Regional Perspective." Pp. 3-12 in *The Situation of the Elderly in Botswana*, edited by F. J. Bruun, M. Mugabe, and Y. Coombes. Oslo/Gaborone: NIR-SUM Programme on Health, Population and Development.

Keck, Verena. 1999. "Colder Than Cool: Disability and Personhood among the Yupno in Papua New Guinea. *Anthropology & Medicine* 6 (2): 261-84.

Kleinman, Arthur and Joan Kleinman. 1996. "The Appeal of Experience: The Dismay of Images: Cultural Appropriations of Suffering in Our Times." *Dædalus:* 125 (1): 1-24.

Leavitt, Ronnie L., ed. 1999. *Cross-Cultural Rehabilitation: An International Perspective.* London: W. B. Saunders.

Miles, M. 1985. *Where There Is No Rehabilitation Plan.* Peshawar, Pakistan: Mental Health Centre.

———. 1996. "Community, Individual of Information Development? Dilemmas of Concept and Culture in South Asian Disability Planning." *Disability & Society* 11 (4): 485-500.

———. 1999. "Some Influences of Religions on Attitudes towards Disabilities and People with Disabilities." Pp. 49-58 in *Cross-Cultural Rehabilitation: An International Perspective,* edited by Ronnie Leavitt. London: W. B. Saunders.

Nuttal, Mark. 1998. "States and Categories: Indigenous Models of Personhood in Northwestern Greenland." Pp. 176-93 in *Questions of Competence: Culture, Classification and Intellectual Disability,* edited by R. Jenkins. Cambridge, UK: Cambridge University Press.

Okunda, A. D. 1981. "Visual, Auditory and Physical Handicaps in Nigerian Children." *International Nursing Review* 28 (6): 176-77.

Pfeiffer, D. 1998. "The ICIDH and the Need for Its Revision, 1998." *Disability & Society* 13 (4): 503-23.

Rapp, Reyna. 1998. "The Uneven Meanings of Bioscience in a Mulitcultural World." Pp. 143-67 in *Cyborg Babies. From Techno-Sex to Techno-Tots,* edited by R. Davis-Floyd and J. Dumit. New York: Routledge.

United Nations. 1971. *Declaration on the Rights of Mentally Retarded Persons.* New York: Author.

———. 1975. *Declaration on the Rights of Disabled Persons.* New York: Author.

———. 1983. *World Programme of Action Concerning Disabled Persons.* New York: Author.

———. 1990. *Disability Statistics Compendium.* New York: United Nations Statistical Office, Statistics on Special Population Groups.

———. 1994. *The Standard Rules on the Equalization of Opportunities for Persons with Disabilities.* New York: Author.

United Nations Educational, Scientific, and Cultural Organization (UNESCO). n.d. *Making It Happen: Examples of Good Practice in Special Needs Education & Community-Based Programmes.* Paris: Author.

United Nations Educational, Scientific, and Cultural Organization (UNESCO)/Ministry of Education and Science, Spain. 1994. *The Salamanca Statement and Framework for Action on Special Needs Education.* Paris: Author.

Vaughan, M. 1991. *Curing Their Ills: Colonial Power and African Illness.* Cambridge, UK: Polity.

Weiss, Meira. 1998. "Ethical Reflections: Taking a Walk on the Wild Side." Pp. 149-62 in *Small Wars: The Cultural Politics of Childhood,* edited by Nancy Sheper-Hughes and Carolyn Sargent. Berkeley: University of California Press.

Werner, David. 1987. *Disabled Village Children: A Guide for Community Health Workers, Rehabilitation Workers, and Families.* Palo Alto, CA: Hesperian Foundation.

———. 1993. *Where There Is No Doctor: A Village Health Care Handbook for Africa.* London: Macmillan.

———. 1998. *Nothing about Us without Us: Developing Innovative Technologies for, by, and with Disabled Persons.* Palo Alto, CA: HealthWrights.

Whyte, Susan R. 1991a. "Family Experience with Mental Health Problems in Tanzania." *Acta Psychiatrica Scandinavica* 83:77-111.

———. 1991b. "Attitudes towards Mental Health in Tanzania." *Acta Psychiatrica Scandinavica* 83:153-75.

———. 1998. "Slow Cookers and Madmen: Competence of Hearth and Head in Rural Uganda." Pp. 153-75 in *Questions of Competence: Culture, Classification and Intellectual Disability,* edited by R. Jenkins. Cambridge, UK: Cambridge University Press.

World Bank. 1993. *World Development Report: Investing in Health.* New York: Oxford University Press.

World Health Organization (WHO). 1980. *International Classification of Impairments, Disabilities, and Handicaps: A Manual of Classification Relating to the Consequences of Disease.* Geneva: Author.

———. 1982. *Community-Based Rehabilitation.* Geneva: Author.

Author Index

Kazak, A. E., 385
Keck, V., 774
Keith, K., 49
Keith, L., 530, 739
Keller, E. F., 669-670
Kellner, D., 516
Kelly, A., 412
Kelly, M. P., 399, 400, 401, 402, 404, 407
Kelman, S., 100
Kemp, S. P., 173
Kennedy, J., 715
Kennedy, J. F., 46
Kennisto, M., 363
Kent, D., 199, 519
Kerlin, I. N., 36, 38
Kevles, D. J., 40
Khoury, M., 767
Kielhofner, G., 174
Kiernan, C., 278
Kiernan, P., 363, 367
Kiesler, D. J., 86
Kiger, G., 548
Kimmick, M., 714
King, A., 736
Kinsman, S. L., 766
Kipp, R. S., 20
Kirchner, C., 48, 153
Kirk, N., 417
Kirkbride, T., 32, 33
Kirkman Gray, B., 415
Kirkmayer, J., 140
Kirkpatrick, C., 597
Kita, M. W., 73
Kitzinger, J., 522
Klapwijk, A., 746
Klein, B. S., 366
Klein, S., 332
Kleinfield, S., 437, 530
Kleinman, A., 257, 479, 774
Kleinman, J., 257, 774
Klobas, L. E., 518
Knight, G. H., 35, 36, 37
Knoke, D., 481
Knoll, J., 386
Knowles, J., 598-599
Knox, M., 290
Koegel, L. K., 46
Koegel, R. L., 46
Koestler, F. A., 44
Kohl, M., 303
Kokkonen, J., 386
Koperski, M., 616, 620, 629
Kourilsky-Belliard, F., 173
Koven, S., 39
Kramer, S., 91
Krane, N., 48
Krause, J. S., 761
Krauss, C., 596
Krauss, M. W., 384, 386
Kriegel, L., 197, 199, 518-519
Krishnan, B., 553, 714

Kroll, J., 17, 18
Kronenfeld, J. J., 481
Krugman, P., 604
Kruse, D. L., 434
Kuhlmann, F., 37
Kuhn, T., 667
Kuhn, T. S., 153, 175
Kuhse, H., 235, 282-283, 304
Kuipers, L., 469
Kurtz, R., 518
Kuttner, R., 602
Kymlicka, W., 508, 509

LaCom, C., 203
Lakey, J., 412, 417, 420
Lakin, K., 41, 275
Lamb, B., 423
Landau, E., 362
Lane, H., 28, 30, 35, 39, 224, 320, 498, 526, 527
Lane, J. P., 664
Lane, R., 596
Langdon-Down, G., 421
LaPlante, M. P., 643, 763
LaPorte, V., 637
Laqueur, T., 254
Lasch, C., 377, 379
Latham, M., 290-291
Law, M., 172, 174
Lawton, M. P., 173
Lazar, I., 43
Lazarus, R., 403
Le Grand, J., 699
Leaman, D., 746
Leavitt, R. L., 790
Leech, P., 712
Lefley, H., 41, 45
LeGrand, J., 618, 620
Leik, R. K., 484
Lembke, D., 439
Lemert, E., 397, 412
Lende, H., 42
Leonard, J. S., 638
Leonard-Barton, D., 333
Leplege, A., 363, 367
Lerner, R. M., 174
Leutz, W. N., 629
Levin, B., 698
Levin, H., 23, 42
Levine, C., 587
Levitas, R., 694
Leviton, G. L., 354
Levy, F., 601
Levy, J., 360, 418
Levy, L., 418
Levy, R. M., 41, 46, 47
Lewis, J., 414
Lewis, M., 601
Lewis, V., 358
Li, L., 360
Liachowitz, C. H., 565
Lie, H. R., 386

Subject Index

About the Contributors

Gary L. Albrecht is Professor of Public Health and of Disability and Human Development at the University of Illinois at Chicago. His current work focuses on the quality of life of persons with disabilities based on National Institutes of Health–funded studies of disabled women experiencing the menopausal transition, a three-nation study of risk, and two studies of disability in the inner city. He is past Chair of the Medical Sociology Section of the American Sociological Association and a member of the Executive Committee of the Disability Forum of the American Public Health Association. He has received the Award for the Promotion of Human Welfare and the Eliot Freidson Award for the book *The Disability Business: Rehabilitation in America*. He also has received a Switzer Distinguished Research Fellowship, Kellogg Fellowship, World Health Organization Fellowship, Schmidt Fellowship, New York State Supreme Court Fellowship, the Lee Founders Award from the Society for the Study of Social Problems, the Licht Award from the American Congress of Rehabilitation Medicine, and the University of Illinois at Chicago Award for Excellence in Teaching. He was a Visiting Fellow at the University of Oxford and Maison des Sciences de l'Homme, Paris. He has led scientific delegations in rehabilitation medicine to the Soviet Union and the People's Republic of China. His most recent book is *The Handbook of Social Studies in Health and Medicine* (2000, edited with Ray Fitzpatrick and Susan Scrimshaw).

Barbara M. Altman is Senior Research Fellow with the Agency for Healthcare Research and Quality and an Adjunct Associate Professor at the University of Maryland, Baltimore County. She is a past president of the Society for Disability Studies and served on the founding board of directors of that organization. her disability research interests focus on three areas: operationalization of disability definitions/measures in survey data; access to, financing, and use of health care services by persons with disabilities, particularly working-age persons and women with disabilities; and the impact of primary, secondary, and tertiary resources on disability outcomes. She is the author of a number of articles and book chapters on disability topics and has served as editor of special issues of *Disability Studies Quarterly* and *Journal of Disability Policy Studies*. She is coeditor of the new series, *Research in Social Science and Disability*.

Felicity Armstrong is Lecturer at the Department of Educational Studies, University of Sheffield, England. She is codirector of the M.Ed. in Special and Inclusive Education. Her research interests include curriculum, culture and diversity, and cross-cultural issues in policy and difference. She has recently coedited two books with Len Barton—*Disability, Human Rights and Education* and *Inclusive Education: Policy, Contexts and Comparative Perspectives*.

Adrienne Asch is the Henry R. Luce Professor in Biology, Ethics, and the Politics of Human Reproduction at Wellesley College. She came to Wellesley from Boston University, where she taught at the School of Social Work. From 1987 to 1990, she served as an Associate in Social Science and Policy with the New Jersey Bioethics Commission and during 1993 was a member of the Clinton Task Force on Health Care Reform. Most recently, her work has focused on the ethical, political, psychological, and social implications of human reproduction and the family. She has been involved with the disability rights movement and disability studies for 30 years and is a past president of the Society for Disability Studies.

Sharon Barnartt is Professor of Sociology at Gallaudet University. Coauthor of *Deaf President Now: The 1988 Revolution at Gallaudet University* (1995) and also of *Contentious Politics in the Disability and Deaf Communities* (forthcoming), she has also published widely in the area of socioeconomic status and disability/deafness, legal and disability policy issues, and social movements in the deaf and disability communities.

Colin Barnes is a disabled writer and activist. A committed advocate of user-led research initiatives and methodologies, he has conducted studies on a whole range of disability-related issues, including the social construction of dependence, institutional discrimination and disabled people, disabling imagery and the media, independent/integrated living, and user-led services. He has authored and coauthored several books and articles in the general area of disability studies and is founder and Director of the Disability Research Unit (DRU) in the Department of Sociology and Social Policy at the University of Leeds, England.

Len Barton is Professor in the Department of Educational Studies at the University of Sheffield, England. He is the Director of an Inclusive Education Research Centre. His main interests are in a sociopolitical approach to disability issues, cross-cultural insights and relationships on questions of disability policy and practice, and the position and perspectives of disabled people, both individually and as a collective. He is also the founder and editor of *Disability and Society,* the world's leading journal in the field of disability studies. He has published extensively on these issues, and his latest publication is *Disability, Human Rights and Education. Cross-Cultural perspectives* (coedited with F. Armstrong, 1999).

Ian Basnett is a physician and the Deputy Director of Public Health for Camden and Islington Health Authority in central London. In 1997 and 1998, he was a Harkness Fellow sponsored by the Commonwealth Fund and based at the University of California at San Francisco, where he focused on issues related to managed health care, disability, and long-term care. He retains a broad interest in issues related to health and disability policy, personal assistance, and disability advocacy. As an individual with a disability, he works on disability issues with both the national and local disability organizations. He is an honorary senior lecturer at the London School of Hygiene and Tropical Medicine and is a member of the Royal College of Physicians. He also has a background in public health.

Line Beauregard is a research assistant at the Institute of Rehabilitation of Quebec City. She is completing a Ph.D. in social work at the Laval University. Her research focuses on aging with a disability. She also studies the interactive person-environment process.

Monroe Berkowitz is Professor of Economics, Emeritus, Rutgers University; Director of Disability and Health Economics Research of the Bureau of Economic Research; and Director of Research, Rehabilitation International. He has published extensively in the area of economics of disability, with particular emphasis on work-related disability. He has authored or coauthored numerous books and journal articles, including *Permanent Partial Disability and Workers' Compensation.* He is the editor of the book *Measuring the Efficiency of Public Programs* and coauthor of *The Economic Consequences of Traumatic Spinal Cord Injury and Spinal Cord Injury: An Analysis of Medical and Social Costs.* His current research interests include a study of the full costs of disability in a selected sample of firms, a study of mobility devices, and studies of work injuries and rehabilitation here and abroad. He has served as a consultant to various workers' compensation agencies and organizations such as the U.S. Department of Health and Human Services, U.S. Department of Education, U.S. Department of Labor, Social Security Administration, the International Labor Organization, and the World Health Organization. He is also a member of the National Academy of Arbitrators, having served as an arbitrator in management-labor disputes since 1946.

Jerome E. Bickenbach is Professor in the Department of Philosophy and Faculties of Law and Medicine at Queen's University, Kingston, Ontario, Canada. He is the author of *Physical Disability and Social Policy* (1993) and coeditor of *Introduction to Disability* (1998) and many articles in disability studies, focusing on the nature of disability and disability law and policy. His research is entirely within disability studies and more recently includes disability epidemiology, disability and health issues, the ethics and policy of summary health measures, and health law generally. Since 1995, he has been a consultant with the World Health Organization working on the revision of the *ICIDH-2*.

Ellen Liberti Blasiotti is Manager of the Information Dissemination and Utilization Program and Director of the Mary E. Switzer Fellowship Program at the National Institute on Disability and Rehabilitation Research (NIDRR). She is a national expert in information dissemination and utilization and has a chapter published in *Knowledge: Creation, Diffusion, Utilization*. She has 30 years of experience in rehabilitation research, research information dissemination and utilization, and public affairs. She has directed national information clearinghouses, a national rehabilitation research library, information services, databases, media outreach projects, and technical assistance efforts. She has served as a delegate to U.S.-Japan Common Agenda conference and has been a NIDRR Fellow to India. She is the winner of a prestigious Hammer Award from the Vice-President's National Performance Review and the Deputy Secretary's Reinvention Award. Prior to her service in helping to establish the NIHR (now NIDRR), she held various public affairs positions at the U.S. Information Agency and the U.S. Department of State.

David L. Braddock is Professor of Human Development and Public Health, Head of the Department of Disability and Human Development, and founding Director of the Institute on Disability and Human Development at the University of Illinois at Chicago. His research has focused on the comparative study of the provision and financing of services for people with developmental disabilities in the 50 American states. This work has been published in six editions as the "State of the States in Developmental Disabilities." In addition to his work on deinstitutionalization, he has also published research on health promotion and disease prevention for persons with disabilities, compensation and turnover in residential facilities, and federal policy toward mental retardation and developmental disabilities. He was instrumental in establishing the University of Illinois at Chicago's interdisciplinary Ph.D. degree program in disability studies, the nation's first. He has received Career Research Awards from the American Association on Mental Retardation, the Association for Retarded Citizens of the United States, and the University of Illinois. He is a former president of the American Association on Mental Retardation.

Scott Campbell Brown is Educational Research Analyst in the Office of Special Education Programs, Office of Special Education and Rehabilitation Services, Department of Education. His background includes posts as a consultant to the United Nations and the International Labour Organization on disability issues and as a research scientist at Gallaudet University, where he codesigned the United Nations Disability Statistics Database.

Michael Bury is coeditor of the international journal *Sociology of Health and Illness*. He was educated at the University of Sussex and then at Bristol, where he did postgraduate work on mental health. In the 1970s, he worked with Philip Wood in Manchester on sociological aspects of chronic illness and disability and helped to write the WHO's *International Classification of Impairments, Disabilities, and Handicaps.* In the early 1980s, he moved to London to work with Margot Jefferys at Bedford College and teach on the M.Sc. in Medical Sociology. With the merger of Bedford College with Royal Holloway in 1985 (still within London University), he moved his activities to the Royal Holloway site. He has been published widely in the fields of chronic illness, disability, and aging. His latest book, *Health and Illness in a Changing Society,* was published in 1997.

Lennard J. Davis is Professor of Disability and Human Development and Professor and Chair of the Department of English at the University of Chicago, Illinois. He is the author of two works on the novel: *Factual Fictions: The Origins of the English Novel* (1983, reprinted in 1996) and *Resisting Novels: Fiction and Ideology* (1987). He is also coeditor of *Left Politics and the Literary Profession.* His works on disability include *Enforcing Normalcy: Disability, Deafness, and the Body* (1995), which won the 1996 Gustavus Myers Center for the Study of Human Rights' annual award for the best scholarship on the subject of intolerance in North America, and *The Disability Studies Reader* (1996). He has also written a memoir *My Sense of Silence* (2000) about growing up in a deaf family and edited his parents' correspondence *Shall I Say a Kiss: The Courtship Letters of a Deaf Couple, 1936-38* (1999). He was a founding member of the Modern Language Associations Committee on Disability Issues in the Profession and is an active member of Children of Deaf Adults (CODA). His current projects are *Novel Theory* (2001) and *Obsession: The History of Fascination and the People Who Made It a Disease.*

Gerben DeJong is Director of the National Rehabilitation Hospital (NRH) Center on Health and Disability Research (formerly NRH Research Center) in Washington, D.C. In this capacity, he also serves as Director of the Center's federally funded Research and Training Center (RTC) on Managed Care & Disability. He is Professor in the Department of Family Medicine and Adjunct Professor in the Georgetown Public Policy Institute at Georgetown University. In 1984, he was a Fulbright Scholar in the Netherlands, serving with the research staff of the Social Security Council. He is the author or coauthor of more than 180 papers on health, income maintenance, and disability issues. He is perhaps best known for his seminal work on disability and health policy and the independent living movement. He is an ardent student of health care reform and health system change and their impact on individuals with disabilities. He has had an abiding interest in the consumer side of health markets and the ability of consumers to make informed decisions about their health care needs. Dr. DeJong is also one of the few analysts, apart from Wall Street, tracking the rapid consolidation of American postacute care through mergers and acquisitions.

Robert F. Drake is Lecturer in Social Policy at the University of Wales, Swansea, in the United Kingdom. For several years, he worked in voluntary sector management for a number of nongovernmental organizations. He also provides consultancy services to governments and major voluntary bodies on disability and equal opportunity policies, and he has published widely on both these topics. He has recently completed a review of the position of disabled people in Northern Ireland (for Pricewaterhouse-Coopers) and is currently writing a major text on the principles of social policy.

Alexandra Enders is Senior Research Associate at the Research and Training Center on Rural Rehabilitation, Rural Institute on Disabilities at the University of Montana, where she has also been Director of Training and Associate Director for Information Dissemination. For more than 25 years, she has been involved with service delivery systems and networks, public policy, funding and quality assurance issues, program development and training activities, information services, independent living program development, and technology evaluation and effectiveness studies at the Electronic Industries Foundation in Washington, D.C., the Rehabilitation Engineering Center at Children's Hospital at Stanford, and the Center for Independent Living in Berkeley, California. She has published widely, including three editions of the *Assistive Tech-*

nology Sourcebook. She is the current president of RESNA, the Rehabilitation Engineering and Assistive Technology Association of North America.

Philip M. Ferguson is Associate Professor and Senior Research Associate in the Department of Special Education and Community Resources at the University of Oregon. His research focuses on the areas of family and professional interaction and support policy, social policy and history in disability studies, and qualitative research methods in disability studies and education. In addition to numerous articles and book chapters, he has published a book on the history of disability policy and coedited a popular reader in qualitative research in disability studies.

Patrick Fougeyrollas is a social anthropologist and scientific director at the University Institute of Rehabilitation of Quebec City and Associate Professor in the Department of Rehabilitation and in the Department of Sociology at Laval University. He is a founding member and president of the International Network on the Disability Creation Process; president of the Canadian Society on the Classification of Impairments, Disabilities and Handicaps; and an active member of committees related to rehabilitation, social integration, and issues related to the disability process for the World Health Organization and the Council of Europe. He is a social researcher specializing in the study of the interactive person-environment process, determining the quality of social participation of persons with organic or functional differences. He is an active advocate in the international disability movement for the exercise of human rights and equalization of opportunities for people with disabilities. With his team in Quebec, he developed the classification "Disability Creation Process," which was innovative by its full recognition of environmental factors and clarification of personal factors from extrinsic factors in the international debate around the revision of the WHO's *ICIDH*. He also developed new measurement tools for measuring the quality of social participation and their environmental, physical, and social determinants.

Sally French is a lecturer in social care at the Open University, United Kingdom. She has written and edited numerous articles and books on psychosocial issues relating to health, illness, and disability. Her publications include *On Equal Terms: Working with Disabled People* and *Physiotherapy: A Psychosocial Approach and Disability Discourse.* She has a background in physiotherapy and teaching.

Glenn T. Fujiura is Associate Professor of Human Development at the Department of Disability and Human Development at the University of Illinois at Chicago. His research has focused on the fiscal structure and demography of the developmental disability service system, on family policy, and on evaluation of long-term care services. He is the principal investigator of studies on demography and economics of families and disability; the intersection of poverty, race, and disability; institutional closure; and demographic analyses of trends in disability populations. Prior to his academic career, he worked in work rehabilitation programs, schools, and long-term care residential settings. He is a 1999 National Rehabilitation Association Switzer Scholar and currently Chair of the U.S. Administration on Developmental Disabilities Multicultural Advisory Committee.

Carol J. Gill is a clinical and research psychologist specializing in health and disability. She is Assistant Professor in the Department of Disability and Human Development at the University of Illinois at Chicago (UIC), where she teaches and provides leadership in disability studies curriculum development. She also directs the department's Chicago Center for Disability Research, through which she and colleagues conduct research, training, and community service projects in the social sciences, emphasizing a disability studies approach and substantive direction by persons with disabilities at all levels. Since 1998, she has served as Executive Officer of the Society for Disability Studies. Her research interests include disability identity development, health concerns and health service experiences of women with disabilities, disability bioethical issues and professional training. Her conceptual and research articles have been widely published in both professional journals and in the popular disability press.

Benedicte Ingstad is Professor of Medical Anthropology at the Department of General Practice and Community Medicine, University of Oslo, Norway. She was a Visiting Fulbright Scholar at the Department of Anthropology, University of California, Berkeley (1999-2000). She is trained as a social anthropologist with fieldwork done in Greenland, Botswana, Gambia, and Norway. Her main areas of research include disability in an international and cross-cultural perspective, aging in a cross-cultural perspective, family care for dependent members, traditional healers and healing systems, AIDS in Southern Africa, and the concept of "good health" in Norway. She was born in Norway 1943 and is a widow and mother of five children, one of them severely physically and mentally handicapped.

Michael P. Kelly is Head of School and Professor of Social Sciences at the University of Greenwich, London. He is also Director of the Centre for Research in Human Sciences and Business at that university. He is a medical sociologist with particular interests in the sociology of chronic illness and surgery. His work in this field has been concerned with the effects on self and identity of illness and surgery. He has also written about coronary heart disease prevention, health promotion, labeling theory, alcoholism, and the implications of postmodern theory for medical sociology. He previously taught at the Universities of Glasgow, Dundee, Abertay, and Leicester.

Iwao Kobayashi is a lecturer in Faculty of Software and Information Science, Iwate Prefectural University in Japan. In April 1999, he worked in the General Secretariat of Special Education, Ministry of Education, Kingdom of Saudi Arabia as an expert of Japan International Cooperation Agency (JICA). His research interests include the use of information technology by and for people with disabilities.

Simi Litvak is Senior Research and Policy Analyst at the World Institute on Disability (WID), Oakland, California. She is a former director of both the Rehabilitation Research and Training Center (RRTC) on Personal Assistance Services (PAS) and of the RRTC on Independent Living and Disability Policy at WID. She has done extensive research in the area of independent living and is a nationally known expert in independent living, PAS, income supports, and health care access for people with disabilities. She has more than 35 years of experience in the disability field as an educator, researcher, policy analyst, policymaker, author, speaker, and rehabilitation professional. She served as a member of President Clinton's 1993 Health Care Reform Task Force. Her hidden disabilities result from back injury and environmental illness.

Donald J. Lollar is Chief, Disability and Health Branch, at the Centers for Disease Control and Prevention (CDC). He has spent the past 5 years helping develop the science and programs to improve the health of people with disabilities, prevent secondary conditions, and increase full participation. Prior to joining CDC, he practiced rehabilitation psychology for 25 years, working with children, adults, and families across ages and conditions. His primary scientific emphasis has been the development of instruments to measure variables such as need satisfaction, pain perception among children, and independent functioning. His clinical interests have focused emotional balance and helping coordinate services needed for individuals and their families. He is currently on the Research Advisory Committee for Special Olympics and Very Special Arts.

Geoff Mercer is Senior Lecturer in the Department of Sociology and Social Policy and a member of the Disability Research Unit, University of Leeds. He has published widely on disability theory and research, including editing (with Colin Barnes) two major collections: *Exploring the Divide: Illness and Disability* (1996) and *Doing Disability Research* (1997). He is coauthor (with Colin Barnes and Tom Shakespeare) of *Exploring Disability: A Sociological Introduction*

(1999). His current disability research projects include a study of centers for independent/ integrated living and of people with severe aphasia.

David T. Mitchell is Associate Professor of English and Cultural Studies at Northern Michigan University. He has served as president of the Society for Disability Studies and chair of the Committee on Disability Issues in the Academy and the Disability Studies Discussion Group in the Modern Languages Association (MLA). He was also one of the founders of both of these MLA groups. He is coproducer and codirector of the award-winning video, *Vital Signs: Crip Culture Talks Back*. In addition, he has published numerous essays on disability studies in the humanities and was the coeditor of the anthology, *The Body and Physical Difference: Discourses of Disability*. He is the editor of a book series, titled *Corporealities: Discourses of Disability*, for the University of Michigan Press. His most recent book (coauthored with Sharon Synder) is *Narrative Prosthesis: Disability and the Dependencies of Discourse* (2000).

Bonnie O'Day is Senior Research Associate at Cherry Engineering and Support Services, Inc. (CESSI). She formerly served as the Director of Disability Research at the National Rehabilitation Hospital Research Center. She is the principal investigator on several research projects, including *Policy Barriers for People with Long-term Mental Illness Who Want to Work*. Other projects include several research and training projects in the areas of managed care, which use qualitative and quantitative methods to examine access to and quality of care for people with disabilities. She has also been appointed by President Clinton to the National Council on Disability, an advisory body to Congress and the president on disability-related issues. She has served as research associate on several projects, including *From Institutions to Independence*, an examination of the policy-level barriers people with disabilities face in moving from nursing homes into the community, and the strategies that independent living centers use to assist people in making this transition.

Susan L. Parish is Associate Project Director of the State of the States in Developmental Disabilities, a longitudinal research project examining state and national trends in financing and services for persons with developmental disabilities. She is a doctoral candidate in Public Health at the University of Illinois at Chicago.

Trevor R. Parmenter holds a joint appointment as Foundation Professor of Developmental Disability in the Faculty of Medicine at the University of Sydney and Director of the Centre for Developmental Disability Studies (CDDS). Prior to his appointment at CDDS in 1997, he held the position of Professorial Fellow in the School of Education, Macquarie University and Director of the Unit for Community Integration Studies. Previous to his appointment to Macquarie University in 1974, he held teaching and administrative positions with the New South Wales Department of Education (1953-1973). Among his honors and awards are fellowships from the Australian College of Education, the American Association on Mental Retardation, and the International Association for the Scientific Study of Intellectual Disabilities. He has received distinguished international researcher awards from the American Association on Mental Retardation and the American Association of University Affiliated Programs. He also received the Distinguished Service Citation from the Australian Society for the Study of Intellectual Disability. He is presently serving a four-year term as the president of the International Association for the Scientific Study of Intellectual Disabilities. He is a member of the Division of International Special Education and Services International Liaison Network of the Council for Exceptional Children and a foundation member of the Global Applied Disability Research and Information Network on Employment & Training (GLADNET).

Bernice A. Pescosolido is Chancellors' Professor of Sociology at Indiana University and Director of the Indiana Consortium for Mental Health Services Research. Her areas of research target issues of the role of social networks in health, illness, and healing. She received an Independent Scientist Award from the National Institute of Mental Health. She has served as the chair of the Medical Sociology Section of the American Sociological Association and has participated in the development of research agendas on the social and behavioral sciences for the National Cancer Institute; the National Institute of Heart, Lung and Blood; and the National Institute of Mental Health. Her current projects focus on the larger public climate toward persons with mental illness, a longitudinal study of the service utilization of persons newly diagnosed with mental illness, and the role of community networks in recognizing and coping with mental health problems in Puerto Rico.

Jean-François Ravaud is a research director in public health at INSERM (Institut national de la santé et de la recherche médicale, the French National Institute of Health and Medical Research). He is active at CERMES (Centre de recherche médecine, sciences, santé et société), a research unit associated with INSERM), CNRS (Centre national de la recherche scientique, the national French Center of Scientific Research), and EHESS (École des hautes études en sciences sociales, the Institute for Advanced Studies in the Social Sciences). After studies in psychiatry, he specialized in social epidemiology and has been engaged for more than 15 years in research on the social integration of disabled persons. He is a codirector of RFRH (Réseau federatif de recherche sur le handicapé), which brings together French research teams specialized in rehabilitation, technological research, public health, and the social sciences, and he oversees the main thrust of such activity. His research has led to publications in various international journals such as *Social Science and Medicine, Sociology of Health and Illness, Disability and Rehabilitation,* and *International Journal of Rehabilitation Research.*

Violet Rutkowski-Kmitta is a research specialist in the Department of Disability and Human Development at the University of Illinois at Chicago. She is a recent graduate from Saint Louis University School of Public Health in Saint Louis, Missouri with a concentration in epidemiology. She has been involved in research on health-related quality-of-life measures and with measurement development projects involving the *International Classification of Impairments, Disabilities, and Handicap (ICIDH-2).* She is working with Glenn Fujiura, conducting disability epidemiological research using state public health surveillance systems.

Kay Schriner is Research Professor in the Department of Political Science and Research Fellow in the Fulbright Institute of International Relations at the University of Arkansas. She is the founding editor of the *Journal of Disability Policy Studies.* Her research interests are in disability politics and policies both domestically and internationally.

Richard Scotch is Professor of Sociology and Political Economy at the University of Texas at Dallas. He is the author of *From Good Will to Civil Rights: Transforming Federal Disability Policy* and coauthor of the forthcoming *Contentious Politics in the Disability and Deaf Communities.* He has published numerous articles and monographs on the conceptual basis for social policy reform and social movements in disability, health care, education, and human services.

Katherine D. Seelman was named by President Clinton in 1994 as the Director of the National Institute of Disability and Rehabilitation Research (NIDRR). She chairs the Interagency Committee on Disability Research, which promotes coordination and cooperation among federal agencies supporting rehabilitation research. During her tenure as Director of NIDRR, she has advanced scientific endeavor in many areas, especially in applications of rehabilitation technology to advance the independence of people with disabilities. Dr. Seelman is a member of a number of National Science Foundation (NSF) and National Institutes of Health (NIH) committees, including the National Center for Medical Rehabilitation Research (NCMRR). She is co-chair of the U.S.-Japan Common Agenda steering committee in educational and assistive technology and was co-chair of the Research Committee for the 1996 Paralympic Games in Atlanta. Dr. Seelman, who is hard of hearing, has held leadership positions at the National Council on Disability, the Administration on Developmental Disabilities, and the Massachusetts Commission for the Deaf and Hard of Hearing. During her career, she has received numerous awards, including an honorary fellow Rehabilitation Engineering and Assistive Technology Society of North America (RESNA), a National Science Foundation Assistantship, and a distinguished Switzer Fellowship.

Tom Shakespeare works to develop research and public debate on the social aspect of the new genetics at the PEALS Research Institute, Newcastle. He has been active in the U.K. disability movement since 1986 and has been involved with disability studies since 1989. His publications include *The Sexual Politics of Disability* (1996), *Exploring Disability* (1999), and *The Disability Reader* (1998). His most recent research has been with disabled children and on disabled people's views of the new genetics.

Sharon L. Snyder is Assistant Professor in Film Studies and Literature in Northern Michigan University. Most recently, she coedited *Enabling the Humanities: A Sourcebook in Disability Studies*. She is a series editor of *Corporealities: Discourses of Disability,* coauthor of *Narrative Prosthesis: Disability and the Dependencies of Discourse,* coeditor of *The Body and Physical Difference: Discourses of Disability,* and a founding member of the Modern Language Asssociation's Committee on Disability Issues. Her film, *Vital Signs: Crip Culture Talks Back,* has received many awards, including Grand Prize from Rehabilitation International.

Henri-Jacques Stiker is Director of Research at the Laboratoire Histoire et Civilisations des Societes Occidentales at the Université Denis Diderot in Paris. After a doctoral dissertation in philosophy and appointment to a research position in semiotics at EHESS, he specialized in the historical anthropology of disability. He has written several books and numerous articles, which have resulted in his being invited to lecture at a number of French, American, and Canadian universities, as well as to join the editorial boards of journals and the science councils of several institutions. He is the president of an international learned society devoted to the history of disability (ALTER). One of his now standard works, *Corps infirmes et societes* (1982, reprinted 1997) appeared in English in late 1999 under the title *A History of Disability.* He is also the author of *Culture brisée, culture a naitre* (1979) and of chapters in works such as *Handicap vecu et evalue* (1987), *Fragments pour une histoire, notions et acteurs* (1996), and *L'exclusion l'etat des savoirs* (1996).

John Swain is a principal lecturer in research and a reader in Disability Studies at the University of Northumbria at Newcastle, United Kingdom. He has researched and published widely in the field of disability studies. He has a background in psychology and teaching young people with special educational needs. With Sally French, he coedited *Therapy and Learning Difficulties: Advocacy, Participation, and Partnership.* He has worked as a consultant on a number of disability studies courses at the Open University, United Kingdom, and is coeditor of a course setbook, *Disabling Barriers—Enabling Environments.*

Bryan S. Turner is Professor of Sociology at the University of Cambridge, England. He has held professorial chairs in Australia, Britain, and the Netherlands, and he was the Morris Ginsberg Fellow at the London School of Economics (1981) and an Alexander von Humboldt Professorial Fellow at Bielefeld University, Germany (1986-1987). He is founding coeditor of the journal *Body & Society,* founding editor of *Citizenship Studies,* and founding coeditor of the *Journal of Classical Sociology.* His current research interests include (1) voluntary associations, the privatization of the welfare state, and the remaking of civil society and (2) the culture and politics of postwar generations. He has published extensively in medical sociology, the sociology of religion, and political sociology. His recent publications include *The Blackwell Companion to Social Theory* (1999), *The Talcott Parsons Reader* (1999), and *Classical Sociology* (1999).

David Wasserman is a research scholar at the Institute for Philosophy and Public Policy in the University of Maryland's School of Public Affairs. He has written about the moral underpinnings of criminal law and legal practice, the concept of discrimination, and issues in procedural and distributive justice. His present research focuses on ethical and policy issues in disability, health care, reproduction, and genetic technology. In addition to numerous articles and book chapters, he has published *A Sword for the Convicted: Representing Indigent Defendants on Appeal* (1990). He has coauthored *Disability, Difference, Discrimination* with Anita Silvers and Mary Mahowald (1998) and coedited *Genetics and Criminal Behavior: Methods, Meanings, and Morals* with Robert Wachbroit (forthcoming).

Nick Watson is a lecturer in the sociology of health and illness in the Department of Nursing Studies, University of Edinburgh. He has published research on a wide range of disability issues, and his most recent work has involved research with disabled children. He is coeditor of two forthcoming collections on the sociology of the body (*Organising Bodies: Policy, Institutions* and *Work and Reframing the Body*). He is active in the disabled people's movement and is convenor of Access Ability, Lothian.

John D. Westbrook is Manager of the Special Education and Rehabilitation Services Program at the Southwest Educational Development Laboratory in Austin, Texas. He is also director of the National Center for the Dissemination of Disability Research, funded by a grant from the National Institute on Disability and Rehabilitation Research in the U.S. Department of Education. He has written numerous, articles, reports, monographs, guides, articles, and chapters in the knowledge dissemination and utilization area. He has directed a variety of federally funded projects in the knowledge development and dissemination areas focusing on wide-ranging issues surrounding disability, vocational rehabilitation, special education, and research. He also has extensive experience in the provision of technical assistance and training services at the state, regional, and national levels; he has facilitated numerous technical assistance brokerages to federal grantees, disability consumer groups, and service provider agencies and organizations. He was selected as a Mary E. Switzer Scholar in 1998 by the National Rehabilitation Association. He has had a variety of employment experiences, including special education teacher and supervisor, state education agency consultant, staff development specialist, continuing medical education specialist, and university student teacher trainer. He has also held a variety of public service posts, including service on the board of a community-based independent living center and state committee planning for classroom computer capacity building.

Gareth Williams is Research Professor in the School of Social Sciences at Cardiff University in Wales and is the School's Director of Research. He was previously Professor of Sociology at the University of Salford, England. He has published widely in academic and professional journals and is coauthor and coeditor of a number of books, including *Researching the People's Health* (1994), *Challenging Medicine* (1994), *Markets and Networks* (1996), *Understanding Rheumatoid Arthritis* (1996), and *Contracting for Health* (1997). His published work is mainly in the areas of disability and chronic illness, lay and expert knowledge, and public health and health policy. He is currently one of the principal researchers on a study of inequalities in health in England, funded by the Economic and Social Research Council as part of its Health Inequalities Programme.

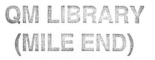